Immunology of the Nervous System

Immunology of the Nervous System

Edited by

Robert W. Keane, Ph.D.
Department of Physiology and Biophysics
University of Miami School of Medicine

William F. Hickey, M.D.
Department of Pathology
Dartmouth Medical School

New York   Oxford
OXFORD UNIVERSITY PRESS
1997

Oxford University Press

Oxford   New York
Athens   Auckland   Bangkok   Bogota
Bombay   Buenos Aires   Calcutta   Cape Town
Dar es Salaam   Delhi   Florence   Hong Kong   Istanbul
Karachi   Kuala Lumpur   Madras   Madrid
Melbourne   Mexico City   Nairobi   Paris
Singapore   Taipei   Tokyo   Toronto

and associated companies in
Berlin   Ibadan

Library of Congress Cataloging-in-Publication Data
Immunology of the nervous system /
edited by Robert W. Keane, William F. Hickey.
p. cm.   Includes bibliographical references and index.
ISBN 0-19-507817-9
1. Neuroimmunology.   2. Nervous system—Diseases—Immunological aspects.
I. Keane, Robert W.   II. Hickey, William F., 1949–.
[DNLM: 1. Nervous System—immunology.
2. Nervous System Diseases—immunology.
3. Neuroimmunomodulation.
WL 102 I33 1997]   QP356.47.I46   1997
612.8—dc20   DNLM/DLC for Library of Congress   96-24678

9 8 7 6 5 4 3 2 1

Printed in the United States of America
on acid-free paper

Contents

Foreword   ix
Preface   xiii
Abbreviations   xv

I   HISTORY OF NEUROIMMUNOLOGY

1. A Brief History of Neuroimmunology   3
   Byron H. Waksman

II   BASIC CONCEPTS

2. A Review of the Immune System   69
   Emil R. Unanue

3. Immunologic Principles Related to the Nervous System and the Eye:
   Concerning the Existence of a Neural-Ocular Immune System   99
   J. Wayne Streilein and Andrew W. Taylor

4. Cervical Lymphatics, the Blood-Brain Barrier, and Immunoreactivity
   of the Brain   134
   Helen F. Cserr and Paul M. Knopf

III   IMMUNOLOGICALLY ACTIVE CELLS

5. Microglia and Macrophages   155
   V. Hugh Perry and Siamon Gordon

6. Astrocytes: Normal Aspects and Response to CNS Injury   173
   Michael D. Norenberg

7. Lymphocyte Entry and the Initiation of Inflammation
   in the Central Nervous System   200
   William F. Hickey, Hans Lassmann, and Anne H. Cross

8. Innervation of Lymphoid Organs and Neurotransmitter–Lymphocyte
   Interactions   226
   Denise L. Bellinger, Suzanne Y. Felten, Dianne Lorton, and David L. Felten

IV   CELLULAR AND HUMORAL IMMUNE RESPONSES IN THE NERVOUS SYSTEM

9. Autoantigens of the Nervous System   333
   Lou Ann Barnett and Robert S. Fujinami

10. Antigen Presentation in the Central Nervous System   364
    Jonathon D. Sedgwick and William F. Hickey

11. Cytokine Expression in the Nervous System   419
    Etty N. Benveniste

12. CD4 Effector Cells in Autoimmune Diseases
    of the Central Nervous System   460
    Hartmut Wekerele

13. Direct Cell-Mediated Responses in the Nervous System: CTL vs. NK Activity,
    and Their Dependence Upon MHC Expression and Modulation   493
    Wendy S. Armstrong and Lois A. Lampson

14. Neuroendocrine–Immune Interactions   548
    Douglas A. Weigent and J. Edwin Blalock

15. Establishment and Control of Viral Infections
    of the Central Nervous System   576
    *Jürgen Schneider-Schaulies, Uwe G. Liebert, Rüdiger Dörries,
    and Volker ter Meullen*

16. Transplantation into the Central Nervous System   611
    Maciej Poltorak and William J. Freed

17. Immunosuppression: CNS Effects   642
    Robert W. Keane

18. Immunology of the Eye   668
   Scott W. Cousins and Richard D. Dix

V   NEUROIMMUNOLOGY OF DISEASE

19. Autoimmune Demyelinating Diseases of the Central Nervous System   703
   Claude P. Genain and Stephen L. Hauser

20. AIDS and the Nervous System   727
   Lawrence S. Honig

21. Tumors of the Central Nervous System   760
   Carol J. Wikstrand and Darell J. Bigner

22. Immunology of the Peripheral Nervous System   785
   Rachel George, Judith Spies, and John W. Griffin

Foreword

CEDRIC S. RAINE

As one of a proud group of investigators who has endeavored over the past three decades to carve a niche for neuroimmunology, I count it an honor and a singular privilege to write the Foreword to this, the latest and probably most comprehensive, tome on the subject. To begin by defining what we mean by neuroimmunology is no longer necessary (not that any reader studying this book would require a definition), first because it has already been done quite eloquently elsewhere, and second, because as we dissect more the montage of molecules and responses associated with nervous and immune interactions, the lines of distinction between the two systems become less clear and definition becomes a little hazardous. Indeed, it is precisely within the purview of the present volume to spell out in succinct terms where the two systems differ and where they overlap. One should note that to achieve their goal, the editors have assembled a diverse team of authors, many of them relatively new to the field with fresh outlooks, a laudable accomplishment. Speaking as the founding editor of what may well be the major journal on the subject of neuroimmunology and president of its international society, I can say with considerable hindsight that no matter how hard one tries to cover the many topics that fall under the dome of neuroimmunology, it will be impossible to satisfy all readers. The topics to be covered range in nature from basic to clinical, structural to behavioral, classifiable to unclassifiable, and tangible to intangible, yet all lean toward the understanding of immune system interactions with nervous tissue in health and disease. The irony seems to be that, although most neuro-immunologists were weaned on the dogma that the brain is immunologically privileged terrain, the more we investigate the differences between the nervous and immune systems, the more similarities we find. These issues are addressed in a scholarly fashion in the following twenty-three chapters, which carefully embody most current neuroimmunologic problems.

Precisely what the editors had in mind when they invited me to write a Foreword was not immediately clear, but I assume it was related to my role in the evolution of the field. Therefore, I shall frame the following paragraphs in the context of a brief history by one who has lived through (and perhaps even participated in) the veritable explosion of knowledge on the immunology of the nervous system over the past two decades, and the manner in which this prestigious volume presents our current understanding of the resultant diaspora which has become known as "Neuroimmunology."

While currency was given to the term many years earlier by pioneers like Rivers, Waksman (featured in this volume), Witebsky, Adams, Kabat, Koprowski, *inter alia,* in my mind, "Neuroimmunology" did not really become legal tender until the early 1970s. Recognizing its potential, Don Tower in 1974, the Director of NINCDS at that time, created a Neuroimmunology Branch at the National Institutes of Health. This was to be a clinically oriented research entity, with Dale McFarlin at its helm and was probably the first of its kind in the world. The research charter of the Branch targeted multiple sclerosis and its experimental models, conditions with a unifying pathology— immune-mediated destruction of myelin. However, at that time, the thrust of most research on multiple sclerosis was more focused on a viral etiology than on the immunologic (or autoimmune) aspect of the pathology. Thus, since Dale's area of interest was immunology, Don Tower's new Branch may have at first been perceived as something of an academic gamble. Nevertheless, his insight was brought to fruition when the Branch, under Dale's leadership, grew into an international multidisciplinary powerhouse serving as both a major training resource and a launching pad for today's key players in the field. Subsequently, neuroimmunology groups were spawned world-wide, giving rise to the present situation whereby almost every center for research in the neurological sciences embraces a section devoted to the subject. The field owes a debt of gratitude to the foresight of Don Tower and the efforts of Dale McFarlin.

In former times, tracing the literature on the history of neuroimmunology was always an arduous task since works on the subject were disseminated across a broad array of journals aimed at immunologists, neurologists, neuropathologists, and neuro-biologists. Most of the early reports were disease-oriented and stemmed from work on multiple sclerosis and related conditions and the recognition that an inflammatory response within the nervous system was an abnormal event, usually the harbinger of clinical manifestations and tissue damage. It was clear from the outset that a breach in the blood-brain barrier was integral in such instances. As a consequence, many pioneer works were dedicated to alterations in CNS permeability and the analysis of inflamma-tory responses in the nervous system generated by a variety of antigenic mixtures. These approaches had at their roots a need to understand the etiology of the acute disseminated encephalomyelitides and multiple sclerosis. Books like *Allergic Encepha-lomyelitis* by Kies and Alvord (Thomas, Springfield, IL, 1959), and *Research in De-myelinating Diseases* by Scheinberg, Kies, and Alvord (NY Academy of Sciences, 1965) provide images of the early status of the field.

The first real step towards neuroimmunology acquiring its own identity occurred with the inception of the *Journal of Neuroimmunology* in 1981, an event that has since been endorsed by the appearance of other journals on the same and similar subjects, viz. psychoneuroimmunology, neuroendocrinology, and neuroimmunomodulation. As neuroimmunology grew in the 1980s, so did the number of reference books dedicated to it and its subspecialities. It might be of interest to survey briefly some of these chronologically since they appear to reflect the metamorphosis of the field from one with a disease bias, to one with basic neurobiology tagged on, and ultimately to the one we recognize today, covering not only disease and basic mechanisms, but also immunogenetics; neuroimmune interactions; the effects of neuropeptides, neuroendocrine products, and behavior on the immune system; developmental problems dictated by immune system molecules; and the ability of nervous system elements to function as cells of the immune system. Peruse, for example, *Neuroimmunology*, edited by Brockes in 1982 (Plenum), a mixed collection of articles dedicated largely to the analysis of nervous system elements with immunologic markers, a landmark publication at the time. Then survey *Neuroimmunology*, edited by Behan and Spreafico in 1984 (Raven), representing the proceedings of the First International Congress of Neuroimmunology (Stresa, Italy, 1982). Significantly, this book was the first serious attempt to bring together the emerging diverse topics embraced by neuroimmunology. However, even in 1982, a heavy bias towards CNS disease mechanisms was still apparent. Lastly, examine the proceedings of the Second International Congress of Neuroimmunology published under the title *Advances in Neuroimmunology*, edited by Raine (NY Academy of Sciences, 1988). This was probably the first volume to give an overall view of the breadth of the neuroimmunologic landscape.

Certainly, there has been no shortage of reading material since 1988, with the several journals on the subject increasing steadily their annual page allocations and circulation. Nevertheless, with the exception of a few volumes focused on specific areas of neuroimmunology, the book scene has been relatively quiet. Thus, the present work edited by Keane and Hickey, comes at an opportune moment after a book-free period, a period during which we have been deluged with the identification of a host of soluble and membrane-bound immune mediators and their receptors, with molecular sequencing, and with the development of some spectacularly sophisticated probes and methods to identify and analyze nervous and immune system components in situ, approaches that have not yet appeared in a reference text.

Immunology of the Nervous System is not only a book for the specialist but one that will also serve as an essential text for the graduate, the postdoctoral fellow, and the nonspecialist seeking enlightenment. It is divided into useful sections intended to cover distinct arenas. There is inevitably some repetition and overlap in places, particularly in the area of myelin autoimmunity, lymphocyte trafficking, and inflammation, and some topics are not covered in exhaustive fashion (e.g., latest technologies). Nevertheless, one can rest assured that this book is going to provide a key reference on the field. Refreshing it is to see that interspersed among a more traditional assemblage of topics on basic immunology, lymphocyte trafficking, cytokines, and autoimmunity, there is competent coverage of cerebral lymphatics, lymphoid organ innervation, neuroendocrine feedback mechanisms, and ophthalmologic neuroimmunology. All too often, the latter areas are deemphasized at our meetings, and when they are included on the program, presenters may justifiably feel a little out of place. This is not a problem in the present text where the contributors have been carefully screened and where the charge of each author has been clearly assigned and executed. In this regard, the editors are to be congratulated.

From these pages, it will also be clear that neuroimmunology is still an evolving field. To say that this volume is the last word on the subject would be frivolous. This book fills a much needed niche inasmuch as it provides a valuable update and lays out clearly the breadth of today's neuroimmunologic terrain. Indeed, it does so in such a fashion that another volume on the subject will not be necessary for several years to come. With this book, the editors might well have generated a scaffold to which new areas can be appended and which can be periodically updated as the subject continues to evolve.

Preface

Neuroimmunology is an emerging discipline whose subject matter is drawn from the overlapping areas of neuroscience and immunology, two of today's largest and most rapidly advancing scientific arenas. As such, the purview of neuroimmunology is wide, complex, and constantly growing. Over the past decade it has become increasingly clear that the general principles of immunology must be applied in a highly specialized fashion when dealing with immunologic reactions in the nervous system. The concepts of immunologic privilege of the nervous system, the blood brain barrier, immunologic surveillance of the nervous system, as well as infectious, autoimmune, and neoplastic diseases of the nervous system must all be carefully scrutinized. Likewise, in neuroscience there is a growing awareness that the cells and substances well known in immunology can play critical roles in specific responses of the nervous system and its constituent elements. Issues relating to neural innervation of organs of the immune system, feedback mechanisms for neuroendocrine hormones and immunologic cytokines on brain nuclei, and the effects of trauma, stress, or depression on specific neural circuits also merit special attention. Therefore, the field of neuroimmunology fills a vital gap by analyzing and explaining phenomena that occur in either the nervous or immune systems in response to manipulations or perturbations in the other system.

The first section of this book sketches the development of neuroimmunology from a series of disease related observations to the scientific specialty it now is. The second section provides an overview of the elements and principle functions of the immune system and problems confronting the experimentalist and clinician in examination of immunologic responses within the the nervous system. In the third section, the cellular elements of the immunologic and nervous systems active in neuroimmunologic events are set forth in detail. The fourth and largest section deals with the basic physiologic and pathologic processes central to the interactions between these two disparate systems. The final section considers the pathogenesis and therapy of the spectrum of diseases in which neuroimmunologic phenomena are active. In aggregate, the majority of areas and topics currently comprising neuroimmunology will be considered; some— such as autoimmune neurologic diseases—will be examined from a variety of viewpoints.

This volume is intended to survey the field of neuroimmunology in a broad manner. The chapters have been written so that the reader can understand how a specific area has evolved, learn of the critical experiments and seminal observations relative to that topic, become familiar with the current hypotheses and problems guiding ongoing investigations, and be directed to the important publications that have framed an issue. While some basic knowledge of immunology and neuroscience is assumed, all of the chapters are intended to be accessible to any scientist wanting to gain insight into the complex interactions occurring between two of the most intricate mammalian systems. It is the aim of the editors and authors that this text should be the starting point for any scholar wishing to learn about neuroimmunology or its disparate parts.

R.W.K.
W.F.H.

Abbreviations

AbSC	antibody-secreting cell
AC	anterior chamber
AC	adenylate cyclase
ACAID	anterior chamber–associated immune deviation
ACh	acetylcholine
AChE	acetylcholinesterase
AChR	acetylcholine receptor
ACTH	adrenocorticotropin
AD	Alzheimer's disease
ADC	AIDS dementia complex
ADCC	antibody-dependent complement-mediated cytotoxicity
ADCC	antibody-dependent cell-mediated cytotoxicity
ADE	antibody-dependent enhancement
ADE	acute disseminated encephalitis
ADEM	acute disseminated encephalomyelitis
Ag	antigen
AHL	acute hemorrhagic encephalomyelitis
AIDP	acute inflammatory demyelinating polyneuropathy
AIDP	acute inflammatory demyelinating polyradiculoneuropathy
AIDS	acquired immunodeficiency syndrome
A-LAK	adherent lymphokine-activated killer (cell)
α-MSH	α-melanocyte-stimulating hormone
ALS	amyotrophic lateral sclerosis
AMAN	acute motor axonal neuropathy
AMSAN	acute motor sensory axonal neuropathy
APC	antigen-presenting cell
ARN	acute retinal necrosis
ARV	AIDS-associated retrovirus
ATL	acute T-cell leukemia
ATP	adenosine triphosphate autoantigen
AVP	arginine vasopressin

AZT	azidothymidine
BALT	bronchial-associated lymphoid tissue
BBB	blood-brain barrier
BDNF	brain-derived neurotrophic factor
BDV	Borna disease virus
b-gal	b-galactosidase
β2M	β2-microglobulin
BIV	bovine immunodeficiency virus
BN	brown Norway (mouse)
C	complement
C	constant (region)
CA	catecholamine
CAEV	caprine arthritis-encephalitis virus
CCK	cholecystokinin
CD	cluster of differentiation
CDR	complementary determining region
CDV	canine distemper virus
CGRP	calcitonin gene-related peptide
ChAT	choline acetyltransferase
CIDP	chronic inflammatory demyelinating polyradiculoneuropathy
CIDP	chronic inflammatory demyelinating polyneuropathy
CLL	chronic lymphocytic leukemia
CLN	cervical lymph node
CMI	cell-mediated immunity
CMV	cytomegalovirus
CNS	central nervous system
CPEC	choroid plexus epithelial cell
CR	complement receptor
CR-LR	cysteine-rich, leucine-rich
CRE	cumulative radiation effect
CREAE	chronic relapsing experimental allergic encephalomyelitis
CRF	corticotropin-releasing factor
CRH	corticotropin-releasing hormone
CSF	colony-stimulating factor
CSF	cerebrospinal fluid
CT	computed tomography
CTL	cytotoxic T lymphocyte
CTNF	ciliary neurotrophic factor
CVO	circumventricular organ

DAF	decay-accelerating factor
DC	dendritic cell
ddC	dideoxycytidine
ddI	dideoxyinosine
DSPN	distal symmetric polyneuropathy
DTH	delayed-type hypersensitivity
EAE	experimental allergic (autoimmune) encephalomyelitis
EAMG	experimental allergic (autoimmune) myasthenia gravis
EAN	experimental allergic (autoimmune) neuritis
EAU	experimental allergic (autoimmune) uveitis
EBV	Epstein-Barr virus
EC	endothelial cell
EGF	epidermal growth factor
EGFR	epidermal growth factor receptor
EIAV	equine infectious anemia virus
ELISA	enzyme-linked immunoassay
EM	electron microscopic
EP	epinephrine
ER	endoplasmic reticulum
F	fusion
FACS	fluorescence-activated cell sorter
Fc	crystallizable fragment (of immunoglobulin)
FCA	Freund's complete adjuvant
FGF	fibroblast growth factor
FIV	feline immunodeficiency virus
G-CSF	granulocyte colony-stimulating factor
GABA	γ-aminobutyric acid
Gal	galactose
galC	galactocerebroside
GALT	gut-associated lymphoid tissue
GBS	Guillain-Barré syndrome
GCV	ganciclovir
GFAP	glial fibrillary acidic protein
GH	growth hormone
Glu	glutamate
GM-CSF	granulocyte-macrophage colony-stimulating factor
gp	glycoprotein
GvHD	graft-versus-host disease

h	human
H	hemagglutinin
HAM	HTLV-1-associated myelopathy
HAM/TSP	HTLV-1-associated myelopathy/tropical spastic paraparesis
HEV	high endothelial venules
Hh	hematopoietic histocompatiblity
HIV	human immunodeficiency virus
HLA	human leukocyte antigen
HLA	histocompatibility leukocyte antigen
HPA	hypothalamic–pituitary–adrenal
HPB	human peripheral blood
HPLC	high-pressure liquid chromatography
HRP	horseradish peroxidase
HSA	human serum albumin
HSV	herpes simplex virus
HTLV	human T-cell lymphotropic virus
IC	intracerebral
IC	immune complex
ICAM	intercellular adhesion molecule
ICC	immunocytochemistry
ICS	intercellular space
IFN	interferon
IFNNEX	interferon-γ-enhanced factor X
Ig	immunoglobulin
IL	interleukin
INO	internuclear opthalmoplegia
IP	interferon-γ-inducible protein
ir	immunoreactive
IRBP	interphotoreceptor retinoid-binding protein
ISF	interstitial fluid
JHMV	J. Howard Mueller virus
kDA	kilodalton
LAK	lymphokine-activated killer (cell)
LAT	latency-associated transcript
LAV	lymphadenopathy-associated virus
LCA	leukocyte common antigen
LCM	lymphocytic choriomeningitis
LCMV	lymphocytic choriomeningitis virus

LEMS	Lambert-Eaton myasthenic syndrome
LEW	Lewis (rat)
LFA	lymphocyte function–associated antigen
LGL	large granular lymphocyte
LHRH	luteinizing hormone–releasing hormone
LPS	lipopolysaccharide
mAB	monoclonal antibody
MAG	myelin-associated glycoprotein
MAI	Mycobacterium avium intracellulare
MAIDS	murine AIDS
MALT	mucosa-associated lymphoid tissue
MBP	myelin basic protein
M-CSF	macrophage colony-stimulating factor
MCMV	murine cytomegalovirus
MCP	monocyte chemoattractive protein
MePDN	methylprednisone
MG	myasthenia gravis
MG	microglia
MGC	multinucleated giant cell
MHC	major histocompatibility complex
MIP	macrophage inhibitory protein
MLR	mixed leukocyte response
MLR	mixed leukocyte reaction
MMTV	mouse mammary tumor virus
MND	motor neuron disease
MOG	myelin-oligoglycoprotein
MRI	magnetic resonance imaging
MS	multiple sclerosis
MV	measles virus
MW	molecular weight
N	nucleocapsid
NA	noradrenergic
NC	natural cytotoxic (cell)
N-CAM	nerve cell adhesion molecule
NE	norepinephrine
NF-κB	nuclear factor kappa B
NGF	nerve growth factor
NIS	neural–ocular immune system
NK	natural killer (cell)
NKTS	natural killer target structure

NO	nitric oxide
NO	nitrate
NOS	nitrate synthase
NPY	neuropeptide Y
NT	neurotensin
NTR	nontranslated region
NZB	New Zealand black (mouse)
NZW	New Zealand white (mouse)

OB	oligoclonal band
ODC	oligodendrocyte
OPPV	ovine progressive pneumonia virus
OV, OVA	ovalbumin

PALS	periarteriolar lymphatic sheath
PBL	peripheral blood lymphocyte
PCD	paraneoplastic cerebellar degeneration
PCD-AA	paraneoplastic cerebellar degeneration–associated antigen
PCR	polymerase chain reaction
PDGF	platelet-derived growth factor
PECAM	peritoneal exudate cell adhesion molecule
PFC	plaque-forming cell
PGE2	prostaglandin E2
PHA	phytohemagglutinin antigen
PHI	peptide histidine isoleucine
PIE	postinfectious/parainfectious encephalomyelitis
PKC	protein kinase C
PLP	proteolipid protein
PMA	phorbol myristate acetate
PML	progressive multifocal leukoencephalopathy
PMN	polymorphonuclear leukocyte
PNS	peripheral nervous system
POEMS	*p*olyneuropathy, *o*rganomegaly, *e*ndocrinopathy, *m*yeloma, *s*kin changes (syndrome)
POMC	proopiomelanocortin
PPD	purified protein derivative
PRL	prolactin
PRP	progressive rubella panencephalitis
PVC	perivascular cell
PVE	postvaccinal encephalomyelitis

R	receptor

RANTES	regulated on activation normal T-cell expressed and secreted
RIA	radioimmunoassay
RISA	radioiodinated serum albumin
ROS	reactive oxygen species
RPE	retinal pigment epithelium
RT-PCR	reverse transcription polymerase chain reactions
RV	rabies virus
SAME	subacute measles encephalomyelitis
S-antigen	soluble antigen
SC	subcutaneously
SCG	superior cervical ganglia
SCID	severe combined immunodeficiency disease
SCLC	small-cell lung cancer
SDE	subacute demyelinating encephalomyelitis
SEA	Staphylococcus enterotoxin A
SFV	Semliki Forest virus
SGLPG	sulfated glucoronic acid lactosaminyl paragloboside
SGPG	sulfated glucoronic acid paragloboside
SIV	Simian immunodeficiency virus
SLE	systemic lupus erythematosus
SMCG	superior mesenteric-celiac ganglionic complex
SM/P	smooth muscle cell/pericyte
SOM	somatostatin
SP	substance P
SPN	suppressin
SRBC	sickle red blood cell
SSPE	subacute sclerosing panencephalitis
T3	triiodothyronine
TcR	T-cell receptor
Th, TH	T helper (cell)
TH	tyrosine hydroxylase
THF	thymic humoral factor
TIC-X	tumor necrosis factor-α-induced complex X
TIL	tumor-infiltrating lymphocyte
TK	tachykinin
TMEV	Theiler's murine encephalitis virus
TNF	tumor necrosis factor
Tpo	thymopoietin
Ts	T suppressor (cell)
TSH	thyroid-stimulating hormone

TSP	tropical spastic paraparesis
UV	ultraviolet
V	variable (region)
VCAM	vascular cell adhesion molecule
VIP	vasoactive intestinal peptide
VLA	very late antigen
VMV	(ovine) Visna-Maedi virus
WGA	wheat germ agglutinin
WHO	World Health Organization
YFV	yellow fever virus
ZDF	zidovudine

I

HISTORY OF NEUROIMMUNOLOGY

1

A Brief History of Neuroimmunology

BYRON H. WAKSMAN

Neuroimmunology was originally concerned with diseases of the nervous system, caused or modulated by immune mechanisms, and with a series of animal models of disease, both those involving exogenous antigens and those which proved to be auto-immune (454). Many of the latter were postinfectious, but later the category of para-neoplastic disorders of the nervous system has assumed increasing importance. To-day neuroimmunology also encompasses the study of neural antigens, cellular immunology, antibodies, and products of the complement cascade; neurotransmitters and neuropeptides; cytokines and more conventional hormones and growth factors, and their binding to specific and nonspecific receptors in the cell membrane; the intervention of other membrane recognition elements, such as major histocom-patibility complex (MHC) and a variety of adhesion molecules; signal transduction and activation of second messenger systems; gene regulation; and finally, the produc-tion and expression or secretion of significant gene products. The companion field of psychoneuroimmunology, or neuroendocrinimmunology, deals with actions of the nervous system on the immune system at the level of the central and peripheral lymphoid organs, including mature lymphocytes and their functions, and inflamma-tory processes; with the production and use of neurotransmitters and neuropeptides as mediators in the immune system and of cytokines in the nervous system; and finally with the interaction of the immune and nervous systems with the hypothalamic–pituitary–adrenal (including thyroid and gonadal) axes. In contrast to neuroimmunology, as a field, psychoneuroimmunology has undergone a similar but somewhat later growth.

Role of Neural Elements in Immune Responses

Antigen presentation in the induction of the immune response takes place primarily in the spleen, lymph nodes, and mucosa-associated lymphoid tissues. However, Silverstein and Lukes, in 1962, observed massive plasma cell infiltrates in the Virchow-Robin spaces of the brain in neonates with congenital syphilis or toxoplasmosis (403). More recently, Prineas reported that lymphoid aggregates resembling immunocompetent peripheral lymphoid tissue form about vessels within multiple sclerosis (MS) plaques in the brain (343). These appear comparable to the lymphoid aggregates found in the thyroid in Hashimoto's thyroiditis and represent an end stage of the "progressive immunization reaction" occurring at sites of elicitation of inflammatory (antibody or cell-mediated) immunologic reactions in target organs (404).

It seems clear that neural elements play a significant role when immunologic events are enacted within the central (CNS) or peripheral nervous system (PNS), whether involving autoimmune responses or responses to exogenous infectious agents, tumors, or grafts. In the normal CNS, there is limited expression of MHC class I, mainly on glial cells and endothelium, while MHC-II and the various immunoactive adhesion molecules are not constitutively expressed. In 1981, Fontana and colleagues first called attention to the ability of such cytokines as interferon-γ (IFN-γ) to up-regulate the astrocytes' ability to express MHC class II, to secrete cytokines (interleukin-1 [IL-1], IL-3, tumor necrosis factor alpha [TNF α]), and to present antigens like myelin basic protein (MBP) to specific T-cell lines (118,120,264). This work was amply confirmed (reviews in 31,119,122,227,263,351) and the level of MCH-II expression was found to parallel susceptibility to experimental autoimmune encephalomyelitis (EAE) in a comparison of mouse strains (264). In 1986 attention turned to microglia, which were also found to respond to IFN-γ with up-regulation of MHC-II (see 122). Introduction of IFN-γ or IFN-γ + TNF-α directly into the CNS results in progressive, independent up-regulation of the two classes of MHC and of adhesion molecules, such as intracellular adhesion molecule I (ICAM-I) and their expression—first, on perivascular macrophages (164), then on macrophages and microglia throughout the CNS, and lastly, on astrocytes (226,262). In the PNS, there may be comparable up-regulation and expression of MHC-II on Schwann cells. In muscle, myoblasts stimulated by IFN-γ or IFN-γ + TNF-α express MHC-II and various adhesion molecules and can present antigen to T cells (132).

In the induction and elicitation of EAE, the main presentation of CNS antigens to circulating specific T cells appears to be by perivascular macrophages (163–165). The role of astrocytes is now felt to be ambiguous. These cells are actually lysed when they present antigen to specific T cells in vitro, and it is not clear whether the T cells are stimulated to proliferate and/or release inflammatory cytokines or are turned off because of the absence of suitable costimulatory signals, or so-called clonal anergy. The role of cerebral vascular endothelium in antigen presentation within the CNS is similarly ambiguous. The demonstration in 1986 that these cells could be stimulated in vitro by IFN-γ to express MHC-II and to present MBP or other proteins to specific T cells (269,407) was followed by the finding that the endothelial cells themselves might be lysed in the process (363) and the T cells were rendered anergic rather than stimulated. Thus the relative importance of these "nonprofessional antigen-presenting cells" and the significance of various adhesion molecules, cytokines, and other costimulatory signals in relation to the various outcomes of antigen presentation (proliferation, cytokine production, immune deviation from TH1 to TH2, anergy, and lysis) remain unclear.

The Brain as an Immunologically Privileged Site

In 1948 Medawar described the brain as an immunologically privileged site after observing that skin allografts placed in this organ failed to induce the usual transplant rejection response (275). Such transplants were nevertheless rejected if the graft recipient was immunized by an orthotopically placed skin graft from the same (or a syngeneic) donor. These contrasting results could be related to the absence of conventional lymphatic drainage, i.e., an afferent immunizing pathway, from the brain and to the presence of a conventional vasculature, the efferent pathway for transplant rejection. On the other hand, many people incorrectly inferred a relationship between immunologic privilege and the separation of the CNS from the blood stream by the blood-brain barrier. The blood-brain barrier concept originated in Ehrlich's observation of 1885 that certain aniline dyes failed to stain the CNS, but the existence of a barrier remained in doubt as late as 1961 (97). This doubt was finally laid to rest by the ultrastructural studies of Reese and Karnovsky in 1967 (357).

Investigation of other organs showing peculiarities of transplant rejection, such as the eye and the testis (275), supported the notion that deficiencies affecting either the afferent or efferent pathways of the immune response always led to some degree of immunologic privilege. This property had the practical consequences that tissue allografts or even xenografts to the brain or eye would remain more or less normal and could serve as experimental substrate, in studies of normal development and regulation or of neurological disease. In 1979, Aguayo spliced normal peripheral nerve into trembler mouse sciatic in a study of axon-glial relationships (6) and soon after extended this approach to the CNS. By 1983 Gumpel and colleagues were grafting oligodendrocytes from normal donors into the CNS of shiverer mutants—these migrated widely and produced normal myelin; they were not rejected (142). These studies were subsequently extended to studies of astrocyte transplants and finally of neurons. The transplantation to the brain of dopamine-producing adrenal tissue, with long survival of the transplanted cells in a fully functional state, is now the basis of an effective therapy in advanced parkinsonism. Immunologic tolerance has to be invoked in some of this experimentation. An extreme example of grafting and tolerance is provided by the famous Le Douarin experiment, in which embryonic spinal cord grafts between chicken and quail persist in perfect harmony for 5–7 weeks, followed by the appearance of disease in the grafted core (graft rejection) and later in the host CNS (autoimmunity) (208).

The subject of immunological privilege has acquired new dimensions with Streilein's demonstration that placing protein antigens in the anterior chamber of the eye leads to a qualitative change in the nature of the specific immune response: a significant shift away from the cell-mediated immune response and towards antibody formation occurs, what we have come to think of as a shift from a TH1 to a TH2 type of response (291). It has become clear that in many species, antigens introduced into the brain leave via cerebrospinal fluid drainage over the olfactory nerves and through the cribriform plate within the nose, and enter lymphatics draining the nasal mucosa, finally reaching deep and superficial cervical lymph nodes (169). These nodes, like others draining mucosal sites, make a predominantly TH2 immune response. Not surprisingly, if placed in the cerebrospinal fluid, MBP induces an antibody response within the cervical lymph nodes and renders the treated animal refractory to the induction of EAE (151). This observation forces a reinterpretation of the term immunologically privileged site, as applied to the brain.

In the 1950s and '60s, it was commonly thought that, because the blood-brain barrier prevented escape of antigens or their breakdown products from the CNS, neural antigens never attained high enough concentrations in the blood to induce tolerance by negative selection within the thymus or clonal T-cell anergy in the periphery. As we have seen, antigens in fact leave the CNS readily, so this idea has been abandoned. An unexpected more recent finding is that neural antigens such as (a form of) MBP and S100β are actually formed within the normal thymus (339), yet their presence fails to eliminate the corresponding "autoreactive" T cells.

Psychoneuroimmunology

Selye proposed in the 1930s that stress, operating through neural and endocrine pathways, might affect the function of the immune system (396). The adrenal corticosteroids were shown to be *stress hormones,* with profound lympholytic effects on thymus and secondary lymphoid organs and the ability to suppress immune responses, inhibit lymphocytic functions, and modify inflammation (74). A distinct field of *psychoimmunology* or, as it has more recently been called, *psychoneuroimmunology* (4,411) or *neuroimmunomodulation* (328,349), and the companion field of *neuroendocrinimmunology* (42) did not, however, come into being until the late 1970s and early '80s. Pavlov's brilliant work on conditioned reflexes in the early part of the century had led to a profusion of Russian studies professing to relate the nervous system, and conditioned reflexes in particular, to the functioning of the immune system. Much of this work was poorly controlled and/or unreproducible. Together with what were seen as Selye's exaggerated claims, they cast a shadow on the field for several decades.

The first observations to be accepted scientifically concerned the effect of bereavement on reducing immune responsiveness and increasing morbidity in human subjects (24,415,416) and the similar effect of stress in animal models (198). Ader and Cohen's demonstration in 1975 that immune responses could be reproduced and manipulated by conditioned reflexes (5, see 4) did much to alleviate the earlier skepticism, as did the demonstration that electrolytic lesions in the brain profoundly affected immune responses (369). The introduction of the dexamethasone test in 1981 led to the discovery that the hypothalamic–pituitary–adrenal (HPA) axis is hyperactive in about half of depressed patients; this hyperactivity appears to be causally related to the depressed lymphocytic responses (255).

After isolated publications in the 1960s and '70s (131,358,467), Felten et al. (114), Bullock and Moore (58), and now several other investigators have provided solid morphologic evidence for the autonomic (noradrenergic) innervation of both central (bone marrow, thymus) and peripheral (spleen, lymph nodes, mucosa-associated) lymphoid organs (see 252). In these organs the nerve terminals make direct contact with macrophages, as well as with T and B cells (91). Hadden and others demonstrated receptors for neurotransmitters on lymphoid cells (also on macrophages, granulocytes, and bone marrow stem cells) as early as 1970 (145,253,468). Adrenergic agonists were found to inhibit proliferative responses elicited with mitogens, apparently by elevating cyclic adenosine monophosphate (cAMP) (144), while cholinergic stimuli and elevation of cyclic guanosine monophosphate (cGMP) acted to enhance them. Accordingly, beta-adrenergic agonists enhance immune responses if administered before the immune stimulus and inhibit them if given during the proliferative phase of the response. Adrenergic antagonists have opposite effects. Parasympathetic mediators such as acetylcholine also act on certain T-cell subsets and mediate enhanced proliferative responses (135), and opiates are reported to enhance cytotoxic T lymphocyte (CTL) function (163,316). Surgical and chemical sympathectomy have been found to enhance immune responses (38) and to alter immune regulation (38,67,80,168,278). These effects appear to be mediated by an up-regulation of beta-adrenergic receptors on all lymphocyte subsets but especially on CD8+ suppressor populations (63). Of particular interest is Arnason and Chelmicka-Schorr's demonstration that EAE is enhanced by sympathectomy (68) and inhibited by treatment with beta-adrenergic agonists such as isoproterenol (69). Experimental autoimmune myasthemia gravis (EAMG) is also enhanced by sympathectomy (see 67).

Endocrine influences on immune function have been well recognized since the 1960s (see Ahlqvist's 1976 review, 7). The importance of pituitary growth hormones, prolactin and GH in particular, on the maturation of the lymphoid organs and their functions was already known from the hypertrophy of thymus and lymph nodes in acromegaly and immune deficiency in hypopituitary dwarfs. Hypophysectomy (or blocking prolactin release with bromocriptine) results in reduced immune (including autoimmune) responses; these are restored by the administration of prolactin (294). Similarly, more "peripheral" hormones, such as adrenal corticosteroids, vasopressin, and estrogens, act directly on the survival and function of more mature lymphocytes (376). An increased interest in neuropeptide hormones and their receptors on cells of the immune system was fueled by the work of Blalock and collaborators, starting in 1980 (42,43,406). Their studies have been seminal in focusing attention on the mechanisms by which an individual's psychological state directly influences his or her immunological responses.

The 1980s also saw the unexpected discovery that many of the cytokines playing a role in immune responses act in the CNS as well. The role of interleukin-1 (IL-1) as an "endogenous pyrogen" acting on the hypothalamus to cause fever and sleep and stimulating the HPA (with release of thyroid-stimulating hormone (TSH), growth hormone (GH), prolactin (PRL), and changes in glucose homeostasis) is by now well known (20,37,96). Not only IL-1 (39) but also IL-6, TNF-α, and several of the interferons act on neurons in the organum vasculosum of the lamina terminalis, causing them to release prostaglandins which, in turn, induce cells of the hypothalamic nuclei to release corticoprotein-releasing factor (CRF) and activate the pituitary–adrenal corticosteroid system. In 1986, it was discovered that both IL-1 and TNF-α are actually produced by the neurons of specific nuclei in the hypothalamus and appear to serve as a new class of peptide transmitters (sometimes called *neurokines*) (51,383). Arnason has suggested (74) that cytokine action on hypothalamic nuclei may account for the sleep of advanced trypanosomiasis, the stupor and coma of meningitis, and the characteristic lassitude of multiple sclerosis. Astrocytes, too, produce a variety of cytokines when stimulated and are responsive to IFN-γ (118,119,264), while oligodendryocytes bear receptors for several cytokines.

Autoimmunity and Autoimmune Disease

During the explosion of new immunologic discoveries that took place mainly in France and Germany during the first decade of the present century, the central nervous system was shown to contain multiple "organ-specific" antigens (377). In 1903, the crystalline lens was the first tissue to be recognized as containing potential autoantigens (440). Its protein antigen(s) was shown in 1922 to induce a cell-mediated immunity in human subjects after lens extraction for cataract. This sensitization could be detected by delayed skin reactions and was manifested by the associated disease, phakoanaphylactic endophthalmitis (known today as phakogenic uveitis) (450). The corresponding animal model was produced experimentally by Burky (in rabbits) in 1934, just a year after Rivers' discovery of EAE (59), while experimental autoimmune uveitis, a model for sympathetic ophthalmia in humans, was not obtained in a reproducible form (in guinea pigs) until 1949 (77; see 105).

These early studies were written off by most physicians and scientists as being concerned with tissues completely sequestered from the immune system, notably the lens and ciliary body within the eye, and the brain hiding behind its blood-brain barrier.

A few hardy souls like Dameshek insisted that there were instances of true autoimmunity, principally affecting blood cells (83), but dogmatic resistance to the concept of autoimmunity gave way only after 1956, when experimental autoimmune thyroiditis was established as a model (368) and the similarity could be recognized between the immune responses in this animal model and those in Hashimoto's thyroiditis in humans (367).

The 1920s and '30s saw a series of increasingly thorough serologic studies of CNS glycolipid antigens and their comparison with the Wassermann and Forssman antigens by well-known research groups, such as Brandt, Guth, and Müller; Witebsky and Steinfeld; and Plaut and Kossowitz. These antigens and the corresponding antibodies were never effectively related to autoimmune diseases during the early development of neuroimmunology. They included phospholipids, gangliosides, globosides, other glycosphingolipids, glycoproteins, and a variety of additional "cytolipins" (G, H, K, and R), and their investigation required specialized serological techniques, available to a limited number of laboratories (356). Only in the 1980s have many of these complex CNS antigens been related to disease pathogenesis in systemic lupus erythematosus, neuropathic syndromes associated with gammopathy, and some cases of motor neuron disease (477; see below).

Molecular Mimicry and Related Mechanisms

The first precise observations on molecular mimicry have been attributed (82) to Ajdukewic and colleagues who in 1972 described antibodies to smooth muscle arising in infectious hepatitis patients. In 1976 Husby et al. reported that streptococcal cell membranes carried epitopes cross-reactive with neurons of the caudate and subthalamic nuclei that might play a causative role in Sydenham's chorea (178). However, the mimicry concept could not really be validated until monoclonal antibodies became widely used in the late 1970s and, more to the point, before complete structural information became available on the many candidate viral and bacterial antigens and on the autoantigens that were incriminated in various acute and chronic demyelinating diseases in the 1980s.

Using monoclonal antibodies, in 1983, Dales, Fujinami, and Oldstone showed cross-reactions between vaccinia virus hemaglutinin and intermediate filament vimentin (82) and between measles virus phosphoprotein and a cytokeratin component of human intermediate filaments (126). In 1985 Fujinami and Oldstone published results of the first attempt to scan databases of known viral antigens for peptide sequences identical with or closely similar to those of known encephalitogenic or neuritogenic proteins (125). MBP peptide 66-75 and hepatitis-B virus polymerase peptide 589-598 were found to be almost identical. Fujinami synthesized the viral peptide, which induced mild EAE in about a third of a small group of rabbits, T cells reactive with MBP in half of the group, and antibody reactive with MBP in more than half of the group. Similar results were obtained virtually at the same time by Jahnke et al. (182) for several well-known viruses cross-reactive with MBP, P2, and so on. The Lees group showed the same kind of relationships between viral antigens and proteolipid protein (399).

To prove viral mimicry as a pathogenetic element in a given neurologic disease associated with viral infection, one must obtain individual T-cell clones that recognize both viral and host epitope and show reciprocal blocking by the two epitopes of responses to either. This was carried out first in an isolated observation by Marquardt in the early 1980s and more recently by Martin et al. in a series of patients with rubella panencephalitis: lines or clones could be obtained that were reactive with both virus and MBP (221). On the other hand, in a survey of 500 MBP-specific T-cell clones from MS patients, Pette and Liebert failed to find any clones that recognized measles epitopes! (331). Wucherpfennig and Strominger have now documented extensive cross-reactions between viral peptides and the immunodominant peptide (85-99) of MBP, using MBP-specific T-cell clones from MS patients (474).

The current preoccupation with viruses should not lead us to forget that molecular mimicry can be important when the immunizing event is a bacterial infection, as in the case of Syndenham's chorea following β-hemolytic streptococcal infection (178), or parasitic infestation, as in the neurologic syndrome of Chagas disease (211,405).

Mechanisms other than molecular mimicry may lead to biologically significant cross-reactions. Perhaps the most important one is the incorporation of host antigens into the envelope of a virus actually growing within the nervous system. In 1979 Steck et al. showed that purified vaccinia virus grown in brain can produce EAE (413). Conversely, myelinated tissue in which virus (vaccinia, rubella) has grown acquires greatly enhanced encephalogenicity (442). In the Semliki Forest virus model, antibodies reactive with myelin glycolipids cross-react only with brain-passaged virus (464); i.e., there is no mimicry between these lipids and antigen encoded by the viral genome.

Anti-idiotypic networks may also play a role in autoimmunization, since antibody against the binding site of a virus is the structural homologue of the host cell membrane receptor for that virus. The first clear documentation of autoimmunization involving idiotypes was provided by Reovirus hemagglutinin and an oligodendrocyte membrane component, later shown to be a beta-adrenergic receptor (302). The complete network of antigen, antibody, idiotype, autoantigen, and autoantibody can be perturbed at any point to result in increased autoimmunity (334).

Experimental Autoimmune Diseases—The EAE and EAN Models

For many people, the central theme of neuroimmunology is the study of immunologically mediated disease in the nervous system. Autoimmune inflammatory processes have, for the most part, been shown to reflect cell-mediated immunity against neural antigens, mediated largely by TH1 lymphocytes. A second major category is the group of autoimmune processes, mediated primarily by antibody. Finally, infectious agents entering the CNS or PNS frequently elicit inflammatory responses, mediated by cellular (TH1) immunity directed at the agents themselves (not autoimmune).

The first clearly identified neuroimmunologic disease in humans was *post-rabies vaccination encephalomyelitis,* in which repeated injections of homogenized rabbit spinal cord or mouse brain containing inactivated rabies virus led to a disseminated inflammatory demyelinative CNS disease (168). It was assumed that this disease resulted from immunization with antigenic components of the injected neural tissue cross-reactive with homologous components of the host's CNS. This suggestion was confirmed in 1933 with Rivers and his colleagues' demonstration that immunization of experimental animals with myelinated tissue regularly led to what is now called *experimental allergic (or autoimmune) encephalomyelitis (EAE)* (176,275,364).

As the first well-studied animal model of autoimmune disease in the nervous system possessing similarities to human demyelinative disease, particularly multiple sclerosis, EAE has been the subject of literally thousands of scientific papers in the 60 years since its discovery. During this time, the in-depth investigation of EAE has provided a model for investigations of all other organ-specific autoimmune diseases affecting the nervous or other organ systems of the body, both in animals and humans.

Early History

The method used by Rivers et al. to produce EAE in 1933 was long and tedious. In 1947, Kabat et al. and Morgan showed independent of each other that use of Freund's adjuvant (killed mycobacteria in mineral oil) resulted in prompt and rapid development of disease in a high proportion of animals injected once (192,298). Two different protein antigens of CNS myelin, proteolipid protein (PLP) and myelin basic protein were shown in 1954 and 1956, respectively, to induce EAE (460,205). Its course and intensity were shown to reflect the course and intensity of the cell-mediated immune response to those antigens and to have little if any relation to humoral responses against the antigen used for immunization (192,459,460). The use of Freund's adjuvant was shown to be nonessential, as other means of inducing strong cell-mediated immunity (for example intradermal injection of heterologous antigen) were also effective (451).

The next autoimmune model, described in 1955, was one affecting the peripheral nervous system; *experimental allergic (autoimmune) neuritis (EAN)* (455). The similarity of EAN to the Guillain-Barré syndrome (GBS) was duly noted, as was the similarity of its basic lesion to that of EAE. The characteristic albuminocytologic dissociation in the CSF of GBS patients was reproduced in rabbits with EAN.

The 1950s ended with a major symposium on EAE (204) and a major review (451) in which EAE and EAN found their place among a host of new models affecting not only the eye but also the testis, thyroid, and adrenal. In all these it had become clear that the distribution of lesions was determined first, by the distribution of the relevant antigen and second, by the location of small veins. The lesions themselves were perivenous, with diapedesis of lymphocytes and monocytes occurring, as well as destruction of parenchyma in the zone of invasion of these cells.

At a Ciba symposium in 1959 (452), these experimental autoimmune diseases were shown to have all the essential characteristics of the newly recognized group of cell-mediated immune reactions, including a single consistent morphology, *delayed-type hypersensitivity* (DTH) to the specific antigen, and transfer with living lymphoid cells rather than antibody (these results were accomplished for EAE by Paterson, also in 1959 [323]). This comparison was solidified by the demonstration in 1961–62 that the earliest recognizable lesion in EAE was a perivenous mononuclear cell reaction and not myelin breakdown, as previously thought by many neuropathologists (457); that the disease could be prevented and treated by antilymphocyte sera (458) and was therefore mediated by circulating lymphocytes; and that it was prevented by neonatal thymectomy (16), which identified the source of these cells as the thymus. Autoradiography confirmed that both the lymphocytes and monocytes in the lesion were hematogenous and that they proliferated in the lesion (220).

It was now possible to look more closely at the similarities and differences between autoimmune disease models, as exemplified by EAE and EAN, and their apparent human equivalents (364,453). In 1933 Klinge had developed the concept of *hyperergic inflammation* in relation to rheumatic disorders (209), and his concept was applied by Pette to the demyelinative diseases, particularly multiple sclerosis, in his writings during the 1920s and '30s (329). By the late 1940s, the neurology community was poised (276) to assimilate the new ideas that grew out of the research on EAE. Ferraro and Roizin had demonstrated that EAE in animals could take many forms mimicking human disease, including acute monophasic perivenous encephalomyelitis, acute hemorrhagic encephalomyelitis, or chronic progressive or relapsing-remitting disease with large demyelinated plaques resembling MS (116). EAE in humans, produced by rabies vaccination, could be expressed not only as disseminated perivenous encephalomyelitis but also, in a suitably susceptible population (the Japanese), by chronic disease indistinguishable from MS of the brain and/or spinal cord, as shown by Uchimura and Shiraki in 1957 (439).

Thus it was possible in 1962 (453) to make the generalization that the autoimmune model was probably a true model for two classes of human disease: acute monophasic diseases (including hemorrhagic and necrotizing forms), which occur after infection or actual immunization with tissue antigen(s); and chronic progressive or intermittent forms of disease, which usually occur without any clear evidence of antecedent immunization. In the latter forms of illness, one or more genetically determined susceptibility factors predisposed to the occurrence of chronic disease. In some instances, the suggestion that a human disease might be autoimmune actually preceded the production of a satisfactory animal model, as we have seen in the case of the inflammatory eye diseases elicited with uvea and lens.

Two new neuroimmunologic disease models were described in 1965 that affect the sympathetic nervous system (14) and muscle (86). The former received no further study for more than a quarter of a century, when Brimijoin et al. showed it to result from autoimmunization with acetylcholine esterase, followed by antibody-mediated damage of preganglionic nerve terminals in the sympathetic ganglia and death of the corresponding neurons (52). A claim was also made in 1966 that a myasthenic syndrome appeared in guinea pigs immunized with thymus (134); this is discussed further in the section on myasthenia gravis. By 1971 the number of known experimental autoimmune diseases had risen to 18 and later, several more were to be found.

The 1960s saw the introduction of in vitro techniques for studying cell-mediated immune reactions, and each new method was applied to the EAE problem soon after its development. Thus lymphocytes from EAE animals could react in vitro to single myelin antigens by proliferation (218), cytotoxicity (33), and cytokine production (85). These findings essentially confirmed what had already been learned from skin tests with purified antigens and from cell transfer and antilymphocyte serum studies. They also paved the way for subsequent, more basic studies of disease mechanisms.

Genes, Molecules, and Cells

There was a relative lull in research on EAE during the 1960s and early '70s. During this period Levine and Sowinski, working with rats, characterized various inbred strains as to EAE susceptibility or other disease characteristics and initiated work on congenic strains and backcrosses (235). In 1973 Williams and Moore, through studying successive backcrosses of Lewis (susceptible) and brown Norway (BN) (resistant) rats, established that susceptibility was an autosomal dominant characteristic linked to the MHC (469). Within a few years the same relationship was shown to hold in mice (Bernard [34]). Congenic and congenic-recombinant rat and mouse strains were developed, as well as a variety of standardized backcross strains, to elucidate not only the non-MHC associated genetic controls affecting susceptibility but also controls that might affect the character of the disease, e.g., intensity, relapse rate, stress responses (production of adrenal steroids), histologic elements, etc. Knobler and colleagues played an important role in the development of this phase of EAE investigation (210).

At the same time, rapid advances in protein chemistry technology made it possible to refine the study of the antigens responsible for EAE and EAN. In 1977 Chou et al. (202) and almost simultaneously Hashim (155,196) identified p68-88 as the immunodominant epitope for EAE in rats. Fritz and colleagues later showed that the peptides of MBP which were immunodominant in different mouse strains were, in fact, determined (restricted) by the MHC class II background of each strain (123,332). The effective peptides, it appeared, needed to be no longer than 9–12 amino acid residues: p89-101 in SJL/J mice (H-2^s) and pAcl-9 in PL/J (H-2^u) mice (370). In hybrid (SJL $\times$

PL) F1 animals with chronic EAE, McFarlin and colleagues showed a progressive change in both specificity and MHC restriction over time (268).

The encephalitogenicity of PLP (or so-called "lipophilin") was first shown in 1955, and rediscovered by Hashim et al. (156) working with guinea pigs in 1980, and by Lees et al. with rabbits in 1983 (62). PLP was shown to be pathogenic in both rats and mice shortly thereafter. PLP produced more demyelination than MBP (and more axon damage) and tended to induce antibodies which increased during relapses but poorly correlated with clinical or histological scores (106). It also produced chronic progressive disease in guinea pigs and relapsing remitting disease in rats and mice far more readily than MBP. Tuohy demonstrated the same relationship between MHC-II and immunodominant peptide, as had been seen with MBP peptides. In SJL/J mice, p141-149 proved to be immunodominant, as was p105-115 in SWR/J mice (H-2q) (436).

The third important antigen in EAE was myelin-oligoglycoprotein (MOG), a constituent of both myelin and the oligodendrocyte membrane. It was shown to be encephalitogenic by Lebar et al. in 1986 (228) and later studied at some length by Linington. MOG has proven to be a potent encephatiogenic antigen capable of inducing relapsing EAE with significant CNS demyelination.

A pivotal event in the study of EAE (and subsequently in many other animal models) was the ability to produce long-term, MBP-specific T-cell lines, as introduced by Ben-Nun, Wekerle, and Cohen in 1981 (29). Also important was the discovery by the same group, that vaccination with such cells inactivated by various means leads to resistance to EAE (30,236). T-cell lines specific for PLP were developed in the late 1980s by Satoh et al. that confirmed what had been learned about immunodominant epitopes and MHC-restriction (385,444). In the 1990s it has become commonplace to carry out active immunization of thymocytes or peripheral T cells in vitro using whole antigens or arbitrary peptides, to obtain expanded lines or clones and identify the actual corresponding epitopes and finally, to test individual lines or clones for encephalogenicity.

Subsequently, several more antigens have been found to induce EAE, including myelin-associated glycoprotein (MAG), and even astrocytic and axonal constituents such as glial fibrillary acidic protein (GFAP), B-crystallin, and S100β. For each of these protein antigens no more than 5 or 6 epitopes are found that are reactive with T cells in the normal repertoire, and usually no more than 2 or 3 of these have proved to be encephalitogenic in animals of different genetic background.

Mokhtarian, McFarlin, and Raine showed in 1984 that transfer of MBP-specific cells could produce chronic relapsing EAE (286,352) with progressive recruitment of cells recognizing a series of epitopes. In 1987 investigators showed that the largely inflammatory lesions, produced by transferred MBP-specific T cells could be intensified and converted into lesions with extensive demyelination by simultaneous transfer of antibody against MOG or galactocerebroside (386). Varying the quantitative relationship between MBP-specific T cells and MOG-specific antibody varied the balance between inflammation and demyelination and duplicated the full spectrum of lesions seen in early MS (see also 433).

The structure of the T-cell receptor (TcR) peptides and their chromosomal localization in mice and rats were worked out during the early 1980s, but heterogeneity existed between strains. Mouse strains showing heightened susceptibility to autoimmunity (NZW, SJL) were found to have large beta-chain deletions in either the variable (V) or constant (C) regions (27,306). Such deletions may account for their failure to regulate their T cell responses effectively, perhaps because CD8+ cells are unable to recognize the defective TcR of effector CD4+ T cells in these animals. While no single TcR peptide sequence was found that defined reactivity to MBP, certain sequences, notably, V β 8.2, were markedly overrepresented in the responses of both mice and rats (150), and this led to somewhat speculative explanations (160). TcR gene usage in relation to p89-101, for example, is restricted: 50% of cells use V β 8 and 50% use V β 17. It is even more restricted in the case of PAC1-9: 80% use V β 8 and 100% use V α 4.

In the mid 1980s, chimeric animals were developed in which actions of the immune system could be distinguished from local factors. In the radiation chimeras developed by Korngold et al. (215), marrow was provided from susceptible (SJL/J) to resistant (BlO.S) hosts or vice versa (see also 165). Heterotopic grafts of nervous tissue from one animal to another of different genetic background provided an additional means of separating systemic from local factors influencing disease, and grafts to chimeric recipients permitted a three-way split of information. Lublin and colleagues grafted fragments of allogeneic brain under the kidney capsule of recipients or (with better survival) into the anterior chamber of the eye (133), while Arnason and colleagues placed similar grafts into the cerebral ventricles (304). The blood-brain barrier is conserved in such grafts (286), which could be observed for the development of EAE after immunization of the host with myelin antigen (133,305). These experiments showed clearly the existence of a number of susceptibility or resistance genes other than those encoding the specific elements involved in T-cell recognition. Some were systemic and others local; these genes govern the level of expression of MHC in particular types of potential antigen-presenting cells (APC) (microglia, astrocytes, vascular endothelium), the ability of macrophages to produce certain cytokines, sensitivity of the blood vessel wall to vasoamines, adhesion molecule expression in vascular endothelium, efficacy of immunoregulatory systems, etc.

The development of transgenic animals in 1983 and 1986 provided another major technological advance (reviews in 17,149). The MBP gene can, for example, restore normal myelin formation in dysmyelinative mutant mice. The first application of this powerful technology in the EAE field was J.F.A.P. Miller's creation in 1991 of transgenic mice, with the *H-2K^b* gene under the control of the MBP promotor (437). The introduced gene was expressed in oligodendrocytes. The resulting "wonky" mice developed shivering the tonic seizures related to hypomyelination and died in 2–3 weeks. Autoimmunity to MBP was not enhanced in these animals.

Knockout mice, transgenics in whom a single function, such as expression of CD4 of MHC class-II, or production and secretion of IL-2, is inhibited by antisense DNA or RNA transgenes, provide a further technological innovation with great promise for neuroimmunology. A less sophisticated but equally successful method is the use of appropriate monoclonal antibodies to prepare knockouts lacking MHC-I or -II or the CD4 or CD8 molecules. CD8 knockouts show evidence of both T–effector cell deficiency and deficient T-cell-mediated regulation (discussed below under Regulatory Mechanisms).

Cytokines and Other Interactive Molecules

The first cytokines were described in the early 1960s. By 1975 over 100 names existed, all with 2–4 letter acronyms, to describe soluble protein or peptide mediators (excluding antibody and components of complement). In 1979 a new "molecular" approach to the identification and naming (later, the cloning and sequencing) of individual cytokines was introduced. IL-1 and IL-2 replaced endogenous pyrogen or lymphocyte-activating factor and T-cell growth factor and these were followed by TNF-α (former cachectin), TNF-β (former lymphotoxin), and others. In the 1980s specific monoclonal antibodies began to be used both as immunohistochemical reagents and in radioimmunoassay (RIA), enzyme-linked immunosorbent assay (ELISA), or other in vitro tests for identifying cytokines, and the increasing availability of pure recombinant cytokines enabled new types of in vivo and in vitro experimentation. There was a parallel expansion in the field of growth factors and adhesion molecules.

Most of the cytokines detected in EAE and MS lesions, such as IL-2 and IFN-γ, are products of the activated T cells, while others, like IL-1 and TNF-α, come from the macrophages and from activated astrocytes. Astrocytes stimulated by IFN-γ and/ or TNF produce IL-1 and IL-3, TNFα, transforming growth factor beta (TGFβ), granulocyte-macrophage colony-stimulating factor (GM-CSF), and molecules of other types such as prostaglandin E2 (PGE2) (32,237), i.e., the same mediators produced by macrophages and microglia, which are the predominant cells of the EAE/EAN infiltrate. In the late 1980s, Hartung and Toyka demonstrated the generation of reactive oxygen species (ROS) and nitrite (NO) in activated macrophages (see 153); these are also produced by activated astrocytes.

Interferon-γ, IL-1 and -6, and TNF-α (and now the chemokines, ROS, and NO) are properly viewed as effector molecules that contribute to tissue damage and the inflammatory cascade. Among MBP-specific T-cell lines/clones, only those producing TNF are encephalitogenic, and lesion formation is blocked by monoclonal antibodies against TNF (337,374). On the other hand, TGF-β and IL-4, which are strong inhibitors of IFN-γ production by T helper 1 (TH1) cells, have been identified as the main players down-regulating immune responses at the time the acute EAE attack begins to wane (197). Brosnan, Selmaj, Raine, and colleagues, working first in the rabbit eye and then in vitro over most of the last decade, showed that IL-1 and -2, IFN-γ, and TNF produce primary effects on blood vessels and secondary changes in myelin and conduction (as observed, for example, in visual evoked potentials) (54,395). IL-1 and TNF act on endothelial cells to cause expression of the intracellular adhesion molecules (ICAMs) and related adhesion molecules and are thus capable of initiating an inflammatory cascade and getting potentially pathogenic T cells across the blood-brain barrier and into the parenchyma.

McFarlin and Panitch, and Reichert et al. had shown independently in 1977 and 1979, respectively, that specific T-cells required in vitro activation, whether by antigen or nonspecific mitogen, before they could produce disease on transfer (322,361). This requirement was interpreted as the need for IFN-γ production by the transferred cells and the resulting up-regulation of MHC-II in potential APC that they might encounter. In 1986 Wekerle and colleagues (464a) observed that T cells specific for ovalbumen, a non-CNS antigen, could easily gain entrance to the brain if the T cell was activated. This seminal observation was expanded and further parameters for T cell entry delineated by others shortly thereafter (163). The ability of activated T cells to enter the parenchyma implied that the specific recognition event could take place anywhere, studies in chimeras have identified perivascular microglia and macrophages as the effective APC (163,164). The activation requirement may actually have more to do with stimulating TNF production, leading to upregulation of adhesion molecules on vascular endothelium and facilitation of the cells' passage into the parenchyma. Immunological adhesion molecules are in fact elevated in the lesions of EAE (and MS), both at the level of the inflammatory cells and of the vascular endothelium and astrocytes (226,350,409).

The possible role of complement (C) in tissue damage remains unclear. M. Shin and her collaborators, using techniques developed over almost half a century by Mayer and his students, established that normal CNS myelin, in the absence of antibody, activates C by the classical pathway to produce the membrane attack complex (C5b-9) (219,251). This reaction is enhanced by the presence of antibody. Myelin exposed to C5b-9 loses its integrity and becomes more vulnerable to both cell and enzymatic attach. Cultured oligodendrocytes, like myelin, activate the classical C pathway in the absence of antibody (390). Activated C is lytic for oligodendrocytes. However, at sublytic doses it stimulates them to generate leukotriene (LTB4) from arachidonate. C was also shown to participate in demyelination produced by the antibody-dependent complement-mediated cytotoxicity (ADCC) mechanism in intact animals.

Immune Regulation

The mode of resolution of EAE lesions at the end of an acute attack has become the subject of significant new research. Mason and Pender have independently called attention to the sudden appearance of large numbers of apoptotic cells (lymphocytes and some oligodendrocytes) in EAE lesions, just as the disease reaches its peak and the inflammatory process starts to wane (see 326). All three authors attribute this apoptosis to the action of steroids and regard it as the main mechanism that brings the inflammatory process to an end. Mason et al. have shown that the unusually severe EAE of Lewis rats is related to a deficient ability to produce adrenal steroids in response to stress (261). The apoptosis observed may or may not also be related to the function of immunoregulatory cells, for example, cytotoxic CD8+ T cells like those studied by Sun and Wekerle (421). In rats with tolerance for MBP induced by feeding (281,282), cells producing TGF-β and IL-4 are found in the brain; they are not present in the usual EAE infiltrates where IFN-γ and TNF-α production are prominent (201).

The question of lesion resolution is intimately tied to the problem of chronicity and the phenomena of relapse and remission, which are fundamental components of the disease process in MS. Stone's rediscovery of chronic relapsing-remitting EAE in strain-13 guinea pigs 20 years after Ferraro's first description of chronic disease (115,116), and the development and exploitation of chronic relapsing EAE in mice of susceptible strains (SJL, PL/J) by Lublin et al. (256) and by Brown and McFarlin in 1981 (55) opened this problem to deeper investigation. Lyman and Brosnan published several papers in the mid-1980s on suppressor cells found during EAE remission in the spleens of MBP-immunized strain-13 guinea pigs—cells which were absent during relapse (257). These cells responded to the specific antigen, MBP, but they suppressed proliferation of mitogen-stimulated (i.e., unrelated, nonspecific) cells. Another approach grew out of the first vaccination studies with MBP-specific T-cell lines or clones in 1981 (30,76). Sun and Wekerle attempted to clone suppressor cells from the lymphoid organs of Lewis rats after the rats had recovered from EAE induced by an MBP-specific T-cell line known as *S1,* or after vaccination with irradiated, fixed, or lysed S1 cells (421). They obtained CD8+ T cells that responded with proliferation to S1 cells and presumably recognized idiotypic sequences in the MBP-specific TCR, but that were also specifically cytolytic for S1 cells and thus functionally suppressive (422). Swanborg, who also worked with EAE in Lewis rats, identified a CD4+ suppressor T cell that appears during recovery. This cell too recognizes the effector T-cell's TCR, but it reacts by releasing IL-4 and TGF-β, along with suppressing IFN-γ production and release from the CD4+ effector T-cells and suppressing EAE (197). Other laboratories (34) have reported similar findings.

Mak and colleagues reported that in CD8-knockout PL/J mice, there is decreased disease severity accompanied by a markedly increased frequency of relapses, implying loss of an effector cell of CTL type and at least one type of suppressor cell (213). Pernis et al. have obtained a similar result in knockout mice produced with monoclonal antibody against CD8 (184,208). They have presented evidence that the CD8+ suppressor cell recognizes an idiotope of the effector T cell's TcR bound to the MHC-1 alpha chain (476). Another approach is exemplified by Pender's discovery in 1990 that cyclosporin converts the normally monophasic course of EAE and EAN in Lewis rats into a true chronic relapsing-remitting course like that of MS (271,272). One may compare this chronic disease to the GVH-like syndrome seen in rats treated with cyclosporin possible attributable to loss of a suppressor system that normally holds autologous (MLR/GVH)-regulatory T cells in check and that is sensitive to cyclosporin.

Model for Screening New Therapies

Over more than 30 years, EAE has served as a screening device for nonspecific anti-inflammatory and immunosuppressive agents which, it was hoped, would prove effective in MS. Adrenocorticotropic hormone (ACTH) and adrenal steroids head the list, followed by a variety of antimitotic and cytotoxic agents drawn from the cancer field. Virtually all of these turned out to inhibit EAE and moved to clinical trial for MS in due course. Now the molecular mechanisms underlying T-cell recognition provide the targets for possible new therapies. These targets include the MHC; presumed immunodominant epitopes of individual antigens, always with MBP dominating the field, the T-cell receptor; and various adhesion molecules. Therapeutic strategies have included blocking function with monoclonal antibodies or modified peptide sequences of the epitope; down-regulating expression of the target molecule nonspecifically, e.g., by using IFN-β to downregulate MHC-II (e.g., 189); or inducing formation of target-specific regulatory (suppressor) cells (e.g., 392,398). Essentially all these strategies have been reported to inhibit EAE and all have inhibited disease development, and in some instances, disease progression or relapse (e.g., 175). The newest approach to therapy is the attempt to induce a shift of the immune response from TH1 to TH2 (89,291) in the EAE host by oral administration of antigens such as MBP (201,281,282). Effectively, one replaces cells that generate inflammation with cells that suppress it by producing down-regulatory cytokines such as IL-4, IL-10, and TGF-β or one can treat with the mediator (TGF-β) alone (348). Another approach is the generation of regulatory cells by intrathymic injection of MBP (104).

Human Neuroimmunological Diseases: Autoimmunity

Multiple Sclerosis (MS)

The explosion of new immunologic research on MS, growing out of the earlier EAE research and driven by new technology throughout the 1970s and '80s and into the '90s, precludes any but the most superficial review. Only a few high points will be mentioned, with occasional key citations.

Epidemiologic studies provided the earliest insights into determinants of MS susceptibility (review in 98), beginning with migration studies carried out by Geoffrey Dean in South Africa in the 1960s (90). Later came studies of clusters, e.g., in Switzerland and Finland, and studies of point epidemics, e.g., in Iceland, Norway, and the Faeroe Islands; family studies and twin studies, e.g., in Canada, the U.S. and elsewhere; and socioeconomic analyses, in the U.K. in particular. These approaches have been unanimous in pointing to multigenic control of MS susceptibility and the importance of unknown environmental agent(s) acting in early adolescence as precipitating factor(s). An attempt by Mackay and Myrianthopoulos in 1966 to study genetic determinants of

MS susceptibility in twins led to inconclusive results (258). Twenty years later a Canadian population-based family study showed a high rate of concordance (25.9%) in monozygotic twins (103), establishing conclusively both the importance of genetic determinants in susceptibility and that of environmental precipitating factors.

The most obvious candidate genes that might be expected to play a role in susceptibility, following the EAE model, are those governing T-cell recognition, notably MHC class-II and the T-cell receptor (TcR). The first studies of MHC association with MS—and there have been many—date to the early 1970s (183). The consensus now is that MS is most frequently associated with DR2, 4, and 6 and with DQwl. There is a strong suggestion that the DQ association may have special significance (384,447). TcR studies which were first reported in 1989 by Beall et al. and others, uncovered additional associations with peptide isoforms of the TcR-α and -β chains (25). Meticulous family studies of chromosomal inheritance in relation to MS susceptibility have led to essentially the same conclusions (see e.g., 73,391). The 1990s have seen the initiation of broadly based studies of pedigreed MS families to identify additional MS susceptibility genes like those found in animal studies, e.g., genes controlling the expression levels of MHC-II, vascular vasoamine sensitivity, and nonspecific elements of the inflammatory response. Most of the susceptibility genes identified thus far are associated with relative risk figures between 2 and 12 (compared with a relative risk of 250 to 500 in monozygotic twins). In the presence of both the appropriate MHC-II and certain TcR isotypes, however, the relative risk figure may exceed 50. It is not unlikely that as yet unknown genes account for the further susceptibility increment between 50 and 500.

Kurtzke's studies over the last two decades, which are devoted to the Faeroe Islands epidemic of MS, an outbreak apparently precipitated by the arrival of British troops in the early 1940s, provided the basis for an *infectious theory of MS* (223, see also 185). A population-based study by Compston in Wales in the late 1980s suggests strongly that the disease process is triggered by common childhood viral infections (e.g., measles, rubella, mumps, Epstein-Barr virus [EBV]) occurring at or shortly after puberty (see 78). On the other hand, epidemiologic studies over a 10-year period by Sibley et al. have incriminated upper respiratory viral infections as triggering relapses of MS (401). This has been confirmed in Panitch's recent work and in Scandinavian studies which point particularly to adenoviruses as the triggering agent. IFN-γ may serve as an intermediary in this process (321).

A definitive description of the basic lesion of MS was provided by Adams and Kubik in 1952 (3). Nevertheless, the elucidation of lesion pathogenesis awaited the refined morphologic studies of very early lesions carried out in the late 1970s by Prineas (343–346). These studies were quickly complemented by the immunohistochemical investigations, at the light and electron microscopic levels (408) to assess the expression of MHC and (10 years later) adhesion molecules on vascular and glial elements and to characterize the cells invading the parenchyma by subset, activation markers, and the like (226,408,409,432). Traditional serologic studies were replaced by RIA and ELISA tests for antigens released during tissue breakdown and for antibodies, cytokines, released cytokine receptors, and elements of the complement cascade.

Prineas emphasized the essential identity of the MS and EAE lesions, which are characterized by the invasion of the perivascular space and the parenchyma by a mixed population of T-cells and some B cells, accompanied by a massive influx of monocytes and macrophages which serve as the prime agents of myelin destruction. By 1978 he had demonstrated macrophages phagocytosing myelin by way of clathrin-coated pits— a receptor-mediated process (344,346). The finding was followed by the demonstration of immunoglobulin (Ig)G capping on macrophages in the lesion and the presumption that IgG antibody-mediated ADCC is the basis of demyelination (345). By 1985 it became clear that MHC class II is expressed in about 10% of vascular endothelial cells and some astrocytes, that macrophages making up the bulk of the lesion express both MHC-I and MHC-II, and that T cells at the advancing edge of the lesion are predominantly CD4+ and activated (Il-2R+) (132,158). In later studies CD8+ cells were found to be prominent in the lesions while CD4+CD45R+ cells, presumed to be suppressor–inducer cells, were relatively absent (408).

Some research groups found a broad repertoire of TcR Vβ usage in the lesions (473), while Oksenberg, Steinman, and their collaborators found restricted usage of both Vα and Vβ (309). For example, about half of MS brains, all from DR2Dw2 patients, show use of rearranged Vβ5.2 with a common D-J motif that can be related to recognition of peptide 89-106, the "immunodominant epitope" of MBP. The 1990 discovery of γδ T-cells in MS lesions (394) paralleled the demonstration of local heat-shock protein (HSP) formation: HSP65 is up-regulated in oligodendrocytes at the edge of the MS plaque, while HSP72 is found in astrocytes in both MS and normal brains and seems to be unrelated to lesion formation (393). An entirely unexpected new discovery is the presence of nitrite synthase (NOS) in astrocytes rather than in macrophages at the advancing edge of MS plaques (48).

Paralleling these studies of lesions are studies of the blood and CSF. Starting in 1975, Arnason and his colleagues Antel, Reder and Noronha, described several abnormalities of the circulating CD8+CD28− T-cell population that are apparently related to clinical disease activity. First a deficiency in "nonspecific suppressor" activity following antigen, MHC, or mitogen stimulation was found (11,12). The cell functions suppressed included both DNA synthesis and, in the case of B cells, immunoglobulin synthesis. The deficient T cells were shown to express less CD8 than normal and to show up-regulation of cell membrane β-adrenergic receptors (15). In 1988 the subpopulation of suppressor-inducer T cells (CD3+CD4+CD45R+) also was shown to be decreased (290); this decrease was associated with the loss of functional suppressor activity (70,290).

Burns et al. had shown as early as 1983 that CD4+ T cells recognizing MBP could be cloned from the peripheral blood of both MS patients and controls (60). Such clones are quite heterogeneous; Richert et al. identified more than 10 recognition sites distinguished by clones from a single donor (362). (In this work and what has followed, reactivity of CD8+ T cells and cells bearing the γδ receptor have received little attention). In 1990 laboratories at the National Institutes of Health, in Boston, and in Munich simultaneously published the discovery that, in spite of this heterogeneity, a few peptide sequences, so-called immunodominant epitopes, reacted with the majority of the clones (260,314,330), e.g., MBP peptide 84-102 reacted with clones from both patients and disease-free controls carrying human leukocyte antigen (HLA)-DR2. At roughly the same time as these findings, two preliminary studies tackled the question of cloning CD4+ MBP-specific T cells already circulating in the MS patient in an activated (potentially pathogenic) state. One study identified cells carrying a common mutation (8) and the other identified cells expressing the IL-2 receptor (308). Both reported that many activated MBP-specific cells could be retrieved from MS patients but not from controls. High-powered technology has now been applied to rapid cloning and identification of activated MBP- or PLP-specific T cells carrying Il-2R and has confirmed the very marked difference between MS patients (many such cells in the circulation) and normal controls (virtually none) (478).

Cerebrospinal fluid (CSF) which is the most accessible (or easily sampled) element of the nervous system, has always received special attention from immunologists. After Kabat's discovery in 1942 that immunoglobulin is elevated in the CSF of MS patients (191), almost 20 years elapsed before Lowenthal's demonstration that this Ig shows restricted heterogeneity, manifested in the now famous oligoclonal bands (OB) (254). It was another 20 years before Tourtellotte demonstrated that most of the Ig in the OB is synthesized locally within the brain and CSF compartments (429).

Subsequent studies dealt with the altered κ:λ ratio, IgG subclass restriction, etc., of CSF immunoglobulin, and introduced many refinements of technique (446). The OB proved to contain antibodies of all isotypes specific for a variety of autoantigens like MBP (462) and exogenous antigens, but the bulk of the Ig remained unaccounted for. (A recent report claims that antibody to HSP60 is closely tied to the OB [338]). In 1974, Sandberg-Wollheim showed that the CSF contained B cells that could produce Ig with an OB pattern much like that of the whole CSF (380). For the most part, the T-cells proved to be activated cycling cells (307). Like the B cells, many showed specificity for viral and other exogenous antigens (359). They proved to be quite different from the T-cell population of the peripheral blood: most were CD4+CDw29+ and there was a remarkable absence of CD4+CD45R+ suppressor-inducer cells (71,290).

In 1988 Olsson, Link, and colleagues developed a nitrocellulose immunospot test, based on the old plaque-forming cell technique, to identify B cells and the antibodies produced by individual cells (245,246). This technique showed 100% of MS CSF to contain B cells making IgG, 70% making IgA, and 57% making IgM; a high proportion of the IgG cells made antibody against MBP (311). Using a modification of this technique, the same investigators showed that a remarkably high proportion of CSF T cells responded to MBP and PLP by secretion of IFN-γ (246). The cloning techniques developed in the study of peripheral blood T cells have, of course, also been applied to the CSF. Using this technology a very high proportion of activated CD4+ T cells (expressing the Il-2 receptor) specific for MBP and PLP have been demonstrated in MS patients CSF (478). The CSF also serves as an accumulation site for the products of activated T and B cells in the CNS and CSF, notably, such cytokines as IL-1 and TNF and soluble receptors such as IL-2R and TNF-R and for activated complement components (288) and adhesion molecules (ICAM-1). (See 434). The latter, however, may be derived from activated cerebrovascular endothelium (435).

Along with the various studies cited, there has been a stream of publications seeking to relate MS to a viral infection by virologic or immunologic techniques (185). Such claims have been made for over 20 viruses since 1946. Perennial favorite candidates include measles, EBV, coronaviruses, and human T cell lymphotropic virus 1 (HTLV-1) or a similar retrovirus. Virtually all immunologic studies have demonstrated elevated antibodies to the various suspect viruses (see, e.g., 121). Cell studies have tended to give ambiguous results. The single result worth noting here, which was reported in 1985 by Jacobson et al. (179), is the relative absence in MS of a T-cell subpopulation identified as CD4+ measles-specific CTL precursors. No comparable deficit was noted for other viruses (flu, mumps). In later work the abnormality could not be related to any one measles virus antigen, perhaps it involves an as yet undefined regulatory system.

The last point concerns the question of a possible abnormality in immune regulation, which might be responsible for the prolonged course of MS. Arnason and colleagues identified a series of abnormalities of autonomic and neuroendocrine function in MS patients in the 1970s and attempted to determine their reflection in the immune system. The findings thus far include increased beta-adrenergic receptors (approximately three-fold) on T cells of suppressor phenotype (CD8+CD28−) (15) and increased muscarinic (type M2) acetylcholine receptors on helper (CD4+) T cells; decreased sweating in about half the patients tested (195); and hyperactivity of the HPA axis, as shown by an abnormal dexamethasone suppression test (255), which is associated with decreased lymphocytic responses in vitro. These findings are similar to those findings in animals sympathectomized in early life (see Psychoneuroimmunology [5]). The abnormal immunoregulatory activity bears an as yet unknown relation to the reduced level of suppressor–inducer (70,290) and suppressor (11,12) cells, and the autologous mixed-lymphocyte reaction (79,146) referred to previously.

Acute Disseminated (Including Postvaccinal and Postinfectious) Encephalomyelitis (ADE, PVE and PIE)

Neuroparalytic accidents after rabies vaccination (early vaccines contained sheep, goat, or rabbit brain, as well as virus) were known as early as 1889. The disease, now called *postvaccinal encephalomyelitis* (PVE), is usually monophasic but in rare instances may assume a chronic form (for review see 162). The characteristic lesions are small, perivenous, predominantly mononuclear, inflammatory demyelinative lesions, disseminated throughout the white matter of the CNS. The spinal roots and sensory ganglia may also be affected and sometimes are the principal site of disease.

Early investigators found antibody to neural antigens in patients with PVE (see, e.g.,

176). The discovery of EAE and EAN, in 1933 and 1955 respectively, added the suggestion that cell-mediated immunity might equal or exceed humoral antibody as the principal agent of pathogenesis. Refined study had to await the identification and resolution of the many myelin antigens. Such studies, carried out mainly in Thailand in the early and mid-1980s by Johnson and colleagues, particularly Griffin and Hemachudha, showed that patients' high titer of anti-myelin antibody, which is present in both the blood and CSF, is largely directed against MBP (161). Vaccinated individuals not developing PVE make antibody to many myelin antigens: MAG, galactocerebroside, and GMl, GD1a, GD1b, GT1b gangliosides, but not to MBP. These additional antibodies are also made by the PVE patients and may contribute to disease pathogenesis, as they have been shown to do in EAE. The patient's circulating T cells are also specifically reactive with MBP (162). It remains unclear what the relative contributions may be of cell-mediated immunity (CMI) and humoral antibody to lesion pathogenesis.

Postinfectious or parainfectious encephalomyelitis (PIE) occurring during or after measles or infection with other enveloped viruses (influenza, smallpox, vaccinia, rubella, varicella-zoster, mumps) was well recognized as a nosologic entity by 1956 (279) (for review see 186). PIE is also a monophasic disease manifesting disseminated perivenular inflammation and demyelination indistinguishable from the lesions of EAE and PVE, and it has usually been assumed to have the same mechanism. Its close relationship to the immune response against virus was clearly demonstrated by Finley with vaccinia as early as 1938 (117). However, it was only many years later that specific cell-mediated immunity against MBP was demonstrated in PIE. It was first detected by the DTH reaction to skin test with this antigen (26) and later in measles studies by conventional lymphocytic reactions to MBP in vitro (187,250). Antibody to MBP is also produced by PIE patients (187). Thus, as in the case of PVE, the relative roles of these "polar" forms of immune response remain unclear. Also, there has been insufficient testing of other myelin antigens, such as PLP and MOG. No evidence could be uncovered that measles virus enters the brain in association with the development of PIE after measles (129). Genetic studies have failed to uncover a relationship between MHC and susceptibility, but genes encoding the T-cell receptor peptides have not been investigated.

There remains the problem of acute disseminated encephalomyelitis (ADE) cases occurring in the absence of an antecedent infection or immunizing event. It is commonly assumed that these are really cases of PIE in which a triggering viral infection (e.g., subclinical influenza) has taken place but the infection was clinically inapparent.

Animal Models for PIE and ADE

Distemper virus of dogs, which is closely related to the measles virus, was recognized by 1940 as producing typical perivascular inflammatory demyelinative lesions, which are largely limited to the white matter, in some animals (177,207). It has not proved a convenient model for immunopathologic research, simply because of the variability of the experimental animals and the lack of reagents for immunohistochemical and immunogenetic analysis. Dogs with distemper have circulating MBP-sensitized lymphocytes (65a).

In 1978 it was observed that Lewis rats infected as weanlings with the JHM strain of corona virus develop first an acute viral encephalitis and thereafter, a subacute demyelinating encephalomyelitis (SDE), with disseminated perivascular, inflammatory demyelinating lesions throughout the CNS (293). The onset of SDE occurs at any time from 2 weeks to 8 months, and its course is sometimes relapsing. In about 20% of Lewis rats, neurotropic measles strains produce a closely similar subacute measles encephalomyelitis (SAME), with onset at 3 weeks to 3 months (240). In neither disease is virus found in the lesion. In both SDE (463) and SAME (239), T-cell-mediated immunity develops against virus, as well as against MBP (425). The disease process can be transferred to normal Lewis recipients by transfer of T cells in the complete absence of virus and appears to be typical EAE. CD4+ T cells from these animals respond to the same immunodominant epitopes of MBP as T cells from rats immunized directly with MBP (238), but some rats respond also to a second, minor determinant.

A fourth PIE model, which is quite different from the others, is seen in mice infected with Semliki Forest virus (SFV) (see summary in 113,419). The first papers on this disease appeared in the 1970s. The virus produces a peripheral infection in mice, followed by viremia and infection of vascular endothelium in the brain, and finally CNS parenchymal involvement, with focal mononuclear inflammatory lesions and primary demyelination throughout the brain, spinal cord, and optic nerves. Virus ceases to be detectable when the demyelination peaks at 14 days. The demyelination is paralleled by high titers of antiviral antibody which is cross-reactive with myelin glycolipids (464). In immunosuppressed or nude mice, SFV replicates unchecked and reaches high titers; there is no demyelination. The "normal" response, i.e., inflammation, demyelination, and clearance of virus, can be reconstituted in nude mice by an infusion of splenic T cells but not by B cells or antiviral antibody. This intriguing model appears to involve both virus-specific T cells and autoantibody that is reactive with myelin glycolipids, perhaps as a result of the host–antigen-in-viral-envelope mechanism. It closely resembles the EAE model resulting from adoptive transfer of MBP-reactive T cells and antibody to MOG but it is shorter-lived, since the T-cell component depends on a response to the virus, a nonpersisting antigen.

Guillain-Barré Syndrome (GBS, AIDP)

Acute monophasic disease affecting the peripheral nervous system and occurring a few days to several weeks after a viral infection (often cytomegalovirus, EBV, or human immunodeficiency virus [HIV]) is known as the Guillain-Barré syndrome (GBS) or acute inflammatory demyelinating polyneuropathy (AIDP) (see 19,153,154,397 for review). GBS was recognized relatively late as a distinct nosologic entity and was described by Asbury et al. in 1969 as a primary inflammatory demyelinative process that particularly affects the nerve roots and sensory ganglia (18).

Much of the significant research on the pathogenesis of the GBS was done in the 1980s (see 19,153). The response of the disease to steroids and to plasma exchange and the failure to find viral genome (e.g., of HIV) in Schwann cells by sensitive methods were seen as arguments for an immunologic and probably autoimmune etiology. The ability of GBS patients' serum to produce demyelination and conduction block in myelinated peripheral nerve cultures (166) or experimental animals when injected intraneurally (420), argued in favor of a humor mechanism, as did the presence of antibody against neutral glycolipids and the activation of complement in patients' serum and CSF, the finding of activated C neoantigen on myelin sheaths in the lesions, and the frequent success of plasma exchange in ameliorating GBS manifestations. A correlation could be shown between the level of circulating IgM antibody against PNS myelin as a whole and the amount and kinetics of the membrane attack complex (C5b-9) in serum and deposited in the roots and nerves (381).

As early as 1975, Abramsky and colleagues showed DTH responses to PNS antigens in patients with GBS (2). The study of T-cell reactions to various myelin antigens became a popular subject during the 1980s. The lymphocytes of GBS patients were found to react inconsistently with the P2 protein of peripheral myelin (128) but in GBS-like disease after rabies vaccination, to give definite reactions to MBP (161). In more recent studies, most patients' T cells are found to react with either P2, PO, and/or P2 or PO peptides. T-cell lines and clones reactive with these are being actively investigated. No convincing HLA association has been found, although there are reports of a slight association with HLA-B8 and a stronger association with HLA-Cw specificities (448).

An important new development in the early 1990s is the recognition of a childhood form of GBS that occurs during the summer in rural children (mainly in northern China and in Mexico); the lesion affects peripheral motor fibers and is primarily axonal. There is substantial evidence relating such disease (as well as some instances of classical demyelinating GBS) to antecedental infection with *Campylobacter jejuni,* and it has been suggested that IgG or IgA antibodies to the lipopolysaccharide of certain stains of this organism might cross-react with myelin glycolipids such as GMI and GD1a (see 138). No studies have yet appeared on the T cells in this disease.

Chronic Inflammatory Demyelinating Polyradiculoneuropathy (CIDP)

A chronic demyelinating inflammatory disease that resembles MS in its clinical course and main histopathologic characteristics but affects the peripheral nervous system began to be distinguished from the GBS before 1975 (102,200, see 153). Many of its clinical and other features resemble those of the GBS; however, the lesions show less inflammation in relation to the amount of demyelination and scarring (270).

There has been a strong emphasis on possible humoral mechanisms in the pathogenesis of CIDP, encouraged by the finding that plasma exchange ameliorates the disease process. Recently, however, Gregson, Hughes, and collaborators have demonstrated lymphocytic reactions to P2, PO, and their peptides in about half of a small group of CIDP patients. It remains to be determined whether such cells function in their hosts as mediators of cell-mediated inflammatory reactions (TH1) or as helpers (TH2) of pathogenetically important antibody response(s). The recent interest in specific strains of *Campylobacter jejuni* as possible inducers of the acute GBS has led to studies in patients with chronic motor neuropathies. A high proportion of patients tested showed binding (cross-reactive) of IgM, anti-GMI, or asialo-GMI ganglioside with the lipopolysaccharide (LPS) of certain *Campylobacter jejuni* strains.

Animal Models of the GBS/AIDP and CIDP

The description in 1955 of experimental allergic neuritis (EAN), which showed many clinical and morphologic features characteristic of the GBS and similar CSF changes (455), fixed the notion that the GBS might simply be EAN in the human. The whole gamut of studies carried out in EAE has been repeated in EAN (mostly in the 1970s and '80s). These included examinations of dermal DTH reactions to purified PNS myelin antigens and in vitro cellular reactions to those antigens, and studies of cell transfer, neonatal thymectomy, tolerance induction, genetic restrictions, and so on. More recent studies have dealt with T-cell subsets in EAN lesions (first CD4, then CD8, and always many macrophages, which appear to be the main agents of demyelination); local MHC class II (and I) expression on Schwann cells, antigen presentation mechanisms; regulatory mechanisms; electrophysiological issues; immunohistochemical approaches to cytokines; and local production and release of free oxygen radicals, nitrite, eicosanoids, lysosomal proteases, and vasoamines.

EAN can be elicited with purified peripheral myelin proteins such as P2 (193) and PO (280) or their peptides and can now be transferred with lines or clones of CD4+ T cells specific for these proteins of MBP (also known as Pl) (171). As in the case of EAE, the number of immunodominant peptides seems to be very limited. In P2, such a peptide has been identified as 66-78 (277), or more recently as 61-70.

There are also viral models for classical GBS, among them Marek's disease, coonhound paralysis, and inflammatory cauda equina disease in horses (229). The best studied of these is Marek's disease, which affects chickens. The agent, which was isolated in the late 1960s, is a lymphotropic herpes virus, like EBV and cytomegalovirus (CMV), but it also grows in follicle epithelium and is therefore transmitted by feathers, dander, and dust. As originally described by Marek in 1907, the disease begins as a mononuclear inflammatory demyelinating disease of the peripheral nervous system, which is followed by late infiltration with neoplastic lymphoblastoid cells.

By 1972 it became clear that the virus at first produces only latent infection of the T cells and gives rise at the same time to inflammatory lesions indistinguishable from those of EAN in chickens, accompanied by a secondary demyelination with axon-sparing (347). Schmahl et al. showed in 1975 that disease could be transferred to normal chickens with spleen cells from diseased donors (170). Stevens and colleagues established in 1981 that the virus also produces a latent infection in PNS-supporting cells (satellite cells, Schwann cells) and induces both cell-mediated immunity and IgG antibody against PNS myelin (327,417). Typical DTH reactions can be elicited with PNS homogenate in the wattle. On the other hand, antibody titer seemed to bear no evident relation to the disease (417) and neonatal bursectomy failed to inhibit the disease process (352).

The first animal models thought to resemble CIDP were rather mild antibody-mediated lesions observed in rabbits immunized with galactocerebroside in the 1970s (379). This theme has continued in recent studies of other glycolipids that induce a strong, potentially pathogenetic antibody response (214,259). More attention, however, has been devoted to studying chronic variants of EAN, which are felt to be better models. Different methodological approaches (272) include repeated immunization or the use of unusually high doses of inoculum, immunization of juvenile animals, and the use of immunization accompanied by cyclophosphamide or low doses of cyclosporin A. The success of the two immunosuppressants may depend on the elimination of immunoregulatory cells that normally terminate the acute disease process while effector T cells are spared (271).

Myasthenia Gravis and its Models (MG and EAMG)

Myasthenia gravis (MG) is "perhaps the most thoroughly characterized antibody-mediated autoimmune disease" of the nervous system (99) (for recent reviews see 101,244). In contrast to autoimmune inflammatory polymyositis (86,87), wherein inflammatory infiltrates and cell necrosis occur, in MG there is frequently minimal inflammation. As early as 1949 a relationship was recognized between some myasthenia cases and the presence of lymphoid follicles in the thymus (65), a lesion later shown to be associated with the full cellular machinery for antibody formation (follicular dendritic cells, CD4+ T cells, and B-cell blasts), together with actual antibody and local immune complex formation (84,428).

For a quarter century, studies of antibody to muscle constituents and their homologues in myoid cells of the thymus dominated research on MG, and the literature was filled with beautiful immunofluorescence pictures of muscle striations stained with antibodies present in patients' sera (see e.g., 443). Identification of the actual etiologic mechanism and the responsible antigen, however, occurred as a chance byproduct of immunochemical studies by Patrick and Lindström in 1973 (324) of the acetylcholine receptor (AChR) in the myoneural junction (231); AChR could be purified in large amounts from the electric organ of the Torpedo fish with the help of α-bungarotoxin from the venom of the banded krait. Rabbits immunized with this minor component of muscle in Freund adjuvant developed typical, usually fatal myasthenia (324). The discovery of experimental autoimmune myasthenia gravis (EAMG) provided the impetus for a flood of new work on human myasthenia. Fambrough and colleagues (112) showed that the AChR is the molecular target in this disease; it decreases within the neuromuscular junction as the disease progresses. The AChR molecule was found to contain multiple potentially immunogenic epitopes (438,449). Eighty to ninety percent of MG patients had circulating antibody to epitopes of the AChR (243,438), and transfer of the human antibody to mice was effective in transferring physiologically defined myasthenia, a quantitative decrement in neuromuscular transmission (430). Antibody may lead to receptor loss either by cross-linking and down-regulating its production (100,107,157) or by simple complement-mediated lysis (see 107). Finally, reduction of circulating antibody level, for example, by plasma exchange, ameliorates the disease state.

EAMG proved to differ in some details from human MG (83); yet it was immediately accepted as a valid model for the human disease. The earliest emphasis was on humoral antibody as the principal agent damaging the myoneural junction, and the disease could be transferred with antibody (242). Anti-idiotypic responses were shown to play a regulatory role in humorally mediated EAMG (388) and complement to contribute to antibody-mediated damage of the AChR in vivo (233). However, cell-mediated immunity played its own role in pathogenesis (231) and a form of EAMG could be adoptively transferred with lymph node cells. Finally, susceptibility to EAMG was shown to be genetically determined (124) and the MHC clearly makes a major contribution to this susceptibility (72).

All this work was accomplished during a short period between 1973 and 1978. Subsequent developments have largely represented the application of newly evolving immunologic concepts and techniques. Genetic associations were established in the early 1980s for both MG (296) and the related Lambert-Eaton myasthenic syndrome (LEMS) (466) with genes in the immunoglobulin heavy chain region on chromosome 14, one near VH, one near Gm, and one downstream of IgH (92). In 1984 Hohlfeld et al. succeeded in cloning T cells reactive with AChR from the thymus (171) and later also from lymph nodes and peripheral blood of MG patients (172). Both antibody and T cells react with the alpha subunit of the AChR (191).

The use of peptides instead of the complex AChR molecule (241) greatly simplified later studies, as did the use of monoclonal antibodies to single AChR epitopes (230). While the cholinergic binding site has been identified with peptide 185-196 of the alpha subunit, the principal immunogenic region (B-cell epitope?) proved to be at p125-147 of the alpha subunit (232). On the other hand, T-cell responses, both in animals and humans, were heterogenous (303). Immunodominant epitopes were reported at pl25-143 but also at pl69-181, 257-271, and 351-368 (see e.g., 36). Recent studies of TcR Vβ chain gene usage also shows this heterogeneity, with separate reports pointing to Vβ 12 and to Vβ 8 and 5.

After T-cell clones were introduced into the study of EAE, clones specific for the AChR were developed and used to transfer EAMG adoptively (318). Inactivated clones could be used to immunize animals against EAMG. Specific regulatory cells could be isolated and cloned from the spleens of actively immunized mice recovering from EAMG (317). Current studies make use of transgenic animals, including knock-out mice, in which CD4+ or CD8+ cells of IL-2 of IL-4 are not made. SCID mice are also used as recipients in transfer studies, particularly with human cells (387).

Thymic myoid cells carry AChR indistinguishable from that in muscle (194), and in some patients, a major part of the antibody contributing to disease is formed in the thymus, presumably in response to local antigen. Thymectomy leads to improvement in such patients. CD4+ T cells reactive with AChR can be cloned from both the thymus and blood in MG (172). If human AChR rather than Torpedo AChR is used, or even better, an immunodominant peptide (p37-87) of human AChR, such clones appear to be specific for the disease and are absent in control subjects (303). In recent work, MG thymus, i.e., thymus of human origin, transplanted ectopically (under the kidney capsule) in the SCID mouse, has been shown to live for several weeks and to continue producing the crucial autoantibodies (387).

It is pertinent to cite here the 1966 report by Goldstein of an autoimmune thymitis induced by immunizing guinea pigs with thymus (129). Immunized animals show clinical abnormalities resembling those of MG. These were accounted for by the demonstration that the inflamed thymus releases a peptide (thymopoietin, [Tpo]) capable of inhibiting neurotransmission (21), apparently by binding to nicotinic AChR (388). Tpo was later shown to bind to human AChR and myasthenics' sera to bind to the Tpo-AChR complex.

The initial immunization against AChR in the susceptible individual, as in the case of MS, may depend on molecular mimicry, Stefansson and colleagues have shown that common intestinal bacteria *(E. coli, P. vulgaris, K. pneumoniae)* carry epitomes cross-reactive with the human AChR (414).

Paraneoplastic Syndromes

The term paraneoplastic syndromes (141,336) was coined by Denny-Brown to describe rare disorders of the nervous system that occur as nonmetastatic complications of cancer. After 1950 these disorders were subjected to increasingly systematic clinical and pathological study and it became clear that many were probably autoimmune. The first autoimmune animal model, an experimental autonomic neuropathy manifested clinically by abnormal vasomotor responses, was produced in 1965 (14).

The first serious studies of the syndromes' mechanism, however, were not initiated until the 1980s with Newsom-Davis and colleagues' investigation of patients with the Lambert-Eaton myasthenic syndrome (224). The characteristic physiologic abnormality of this disease could be reproduced in mice receiving infusions of IgG from LEMS patients (224,312). At almost the same time, Kornguth and colleagues described an animal model in which blindness associated with large ganglion cell degeneration in the retina was produced by intravitreous injection of heterologous anti-retina antibody (217). They were able to demonstrate a high-titered autoantibody against retinal ganglion cells in a patient with small-cell lung cancer and blindness (216). Studies soon followed examining patients with breast or ovarian cancer who exhibited progressive cerebellar degeneration. High titers of antibody against cytoplasmic Purkinje cell antigens were detected (137,181).

At present, approximately 20 distinct neurological syndromes associated with cancer and presumed to be autoimmune are recognized. What appear to be identical diseases, however, are found relatively commonly in patients unaffected by cancer, and the neurological manifestations often become prominent, even disabling, before a "causative" tumor can be identified. Almost every part of the nervous system may be affected; the list includes cerebellar degeneration, opsoclonus-myoclonus, limbic encephalitis, brain stem encephalitis, optic neuritis, retinal degeneration, myelitis, motor neuron disease, sensory neuropathy, a type of Guillain-Barré syndrome, LEMS, myasthenia gravis, dermato- and polymyositis, and other myopathies. Inflammation that presumably reflects a local T-cell-mediated response may or may not contribute significantly to the basic histopathologic character of the disease.

The finding of autoantibodies in high titer is usually taken to support the autoimmune hypothesis; the best confirmatory evidence remains passive transfer experiments like those carried out by Newsom-Davis et al. with sera of LEMS patients. A variety of nuclear, cytoplasmic, and cell membrane constituents (protein, glycolipid) have been identified in the various syndromes. The extraordinary specificity of the epitopes involved in each case is well brought out in the case of LEMS, where voltage-gated calcium channels of the presynaptic nerve terminal serve as the target for autoantibody elicited by apparently identical calcium channel proteins in the associated tumor, a small-cell lung carcinoma (312). The responsible antigen appears to be synaptotagmin. A mild disease resembling LEMS is induced in rats immunized with this antigen (424). Drachman (99) has proposed the following criteria for recognizing antibody-mediated autoimmune disease:

Antibody is present in patients with the disease.

Antibody interacts with the target antigen.

Passive transfer of the antibody reproduces the principal disease features.

Immunization with the antigen produces a model disease.

Reduction of the antibody ameliorates the disease.

These represent in essence an updating of criteria (intended to resemble Koch's postulates) proposed earlier by Waksman (453) and Witebsky et al. (470) and are applicable not only to paraneoplastic syndromes but also to antibody-mediated diseases triggered by other means, e.g., viral infection, drugs, etc. In inflammatory diseases, where immune T cells may play the principal role as effectors of the autoimmune process, these criteria must be modified by substituting the phrase "specific T lymphocytes" for "antibody" throughout. In most of the paraneoplastic syndromes, the criteria cited have not been fulfilled. Also, for most of these syndromes, meaningful immunologic research at the cellular level is still largely lacking because of the rarity of the cases and because no convenient animal models exist to facilitate such studies.

Neuropathic Syndromes Associated with Monoclonal Gammopathies

Peripheral neuropathies are frequently associated with lymphoproliferative disorders affecting B cell (199). These include benign plasma cell dyscrasias and other nonmalignant B-cell disorders, which are accompanied by IgM, G, or A monoclonal gammopathy. They also occur less frequently with multiple myeloma in which monoclonal IgG or A is produced, or with Waldenstroms's disease, B-cell lymphoma, or chronic lymphocytic leukemia, in which IgM is produced. Peripheral neuropathies differ from paraneoplastic disorders, in that they involve activation and proliferation, i.e., a transformation, of preexisting antibody-forming cells and production of antibody by these cells, whereas paraneoplastic syndromes result from an active immune response against an antigenic component of growing tumor cells.

After isolated case reports in the 1960s, a number of clinical syndromes were defined in the 1970s, that were associated with direct damage to tissue components such as myelin, intravascular deposition of immune complexes or other aggregated materials (e.g., cryoglobuline), and amyloid deposits in tissue. In cases where the principal element of pathogenesis is a pathologically elevated immunoglobulin with tissue specificity, i.e., a true autoantibody, symptoms (and the histologic lesions) are alleviated by removing the pathologic immunoglobulin, where by plasma exchange or by effective therapy to eliminate the proliferating B cells. The most productive research has been done on patients with the diseases in question rather than in animal models.

The best-studied syndrome within this group is a peripheral neuropathy associated with elevated IgM (199). In 1982 Latov and colleagues discovered that this IgM is a specific antibody binding to carbohydrate epitopes shared by myelin-associated glycoprotein (MAG), several other glycoproteins, and two glycolipids: sulfated glucuronic acid paragloboside (SGPG) and sulfated glucuronic acid lactosaminyl paragloboside (SGLPG). The lesion is a relatively noninflammatory demyelination (with a characteristic increase in spacing of the myelin layers), showing deposition of the specific immunoglobulin and of complement components on affected myelin sheaths. The antibody produces demyelination when transferred into cats (159). The B cell that makes the anti-MAG has been cloned; and a mouse model is reported. Somewhat different syndromes are produced when the antibody proves to be directed at chondroitin sulfate, disialoyl-containing gangliosides (GM1, GM2, etc.), or endoneurial constituents.

Monoclonal gammopathies associated with multiple myeloma, and especially with osteosclerotic myeloma, are almost all IgG or IgA and usually have lamda as the principal light chain. They may be associated with endocrine abnormalities, organomegaly, anasarca, gynecomastia, hyperpigmentation, and hirsutism (Crow-Fukase syndrome) (295). The common picture is referred to as the POEMS syndrome: **p**olyneuropathy, **o**rganomegaly, **e**ndocrinopathy, **m**yeloma, and **s**kin changes (23). While the immunoglobulin as antibody may mediate the neuropathologic changes, the other findings are speculatively ascribed to neuropeptides and cytokines released from the malignant lymphoid cells. TNF-α levels are very high in POEMS patients (130). Neuropathy can actually be transferred with multiple myeloma sera to the mouse (40). A mouse model of myeloma with polyneuropathy was developed in 1972 (88), but it has been little exploited.

The further study of SGPG by Yu and colleagues in the late 1980s (e.g., 214,259) has shown that this antigen (or an epitope cross-reactive with SGPG) is expressed on MAG, in axolemma and nerve terminals, and at the same time in human and rat vascular endothelium. Rabbits producing antibody to SGPG (after active immunization) develop noninflammatory demyelinative lesions in the nerve roots associated with complement-dependent demyelination and conduction block. In rats such immunization results in axonal loss in the dorsal columns and endothelial damage in the spinal cord, which suggests a breakdown in the blood-brain and blood-nerve barrier. Intraneural injection of antibody into the rat sciatic nerve produces a demyelinative lesion and conduction block.

Systemic Lupus Erythematosus (SLE)

As many as 75% of patients with SLE show neurological complications. This relationship was first recognized in the 1960s (188), as was the occurrence of similar complications in Sjögren's syndrome (28) and primary vasculitis a decade later (review in 152,249). The neurological manifestations are protean, including meningitis, encephalopathy, myelopathy, mood disturbances, psychosis, seizures, strokes, polyneuropathy, and derangements of hypothalamic function. Neurological textbooks attribute the different changes in SLE largely or entirely to widespread microinfarction of the cerebral cortex and brain stem in the absence of a true vasculitis. However, immunologic investigations during the late 1970s and early '80s and the use of standardized batteries of tests for cognitive dysfunction have made it possible to distinguish several quite different conditions occurring independently of each other.

Through immunofluorescence and cytotoxicity on neuroblastoma cells, Bluestein et al. and Denburg et al. identified antineuronal antibodies as specifically related to cognitive dysfunction and neurophychological abnormalities, even to the level of psychosis (45–47,93,94). Several antigens may be involved, including a ribosomal protein (49) and a membrane component. Circulating immune complexes, e.g., with DNA, in the spinal fluid and deposits of complexes in the choroid plexus show an equally clear-cut relation to membranous and/or vascular choroidopathy (212,389). Antibodies against phospholipids, with anticoagulant activity, can be related to microinfarction and dementia (152, 292, review in 274). Finally, isolated angiitis, e.g., in patients with neuropathy, is an inflammatory, largely monocytic vascular disease, possibly resulting from a cell-mediated immune reactions (249).

A mouse model for cognitive and behavioral dysfunction is available in the SLE-prone New Zealand black-New Zealand white (NZB-NZW) hybrid mouse (203). The clinical disturbance can be quite directly related to high-circulating titers of anti-DNA and anticardiolipin antibodies. The corresponding lesions, however, include mononuclear infiltration around cerebral and hippocampal blood vessels and in the choroid plexus.

Other Autoimmune CNS and PNS Diseases

Additional disorders of the nervous system which may have an autoimmune etiology are listed in Table 1-1. In some of these, the findings suggest an immunological mechanism, but our understanding of the pathophysiology remains rudimentary and the exact role of the immune system can be no more than conjectured. On the other hand, immunologically mediated inflammatory diseases of the eye, loosely grouped under the term uveitis and the idiopathic inflammatory myopathies are well understood, but they do not fall within the scope of the present chapter and are not reviewed here.

Human Neuroimmunological Diseases: Infections

All infections of the CNS and PNS elicit immunopathologic responses. A large proportion of the recognized neuroimmunologic diseases are autoimmune. Many of these, both in humans and experimental animals, are associated with infection and involve immune response to epitopes shared between the infectious agent (bacterial, viral, or parasite) and the host. However, there remain two further disease categories which do *not* primarily involve autoimmunity. In one of these, disease is the consequence of the immune response to antigens of the infectious agent itself that are present in the nervous system, usually expressed as T-cell mediated inflammatory lesions. In Lyme disease and Chagas' disease, however, there may be an important autoimmune component as well. In the other disease category, lesions occur in the absence of a specific T-cell response, whether because of actual destruction of CD4+ T cells, as in AIDS dementia, or because of epitope-specific immunologic tolerance or immune deviation, as in subacute sclerosing panencephalitis (SSPE) and lepromatous leprosy. In terms of

Table 1-1 Autoimmune/Neurologic Disorders with Inadequately Defined Immunopathogenetic Elements[a]

Disease	Principal Findings	Year	Reference(s)
Motor neuron disease (MND) and amyotrophic lateral sclerosis (ALS)	1. Antibody against Ca^{2+} channel protein in motor nerve terminal; intracellular Ig at neuromuscular junction	1992	13,64,371,402
	2. IgM gammopathy. Antibody to gangliosides GM1 and GD1b	1986	400
(Experimental autoimmune MND)	Destruction of motor neurons; antibody against cytoplasmic antigen of motor neurons)	(1986)	(108,110)
(Experimental autoimmune gray matter disease)	(Antibody against cell membrane and cytoplasmic antigens of motor neurons)	(1990)	(109)
(Additional subsets of MND/ALS cases are reported to show genetically determined abnormalities of Cu, Zn superoxide dismutase or of neural growth factors [CNTF, BDNF])			
Adrenoleukodystrophy (rapidly progressive childhood form)	T- and B-cell infiltrates, CNS and CSF	1985	35,140
Narcolepsy/cataplexy (rat model)	All patients HLA-DR2+	1984 (1991)	41,190,225,335 (342)
Obsessive-compulsive disorders	IgG antibody vs. opiates (β-endorphin, dynorphin)	1986	372
Major depression	IgG antibody vs. opiates and somatostatin	1988	373
Sydenham's chorea (with rheumatic fever)	IgG antibody vs. neurones of caudate and subthalamic nuclei	1976	178
Stiff man syndrome	Antibody vs. glutamic acid carboxylase (GAD)	1988	410
Rasmussen's encephalitis (rabbit model)	Antibody vs. glutamate receptor 3 (GluR3)	1994	366
Schizophrenia	↑IL-1a and IL-2 in CSF	1992	267
	Soluble IL-2R in blood	1989,1992	265,354,355
	Serum antibody vs. brain	1989	423
	Serum antibody vs. HSP60	1993	206
	↑CD5+ B cells in blood	1989	266
(Borna disease virus model in tree shrew, rat)	(Behavioral disorder, requires T-cell response)	(1983)	(10,298,412,445)

[a]All items dealing with animal models are shown in parentheses.

the total burden of human suffering, diseases in these two categories may equal or exceed the autoimmune diseases in importance. Better-studied non-autoconditions are listed in Table 1-2.

Following is a more detailed account of viral diseases in each of the two categories and of leprous neuritis. The latter is included because it is bacterial rather than viral and

Table 1-2 Immunopathologic Reactions to Infectious Agents (Bacteria, Viruses, Prozozoa) in the CNS and PNS[a,b]

Disease	Principal Findings	Year	Reference
Acute viral encephalitis (with many viruses) (Sindbis viral encephalitis in mice)	(Specific CD8+ T cells plus B cells and macrophages in CNS and CSF infiltrates)	(1972)	(139,234,286)
HTLV-associated myelopathy/ tropical spastic paraparesis (HAM/TSP)	Inflammation/demyelination; persistent virus in CD4+ T cells; CD8+ T cells cytotoxic for infected CD4+ T cells	1956, 1979	180,441
(Visna/Maedi in sheep)	(Inflammation/demyelination persistent virus in macrophages and oligodendrocytes)	(1958, 1976)	(143,148,297,299, 300,333)
Theiler's virus [TMEV] in mice)	(Specific CD8+ T cells responsible for lesions and immunity)	(1934, 1975)	(75,247,283,353, 365,427)
Lyme disease (with B. burgdorferi)	Inflammation/demyelination; antibody and T-cells specific for parasite; possible autoimmunity.	1977	1,153,319,320
Toxoplasmosis (with T. gondii) (T. gondii in mice)	Persistent infection of macrophages and neurons; resistance involves CD8+ T cells/NK cells, IFN-γ, and macrophage production of NO.	(1991)	(127)
Leprous neuritis (tuberculoid)	Tuberculoid lesions in nerve, CD4 > CD8; few organisms, high CMI, low antibody	1978, 1986	44,111,153,167, 285,315,382, 472
American trypanosomiasis (with T. cruzi)	Peripheral neuropathy; lymphocytic infiltration and destruction of parasympathetic ganglia; secondary cardiomyopathy, megacolon; autoantibody to Schwann cells and nerve sheaths and to neuronal ribosomal phosphoprotein; autoantibody and CM1 to cysteinyl proteinase: all cross-reactive with parasite epitopes		211 127,200,405
(T. cruzi in mice)	(Granulomatous infiltrates in nerves with demyelination and axonal damage; lesion transfer with CD4+ T cells lines; resistance mediated by CD4+ T cells, IFN-γ, and ROS/NO in macrophages; susceptibility mediated by IL-10 and THF-β	(1985)	(127,173,378, 472)
AIDS dementia (with HIV)	Infection of macrophages and infection/destruction of CD4+ T cells	1985	9,57,168,273,301, 340,341,465

(*continued*)

Table 1-2 (*Continued*)

Disease	Principal Findings	Year	Reference
(Feline and simian immunodeficiency virus models)	Viral superantigen; TH1-TH0 shift gp120-toxicity for CD4+ T cells high TNF production in brain		
Progressive multifocal leukoencephalopathy (PML) (with JC virus)	Immunosuppression or sarcoid Hodgkins, CLL, or AIDS; virus in oligos and astrocytes; demyelination (similar)	1959	53,148,360,461
(Coronavirus [JHM] in mice)	Similar	(1949)	(66,418,456)
Subacute sclerosing panencephalitis (SSPE) (with measles virus)	Persistent virus in brain; local antibody synthesis	1933	95,136,148
Progressive rubella pancencephalitis	Immunoglobulin in deposition; chronic inflammation and white matter loss; high antibody, low or absent CMI	1975	471
(Lymphocytic choriomeningitis virus in mice)	Similar	(1936)	(22,56,174)
Leprous neuritis (lepromatous)	Few T cells, foamy macrophages in nerve lesions. CD8 ≫ CD4, IL-4 and IL-10; low CMI, high Ab, many organisms	1978, 1986	310,431,479

[a]This list refers mainly to well-studied cases and ignores African trypanosomiasis (sleeping sickness), cerebral malaria, helminths such as echinococcus, and fungi.

[b]All items dealing with animal models are shown in parentheses.

it affects the PNS, and because it exhibits a complex but by now a well-studied suppressor system in its lepromatous form.

HTLV-1 Associated Myelopathy/Tropical Spastic Paraparesis (HAM/TSP)

Tropical spastic paraparesis was first distinguished as a clinical entity on the island of Jamaica in the early 1960s. Its relationship to the human T-lymphotropic virus-1 (HTLV-1), identified as the cause of acute T-cell leukemia (ATL) in the Caribbean and southern Japan in 1979–80, was first accomplished by serological methods in 1984–85. The disease is widespread in the Caribbean and South America, central Africa, the Seychelles Islands, and southern Japan, and significant numbers of immigrant cases have been identified in the U.S. and western Europe.

HAM/TSP is a lentiviral infection of the CNS, passed by sexual or other intimate contact, by breast milk, blood transfusion, or the use of infected needles in drug abuse. It is a slowly progressive, spastic paraparesis, accompanied by bladder dysfunction, and is difficult to distinguish from MS clinically or by magnetic resonance imaging. Postmortem studies show primarily perivascular inflammatory lesions of the meninges and CNS (mainly the spinal cord). Reports that MS is caused by HTLV-1 were based on false-positive Western blots obtained with MS sera and HTLV-1 on irreproducible data obtained with PCR, and on diagnostic confusion between MS and HAM/TSP. ATL is not present in HAM/TSP patients, but similar antibodies are found in both classes of patients, both in serum and in CSF. The virus can be identified in much mutated form in blood and spinal fluid lymphocytes in HAM/TSP (222).

In high prevalence areas like southern Japan, 97% of the population have antibody to virus but only 1% have the disease. Both, however, have characteristic abnormalities in T lymphocytes containing virus: spontaneous proliferation, increased expression of MHC-II and IL-2 receptor, and failure to differentiate. By 1990 it became clear that HAM/TSP patients have a high level of blood and CSF CD8+ T cells recognizing viral antigen (mainly pX protein) in association with MHC-I on CD4+ cells (180,441). These are not seen in ATL patients or seropositive carriers. The CNS lesions contain many CD8+ cells, and tissue damage appears to result from the activation of these cells. Autoimmunization against myelin antigens is not seen. HAM-TSP shows an HLA association which is lacking in groups of ATL patients (441).

Animal Models for HAM/TSP

HAM/TSP has two models in experimental animals that have shed a good deal of light on its possible pathogenetic mechanisms.

Visna/maedi, a chronic lentiviral infection of sheep, affects the lungs, joints, and nervous system, as well as the hemopoietic and immune systems (reviews in 143,148). This disease, considered by some investigators to be a model for MS, became epizootic in Iceland in the 1940s (see also 81). The term slow infection was introduced in 1954 and the viral etiology of visna established in 1958. Details of visna pathogenesis were well understood by the mid-1970s (333). The organism proliferates in the lung, the usual site of infection, spreading later to the CSF and CNS, where it persists until the animal dies. Antigenic variation contributes significantly to viral persistence and the occurrence of relapses, like those seen in MS (297). Virus persists and is expressed within macrophages throughout the body (300). Indeed, it enters the CNS within infected monocytes like a so-called Trojan horse. Infected macrophages show up-regulated MHC, which stimulates production of a unique interferon capable of restricting the organism's replication (299). The immune response to virus appears to be responsible for the characteristic inflammatory demyelinative lesions; disease is inhibited by immunosuppressive therapy. The mechanism of demyelination is unclear, it may fall into the category of "bystander" demyelination, which is produced by the activated macrophages. In some strains of sheep, the virus fails to invade the CNS, and the pulmonary lesions, the "maedi," dominate the clinical picture. The caprine arthritis-encephalitis virus, a closely related organism, produces similar interstitial pneumonia and encephalitis in goats, as well as a prominent synovitis/arthritis.

The second model is provided by mice infected with Theiler's murine encephalitis virus (TMEV). The inflammatory demyelinative lesions have long been regarded as a model for MS. However, here as in the case of visna, we are dealing with a CNS lesion attributable to the immune response to virus persisting in the CNS, in the absence of autoimmunization to myelin components. TMEV is a picornavirus and is a common mouse pathogen that was described in 1937 and originally regarded as a model for poliomyelitis (427). In the early 1970s Lipton called attention to the fact that the early, polio-like phase may be followed by a chronic demyelinative phase (247). Along with dal Canta, he established that the chronic disease is eliminated by immunosuppressive therapy and must therefore be immunologic (248). Nevertheless, virus persistence could be shown in CNS glial elements throughout the chronic phase. Lipton et al. and independently, Rodriguez et al. established in 1985 that disease could be related to DTH against virus and was MHC I restricted (75,365). Adoptive transfer studies showed that the pathogenic immune response was directed to virus and did not include any autoimmune component (283). This was later borne out by carefully designed reciprocal tolerance–immunization experiments involving TMEV and EAE (475). CD8+ T cells make up the principal reacting cell population, as is also the case in HAM/TSP and visna.

Subacute Sclerosing Panencephalitis (SSPE) and Progressive Rubella Panencephalitis (PRP)

SSPE, which was described in 1933, is characterized by progressive cognitive and motor deficit in children who have survived an uncomplicated measles infection in early childhood (see 136,148). Striking inclusion body encephalitis is accompanied in each case by high levels of intrathecally synthesized anti-measles antibody. This disease is thought to represent measles virus infection in individuals showing T-cell tolerance to the virus after early exposure to measles virus antigen(s), or possibly individuals whose response to measles has shifted from TH1 (associated with cell-mediated immunity responsible for clearing the virus) to TH2 (associated primarily with a humoral response). SSPE has largely disappeared in recent years in countries with an effective measles vaccination program.

Measles virus was first isolated from the brains of children with SSPE in 1969 (148,426). It persists within neurons and oligodendrocytes. Recent molecular studies have shown that the persisting intracellular virus undergoes loss of certain antigens, the viral "M" proteins in particular, and there is reduced expression of virus at the cell surface (147,148). This reduction is all the greater in cells exposed to the abnormally high titers of anti-measles antibody commonly seen in the peripheral blood and CSF of SSPE patients.

Diminished cytoxic CD8+ T-cell responsiveness to measles virus antigen was observed by Dhib-Jalbut and colleagues in 1988 (95). There is no comparable diminution of cytotoxic T-cell responses to influenza or mumps. On the other hand, the high antibody titers imply that TH2 responses are intact or increased.

A disease similar to SSPE but related to rubella virus, PRP, was described in 1975 as a late complication of the congenital rubella syndrome or of typical childhood rubella (see 471). As in SSPE, there is immunoglobulin deposition throughout the cerebral vasculature, with subacute–chronic inflammation in the meninges and perivascular areas in the brain parenchyma. White matter is also destroyed with loss of myelin and severe gliosis. As in SSPE, research findings suggest infection in a host showing tolerance or immune deviation (TH1→TH2) as a result usually of intrauterine exposure to the virus. Since clones have been obtained of CSF T cells that react with both rubella virus and MBP (221), there may be an autoimmune component in the pathogenesis of this disease.

Animal Model for SSPE and PRP

Lymphocytic choriomeningitis (LCM) in mice is the best-studied example of tolerance immunity relationships in an animal model of viral disease of the CNS (review in 56). The virus is a single-stranded Arenavirus and is a common mouse pathogen. In normal adult mice, it produces an acute infection with an immunologically mediated inflammatory reaction that results either in viral clearing or death of the infected mouse. On the other hand, neonatal infection (e.g., by vertical transmission from an infected mother) or infection in immunosuppressed adults results in tolerance, with persistence of virus in neurons throughout the CNS. In tolerant mice there is often a late rise in antiviral antibody to quite high levels and the mice may develop late and sometimes fatal immune complex-mediated renal disease.

As early as 1936, Traub observed the tolerant state in mice infected in utero with LCM, many of whom had persistently high levels of virus in their circulation (431). In later studies, it was found that disease competence was restored to tolerized animals by transfer of normal syngeneic lymphocytes and that disease accelerated with immune lymphocytes. Hotchin and Cintis performed studies of conditions favoring the induction of tolerance: age at induction, dose and route of virus inoculation, state of maternal health, even the role of the thymus all play a role (174).

LCM somewhat resembles Theiler's murine encephalitis virus in that it is MHC-I instead of MHC-II restricted (reviewed in #98). Zinkernagel and Oldstone, along with their respective colleagues, showed in the mid-80s that the disease is actually mediated by activated CD8+ cells and that CD4+ cells seem to play little role in the disease (22,479). The CSF contains macrophages and T cells, most of which are CD8+, and these cells appear to be responsible as well for H-2D restricted DTH (479). Cloned LCM-specific cytotoxic CD8+ cells alone, when transferred to a tolerant, infected host, clear virus efficiently (61,310). The MHC restriction can involve either H-2L or

H-2K, but the relatively greater affinity of viral epitope for the H-2L molecule leads to its being dominant over H-2K when both are present (313).

Leprosy

Mycobacterium leprae produces a chronic granulomatous disease in humans. The organism infects skin and Schwann cells, producing of characteristic skin lesions and neuropathy (reviews in 44,153,375). There is a spectrum of leprosy cases between two immunologically distinct extremes (382). Patients with tuberculoid leprosy show DTH to protein antigens of *M. leprae,* develop a limited number of well-localized inflammatory skin and nerve lesions, and few organisms can be found in the lesions. In patients with lepromatous leprosy, DTH and in vitro cell-mediated immunity to the organism are lacking and there are high titers of antibody. In both skin and nerve lesions, the inflammatory response fails, there is massive invasion by the organisms, and the host may die.

In tuberculoid leprosy, CD4+ T cells greatly outnumber CD8+ cells in the skin lesions. There is general agreement that the skin lesion is essentially a DTH reaction against the organism without any reaction to parenchymal antigen. The nerve trunks and cutaneous nerves are conspicuous by enlarged and are invaded and destroyed by a granulomatous reaction containing many giant cells. The infected Schwann cells show up-regulation of MHC-II expression. By contrast, in lepromatous disease, CD8+ T cells predominate in the lesions. Foamy macrophages full of dividing *M. leprae* invade the endo- and perineurium. These cells are unable to kill the organisms; this has been attributed to the absence of IL-2 and IFN-γ. The high levels of antibody neither protect nor contribute to pathogenesis, although they include antibody to an intermediate filament protein (111).

The nonreactivity of T cells in lepromatous disease is at least in part accounted for by the presence of suppressor T-cell populations. Such suppressor cells have been cloned from both skin and nerve in a variety of conditions by Modlin, Bloom, and Sasazuki, in work first published in 1986 (167, 284, 285, 315, review in 44). The picture of a two-cell system emerged: A CD4+ T cell (suppressor–inducer) that is epitope-specific and restricted by IgVH (on antigen-presenting B cells?); and a CD8+ T cell (suppressor), specific for idiotopes of the suppressor–inducer cell TcR. The nonspecific suppressor factor produced by the system is IL-4, which can effectively suppress the in vitro response of CD4+ cells specific for *M. leprae* to antigen.

Summary

Neuroimmunology has come of age since 1980. Its parent disciplines—immunology, experimental pathology (neuropathology), neurobiology, and neurophysiology—have been virtually transformed into branches of cellular and molecular biology. The interactions of nervous, endocrine, and immune systems and their perturbations in disease have been recognized as an important part of fundamental biology. Throughout its history neuroimmunology has been driven both by technological advances and by new concepts in the parent fields. The application of these concepts and techniques and of insights gained from the study of animal models has proven remarkably fruitful. It has permitted an even deeper understanding of many important inflammatory neurological conditions and has opened the way to rational approaches to prevention and therapy.

References

1. Aberer E, Brunner C, Suchanek G, et al. Molecular mimicry and Lyme borreliosis: a shared antigenic determinant between Borrelia burgdorferi and human tissue. Ann Neurol 26: 732–737, 1989.
2. Abramsky O, Webb C, Teitelbaum D, Arnon R. Cellular hypersensitivity to peripheral nervous antigen in the Guillain-Barré syndrome. Neurology 25:1154–1159, 1975.
3. Adams RD, Kubik CS. The morbid anatomy of the demyelinating diseases. Am J Med 12:510–546, 1952.
4. Ader R, ed. Psychoneuroimmunology. Academic Press, New York, 1981.
5. Ader R, Cohen N. Behaviorally conditioned immunosuppression. Psychosom Med 37:333–340, 1975.
6. Aguayo AJ, Bray GM, Perkins SC. Axon-Schwann cell relationships in neuropathies of mutant mice. Ann NY Acad Sci 317:512–531, 1979.
7. Ahlqvist J. Endocrine influences in lymphatic organs, immune responses, inflammation, and autoimmunity. Acta Endocrinnol 83 (Suppl 206): 1–136, 1976.
8. Allegretta M, Nicklas JA, Sriram S, and Albertini RJ. T cells responsive to myelin basic protein in patients with multiple sclerosis. Science 247:718–721, 1990.
9. Ameisen JC. Programmed cell death and AIDS: from hypothesis to experiment. Immunol Today 13:388–391, 1992.
10. Amsterdam JD, Winokur A, Dyson W, et al. Borna disease virus. A possible etiologic factor in human affective disorders? Arch Gen Psychiatry 42:1093–1096, 1985.
11. Antel JP, Bania MP, Reder A, Cashman N. Activated suppressor cell dysfunction in progressive multiple sclerosis. J Immunol 137:137–141, 1986.
12. Antel JP, Nickolas MK, Bania MB, et al. Comparison of T8+ cell-mediated suppressor and cytotoxic functions in multiple sclerosis. J Neuroimmunol 12:215–224, 1986.
13. Appel S. Amyotrophic lateral sclerosis. Abstracts: 23rd Annual Meeting, Am Soc Neurochem, p 29, 1992.
14. Appenzeller O, Arnason BG, Adams RD. Experimental autonomic neuropathy: an immunologically induced disorder of reflex vasomotor function. J Neurol Neurosurg Psychiatry 28:510–515, 1965.
15. Arnason BGW, Brown M, Maselli R, et al. Blood lymphocyte beta-adrenergic receptors in multiple sclerosis. Ann NY Acad Sci 540:585–588, 1988.
16. Arnason BG, Jankovic BD, Waksman BH. Effect of thymectomy on "delayed" hypersensitive reactions. Nature 194:99–100, 1962.
17. Arnold B, Goodnow C, Hengartner H, Hämmerling G. The coming of transgenic mice: tolerance and immune reactivity. Immunol Today 11:69–72, 1990.

18. Asbury AK, Arnason BG, Adams RD. The inflammatory lesion in idiopathic polyneuritis: its role in pathogenesis. Medicine 48:173–215, 1969.
19. Asbury AK, Gibbs CJ Jr, eds. Autoimmune neuropathies. Guillain-Barré syndrome. Ann Neurol 27 (Suppl): S1–S79, 1990.
20. Atkins E, Wood WB Jr. Studies on the pathogenesis of fever: I. The presence of transferable pyrogen in the blood stream following the injection of typhoid vaccine. J Exp Med 101:519–528, 1955.
21. Audhya T, Schlesinger DH, Goldstein G. Complete amino acid sequences of bovine thymopoietins I, II, and III: closely homologous polypeptides. Biochemistry 20:6195–6200, 1981.
22. Baenziger JH, Hengartner H, Zinkernagel RM, Cole GA. Induction or prevention of immunopathological disease by cloned cytotoxic T cell lines specific for lymphocytic choriomeningitis virus. Eur J Immunol 16:387–393, 1986.
23. Bardwick PA, Zvaifler WJ, Gill GN, et al. Plasma cell dyscrasia with polyneuropathy, organomegaly, endocrinopathy, M protein and skin changes. The POEMS syndrome. Medicine 59:311–322, 1980.
24. Bartrop RW, Luckhurst E, Lazarus L, Kilch LG, Penny R. Depressed lymphocyte functions after bereavement. Lancet i:834–836, 1977.
25. Beall SS, Concannon P, Charmley P, et al. The germline repertoire of T cell receptor beta-chain genes in patients with chronic progressive multiple sclerosis. J Neuroimmunol 21:59–66, 1989.
26. Behan, PO, Geschwind N, Lamarche JB, et al. Delayed hypersensitivity to encephalitogenic protein in disseminated encephalomyelitis. Lancet ii:1009–1012, 1968.
27. Behlke MA, Chou HS, Huppi K, Loh DY. Murine T-cell receptor mutants with deletions of beta-chain variable region genes. Proc Nat Acad Sci 83:767–771, 1986.
28. Bennett RM, Bong DM, Spargo BH. Neuropsychiatric probes in mixed connective tissue disease. Am J Med 65:955–962, 1979.
29. Ben-Nun A, Wekerle H, Cohen IR. The rapid isolation of clonable antigen-specific T lymphocyte lines capable of mediating autoimmune encephalomyelitis. Eur J Immunol 11:195–199, 1981.
30. Ben-Nun A, Wekerle H, Cohen IR. Vaccination against autoimmune encephalomyelitis with T-lymphocyte line cells reactive against myelin basic protein. Nature 292:60–61, 1981.
31. Benveniste EN, Sparacio SM, Bethea JR. Tumor necrosis factor-alpha enhances interferon-gamma-mediated class II antigen expression on astrocytes. J Neuroimmunol 25:209–219, 1989.
32. Benveniste EN, Sparacio SM, Norris JG, et al. Induction and regulation of interleukin-6 gene expression in rat astrocytes. J Neuroimmunol 30:201–212, 1990.
33. Berg O, Källén B. White blood cells from animals with experimental allergic encephalomyelitis tested on glia cells in tissue culture. Acta Path Microb Scand 58:33–72, 1963.
34. Bernard CCA. Suppressor T cells prevent experimental autoimmune encephalomyelitis in mice. Clin Exp Immunol 291:100–109, 1977.
35. Bernheimer H, Budka H, Müller P. Brain tissue immunoglobulins in adrenoleukodystrophy: a comparison with multiple sclerosis and systemic lupus erythematosus. Acta Neuropath 59:95–102, 1983.
36. Berrich-Aknin S, Cohen-Kaminsky S, Neumann D, et al. Proliferative responses to acetylcholine receptor peptides in myasthenia gravis. Ann NY Acad Sci 540:504–505, 1988.
37. Besedovsky H, del Rey A. Neuroendocrine and metabolic responses induced by interleukin-1. J Neurosci Res 18:172–178, 1987.

38. Besedovsky HO, del Rey A, Sorkin E, et al. Immunoregulation mediated by the sympathetic nervous system. Cell Immunol 48:346–355, 1979.

39. Besedovsky HO, del Rey A, Sorkin E, Dinarello CA. Immunoregulatory feedback between interleukin-1 and glucocorticoid hormones. Science 233:652–654, 1986.

40. Bessinger VA, Toyka KV, Anzil AP, et al. Myeloma neuropathy; passive transfer from man to mouse. Science 213:1027–1030, 1981.

41. Billiard M, Seignalet J. Extraordinary association between HLA-DR2 and narcolepsy. Lancet i:226–227, 1985.

42. Blalock JE. Neuroimmunoendocrinology. Chem Immunol 52:1–195, 1992.

43. Blalock JE, Smith EM. Human leukocyte interferon: structural and biological relatedness to adrenocorticotropic hormone and endorphins. Proc Natl Acad Sci USA 77:5972–5974, 1980.

44. Bloom BR, Salgame P, Diamond B. Revisiting and revising suppressor T cells. Immunol Today 13:131–136, 1992.

45. Bluestein HG, Williams GW, Steinberg AD. Cerrebrospinal fluid antibodies to neuronal cells: association with neuropsychiatric manifestations of systemic lupus erythematosus. Am J Med 70:240–246, 1981.

46. Bluestein HG, Woods VL Jr. Antineuronal antibodies in systemic lupus erythematosus. Arthritis Rheum 25:773–778, 1982.

47. Bluestein HG, Zvaifler NJ. Brain-reactive lymphocytotoxic antibodies in the serum of patients with systemic lupus erythematosus. J Clin Invest 57:509–516, 1976.

48. Bö L, Dawson TM, Wesselingh S, et al. Induction of nitric oxide synthase in demyelinating regions of multiple sclerosis brains. Ann Neurol 36:778–786, 1994.

49. Bonfa E, Golombach SJ, Kaufman LD, et al. Association between lupus psychosis and ribosomal protein antibodies. New Engl J Med 317:265–271, 1987.

50. Braun PE, Frail DE, Latov N. Myelin associated glycoprotein is the antigen for a monoclonal IgM in polyneuropathy. J Neurochem 39:1261–1265, 1982.

51. Breder CD, Dinarello CA, Saper CB. Interleukin-1 immunoreactive innervation of the human hypothalamus. Science 240:321–324, 1988.

52. Brimijoin S, Moser V, Hammand P, et al. Death of intermediolateral spinal cord neurons follows selective complement-mediated destruction of peripheral preganglionic sympathetic terminals by acetylcholinesterase antibodies. Neuroscience 54:201–223, 1993.

53. Brooks BR, Walter DL. Progressive multifocal leukoencephalopathy. Neurol Clin 2:299–313, 1984.

54. Brosnan CF, Litwak MS, Schroeder CE, et al. Preliminary studies of cytokine-induced functional effects on the visual pathways in the rabbit. J Neuroimmunol 25:227–239, 1989.

55. Brown AM, McFarlin DE. Relapsing experimental allergic encephalomyelitis in the SJL/J mouse. Lab Invest 45:278–284, 1981.

56. Buchmeier MJ, Welsh RM, Dutko FJ, Oldstone MBA. The virology and immunobiology of lymphocytic choriomeningitis virus infection. Adv Immunol 30:257–331, 1986.

57. Budka H. Multinucleated giant cells in brain: a hallmark of the acquired immune deficiency syndrome (AIDS). Acta Neuropathol 69:253–258, 1986.

58. Bullock K, Moore RY. Innervation of the thymus gland by brain stem and spinal cord in the mouse and rat. Am J Anat 162:157–166, 1981.

59. Burky EL. Experimental endophthalmitis phaco-anaphylactica in rabbits. Arch Ophthalmol 12:536–546, 1934.

60. Burns J, Rosenzweig A, Zweiman B, Lisak R. Isolation of myelin basic protein-reactive T-cell lines from normal human blood. Cell Immunol 81:435–440, 1983.

61. Byrne JA, Oldstone MBA. Biology of cloned cytotoxic T lymphocytes specific for lympho-cytic choriomeningitis virus. Clearance of virus in vivo. J Virol 51:682–686, 1984.

62. Cambi F, Lees, MB, Williams RM, Macklin WB. Chronic experimental allergic encepha-lomyelitis produced by bovine proteolipid apoprotein. Immunological studies in rabbits. Ann Neurol 13:303–308, 1983.

63. Carr DJ, Klimpel GR. Enhancement of the generation of cytotoxic T cells by endogenous opiates. J Neuroimmunol 12:75–87, 1986.

64. Cashman NR, Antel JP. Amyotrophic lateral sclerosis: an immunologic perspective. Immu-nol Allergy Clin N Am 8:331–342, 1988.

65. Castleman B, Norris EH. The pathology of the thymus gland in myasthenia gravis. A study of 35 cases. Medicine 28:27–58, 1949.

65a. Cerruti-Sola S, Kristensen F, Vandevelde M, et al. Lymphocyte responsiveness to lectin and myelin antigens in canine distemper infection in relation to the development of demyelinating lesions. J Neuroimmunol 4:77–90, 1983.

66. Cheever FS, Daniels JB, Pappenheimer AM, Bailey OT. A murine virus (JHM) causing disseminated encephalomyelitis with extensive destruction of myelin. I. Isolation and biological properties of the virus. J Exp Med 90:181–212, 1949.

67. Chelmicka-Schorr E, Arnason BGW. Nervous system–immune system interactions. Res Publ Assoc Res Nerv Ment Dis 68:69–90, 1990.

68. Chelmicka-Schorr E, Checinski M, Arnason BGW. Sympathectomy augments the severity of experimental allergic encephalomyelitis in rats. Ann NY Acad Sci 540:707–708, 1988.

69. Chelmicka-Schorr E, Kwasniewski MN, Thomas BE, Arnason BGW. The beta-adrenergic agonist isoproterennol suppresses experimental allergic encephalomyelitis in Lewis rats. J Neuroimmunol 25:203–207, 1989.

70. Chofflon MM, Weiner HL, Morimoto C, Hafler DA. Loss of functional suppression is linked to decreases in circulating suppressor-inducer (CD4+2H4+) T cells in multiple sclerosis. Ann Neurol 24:185–191, 1988.

71. Chofflon M, Weiner HL, Morimoto C, Hafler DA. Decrease of suppressor inducer (CD4+2H4+) T cells in multiple sclerosis cerebrospinal fluid. Ann Neurol 25:494–497, 1989.

72. Christadoss P, Lennon VA, David C. Genetic control of experimental autoimmune my-asthenia gravis in mice. I. Lymphocyte proliferation response to acetylchholine receptor is under H-2-linked Ir gene control. J Immunol 123:2540–2543, 1979.

73. Ciulla TA, Robinson MA, Seboun E, et al. Molecular genotypes of the T-cell receptor beta chain in families with multiple sclerosis. Ann NY Acad Sci 540:271–276, 1988.

74. Claman HN. How corticosteroids work. J Allergy Clin Immunol 55:145–151, 1975.

75. Clatch JR, Melvold RW, Miller SD, Lipton HL. Theiler's murine encephalomyelitis virus (TMEV)-induced demyelinating disease in mice is influenced by the H-2D region: cor-relation with TMEV-specific delayed type hypersensitivity. J Immunol 135:1408–1414, 1985.

76. Cohen IR, Ben-Nun A, Holoshitz J, et al. Vaccination against autoimmune disease using lines of autoimmune T-lymphocytes. Immunol Today 4:227–230, 1983.

77. Collins RC. Experimental studies on sympathetic ophthalmia. Am J Ophthalmol 32:1687–1699, 1949.

78. Compston DAS. The Langdon-Brown lecture 1989: the dissemination of multiple sclerosis. J R Coll Physicians Lond 24:207–218, 1990.

79. Crisp DT, Greenstein JL, Kleiner JE. Regulation of the autologous mixed lymphocyte response in multiple sclerosis. Ann Neurol 18:129, 1985.

80. Cross RJ, Brooks WH, Roszman TL. Modulation of T-suppressor cell activity by central nervous system catecholamine depletion. J Neurosci Res. 18:75–81, 1987.

81. Cuillé J, Chelle PL. La maladie dite tremblante du mouton est-elle inoculable? C R Acad Sci (Paris) 203:1552, 1936.

82. Dales S, Fujinami RS, Oldstone MBA. Infection with vaccinia favors the selection of hybridomas synthesizing autoantibodies against intermediate filaments, one of them cross-reacting with the virus hemagglutinin. J Immunol 131:1548–1553, 1983.

83. Dameshek W. Hemolytic anemia. Direct and indirect indications, pathogenetic mechanisms and classifications. Am J Med 18:315–325, 1955.

84. Dau PC, ed. Plasmapheresis and the Immunobiology of Myasthenia Gravis. Houghton Mifflin, Boston, 1979.

85. David JR, Paterson PY. In vitro demonstration of cellular sensitivity in allergic encephalomyelitis. J Exp Med 122:1161–1172, 1965.

86. Dawkins RL. Experimental myositis associated with hypersensitivity to muscle. J Pathol Bacteriol 90:619–625, 1965.

87. Dawkins RL, Mastaglia FL. Cell-mediated cytotoxicity to muscle in polymyositis. New Engl J Med 288:434, 1973.

88. Dayan AD, Stokes MI. Peripheral neuropathy and experimental myeloma in the mouse. Nature 236:117–118, 1972.

89. Daynes RA, Araneo BA, Dowell TA, et al. Regulation of murine lymphokine production in vivo. III. The lymphoid tissue microenvironment exerts regulatory influences over T helper cell function. J Exp Med 171:979–996, 1990.

90. Dean G. Annual incidence, prevalence, and mortality of multiple sclerosis in white South-African-born and in white immigrants to South Africa. Br Med J 2:724–730, 1967.

91. De Coursey TE, Chandy KG, Gupta S, Cahalan MD. Voltage-dependent ion channels in T-lymphocytes. J Neuroimmunol 10:71–95, 1985.

92. Demaine A, Willcox N, Welsh, K, Newsom-Davis J. Associations of the autoimmune myasthenias with genetic markers in the immunoglobulin heavy chain region. Ann NY Acad Sci 540:266–268, 1988.

93. Denburg JA, Carbotte RM, Denburg SD. Neuronal antibodies and cognitive function in systemic lupus erythematosus. Neurology 37:464–467, 1987.

94. Dent PB, Liao SK, Denburg JA. Antineuronal antibodies in neuropsychiatric systemic lupus erythematosus. Arthritis Rheum 28:789–795, 1985.

95. Dhib-Jalbut S, Jacobson, S, McFarlin DE, McFarland HF. Impaired measles-specific cytotoxic T-cell responses in subacute sclerosing panencephalitis. Ann NY Acad Sci 540:645–648, 1988.

96. Dinarello CA, Wolff SM. Molecular basis of fever in humans. Am J Med 72:799–819, 1982.

97. Dobbing J. The blood-brain barrier. Physiol Rev. 41:130–188, 1961.

98. Doherty PC. Cell-mediated immunity in virus infections of the nervous system. Ann NY Acad Sci 540:228–294, 1988.

99. Drachman DB. How to recognize an antibody-mediated autoimmune disease: criteria. Res Publ Assoc Res Nerv Ment Dis 68:183–186, 1990.

100. Drachman DB, Adams RN, Stanley EF, Pestronk A. Mechanisms of acetylcholine receptor loss in myasthenia agravis. J Neurol Neurosurg Psychiatry 43:601–610, 1980.

101. Drachman DB, De Silva S, Ramsay D, Pestronk A. Humoral pathogenesis of myasthenia gravis. Ann NY Acad Sci 505:90–104, 1987.

102. Dyck PH, Lais AC, Ohta M, et al. Chronic inflammatory polyradiculoneuropathy. Mayo Clinic Proc. 50:621–637, 1975.

103. Ebers GC, Bulman DE, Sadovnick AD, et al. A population-based study of multiple sclerosis in twins. New Engl J Med 315:1638–1642, 1986.

104. Ellison GW, Waksman BH. Role of the thymus in tolerance. IX. Inhibition of experimental autoallergic encephalomyelitis by intrathymic injection of encephalitogen. J Immunol 105:322–324, 1970.

105. Elschnig A. Ueber Augenerkrankungen durch Autointoxikation. Wien Med Wochenschr 4:2477–2480, 1905.

106. Endoh M, Tabira T, Kunishita T. Antibodies to proteolipid apoprotein in chronic relapsing experimental allergic encephalomyelitis. J Neurol Sci 73:31–38, 1986.

107. Engel AG, Tsujihata MT, Lambert EH, et al. Experimental autoimmune myasthenia gravis. A sequential and quantitative study of the neuromuscular junction, ultrastructural and electrophysiologic correlation. J Neuropathol Exp Neurol 35:563–587, 1976.

108. Engelhardt JI, Appel SH, Killian JM. Experimental autoimmune motoneuron disease. Ann Neurol 26:368–376, 1989.

109. Engelhardt JI, Appel SH, Killian JM. Motor neuron destruction in guinea pigs immunized with bovine spinal cord ventral horn homogenate: experimental autoimmune gray matter disease. J Neuroimmunol 27:21–31, 1990.

110. Engelhardt J, Joo F. An immune-mediated guinea pig model for lower motor neuron disease. J Neuroimmunol 12:279–290, 1986.

111. Estis-Turf EP, Benjamins JA, Lafford MJ. Characterization of the anti-neural antibodies in the sera of leprosy patients. J Neuroimmunol 10:313–330, 1986.

112. Fambrough DM, Drachman DB, Satyamyurti S. Neuromuscular junction in myasthenia gravis: decreased acetylcholine receptors. Science 182:293–295, 1973.

113. Fazakerlyl JK, Khalili-Shirazi A, Webb HE. Semliki Forest virus (A7[74]) infection of adult mice induces an immune-mediated demyelinating encephalomyelitis. Ann NY Acad Sci 540:672–673, 1988.

114. Felten DL, Overhage JM, Felten SY, Schmedtje, JF. Noradrenergic sympathetic innervation of lymphoid tissue in the rabbit appendix—further evidence for a link between the nervous and immune systems. Brain Res Bull 7:595–612, 1981.

115. Ferraro A, Cazzullo CL. Chronic experimental allergic encephalomyelitis in monkeys. J Neuropathol Exp Neurol 7:235–260, 1948.

116. Ferraro A, Roizin L. Neuropathological variations in experimental allergic encephalomyelitis. Hemorrhagic encephalomyelitis, perivenous encephalomyelitis, diffuse encephalomyelitis, patchy gliosis. J Neuropathol Exp Neurol 13:60–89, 1954.

117. Finley KH. Pathogenesis of encephalitis occurring with vaccination, variola, and measles. Arch Neurol Psychiatry 39:1045–1054, 1938.

118. Fontana A, Fierz W, Wekerle H. Astrocytes present myelin basic protein to encephalitogenic T cell lines. Nature 307:273–276, 1984.

119. Fontana A, Frei K, Bodmer S, Hofer E. Immune-mediated encephalitis: on the role of antigen-presenting cells in brain tissue. Immunol Rev 100:185–201, 1987.

120. Fontana A, Kristensen F, Dubs R, et al. Production of prostaglandin E and an interleukin-1 like factor by cultured astrocytes and C-6 glioma cells. J Immunol 129:2413–2419, 1982.

121. Forghani B, Cremer NE, Johnson KP, et al. Viral antibodies in cerebrospinal fluid of multiple sclerosis and control patients: comparison between radioimmunoassay and conventional techniques. J Clin Microbiol 7:63–69, 1978.

122. Frei K, Siepl C, Groscurth P, et al. Antigen presentation and tumor cytotoxicity by interferon-gamma treated microglial cells. Eur J Immunol 17:1271–1278, 1987.

123. Fritz RB, Chou C-HJ, McFarlin DE. Induction of experimental allergic encephalomyelitis

in PL/J and (SJL/J × PL/J) F1 mice by myelin basic protein and its peptides. Localization of a second encephalitogenic determinant. J Immunol 130:191–194, 1983.

124. Fuchs S, Nevo D, Tarrab-Hazdai R, Yaar I. Strain differences in the autoimmune response to acetylcholine receptors. Nature 263:329–330, 1976.

125. Fujinami RS, Oldstone MBA. Amino acid homology between the encephalitogenic site of myelin basic protein and virus. Mechanism for autoimmunity. Science 230:1043–1045, 1985.

126. Fujinami RS, Oldstone MBA, Wroblewska Z, et al. Molecular mimicry in virus infection: cross reaction of measles virus phosphoprotein or of Herpes simplex virus protein with human intermediate filaments. Proc Natl Acad Sci 80:2346–2350, 1983.

127. Gazzinelli RT, Hakim FT, Hieny S, et al. Synergistic role of CD4+ and CD8+ T lymphocytes in IFN-gamma production and protective immunity induced by an attenuated Toxoplasma gondii vaccine. J Immunol 146:286–292, 1991.

128. Geczy C, Raper R, Roberts IM, et al. Macrophage procoagulant activity as a measure of cell-mediated immunity to P2 protein of peripheral nerves in the Guillain-Barré syndrome. J Neuroimmunol 19:179–191, 1985.

129. Gendelman H, Wolinsky JS, Johnson RT, et al. Measles encephalitis. Lack of evidence of viral invasion of the central nervous system and quantitative study of the nature of demyelination. Ann Neurol 15:353–360, 1984.

130. Gherardi RK, Chouaib S, Malapert D, et al. Early weight loss and high serum tumor necrosis factor-alpha levels in polyneuropathy, organomegaly, endocrinopathy, M protein, skin changes syndrome. Ann Neurol 35:501–505, 1994.

131. Giron LT, Crutcher KA, Davis JN. Lymph nodes—a possible site for sympathetic neuronal regulation of immune responses. Ann Neurol 8:520–525, 1980.

132. Goebels N, Michaelis D, Wekerle H, Hohlfeld R. Human myoblasts as antigen-presenting cells. J Immunol 149:661–667, 1992.

133. Goldowitz D, Knobler RL, Lublin FD. Heterotopic brain transplants in the study of experimental allergic encephalomyelitis. Exp Neurol 97:653–661, 1987.

134. Goldstein G, Whittingham S. Experimental autoimmune thymitis, an animal model of human myasthenia gravis. Lancet ii:315–318, 1966.

135. Gordon MA, Cohen JJ, Wilson IB. Muscarinic cholinergic receptors in murine lymphocytes: demonstration by direct binding. Proc Natl Acad Sci 75:2902–2904, 1970.

136. Graves MC. Subacute sclerosing panencephalitis. Neurol Clin 2:267–280, 1984.

137. Greenlee JE, Brashear H. Antibodies to cerebellar Purkinje cells in patients with paraneoplastic cerebellar degeneration and ovarian carcinoma. Ann Neurol 14:609–613, 1983.

138. Griffin JW, Ho TW-H. The Guillain-Barré Syndrome at 75: The *Campylobacter* connection. Ann Neurol 34:125–127, 1993.

139. Griffin DE, Johnson RT. Role of the immune response in recovery from Sindbis virus encephalitis in mice. J Immunol 118:1070–1075, 1977.

140. Griffin DE, Moser HW, Mendoza, Q, et al. Identification of the inflammatory cells in the nervous system of patient with adrenoleukodystrophy. Ann Neurol 18:660–664, 1985.

141. Gulcher JR, Stefansson K. Paraneoplastic syndromes of the nervous system. Immunol Allergy Clin N Am 8:295–314, 1988.

142. Gumpel M, Bauman N, Raoul M, Jaque C. Survival and differentiation of oligolendrocytes from neural tissue transplanted into newborn mouse brain. Neurosci Lett 37:307–311, 1983.

143. Haase AT. Pathogenesis of lentivirus infections. Nature 322:130–136, 1986.

144. Hadden JW. Cyclic nucleotides in lymphocytic function. Ann NY Acad Sci 256:352–363, 1975.
145. Hadden JW, Hadden EM, Middleton E Jr. Lymphocyte blast transformation—I. Demonstration of adrenergic receptors in human peripheral lymphocytes. Cell Immunol 1:583–595, 1970.
146. Hafler DA, Buchsbaum M, Weiner HL. Decreased autologous mixed lymphocyte reaction in multiple sclerosis. J Neuroimmunol 9:339–347, 1985.
147. Hall WW, Kiessling WR, ter Meulen V. Biochemical comparison of measles and subacute sclerosing panencephalitis viruses. In: Negative Strand Viruses and the Host Cell, RD Barry, SW Mahy, eds. Academic Press, New York, 1977.
148. Hall WW, ter Meulen V. Slow virus infections of the nervous system. Virological, immunological, and pathological considerations. J Gen Virol 41:1–25, 1978.
149. Hanahan D. Transgenic mouse models of self-tolerance and autoreactivity by the immune system. Ann Rev Cell Biol 6:403–537, 1990.
150. Happ MP, Heber-Katz E. Differences in the repertoire of the Lewis rat T cell response to self and non-self myelin basic proteins. J Exp Med 167:502–513, 1988.
151. Harling-Berg CJ, Knopf PM, Cserr HF. Myelin basic protein infused in cerebrospinal fluid suppresses experimental autoimmune encephalomyelitis. J Neuroimmunol 35:45–52, 1991.
152. Harris EN, Hughes GRV. Cerebral disease in systemic lupus erythematosus. Springer Semin Immunopathol 8:251–266, 1985.
153. Hartung H-P, Heininger K, Schäfer B, et al. Immune mechanisms in inflammatory polyneuropathy. Ann NY Acad Sci 540:122–161, 1988.
154. Hartung HP, Pollard JD, Harvey GK, Toyka KV. Immunopathogenesis and treatment of the Guillain-Barré syndrome—Part I. Muscle Nerve 18:137–153, 1995.
155. Hashim GA. Molecular bases for the difference in potency of myelin basic protein from different species in Lewis rats. Adv Exp Med Biol 100:289–301, 1978.
156. Hashim GA, Wood DD, Moscarello MA. Myelin lipophilin-induced demyelinating disease of the central nervous system. Neurochem Res 5:1137–1145, 1980.
157. Hayafil F, Morello D, Babinet C, Jacob F. A cell surface glycoprotein involved in the compaction of embryonal carcinoma cells and cleavage stage embryos. Cell 21:927–934, 1980.
158. Hayashi T, Burks JS, Hauser SL. Expression and cellular localization of major histocompatibility complex antigens in active MS lesions. Ann NY Acad Sci 540:301–305, 1988.
159. Hays AP, Latov, N, Takatsu M, Sherman WH. Experimental demyelination of nerve induced by serum of patients with neuropathy and an anti-MAG IgM M-protein. Neurology 37:242–256, 1987.
160. Heber-Katz E. The autoimmune T cell receptor: epitopes, idiotopes, and malatopes. Cell Immunol Immunopathol 55:1–8, 1990.
161. Hemachudha T, Griffin DE, Griffels JJ, et al. Myelin basic protein as encephalitogen in encephalomyelitis and polyneuritis following rabies vaccination. New Engl J Med 316:369–374, 1987.
162. Hemachudha T, Phanuphak P, Johnson RT, et al. Neurological complications of Semple type rabies vaccine: clinical and immunological studies. Neurology 37:550–556, 1987.
163. Hickey WF. Migration of hematogenous cells through the blood-brain barrier and the initiation of CNS inflammation. Brain Pathol. 1:97–105, 1991.
164. Hickey WF, Kimura H. Perivascular microglial cells of the CNS are bone marrow-derived and present antigen in vivo. Science 239:290–292, 1988.

165. Hinrichs DJ, Wegmann KW, Dietsch GN. Transfer of EAE to bone marrow chimeras; endothelial cells are not a restricting element. J Exp Med 166:1906–1911, 1987.

166. Hirano A, Cook SD, Whitaker JN, et al. Fine structural aspects of demyelination in vitro. The effects of Guillain-Barré serum. J Neuropathol Exp Neurol 30:249–265, 1971.

167. Hirayama K, Matsushita S, Kikuchi I, et al. HLA-DQ is epistatic to HLA-DR in controlling the immune response to schistosomal antigen in humans. Nature 327:426–430, 1987.

168. Ho DD, Ropte T, Hirsch M. Infection of monocyte-macrophages by human T-lymphotropic virus type III. J Clin Invest 77:1712–1715, 1986.

169. Hochwald GM, Van Driel A, Robinson ME, Thorbecke JG. Immune response in draining lymph nodes and spleen after intraventricular injection of antigen. Int J Neurosci 39:299–306, 1988.

170. Hoffman-Fezer G, Schmahl W, Hoffman R. Zur Pathogenese der Nervenläsionen bei Marekscher Krankheit des Huhnes. II. Uebertragbarkeit von Nervenveränderungen mit Milzzellen Marek-kranker Tiere. Z. Immunitätsforsh 150:301–308, 1975.

171. Hohlfeld R, Toyka KV, Heininger K, et al. Autoimmune human T lymphocytes specific for acetylcholine receptor. Nature 310:244–246, 1984.

172. Hohlfeld R, Toyka KV, Tzartos SJ, et al. Human T helper lymphocytes in myasthenia gravis recognize the nicotinic receptor a-subunit. Proc Natl Acad Sci 84:5379–5383, 1987.

173. Hontebeyrie-Joskowicz MN, Said G, Milon G, et al. L3T4+ T cells able to mediate parasite-specific delayed-type hypersensitivity play a role in the pathogenesis of experimental Chagas' disease. Eur J Immunol 17:1027–1033, 1987.

174. Hotchin JE, Cintis M. Lymphocytic choriomeningitis infection of mice as a model for the study of latent virus infection. Can J Microbiol 4:149–163, 1958.

175. Howell MD, Winters ST, Olee T, et al. Vaccination against experimental allergic encephalomyelitis with T cell receptor peptides. Science 246:668–670, 1989.

176. Hurst EW. The effects of the injection of normal brain emulsion into rabbits, with special reference to the aetiology of the paralytic accidents of antirabic treatment. J Hygiene 32:3–44, 1932.

177. Hurst EW, Cooke BT, Melvin P. "Nervous distemper" in dogs. A pathological and experimental study, with some reference to demyelinating diseases in general. Aust J Exp Biol Med Sci 21:115–126, 1943.

178. Husby C, Van de Rijn I, Zabriskie MB, et al. Antibodies reacting with cytoplasm of subthalamic and caudate nuclei neurons in chorea and acute rheumatic fever. J Exp Med 144:1094–1110, 1976.

179. Jacobson SJ, Flerlage ML, McFarland HR. Impaired measles virus-specific cytotoxic CD4+ T cell responses in multiple sclerosis. J Exp Med 162:839–850, 1985.

180. Jacobson S, Shida H, McFarlin DE, et al. Circulating CD8+ cytotoxic T lymphocytes specific for HTLV-1 pX in patients with HTLV-1 associated neurological disease. Nature 348:245–248, 1990.

181. Jaeckle KA, Graus F, Houghton AN, Nielsen SL, Posner JB. Autoimmune response of patients with paraneoplastic cerebeller degeneration to a Purkinje cell cytoplasmic protein antigen. Ann Neurol 18:592–600, 1985.

182. Jahnke U, Fischer EH, Alvord EC Jr. Sequence homology between certain viral proteins and proteins related to encephalomyelitis and neuritis. Science 229:282–284, 1985.

183. Jersild C, Svejgaard A, Fog T. HL-A antigens associated with multiple sclerosis. Lancet i:1242–1243, 1972.

184. Jiang HJ, Zhang SI, Pernis B. Role of CD8+ T-cells in murine experimental allergic encephalomyelitis. Science 256:1213–1215, 1992.

185. Johnson RT. Viral Infections of the Nervous System. Raven Press, New York, 1982.

186. Johnson RT, Griffin DE, Gendelman HE. Postinfectious encephalomyelitis. Semin Neurol 5:180–190, 1985.
187. Johnson RT, Griffin DE, Hirsch RL, et al. Measles encephalomyelitis—clinical and immunological studies. New Engl J Med 310:137–141, 1984.
188. Johnson RT, Richardson EP. The neurologic manifestations of systemic lupus erythematosus: a clinical pathological study of 24 cases and review of the literature. Medicine 47:337–369, 1968.
189. Joseph J, d'Imperio C, Knobler RL, Lublin FD. Down-regulation of interferon-induced class-II expression of human glioma cells by recombinant beta-interferon. Ann NY Acad Sci 540:475–476, 1988.
190. Juji T, Satake M, Honda, Y, Doi Y. HLA antigens in Japanese patients with narcolepsy. All the patients were DR2 postive. Tissue Antigens 24:316–319, 1984.
191. Kabat EA, Moore DH, Landow H. An electrophoretic study of the protein components in the cerebrospinal fluid and their relationship to serum proteins. J Clin Invest 21:571–577, 1942.
192. Kabat EA, Wolf A, Bezer AE. The rapid production of acute disseminated encephalomyelitis in rhesus monkeys by injection of heterologous and homologous brain tissue with adjuvants. J Exp Med 85:117–130, 1947.
193. Kadlubowskik M, Hughes RAC. Identification of neuritogen for experimental allergic neuritis. Nature 277:140–141, 1979.
194. Kao I, Drachman DB. Thymic muscle cells bear acetylcholine receptors: possible relation to myasthenia gravis. Science 195:174–175, 1977.
195. Karaszewski JW, Reder AT, Maselli R, et al. Sympathetic skin responses are decreased and lymphocytic beta-adrenergic receptors are increased in progressive multiple sclerosis. Ann Neurol 27:366–372, 1990.
196. Kardys GA, Hashim GA. Experimental allergic encephalomyelitis in Lewis rats: immunoregulation of disease by a single aminoacid substitution in the disease-inducing determinant. J Immunol 127:862–866, 1981.
197. Karpus WJ, Swanborg RH. CD4+ cells differentially affect the production of IFN-gamma by effector cells of experimental allergic encephalomyelitis. J Immunol 143:3492–3497, 1989.
198. Keller SE, Weiss, JM, Schleiffer SJ, et al. Suppression of immunity by stress. Effect of a graded series of stressors on lymphocyte stimulation in the rat. Science 213:1397–1400, 1981.
199. Kelly JJ Jr, Kyle R, Latov N. Polyneuropathies and Plasma Cell Dyscrasias. Martinus Nijhogg, Boston, 1987.
200. Khoury EL, Ritacco V, Cossio PM, et al. Circulating antibodies to peripheral nerve in American trypanosomiasis (Chagas' disease). Clin Exp Immunol 36:8–15, 1979.
201. Khoury SH, Hancock WW, Weiner HL. Oral tolerance to myelin basic protein and natural recovery from experimental autoimmune encephalomyelitis are associated with down-regulation of inflammatory cytokines and differential upregulation of transforming growth factor beta, interleukin 4, and prostaglandin E expression in the brain. J Exp Med 176: 1335–1364, 1992.
202. Kibler RF, Fritz RB, Chou FC-H, et al. Immune response of Lewis rats to peptide C1 (residues 68-88) of guinea pig and rat myelin basic protein. J Exp Med 146:1323–1331, 1977.
203. Kiers AB. Clinical neurology and brain histopathology in NZB/NZW F1 lupus mice. J Comp Pathol 102:165–177, 1990.
204. Kies MW, Alford EC Jr, eds. "Allergic" Encephalomyelitis. C. C. Thomas, Springfield, 1959.

205. Kies MW, Roboz E, Alvord EC Jr. Experimental encephalitogenic activity in a glycoprotein fraction of bovine spinal cord. Federation Proc. 15:288, 1956.

206. Kilidreas K, Latov N, Strauss DH, et al. Antibodies to the human 60 kDa heat-shock protein in patients with schizophrenia. Lancet 340:569–572, 1992.

207. King LS. Moose encephalitis. Am J Pathol 15:445–454, 1939.

208. Kinutani M, Coltey, M, LeDouarin N. Postnatal development of a demyelinating disease in avian spinal cord chimeras. Cell 45:307–314, 1986.

209. Klinge F. Der Rheumatismus. Ergebnisse allgemeine Pathologie pathologiselie Anatomie 27:1–336, 1933.

210. Knobler RL, Linthicum DS, Cohn M. Host genetic regulation of acute MHV-4 viral encephalomyelitis and acute experimental allergic encephalomyelitis in (BALB/cKe × SJL/J) recombinant inbred mice. J Immunol 8:15–28, 1985.

211. Koberle F. Chagas' disease and Chagas syndromes: the pathology of American trypanosomiasis. Adv Parasitol 6:63–115, 1968.

212. Kofe EB, Bardona EF Jr, Harbeck RJ, et al. Lupus meningitis antibodies to deoxyribonucleic acid (DNA): anti-DNA complexes in cerebrospinal fluid. Ann Intern Med 80:58–60, 1974.

213. Koh DR, Fung-Leung WP, Ho A, et al. Less mortality but more relapses in experimental allergic encephalomyelitis in CD8$^{-/-}$ mice. Science 256:1210–1213, 1992.

214. Kohriyama T, Ariga T, Yu RK: Preparation and characterization of antibodies against a sulfated glucuronic acid-containing glycosphingolipid. J Neurochem 51:869–877, 1988.

215. Korngold R, Feldman A, Rourke L, et al. Acute experimental allergic encephalomyelitis in radiation bone marrow chimeras between high and low susceptible strains of mice. Immunogenetics 24:309–315, 1986.

216. Kornguth SE, Klein R, Aspen R, Choate J. Occurrence of anti-retinal ganglion cell antibodies in patients with small cell carcinoma of the lung. Cancer 50:1289–1293, 1982.

217. Kornguth SE, Spear PD, Langer E. Reduction in number of large ganglion cells in cat retina following intravitreous injection of antibodies. Brain Res 245:35–45, 1982.

218. Kornguth SE, Thompson HG Jr. Stimulation of lymph node protein synthesis by a basic protein from brain. Arch Biochem 105:308–314, 1964.

219. Koski CL, Vanguri P, Shin ML. Activation of the alternative pathway of complement by human peripheral nerve myelin. J Immunol 134:1810–1814, 1985.

220. Kosunen T, Waksman BH, Samuelsson IK. Radioautographic study of cellular mechanisms in delayed hypersensitivity. II. Experimental allergic encephalomyelitis in the rat. J Neuropathol Exp Neurol 22:367–380, 1963.

221. Kreth HW, Marquardt P, Martin R. Specificity of clones and T cell lines from cerebrospinal fluid in viral meningoencephalitis and multiple sclerosis. In: Cellular and Humoral Components of Cerebrospinal Fluid in Multiple Sclerosis. J Raus, A Lowenthal, eds. Plenum Press, London, 1987.

222. Kubota R, Umehara F, Izumo S, et al. HTLV-I proviral DNA amount correlates with infiltrating CD4+ lymphocytes in the spinal cord from patients with HTLV-I-associated myelopathy. J Neuroimmunol 53:23–29, 1994.

223. Kurtzke J, Hyllested K. Multiple sclerosis in the Faroe Islands. II. Clinical updates, transmission and the nature of multiple sclerosis Neurology 36:307–328, 1986.

224. Lang B, Newsom-Davis J, Wray D, Vincent A. Autoimmune aetiology for myasthenic (Eaton-Lambert) syndrome. Lancet ii:224–226, 1981.

225. Langdon N, Van Dam M, Welsh KI, et al. Genetic markers in narcolepsy. Lancet ii: 1178–1180, 1984.

226. Lassmann H, Rössler K, Zimprich F, Vass, K. Expression of adhesion molecules and histocompatibility antigens at the blood-brain barrier. Brain Pathol 1:115–123, 1991.

227. Lavi E, Suzumura A, Murasko DM, et al. Tumor necrosis factor induces expression of MHC class I antigens on mouse astrocytes. Ann NY Acad Sci 540:488–489, 1988.

228. Lebar E, Lubetzki C, Vincent C, et al. The M2 autoantigen of central nervous system myelin, a glycoprotein present in oligodendrocyte membrane. Clin Exp Immunol 66:423–443, 1986.

229. Leibowitz A, Hughes RAC. Immunology of the Nervous System. E. Arnold, London, 1983, pp. 101–130.

230. Lennon VA, Lambert EH. Myasthenia gravis induced by monoclonal antibodies to acetylcholine receptors. Nature 285:238–240, 1980.

231. Lennon VA, Lindström JM, Seybold ME. Experimental autoimmune myasthenia: a model for myasthenia gravis in rats and guinea pigs. J Exp Med 141:1365–1375, 1975.

232. Lennon VA, McCormick DF, Lambert EH, et al. Region of peptide 125-147 of acetylcholine receptor alpha subunit is exposed at neuromuscular junction and induces experimental autoimmune myasthenia gravis. Proc Natl Acad Sci 82:8805–8809, 1985.

233. Lennon VA, Seybold ME, Lindstöm JM, et al. Role of complement in the pathogenesis of experimental autoimmune myasthenia gravis. J Exp Med 146:973–983, 1978.

234. Levine B, Hardwick JM, Trapp BD, et al. Antibody-mediated clearance of alphavirus infection from neurons. Science 254:856–860, 1991.

235. Levine SD, Sowinski R. Experimental allergic encephalomyelitis in congenic strains of rats. Immunogenetics 1:352–356, 1974.

236. Lider O, Baharav E, Reshef T, Cohen IR. Vaccination against experimental autoimmune encephalomyelitis using a subencephalitogenic dose of autoimmune effector cells. (1) Characteristics of vaccination. J Autoimmun 2:75–86, 1989.

237. Lieberman AP, Pitha PM, Shin HS, Shin ML. Production of tumor necrosis factor and other cytokines by astrocytes stimulated with lippolysaccharide or a neurotropic virus. Proc Natl Acad Sci 86:6348–6352, 1989.

238. Liebert UG, Hashim GA, ter Meulen V. Characterization of measles virus-induced cellular autoimmune reactions against myelin basic protein in Lewis rats. J Neuroimmunol 29:139–147, 1990.

239. Liebert UG, Linington C, ter Meulen V. Induction of autoimmune reactions to myelin basic protein in measles virus encephalitis in Lewis rats. J Neuroimmunol 17:103–118, 1988.

240. Liebert UG, ter Meulen V. Virological aspects of measles virus induced encephalomyelitis in Lewis and BN rats. J Gen Virol 68:1715–1722, 1987.

241. Lindström J, Einarson B, Merlie J. Immunization of rats with polypeptide chains from torpedo acetylcholine receptor causes an autoimmune response to receptors in rat muscle. Proc Natl Acad Sci 75:769–773, 1978.

242. Lindström JM, Engle AG, Seybold ME, Lennon VA, Lambert EH. Pathological mechanisms in experimental autoimmune myasthenia gravis. II. Passive transfer of experimental autoimmune myasthenia gravis in rats with anti-actylcholine receptor antibodies. J Exp Med 144:739–753, 1976.

243. Lindström J, Seybold ME, Lennon VA, et al. Antibody to acetylcholine receptor in myasthenia gravis: prevalence, clinical correlates, and diagnostic value. Neurology 26:1054–1959, 1976.

244. Lindström J, Shelton D, Fuji Y. Myasthenia gravis. Adv Immunol 42:233–284, 1988.

245. Link H, Baig, S, Olsson T, Zachau Z. A new principle for evaluation of B-cell response in inflammatory nervous system diseases. Ann NY Acad Sci 540:277–281, 1988.

246. Link H, Olsson T, Wang WZ, et al. Autoreactive T cells in multiple sclerosis and controls. Neurology 40 (Suppl 1):283, 1990.

247. Lipton HL. Theiler's virus infection in mice: an unusual biphasic disease process leading to demyelination. Infect Immun 11:1147–1155, 1975.

248. Lipton HL, Dal Canto MC. Theiler's virus-induced demyelination: prevention by immunosuppression. Science 192:62–64, 1976.

249. Lisak RP, Moore PM, Levinson AI, Zweiman B, Neurologic complications of collagen vascular diseases. Ann NY Acad Sci 540:115–121, 1988.

250. Lisak RP, Sweiman B. In vitro cell-mediated immunity of cerebrospinal fluid lymphocytes to myelin basic protein in primary demyelinating diseaes. New Engl J Med 297:850–853, 1977.

251. Liu WT, Vanguri P, Shin ML, Studies of demyelination in vitro: the requirement of membrane attack components of the complement system. J Immunol 131:778–782, 1983.

252. Livnat S, Felten SY, et al. Involvement of peripheral and central catecholamine systems in neural-immune interactions. J Neuroimmunol 10:5–30, 1985.

253. Lopker A, Abood LG, Hoss W, Lionetti FJ. Stereoselective muscarinic acetylcholine and opiate receptors in human phagocytic leukocytes. Biochem Pharmacol 29:1361–1365, 1980.

254. Lowenthal A, Vansande M, Karcher D. The differential diagnosis of neurological disease by fractionating electrophoretically the CSF-globulins. J Neurochem 6:51-56, 1960.

255. Lowy MT, Reder AT, Antel JP, Meltzer HY. Glucocorticoid resistance in depression: the dexamethasone suppression test and lymphocytic sensitivity to dexamethasone. Am J Psychiatry 141:1365–1370, 1984.

256. Lublin FD, Maurer PH, Berry RG, Tippett D. Delayed, relapsing experimental allergic encephalomyelitis in mice. J Immunol 126:819–822, 1981.

257. Lyman WD, Brosnan CF, Raine CS. Chronic relapsing experimental autoimmune encephalomyelitis: myelin basic protein induces suppression of blastogenesis during remissions but not during exacerbations. J Neuroimmunol 7:345–353, 1985.

258. Mackay RP, Myrianthopoulos NC. Multiple sclerosis in twins and their relatives. Arch Neurol 15:449–462, 1966.

259. Maeda Y, Brosnan CF, Miyatani N, Yu RK. Preliminary studies on sensitization of Lewis rats with sulfated glucuronyl paragloboside. Brain Res 541:257–264, 1991.

260. Martin R, Jaraquemada D, Flerlage M, et al. Fine specificity and HLA restriction of myelin basic protein specific cytotoxic T cell lines from multiple sclerosis patients and healthy individuals. J Immunol 145:540–548, 1990.

261. Mason D, McPhee I, Antoni F. The role of the neuroendocrine system in determining genetic susceptibility to experimental allergic encephalomyelitis in the rat. Immunology 70:1–5, 1990.

262. Massa PT, Dörries R, ter Meulen V. Viral particles induce Ia antigen expression on astrocytes. Nature 320:543–546, 1986.

263. Massa PT, Schimpl A, Wecker E, ter Meulen V. Tumor necrosis factor amplifies measles virus-mediated Ia induction on astrocytes. Proc Natl Acad Sci 84:7242–7245, 1987.

264. Massa PT, ter Meulen V, Fontana A. Hyperinducibility of Ia antigen on astrocytes correlates with strain specific susceptibility to experimental autoimmune encephalomyelitis. Proc Natl Acad Sci 84:4219–4223, 1987.

265. McAllister CG, Rapaport MH, Pickar D, Paul SM. Autoimmunity and schizophrenia. In: Schizophrenia Research, CA Tamminga and SC Schulz, eds. Raven Press, New York, 1991, pp 111–118.

266. McAllister CG, Rapaport MH, Pickar D, et al. Increased numbers of CD5+ lymphocytes in schizophrenic patients. Arch Gen Psychiatry 46:890–894, 1989.

267. McAllister CG, van Kammen DP, Rehn TJ, et al. Increases in CSF levels of interleukin-2 in schizophrenia patients: effect of recurrence of psychosis and medication status. Amer J Psychiatry 152:1291–1297, 1995. submitted, 1992.

268. McCarron RM, Fallis RJ, McFarlin DE. Alterations in T cell antigen specificity and class II restriction during the course of chronic relapsing experimental allergic encephalomyelitis. J Neuroimmunol 29:73–79, 1990.

269. McCarron RM, Spatz M, Kempski O, et al. Interaction between myelin basic protein-sensitized T lymphocytes and murine cerebral vascular endothelial cells. J Immunol 137:3428–3435, 1986.

270. McCombe PA, Pollard JD, McLeod JG. Chronic inflammatory demyelinating polyneuropathy. Brain 110:1617–1630, 1987.

271. McCombe PA, van der Kreek SA, Pender MP. The effects of cyclosporin A on experimental allergic neuritis (EAN) in the Lewis rat. Induction of relapsing EAN using low dose cyclosporin A. J Neuroimmunol 28:131–140, 1990.

272. McCombe PA, van der Kreek SA, Pender MP. Neuropathological findings in chronic relapsing experimental allergic neuritis induced in the Lewis rat by inoculation with intradural root myelin and treatment with low dose cyclosporin A. Neuropathol Appl Neurobiol 18:171–187, 1992.

273. McDougal JS, Kennedy MS, Sligh JM, et al. Binding of HTLV-III/LAV to T4+ T cells by a complex of the 110K viral protein and the T4 molecule. Science 231:382–385, 1986.

274. McNeil HP, Chesterman CN, Krilis SA. Immunology and clinical importance of antiphospholipid antibodies. Adv Immunol 49:193–279, 1991.

275. Medawar PB. Immunity of homologous grafted skin. III. The fate of skin homografts transplanted to the brain, to subcutaneous tissue and to the anterior chamber of the eye. Br J Exp Pathol 29:58–69, 1948.

276. Merrit HH, Wortis SB, Woltman HW, eds. Multiple Sclerosis and the Demyelinating Diseases. Res. Publ Assoc Res Nerv Ment Dis Vol 28, 1950.

277. Milek DH, Cunningham JM, Powers JM, Brostoff SW. Experimental allergic neuritis: humoral and cellular immune responses to the cyanogen bromide peptides of the P2 proteins. J Neuroimmunol 4:105–117, 1983.

278. Miles K, Quintans J, Chelmicka-Schorr E, Arnason BGW. The sympathetic nervous system modulates antibody response to thymus-independent antigens. J Neuroimmunol 1:101–105, 1981.

279. Miller A, Lider O, Roberts AB, et al. Suppressor T cells generated by oral tolerization to myelin basic protein suppress both in vitro and in vivo immune responses by the release of transforming growth factor-beta after antigen specific triggering. Proc Natl Acad Sci 89:421–425, 1992.

280. Miler A, Lider O, Weiner HL. Antigen-driven bystander suppression following oral administration of antigen. J Exp Med 174:791–798, 1991.

281. Miller HG, Stanton JB, Gibbons JL. Para-infectious encephalomyelitis and related syndromes: a critical review of the neurological complications of certain specific fevers. Q J Med 25:427–505, 1956.

282. Miller SD, Clatch RJ, Pevear CD, et al. Class II-restricted T cell responses in Theiler's murine encephalomyelitis virus (TMEV)-induced demyelinating disease. I. Cross-specificity among TMEV substrains and related picornavirusese but not myelin proteins. J Immunol 138:3776–3784, 1987.

283. Milner PC, Lovelidge A, Taylor WA, Hughes RAC. Po myelin protein produces experimental allergic neuritis in Lewis rats. J Neurol Sci 79:275–285, 1987.

284. Modlin RL, Kate H, Mehra V, et al. Genetically restricted suppressor T-cell clones derived from lepromatous leprosy lesions. Nature 322:459–461, 1986.
285. Modlin RL, Mehra V, Wong L, et al. Suppressor T lymphocytes from lepromatous leprosy skin lesions. J Immunol 137:2831–2834, 1986.
286. Moench TR, Griffin DE. Immunocytochemical identification and quantitation of the mononuclear cells in the cerebrospinal fluid, meninges, and brain during acute viral meningoencephalitis. J Exp Med 159:77–88, 1984.
287. Mokhtarian F, McFarlin DE, Raine CS. Adoptive transfer of myelin basic protein-sensitized T cells produces chronic relapsing demyelinative disease in mice. Nature 309:356–358, 1984.
288. Morgan BP, Campbell AK, Compston DAS. Terminal components of complement (C9) in cerebrospinal fluid of patients with multiple sclerosis. Lancet ii:251–254, 1984.
289. Morgan IM. Allergic encephalomyelitis in monkeys in response to injection of normal monkey nervous tissue. J Exp Med 85:131–140, 1947.
290. Morimoto C, Hafler DA, Weiner HL, et al. Selective loss of the suppressor inducer T-cell subset in progressive multiple sclerosis: analysis with anti-2H4 monoclonal antibody. New Engl J Med 316:67–72, 1987.
291. Mossman TR, Coffman RL. Th1 and Th2 cells: different patterns of lymphokine secretion lead to different functional properties. Annu Rev Immunol 7:145–173, 1989.
292. Mueh JR, Herbert KD, Rapaport SI. Thrombosis in patients with lupus anticoagulant. Ann Intern Med 92:156–159, 1980.
293. Nagashima K, Wege H, Meyermann R, ter Meulen V. Coronavirus induced subacute demyelinating encephalomyelitis in rats. A morphological analysis. Acta Neuropathol 44:63–70, 1978.
294. Nagy E, Berczi I. Immunodeficiency in hypophysectomized rats. Acta Endocrinol 89:530–537, 1978.
295. Nakanishi T, Sobue I, Toyokura Y, et al. The Crow-Fukase syndrome: a study of 102 cases in Japan. Neurology 34:712–720, 1984.
296. Nakao Y, Matsumoto H, Miyazaki T, et al. IgG heavy chain allotypes (Gm) in auto-immune diseases. Clin Exp Immunol 42:20–26, 1980.
297. Narayan O, Griffin DE, Chase J. Antigenic drift of visna virus in persistently infected sheep. Science 197:376–378, 1977.
298. Narayan O, Hertzog S, Frese K, et al. Behavioral disease in rats caused by immunopathological response to persistent Borna virus in the brain. Science 220:1401–1403, 1983.
299. Narayan O, Sheffer D, Clements JE, Tennekoon G. Restricted replication of lentiviruses. Visna viruses induce a unique interferon during interaction between lymphocytes and infected macrophages. J Exp Med 162:1954–1969, 1985.
300. Narayan O, Wolinsky JS, Clements JE, et al. Slow virus replication: the role of macrophages in the persistence and expression of visna virus in sheep and goats. J Gen Virol 59:345–356, 1982.
301. Navia BA, Cho E-S, Petito C, Price RW. The AIDS dementia complex. II. Neuropathology. Ann Neurol 19:525–535, 1986.
302. Nepom JT, Weiner HL, Dichter MA, et al. Identification of a hemagglutinin-specific idiotype associated with reovirus recognition shared by lymphoid and neural cells. J Exp Med 155:155–167, 1982.
303. Newsom-Davis J, Harcourt G, Sommer N, et al. T cell reactivity in myasthenia gravis. J Autoimmun 2 (Suppl): 101–108, 1989.
304. Nicholas MK, Sagher O, Hartley JP, et al. A phenotypic analysis of T lymphocytes isolated

from the brains of mice with allogeneic neural transplants. Prog Brain Res 78:249–259, 1988.

305. Nicholas MK, Stefansson K, Antel JP, Arnason BG. An in vivo and in vitro analysis of systemic immune function in mice with histologic evidence of neural transplant rejection. J Neurosci Res 18:245–257, 1987.

306. Noonan DJ, Kofler R, Singer PA, et al. Delineation of a defect in T cell receptor beta genes of NZW mice predisposed to autoimmunity. J Exp Med 163:644–653, 1986.

307. Noronha ABC, Richman DP, Arnason BGW, Detection of in vivo stimulated cerebrospinal fluid lymphocytes by flow cytometry in patients with multiple sclerosis. New Engl J Med 303:713–717, 1980.

308. Ofosu-Appiah W, Mokhtarian F, Miller A, Grob D. Characterization of in vivo-activated T cell clones from peripheral blood of multiple sclerosis patients. Cell Immunol Immunopathol 58:46–55, 1991.

309. Oksenberg JR, Stuart S, Begovich AB, et al. Limited heterogeneity of rearranged T-cell receptor V alpha transcripts in brains of multiple sclerosis patients. Nature 345:344–346, 1990 [erratum in Nature 353:94, 1991].

310. Oldstone MBA, Blount P, Southern PJ, Lampert PW. Cytoimmunotherapy for persistent virus infection reveals in unique clearance pattern from the central nervous system. Nature 321:239–243, 1986.

311. Olsson T, Baig S, Höjeberg B, Link H. Antimyelin basic protein and antimyelin antibody-producing cells in multiple sclerosis. Ann Neurol 27:132–136, 1990.

312. O'Neill JH, Muray NMF, Newsom-Davis J. The Lambert-Eaton myasthenic syndrome: a review of 50 cases. Brain 111:577–596, 1988.

313. Orn A, Goodenow RS, Hood L, et al. Product of a transferred H-2L^d gene acts as a restriction element for LCMV-specific killer T cells. Nature 297:415–417, 1982.

314. Ota K, Matsui M, Milford EL, et al. T cell recognition of an immunodominant myelin basic protein epitope is associated with DR2. Nature 346:183–187, 1990.

315. Ottenhof THM, Elferink DG, Klatser PR, de Vries RP. Cloned suppressor T cells from a lepromatous leprosy patient suppress Mycobacterium leprae reactive helper T cells. Nature 322:462–464, 1986.

316. Ovadia H, Abramsky O. Dopamine receptors on isolated membranes of rat lymphocytes. J Neurosci Res 18:70–74, 1987.

317. Pachner AR, Kantor FS. In vitro and in vivo actions of acetylcholine receptor educated suppressor T cell lines in murine experimental autoimmune myasthenia gravis. Clin Exp Immunol 56:659–668, 1984.

318. Pachner AR, Kantor FS. Helper T-cell lines specific for the acetylcholine receptor: induction, characterization, and in vitro effects. Clin Immunol Immunopathol 35:245–251, 1985.

319. Pachner AR, Steere AC. The triad of neurologic manifestations of Lyme disease: meningitis, cranial neuritis and radiculoneuritis. Neurology 35:47–53, 1985.

320. Pachner AR, Steere AC, Sigal SH, Johnson CH. Antigen-specific proliferation of CSF lymphocytes in Lyme disease. Neurology 35:1642–1644, 1985.

321. Panitch HS, Hirsch RL, Haley AS, Johnson KP. Exacerbations of multiple sclerosis in patients treated with gamma-interferon. Lancet 1:893–895, 1987.

322. Panitch HS, McFarlin DE. Experimental allergic encephalomyelitis: enhancement of cell-mediated transfer by concanavalin A. J Immunol 119:1134–1137, 1977.

323. Paterson PY. Transfer of allergic encephalomyelitis in rats by means of lymph node cells. J Exp Med 111:119–135, 1960.

324. Patrick J, Lindstöm J. Autoimmune response to acetylcholine receptor. Science 180:871–872, 1973.

325. Payne LN, Frazier JA, Powell PC. Pathogenesis of Marek's disease. Int Rev Exp Pathol 16:59–154, 1976.

326. Pender MP, Nguyuen KB, McCombe PA, Kerr JFR. Apoptosis in the nervous system in experimental allergic encephalomyelitis. J Neurol Sci 14:81–87, 1991.

327. Pepose JS, Stevens JG, Cook ML, Lampert PW. Marek's disease as a model for the Landry-Guillain Barré syndrome: latent viral infection is restricted to nonneuronal cells accompanied by specific immune responses to peripheral nerve and myelin. Am J Pathol 103:309–320, 1981.

328. Perez-Polo JR, Bulloch K, Angeletti RH, et al. Neuroimmunomodulation. J Neurosci Res 18, No. 1 (special issue):1–257, 1987.

329. Pette H. Klinische und anatomische Studien und die Pathogenese der multiplen Sklerose. Dtsch Z Nervenkeilk 105:76–132, 1928.

330. Pette M, Fujita K, Wilkinson D, et al. Myelin autoreactivity in multiple sclerosis; recognition of myelin basic protein in the context of HLA-DR2 products by T lymphocytes of multiple sclerosis patients and healthy donors. Proc Natl Acad Sci 87:7968–7972, 1990.

331. Pette M, Liebert UG, Göbel U, et al. Measles virus-directed responses of CD4+ T lymphocytes in MS patients and healthy individuals. Neurology 43:2019–2025, 1993.

332. Pettinelli CB, Fritz, RB, Chou C-HJ, McFarlin DE. Encephalitogenic activity of guinea myelin basic protein in the SJL mouse. J Immunol 129:1209–1211, 1982.

333. Petursson G, Nathanson N, Georgsson G, et al. Pathogenesis of visna. I. Sequential virologic, serologic, and pathologic studies. Lab Invest 35:402–412, 1976.

334. Plotz PH. Autoantibodies are anti-idiotype antibodies to antiviral antibodies. Lancet ii:824–826, 1983.

335. Polimacher T, Schulz H, Geisler P, et al. DR2-positive monozygotic twins discordant for narcolepsy. Sleep 13:336–343, 1990.

336. Posner JB, Furneaux HM. Paraneoplastic syndromes. Res Publ Assoc Res Nerv Ment Dis 68:187–219, 1990.

337. Powell MB, Mitchell D, Lederman J, et al. Lymphotoxin and tumor necrosis factor alpha production by myelin basic protein-specific T cell clones correlates with encephalitogenicity. Immunol 2:539–544, 1990.

338. Prabhakar S, Kurien E, Gupta RS, et al. Heat shock protein immunoreactivity in CSF: correlation with oligoclonal banding and demyelinating disease. Neurology 44:1644–1648, 1994.

339. Pribyl TM, Campagnoni CW, Kampf K, et al. The human myelin basic protein gene is included within a 179-kilobase transcription unit: expression in the immune and central nervous systems. Proc Natl Acad Sci 90:10695–10699, 1993.

340. Price RW, Brew B. Infection of the central nervous system by human immunodeficiency virus. Role of the immune system in pathogenesis. Ann NY Acad Sci 540:162–175, 1988.

341. Price RW, Brew B, Sidtis J, et al. The brain in AIDS dementia complex. Science 239:586–592, 1988.

342. Prieto GJ, Urba-Holmgren R, Holmgren B. Sleep and EEG disturbances in a rat neurological mutant (taiep) with immobility episodes: a model of narcolepsy-cataplexy. Electroencephalogy Clin Neurophysiol 79:141–147, 1991.

343. Prineas JW. Multiple sclerosis: presence of lymphatic capillaries and lymphoid tissue in the brain and spinal cord. Science 203:1123–1125, 1979.

344. Prineas JW, Connell F. The fine structure of chronically active multiple sclerosis plaques. Neurology 28 (9, part 2):68–75, 1978.

345. Prineas JW, Graham JS. Multiple sclerosis: capping of surface immunoglobulin G on macrophages engaged in myelin breakdown. Ann Neurol 10:149–158, 1981.

346. Prineas JW, Kwon EE, Cho E, Sharer LR. Continual breakdown and regeneration of myelin in progressive multiple sclerosis plaques. Ann NY Acad Sci 436:11–32, 1984.

347. Prineas JW, Wright RG. The fine structure of peripheral nerve lesions in a virus-induced demyelinating disease in fowl (Marek's disease). Lab Invest 26:548–557, 1972.

348. Racke MK, Dhib-Jalbut S, Cannella S, et al. Prevention and treatment of chronic relapsing experimental allergic encephalomyelitis by transforming growth factor-beta 1. J Immunol 146:3012–3017, 1991.

349. Raine CS, ed. Neuroimmunomodulation. J Neuroimmunol 10, No. 1 (special issue):1–100, 1985.

350. Raine, CS. Adhesion molecules on endothelial cells in the central nervous system: an emerging area in the neuroimmunology of multiple sclerosis. Cell Immunol Immunopathol 57:173–187, 1990.

351. Raine, CS, Multiple sclerosis: immunopathologic mechanisms in the progression and resolution of inflammatory demyelination. Res Publ Assoc Res Nerv Ment Dis 68:37–54, 1990.

352. Raine CS, Mokhtarian F, McFarlin DE. Adoptively transferred chronic relapsing experimental autoimmune encephalomyelitis in the mouse. Lab Invest 51:531–546, 1984.

353. Raine CS, Traugott U. Chronic relapsing experimental autoimmune encephalomyelitis: ultrastructure of the central nervous system of animals treated with combinations of myelin components. Lab Invest 48:275–284, 1983.

354. Rapaport MH, McAllister CG. Neuroimmunologic factors in schizophrenia. In: Psychoneuroimmunology Update, JM Gorman, RM Kertzner, eds. American Psychiatric Press, Inc., Washington, 1991, pp 31–54.

355. Rapaport MH, Torrey EF, McAllister CG, et al. Increased serum soluble interleukin-2 receptors in schizophrenic monozygotic twins. Eur Arch Psychiatry Clin Neurosci 243:7–10, 1993.

356. Rapport MM, Graf L. Immunochemical reactions of lipids. Prog Allergy 13:273–331, 1969.

357. Reese TS, Karnovsky MJ. Fine structural localization of a blood-brain barrier to exogenous peroxidase. J Cell Biol 34:207–217, 1967.

358. Reilly FD, McCluskey RS, Meineke HA. Studies of the hemopoietic microenvironment. VIII. Adrenergic and cholinergic innervation of the murine spleen. Anat Rec 105:100–117, 1976.

359. Reunanen M, Ilonen J, Arnadottir T, et al. Mitogen and antigen stimulation of multiple sclerosis cerebrospinal fluid lymphocytes in vitro. J Neurol Sci 58:211–221, 1983.

360. Richardson EP. Progressive multifocal encephalopathy. New Engl J Med 265:815–823, 1961.

361. Richert JR, Driscoll BF, Kies MW, Alvord EC Jr. Adoptive transfer of experimental allergic encephalomyelitis: incubation of rat spleen cells with specific antigen. J Immunol 122:494–496, 1979.

362. Richert JR, Reuben-Burnside CA, Deibler GE, Kies MW. Fine specificities of myelin basic protein-specific human T-cell clones. Ann NY Acad Sci 540:345–348, 1988.

363. Risau W, Engelhardt B, Wekerle H. Immune function of the blood brain barrier: incomplete presentation of protein (auto-) antigens by rat brain microvascular endothelium in vitro. J Cell Biol 110:1757–1766, 1990.

364. Rivers TM, Sprunt DH, Berry GP. Observations on attempts to produce acute disseminated encephalomyelitis in monkeys. J Exp Med 58:39–53, 1933.

365. Rodriguez M, Leibowitz J, David CL. Susceptibility to Theiler's virus-induced demyelination. Mapping of the gene within the H-2D region. J Exp Med 163:620–631, 1986.

366. Rogers SW, Andrews PI, Cahring LC, et al. Autoantibodies to glutamate receptor GluR3 in Rasmussen's encephalitis. Science 265:648–651, 1994.

367. Roitt IM, Doniach D, Campbell PN, Hudson, RV. Auto-antibodies in Hashimoto's disease (lymphadenoid goitre). Lancet ii:820–821, 1956.

368. Rose NR, Witebsky W. Studies on organ specificity. V. Changes in the thyroid glands of rabbits following active immunization with rabbit thyroid extracts. J Immunol 76:417–427, 1956.

369. Roszman TL, Brooks WH. Neural modulation of immune function. J Neuroimmunol 10: 59–69, 1985.

370. Rothbard B, Steinman L. Characterization of a major encephalitogenic T cell epitope in SJL/J mice with synthetic oligopeptides of myelin basic protein. J Neuroimmunol 19:21–32, 1988.

371. Rowland LP. Amyotrophic Lateral Sclerosis and Other Motor Neuron Diseases. Raven Press, New York 1991.

372. Roy BF, Rose JW, McFarland HF, et al. Anti-beta-endorphin immunoglobulin G in humans. Proc Natl Acad Sci 83:8739–8743, 1986.

373. Roy BF, Rose JW, Sunderland T, et al. Anti-somatostatin immunoglobulin G in major depressive disorder: a preliminary study with implications for an autoimmune mechanism of depression. Arch Gen Psychiatry 45:924–928, 1988.

374. Ruddle NH, Bergman CM, McGrath KM, et al. An antibody to lymphotoxin and tumor necrosis factor prevents transfer of experimental allergic encephalomyelitis. J Exp Med 172:1193–1200, 1990.

375. Sabin TD, Swift TR. Leprosy. In: Peripheral Neuropathy, 2nd ed, Vol 2, Dyck, PJ, et al, eds. Saunders, Philadelphia, 1984, pp 1955–1987.

376. Sacerdote P, Ruff MR, Pert CB. Vasoactive intestinal peptide 1-12: a ligand for the CD4 (T4)/human immunodeficiency virus receptor. J Neurosci Res 18:102–107, 1987.

377. Sachs H. Die Cytotoxine des Blutserums. Biochem Zentralblatt 1:573–578, 613–618, 653–656, 693–698, 1903.

378. Said G, Joskowicz M, Barreira AA, Eisen H. Neuropathy associated with experimental Chagas' disease. Ann Neurol 18:676–683, 1985.

379. Saida T, Saida K, Dorfman SH. Experimental allergic neuritis induced by sensitization with galactocerebroside. Science 204:1103–1106, 1979.

380. Sandberg-Wollheim M. Immunoglobulin synthesis in vitro by cerebrospinal fluid cells in patients with multiple sclerosis. Scand J Immunol 3:717–730, 1974.

381. Sanders ME, Koski CL, Robbins D, et al. Activated terminal complement in cerebrospinal fluid in Guillain-Barré syndrome and multiple sclerosis. J Immunol 136:4456–4459, 1986.

382. Sansonetti P, Lagrange PH. The immunology of leprosy: speculations on the leprosy spectrum. Rev Infect Dis 3:422–469, 1981.

383. Saper CB, Breder CD. Endogenous pyrogens in the CNS: role in the febrile response. Prog Brain Res 93:419–428, 1992.

384. Sasazuki T, Kaneoka H, Nishimura Y, et al. An HLA-linked immune suppression gene in man. J Exp Med 152 (Suppl): 297s–313s, 1980.

385. Satoh J, Sakai K, Endoh M, et al. Experimental allergic encephalomyelitis by murine encephalitogenic T cell lines specific for myelin proteolipid apoprotein. J Immunol 138:179–184, 1987.

386. Schluesener HJ, Sobel RA, Linington C, Weiner HL. A monoclonal antibody against a myelin oligodendrocyte glycoprotein induces relapses and demyelination in central nervous system autoimmune disease. J Immunol 139:4016–4021, 1987.

387. Schönbeck S, Padberg F, Hohlfeld R, Wekerle H. Transplantation of autoimmune microenvironment to severe combined immunodeficiency mice. A new model of myasthenia gravis. J Clin Invest 90:245–250, 1992.

388. Schwartz M, Novick D, Givol D, Fuchs S. Induction of anti-idiotypic antibodies by immunization with syngeneic spleen cells educated with acetylcholine receptor. Nature 273: 543–545, 1978.

389. Schwartz MM, Roberts JL. Membranous and vascular chroidopathy: two patterns of immune deposits in systemic lupus erythematosus. Clin Immunol Immunopathol 29:369–380, 1983.

390. Scolding NJ, Morgan BP, Campbell AK, Compston DAS. Complement mediated serum cytotoxicity against oligodendrocytes: a comparison with other cells of the oligodendrocyte-type 2 astrocyte lineage. J Neurol Sci 97:155–162, 1990.

391. Seboun E, Robinson MA, Doolittle TH, et al. A susceptibility locus for multiple sclerosis is linked to the T cell receptor beta chain complex. Cell 57:1095–1100, 1989.

392. Sedgwick JD, Mason DW. The mechanism of inhibition of experimental allergic encephalomyelitis in the rat by monoclonal antibody against CD4. J Neuroimmunol 13:217–232, 1986.

393. Selmaj K, Brosnan CF, Raine CS. Expression of heat shock protein-65 by oligodendrocytes in vivo and in vitro: implications for multiple sclerosis. Neurology 42:795–800, 1992.

394. Selmaj C, Cannella B, Brosnan CF, Raine CS. TCR gamma delta cells: a new category of T cells in multiple sclerosis lesions. J Neuropathol Exp Neurol 49:288, 1990 [Abstract].

395. Selmaj K, Raine CS. Tumor necrosis factor mediates myelin damage in organotypic cultures of nervous tissue. Ann NY Acad Sci 540:568–570, 1988.

396. Selye H. Thymus and adrenals in the response of an organism to injuries and intoxication. Br J Exp Pathol 17:234–248, 1936.

397. Server AC, Johnson RT. Guillain-Barré syndrome. In: Current Clinical Topics in Infectious Diseases, JS Remington, MN Swartz, eds, Vol 3. McGraw-Hill, New York, 1982, pp 74–96.

398. Sharma SD, Nag B, Su X-M, et al. Antigen-specific therapy of experimental allergic encephalomyelitis by soluble class II major histocompatibility complex-peptide complexes. Proc Natl Acad Sci 88:11465–11469, 1991.

399. Shaw, SY, Laursen RA, Lees MB. Analogous amino acid sequences in myelin proteolipid and viral proteins. FEBS Lett 207:266–270, 1986.

400. Shy ME, Rowland LP, Smith T, et al. Motor neuron disease and plasma cell dyscrasia. Neurology 36:1429–1436, 1986.

401. Sibley WA, Bamford CR, Clark K. Clinical viral infections and multiple sclerosis. Lancet i:1313–1315, 1985.

402. Sillevis Smitt PA, de Jong JM. Animal models of amyotrophic lateral sclerosis and the spinal muscular atrophies. J Neurol Sci 91:231–258, 1989.

403. Silverstein AM, Lukes RJ. Fetal responses to antigenic stimulus. I. Plasmacellular and lymphoid reactions in the human fetus to intrauterine infection. Lab Invest 11:918–932, 1962.

404. Silverstein AM, Welter S, Zimmerman LE. Progressive immunization reaction in the rabbit eye. J Immunol 86:312–323, 1961.

405. Skeiky YA, Benson DR, Parsons M, et al. Cloning and expression of Trypanosoma cruzi ribosomal protein Po and epitope analysis of anti-Po autoantibodies in Chagas' disease patients. J Exp Med 176:201–211, 1992.

406. Smith, EM, Morrill AC, Meyer WJ, Blalock JE. Corticotropin releasing factor induction of leukocyte derived immunoreactive ACTH and endorphins. Nature 321:881–882, 1986.

407. Sobel RA, Blanchette BW, Bhan AK, Colvin RB. The immunopathology of experimental allergic encephalomyelitis. II. Endothelial cell Ia increases prior to inflammatory cell infiltration. J Immunol 132:2402–2407, 1984.

408. Sobel RA, Hafler DA, Castro EE, et al. Immunohistochemical analysis of suppressor-inducer and helper-inducer T cells in multiple sclerosis brain tissue. Ann NY Acad Sci 540:306–308, 1988.

409. Sobel RA, Michell ME, Fondren G. Intercellular adhesion molecule-1 (ICAM-1) in cellular immune reactions in the human central nervous system. Am J Pathol 136:1309–1316, 1990.

410. Solimena M, Folli F, Denis-Donini S, et al. Autoantibodies to glutamic acid decarboxylase in a patient with stiff-man syndrome, epilepsy, and type I diabetes mellitus. New Engl J Med 318:1012–1020, 1988.

411. Solomon GF. Psychoneuroimmunology: interactions between central nervous system and immune system. J Neurosci Res 18:1–8, 1987.

412. Sprankel H, Richarz K, Ludwig H, Rott R. Behavior alterations in tree shrew (Tupaia glis, Diard 1820) induced by Borna disease virus. Med Micr Immunol 165:1–18, 1978.

413. Steck AJ, Tschannen R, Schäfer R. Interactions of vaccinia virus with the myelin membrane. In: Humoral Immunity in Neurological Diseases, D Karcher, A Lowenthal, AD Strosberg, eds. Plenum Press, New York 1979, pp 493–497.

414. Stefansson K, Dieperink ME, Richman DP, et al. Sharing of antigenic determinants between the nicotinic acetylcholine receptor and proteins in E. coli, P. vulgaris, and K. pneumoniae: possible role in the pathogenesis of myasthenia gravis. New Engl J Med 312:221–225, 1985.

415. Stein M, Keller SE, Schleifer SJ. Stress and immunomodulation: the role of depression and neuroendocrine function. J Immunol 135:827–833, 1985.

416. Stein M, Schiavi RC, Camerino M. Influence of brain and behavior on the immune system. Science 191:437–440, 1976.

417. Stevens JG, Pepose JS, Cook ML. Natural model for the Landry-Guillain-Barré syndrome. Ann. Neurol 9 (Suppl): 102–106, 1981.

418. Stohlmann SA, Weiner LP. Chronic central nervous system demyelination in mice after JHM virus infection. Neurology 31:38–44, 1981.

419. Suckling AJ, Jagelman S, Illavia S, Webb HE. The effect of mouse strain on the pathogenesis of the encephalitis and demyelination induced by avirulent Semliki Forest Virus infections. Br J Exp Pathol 61:281–284, 1980.

420. Sumner A, Said G, Idy I, Metral S. Syndrome de Guillain Barré Effets électrophysiologiques et morphologiques du serum humain introduit dans l'espace endoneural du nerf sciatique du rat: résultats préliminaires. Rev Neurol (Paris) 138:17–24, 1982.

421. Sun D, Ben-Nun A, Wekerle H. Regulatory circuits in autoimmunity: recruitment of counter-regulatory CD8+ T cells by encephalitogenic CD4+ T line cells. Eur J Immunol 18:1993–1999, 1988.

422. Sun D, Qin Y, Chluba J, et al. Suppression of experimentally induced autoimmune encephalomyelitis by cytolyic T-T cell interactions. Nature 332:834–835, 1988.

423. Sundin U, Thelander S. Antibody reactivity to brain membrane proteins in serum from schizophrenic patients. Brain Behav Immun 3:345–358, 1989.

424. Takamori M, Hamada T, Komai K, et al. Synaptotagmin can cause an immune-mediated model of Lambert-Eaton myasthenic syndrome in rats. Ann Neurol 35:74–80, 1994.

425. ter Meulen V. Autoimmune reactions against myelin basic protein induced by corona and measles viruses. Ann NY Acad Sci 540:202–209, 1988.

426. ter Meulen V, Katz M, Miller D. Subacute sclerosing panencephalitis. Curr Top Microbiol Immunol 57:1–38, 1972.

427. Theiler M. Spontaneous encephalomyelitis of mice, a new virus disease. J Exp Med 65:705–719, 1937.

428. Thomas JA, Willcox N, Newsom-Davis J. Immunohistological studies of the thymus in myasthenia gravis. Correlation with clinical state and thymocyte culture response. J Neuroimmunol 3:319–335, 1982.

429. Tourtellotte WW, Walsh, MJ, Baumhefner MW. The current status of multiple sclerosis intra-blood-brain-barrier IgG synthesis. Ann NY Acad Sci 436:52–67, 1984.

430. Toyka KV, Drachman DB, Pestronk A, Kao I. Myasthenia gravis: Passive transfer from man to mouse. Science 190:397–399, 1975.

431. Traub E. Persistence of lymphocytic choriomeningitis virus in immune animals and its relation to immunity. J Exp Med 63:847–861, 1936.

432. Traugott, U., Scheinberg LC, Raine CS. On the presence of Ia-positive endothelial cells and astrocytes in multiple sclerosis lesions and its relevance to antigen presentation. J Neuroimmunol 8:1–14, 1985.

433. Trotter J, De Jong LJ, Smith ME. Opsonization with antimyelin antibody increases the uptake and intracellular metabolism of myelin in inflammatory macrophages. J Neurochem 47:779–789, 1986.

434. Tsukada N, Matsuda M, Miyagi K, Yanagisawa N. Increased levels of intercellular adhesion molecule-1 (ICAM-1) and tumor necrosis factor receptor in the cerebospinal fluid of patient with multiple sclerosis. Neurology 43:2679–2682, 1993.

435. Tsukada N, Matsuda M, Miyagi K, Yanagisawa N. In vitro intercellular adhesion molecule-1 expression on brain endothelial cells in multiple sclerosis. J Neuroimmunol 49:181–187, 1994.

436. Tuohy VK, Laursen RA, Lees MB. Acute experimental allergic encephalomyelitis in SJL/J mice induced by a synthetic peptide of myelin proteolipid protein. J Neuropathol Exp Neurol 49:468–479, 1990.

437. Turnley AM, Morahan G, Okano H, et al. Dysmyelination in transgenic mice resulting from expression of class I histocompatibility molecules in oligodendrocytes. Nature 353:566–569, 1991.

438. Tzartos SJ, Lindström JM. Mononclonal antibodies used to probe acetylcholine receptor structure: localization of the main immunogenic region and detection of similarities between subunits. Proc Natl Acad Sci 77:755–759, 1980.

439. Uchimura I, Shiraki H. A contribution to the classification and the pathogenesis of demyelinating encephalomyelitis, with special reference to the central nervous system lesions caused by preventive inoculation against rabies. J Neuropathol 16:139–203, 1957.

440. Uhlenhuth P. Zur Lehre von der Unterscheidung verschiedener Eiweissarten mit Hilfe specifischer Sera. In: Festschrift Robert Koch, Fischer, Jena, 1903, pp 49–74.

441. Usuku K, Sonoda S, Osame M, et al. HLA haplotype-linked high immune responsiveness against HTLV-1 in HTLV-1-associated myelopathy: comparison with adult T-cell leukemia/lymphoma. Ann Neurol 23 (Suppl): S143–S150, 1988.

442. Van Alstyne D, Dyck IM, Berry K, Paty DW. Accelerated EAE in SJL mice by use of virus-infected brain as encephalitogen. Neurology 33 (Suppl 2): 195, 1984 [Abstract].

443. Van der Geld TEW, Feltkamp H, Oosterhuis HJGH. Reactivity of mysthenia gravis serum globulin with skeletal muscle and thymus demonstrated by immunofluorescence. Proc Soc Exp Biol Med 115:782–785, 1964.

444. Van der Veen, RC, Trotter, JL, Hickey WF, Kapp JA. The development and characterization of encephalitogenic cloned T cells specific for myelin proteolipid protein. J Neuroimmunol 26:139–145, 1990.

445. VandeWoude S, Richt JA, Zink MC, et al. A Borna virus cDNA encoding a protein

recognized by antibodies in humans with behavioral diseases. Science 250:1278–1281, 1990.

446. Vandvik B, Natvig JB, Winger D. IgG1 subclass restriction of oligoclonal IgG from cerebrospinal fluids and brain extracts in patients with multiple sclerosis and subacute encephalitides. Scand J Immunol 5:427–436, 1976.

447. Vartdal F, Sollid LM, Vandvik B, et al. Patients with multiple sclerosis carry DQB1 genes which encode shared polymorphic aminoacid-sequences. Hum Immunol 25:103–110, 1989.

448. Vaughan RW, Adam AM, Gray IA, et al. Major histocompatibility complex class I and class II polymorphism in chronic idiopathic demyelinating polyradiculoneuropathy. J Neuroimmunol 27:149–153, 1990.

449. Venkatasubramanian K, Audhya T, Goldstein G. Binding of thymopoietin to the acetylcholine receptor. Proc Natl Acad Sci 83:3171–3174, 1986.

450. Verhoeff FH, Lemoine AN. Endophthalmitis phacoanaphylactica. Am J Ophthalmol 5:737–745, 1922.

451. Waksman BH. Experimental Allergic Encephalomyelitis and the "Auto-Allergic" Diseases. Int Arch Allergy Appl Immunol Vol 14 (Suppl), 1959.

452. Waksman BH. A comparative histopathological study of delayed hypersensitive reactions. Ciba Found Symp Cell Aspects Immun 280–322, 1960.

453. Waksman BH. Autoimmunization and the lesions of autoimmunity. Medicine 41:93–141, 1962.

454. Waksman BH, ed. Immunologic Mechanisms in Neurologic and Psychiatric Disease. Res Publ Assoc Res Nerv Ment Dis 68:1–336, Raven Press, New York, 1990.

455. Waksman BH, Adams RD. Allergic neuritis: an experimental disease of rabbits induced by the injection of peripheral nervous tissue and adjuvants. J Exp Med 102:213–216, 1955.

456. Waksman BH, Adams RD. A critical comparison of certain experimental and naturally occurring viral leukoencephalitides with experimental allergic encephalomyelitis. J Neuropathol Exp Neurol 21:491–518, 1962.

457. Waksman BH, Adams RD. A histological study of the early lesion in experimental allergic encephalomyelitis in the guinea pig and rabbit. Am J Path 41:135–162, 1962.

458. Waksman BH, Arbouys S, Arnason BG. The use of specific "lymphocyte" antisera to inhibit hypersensitive reactions of the "delayed" type. J Exp Med 114:997–1022, 1961.

459. Waksman BH, Morrison LR. Tuberculin type sensitivity to spinal cord antigen in rabbits with isoallergic encephalomyelitis. J Immunol 66:421–444, 1951.

460. Waksman BH, Porter H, Lees MD, Adams RD, Folch J. A study of the chemical nature of components of bovine white matter effective in producing allergic encephalomyelitis in the rabbit. J Exp Med 100:451–471, 1954.

461. Walker DL. Progressive multifocal leukoencephalopathy. In: Handbook of Clinical Neurology Vol 3, PJ Vinken, GW Bruyn, HL Klawans, DMD Koetsier, eds. Elsevier, Amsterdam, 1985, pp 503–524.

462. Warren KG, Catz I. Diagnostic value of cerebrospinal fluid anti-myelin basic protein in patients with multiple sclerosis. Ann Neurol 20:20–25, 1986.

463. Watanabe R, Wege H, ter Meulen V. Adoptive transfer of EAE-like lesions by MBP-stimulated lymphocytes from rats with coronavirus-induced demyelinating encephalomyelitis. Nature 305:150–153, 1983.

464. Webb HE, Mehta S, Gregson NA, Leibowitz S. Immunological reaction of the demyelinating Semliki Forest virus with immune serum to glycolipids and its possible importance to central nervous system viral auto-immune disease. Neuropathol Appl Neurobiol 10:77–84, 1984.

464a. Wekerle H, Linington C, Lassmann H, Meyermann R. Cellular immune reactivity within the CNS. TINS 9:271–276, 1986.

465. Wiley CA, Schrier RD, Nelson JA, et al. Cellular localization of human immunodeficiency virus infection within the brains of acquired immune deficiency syndrome patients. Proc Natl Acad Sci 83:7089–7093, 1986.

466. Willcox N, Demaine AG, Newsom-Davis J, et al. Increased frequency of IgG heavy chain marker G1m (2) and of HLA-B8 in Lambert-Eaton myasthenic syndrome with and without associated lung carcinoma. Hum Immunol 14:29–36, 1985.

467. Williams JM, Peterson RG, Shea PA, et al. Sympathetic innervation of murine thymus and spleen. Evidence for a functional link between the nervous and immune systems. Brain Res Bull 6:83–94, 1981.

468. Williams LT, Snyderman R, Lefkowitz RJ. Identification of beta-adrenergic receptors in human lymphocytes by (−) [³H] alprenolol binding. J Clin Invest 57:149–155, 1976.

469. Williams RM, Moore MJ. Linkage of susceptiblity to experimental allergic encephalomyelitis to the major histocompatibilitiy locus in the rat. J Exp Med 138:175–183, 1973.

470. Witebsky E, Rose NR, Terplan K, et al. Chronic thyroiditis and autoimmunization. JAMA 164:1439–1447, 1957.

471. Wolinsky JS. Rubella virus and its effect on the developing nervous system. In: Viral Infections of the Developing Nervous System, RT Johnson, G Lyon, eds. MTP Press, Lancaster, 1988, pp. 125–142.

472. Wood, JN, Hudson L, Jessell TM, Yamamoto M. A monoclonal antibody defining antigenic determinants on subpopulations of mammalian neurones and Trypanosoma cruzi parasite. Nature 296:34–38, 1982.

473. Wucherpfennig KW, Ota K, Endo N, et al. Shared human T cell receptor V beta usage to immunodominant regions of myelin basic protein. Science 248:1016–1019, 1990.

474. Wucherpfennig KW, Strominger JL. Molecular mimicry in T cell-mediated autoimmunity: viral peptides activate human T cell clones specific for myelin basic protein. Cell 80:695–705, 1995.

475. Yamada M, Zurbriggen A, Fujinami RS. Monoclonal antibody to Theiler's murine encephalitis virus defines a determinant on myelin and oligodendrocytes and augments demyelination in experimental allergic encephalomyelitis. J Exp Med 171:1893–1907, 1990.

476. Yamane Y, Perez, M, Edelson R, et al. Endocytosis of TCR/CD3 complex and the class I major histocompatibility complex in a human T cell line. Cell Immunol 136:496–503, 1991.

477. Yu RK, Saito M. Structure and localization of gangliosides. In: Neurobiology of Glycoconjugates, RU Margolis, RK Margolis, eds. Plenum, New York, 1989, pp 1–42.

478. Zhang J, Markovic-Plese S, Lacet B, et al. Increased frequency of interleukin 2-responsive T cells specific for myelin basic protein and preteolipid protein in peripheral blood and cerebrospinal fluid of patients with multiple sclerosis. J Exp Med 179:973–984, 1994.

479. Zinkernagel RM, Leist T, Hengartner H, Althage A. Susceptibility to lymphocytic choriomeningitis correlated directly with early and high cytotoxic T cell activity, as well as with footpad swelling reaction, and all three are regulated by H-2D. J Exp Med 162:2125–2141, 1985.

II

BASIC CONCEPTS

2

A Review of the Immune System

EMIL R. UNANUE

This chapter considers some of the basic properties of the immune system and introduces their component cells and molecules. It is slightly modified from one published in *Samter's Immunologic Disease,* Fifth Edition (Little, Brown, 1995, edited by M. M. Frank, H. Claman, K. F. Austen, and E. R. Unanue). The carefully orchestrated cellular immune system operates physiologically as the major impediment to infections and, consequently, has a major survival value for the species. Without immunity the individual ultimately succumbs to infections with one or another of microbial agents. The immune system, however, like many cellular systems, can be involved in disease, including neurological diseases, the major theme of this book. Immunological diseases in general result from specific cellular and/or molecular aberrations, or from encounters with foreign materials that, under particular conditions, create pathology.

The immune system functions through a critically regulated series of cellular interactions. These cellular interactions display at the same time a marked and exquisite specificity—the well-known specificity of antigen recognition—and also a wide range of nonspecificity, the nonantigen specificity of the effector functions of immunity that result in the acute or chronic inflammation. Both functions are highly integrated to bring about an early recognition and fast elimination of an antigen.

Here we first comment on general properties of the immune system. We then discuss the cells of the system and their main interactions, and finally examine the effector reactions and their role in disease. References are not comprehensive but are selected for key studies. Some of the major findings in immunology are also summarized briefly in the context of their historical background.

General Properties of the Immune System and Their Cellular Basis

The major properties of the immune system are

1. its specificity of recognition and discrimination among antigen molecules;
2. its capacity to identify a very large number of foreign structures, that is, the immune system has a wide library of recognition;
3. the memory response;
4. the capacity to discriminate between foreign, or non-self-determinants, and autologous, or self-determinants.

The cellular foundation of these four properties and how each has been examined and exploited by immunologists will be discussed here.

Specificity: the Cellular and Biochemical Basis of Specific Antigen Recognition

The *specificity* of the immune system is one of its highly distinguishing features. Specificity means the property of the immune system to discriminate among various chemical entities, i.e., antigens. The immune system can resolve and distinguish chemical entities that are closely similar to each other, for example, the position of a chemical group in a ring structure or one amino acid side chain in a peptide, or the number of monosaccharides in a complex polysaccharide (11,62,86,105). The cellular basis of such specificity resides on the lymphocyte, which is endowed with specific and unique antigen receptors.

The two major sets of lymphocytes, the B and T lymphocytes, have distinct receptors for antigen. The antigen receptor of the B lymphocyte is an antibody molecule, an immunoglobulin (Ig) inserted in its membrane (141,144,155,177). The major product of the activated or differentiated B lymphocyte is the secreted antibody molecule found in blood and tissue fluids, which has the same specificity for antigen as that found on the surface immunoglobulin of the B cell. In the resting B lymphocyte, the immunoglobulins represented on their plasma membrane are IgM and IgD.

The receptor for antigen on the T lymphocyte is a unique protein distinct from immunoglobulin but with properties akin to it (28,73,151,192). In contrast to the B cell, the receptor for antigen of T cells is exclusively membrane bound. There are a number of important membrane molecules that associate with the T-cell antigen receptor. For example, the CD3 complex regulates the whole process of signal transduction following the engagement of the receptor (17,118,119,152). The CD4 molecule, a protein that distinguishes one of the two major stable subsets of peripheral T cells, binds to class II MHC molecules and also transduces metabolic signals. The CD8 molecule, which distinguishes the second subset of peripheral T cells, binds to cells displaying class I MHC molecules (120,162).

In contrast to the B cell, the major product of secretion of activated T cells is not a secreted form of the receptor, rather, it is represented by a wide number of biologically active proteins, the cytokines, which are not antigen specific. Cytokines are important regulators of the immune system and represent one of the ways in which information is communicated among cells in immunity.

The B lymphocyte uses the exquisite specificity of its receptors to carry out two sets of reactions. One set is intimate, in which close cell-to-cell interactions characteristic of the cellular inductive events involving B cells, T cells, and accessory cells occur (comments on these will be made in the next section). The second kind of reaction is carried out at a distance by the secreted antibody molecule. The secreted antibody molecule binds antigen molecules forming antigen–antibody complexes that are rapidly eliminated from blood and tissues.

The biochemical analysis of the immunoglobulin molecule and of its interaction with antigen was a major and dominant feature of research in immunology from its foundation at the end of the 19th century (6) to about the first half of this century (3,74,88,103,114,166). The antibody molecule has a dual role—one of antigen-binding (87), the other of modulating different effector functions. These properties are associated with distinct regions of the molecule as its constituents heavy and light chains assemble into two distinct and identical half-molecules (42,142). Each of the five major antibody classes, or isotypes, have unique properties in the constant domains of their heavy chain which allow them to carry out their specific effector functions. These effector functions are essential for the antimicrobial response, particularly to pyogenic organisms and to toxin-producing bacteria, and to some viruses. The specific effector functions include opsonization (i.e., the binding to an antigen favoring its high rate of uptake by phagocytes), interactions with complement proteins (inducing a cascade of inflammatory and cytolytic reactions), transplacental passage (protecting the fetus and newborn during early stages of life), and mucosal immunity (represented by the IgA molecules produced in the gastrointestinal and respiratory tracts) (167).

Because of its specificity for antigen, the antibody molecule in serum has been utilized extensively as a reagent for diagnosis, or in clinical medicine as a therapeutic device. Transfusions of immunoglobulins are used in the treatment of B-cell immunodeficiencies, but another therapeutic application uses specific antibodies. It was von Behring, following his discovery of anti-diphtheria toxins with Kitasato (6), who introduced serotherapy as a mode of treatment of infectious diseases (70). (In 1901 von Behring was awarded the first Nobel Prize for physiology or medicine for this accomplishment.) A highly successful use of specific antibodies is in the prevention of hemolytic disease in the newborn caused by Rh incompatibility (47,49,108). Here, giving anti-D(Rho) antibody to an Rh-negative woman who has just delivered an Rh-positive baby will prevent her from developing the anti-D(Rho) antibodies that cause erythroblastosis fetalis. Although the antigen, dose, isotype, etc., may vary, the point is that antibody molecules can be used as an agent to inhibit the specific development of immune responses (170,171).

A modern form of serotherapy uses monoclonal antibodies. Monoclonal antibodies are produced from hybridomas resulting from the fusion of a selected myeloma cell with a B cell producing a specific antibody (101). Monoclonal antibodies are unique products because of their homogeneity, their very fine specificity, and their unending availability. As our understanding of immunity and immunopathology increases, it is clear that monoclonal antibodies will be used more and more in clinical medicine, for example, to neutralize cytokines, to bind to and inhibit specific surface molecules of cells, to inhibit microbial phlogogenic molecules (like endotoxins), and to kill tumor cells, as in the case of antibodies coupled directly to toxins (these are now called *immunotoxins*) (178).

Monoclonal antibodies, therefore, will be used to control transplantation reactions and autoimmune and allergic diseases, cancer growth, and to prevent the sequelae of microbial infections. (In the context of this book, monoclonal antibodies to CD4 T cells and to adhesion molecules and cytokines have been successfully employed to modulate experimental allergic encephalomyelitis, the animal model of multiple sclerosis. See Chapter 7.) Methods to engineer murine monoclonal antibody molecules (the usual antibodies that are now available) to produce chimeric molecules containing portions of the human molecule, most likely will become available in the future (187). Regardless, the usefulness of monoclonal antibodies in diagnosis is immense. For example, monoclonal antibodies coupled to fluorescent-tagged reagents now constitute the best way to apply the fluorescent antibody methods originally devised by Coons (31). As used in flow cytometry (71), antibodies tagged to fluorescent compounds have resulted in a powerful method to quantitate leukocyte subsets and show their differential expression of various molecules.

The T-cell receptor shows, like the immunoglobulin molecule, a high degree of specificity and a fine capacity to discriminate antigen molecules. However, there are major differences in the molecular basis of antigen recognition by B and T cells which underline the teleological reasons for their existence as distinct cellular lineages. B cells bind directly to protein or to polysaccharide antigen molecules through their surface Ig. Despite such direct recognition, B cells for the most part are not triggered to grow and differentiate from such interactions, and, in fact, depend on T cells for their stimulation, an issue discussed in the next section. In contrast, T cells will not interact directly with antigens. The T-cell antigen receptor binds only to peptides or unfolded proteins that are bound to histocompatibility molecules, those molecules encoded in the major histocompatibility gene complex (MHC) of the species. T-cell recognition therefore requires that a protein be taken up and biochemically degraded or denatured by antigen handling or presenting cells (APC) that bear MHC molecules (173,193). Moreover, T cells also recognize part of "self", in that both the MHC molecule and the peptide constitutes the antigenic determinant. This dual specificity of the T-cell receptor explains the phenomenon of *MHC restriction,* discovered in 1973 and 1974

(93,95,150,194,195). This concept in its simple definition states that T cells recognize and have specificity to foreign determinants that are displayed *always* in the context of self-MHC molecules. Thus, here is a major curiosity in how the immune system is built: on the one side, B cells show the fine recognition by antibody of polysaccharides and proteins in their tertiary configuration, while on the other, the T cells are dependent on another cellular system (the APC system), recognizing *only* linear sequences of amino acids. The differences in recognition between B and T cells explain the observation that antibody responses to protein antigens are directed to epitopes in the intact unfolded proteins. In contrast, those T-cell responses are to linear sequences of amino acids. It should also be noted that pure polysaccharides do not bind to MHC proteins and do not elicit T-cell responses.

These differences in the specificity of recognition by B and T cells constituted a major puzzle for immunologists, until the time of the discovery of B and T cells, the two major cellular lineages. Indeed, there is quite an extensive early literature comparing two kinds of reactions to protein antigen (for example, 19,54,154, reviewed in 9,172). One kind of reaction was examined by antibodies, which were easy to directly measure in the test tube. Alternatively, antibody-mediated reactions could be measured in vivo, by studying the inflammatory reactions such as the Arthus reaction and the acute anaphylactic reaction. The second set of reactions involved delayed hypersensitivity skin reactions. These reactions were first identified in the early studies of Robert Koch with tuberculin (99). It was Chase and Landsteiner who first called attention to the transfer of these reactions by lymphoid cells (27,106). Subsequently, many investigators explored their fine specificity. Delayed reactions were "carrier dependent" and did not discriminate between denatured and native protein antigens (53). We now know the reasons for it.

In summary, then, the specificity of the immune response lies in the two major families of lymphocytes bearing specific receptors—B and T cells. A single lymphocyte exhibits only one set of receptors, i.e., each lymphocyte is equivalent to the recognition of a unique antigenic determinant. The activation of such a lymphocyte results in the production of a clone of cells with the same antigenic specificity. The cellular immune system is therefore made up of multiple clones and the stimulation of the system is through a selection of those clones with higher specificity and/or affinity for the antigen. It is noteworthy that the first cellular explanation for antibody production was made by Paul Ehrlich with his side-chain theory of 1900 (43,44). He postulated side chains as extension of the cell's protoplasm that would capture the toxins but which, when produced in excess, would spill out of the cell to represent the antitoxins found in blood. In his own words, "the antitoxins represent nothing more than the side-chains reproduced in excess during regeneration, and therefore pushed off from the protoplasm, and so coming to exist in a free state". This is a remarkable theory made at a time when there was little if any information on cellular immunity. Curiously, the first direct demonstration that Ig was a component of the B-cell surface did not take place until the late 1960s and early 1970s (141,144,155,177).

Diversity

The library of specific receptors available to the cellular immune system is extensive, estimated to recognize 10^9 or more specificities. The molecular basis of diversity has been much debated since the establishment of foundations of immunological concepts at the turn of the century. Explanations of diversity developed with the template theories, which gave the antigen molecule a direct role in the folding of the antibody molecule (157). Of course, these theories were later discarded as information on the molecular and genetic properties of protein molecules was established. The selective theories explained the immune response on the basis of the antibody molecule itself (85,164). Niels Jerne made a major theoretical advance in 1955 by postulating that the selection for antigen was through the antibody molecule: "The role of the antigen is neither that of a template nor that of an enzyme modifier. The antigen is solely a selective carrier of spontaneously circulating antibody to a system of cells that can reproduce this antibody" (85). As an important extension, the clonal selection theory was formulated and championed, particularly by F. MacFarland Burnet and associates, as the Hall Institute in Melbourne (23,24). This theory explained antigenic specificity at the cellular level, at the level of the lymphocyte through a cell-bound antibody. The clonal selection theory has dominated much of the thinking in cellular immunology during the last three decades and has served to guide much of the research during this period.

One lymphocyte clone is equivalent to the recognition of one antigenic specificity. Thus the system operates by having multiple clones. But how does diversity arise? Is each specificity encoded in one gene or is it the result of mutations in a selected number of germ-line encoded genes? And how does one explain immunoglobulin class switching in which the antibody-combining site is preserved, yet expressed in the various isotypes (38)? The introduction of molecular biology into immunology caused a major revolution and answered these fundamental questions. First, the molecular identification of the genomic organization of the immunoglobulin gene locus was accomplished and shown to contain a finite number of germ-line encoded segments. The seminal discovery was made that the antigen-combining segments of the antibody molecule were formed and, as a result of rearrangements of these germ-line genes, encoded in different segments of the DNA. These findings eventually brought the molecular explanation for diversity as well as for immunoglobulin class switch and allelic exclusion (10,41,153,168,169,186). Rearrangement of immunoglobulin genes thus creates in a stochastic fashion the wide library of antigen recognition.

Memory

The introduction of antigen imprints a long-lasting reaction in the immune system so that a subsequent challenge, from days to sometimes months or even years later, results in an accelerated response. In its classical description, the memory or secondary response shows a short period of latency (the interval between antigen introduction and a detectable response), followed by a high antibody titer, a high affinity of antibodies for antigen, a large titer of IgG or its subclasses, and prominent T-cell reactivities. Memory in the T-cell system is evident by increased proliferation, the generation of effector cells capable of cytokine secretion and of killing nucleated cells, and delayed hypersensitivity. For the B cell, the memory response involves isotype class switching, where the secreted antibody molecule now expresses other heavy-chain isotypes, together with the same variable region of the molecule. At the DNA level, the memory response of the B cell involves mutations in the variable region genes, resulting in a variety of different but related clones (52,183, reviewed in 100). Those clones with high-affinity receptors for the antigen are eventually selected. This is the molecular explanation for the initial observations made in the analysis of the antihapten antibody responses, which showed high-affinity antibodies appearing in the serum as the response matured with time (45,158). (*Haptens* are classically defined as small molecules that by themselves are unable to stimulate immunity, although these compounds are capable of binding to antibodies. However, haptens bound to carrier molecules represented by foreign proteins are strongly immunogenic. Haptens such as dinitrophenol are particularly useful because, by equilibrium dialysis methods, the primary strength of the binding can be measured [45,86]). Despite much research, the entire explanation for the various cellular components of the memory response is not entirely elucidated. Undoubtedly playing a role are the contributions of clonal expansion, of antigen retention, and the long (or short) life of the memory B and T cells.

The memory, secondary, or anamnestic response is the basis for prophylactic immunization—undoubtedly the greatest benefit of immunology to humankind. It was through the analysis of this memory response that many of the immunological phenomena were first discovered. This analysis started in antiquity with the appreciation that individuals who survived an infectious disease were protected from a second exposure and could participate in the care of the sick. The effect of contact of unexposed populations to smallpox and other infectious agents was pointedly shown 500 years ago by the arrival of the Europeans to the American continents (32); the major cause of devastation of the indigenous populations of Central and South America was infection of an adult population unexposed to infectious agents during childhood.

Through the analysis of smallpox, with its major effects on populations, vaccination was developed. In the 18th century protection from smallpox was accomplished by inducing a mild disease through the process known as variolation, i.e., by applying a small inoculum from the blister of a smallpox lesion onto the hands of the individual. When done carefully, this produced a milder disease limited to the presence of a few pox lesions on the hands. However, variolation was a dangerous procedure that frequently resulted in serious illness. Edward Jenner made the seminal observation in 1788 that exposure to a limited pox disease, that of cowpox, resulted in cross-protection against smallpox (84). It was an astute clinical observation, one of the many that have influenced our discoveries and understanding of immunological phenomena. Rapidly, usage of the Jennerian procedure became widespread, effecting a major decrease in the incidence of smallpox. Eventually, vaccination led to the extermination of smallpox; the last case was reported in 1972. Vaccination was later developed and encouraged by Pasteur with his studies on the germ basis of disease and his experiments on vaccination against chicken cholera (138) and, particularly, against rabies (139).

Vaccination is now carried out primarily in early childhood and represents one of the most, if not *the* most efficient preventive measure in medicine. The crux of vaccination is how to immunize optimally and long-lastingly against an infectious agent. Curiously, the science of vaccination has lagged, only to be revived with great interest, particularly with the advent of infections with the human immunodeficiency virus (HIV). At this point, however, the stage is set for a more rational approach to vaccine production, as our molecular understanding of antigenicity continues to progress. The fact that the precise epitopes reactive with B and/or T cells can now be identified and engineered into different immunizing vectors means that some new approaches will be provided that will be employed much more in the near future.

Self vs. Non-self Discrimination

A distinguishing feature of immunity is the capacity to discriminate self versus nonself, that is, autologous from foreign molecules. During their differentiation, B and T cells develop with receptors reactive with self molecules. The price paid for the development of a wide diversity of antigen-specific receptors is that many of the receptors on the early differentiating B and T cells have specificity directed toward an autologous component, i.e., self-reactivity. Hence, a number of critical control steps need to be superimposed on the system to ensure the dormancy or elimination of these self-reactive clones. The reason for the many control mechanisms centers clearly on the need to control self-reactivity. Regulatory events that control self-reactivity include the elimination of part of self-reactive T cells during thymus differentiation (76,90,91,96,111,156) and the inactivation of mature self-reactive B and T lymphocytes that bind to self-antigen molecules.

Autoimmunity was first discussed by Ehrlich with his famous term, *horror autotoxicus* (43), and became apparent in the clinical findings of the antibodies of paroxysmal cold hemoglobinuria in 1904 (37). The early descriptions of autoimmune reactions perturbed immunobiologists until relatively recently when this phenomenon became accepted. The history of these early debates has been cogently analyzed by Arthur Silverstein (157, p. 160). Autoimmunity became evident when experimental animals were immunized against brain matter (89,147; see Chapter 1), testicular antigens (51), and thyroid (149). Such immunizations resulted in encephalomyelitis, aspermatogenesis, and thyroiditis, respectively. The first studies on clinical autoimmunity were made on thyroid diseases (148,188) and subsequently were applied to numerous neurological diseases, especially multiple sclerosis.

At present, the analysis of autoimmune diseases has become a central area of investigation that brings together the studies on T- and B-cell differentiation with those on tolerance and experimental and clinical diseases. A surprising number of diseases show a component of autoimmunity. Some, like multiple sclerosis, insulin-dependent diabetes mellitus, systemic lupus erythematosus, and allied "connective tissue" diseases, such as rheumatoid arthritis, constitute major diseases. Reacting against self, however, does not mean that pathology develops. In fact, some autoimmune reactions follow injury and/or death of cells in tissues. These reactions are not pathogenic as, for example, when antimyosin antibodies are made in patients with myocardial infarctions.

Vital to the concept of autoimmunity and to our understanding of it is acquired immunological tolerance, which was championed in the 1940s by Owen's studies on chimeric cattle twins (187) and by the pioneering studies of the Medawar (12) and Hasek laboratories (72). It was Medawar and associates, however, who brought out the fundamental principles of tolerance at the level of the lymphocyte. Clearly, exposure to antigen during embryonic or early postnatal life, at a time when the immune system is not fully developed, results in a lack of responsiveness and an acceptance of the foreign antigen as self. As Medawar and colleagues noted in their classic paper: "This phenomenon is the exact inverse of 'activity acquired immunity' and we therefore propose to describe it as 'actively acquired tolerance'" (12). Prior to these studies, the response to polysaccharides was shown to "paralyze" the immune system, depending on the dose (46), as was the case with certain skin sensitizers. Recently, foreign antigens have been introduced into the genome of mice by using transgenic methodology (128). As expected, such foreign proteins are recognized as self.

All these studies have led to the fundamental concept that the immune system has two different ways to react toward antigens: one is a positive response and the other a negative response. Much research has gone into explaining the cellular basis of tolerance, and many controversies have ensued. Along these lines, the role of a specific suppressor cellular lineage polarized immunologists for a great part of the late 1970s and early 1980s, following Gershon's introduction of the concept of specific T-cell suppression to explain tolerance (57). This very provocative idea has now been redefined without having to postulate the presence of a specific cellular lineage to control the negative response.

There is more than one pathway to immunological tolerance. Tolerance can be central, i.e., it can occur in the thymus, or it can take place in peripheral tissues. The understanding of tolerance in the thymus was revolutionized by the finding that sets of lymphocytes can be eliminated during their differentiation, or negative selection (76,90,91,96,111,156). Tolerance in mature B and T cells seems to be more complex and in need of further evaluation, although substantial progress has recently been made (63,132). Here the role of clonal anergy (i.e., unresponsiveness when lymphocytes interact with antigen in the absence of costimulatory signals) or of clonal elimination will need to be ultimately defined. Likewise, the role of cytokines that inhibit some aspects of antigen presentation and T-cell stimulation, such as IL-10, IL-4 or transforming growth factor β, is currently being evaluated (see for example, 48).

The full understanding of the cellular basis of immunological tolerance will, of course, take us a step further toward explaining, and ultimately controlling, autoimmunity. It may also lead us into ways to specifically eliminate or inactivate lymphocytes for the control of transplantation reactions. Indeed, since Medawar's findings, transplantation tolerance has been a major focus of research, albeit difficult and frustrating, particularly because the surgical component of organ transplantation has advanced so rapidly (165). The control of organ transplantation reactions with cyclosporin (16) has been a major breakthrough, but still the ultimate goal is clearly that of specific clonal elimination. This will be the ultimate therapeutic modality, for example, to control neuroimmune diseases.

Cells of the Immune System: Their Responses and Interactions

Regulation of the Lymphocyte: to Grow or Die

In this section the major characteristics of the cellular immune system will be considered briefly, providing further comment on the points raised in the previous section.

Clearly, the cellular immune system operates through close cell-to-cell interactions triggered by antigen, involving more than one cell type. Antigens introduced in an individual induce different types of responses. The outcome of these responses depends critically on the form and type of antigen, its dose, route, and frequency of administration. The form in which the antigen is presented, whether soluble or incorporated in adjuvants, is critical, but an individual's response depends even more on the intrinsic immunogenic strength of the antigen. The dose of antigen, that is, the amount that is able to engage the B- or T-cell receptors, is likewise important. At the level of B and T cells, indications are that the amount needed is very low, or on the order of a few hundred molecules reactive per lymphocyte. To obtain such responses in the whole individual, the antigen molecules need to be focussed or concentrated in lymphoid tissues, particularly by the APC system, to initiate the cellular interactions. Finally, the site where antigen is trapped is also important. Indeed, certain tissues, like those of the central nervous system, do not foster effective responses, most likely because of their inaccessibility to circulating lymphocytes (see Chapter 7).

The response of the lymphocytes to antigen varies. The remarkable cellular transformation of the "small" lymphocyte upon stimulation was not recognized by the early researchers who studied the immune system using morphological approaches. Two seminal findings in the 1960s changed this. One was the discovery that phytohemagglutinin induced quiescent lymphocytes to enter the DNA cycle and to proliferate vigorously and synthesize proteins (134). (The results with phytohemagglutinin led to the concept of polyclonal stimulators, or molecules that stimulate more than one clone of lymphocyte. This concept of polyclonal stimulation has recently been extended to the superantigens, that is, bacterial and viral products that also engage more than one T cell and which may be highly relevant in clinical diseases [77,185]).

The other finding that called attention to the remarkable virtuousity of lymphocytes was that pure populations of small lymphocytes were capable of transferring all manifestations of specific immunity into irradiated syngeneic recipients (66,69). Of course, the capacity to reproduce cellular immunity in culture left no doubt about the role of different lymphocytes and accessory cells in cellular interactions (124).

Under optimal conditions of antigenic stimulation, the lymphocyte will enter the cell cycle and multiply, expanding the number of reactive cells (clonal expansion). At the same time, some of the expanding cells undergo programs of differentiation that are still in the midst of being defined from a molecular standpoint. For B cells, differentiation involves the secretion of immunoglobulin and isotype switching, which are mediated to a great extent by cytokines. For the CD4 T cell, differentiation involves the expression of various cytokine genes, thus making this subset of T cells central to regulating immunity. This happens, for example, by releasing several cytokines, such as IL-2, the major growth-promoting protein (59,129), IL-4, a key cytokine inducing B-cell growth and differentiation (78), and/or interferon-γ, which induces activation of macrophages (161,21), and other cytokines. Finally, the CD8 T-cell differentiation involves not only expression of some cytokine genes, particularly interferon-γ, but also the capacity to produce cytolysis, i.e., a lesion in the target cells that leads to death.

A major issue of present analysis is the regulation of cytokine gene expression by CD4 and CD8 T cells. This issue has now become critical because, in the mouse, different subsets of CD4 T cells develop during antigen stimulation (130). The TH1 subset releases IL-2 and interferon-γ, while the TH2 subset releases IL-4, IL-5, and IL-10. The ratio of these two subsets may vary, depending on unknown variables (but probably centering on the APC) and, importantly, may be reflected in disease states. The most striking example is the response of inbred strains of mice to Leishmania major, where one strain makes a predominant TH1 response that induces resistance, while a second strain induces a TH2 response that does not curb Leishmania growth (75). This dichotomy now needs to be critically evaluated in the context of human diseases (30,191).

In all cases, however, more than engagement of the antigen receptor is required for lymphocyte stimulation, an issue that is relevant to the discussion on peripheral tolerance made in the previous section. Indeed, there are a number of critical molecular interactions involved in the B–T cell interactions and in the APC–T cell interactions that extend beyond T-cell receptor recognition of the MHC-peptide complex. These interactions are at the level of the lymphocyte and the tissue microenvironment. For the lymphocyte, these second interactions are represented in the two-signal model of cell activation (18,137). The two-signal model, stated at its simplest, means that for a lymphocyte to be effectively stimulated, the antigen receptor must be specifically engaged at the same time as it receives a "second signal" represented by growth or differentiating molecules. An extension of this concept is that if the second signal is not displayed, then the lymphocyte goes through an inactivation or unresponsive stage. This is the state of anergy, considered by many to be a major component in peripheral tolerance (104,131).

The second-signal concept is most likely correct. For example, powerful costimulatory molecules like the B7 protein have now been identified that, upon interaction with receptors on lymphocytes, regulate the expression of cytokine genes (109). The most powerful of these costimulator molecules are represented by the B7 molecule of the APC and the CD28 molecule of the T cell. Probably more than one costimulatory molecule is operative. Included among them are most likely some of the early cytokines released by APC such as IL-1. IL-1 not only acts on lymphocytes but also on the vascular microenvironment. Thus, its role extends to the tissue level.

A critical question that needs to be answered is, what turns on the costimulatory and early cytokine molecules? Here only partial answers are known at present, but attention needs to be focussed on the concept of adjuvants (50). *Adjuvants* are molecules that, when mixed with the antigen, enhance the immune response. These molecules may not be anything more than stimulatory molecules that regulate the tissue environment and/or its cells to foster an immune response. For example, many foreign serum proteins require their incorporation into adjuvants to become immunogenic. Perhaps a lesson in what the foreign serum proteins lack for immunogenicity can be gathered from an analysis of the strong antigens. Strong antigens are those that are powerful at immunizing, by themselves, without the need of adjuvants. The most powerful antigens are microorganisms that usually have three components: 1) many proteins which, upon processing, will engage multiple T-cell clones; 2) a high uptake into APC, and 3) content of phlogogenic molecules (for example, the lipopolysaccharides of Gram-negative bacteria and the muramyl peptides of *M. tuberculosis*). These latter molecules stimulate the expression of costimulatory molecules and the release of early cytokines, both of which then activate the immune system.

We have underscored the point that not all responses of lymphocytes result in clonal expansion and differentiation. Indeed, during their normal program of activation, many of the cells of the immune system undergo programmed cell death or apoptosis (40). Cell death programs represent an integral part of the immune response, perhaps as part of the normal homeostasis that takes place following stimulation. Apoptosis forms part of the differentiation and negative selection responses in the thymus, in the B-cell response in germinal centers, and in the response of neutrophils and macrophages during inflammation.

Some of the genes involved in apoptosis are now being defined. Two noted experiments called attention to molecules involved in apoptosis. One was the finding that giant follicular lymphoma involved the chromosomal translocation of the *bcl-2* gene close to the Ig heavy-chain gene. The *bcl-2* is now known to regulate programmed cell death by blocking some forms of it (135,176). The second experiment produced the recognition that excessive lymphocyte growth, which occurs in the lpr mouse strain as it develops a lupus-like syndrome, is caused by a lack of the protein fas. This surface protein modulates apoptosis (182).

B–T Cell Cooperation

The dichotomy of two sets of lymphocytes, each with different recognition systems, was one of the seminal findings of the late 1960s and early 1970s. The observation pointed to how the immune system operates: as a close, interdependent network of cells; cell-to-cell interaction is the rule. The discovery of B–T interactions not only underlined their importance but indicated which cellular and functional components of the system were separate from each other and which were interdependent.

It is informative to recapitulate how disparate clinical and experimental observations resulted in the discovery of B and T cells and their interactions. These observations indicated a functional and anatomical separation of two sets of immune responses: that of the *humoral* (antibody-forming) system, which is responsible for resistance to pyogenic organisms, and the immune response of the cellular system, which is responsible for resistance to intracellular pathogens and for contact sensitivity. First, patients with x-linked agammaglobulinemia were found to lack gamma globulin and to exhibit severe infections with pyogenic organisms (20). Such patients, however, resisted many viral infections and showed skin delayed hypersensitivity reactions.

The second set of observations were experimental, consisting of the surgical or hormonal deletion of primary lymphoid organs. A primary lymphoid organ is one where differentiation of stem cells to either B or T cells takes place, in a process that is independent of antigen stimulation. Initially, studies by Jacques Miller (121,122) using neonatally thymectomized mice pointed out the role of the thymus in the control of some elements of lymphopoiesis. The neonatally thymectomized mouse is lymphopenic, does not develop protective immunity to intracellular pathogenic microorganisms, and shows weak antibody responses to protein antigens (2,61,121,122). The lymph nodes are tiny; the lymphocytes, however, are deleted from selected areas, named the *T-dependent areas* of the deep cortex. But the follicles, which are constituted by B cells are present. In fact, the thymectomized mouse makes an antibody response to polysaccharide antigens (82). These observations indicate the compartmentalization at the level of the lymphoid tissue between cellular T- and B-cell responses. For a highly interactive system, this compartmentalization has always been a puzzle and speaks to the various local cellular microenvironments, each of which may be regulated in different ways (81). Thus, the interactions taking place in follicles and germinal centers of a lymph node involve primarily B cells. These interactions are very different from those in the deep cortex, which involve primarily T cells and APC (133).

The studies on the immune response of birds has also been important for our understanding of B- and T-cell responses because birds, in contrast to mammals, have two primary lymphoid organs—the bursa of Fabricius and the thymus. The bursa is a lymphoepithelial organ situated in the posterior wall of the cloacae, controlling the generation of early B cells. By contrast, the thymus is the only defined primary lymphoid organ in mammals. Bursectomized birds are agammaglobulinemic and are impaired in antibody responses (60,181), while thymectomized birds exhibit impairment of allograft rejection, since they have normal levels of immunoglobulins (181).

Finally, a third series of studies needs to be mentioned because they directly delineated the cooperation of B and T cells following adoptive transfer of separate or mixed populations of lymphocytes into irradiated recipients, using inbred mouse strains (159). Transfer into irradiated recipients of bone marrow cells (a source of B cells) did not result in antibody formation to a protein unless thymocytes or purified T cells were cotransferred (29,35,123,125,126). Included in these analyses (127) were the interactions with haptens, the chemical compounds introduced by Landsteiner. Hapten-carrier conjugates are immunogenic. The secondary or memory response to the hapten depends on boosting with the same carrier molecule used in the primary immunization (136). These results are now clearly explained by the dependency of B cells (to which the haptens bind) on T-cell stimulation (i.e., dependent on recognition of the carrier protein displaying, after its processing, a linear sequence of amino acids). The concept of hapten-carrier leads to a very practical application: in order to produce good antibodies to weak immunogens it is useful to couple the weak immunogen to a strong carrier protein. In essence, all these studies called direct attention to cellular interactions as a major step in immune responses to proteins, and to the dependency of B cells on help by T cells.

Localization and Migration of Lymphocytes

Lymphocytes are lodged in the secondary lymphoid tissues, represented by the lymph nodes and the spleen, and in the disseminated lymphoid tissue of the gastrointestinal and respiratory tract. But lymphoid tissue is not static. Lymphocytes are found in blood in a continuous recirculation with the lymphatic tissues (67,68,113). Through the process of recirculation the lymphocytes continuously sample the environment, searching for the antigen that will select and trigger them. The T cells are the major component of the recirculating pool of lymphocytes. The localization or homing of a lymphocyte to a particular vascular bed takes place by way of ligand–receptor interactions involving one or more components of the lymphocyte plasma membrane with complementary structures on the endothelium (25,160,189). Normally, lymphocytes bind only to the high endothelium of the postcapillary venules of lymph nodes, which is the site of crossing from blood into lymphatic tissues. In inflammation, however, endothelia acquire and/or reexpress novel adhesive molecules that will bind to neutrophils, monocytes, and lymphocytes. (See Chapter 7). The number of adhesion molecules regulating endothelium-leukocyte interactions is large and includes the selectins, intracellular (ICAM) and vascular adhesion molecules (VCAM) series of molecules (39). These observations on adhesion molecules explain the old observations of classic pathology indicating the importance of margination and sticking of leukocyte to vessels at the sites of inflammation. As adhesion molecules are defined and the regulation of their expression is understood, it may be possible to block, control, and/or inhibit their expression at times of unwanted inflammation, for example, during acute homograft rejection, or following vascular injury.

Cellular Interactions and the APC System

Each set of B and T cells has defined subsets with particular functions (26). These major subsets were first recognized for T cells with the discovery of CD4 and CD8 molecules and their role in fostering interaction with class II MHC or class I MHC molecules, respectively (120,162). CD4 and CD8 molecules define stable T cell subsets that show overlapping and distinct functions. CD4 and CD8 T cells have close interaction with APC. The major APCs are the mononuclear phagocytes (the monocyte–macrophage lineage), the Langerhans-dendritic family of cells, and the B cell during its early phase of interaction with antigen and T cells. The interactions between APCs and T cells are in fact truly symbiotic and indicate how nonspecific immune reaction and specific immunological reactions are simply part of a whole continuum of cellular interactions. In the central and peripheral nervous systems, the mononuclear phagocyte lineage constitute the major APCs.

Non specific or *innate immunity* is the term indicating those cellular reactions not involving lymphocytes, particularly those involving macrophages and natural killer (NK) cells (94). The discovery of phagocytosis by Metchnikoff in 1882 constituted a major finding for our understanding of immunity, inflammation, and pathology (117). The impact of Metchnikoff's work was to call attention to the function of phagocytosis as a major element of defense. The macrophage, together with the netruophil, are the two major phagocytic cells in inflammation, but each perform distinct functions and are modulated by different sets of external signals. The neutrophils are the predominant cells of the acute inflammatory reactions and are particularly adept at handling pyogenic organisms. The macrophages are the typical cells of the chronic reactions and are highly effective in phagocytosis and in modulating their surrounding cells by way of numerous biologically active secretory products. Furthermore, macrophages have the important property of becoming "activated" (110,112). *Activated macrophages* indicates a macrophage that responds to cytokines, particularly interferon-γ, displaying a highly effective cytocidal system (92). This cytocidal system involves reactive oxygen and nitrogen derivatives.

Shortly after Metchnikoff's seminal observation, the first major controversy in immunology developed between those who favored the macrophage as a key cell and those who saw humoral components as the major elements for defense. The discovery of opsonization by Wright and Douglas (190) put an end to this debate by indicating the tight relationship between the scavenging macrophage and specific immunity. The cellular basis of opsonization is now recognized through the findings of the family of Fc receptors and C3 receptors (102,145).

The relationships between phagocytic cells and phagocytosis (or the internalization of extracellular molecules) and lymphocytes became clearer with the discovery of APC–T cell interactions and the processing of antigen (173). Indeed, it is surprising that immune recognition is dependent on the function of intracellular catabolism or degradation of the protein antigen; if there is no proteolytic processing to peptides, there is no T-cell recognition of most proteins. This concept was difficult to envisage until the discovery of the function of MHC molecules and MHC restriction.

MHC molecules are key proteins involved in APC–T cell interactions. They are peptide-binding proteins that rescue peptides from intracellular digestion (5, reviewed in 172). Together with the peptide, MHC molecules form the epitope that engages the T-cell receptor. MHC molecules were first discovered by those studying transplantation reactions. These molecules were first found to constitute a highly complex serological system explained by their great degree of genetic polymorphism (64,65,159). The human leukocyte antigen (HLA) system was discovered through the analysis of leuko-agglutinins in sera from transfused patient or multiparous women (33,140,174,175). Like many discoveries in biology, the recognition that MHC molecules played a *physiological* role in immunity occurred through serendipity (80). Fortunately, the astute scientists who were involved in these studies were ready to follow the surprising and unexpected results and made critical efforts to explain them (7,8,107,115,116).

The MHC is the most polymorphic gene locus of the species. Its polymorphism may relate to its role in protecting the species against infectious agents (97,98). As mentioned, the major function of MHC molecules is to present peptides, the only way to bring about protective immunity. The site of amino acid differences responsible for allelic polymorphisms is precisely in the combining site of the MHC molecule (13). As Benacerraf stated in summarizing his work in 1980 (7):

> The evolutionary significance of the commitment of T cells to MHC antigens should be assessed from several vantage points. From the point of view of the individual concerned, the existence of such a broadly polymorphic system to determine specific responsiveness and suppression will inescapably result in individuals with different immunological potential to a given challenge. Some will clearly be at greater risk, whereas others will be better prepared to resist certain infectious agents, and it is not surprising that immunological diseases are linked to the MHC. As far as the species is concerned, this polymorphic defense system results in a very significant survival advantage to unforeseen challenges and a better possibility for the immune system to adapt to evolutionary pressures.

Understanding the function of MHC molecules and the structure of the peptides that bind to them will permit the identification of relevant peptides that cause autoimmunity, tumor immunity, and microbial immunity. Progress in this area should be forthcoming.

Effector Reactions, Inflammation, and Immunopathology

A wide range of complex effector mechanisms are put into action when the immune response sets in. These are directed at meeting the many diverse antigenic challenges facing an individual throughout its natural history. These effector mechanisms are part of the inflammatory reaction that prominently involves vascular and cellular changes in tissue. Inflammation involves stereotypic responses that do not distinguish between a beneficial effect from a harmful one. In fact, the effector mechanisms of immunity were identified in the course of examining pathological reactions like allergies, ana-phylaxis, vasculitis, etc.

Effector reactions can be initiated and modulated by the two specific recognition systems of the cellular system, that of the B cells by way of antibody molecules, and that of T cells, in large part through the release of cytokines. It should be noted that part of the inflammatory components can also be induced early, independent of lymphocytes, by the response of macrophages, neutrophils, and/or mast cells to foreign material.

The reactions modulated by antibodies include the activation of the complement system. The complement system was described at the turn of the century as a lytic activity in serum against microorganisms (15,22). Study of this activity over the years (88) resulted in the identification and biochemical purification of the component proteins and their regulatory proteins. Early investigators did not expect the scope of inflammatory reactions triggered as the complement proteins are activated in a cascade of protein-protein effects. These include vasodilatation, neutrophil activation and infiltration, opsonization, and cell lysis, in essence, all the hallmarks of inflammation. Complement is involved in resistance to microbial infections, in the clearing of immune complexes, and perhaps in immune regulation. Abnormalities or deficiencies in complement proteins can result in serious to mild immunodeficiency, depending on which protein is involved. Curiously, some inherited complement deficiencies can also prompt autoimmune reactions akin to systemic lupus erythematosus.

The other major inflammatory effect of antibody is modulated by IgE binding to its specific receptor on mast cells and basophils (83). This leads to degranulation and the release of powerful vasoactive amines that have their effect on vessels and smooth muscles. Although the role of mast-cell degranulation in allergic disease is not disputed, its precise *physiological* significance is still the subject of debate. Most likely, the mast-cell mediators are involved in the vascular changes that take place in the early stages of immunity.

A major component of the cellular immune system is its mode of communication through cytokines, particularly as regards the control of growth and differentiation of leukocytes, and inflammatory reactions (see Chapter 11). Cytokines not only participate in effector reactions but also in the initiation of cellular responses. Cytokines were first described by the finding that macrophages from guinea pigs sensitized to tuberculin were inhibited in their normal patterns of migration in culture when tuberculin was added (55,146). The significance of this assay was not understood, but the observations pointed out for the first time that lymphocytes secreted molecules other than antigen-specific antibody molecules (14,34). Migration inhibitory factor was initially difficult to define chemically, and its presence was under some dispute until its molecular cloning (184). However, soon other biological activities were identified. The first activity on lymphocytes was the lymphocyte-activating factor, now named *IL-1* (58), and the T-cell growth factor, now named *IL-2* (59,129). The number of cytokines operating in the immune system is large, with close to 20 molecules identified and cloned, each with specific receptors. The development of the cytokine field was highly dependent on molecular biological approaches that allowed the cloning of powerful biologically active proteins found in trace amounts in body fluids.

Cytokines are usually produced by more than one cell and their mechanism of action is pleiotropic; and most likely, they play a major role in the entire immune response. For example, their role from a distance alerts the entire individual to an antigen challenge. Thus, the early cytokines like IL-1, tumor necrosis factor (TNF), and IL-6, program the acute phase response in which liver cells release particular sets of protein and the central nervous system responds by fever and by the release of some key hormones. At the local level, cytokines program the reorganization of the tissue during inflammation, including the margination and entry of leukocytes, and they regulate individual cellular activities. The present challenge is to integrate and examine critically how each cytokine operates, in what form and how they are triggered and regulated. In vivo the issues of integrating the cascade of cytokines will be more difficult to assess. But the scenario is set up by the uses of gene ablation approaches or of transgenic mice expressing a given cytokine gene, or by employing neutralizing monoclonal antibodies. These approaches used in a judicious way should resolve the mechanisms of action of cytokines and their biological relevance. The identity of cytokine-producing cells should be elucidated, in the nervous system.

Immunological diseases result from the aberrant or exaggerated interaction of the immune system with antigens of or in the host. From the pathogenetic point of view, several well-defined mechanisms operate in producing pathology. Many of these pathogenetic mechanisms were defined by clinical observations and later established in experimental models of disease. Particularly, the accelerated response to a second injection of antigen was noted by the early students of immunology to cause rapid, untoward reactions in the matter of minutes or days, depending on the type of antigen, amount and form given, route of inoculation, etc. Indeed, much of the current study of immunopathologies and immunological diseases centers on the four observations made by the pioneering studies carried out when immunology was defined as a field of biology. Koch defined the accelerated reaction to tuberculin in the infected guinea pig, which is in great part an accelerated delayed hypersensitivity reaction involving T cells and prominently figuring the activated macrophage (99). Portier and Richet identified anaphylaxis by experimenting on immunized dogs that were boosted with the poison of sea anemones (Richet was Nobel Laureate in 1911) (143). This work initiated decades of studies attempting to define anaphylaxis, the allergic responses, the biochemistry of anaphylactic antibodies, the cell biology of mast cells, and the chemistry of their granules. Indeed, most of the biochemical and cellular protagonists of the IgE-mediated responses have been defined, but a central question still remains. What are the clinical circumstances that lead to or regulate class switch to, and production of, IgE by an activated B cell?

The third set of immunopathologies were reported by Arthus and von Pirquet. Arthus studied the effects of multiple subcutaneous injection of antigen (4). He defined a hemorrhagic lesion, now known to be a local immune complex vasculitis. Von Pirquet reported on "serum disease" in individuals and later, in experimental animals, that was injected (Figs. 2-1, 2-2) systemically with a large bolus of foreign serum (179,

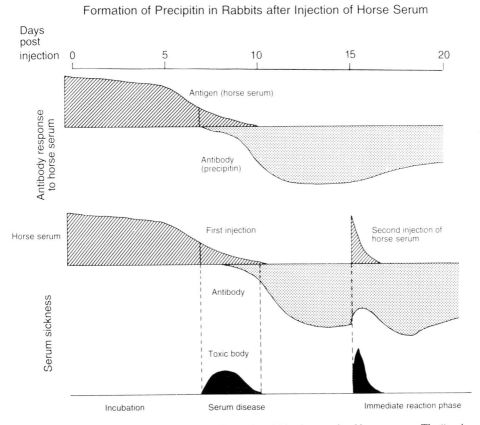

Fig. 2-1. von Pirquet's depiction of serum disease in rabbits that received horse serum. The "toxic body" refers to the antigen–antibody complexes. (From von Pirquet, C, Allergie, Munch Med Wochenschr 53:1457–1466, 1906 (179); Arch Intern Med 7:259–265, 1911 (180) with permission.)

Elimination of I^{131} Labeled BSA Relative to Antibody Response and Development of Lesions

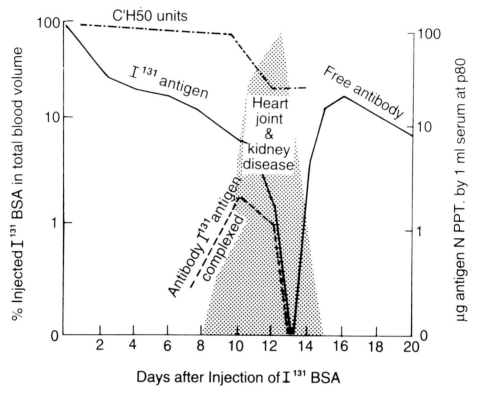

Fig. 2-2. The modern evaluation of von Pirquet's experiment in rabbits infected with a purified antigen (bovine albumin). Antigen–antibody complexes appear at the time of disease and prior to the presence of free antibody. (From Dixon, F J et al., Pathogenesis of serum sickness, AMA Arch Pathol 65:18–22, 1957 (36) with permission.)

180). Both investigators were defining immune complex disease, one of the best studied experimental models of diseases in which most of the steps have been defined: deposition of antigen–antibody complexes → activation of complement and other mediators → neutrophil attraction and degranulation → vascular derangement (36,56,79).

Immunological diseases also result from a genetic loss of key regulatory proteins and/or cells. Many of these diseases translate into immunodeficiencies studied primarily by pediatric immunologists. For example, genetic alterations of the β_2 integrins result in profound deficits in neutrophil and mass functions that translate into severe infections with pyogenic organisms (1). These unfortunate experiments of nature have yielded a wealth of information on how the immune system functions. In a way, they are the equivalent of the gene ablation experiments now beginning to be analyzed and which are revolutionizing our understanding of immunity.

Finally, concerning the nervous system, there is considerable debate over the process of T-cell recognition of antigen. Which cells express MHC molecules, how is this expression regulated, and where does antigen processing take place? Chapters 3 and 10 will address these questions.

Concluding Remarks

David Talmage, who has studied the immune system for a long time, speculated in his presidential address to the American Association of Immunologists in 1988, that the next growth area of immunology would be clinical (163). This certainly appears to be prophetic for the field of neuroimmunology. The extensive progress of the last two decades will indeed allow for a much better and rational understanding of immunological diseases. The expectation is that at last, the molecular and cellular basis of many will be known. The major hurdle will still be putting together all our information of cells and molecules of this complex, multicellular system, which has been so successfully analyzed by the reductionist approaches, into an operating whole. The basic challenge will clearly be to understand immune regulation. For example, in the nervous system, what exactly starts the process and how is it terminated? How are specific lymphocytes recruited to depots of antigen located behind a formidable blood-tissue barrier? How do the various APCs interact, and how is each lymphocyte subset operating in the nervous system's microenvironment? What is the regulatory role of idiotypes and anti-idiotypes? Is there a programmed cascade of cytokines, and which follows which? Are the immunological reactions of the nervous system similar to those in other tissues or are they governed by a unique set of rules? The reductionist approaches caused a revolution in immunology, enabling the identification of key molecules and cells. For example, there is no other cell in biology for which we have as much information on its membrane components as on the lymphocyte. More than 100 CD molecules are now identified. Holistic understanding of the immune system will result now, more than ever, from the tools of gene manipulation in the whole animal.

References

1. Anderson DC, Springer TA. Leukocyte adhesion deficiency—an inherited defect in the Mac-1, LFA-1 and p159,95 glycoproteins. Annu Rev Med 38:175–181, 1987.
2. Arnason BG, Jankovic BD, Waksman BH, Wennersten C. Role of the thymus in immune reactions in rats. II. Suppressive effect of thymectomy at birth on reactions of delayed (cellular) hypersensitivity and the circulating small lymphocyte. J Exp Med 116:177–185, 1962.
3. Arrhenius S. Immunochemistry. MacMillan, New York, 1907.
4. Arthus NM. Injection repetées de serum du cheval chez le lapin. CR Soc Biol Sciences Fil (Paris) 55:817, 1903.

5. Babbitt BP, Allen PM, Matsueda G, Haber E, Unanue ER. Binding of immunogenic peptides to Ia histocompatibility molecules. Nature 317:359–362, 1985.

6. Behring E von, Kitasato S. Über das Zustandekommen der Diphtherie-Immunität und der Tetanus-Immunität bei Thieren. Dtsch Med Wochenschr 16:1113–1119, 1890.

7. Benacerraf B. Role of MHC gene products in immune regulation. Science 212:1229–1231, 1981.

8. Benacerraf B, McDevitt HO. Histocompatibility-linked immune response genes. Science 175:273–275, 1972.

9. Benjamin DC, Berzofsky JA, East IJ, et al. The antigenic structure of proteins: a reappraisal. Annu Rev Immunol 2:67–101, 1984.

10. Bernard O, Hozumi N, Tonegawa S. Sequences of mouse immunoglobulin light chain genes before and after somatic changes. Cell 15:1133–1338, 1978.

11. Berzofsky JA, Berkower IJ. Immunogenicity and antigen structure. In: Fundamental Immunology, WE Paul, ed. Raven Press, New York, 1989, p. 169.

12. Billingham RE, Brent L, Medawar PB. Actively acquired tolerance of foreign cells. Nature 172:603–605, 1953.

13. Bjorkman PJ, Saper MA, Samraoui B, Bennett WS, Strominger JL, Wiley DC. The foreign antigen binding site and T cell recognition regions of class I histocompatibility antigens. Nature 329:512–515, 1987.

14. Bloom BR, Bennett B. Mechanism of a reaction in vitro associated with delayed-type hypersensitivity. Science 153:80–84, 1966.

15. Bordet J, Gengou O. Sur l'existence des substances sensililitrices dans la plupart des serums antimicrobiennes. Ann Inst. Pasteur 15:289–295, 1901.

16. Borel JF, Feurer C, Tubler HU, Stahelin H. Biological effects of cycosporin A—a new antilymphocytic agent. Agents Actions 6:468–472, 1976.

17. Borst J, Alexander S, Elder J, Terhorst C. The T3 complex on human T lymphocytes involves four structurally distinct glycoproteins. J Biol Chem 258:5135–5144, 1983.

18. Bretscher P, Cohn MO. A theory of self-nonself discrimination. Science 169:1042–1046, 1970.

19. Brown RK, Delaney R, Levine L, van Vorakis H. Studies on the antigenic structure of ribonuclease. J Biol Chem 234:2043–2051, 1959.

20. Bruton OC. Agammaglobulinemia. Pediatrics 9:722–731, 1952.

21. Buchmeier NA, Schreiber RD. Requirement of endogenous interferon-gamma production for resolution of Listeria monocytogenes infection. Proc Natl Acad Sci USA 82:7404–7408, 1985.

22. Buchner H. Ueber Bacteriengifte und Gegengifte. Munch Med Wochenschr. 40:449–455, 1893.

23. Burnet FM. The Clonal Selection Theory of Acquired Immunity. Cambridge University Press, London, 1959.

24. Burnet FM. Modification of Jerne's theory of antibody production using the concept of clonal selection. Aust J Sci 20:67–74, 1957.

25. Butcher E, Scollay R, Weissman I. Evidence of continuous evolutionary changes in structures mediating adherence of lymphocytes to specialized venules. Nature 280:496–499, 1979.

26. Cantor H, Boyse EA. Functional subclasses of T lymphocytes bearing different Ly antigens. I. The generation of functionally distinct T cell subclasses is a differentiative process independent of antigen. J Exp Med 141:1376–1389, 1975.

27. Chase MW. The cellular transfer of cutaneous hypersensitivity to tuberculin. Proc Soc Exp Biol Med 59:134–140, 1945.

28. Chien Y, Becker DM, Lindsten T, Okamura M, Cohen DI, Davis MM. A third type of murine T-cell receptor gene. Nature 312:31–33, 1984.
29. Claman HN, Chaperon EA, Triplett RF. Thymus-marrow cell combinations. Synergism in antibody production. Proc Soc Exp Biol Med 122:1167–1174, 1966.
30. Clerici M, Hakim FT, Venzon DJ, Blatt S, Hendrix CW, Wynn TA, Shearer GM. Changes in interleukin-2 and interleukin-4 production in asymptomatic human immunodeficiency virus–seropositive individuals. J Clin Invest 91:759–766, 1993.
31. Coons AH, Creech HJ, Jones RN. Immunological properties of an antibody containing a fluorescent group. Proc Soc Exp Biol Med 47:200–205, 1941.
32. Crosby AW. The Columbian Exchange: Biological and Cultural Consequences of 1492. Greenwood Press, Westport, Conn, 1972.
33. Dausset J. Leuco-agglutinins. Vox Sang 6:190–195, 1954.
34. David JR. Delayed hypersensitivity in vitro: its mediation by cell-free substances formed by lymphoid cell-antigen interaction. Proc Natl Acad Sci USA 56:72–76, 1966.
35. Davies AJS, Leuchars E, Wallis V, Marchant R, Elliott EV. The failure of thymus-derived cells to produce antibody. Transplantation 5:222–228, 1967.
36. Dixon FJ, Vazquez JJ, Weigle WO, Cochrane CG. Pathogenesis of serum sickness. AMA Arch Pathol 65:18–22, 1957.
37. Donath J, Landsteiner K. Über paroxysmale hemoglobinurie. Munch Med Wochenschr 51:1590–1597, 1904.
38. Dreyer WJ, Bennett JC. The molecular basis of antibody formation. Proc Natl Acad Sci USA 54:864–868, 1965.
39. Dustin ML, Springer TA. Role of lymphocyte adhesion receptors in transient interactions and cell locomotion. Annu Rev Immunol 9:27–35, 1991.
40. Duvall E, Wyllie AH. Death and the cell. Immunol Today 7:115–121, 1986.
41. Early P, Huang H, Davis M, Calame K, Hood L. An immunoglobulin heavy chain variable region gene is generated from three segments of DNA: VH, D and JH. Cell 19:981–989, 1980.
42. Edelman GM. Dissociation of γ-globulin. J Am Chem Soc 81:3155–3159, 1959.
43. Ehrlich P. Collected Studies in Immunity. Wiley, New York, 1905.
44. Ehrlich P. The Croonian lecture: on immunity with special reference to cell life. Proc R Soc Lond (Biol) 66:424–431, 1900.
45. Eisen HN, Siskind GW. Variations in affinities of antibodies during the immune response. Biochemistry 3:996–1002, 1964.
46. Felton LD. The significance of antigen in animal tissue. J Immunol 61:107–111, 1949.
47. Finn R, Clarke CA, Donohoe WTA, McConnell RB, Sheppard PM, Lehane D, Kulke W. Experimental studies on the prevention of Rh haemolytic disease. Br Med J 12:1486–1492, 1961.
48. Fiorentino DF, Zlotnick A, Vieira P, Mosman TR, Howard M, Moore K, O'Garra A. IL-10 acts on the antigen-presenting cell to inhibit cytokine production by Thl cells. J Immunol 146:3444–3452, 1991.
49. Freda VJ, Gorman JG, Pollack W. Successful prevention of sensitization with an experimental anti-Rh gamma globulin. Transfusion 4:26–30, 1964.
50. Freund J, McDermott K. Sensitization to horse serum by means of adjuvants. Proc Soc Exp Biol Med 49:548–553, 1942.
51. Freund J, Thompson GE, Lipton MM. Aspermatogenesis, anaphylaxis and cutaneous sensitization induced in the guinea pig by homologous testicular extract. J Exp Med 101:591–604, 1955.

52. Gearhart PJ, Johnson ND, Douglas R, Hood L. IgG antibodies to phosphorylcholine exhibit more diversity than their IgM counterpart. Nature 291:29–34, 1981.

53. Gell PGH, Benacerraf B. Delayed hypersensitivity to simple protein antigens. Adv Immunol 1:319–325, 1963.

54. Gell PGH, Benacerraf B. Studies on hypersensitivity to denatured proteins in guinea pigs. Immunology 2:64–70, 1959.

55. George M, Vaughan JH. In vitro cell migration as a model for delayed hypersensitivity. Proc Soc Exp Biol Med 111:514–520, 1962.

56. Germuth FG Jr, McKinnon GE. Studies on the biological properties of antigen-antibody complex. I. Anaphylactic shock induced by soluble antigen-antibody complexes in unsensitized guinea pigs. Bull Johns Hopkins Hosp 101:13–18, 1957.

57. Gershon RK. A disquisition on suppressor T cells. Transplant Rev 26:170–177, 1975.

58. Gery I, Gershon RK, Waksman BH. Potentiation of T-lymphocyte responses to mitogens. I. The responding cell. J Exp Med 136:128–133, 1972.

59. Gillis S, Smith KA. Long-term culture of cytotoxic T-lymphocytes. Nature 268:154–157, 1977.

60. Glick B, Chang TS, Jaap RG. The bursa of Fabricius and antibody production. Poul Sci 35:224–229, 1956.

61. Good RA, Dalmasso AO, Martinez C, Archer OK, Pierce JC, Papermaster BW. The role of the thymus in development of immunologic capacity in rabbits and mice. J Exp Med 116:773–779, 1962.

62. Goodman JW. Antigenic determinants and antibody combining sites. In: The Antigens, M Sela, ed, vol 3. Academic Press, New York, 1975, pp 127–187.

63. Goodnow CG, Crosbie J, Jorgensen H, Brink RA, Basten, A. Induction of self-tolerance in mature peripheral B lymphocytes. Nature 342:385–390, 1989.

64. Gorer PA. Antigenic basis of tumour transplantation. J Pathol Bacteriol 36:268–275, 1938.

65. Gorer PA. The detection of antigenic differences in mouse erythrocytes by the employment of immune sera. Br J Exp Pathol 17:42–49, 1936.

66. Gowans JL. The life history of lymphocytes. Br Med Bull 15:50–58, 1959.

67. Gowans JL. The recirculation of lymphocytes from blood to lymph in the rat. J Physiol 14:654–660, 1959.

68. Gowans JL, Knight, EJ. The route of recirculation of lymphocytes in the rat. Proc R Soc Lond Series B Biol Sci 159:257–264, 1964.

69. Gowans JL, McGregor DD, Cowen DM, Ford CE. Initiation of immune response by small lymphocytes. Nature 196:651–653, 1962.

70. Grundbacher FJ. Behring's discovery of diphtheria and tetanus antitoxins. Immunol Today 13:188–192, 1992.

71. Halet HR, Bonner WA, Barret J, Herzenberg LA. Cell sorting: automated separation of mammalian cells as a function of intracellular fluorescence. Science 166:747–748, 1969.

72. Hasek M. Parabiosis of birds during embryonic development. Cesk Biol 2:265–272, 1953.

73. Hedrick SM, Nielsen EA, Kavaler J, Cohen DI, Davis MM. Sequence relationships between putative T-cell receptor polypeptides and immunoglobulins. Nature 308:153–155, 1984.

74. Heidelberger M, Kendall FE. A quantitative study of the precipitin reaction between type III pneumococcus polysaccharide and purified homologous antibody. J Exp Med 50:809–817, 1929.

75. Heinzel FP, Sadick MD, Mutha SS, Locksley RM. Production of IFN-γ, IL-2, IL-4, and IL-10 by CD$^+$ lymphocytes in vivo during healing and progressive murine leishmaniasis. Proc Natl Acad Sci USA 88:77011–77016, 1991.

76. Hengartner H, Odermatt B, Schneider R, Schreyer M, Walle G, MacDonald HR, Zinkernagel RM. Deletion of self-reactive T cells before entry into the thymus medulla. Nature 336:388–393, 1988.

77. Herman A, Kappler JW, Marrack P, Pullen AM. Superantigens: mechanisms of T-cell stimulation and role in immune responses. Annu Rev Immunol 9:745–756, 1992.

78. Howard M, Paul WE. Regulation of B-cell growth and differentiation by soluble factors. Annu Rev Immunol 1:307–314, 1983.

79. Humphrey JH. The mechanism of Arthus reactions. I. The role of polymorphonuclear leucocytes and other factors in reversed passive Arthus reactions in rabbits. Br J Exp Pathol 36:268–275, 1955.

80. Humphrey JH. Serendipity in immunology. Annu Rev Immunol 2:1–12, 1984.

81. Humphrey JH, Grennan D. Different macrophage populations distinguished by means of fluorescent polysacchrides. Recognition and properties of marginal-zone macrophages. Eur J Immunol 11:221–230, 1981.

82. Humphrey JH, Parrot DMV, East J. Studies on globulin and antibody responses in mice thymectomized at birth. Immunology 7:419–422, 1964.

83. Ishizaka K, Ishizaka T, Hornbrook MJ. Physiocochemical properties of human reaginic antibody. V. Correlation of reaginic activity with γE globulin antibody. Immunology 97:840–847, 1966.

84. Jenner E. An Inquiry into the Causes and Effects of the Variolae Vaccinae, a Disease Discovered in Some of the Western Counties of England, Particularly Gloucestershire, and Known by the Name of the Cow Pox. Sampson Low, Soho, London, 1798.

85. Jerne NK. The natural-selection theory of antibody formation. Proc Natl Acad Sci USA 41:849–855, 1955.

86. Kabat EA. Structural Concepts in Immunology and Immunochemistry, 2nd ed. Holt, Rinehart and Winston, New York, 1976.

87. Kabat EA. The upper limit for the size of the human antidextran combining site. J Immunol 84:82–88, 1960.

88. Kabat EA, Mayer MM, ed. Experimental Immunochemistry. CC Thomas, Springfield, Ill, 1948.

89. Kabat EA, Wolf A, Bezer AE. The rapid production of acute disseminated encephalomyelitis in rhesus monkeys by injection of heterologous and homologous brain tissue with adjuvants. J Exp Med 85:117–125, 1947.

90. Kappler JW, Roehm N, Marrack P. T cell tolerance by clonal elimination in the thymus. Cell 49:273–280, 1987.

91. Kappler JW, Wade T, White J, Kushnir E, Blackman M, Bill J, Roehm N, Marrack P. A T cell receptor Vβ segment that imparts reactivity to a class II major histocompatibility complex product. Cell 49:263–271, 1987.

92. Karnovsky ML, Lazdins JK. Biochemical criteria for activated macrophages. J Immunol 121:809–814, 1978.

93. Katz DH, Hamaoka T, Dorf ME, Maurer PH, Benacerraf B. Cell interactions between histoincompatible T and B lymphocytes. IV. Involvement of immune response (Ir) gene control of lymphocyte interaction controlled by the gene. J Exp Med 138:734–740, 1973.

94. Kiessling R, Petranyi G, Klein G, Wigzell H. Non-T-cell resistance against a mouse Moloney lymphoma. Int J Cancer 17:1–7, 1976.

95. Kindred B, Shreffler DC. H-2 dependence of co-operation between T and B cells in vivo. J Immunol 109:940–947, 1972.

96. Kisielow P, Bluthman H, Staerz UD, Steinmetz M, von Boehmer H. Tolerance in T cell

receptor transgenic mice involves deletion of nonmature CD4$^+$8$^+$ thymocytes. Nature 333:742–747, 1988.

97. Klein J, Satta Y, O'Huigin C. The molecular descent of the major histocompatibility complex. Annu Rev Immunol 11:269–278, 1993.

98. Klein J, Takahata N. The major histocompatibility complex and the quest for origins. Immunol Rev 113:5–27, 1990.

99. Koch R. Fortsetzung der Mitteilungen über ein Heilmittel gegen Tuberkulose. Dtsch Med Wochenstr 9:101–108, 1891.

100. Kocks C, Rajewsky K. Stable expression and somatic hypermutation of antibody regions in B cell developmental pathways. Annu Rev Immunol 7:537–549, 1989.

101. Kohler G, Milstein C. Continuous culture of fused cells secreting antibody of predefined specificity. Nature 256:495–497, 1975.

102. Krych M, Atkinson JP, Holers VM. Complement receptors. Curr Opin Immunol 4:8–12, 1992.

103. Kunkel HG, Slater RJ, Good, RA. Relation between certain myeloma proteins and normal gamma globulin. Proc Soc Exp Bill Med 76:190–195, 1951.

104. Lamb JR, Feldmann M. Essential requirement for major histocompatibility complex recognition in T cell tolerance induction. Nature 308:72–74, 1984.

105. Landsteiner K. The Specificity of Serological Reactions, Rev ed. Harvard University Press, Cambridge, Mass, 1945.

106. Landsteiner K, Chase MW. Experiments on transfer of cutaneous sensitivity to simple compounds. Proc Soc Exp Biol Med 49:688–692, 1942.

107. Levine BB, Ojeda A, Benacerraf B. Studies on artificial antigens. III. The genetic control of the immune response to hapten poly-L-lysine conjugates in guinea pigs. J Exp Med 118:953–58, 1963.

108. Levine P. The protective action of ABO incompatibility on Rh isoimmunization and Rh hemolytic disease—theoretical and clinical implications. Am J Hum Genet 11:418–425, 1959.

109. Linsley PS, Clark EA, Ledbetter JA. T cell activation antigen CD28 mediates adhesion with B cells by interacting with activation antigen B7/BB1. Proc Natl Aca Sci USA 87:5031–5041, 1990.

110. Lurie MB. Resistance to tuberculosis: experimental studies in native and acquired defensive mechanisms. Cambridge, Mass, Harvard University Press, 1964.

111. MacDonald HR, Schneider R, Lees RK, Howe RC, Acha-Orbea H, Festenstein H, Zinkernagel RM, Hengartner H. T-cell receptor Vb use predicts reactivity and tolerance to Mls^a-encoded antigens. Nature 332:40–43, 1988.

112. Mackaness GB. The immunology of antituberculosis immunity. Am Rev Respir Dis 97:337–342, 1968.

113. Marchesi VT, Gowans JL. The migration of lymphocytes through the endothelium of venules in lymph nodes—an electron microscopic study. Proc R Soc Lond Series B Biol Sci 159:283–290, 1964.

114. Marrack JR. The chemistry of antigens and antibodies. Special Report Series No. 194. Medical Research Council, London, 1934.

115. McDevitt HO, Chinitz A. Genetic control of the antibody response: relationship between immune response and histocompatibility (H-2) type. Science 163:1207–1210, 1969.

116. McDevitt HO, Sela M. Genetic control of the antibody response. I. Demonstration of determinant-specific differences in response to synthetic polypeptide antigens in two strains of inbred mice. J Exp Med 122:517–524, 1965.

117. Metchnikoff E. Lectures on the Comparative Pathology of Inflammation, 1893. Reprinted by Dover Publications, New York, 1968.

118. Meuer SC, Acuto O, Hussey RE, Hodgdon JC, Fitzgerald KA, Schlossman SF, Reinherz EL. Evidence for the T3-associated 90K heterodimer as the T-cell antigen receptor. Nature 303:808–810, 1983.

119. Meuer SC, Fitzgerald KA, Hussey RE, Hodgen JC, Schlossman SF, Reinherz EL. Clonotypic structures involved in antigen specific human T cell function: relationship to the T3 molecular complex. J Exp Med 157:705–710, 1983.

120. Meuer SC, Schlossman SF, Reinherz E. Clonal analysis of human cytotoxic T lymphocytes: T4+ and T8+ effector T cells recognize products of different major histocompatibility complex regions. Proc Natl Acad Sci USA 79:4395–4399, 1982.

121. Miller JFAP. Effect of thymectomy on the immunological responsiveness of the mouse. Proc R Soc Lond Ser B Biol Sci 156:415–422, 1962.

122. Miller JFAP. Immunological function of the thymus. Lancet 2:748–751, 1961.

123. Miller JFAP, Mitchell GM. Cell to cell interaction in the immune response. I. Hemolysin-forming cells in neonatally thymectomized mice reconstituted with thymus or thoracic duct lymphocytes. J Exp Med 128:801–810, 1968.

124. Mishell RI, Dutton RW. Immunization of normal mouse spleen cells suspensions in vitro. Science 153:1004–1007, 1966.

125. Mitchell GM, Miller JFAP. Cell to cell interaction in the immune response. II. The source of hemolysin-forming cells in irradiated mice given bone marrow and thymus or thoracic duct lymphocytes. J Exp Med 128:821–832, 1968.

126. Mitchell GM, Miller JFAP. Immunological activity of thymus and thoracic duct lymphocytes. Proc Natl Acad Sci USA 59:296–301, 1968.

127. Mitchison NA. The carrier effect in the secondary response to hapten-protein conjugates. II. Cellular cooperation. Eur J Immunol 1:18–24, 1971.

128. Moller G. Transgenic Mice and Immunological Tolerance, Immun Rev 122:204–213, 1991.

129. Morgan DA, Ruscetti FW, Gallo RC. Selective in vitro growth of T lymphocytes from normal human bone marrow. Science 193:1007–1010, 1976.

130. Mosman TR, Cherwinski H, Bond M, Giedlin MA, Coffman RL. Two types of murine helper T cells clones. 1. Definition according to profiles of lymphokine activities and secreted proteins. J Immunol 136:2348–2352, 1986.

131. Mueller DL, Jenkins MK, Schwartz RH. Clonal expansion versus functional clonal inactivation—a costimulatory signalling pathway determines the outcome of T cell antigen receptor occupancy. Annu Rev Immunol 7:445–459, 1989.

132. Nemazee D, Burki K. Clonal deletion of B lymphocytes in a transgenic mouse bearing anti-MHC class I antibody genes. Nature 337:562–564, 1989.

133. Nossal GJV, Ada GL. Antigens, Lymphoid Cells, and the Immune System. Academic Press, 1971.

134. Nowell PC. Phytohemagglutinin: an initiator of mitosis in cultures of normal human leucocytes. Cancer Res 20:462–469, 1960.

135. Nunez G, London L, Hockenbery D, Alexander M, McKearn JP, Korsmeyer SJ. Deregulated bcl-2 gene expression selectively prolongs survival of growth factor-deprived hemopoietic cell lines. J Immunol 144:3602–3606, 1990.

136. Ovary Z, Benacerraf B. Immunological specificity of the secondary response to dinitrophenylated proteins. Proc Soc Exp Biol Med 114:72–77, 1963.

137. Owen RD. Immunogenetic consequences of vascular anastomoses between bovine twins. Science 102:400–404, 1945.

138. Pasteur L. De l'attenuation du virus du cholera des poules. C R Acad Sci (Paris) 91:673–680, 1880.

139. Pasteur L. Methode pour prevenir la rage apres morsure. C R Acad Sci (Paris) 101:765–770, 1885.

140. Payne R. Leukocyte agglutinins in human sera. Arch Intern Med 99:587–594, 1957.

141. Pernis B, Forni L, Amante L. Immunoglobulin spots on the surface of rabbit lymphocytes. J Exp Med 132:1001–1009, 1970.

142. Porter RR. The hydrolysis of rabbit γ-globulin and antibodies with crystalline papain. Biochem J 73:119–125, 1959.

143. Portier P, Richet C. De l'action anaphylactique de certain venims. C R Soc Biol 54:170–177, 1902.

144. Raff MC, Sternberg M, Taylor RB. Immunoglobulin determinants on the surface of mouse lymphoid cells. Nature 225:553–562, 1970.

145. Ravetch JV, Kinet J-P. Fc receptors. Annu Rev Immunol 9:457–466, 1991.

146. Rich AR, Lewis MR. The nature of allergy in tuberculosis as revealed by tissue culture studies. Bull Johns Hopkins Hosp 50:115–117, 1932.

147. Rivers TM, Sprent DH, Berry GP. Observations on attempts to product acute disseminated encephalomyelitis in monkeys. J Exp Med 58:39–45, 1933.

148. Roitt IM, Doniach D, Campbell R, Hudson RV. Autoantibodies in Hashimoto's disease (lymphadenoid goitre). Lancet 2:820–824, 1956.

149. Rose NR, Witebsky E. Studies on organ specificity V. Changes in the thyroid gland of rabbits following active immunization with rabbit extract. J Immunol 76:417–422, 1956.

150. Rosenthal AS, Shevach EM. Function of macrophages in antigen recognition by guinea pig T lymphocytes. J Exp Med 138:1194–1199, 1973.

151. Saito H, Kranz D, Takagai Y, Hayday A, Eisen H, Tonegawa S. A third rearranged and expressed gene in a clone of cytotoxic T lymphocytes. Nature 312:36–42, 1984.

152. Samelson LE, Harford HB, Klausner RD. Identification of the components of the murine T cell antigen receptor complex. Cell 43:223–230, 1985.

153. Seidman JG, Leder A, Nau M, Norman B, Leder P. The structure of cloned immunoglobulin genes suggests a mechanism for generating new sequences. Science 202:11–15, 1978.

154. Sela M. Antigenicity: some molecular aspects. Science 166:1365, 1969.

155. Sell S, Gell PGH. Studies on rabbit lymphocyte in vitro. I. Stimulation of blast transformation with an anti-allotype serum. J Exp Med 122:483–490, 1965.

156. Sha WC, Nelson CA, Newberry RD, Kranz DM, Russell JH, Loh DY. Positive and negative selection of an antigen receptor on T cells in transgenic mice. Nature 336:73–77, 1988.

157. Silverstein AM. A history of immunology. Academic Press, New York, 1989.

158. Siskind GW, Benacerraf B. Cell selection by antigen in the immune response. Adv Immunol 10:1–10, 1969.

159. Snell GD. Methods for the study of histocompatibility genes. J Genet 49:87–93, 1948.

160. Stamper HB Jr, Woodruff JJ. Lymphocytes homing into lymph nodes—in vitro demonstration of the selective affinity of recirculating lymphocytes for high endothelial venules. J Exp Med 144:828–834, 1976.

161. Steeg PS, Moore RN, Johnson HM, Oppenheim JJ. Regulation of murine Ia antigen expression by a lymphokine with immune interferon activity. J Exp Med 156:1780–1786, 1982.

162. Swain SL. Significance of Lyt phenotypes: Lyt 2 antibodies block activities of T cells that recognize class I major histocompatibility complex antigens regardless of their function. Proc Natl Acad Sci USA 78:7101–7109, 1981.

163. Talmage DW. A century of progress: beyond molecular immunology. J Immunol 141:S5–S16, 1988.

164. Talmage DW. Immunological specificity. Science 129:1643–1646, 1959.
165. Terasaki PI, ed. History of transplantation—thirty-five recollections. UCLA Tissue Typing Lab, Los Angeles, 1991.
166. Tiselius A, Kabat EA. An electrophoretic study of immune sera and purified antibody. J Exp Med 69:119–130, 1939.
167. Tomasi TB, Tan EM, Salomon A, Prendergast RA. Characteristics of an immune system common to certain external secretions. J Exp Med 121:101–110, 1965.
168. Tonegawa S, Brack C, Hozumi N, Schuller R. Cloning of an immunoglobulin variable region gene from mouse embryo. Proc Natl Acad Sci USA 74:3518–3524, 1977.
169. Tonegawa S, Maxam AM, Tizard R, Bernard O, Gilbert W. Sequence of a mouse germline gene for a variable region of an immunoglobulin light chain. Proc Natl Acad Sci USA 75:1485–1489, 1978.
170. Uhr JW, Bauman JB. Antibody formation. I. The suppression of antibody formation by passively administered antibody J Exp Med 113:935–940, 1961.
171. Uhr JW, Moller G. Regulatory effect of antibodies on the immune response. Adv Immunol 8:81–89, 1968.
172. Unanue ER. Antigen-presenting function of the macrophage. Annu Rev Immunol 1:395–405, 1984.
173. Unanue ER. The regulatory role of macrophages in antigenic stimulation. Part two: symbiotic relationship between lymphocytes and macrophages. Adv Immunol 31:1–7, 1981.
174. van Loghem JJ, van der Hart M, Hijmans W, Schuit HRE. The incidence and significance of complete and incomplete white cell antibodies with special reference to the use of the Coombs consumption test. Vox Sang 3:203–212, 1958.
175. van Rood JJ, Eernisse JG, van Leeuwen A. Leukocyte antibodies in sera from pregnant women. Nature 181:1735–1736, 1958.
176. Vaux DL, Cory S, Adams JM. Bcl-2 gene promotes hemopoietic cell survival and cooperates with c-myc to immortalize pre-B cells. Nature 335:440–443, 1988.
177. Vitetta ES, Baur S, Uhr JW. Cell surface immunoglobulin. II. Isolation and characterization of immunoglobulin from mouse splenic lymphocytes. J Exp Med 134:242–249, 1971.
178. Vitetta ES, Wu JW. Immunotoxins. Annu Rev Immunol 3:197–205, 1985.
179. von Pirquet C. Allergie. Munch Med Wochenschr 53:1457–1466, 1906.
180. von Pirquet C. Allergie. Arch Intern Med 7:259–265, 1911.
181. Warner NL, Szenberg A, Burnet FM. The immunological role of different lymphoid organs in the chicken. I. Dissociation of immunological responsiveness. Aust J Exp Biol Med Sci 40:373–380, 1962.
182. Watanabe-Fukunaga R, Brannan CI, Copeland NG, Jenkins NA, Nagata S. Lymphoproliferation disorder in mice explained by defects in fas antigen that mediates apoptosis. Nature 356:314–316, 1992.
183. Weigert MG, Cesari IM, Yonkovich SJ, Cohn M. Variability in the lambda light chain sequences of mouse antibodies. Nature 228:1045–1049, 1970.
184. Weiser WY, Temple PA, Witek-Giannotti JS, Remold HG, Clark SC, David JR. Molecular cloning of a cDNA encoding a human macrophage migration inhibitory factor. Proc Natl Acad Sci USA 86:7522–7527, 1989.
185. White J, Herman A, Pullen AM, Kubo R, Kappler J, Marrack P. The V_b-specific superantigen Staphylococcal enterotoxin B: stimulation of mature T cells and clonal deletion in neonatal mice. Cell 56:27–35, 1989.
186. Wilson R, Miller J, Storb U. Rearrangements of immunoglobulin genes. Biochemistry 18:5913–5918, 1979.

187. Winter G, Ward S. Antibody Engineering in Clinical Aspects of Immunology, Lachmann PJ, Peters K, Rosen FS, Walport MJ, eds. Blackwell Scientific Publishers, Boston, 1993, p 817.

188. Witebsky E, Rose NR, Kerplan K, Egan RW. Chronic thyroiditis and autoimmunization. JAMA 164:1439–1444, 1957.

189. Woodruff JJ, Clarke LM. Specific cell-adhesion mechanisms determining migration pathways of recirculating lymphocytes. Annu Rev Immunol 5:201–207, 1987.

190. Wright AE, Douglas SR. An experimental investigation of the role of the blood fluids in connection with phagocytosis. Proc R Soc Lond Series B 72:364–374, 1903.

191. Yamamura M, Uyemura K, Deans RJ, Weinberg K, Rea TH, Bloom BR, Modlin RL. Defining protective responses to pathogens—cytokine profiles in leprosy lesions. Science 254:277–281, 1992.

192. Yanagi Y, Yoshikai Y, Leggett K, Clark SP, Aleksander I, Mak TW. A human T cell-specific cDNA clone encodes a protein having extensive homology to immunoglobulin chains. Nature 308:145–149, 1984.

193. Ziegler K, Unanue ER. Decrease in macrophage antigen catabolism by ammonia and chloroquine is association with inhibition of antigen presentation to T cells. Proc Acad Sci USA 78:175–180, 1982.

194. Zinkernagel RM, Doherty PC. Activity of sensitized thymus-derived lymphocytes in lymphocytic choriomeningitis reflects immunological surveillance against altered self components. Nature 251:547–552, 1974.

195. Zinkernagel RM, Doherty PC. Restriction of in vitro T cell-mediated cytotoxicity in lymphocytic choriomeningitis within a syngeneic or semiallogeneic system. Nature 248:701–704, 1974.

3

Immunologic Principles Related to the Nervous System and the Eye: Concerning the Existence of a Neural-Ocular Immune System

J. WAYNE STREILEIN
ANDREW W. TAYLOR

In order to protect the vertebrate host from invasion and infection by the enormous diversity of potentially pathogenic microorganisms that inhabit the earth's surface, the immune system has evolved *(a)* two extraordinarily diverse sets of antigen-specific receptors for use by T and B lymphocytes, and *(b)* a diverse set of effector modalities with functionally distinct properties. The generic mechanisms by which the immune response is mounted and directed at exogenous pathogens are described in the previous chapter. The need for the immune system to produce more than one type of effector modality derives in part from the fact that microbial pathogens that invade the host via the skin utilize different molecular mechanisms than those of organisms that invade surfaces lined by mucous membranes. Not surprisingly, the effector mechanisms that protect the skin differ from the effector mechanisms that protect the gastrointestinal tract. Another reason for the creation of functionally distinct effector modalities is the diversity of cellular and molecular mechanisms by which different microorganisms establish productive infections and cause disease in various organs and tissues. From these considerations it is obvious that only a subset of the immune effector modalities may actually be appropriate for any particular pathogen in any particular tissue.

Many years ago it was realized that not all immune effectors produced in response to an antigenic challenge provide a similar level of protection. For example, protection against infections by certain pathogens (mycobacterium tuberculosis, leishmania) is mediated primarily by T cells that effect delayed hypersensitivity (DH). In fact, specific antibodies directed at antigens expressed on pathogens can often interfere with T-cell mediated protection (21,51). The reverse situation has also been described wherein antibodies are chiefly responsible for providing immune protection, whereas

effector T cells are at best irrelevant, and at worst capable of causing immunopathogenic disease that aggravates the morbidity of the infection (159). From these
considerations it is apparent that the immune system's response to any particular
infectious agent can and must be regulated in order to provide adequate protection
without immunogenic toxicity at the local tissue level.

These issues are crucially important to keep in mind when immunology of the
nervous system—the brain, eyes, and peripheral nerves—is considered. Each of these
components of the neural-ocular system resides behind a specialized set of tissue
barriers that limit the exchange, both ingress and egress, of molecules and cells with the
systemic circulation and therefore, with the remainder of the body. Many reasons have
been advanced to explain the need for the special anatomic arrangements that separate
the neural-ocular system from the rest of the body, and it is beyond the scope of this
chapter to describe these reasons. However, with respect to the goals and content of this
book, one reason that the neural-ocular system exists behind a set of barriers is that
accessibility of immune effectors to the nervous compartments of the body must be
highly regulated. To this end, certain immune effectors, such as complement-fixing
antibodies and T cells that mediate DH, eliminate target organisms by evoking an
intense local inflammatory response. During this process, the competency of the local
vascular bed is compromised, and inflammatory cells and molecules are recruited from
the systemic circulation. These agents of host defense can have a detrimental effect on
the proper biologic functions of the cells and tissues that comprise the neural-ocular
system. It has been speculated that in order to prevent disruption of brain function, it
has been necessary for the brain and other neural tissues to develop strategies for
influencing immune responses qualitatively. The presumed goal of these strategies is to
obtain immune protection that is not deleterious to the aggregate functions of neural-
ocular tissues. This chapter, as well as subsequent chapters on immunology of the eye
and CNS immunosuppression, emphasize this aspect of immunity in the neural-ocular
system.

The Concept of Regional Specialization in Immune Responses

To understand the unique features of immunity within the neural-ocular system, it is
informative to introduce the concept of regional specialization of immune responses,
and to review the specializations that are characteristic of immunity that is fashioned
for other non-neural organs and tissues: the mucosal surfaces and the skin (116).

The theory upon which the concept of regional specialization of immune responses
is based begins with the realizations that (a) the uniqueness of distinct organs and
tissues extends to the range of pathogens to which each is vulnerable, and (b) different
organs and tissues are differentially vulnerable to the injurious side effects of immune-
mediated protection. In order to accommodate these differences, the generic immune

response is subject to tissue-specific modifications that provide protection against pathogens of significance by immune mediators that are consistent with, and not deleterious to, the function of the tissue in question.

Features of Specialized Immune Responses

As in all immune responses to exogenous antigens, the elements that are required for specialized immune responses within a particular organ or tissue include *(a)* antigen-presenting cells (APC), *(b)* antigen-specific lymphocytes, and *(c)* access via lymph and blood vasculature to *(d)* an organized lymphoid tissue (such as lymph node or spleen) where immune recognition, and differentiation leading to the generation of specific effectors, takes place. In addition, *(e)* the parenchymal cells that carry out the differentiated function of a particular tissue or organ create a unique microenvironment by virtue of cytokines and other mediators that they constitutively release (see Table 3-1). In large measure, it is the quality of this microenvironment that dictates the specialized fashion in which antigens are detected, recognized, and eliminated by specific immune effectors in different regions of the body. Each component of regional immune responses will be considered briefly in this section.

Tissue-Restricted APC

It is generally believed that the initial encounter between naive antigen-specific lymphocytes and a new antigen *that leads to specific sensitization* takes place within lymph nodes and/or spleen—not within the parenchyma or stroma of nonlymphoid organs. Therefore, antigen must flow or be carried from the tissue site of introduction to a draining lymphoid organ. In the case of particulate antigens, such as bacteria, the particles may be carried by lymph flow directly to the node, or they may first be

Table 3-1 Components of Regional Specializations of the Immune Response

Regionally distributed APC
Selective tisue-specific lymphocyte homing
Exit pathway for afferent immunogenic signals
Entry route for immune effector modalities
Regional lymphoid organ/compartment
Unique regionally specific microenvironment that regulates induction and expression of immunity

phagocytized by local macrophages and then carried to the node. Soluble antigens or antigenic membrane fragments are thought to be delivered to the draining lymph node primarily by APC, rather than by simple diffusion (78,89). Accordingly, most if not all nonlymphoid organs and tissues contain a population of bone marrow-derived cells of the dendritic cell lineage (113). These cells are found within the stroma and connective tissue, and even adjacent to and among parenchymal cells (73). These cells are capable of endocytosis, constitutively express both class I and class II major histocompatibility complex (MHC) molecules, and are therefore equipped to deliver antigen-specific, MHC-restricted signals to naive T cells. Dendritic cells also display cell surface molecules (such as intercellular adhesion molecule-1 [ICAM-1]) and can secrete cytokines (such as interleukin 1β [IL-1β]) that convey accessory signals required for effective T-cell priming (84). The mobility of dendritic cells insures that delivery of their antigenic signals to T cells takes place in appropriate compartments provided by the deep cortex of the lymph node. From this interaction an array of antigen-specific immune effectors emerges and disseminates systemically.

Resident APC also play an important role during the expression of T-cell mediated immunity in somatic tissues. Once again, the effectiveness with which antigens are presented locally is dictated by cytokines and other mediators that exist within the local microenvironment. Moreover, antigen-activated effector lymphocytes secrete lymphokines into the local environment, and these in turn can endow local parenchymal cells with antigen-presenting capabilities, thereby amplifying the level of T-cell activation. However, responding lymphocytes within a tissue are *also* susceptible to the pharmacologic effects of tissue-derived cytokines and mediators. Therefore, the tissue-restricted microenvironment can reciprocally regulate and modify T-cell function during the expression of immunity.

Tissue-tropic Lymphocytes

Recirculating lymphocytes have the potential of leaving the blood stream and entering somatic tissues by several different mechanisms (20). In the first, the relatively passive process of diapedesis permits small numbers of circulating leukocytes to penetrate through fenestrations of capillaries and postcapillary venules of normal tissues and organs. During inflammatory responses, this process is considerably amplified, and large numbers of circulating cells are permitted to escape into extravascular tissue spaces. As inflammation proceeds, endothelial cells express novel cell surface molecules that serve as coreceptors for cell adhesion molecules expressed on circulating leukocytes. Interactions between these molecules markedly enhance the adherence of blood cells to the endothelial surfaces and lead to transmigration of the cells across the vessel wall into the extravascular compartment.

The field of lymphocyte ecotaxis has blossomed over the past few years. A more detailed consideration of recent findings pertinent to immunity in the nervous system is included in Chapter 4. At this point in time, it is by no means clear that the full range of cell adhesion molecule–ligand interactions that influence lymphocyte migration has been described. It is known that subsets of lymphocytes use unique receptors to enter the lymphoid tissues that drain the mucosal surfaces (20), and that a different set of receptors guide other lymphocyte subsets into the lymph nodes that drain the integument. In addition, some circulating lymphocytes display an affinity for the vessels of the skin (at least for inflamed skin), indicating that tissue-tropism of lymphocytes may be highly selective and organ-specific (11). It remains to be determined whether other tissues, including the neural-ocular system, are represented by unique, tissue-specific receptor–ligand interactions that promote the immigration of subsets of lymphocytes.

The manner is not known by which lymphocytes acquire cell surface molecules that confer upon them tissue-tropism. One view is that as mature, naive lymphocytes are generated, they are not equipped with any particular tissue-tropism. According to this view, the acquisition of tissue-tropism is "imprinted" (in some manner) upon cells that recognize and respond to antigens derived from a particular organ or tissue. Thus, lymphocytes that eventually display "skin-seeking" properties may have acquired these properties during their initial encounter with antigen(s) from skin. The alternative view is that tissue-tropism is conferred upon lymphocytes during their ontogenetic development and that expression of this genetic program is triggered by an encounter with antigen in a particular organ or tissue. While it is apparent that the phenomenon of tissue-tropism is likely to play an important role in the expression of immunity in a particular organ or tissue, it is not clear that the phenomenon is important during the induction of immunity to antigens first introduced through a particular organ or tissue. It is possible (some would say likely) that T and B lymphocytes exist in adult individuals that have a unique affinity for the endothelial cells of vessels in the central nervous system, the eye, and/or the brain. Evidence in favor of this possibility has yet to be produced.

Tissue-serving Vascular Networks

With respect to the concept of regional immunity, the supporting vasculature must accomplish two rather different tasks. In the first, new antigen introduced for the first time into the body must be carried from the site of introduction to a draining lymphoid organ where it can be presented to naive, antigen-specific T and B lymphocytes. This pathway represents the afferent arm of the immune reflex arc. In the second, when antigen is reintroduced into an already sensitized individual, immune effectors must be delivered via the blood to the site of antigen introduction. This pathway represents the efferent arm of the immune reflex arc.

Consider first the afferent limb. The parenchyma and connective tissue stroma of most tissues and organs of the body are elaborately supplied with lymphatic channels. When antigens are introduced (or arise within) these sites, the local lymphatic vessels serve as conduits that deliver antigen and/or antigen-bearing cells (APC) to the draining lymph nodes—an essential step in the induction of immunity. However, not all tissues possess such elaborate lymphatic drainage pathways. The central and peripheral nervous systems, as well as the eye, belong to this latter category. Although this is a somewhat controversial subject, we will take the liberty of presenting our own synthesis of the relevant experimental evidence. Under most conditions, the extracellular fluids of the internal compartments of the eye, and most (but not all!) portions of the brain do not escape the organ via lymphatics, or they do so at a very slow rate (12,27). Instead, bulk flow of extracellular fluid from the eye passes through specialized filtering devices directly into the blood. In the case of the brain, the arachnoid villae serve the filtering function, whereas in the eye, this function is provided by the trabecular meshwork. As a consequence of these specialized anatomic and vascular considerations, the major lymphoid organ for antigenic materials derived from the eye and brain is the spleen, whereas for most other somatic tissues, lymph nodes receive virtually all organ-derived antigenic signals.

For all tissues of the body, immune effectors designed to eliminate antigen are delivered to the antigen-containing site via the blood. In order to accomplish this task, the microvasculature is able to adopt a variety of phenotypic properties, depending upon which tissue or organ it supplies. The most obvious example of this principle is the specialized blood-tissue barrier properties that distinguish fenestrated vessels of the skin from the nonfenestrated vessels of the brain and the eye (14,33). Microvessels, especially postcapillary venules, have the capacity to respond to factors elaborated by lymphocytes, macrophages, mast cells and other stromal cells, factors that promote local inflammation. This capacity results from the ability of endothelial cells of vessels of this type to respond to factors by contracting their cytologic margins, thereby widening the effective pore size for cells and molecules to diffuse from the lumen into the extracellular space. Of perhaps more importance is the ability of stimulated endothelial cells to display several different types of ligands for complementary leukocyte cell adhesion molecules (47), the net result of which is promotion of migration of activated lymphocytes and other leukocytes across the lumen into the extravascular space. In this manner, "tissue-seeking" lymphocytes are recruited to the site, along with macrophages and other leukocytes that can be incorporated into the developing inflammatory response. It is of interest that not all microvessels possess these properties, or at least they resist undergoing these changes until the stimulus is severe or extreme. The vessels of the brain and eye fit this latter description (47). Thus, it is apparent that the types of microvasculature that support different organs and tissues play important roles in both the induction and expression of immunity at these sites.

Draining Lymphoid Organs

The peripheral lymphoid organs—spleen, lymph nodes, and mucosa-associated lymphoid tissues—are designed anatomically and functionally to accept antigenic signals from different regions of the body and to transduce these signals into the antigen-specific immune effectors—sensitized cells and antibodies—which are eventually disseminated through the blood to the entire body. Certain features are common to all peripheral lymphoid organs: follicles and germinal centers where B lymphocytopoiesis occurs and from which antibodies and plasma cells emerge; and parafollicular areas (of the nodal cortex, or splenic periarteriolar sheath) where antigenic signals arrive or are carried by migrating, tissue-derived APC. Memory B cells and plasma cell precursors arise from the follicles. A steady stream of lymphocytes is provided to this parafollicular cortical region via high endothelial venules. Lymphocytes in lymph nodes and mucosal-associated lymph organs encounter their specific antigen, clonally expand, and differentiate into effector and memory T cells. These cellular progeny then enter efferent lymphatic channels which eventually deposit the cells into the venous circulation.

Beyond these common features, the type and range of immune effectors produced by the different peripheral lymphoid organs are not exactly the same. For example, sensitized lymphocytes generated in lymph nodes that drain skin display the property of dermal and epidermal tropism (20), whereas sensitized lymphocytes generated in the lymphoid tissues that drain mucosal surfaces migrate preferentially to mucosal surfaces (20). In addition, immune responses generated in skin-draining lymph nodes tend to be dominated by cell-mediated immunity, whereas immune responses that are initiated in the spleen tend to be dominated by humoral immunity (97,101,105). Moreover, the spleen is thought to have a special role to play in the generation of suppressor lymphocytes (125), and therefore may be especially important in the regulation of immune responses, including those generated toward antigens within the neural-ocular system.

Tissue-restricted Microenvironments

The differentiated cells that comprise the parenchyma of organs and tissues carry out their specialized functions in part by secreting cellular products (cytokines, mediators, hormones) into the extracellular space. As a consequence, the microenvironment created within a specialized organ or tissue may be distinctive, owing to the unique functional properties of the parenchymal cells. While the major purpose of locally produced factors may be to serve as a means of communication between and among parenchymal cells and their supporting connective tissue cells, the factors themselves are usually neither tissue restricted nor unique. That is, many cells of the body, including lymphocytes and other blood-borne leukocytes, may express receptors for factors found in different organs and tissues. Therefore, migrating leukocytes that enter a particular tissue or organ may come under the influence of that tissue's microenvironment, as do the bone marrow–derived resident APC. Not surprisingly, the quality of immune responses elicited by antigens introduced into a tissue or organ are materially influenced by that tissue's unique microenvironment.

We are only beginning to describe the patterns of cytokines, mediators, and other factors that characterize tissue-restricted microenvironments, such as those found in the skin, the gut, and the brain. But even at this early stage of our understanding, examples have been found in which microenvironmental factors modify functions of immigrant cells of the immune system. Release of tumor necrosis factor alpha (TNF-α) in the skin following irradiation with ultraviolet B radiation acts directly on resident Langerhans cells, altering their cytoskeleton and transiently immobilizing them within the epidermis (137,161). This is one important reason why the induction of contact hypersensitivity is significantly impaired when a highly reactive hapten (such as dinitrofluorobenzene) is painted on ultraviolet B–exposed skin (117,131).

The microenvironments of the central and peripheral nervous systems and the eye are distinctly different from other tissues, and contain novel cytokines and factors that are either not present at other body sites or are present in very different concentrations and proportions. This implies that the functions of lymphocytes, APC, and other immune-related cells that intrude into neural-ocular microenvironments may be significantly modified. As described below, the unique molecular features of the fluids that fill the extracellular spaces of the brain and eye play a major role in dictating the special characteristics of immune responses within these organs.

Manifestations of Regional Immune Responses

When the individual components that participate in a regional immune response act in an integrated and physiologic fashion, the response itself is stereotypic and similar for most (if not all) antigens that are introduced into that region. The immune effectors that comprise the response represent a subset of the armory of possible effectors that the immune system can produce. Thus, the net effect of the regional immune process is to *select* an appropriate set of antigen-specific effector modalities from a broader menu.

Each of the two major epithelial surfaces of the body, the integument and the mucosal surfaces, have been recognized and defined as "regions" of the immune system. The mucosa-associated lymphoid tissues (MALT, originally described as gut-associated lymphoid tissues) (1,15,132), in conjunction with the surface epithelial cells of the mucosa and their supporting stroma, represent an integrated response unit for antigens and pathogens that are first encountered at mucosal surfaces: the gastrointestinal tract, the upper and bronchiolar portions of the respiratory tract, the urogenital tract, and the ocular surface. It is now well understood that IgA antibodies are essential features of mucosal immunity (1,15) and that these antibodies are uniquely designed to provide immune protection at the interface between the mucosa and the external environment. Immune responses to mucosally derived antigens also include lymphokine-secreting CD4+ T cells that induce the microbicidal activities of recruited eosinophils that eradicate parasitic infections from the gut. However, regionally dictated immune responses to mucosal pathogens do not usually include significant titers of IgG antibodies in the serum, nor are they represented by T cells that mediate delayed hypersensitivity at cutaneous challenge sites. In fact, these latter activities are actually suppressed (80). Thus, the mucosal immune system selects from the immune effector menu those T- and B-cell mediators that are "appropriate" for protection against pathogens at mucosal surfaces. The economy of this process is evident in the observation that once mucosal immunity has been initiated by an antigen at one mucosal surface (for example, the buccal mucosa of the mouth), it is able to be expressed at other mucosal surfaces and thus confers protection well beyond the original site of antigenic encounter.

The skin associated lymphoid tissues (SALT) (115), represented by the lymph nodes that drain the cutaneous surfaces, combined with the epithelial cells, vascular elements, and bone marrow–derived cells of the epidermis and dermis, comprise the immune response elements that detect antigens and pathogens that are first encountered through the skin. When acting in an orchestrated fashion, the skin immune system generates immune responses that are dominated by delayed and contact hypersensitivity, as well as by immunogenic inflammation mediated by complement-fixing antibodies (arthus-type reactions). Unlike in MALT, IgA antibodies, specific for antigens encountered via the skin, are not observed, nor do such antibodies appear in mucosal secretions. However, delayed hypersensitivity elicited by immunization through the skin at one site can be displayed at any other cutaneous site of the body to which the same antigen is applied, demonstrating protection beyond the original site of infection.

Regional Specializations of the Neural-ocular Immune System (NIS)

Since this book is devoted to one or another aspect of specialization of the immune response in the nervous system, the aim of this section will be to provide a brief survey and summary of existing information concerning the components of regional immune systems as they exist within the neural-ocular system (see Table 3-2). The special issues raised by expression of immunity in the central nervous system have been addressed previously by Waksman (140).

Features of Neural-ocular System Immunity

Nervous System–restricted APC

The search for APC within the brain and eye has been both frustrating and illuminating. Surveys of the nervous system for the presence, density, and distribution of bone marrow–derived cells that express class II MHC molecules (and are therefore candidates for APC) have generally come to the conclusion that conventional APC are poorly represented, if at all, in the neuropil and in the retina (3,46,99,110). However, it is known that neuronal tissues such as these are infiltrated with microglia, which are

Table 3-2 Components of Neural-Ocular Immune System

Bone-marrow–derived dendritic APC (microglia) in neuropil and secretory organs (choroid plexus and iris and ciliary body)

Brain- and eye-seeking lymphocytes (speculative)

Cerebrospinal fluid and aqueous humor that escape primarily via specialized filtration mechanisms (arachnoid villae and trabecular meshwork). To a variable extent, lymphatic pathways also exist (in the brain, cribriform plate, cranial nerve termini; in the eye, uveoscleral pathway)

Blood-brain and blood-ocular barriers limit access of blood-borne cells and molecules to these compartments

Spleen, rather than lymph nodes, is primary central processing mechanism for neural-ocular system-derived antigenic signals

Intracranial and intraocular microenvironments uniquely contain immunosuppresssive cytokines, neuropeptides, and mediators

bone marrow–derived (4,52). Yet there is little evidence that these cells can function as conventional APC within the normal, unperturbed brain (106). However, cells with surface markers that suggest an APC function as well as macrophages have been described in the stroma of the choroid plexus of the brain (107,110) and of the iris and ciliary body of the eye (68,81,155). When putative APC of the iris and ciliary body stroma have been studied in vitro, they have been found to be lacking in the ability to support mitogen-driven T-cell activation, and they fail to stimulate proliferation and lymphokine secretion among alloreactive T cells (119). Moreover, the cornea, which provides the anterior surface of the anterior chamber, is virtually devoid of professional APC (Langerhans cells) (123,155). Thus, at least within the eye, cells with functional properties usually equated with *conventional* APC do not appear to exist. However, there is strong circumstantial evidence that bone marrow–derived cells within these ocular tissues *can* acquire antigens placed in the anterior chamber of the eye. Cells of ocular origin have been found in the blood after antigen is placed in the eye (146,151), and these cells have been demonstrated to carry an antigen-specific signal to the spleen (154) that results eventually in the generation of a deviant, rather than a conventional, form of systemic immunity (146,151). That is, antigens injected into the eye elicit a stereotypic and unconventional systemic immune response that is selectively deficient in T cells that mediate delayed hypersensitivity and in B cells that secrete complement-fixing antibodies (93,114,124). Since present evidence indicates that bone marrow–derived cells with antigen-presenting potential (albeit of an unusual functional type) are normally deployed in the internal structures of the eye, this immune-privileged site contains cells that *can* carry antigen-specific signals to draining lymphoid organs for presentation to T and B cells, indicating that this component of a regional immune system is present in the eye. It needs to be determined whether these types of cells reside within the central and peripheral nervous system.

Once the neuronal components of the nervous system, including the retina, have become involved in a toxic, degenerative, or inflammatory process, mononuclear cells from the blood can readily be recruited. Under these circumstances, cells can be experimentally harvested that display conventional APC function in vitro (35,88,107). While this is undoubtedly important in the immunopathogenesis of inflammatory diseases of the brain and eye, detection of such cells in neural-ocular tissues undergoing inflammation should not be construed to mean that conventional antigen-presenting potential exists within the *unperturbed* brain and eye.

It is well recognized that resident cells (non-bone marrow–derived) of the brain and eye, such as astrocytes, Müller's cells, and epithelial cells of the choroid plexus and ciliary body, are susceptible to the actions of inflammogenic cytokines (129), of which interferon-γ (IFN-γ) is the best example. As will be discussed in subsequent chapters, glial and epithelial elements of the brain and eye can be induced to express class II MHC molecules by cytokine treatment (88,120,126). In this state of activation, antigen-pulsed glial cells can stimulate antigen-specific, primed T lymphocytes (35). However, IFN-γ does not have this positive effect on all glial elements. For example, IFN-γ treatment of Müller cells, the glial cells of the retina, induces class II MHC expression but fails to equip these cells with the ability to activate T cells (19,49). In fact, IFN-γ exposed Müller cells actually prevent T-cell activation, in part through inhibitory mediators that they secrete.

Under normal circumstances, neurons, which are the primary parenchymal cells of the brain and retina, express no class II MHC molecules and little, if any, class I molecules (74,75,143). Upon exposure to IFN-γ, some up-regulation of class I has been observed, but no class II molecules are expressed under these or any other circumstances (75,76,108,158). Therefore, unlike the parenchymal cells of the skin, kidney, and most other organs, neurons exposed to an inflammogenic stimulus cannot function as APC for CD4+ T cells, nor can they serve as targets of specific attack by effector T cells (64).

To summarize, bone marrow–derived cells found within the normal neural-ocular system have been demonstrated to display antigen processing and presenting potential, but under physiologic conditions, the range of their activities may well be limited to that which gives rise to deviant systemic immunity. Moreover, even when immunogenic inflammation has been induced within the brain and eye, conventional antigen presentation may not reach the full potential that is achieved when inflammation is expressed at non-neural-ocular sites in the body, and the parenchymal cells cannot be forced to expand the antigen presentation substrate by expressing class II MHC molecules.

Neural-ocular Tissue-tropic Lymphocytes

There is actually no formal evidence to suggest that, under normal circumstances, any circulating lymphocytes preferentially bind to and migrate through endothelial cells of the microvasculature into the central nervous system and retina. To the contrary, because of the existence of a blood-brain barrier, it is usually stated that far fewer lymphocytes enter the nervous system under resting conditions than enter into other somatic tissues. Surprisingly, little evidence exists to support or refute this quantitative statement (102). However, brain-seeking cells have been postulated to exist, in part because there is impressive localization within the brain of T cells that effect experimental allergic encephalomyelitis (EAE). In fact, the finding in rats that EAE-mediating T cells typically utilize Vα5 elements in composing their receptors for antigen has given rise to the suspicion that T-cell receptors utilizing this element may actually function as cell adhesion molecules that promote the binding of T cells to cerebral endothelial cells, thereby promoting their entry into the very tissues that express the EAE-inducing antigens (17). Based on these types of experimental evidence, there seems little question that lymphocytes can migrate across the blood microvasculature to participate in and mediate immunogenic inflammation within the brain and the eye. However, it remains to be determined whether this migration is promoted by molecules that direct subsets of lymphocytes *preferentially* into the brain and retina. The interesting possibility that neural-ocular system–seeking lymphocytes exist in the peripheral circulation, even in the absence of neural or ocular inflammation, needs to be explored experimentally.

Vascular Networks of the Neural-ocular System

Two features of the vascular supply of the brain and eye are particularly important when one considers *(a)* the route by which antigenic signals might escape from these organs, and *(b)* the route(s) by which immune effector cells and molecules gain access to these organs. On the one hand, the brain and the eye lack a conventional lymphatic drainage pathway. This statement does not mean that there is absolutely no opportunity for intracranial and intraocular antigens to gain access to draining lymph nodes. In fact, given sufficient time, antigens or other molecules placed within the eye and brain can be found in draining lymphoid organs (27,160). However, compared to non-neural tissues, the rapidity with which antigen arrives at the regional nodes is drastically reduced compared to non-neural tissues (28), although the amount of antigen may be considerable (148). Wilbanks et al. have demonstrated that >99% of soluble protein antigen injected into the anterior chamber escapes into the blood within 24 hours. Interestingly, a small amount of this antigen actually remains, trapped within the eye, and can still be detected at least 4 weeks later. This evidence suggests that the anterior chamber can function as an "antigen depot," although the physiologic significance of this finding has yet to be determined. The important dimension to these facts, which bear on the ability of the immune system to recognize intracranial and intraocular antigens, is that under normal conditions, antigen and antigen-bearing cells escape from the brain and eye directly into the blood vasculature—via the arachnoid villae and the trabecular meshwork, respectively. This means that antigen reaches the spleen *before* it reaches the draining lymph node. It is generally recognized that when an antigen is first administered via the blood, the quality of the resulting immune response is different from that which results from antigen administration by intradermal, intra-cutaneous, or other, non-neural routes (101,105). In support of this idea, it has already been mentioned that antigenic signals that escape from the anterior chamber elicit anterior chamber–associated immune deviation (ACAID), rather than conventional immunity. Thus, the fact that antigens from the brain and eye can address the systemic immune apparatus by a direct blood vascular pathway means that immune response to antigens in these organs can be expected to be unconventional. At present, our knowl-edge of the extent to which antigens escape from the brain and the eye via blood, rather than lymphatic, vascular pathways needs to be expanded so that this component of regional immunity can be placed in perspective.

On the other hand, the brain and the eye are supplied by a blood vasculature that erects a significant barrier to the passage of molecules and cells (14,16,33,91,130). This barrier undoubtedly plays a major role in preventing blood-borne immune effector cells and molecules from penetrating into the neuronal tissues of these organs. Yet, this barrier is not complete. The existence of animal models of experimental autoimmune encephalitis (98) and uveitis (18,37) mediated by T cells directed at brain and ocular autoantigens reveals that, at least under pathologic conditions, the blood-brain and blood-retina barriers can be breached. Subsequent chapters will describe in detail the cellular and molecular mechanisms that alter the cerebral and ocular microvasculature, permitting immune effectors and inflammatory agents to enter these compartments and to eliminate pathogens, as well as to mediate immunopathogenic diseases.

The idea that integrity of the blood-brain barrier can influence the character of immune responses to intracranial antigens has been dramatically demonstrated by the recent work of Cserr and colleagues. These investigators have taken pains to develop experimental strategies that permit intracerebral and intraventricular injections of anti-gens under circumstances in which the blood:brain barrier is preserved. When these conditions are met, a deviant systemic immunity is generated and levels of circulating antibodies are greatly enhanced (39,45). Moreover, when myelin basic protein is in-jected intracranially under these conditions, rats are rendered resistant to the subse-quent induction and development of experimental allergic encephalomyelitis (44). These vascular networks of the neural-ocular system play a major role in molding the unique properties of immunity that is eventually expressed in these tissues.

Draining Lymphoid Organs

The observation that antigenic signals escape from the eye (and probably the brain) primarily by a blood vascular route means that the primary draining lymphoid organ is more likely to be the spleen than the lymph nodes. It has long been known that the spleen responds to antigenic stimuli by producing a rather unique set of immune effectors. In general, spleen-dominated immune responses lack delayed hypersen-sitivity but display enhanced antibody formation (101,105). For soluble antigens, the specific antibodies that are produced are primarily of the isotype varieties that do *not* fix complement (34). In addition, immune responses that are initiated first within the spleen are often dominated by regulatory T cells, and these cells have been demonstrated to suppress both induction and expression of antigen-specific immunity (31,125). The cellular and molecular mechanisms that equip the spleen with these special immunologic properties are very poorly understood. Nonetheless, since we suspect that the spleen is the dominant lymphoid organ shaping systemic immune responses to antigens introduced into or arising from the brain and eye, it is anticipated that the special features of spleen-influenced immunity should dominate systemic immunity elicited by antigens from neural tissues. Experiments bearing on this point have already been conducted in mice and reveal that the spleen plays a definitive role in shaping systemic immune responses to ocular antigenic challenges. When antigens were injected into the eyes of mice from which the spleen had been extirpated, they failed to induce ACAID; asplenic animals responded subsequently to intraocular antigens with conventional immunity (61,121,146,151). Whether a similar situation applies to antigens injected into the central or peripheral nervous system remains to be experimentally determined.

Neural-ocular Tissue-restricted Microenvironment

The brain and the internal components of the eye are bathed in highly distinctive fluids—cerebrospinal fluid and aqueous humor/vitreous body. To only a very limited degree are plasma proteins and molecules represented qualitatively and quantitatively in these fluids. Moreover, these fluids contain unique cytokines and other macromolecules with a range of pharmacologic activities found nowhere else in the body. Thus, these specialized fluids are representative of the unique microenvironment of the neural-ocular tissues. Since both induction and expression of immunity depend heavily upon characteristics of the tissue microenvironment in which immunocompetent cells reside, one would expect that the unique microenvironments of the brain and eye would influence both afferent and efferent aspects of immunity to antigens introduced into these organs. And such appears to be the case!

Because of its accessibility, the anterior chamber of the eye represents an ideal microenvironment to sample and study experimentally. The aqueous humor which fills this chamber has been subjected to experimental analysis with respect to its immunologic properties. Whole aqueous humor, from many different species, has been found to be profoundly suppressive when added to in vitro assays of lymphocyte activation. Specifically, normal aqueous humor can inhibit antigen-, mitogen-, and growth factor-driven T-cell proliferation and lymphokine production (59,127). Moreover, when aqueous humor is mixed with effector cells at the time of skin testing, this fluid has even been found to inhibit the in vivo expression of delayed hypersensitivity (24,25). However, aqueous humor is not a universal cell toxin, nor does it inhibit all aspects of immune function. For example, fully functional cytotoxic T cells are readily able to lyse their specific targets in the presence of aqueous humor (59,83). In addition to inhibiting certain T-cell functions, aqueous humor has been found to alter the functional properties of professional APC (macrophages, dendritic cells) (147). As discussed below and in detail in Chapter 20, aqueous humor converts conventional APC into cells that induce deviant systemic immunity (93,114,124). In addition, aqueous humor suppresses the production of reactive oxygen and nitric oxide intermediates by activated macrophages (AW Taylor, personal observations). Thus, aqueous humor is suppressive to T cells, to APC, and to macrophages. Although much remains to be learned about this fascinating fluid, it is already apparent that aqueous humor possesses potent immunosuppressive properties.

The choroid plexus secretes cerebrospinal fluid (26), and the epithelial cells of ciliary body and iris are the primary sources of aqueous humor (36). It is relevant that cells from these intraocular tissues are themselves capable of suppressing T-cell activation in vitro, and that they do so by secreting inhibitory factors into the culture supernatant (53,119,155). Cultured corneal endothelial cells, retinal pigment epithelial cells, and retinal Müller cells have also been reported to secrete suppressive factors (19,49,50,69,119). Since these secretions appear to be a constitutive property of these cells (i.e., the cultured cells do not need any additional cognate stimulation for secretion to be observed), it is tempting to conclude that under physiologic conditions, the parenchymal cells of tissues of the internal compartments of the eye create an immunosuppressive microenvironment that can markedly alter both the induction and expression of immunity in this organ.

Our laboratory as well as others have begun to identify the molecules within aqueous humor that confer upon it immunosuppressive properties. The first factor to be identified was transforming growth factor beta (TGF-β), chiefly the beta-2 isoform (23,40,50,55). More recently, Taylor et al. (127,128) have detected alpha-melanocyte stimulating hormone (α-MSH), and vasoactive intestinal peptide (VIP) in aqueous humor, while other investigators have found calcitonin gene-related peptide (138). While these cytokines may generally share properties that inhibit immune-mediated inflammation, each carries out its functions in somewhat different ways. TGF-β, at the concentration that it is constitutively present in aqueous humor, inhibits T-cell proliferation and activation (23,40) and is also responsible for altering the functional properties of professional APC (29). The concentration of the other cytokines in aqueous humor are too low to inhibit all aspects of T-cell functions in this manner. However, at the physiologic levels found within aqueous humor, α-MSH and VIP (as well as TGF-β) can inhibit IFN-γ secretion by activated T cells (127,128). Moreover, the concentrations of TGF-β and α-MSH in aqueous humor are sufficient to account for the fluid's ability to inhibit reactive oxygen and nitric oxide intermediate production by macrophages (AW Taylor, personal observations). Finally, incubation of normal macrophages and dendritic cells in aqueous humor or supernatans of cultured cells from iris and ciliary body enforces upon the cells a unique pattern of migration. When injected intravenously into normal mice, treated macrophages and dendritic cells traffic exclusively to the spleen. With this in mind, it is now clear why they can only deliver antigen-specific signals acquired in the eye to the spleen (43,151). In the aggregate, the factors in aqueous humor can suppress immunogenic inflammation at multiple stages in its formation and evolution: induction of cell-mediated immunity, activation of effector T cells, and suppression of lymphokine-dependent macrophage effector mechanisms.

It is not only important to describe the constitutive existence of immunosuppressive factors in aqueous humor but also to recognize that this unique microenvironment is profoundly deficient in certain proteins normally found in plasma and in other tissues. A similar description applies to cerebrospinal fluid (130). Serum proteins, including alpha$_2$-macroglobulin, are virtually nonexistent in aqueous humor—undoubtedly a reflection of the integrity of the blood-ocular barrier (8). The absence of these proteins deprives this microenvironment of the types of serum protease activity that can degrade immunosuppressive cytokines, especially the highly sensitive neuropeptides. Alpha$_2$-macroglobulin acts as a carrier and has the potential to bring into the ocular microenvironment proinflammatory cytokines, such as IL-1 and IL-6, which would drastically change the microenvironment's immunosuppressive capabilities (13,79). Moreover, alpha$_2$-macrolobulin binds and neutralizes TGF-β (96). By isolating the anterior chamber from the blood, the blood-ocular barrier allows the accumulation of immunosuppressive cytokines in the aqueous humor and ensures the preservation of their bioactivity and bioavailability.

This discussion has focussed on features of the ocular microenvironment rather than the microenvironment of the central nervous system because much less is known about putative immunoreactive or immunosuppressive properties of cerebrospinal fluid (CSF). There are few published reports concerning the ability of CSF to influence lymphocyte responses in vitro, although there are unconfirmed reports that CSF may be stimulatory to T cells. In our laboratory, we have documented that CSF contains significant amounts of TGF-β (153). Moreover, we have found that CSF from normal mice, rats, and humans can alter the functional properties of professional APC in a manner identical to that ascribed to aqueous humor and to TGF-β (152). Despite the anatomical barriers to the study of CSF and the brain microenvironment, there is sufficient evidence to encourage investigators to probe in this direction. It is likely that the microenvironment of the brain will resemble that of the eye in providing an inhospitable site for the expression of immunogenic inflammation.

Manifestations of Immunity in the Neural-ocular System

Immune Privilege in the Brain and the Eye

For more than 100 years, the anterior chamber of the eye has been considered an immune privileged site, and for more than 50 years, the same designation has been made for the brain (7,48,60,133). The term *immune privilege* refers to the experimental observation that foreign tissue grafts placed in the anterior chamber or in the brain survive for a longer period of time than if the same grafts were placed at conventional body sites, such as the subcutaneous space or the peritoneal cavity. The modern, experimental description of immune privilege in the eye and the brain was the work of Sir Peter Medawar and his collaborators (82); these investigators cognized that other workers had failed to demonstrate a lymphatic drainage pathway for either the eye or the brain (141). At the time (late 1940s, early 1950s), it was first appreciated that lymph nodes that drained sites into which histoincompatible grafts had been placed were critical to the immune process by which the grafts were eventually destroyed (82). Moreover, it had been demonstrated that transplantation antigens from the implanted grafts were carried by lymph flow to the draining node, and that sensitization of graft-destroying lymphocytes occurred in this organ. Based on this knowledge, Medawar reasoned that if lymph nodes are required for the development of allograft immunity, and if the brain and eye lack lymphatic drainage routes, then the failure to reject foreign grafts placed at these sites could be ascribed to a failure of the immune system to become aware of the relevant transplantation antigens. For many years thereafter, it was widely believed that immune privilege results from the isolation of the immune system from grafts at such sites. This idea was first challenged more than 20 years ago by Raju and Grogan (103) who, on the one hand, reaffirmed the statement that the brain and the eye are privileged sites, since skin grafts from Brown Norway rats transplanted into the brain and anterior chamber of Lewis rats were accepted for prolonged intervals. On the other hand, these investigators also demonstrated that the immune system of the recipients was cognizant of the presence of the grafts in the brain and eye, since antibodies specific for antigens on the grafts were detected in the peripheral blood. Raju and Grogan thus raised the paradox of immune privilege: the immune system is aware of and responds to antigens on the foreign grafts, but it is unable to mount a destructive immune attack. Similar studies by Kaplan and Streilein (62,63) confirmed that rats exposed via the anterior chamber of the eye to alien transplantation antigens produced serum antibodies specific for the graft. Moreover, these investigators demonstrated that rats that were first exposed to transplantation antigens via the eye were impaired subsequently in their ability to respond to those same antigens expressed on a skin graft placed at a conventional body site.

The phenomenon of immune privilege has been rediscovered numerous times over the past 30 years and has been a subject of considerable controversy. In part, resistance to the notion of immune privilege has stemmed from the common observation that not all grafts placed in so-called privileged sites are accepted indefinitely. There is now considerable evidence that the phenomenon of immune privilege is not a passive failure of the immune system but an active process that regulates the nature of the immune response in qualitative and quantitative terms (124). This evidence strongly suggests that immune privilege results from unique features of the immune reflex arc's afferent limb, by which antigens in privileged sites gain access to the immune system, and of its efferent limb, in which expression of immunity in a privileged site is altered.

Immune Deviation and the Afferent Limb
of Neural-ocular System Immunity

The introduction of antigenic material into the brain, the subarachnoid space, and the anterior chamber of the eye, leads eventually to the elicitation of a systemic immune response that is deviant, i.e., a response that is somewhat different from that elicited by introduction of antigens by more conventional routes (93,114); see Table 3-3). This summary statement is based on the reported results of experiments conducted in such a manner that antigen was introduced into the brain and into the eye *while retaining the integrity of the blood-tissue barrier.* The resulting immune response is unique in several different ways. First, there is a remarkable failure of cell-mediated immunity, especially that elicited by T cells that mediate delayed hypersensitivity (93,114,156). This failure results in part from the generation of several distinctive sets of regulatory T cells that suppress the induction and expression of delayed hypersensitivity (122,139,149). Second, the serum contains copious amounts of specific antibodies. Following injection of soluble antigen into the anterior chamber of the eye, the antibodies are almost exclusively of the isotypes that do *not* fix complement (150). Following injection of antigen into the subarachnoid space, the magnitude of the serum antibody response is much greater than that elicited by antigen injected by more conventional routes (39,45). Description of the cellular and molecular basis for the development of a deviant response following injection of antigen into the anterior chamber is beyond the scope of this chapter, but is presented in detail in Chapter 18.

A wide variety of antigens, ranging from soluble proteins to transplantation antigens, have been tested for their capacity to induce ACAID. The general conclusion that emerges from these studies is that ACAID is the most invariable outcome if an animal's initial experience with an antigen occurs via the anterior chamber. However, this conclusion must be modified on two accounts: first, strong transplantation antigens induce antigen-specific ACAID, but the phenomenon proves to be transient, rather than permanent. The impermanence of ACAID undoubtedly accounts for the initial growth, but eventual rejection of intracamerally injected MHC-incompatible tumor cells and tumor cells that express strong tumor-specific antigens (70,95). Second, Benson et al. (10) have demonstrated that implantation in the anterior chamber of tumor cells that

Table 3-3 Unique Features of Neural-Ocular Immune System

APC that induce deviant, rather than conventional immunity

Lack of expression of class I and class II MHC molecules on many, if not all, parenchymal cells

Inability to up-regulate MHC expression by IFN-γ treatment of neurons

Presence of immunosuppressive microenvironment that interferes with expression of immunogenic inflammation

Barrier to immigration of blood-borne lymphocytes and mononuclear cells

Immune privilege

express both strong tumor-specific antigens along with minor histocompatibility antigens leads to the induction of ACAID to the latter, but systemic delayed hypersensitivity to the former. The reasons for this paradoxical result have not been identified, or do we understand why strong antigens elicit only a transient form of ACAID.

There is good reason to believe that the deviant immune responses to antigens placed in the eye and the brain are dictated in part by the unique fashion in which antigens reach the immune system from these organs. As mentioned previously, antigen can escape from the eye and the brain directly into the blood vasculature by traversing the specialized filtering devices of the trabecular meshwork and the arachnoid villae. Even though some antigen may also escape by lymphatic routes, that which enters the blood is delivered rapidly to the spleen, permitting this organ to respond before antigen has reached draining lymph nodes. The deviant immune response that characteristically follows intracranial and intracameral antigen injections reflects the splenic dominance of the immune response, favoring humoral rather than cell-mediated immunity.

Local Immunosuppression and the Efferent Limb of Neural-ocular System Immunity

The microenvironments of the brain and the eye have the potential to influence markedly the *local* expression of immunity (see Table 3-3). Cousins et al. (9,24,25) and Niederkorn et al. (94) have recently reported that it is virtually impossible to elicit delayed hypersensitivity reactions in the anterior chamber of the eye, even if the test animal is demonstrably immune, and even if the intracameral inoculum contains antigen, effector T cells and conventional APC. Ksander and his collaborators (71,72) have determined that the anterior chamber (AC) microenvironment inhibits precursor cytotoxic T cells from acquiring their full cytolytic potential in vivo and prevents the accumulation of T cells that mediate AC tumor graft-specific delayed hypersensitivity. These results reveal the anterior chamber to be an inhospitable site for the expression of this type of cell-mediated immunity. As described in more detail in Chapters 17 and 18, cytokines present in the aqueous humor of normal eyes, such as TGF-β (23,40), strongly inhibit delayed hypersensitivity expression by directly suppressing T-cell activation and by counteracting the inflammogenic properties of lymphokines (IFN-γ, tumor necrosis factor alpha [TNF-α). It seems reasonable to conclude that cytokines constitutively present in aqueous humor, including TGF-β, α-MSH (127), VIP (128), and calcitonin gene-related peptide, account for the profoundly immunosuppressive properties of this tissue fluid. Since at least some of these factors are known to be present in cerebrospinal fluid, one might expect this fluid also to possess immunosuppressive features. Thus, the microenvironment of the eye (and presumably the brain) constitutively displays the capacity to down-regulate cell-mediated immunity of the delayed type (24). Reports from the earlier literature suggest that aqueous humor also inhibits the activation of complement (87). Although this issue needs to be reexplored in contemporary terms, the finding indicates that the immunosuppressive features of the ocular microenvironment may also act on those forms of antibody-mediated immunity that give rise to immunogenic inflammation via complement activation.

It is important to point out that not all immune effector modalities are suppressed by aqueous humor or the ocular microenvironment. For example, cytotoxic T cells are not inhibited from lysing target cells in the presence of aqueous humor (59,83). This indicates that the suppressive properties of the ocular microenvironment are selective in their range of action. The emphasis appears to be on the suppression of immune effectors that act by releasing biologically active and inflammatory molecules and mediators.

Findings which reveal the ocular microenvironment to be profoundly immunosuppressive seem to be at variance with the fact that immunopathogenic processes, triggered by microbial or autoantigens, occur within the brain and the eye; lymphocytic choriomeningitis (3) and experimental autoimmune encephalomyelitis (EAE) (98) and uveoretinitis (EAU) (18,22,37) are examples. However, the two lines of experimental inquiry do not yield data that are necessarily at odds. When neural or ocular tissues of experimental animals are infected with appropriate pathogenic organisms, immunogenic inflammation ensues that can lead to severe pathologic consequences. This outcome does not negate the existence of a constitutive immunosuppressive local microenvironment, but it does indicate that local microenvironments, which are maintained actively, are subject to modification when experimentally manipulated or attacked by pathogenic agents. When invaded by an infectious agent, neural-ocular microenvironments can be altered, and expression of conventional immunity and inflammation becomes possible. Similarly, when experimental animals are immunized with autoantigens derived from nervous or ocular tissues, autoimmune diseases ensue in a fashion that strongly suggests that the local microenvironment is no longer immunosuppressive.

We should keep in mind that expression of these autoimmune diseases is dictated by genetic factors. It is possible that the ability of the eye and brain to create and maintain a stable, resilient local immunosuppressive microenvironment is determined by polymorphic alleles at gene loci governing the local production of immunosuppressive factors. Therefore, the emergence of autoimmune or immunopathogenic diseases in the neural-ocular system may depend upon as yet unidentified polymorphic genetic loci that regulate differentially the cytokine content of the microenvironment.

In summary, there is good experimental evidence that the local microenvironments created within the nervous and ocular systems possess immunosuppressive properties. As a consequence, both the induction and the expression of immunity to antigens occurring within these tissues can be expected to be substantially different from that found elsewhere. We believe that the expression of immunopathogenic disease processes within these organs occurs only after the inherently immunosuppressive microenvironment has been overcome. This belief strengthens our hope that elucidation of the molecular and cellular bases for local immunosuppression may make it possible to alleviate or prevent similar types of disease in humans.

Local Production of Immunoglobulins

Under normal circumstances, there is a measurable amount of IgG in aqueous humor and cerebrospinal fluid (2–3 mg/dl), but these concentrations are dramatically lower than IgG levels found in serum (1000–2000 mg/dl) (32,142). Although there may also be trace amounts of IgA in the fluids of the neural-ocular system (0–1 mg/dl, compared to 151–250 mg/dl in serum), other isotypes are virtually undetectable (32,142). It is generally believed that the immunoglobulins found in aqueous humor and cerebrospinal fluid *in the absence of disease* represent the simple diffusion of these antibodies across the local blood-tissue barriers. Breaches in these barriers exist normally among the circumventricular organs of the brain and at the root of the iris in the eye, and these breaches probably account for the small amounts of immunoglobulins detected normally in intracranial and intraocular fluids.

However, when the blood-brain and blood-ocular barriers are compromised, for example, when intracranial or intraocular infection and inflammation develop, significantly greater quantities of immunoglobulins are found in cerebrospinal fluid and aqueous humor (38,41,142). To a certain extent, immunoglobulins, along with other plasma proteins, leak directly across the endothelium of the damaged and inflamed brain and ocular microvasculature, making an important contribution to the finding of increased antibody levels. However, this passive process alone is insufficient to account for the high levels of immunoglobulins sometimes found in the cerebrospinal fluids of patients with multiple sclerosis or the aqueous humor of patients with chronic uveitis (41,90,142). In these latter instances, as well as in other inflammatory diseases of the eye and brain, circumstantial evidence suggests that there is actually de novo synthesis of immunoglobulins *behind* the blood-tissue barrier, i.e. within the internal compartments of the brain and eye. In these instances, the levels of immunoglobulins in cerebrospinal fluid and aqueous humor are not only elevated, but the levels exceed expectations based on the plasma as the only source of immune-related macromolecules. Measurements of specific IgG antibodies directed at human immunodeficiency virus (HIV), herpes simplex virus (HSV), *Toxoplasma gondii,* and *Onchocerca volvulus* have revealed concentrations in cerebrospinal fluid or aqueous humor considerably in excess of the levels of these same antibodies found in the peripheral blood of patients with intracerebral or intraocular infections (2,6,30,65,136,142). Several different mathematical formulae have been used to gain statistical evidence of intracranial or intraocular immunoglobulin synthesis (104,134). Often IgM and IgA antibodies are elevated as well. With respect to the latter, the constitutive presence of TGF-β in cerebrospinal fluid and aqueous humor may serve to encourage local antigen-reactive B cells to switch from IgM to IgA, rather than to IgG. It is known that TGF-β plays a similar role in promoting IgA-producing B cells in the mucosal immune system (66).

Few studies have attempted to identify the antigenic specificities of antibodies found in brain and ocular fluids. Moreover, only in rare instances have investigators successfully isolated immunoglobulin-secreting B lymphocytes from the brain and eye (2).

Based on the results of these studies, it appears that there is no significant impairment of the ability of B cells and plasma cells to produce immunoglobulins directed at antigens located in the microenvironments of the brain and eye.

Thus, the evidence is strong that under pathologic circumstances, B cells can come to reside beyond the blood-brain and blood-ocular barriers, and that the cells can secrete immunoglobulins at these sites. It is important to point out that in organized lymphoid tissues (such as spleen, lymph nodes, Peyer's patches, etc.), as well as in the lamina propria of mucosal surfaces, the recirculating B cells that come to rest locally must then terminally differentiate into antibody-secreting cells. This process occurs under the influence of helper T cells that also occupy the same microenvironment. What remains unclear is whether the B cells that secrete immunoglobulins in the diseased brain and eye also require T-cell help, or whether their terminal differentiation is T-cell independent. If the former is the case, then no information exists to implicate the presence of helper T cells in the brain and eye.

It is worth mentioning that although immunoglobulins may be secreted by B cells located beyond the blood-brain and blood-ocular barrier, the intraocular and intracranial microenvironments offer formidable barriers to the full functional expression of antibody molecules; this is particularly true for complement-fixing antibodies. The only complement components found in normal aqueous humor are C2, C6, C7, and factor B, and these are present in markedly reduced concentrations compared to plasma (87). As expected, inflammation within the anterior segment of the eyes leads to a local increase in complement components in the aqueous humor. Moreover, decay-accelerating factor (DAF) is highly expressed on the cells of the eye, including corneal endothelium, trabecular meshwork, and retina, and the soluble form of DAF is present in high concentration in aqueous humor (77). As a membrane-bound molecule, DAF protects cells from complement-mediated lysis, and as a soluble molecule, DAF suppresses the formation of C3 convertase of the classical complement pathway. By contrast, other complement-independent, antibody-dependent reactions can proceed within ocular and nervous system compartments, such as opsonization mediated by IgG and C3b deposition (54,109). In fact, retinal pigment epithelial cells display receptors for the Fc component of IgG and are able to phagocytize and degrade IgG-antigen complexes (100,135). It is pertinent to a consideration of the intraocular compartment as immunosuppressive that the process of clearing these complexes reduces the threat of inflammation indirectly by limiting activation of complement-derived inflammatory factors (C3a, C5a).

As mentioned elsewhere in this chapter, injection of antigen into the anterior chamber of the eye results in a selective systemic immune deficiency in which complement-fixing antibodies are excluded from production. It is satisfying that the internal microenvironment of the eye is also extremely inhospitable to the antibody-dependent activation of complement. We interpret this to mean that complement activation within the eye is detrimental to the visual axis, and the eye and the immune system have arranged both afferent and efferent mechanisms to cope with this exigency. At present, it is unknown whether a similar set of mechanisms protect the brain from complement-mediated injury.

The Neural-ocular Immune System (NIS)—A Proposal

In concluding this chapter, we have elected to develop a synthetic description of the neural-ocular immune system that is admittedly hypothetical, but is based on experimental information derived largely, although not exclusively, from the study of immune responses elicited by antigens placed within the eye. The ocular system has received considerable experimental scrutiny and is close to our own experimental interests. Our hope is that this attempt at synthesis will provide a framework within which the neural-ocular immune system can be considered as an integrated entity, and we hope our construction provides impetus for new and informative experiments that will serve to advance understanding in this field.

To that end, we make the following proposals. The nervous system and the eye are served by a (similar or identical) highly distinctive regional immune system (see Fig. 3-1). This system displays several discrete elements usually found in regional immune systems, even though these particular elements may function differently from their counterparts elsewhere: *(1)* a specialized set of APC that create unique antigenic signals from local molecules and antigens; *(2)* an outflow pathway that delivers anti-

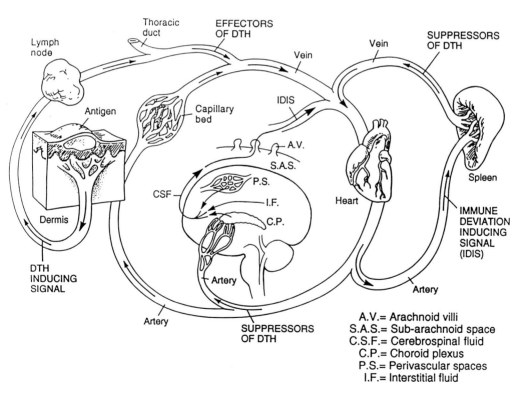

Fig. 3-1. Graphic illustration of the blood vascular connections that concern the proposed neural-ocular immune system.

genic information and migratory APC predominately into the blood vasculature, rather than into lymphatics; *(3)* the spleen, which is the predominant recipient of antigenic signals and cells carried via the blood, and which transduces unique signals borne by neural-ocular tissue–derived APC into the deviant form of systemic immunity typified by ACAID; *(4)* a local blood microvasculature that stringently limits the passage of immune effectors and inflammatory mediators from the blood into the extravascular compartments of the brain and the eye; and *(5)* a local immunosuppressive microenvironment that modifies the immune response during both its afferent phase (where the immunosuppressive microenvironment confers immune deviation–inducing properties on indigenous APC) and its efferent phase (where the microenvironment suppresses antigen-driven activation of effector T cells that gain access to the local environment and antagonizes the inflammogenic effects of lymphokines released from activated immune effectors).

In the aggregate, when the components of the neural-ocular immune system are confronted by a local antigenic challenge, they conspire to produce a stereotypic, systemic immune response that is distinctive, deviant, and largely devoid of T cells that mediate delayed hypersensitivity and of antibodies that fix complement. In addition, the components of this regional immune system create an immunosuppressive microenvironment that mitigates against expression within the nervous system and the eye of the very same set of potentially pathogenic immune effector modalities. It is curious, and undoubtedly important, that other immune effectors (cytotoxic T cells and non-complement-fixing antibodies) that do not promote immunogenic inflammation are well represented in the stereotypic systemic immune response and are readily able to eliminate antigenic targets within the neural and ocular microenvironments. The avoidance of immunogenic inflammation at both local and systemic levels by the neural-ocular immune system is not only striking but also probably accounts for several immune phenomena and features that are uniquely found in the nervous system and the eye.

The experimentally described phenomenon of immune privilege in the eye and the brain is undoubtedly the consequence of the unique attributes of the neural-ocular immune system. Based on the results of recent experiments in which allogeneic tumor cells (56,71) and neonatal retinal tissues (57,58) have been grafted into various compartments of the eye, it appears that prolonged, even indefinite acceptance of intraocular allografts results in part from the induction of alloantigen-specific ACAID. In other body sites, rejection of allografts is usually mediated by T cells of the delayed hypersensitivity type. Thus, the capacity of the neural-ocular immune system to arrange for the development of deviant immunity—devoid of delayed hypersensitivity—is directly responsible for the phenomenon of immune privilege. By the same token, it is well established that some allogeneic tissues and grafts placed in putative neural and ocular privileged sites do *not* survive indefinitely (70,95). We believe that these observations do not refute the existence of privilege, nor do they necessarily reduce the importance of immune deviation. As one might expect from an actively maintained phenomenon, immune privilege is not absolute and can be overwhelmed when one or another component of this regional immune system is compromised: when a graft is implanted at a site where the blood-brain or -ocular barrier has been destroyed; when the strength of the antigen is particularly great, as with major histocompatibility antigens; or when different immune effectors, such as cytotoxic T cells, intervene and secure graft rejection.

Immune privilege is also promoted by the indigenous immunosuppressive microenvironments of the eye and brain. For example, orthotopic corneal allografts are frequently accepted, even when placed in eyes of animals that have been previously sensitized to the antigens expressed on the grafts (112). Recent evidence indicates that this is a direct consequence of the immunosuppressive properties of the aqueous humor in normal eyes. Thus, much more than a laboratory curiosity, immune privilege is the direct expression of the dual capacities of the neural-ocular immune system to inhibit selectively immunogenic inflammation at its induction and at its expression (111).

We have wondered whether the phenomenon of ACAID is relevant to any ocular diseases, particularly those with a known or suspected immunopathogenic basis. Our laboratory and those of our collaborators have explored the possible relationships between the induction of ACAID by ocular antigens and (a) infections of the eye with herpes simplex virus 1, and (b) the induction of experimental autoimmune uveoretinitis with retina-specific antigens. It has been determined that infection of the anterior chamber of mouse eyes with HSV-1 leads to HSV-1-specific ACAID (145). Moreover, in this setting, a majority of animals with ocular HSV-1 develop a devastating and acute retinal necrosis in the contralateral eye (5,144). It is pertinent to note that if intraocular infection with HSV-1 takes place under circumstances in which ACAID induction is prevented, no retinal necrosis is observed (118). Thus, although the precise mechanisms remain to be elucidated, there is a close correlation between the ability of viral antigens to induce ACAID and the vulnerability of the retina to destructive infection with the virus.

It is important to extend these lines of investigation to the central nervous system. At the moment, it appears that introduction of soluble antigen into the ventricular system of the brain with an intact blood-brain barrier produces systemic immunologic effects that are similar if not identical to ACAID (39,45). Moreover, as mentioned above, this maneuver can ameliorate the expression of EAE in susceptible Lewis rats. It is not currently known whether, when the integrity of the blood-brain barrier is maintained, experimental introduction of viruses or allogeneic tumor cells into the brain or its ventricular system will produce immune outcomes similar to those described with the eye. Only when these experiments are conducted will we know whether the eye represents a faithful model of the immune system that serves the entire nervous system.

It has been reported that inoculation of retinal autoantigens into the anterior chamber of the eye induces ACAID in mice (42) and rats (86). Moreover, in strains that are susceptible to experimental autoimmune uveitis, pretreatment with an intraocular injection of a retinal autoantigen prevents or greatly limits the expression of uveoretinitis in these animals (42,85). Thus, ACAID appears to be able to thwart the development and/or expression of ocular autoimmunity.

A Rationale for the Existence of a Neural-ocular Immune System

If the theme of the neural-ocular immune system is to avoid immunogenic inflammation, and if it has required elaborate intracranial and intraocular specializations in order to create this special brand of immunity, one has to wonder why this is so. While immunity that is accomplished with the aid of nonspecific and intense inflammation is important and clearly essential for protection against certain types of pathogens, there are disadvantages to the expression of immunity of this type. On the one hand, delayed hypersensitivity and complement fixation often occur in a setting that leads to "innocent-bystander" injury to surrounding tissues (157). The injury may take the form of outright necrosis of cells that happen to be in the vicinity or, in the case of myelinated neurons, demyelinization may be the consequence. In addition, damage may result from the disruption of the integrity of the local microvasculature, leading to edema formation (which can distort critical microanatomical arrangements) and to the entry of potentially noxious molecules and cells from the blood. On the other hand, immunogenic inflammation—especially if it is extended or chronic in form—has the propensity to produce scarring and permanent damage (67,92). This is particularly important to structures whose function depends upon the maintenance of precise microanatomy. Based on these considerations, one can easily visualize the threat that immunogenic inflammation represents to the nervous system and the eye. In the case of the brain and the retina, any process that nonspecifically eliminates neurons has serious consequences for the individual, because these cells are incapable of regeneration. Moreover, unique functional activities are often invested in only a handful of cells, and the loss of a few can have devastating consequences.

The visual axis is a precise, yet delicate anatomical apparatus that can be easily distorted. Processes such as edema and scar formation, which have minor consequence when expressed in tissues such as the skin, can lead to blindness when they occur in the eye. There are similarly crucial microanatomical arrangements in the central nervous system where a small amount of edema and hemorrhage, that would be trivial elsewhere, can be profoundly disruptive of neural function. Moreover, the unselected delivery of plasma contents into the substance of the brain and eye during inflammation has the potential to interfere with transmission of synaptic signals and to alter the glial-dependent microenvironment that is essential for proper neuronal functioning. We mention these potential consequences of immunogenic inflammation in the nervous system because we believe that the unique attributes of the neural-ocular immune system are not accidents of biology. Rather, we propose that the neural-ocular system and the immune system have developed mechanisms that provide the former with immune protection from invading pathogens, and that these mechanisms insure that the type of immune effectors that are produced mediate protection with minimal disruption to neural-ocular function. Because of the compromise reached between these two very different organ systems, the potential exists for pathologies of two rather different types. Considered from the vantage point of the immune system and its general responsibility to protect the body against all potential pathogens, the deviant immunity elicited by antigens introduced via the neural-ocular system has been demonstrated to be *systemic*. Therefore, the individual with deviant immunity is unable to mobilize delayed hypersensitivity responses, even if the antigen is introduced elsewhere in the body. Since the elimination of certain pathogens requires the participation of delayed hypersensitivity, an individual with deviant immunity is rendered vulnerable to attack by pathogens which cannot be defended. Thus, success of the neural-ocular immune system may place the viability of the host at risk. Alternatively, when the neural-ocular immune system fails in its efforts to fashion a deviant immune response to local antigens, conventional systemic immunity emerges. As described above, under this circumstance the potential for severe disruption of visual and neural functions is great. Therein lies the price of the special compromise between the immune system and the neural-ocular system.

There is, however, another dimension to this issue. The threat of autoimmunity and autoimmune disease hangs heavily over the tissues of the neural-ocular system. The brain and the eye are replete with tissue-restricted molecules (antigens) that appear not to be expressed at other sites in the body, have apparently not been incorporated into the immune system's definition of "self," and are therefore readily able to induce immunity in adult individuals, thereby producing local tissue injury and destruction. The inherently autoantigenic nature of the nervous system and the eye may be dictated in part by the temporal differentiation of these organs *after* the immune system has distinguished "self" from "non-self" during ontogeny. It may therefore have been an important evolutionary advance for the nervous system to develop strategies designed to "fool" the immune system into thinking that the unique molecules of the brain and the eye are "self." Viewed in this context, immune deviation may represent a reasonably effective mechanism for including neural-ocular molecules, *as an addendum,* into the immunologic definition of "self."

References

1. Alley CD, Mestecky J. The mucosal immune system. In: B Lymphocytes in Human Disease, G Bird, JE Calvert, eds. Oxford University Press, Oxford, pp 222–254, 1988.
2. Amadori A, De Rossi A, Gallo P, Tavolato B, Chieco-Bianchi L. Cerebrospinal fluid lymphocytes from HIV-infected patients synthesize HIV-specific antibody in vitro. J Neuroimmunol 18:181–186, 1988.
3. Anderssen IH, Marker O, Thomsen AR: Breakdown of the blood-brain barrier function in the murine lymphocyte choriomeningitis virus infection by virus-specific CD8$^+$ T cells. J Neuroimmunol 31:156–163, 1991.
4. Andersson P-B, Perry VH, Gordon S. Intracerebral injection of proinflammatory cytokines

or leukocyte chemotaxins induces minimal myelomonocytic cell recruitment to the parenchyma of the central nervous system. J Exp Med 176:255–259, 1992.

5. Atherton SS, Streilein JW. Virus-specific DTH prevents contralateral retinitis following intracameral inoculation of HSV-2. Curr Eye Res 6:134–140, 1987.

6. Baarsma GS, Luyendijk L, Kjilstra A, de Vries J, Peperkamp E, Mertens DA, van Meurs JC. Analysis of local antibody production in the vitreous humor of patients with severe uveitis. Am J Opthalmol 112:147–151, 1991.

7. Barker CF, Billingham RE. Immunologically privileged sites. Adv Immunol 25:1–54, 1977.

8. Bengtsson E. Studies on the mechanism of the breakdown of the blood-aqueous barrier in the rabbit eye. Acta Ophthalmol Suppl 131:3–33, 1977.

9. Benson JL, Niederkorn JY. In situ suppression of delayed-type hypersensitivity: another mechanism for sustaining the immune privilege of the anterior chamber. Immunology 74:154–160, 1991.

10. Benson JL, Niederkorn JY. Immune privilege in the anterior chamber of the eye: alloantigens and tumour-specific antigens presented into the anterior chamber simultaneously induce suppression and activation of delayed hypersensitivity to the respective antigens. Immunology 77:189–195, 1992.

11. Berg EL, Yoshino T, Rott LS, Robinson MK, Warnock A, Kishimoto TK, Picker LJ, Butcher EC. The cutaneous lymphocyte antigen is a skin lymphocyte homing receptor for the vascular lectin endothelial cell-leukocyte adhesion molecule-1. J Exp Med 174:1471–1476, 1991.

12. Bill A. The role of ciliary blood flow and ultrafiltration in aqueous humor formation. Exp Eye Res 16:287–299, 1973.

13. Borth W, Urbanski A, Prohaska R, Susani M, Lugar RA. Binding of recombinant interleukin-1β to the third complement component and α-$_2$-macroglobulin after activation of serum by immune complexes. Blood 75:2388–2395, 1990.

14. Bradbury M. The structure and function of the blood-brain barrier. Federation Proc 43:186–190, 1984.

15. Brandtzaeg P. Overview of the mucosal immune system. Curr Top Microbiol Immunol 147:13–25, 1989.

16. Broadwell RD, Brightman MW. Entry of peroxidase into neurons of the central and peripheral nervous systems from extracerebral and cerebral blood. J Comp Neurol 166:256, 1976.

17. Burns FR, Li X, Shen N, Offner H, Chou YK, Vandenbark AA, Heber-Katz E. Both rat and mouse T cell receptors specific for the encephalitogenic determinant of myelin basic protein use similar Vα and Vβ chain genes even though the major histocompatibility complex and encephalitogenic determinants being recognized are different. J Exp Med 169:27–39, 1989.

18. Caspi RR. Basic mechanisms in immune-mediated uveitic disease. In: Immunology of Eye Disease, SL Lightman, ed. MTP Press, London, pp 61–86, 1989.

19. Caspi RR, Roberge FG, Nussenblatt RB: Organ-resident, nonlymphoid cells suppress proliferation of autoimmune T helper lymphocytes. Science 237:1029, 1987.

20. Chin H-Y, Falanga V, Streilein JW, Sackstein R. Specific lymphocyte-endothelial cell interactions regulate migration into lymph nodes, Peyer's patches, and skin. Regional Immunology 1:78–83, 1988.

21. Clark WR. The Experimental Foundations of Modern Immunology, fourth ed. Wiley, New York, pp. 359–379, 1991.

22. Cousins SW. T cell activation within different intraocular compartments during experimental uveitis. Dev Ophthalmol 23:151–156, 1992.

23. Cousins S, McCabe M, Danielpour R, Streilein JW. Identification of transforming growth factor-beta as an immunosuppressive factor in aqueous humor. Invest Ophthalmol Vis Sci 32:2201–2211, 1991.

24. Cousins SW, Streilein JW. Flow cytometric detection of lymphocyte proliferation in eyes with immunogenic inflammation. Invest Ophthalmol Vis Sci 31:2111–2122, 1990.

25. Cousins S, Trattler W, Streilein JW. Immune privilege and suppression of immunogenic inflammation in the anterior chamber of the eye. Curr Eye Res 10:287–297, 1991.

26. Cserr H. Physiology of the choroid plexus. Physiol Rev 51:273–311, 1971.

27. Cserr HF, Harling-Berg C, Ichimura T, Knopf PM, Yamada S. Drainage of cerebral extracellular fluids into cervical lymph: an afferent limb in brain/immune system interactions. In: Pathophysiology of the Blood-Brain Barrier, BB Johansson, C Owman, H Widner, eds. Elsevier Science Publishers (Biomedical Division), pp 413–420, 1990.

28. Cserr HF, Knopf PM. Cervical lymphatics, the blood-brain barrier and the immunoreactivity of the brain: a new view. Immunol Today 13:507–512, 1992.

29. Demidem A, Taylor JR, Grammer SF, Streilein JW. Comparison of effects of transforming growth factor-beta and cyclosporin A on APC of blood and epidermis. J Invest Dermatol 96:401–407, 1991.

30. Dix RD, Resnick L, Culbertson W, Dickinson G, Fisher EMS. Intraocular HIV-1-specific IgG synthesis in a patient with CMV retinits. Reg Immunol 2:1–6, 1989.

31. Dorf ME, Kuchroo VK, Steele JK, O'Hara RM. Understanding suppressor cells: where have we gone wrong? Int Rev Immunol 3:375–392, 1988.

32. Feilder AR, Rahi AHS. Immunoglobulins of normal aqueous humor. Trans Opthalmologr Soc United Kingdom 99:120–125, 1979.

33. Fenstermacher JH, Rapoport SI. Blood-brain barrier. In: Handbook of Physiology. The Cardiovascular System, Vol. IV, Microcirculation, EM Ranken, CC Michel, eds. Am Physiol Soc Bethesda, MD, 1984, part 2, chapt. 21, pp. 969–1000.

34. Ferrer JF. Role of the spleen in passive immunological enhancement. Transplantation 6:167, 1968.

35. Fontana A, Fierz W, Wekerle H. Astrocytes present myelin basic protein to encephalitogenic T cell lines. Nature 307:273–276, 1984.

36. Freddo T, Bartels S, Baersotti M, Kamm R. The source of proteins in aqueous humor of the normal rabbit. Invest Ophthalmol Vis Sci 31:125–138, 1990.

37. Gery I, Mochizuki M, Nussenblatt RB. Retinal specific antigens and immunopathogenic processes they provoke. Prog Retinal Res 5:75–109, 1986.

38. Ghose T, Quigley JH, Landrigan PL, Asif A. Immunoglobulins in aqueous humor and iris from patient with endogenous uveitis patients with cataract. Br J Opthalmol 57:897–903, 1973.

39. Gordon LB, Knopf PM, Cserr HF. Ovalbumin is more immunogenic when introduced into brain or cerebrospinal fluid than into extracerebral sites. J Neuroimmunol 40:81–88, 1992.

40. Granstein R, Stszewski R, Knisely, T, Zeira E, Nazareno R, Latina M, Albert D. Aqueous humor contains transforming growth factor-β and a small (<3500 daltons) inhibitor of thymocyte proliferation. J Immunol 145:3021–3027, 1990.

41. Hamel CP, De Luca H, Billotte C, Offret H, Bloch-Michel E. Nonspecific immunoglobulin E in aqueous humor: evaluation in uveitis. Graefes Arch F Clin Exp Opthalmol 227:489–493, 1989.

42. Hara Y, Caspi R, Wiggert B, Chan CC, Wilbanks GD, Streilein JW. Suppression of experimental autoimmune uveitis in mice by induction of Anterior Chamber Associated Im-

mune Deviation with interphotoreceptor retinoid binding protein. J Immunol 149:1685–1692, 1992.

43. Hara Y, Caspi RR, Wiggert B, Dorf M, Streilein JW. Analysis of an in vitro-generated signal that induces systemic immune deviation similar to that elicited by antigen injected into the anterior chamber of the eye. J Immunol 150:1541–1548, 1992.

44. Harling-Berg C, Knopf PM, Cserr HF. Mylein basic protein infused into cerebrospinal fluid suppresses experimental autoimmune encephalomyelitis. J Neuroimmunol 35:45–51, 1991.

45. Harling-Berg C, Knopf PM, Merriam J, Cserr HF. Role of cervical lymph nodes in the systemic humoral immune response to human serum albumin microinfused into rat cerebrospinal fluid. J Neuroimmunol 25:185–193, 1989.

46. Hart DNJ, Fabre JW. Demonstration and characterization of Ia-positive dendritic cells in the interstitial connective tissues of rat heart and other tissues, but not brain. J Exp Med 154:347–361, 1981.

47. Hart MN, Fabry Z, Waldschmidt M, Sandor F. Lymphocyte interacting adhesion molecules on brain microvascular cells. Mol Immunol 27:1365–1369, 1990.

48. Head JR, Griffin WST. Functional capacity of solid tissue transplants in the brain: evidence for immunological privilege. Proc R Soc Lond B Biol Sci 224:375–387, 1985.

49. Helbig H, Gurley RC, Palestine AG, Nussenblatt RB, Caspi RR. Dual effect of ciliary body cells on T lymphocyte proliferation. Eur J Immunol 20:2457–2463, 1990.

50. Helbig H, Kittredge K, Coca-Prados M, Davis J, Palestine A, Nussenblatt R. Mammalian ciliary body epithelial cells in culture produce transforming growth factor-beta. Graefes Arch Clin Exp Ophthalmol 229:84–87, 1991.

51. Hellstrom KE, Hellstrom I. Lymphocyte-mediated cytotoxicity and blocking serum activity to tumor antigens. Adv Immunol 18:209–277, 1974.

52. Hickey WF, Kimura H. Perivascular microglial cells of the CNS are bone marrow-derived and present antigen in vivo. Science 239:290–292, 1988.

53. Hooper P, Bora NS, Kaplan HJ, Ferguson TA. Inhibition of lymphocyte proliferation by resident ocular cells. Curr Eye Res 10:363–372, 1991.

54. Hou SC, Ho ST, Shaio MF. Opsonizing effect of normal cerebrospinal fluid on Staphylococcus aureus. J Formos Med Assoc 89:977–981, 1990.

55. Jampel HD, Roche N, Stark WJ, Roberts AB. Transforming growth factor-β in human aqueous humor. Curr Eye Res 9:963–969, 1990.

56. Jiang LQ, Streilein JW. Immune privilege extended to allogeneic tumor cells in the vitreous cavity. Invest Ophthalmol Vis Sci 32:224–228, 1991.

57. Jiang LQ, Streilein JW. Immunologic privilege evoked by histoincompatible intracameral retinal transplants. Reg Immunol 3:121–131, 1991.

58. Jiang LQ, Streilein JW. Immunity and immune privilege elicited by autoantigens expressed on syngeneic neonatal neural retina grafts. Curr Eye Res 11:697–709, 1992.

59. Kaiser C, Ksander B, Streilein JW. Inhibition of lymphocyte proliferation by aqueous humor. Reg Immunol 2:42–49, 1989.

60. Kaplan HJ, Stevens TR. A reconsideration of immunologic privilege within the anterior chamber of the eye. Transplantation 19:302–309, 1974.

61. Kaplan HJ, Streilein JW. Do immunologically privileged sites require a functioning spleen? Nature 251:553–554, 1974.

62. Kaplan HJ, Streilein JW. Immune response to immunization via the anterior chamber of the eye. I. F_1 lymphocyte induced-immune deviation. J Immunol 118:809–814, 1977.

63. Kaplan HJ, Streilein JW, Stevens TR. Transplantation immunology of the anterior chamber of the eye. II. Immune response to allogeneic cells. J Immunol 115:805–910, 1975.

64. Keane RW, Tallent MW, Podack ER. Resistance and susceptibility of neural cells to lysis by cytotoxic lymphocytes and by cytolitic granules. Transplantation 54:520–526, 1992.

65. Kijlstra A, Luyendijk L, Baarsma GS, Rothova A, Schweitze CM, Timmerman Z, de Vries J, Breebaart A. Aqueous humor analysis as a diagnostic tool in toxoplasma uveitis. Int Opthalmol 13:383–386, 1989.

66. Kim P-H, Kagnoff MF. Transforming growth factor β1 increases IgA isotype switching at the clonal level. J Immunol 146:3773–3778, 1990.

67. Kimura R, Hu H, Stein-Streilein J. Delayed-type hypersensitivity responses regulate collagen deposition in the lung. Immunology 77:550–555, 1992.

68. Knisely TL, Bleicher PA, Vibbard CA, Granstein RD. Morphologic and ultrastructural examination of I-A$^+$ cells in the murine iris. Invest Ophthalmol Vis Sci 32:2423–2431, 1991.

69. Knisely TL, Bleicher PA, Vibbard CA, Granstein RD. Production of latent transforming growth factor-beta and other inhibitory factors by cultured murine iris and ciliary body cells. Curr Eye Res 10:761, 1991.

70. Ksander BR, Mammolenti MM, Streilein JW. Immune privilege in the anterior chamber of the eye terminates when tumor infiltrating lymphocytes acquire cytolytic function. Transplantation 52:129–133, 1991.

71. Ksander BR, Streilein JW. Immune privilege to MHC disparate tumor grafts in the anterior chamber of the eye. I. Quantitative analysis of intraocular tumor growth and the corresponding delayed hypersensitivity response. Transplantation 47:661–667, 1989.

72. Ksander BR, Streilein JW. Failure of infiltrating precursor cytotoxic T cells to acquire direct cytotoxic function in immunologically privileged sites. J Immunol 146:2057–2063, 1991.

73. Kupiec-Weglinski, JW, Austyn JM, Morris PJ. Migration patterns of dendritic cells in the mouse. J Exp Med 167:632–645, 1988.

74. Lampson L. Molecular bases of the immune response to neural antigens. Trends Neurosci 10:211–216, 1987.

75. Lampson LA. MHC regulation in neural cells. J Immunol 145:512–520, 1990.

76. Lampson LA, George DL. Interferon-mediated induction of class I MHC products in human neuronal cell lines: analysis of HLA and β2-m RNA, and HLA-A and HLA-B proteins and polymorphic specificities. J Interferon Res 6:257–265, 1986.

77. Lass JH, Walter EI, Burris TE, Brossniklaus HE, Roat MI, Skelnik DL, Needham L, Singer M, Medof, ME. Expression of two molecular forms of the complement decay-accelerating factor in the eye and lacrimal gland. Invest Opthalmol Vis Sci 31:1137–1149, 1990.

78. Macatonia S, Knogith SC, Edwards AJ, Griffiths S, Fryer P. Localization of antigen on lymph node dendritic cells after exposure to the contact sensitizer fluorescein isothiocyanate. J Exp Med 166:1654–1667, 1987.

79. Matsuda T, Hirano T, Nagasawa S, Kishimoto T. Identification of α$_2$-macroglobulin as a carrier protein for IL-6. J Immunol 143:149–153, 1989.

80. Mattingly JA, Waksman BH. Immunologic suppression after oral administration of antigen. Specific suppressor cells formed in rat Peyers' patches after oral administration of sheep erythrocytes. J Immunol 121:1878–1883, 1978.

81. McMenamin PG, Holthouse I, Holt PG. Class II major histocompatibility complex (Ia) antigen-bearing dendritic cells within the iris and ciliary body of the rat eye: distribution, phenotype and relation to retinal microglia. Immunology 77:385–393, 1992.

82. Medawar P. Immunity to homologous grafted skin. III. The fate of skin homografts transplanted to the brain, to subcutaneous tissue, and to the anterior chamber of the eye. Br J Exp Pathol 29:58–69, 1948.

83. Miki S, Ksander B, Streilein JW. Studies on minimum requirements for in vitro "cure" of tumor cells by cytotoxic T lymphocytes. Reg Immunol 4:352–362, 1992.

84. Mizel SB. Interleukin-1 and T-cell activation. Immunol Rev 63:51–72, 1982.

85. Mizuno K, Clark AF, Streilein JW. Ocular injection of retinal S antigen: suppression of autoimmune uveitis. Invest Ophthalmol Vis Sci 30:772–774, 1989.

86. Mizuno K, Clark AF, Streilein JW. Anterior chamber associated immune deviation induced by soluble antigens. Invest Ophthalmol Vis Sci 30:1112–1119, 1989.

87. Mondino BJ, Phinney R. The complement system in ocular allergy. Int Ophthalmol Clin 28:329–331, 1988.

88. Mucke L, Oldstone MB. The expression of major histocompatibility complex (MHC) class I antigens in the brain differs markedly in acute and persistent infections with lymphocytic choriomeningitis virus (LCMV). J Neuroimmunol 36:193–198, 1992.

89. Munn CG, Bucana C, Kripke ML. Antigen-binding cells from lymph nodes of mice sensitized epicutaneously with hapten have features of epidermal Langerhans cells. J Invest Dermatol 92:487–489, 1989.

90. Murray PI, Hoekzema R, Luyendijk L, Koning S, Kijlstra A. Analysis of aqueous humor immunoglobulin G in uveitis by enzyme-linked immunosorbent assay, isoelectric focusing, and immunoblotting. Invest Opthalmol Vis Sci 31:2130–2136, 1990.

91. Nathanson JA, Chun LY. Immunological function of the blood-cerebrospinal fluid barrier. Proc Natl Acad Sci USA 86:1684–1688, 1989.

92. Neilson EG, Jimenez SA, Phillips SM. Cell mediated immunity in interstitial nephritis. 3.T lymphocyte-mediated fibroblast proliferation and collagen synthesis: an immune mechanism for renal fibrogenesis. J Immunol 125:1708–1714, 1980.

93. Niederkorn JY. Immune privilege and immune regulation in the eye. Adv Immunol 48:191–226, 1990.

94. Niederkorn JY, Benson JL, Mayhew E. Efferent blockade of delayed-type hypersensitivity responses in the anterior chamber of the eye. Reg Immunol 3:349–354, 1991.

95. Niederkorn JY, Streilein JW. Immunogenetic basis for immunologic privilege in the anterior chamber of the eye. Immunogenetics 13:227–236, 1981.

96. O'Connor-McCourt MD, Wakefield LM. Latent transforming growth factor-β in serum: a specific complex with α_2-macroglobulin. J Biol Chem 262:14190–14199, 1987.

97. Parish C: The relationship between humoral and cell-mediated immunity. Transplant Rev 13:35–66, 1982.

98. Paterson P. Experimental allergic encephalomyelitis and autoimmune disease. Adv Immunol 5:132–208, 1966.

99. Perry VH, Hume DA, Gordon S. Immunohistochemical localization of macrophages and microglia in the adult and developing mouse brain. Neuroscience 15:313–326, 1985.

100. Peress NS, Perillo E. Immunoglobulin G receptor-mediated phagocytosis by the pigmented epithelium of the ciliary processes. Invest Opthalmol Vis Sci 32:78–87, 1991.

101. Prehn RT. The immunity-inhibiting role of the spleen and the effect of dosage and route of antigen administration in a homograft reaction. Biological Problems of Grafting. Les Congres et Colloques de l'Universite de Liege. 12:163, 1959.

102. Pryce G, Male DK, Sarkar C. Control of lymphocyte migration into brain: selective interactions of lymphocyte subpopulations with brain endothelium. Immunology 72:393–398, 1991.

103. Raju S, Grogan J. Immunological study of the brain as a privileged site. Transplant Proc 9:1187–1191, 1977.

104. Reiber H, Felgenhauer K. Protein transfer at the blood cerebrospinal fluid barrier and the

quantification of the humoral immune response within the central nervous system. Clin Chim Acta 163:319–328, 1987.

105. Romball CG, Weigle WO. Splenic role in the regulation of immune responses. Cell Immunol 34:376–384, 1977.

106. Sedgwick JD, Moffner R, Schwender S, Ter Meulen V. MHC-expressing non-hematopoietic astroglial cells prime only CD8+T lymphocytes. J Exp Med 173:1235–1246, 1991.

107. Sedgwick JD, Schwender S, Imrich HJ, Dories R, Butcher GW, Ter Meulen V. Isolation and direct characterization of resident microglial cells from the normal and inflamed central nervous system. Proc Natl Acad Sci USA 88:7438–7442, 1991.

108. Sethna MP, Lampson LA. Immune modulation of the brain: transient and long-lasting, restricted and widespread effects of intracerebral IFNγ on MHC expression, and on infiltration of leukocyte subpopulations. J Neuroimmunol 34:121, 1992.

109. Siegelman J, Peress NS. Fc receptor-mediated binding and ingestion of immunoglobulin G-coated erythrocytes by the epithelium of the posterior ciliary processes: an in-vitro study. Exp Eye Res 47:361–367, 1988.

110. Sminia T, deGroot JA, Dijkstra CD, Koetsier JC, Polman CH. Macrophages in the central nervous system of the rat. J Immunol 174:43–50, 1987.

111. Sonoda Y, Ksander B, Streilein JW. Evidence that active suppression contributes to the success of H-2-incompatible orthotopic corneal allografts in mice. Transplant Proc 25:1384–1386, 1993.

112. Sonoda Y, Streilein JW. Orthotopic corneal transplantation in mice. Evidence that the immunogenetic rules of rejection do not apply. Transplantation 54:694–703, 1992.

113. Steinman, RM, Van Voorhis WC, Spalding DM. Dendritic cells. In: DM Weir, C Blackwell, LA Herzenberg, eds. Handbook of Experimental Immunology, 4th ed, Blackwell Scientific, Oxford, 1986, p 49.

114. Streilein JW. Immune regulation and the eye: a dangerous compromise. FASEB J 1:199–208, 1987.

115. Streilein JW. Skin associated lymphoid tissues (SALT): the next generation. In: The Skin Immune System (SIS), J Bos, ed. CRC Press, 1990, pp 26–48.

116. Streilein JW. Regional immunology. In Encyclopedia of Human Biology, R. Dulbecca, ed. Academic Press, New York, 1991, pp 391–440.

117. Streilein JW. Sunlight and SALT: If UVB is the trigger, and TNFα is its mediator, what is the message? J Invest Dermatol 11:47S–52S, 1993.

118. Streilein JW, Atherton S, Vann VA. Critical role for ACAID in the distinctive pattern of retinitis that follows anterior chamber inoculation of HSV-1. Curr Eye Res 6:127–133, 1987.

119. Streilein JW, Bradley D. Analysis of immunosuppressive properties of iris and ciliary body cells and their secretory products. Invest Ophthalmol Vis Sci 32:2700–2710, 1991.

120. Streilein JW, Cousins S, Bradley D. Effect of intraocular gamma interferon on immunoregulatory properties of iris and ciliary body cells. Invest Ophthalmol Vis Sci 33:2304–2315, 1992.

121. Streilein JW, Niederkorn JY. Induction of anterior chamber-associated immune deviation requires an intact, functional spleen. J Exp Med 154:1058–1067, 1981.

122. Streilein JW, Niederkorn JY. Characterization of the suppressor cell(s) responsible for Anterior Chamber Associated Immune Deviation (ACAID) induced in BALB/c mice by P815 cells. J Immunol 135:1391–1397, 1985.

123. Streilein JW, Toews GB, Bergstresser PR. Corneal allografts fail to express Ia antigens. Nature 282:326–327, 1979.

124. Streilein JW, Wilbanks GA, Cousins SW. Immunoregulatory mechanisms of the eye. J Neuroimmunol 39:185–200, 1992.

125. Sy M-S, Miller SD, Kowach HW, Claman HM. A splenic requirement for generation of suppressor T cells. J Immunol 119:2095–2099, 1977.

126. Takiguchi M, Frelinger JA. Induction of antigen presentation ability in purified cultures of astroglia by interferon-γ. J Mol Cell Immunol 2:269–280, 1986.

127. Taylor AW, Streilein JW, Cousins SW. Identification of alpha-melanocyte stimulating hormone as a potential immunosuppressive factor in aqueous humor. Curr Eye Res 11:1199–1206, 1992.

128. Taylor AW, Streilein JW, Cousins SW. Immunoreactive vasoactive intestinal peptide contributes to the immunosuppressive activity of normal aqueous humor. J Immunol 154:1080–1086, 1994.

129. Tedeschi B, Barrett JN, Keane RW. Astrocytes produce interferon that enhances the expression of H-2 antigens on a subpopulation of brain cells. J Cell Biol 102:2244–2253, 1986.

130. Thompson E. Differences in CSF versus serum proteins. In: The CSF Proteins: A Biochemical Approach, E Thompson, ed. Elsevier, Oxford, UK, 1988, pp 27–34.

131. Toews GB, Bergstresser PR, Streilein JW. Epidermal Langerhans cell density determines whether contact sensitivity or unresponsiveness follows skin painting with DNFB. J Immunol 124:445–453, 1980.

132. Tomasi TB. The discovery of secretory IgA and the mucosal immune system. Immunol Today 13:416–418, 1992.

133. Tompsett E, Abi-Hanna D, Wakefield D. Immunological privilege in the eye: a review. Curr Eye Res 9:1141–1145, 1990.

134. Tourtellotte WW, Staugaitis SM, Walsh MJ, Shapshak P, Baumhefner RW, Potvin AR, Syndulko K. The basis of intra-blood: brain barrier IgG synthesis. Ann Neurol 17:32–27, 1985.

135. Tripathi RC, Borisuth NSC, Tripathi BJ. Mapping of Fc gamma receptors in the human and porcine eye. Exp Eye Res 53:647–656, 1991.

136. Van der Lelij A, Rothova A, De Vries JP, Vetter JC, Van Haren MA, Stilman JS, Kijlstra A. Analysis of aqueous humour in ocular onchocerciasis. Curr Eye Res 10:169–176, 1991.

137. Vermeer M, Streilein JW. Ultraviolet-B light induced alterations in epidermal Langerhans cells are mediated by tumor necrosis factor-alpha. Photodermatol Photoimmunol Photomed 7:258–265, 1990.

138. Wahlestedt C, Beding B, Ekman R, Oksala O, Stjernschantz J, Hakanson R. Calcitonin gene-related peptide in the eye: release by sensory nerve stimulation and effects associated with neurogenic inflammation. Regul Pep 16:107–115, 1986.

139. Waldrep JC, Kaplan HJ. ACAID induced by TNP-splenocytes (TNP-ACAID), I. Systemic tolerance mediated by suppressor T cells. Invest Ophthalmol Vis Sci 24:1086–1092, 1983.

140. Waksman BH. Immunity and the nervous system: basic tenets. Ann Neurol 13:587–591, 1983.

141. Weed LH. The cerebrospinal fluid. Physiol Rev 171:171–203, 1922.

142. Weller M, Stevens A, Sommer N, Wiethölter H, Dichgans J. Cerebrospinal fluid interleukins, immunoglobulins, and fibronectin in neuroborreliosis. Arch Neurol 48:837–841, 1991.

143. Whelan JP, Eriksson U, Lampson LA. Expression of mouse α2-microglobulin in frozen and formaldehyde-fixed central nervous tissues: comparison of tissue behind the blood-brain barrier and tissue in a barrier-free region. J Immunol 138:2561–2566, 1986.

144. Whittum JA, McCulley JP, Niederkorn JY, Streilein JW. Ocular disease induced in mice by

anterior chamber inoculation of herpes simplex virus. Invest Ophthalmol Vis Sci 25:1065–1073, 1984.

145. Whittum JA, Niederkorn JY, McCulley JP, Streilein JW. Intracameral inoculation of herpes simplex virus type 1 induces anterior chamber associated immune deviation. Curr Eye Res 2:691–697, 1983.

146. Wilbanks GA, Mammolenti MM, Streilein JW. Studies on the induction of Anterior Chamber Associated Immune Deviation (ACAID). II. Eye-derived cells participate in generating blood borne signals that induce ACAID. J Immunol 147:3018–3024, 1991.

147. Wilbanks GA, Mammolenti MM, Streilein JW. Studies on the induction of Anterior Chamber-Associated Immune Deviation (ACAID) III. Induction of ACAID depends upon intraocular transforming growth factor-β. Eur J Immunol 22:165–173, 1992.

148. Wilbanks GA, Streilein JW. The differing patterns of antigen release and local retention following anterior chamber and intravenous inoculation of soluble antigen. Evidence that the eye acts as an antigen depot. Reg Immunol 2:390–398, 1989.

149. Wilbanks GA, Streilein JW. Characterization of suppressor cells in Anterior Chamber Associated Immune Deviation (ACAID) induced by soluble antigen. Evidence of two functionally and phenotypically distinct T-suppressor cell populations. Immunology 71:383–389, 1990.

150. Wilbanks GA, Streilein JW. Distinctive humoral responses following anterior chamber and intravenous administration of soluble antigen. Evidence for active suppression of IgG$_{2a}$-secreting B-cells. Immunology 71:566–572, 1990.

151. Wilbanks GA, Streilein JW. Studies on the induction of Anterior Chamber Associated Immune Deviation (ACAID). I. Evidence that an antigen-specific, ACAID-inducing, cell-associated signal exists in the peripheral blood. J Immunol 147:2610–2617, 1991.

152. Wilbanks GA, Streilein JW. Fluids from immune privileged sites endow macrophages with capacity to induce antigen-specific immune deviation via a mechanism involving transforming growth factor-beta. Eur J Immunol 22:1031–1036, 1992.

153. Wilbanks G, Streilein JW. Macrophages capable of inducing anterior chamber associated immune deviation demonstrate spleen-seeking migratory properties. Reg Immunol 4:131–138, 1992.

154. Williamson JSP, Bradley D, Streilein JW. Immunoregulatory properties of bone marrow-derived cells in the iris and ciliary body. Immunology 67:96–102, 1989.

155. Williamson JSP, DiMarco S, Streilein JW. Immunobiology of Langerhans cells on the ocular surface. I. Langerhans cells within the central cornea interfere with induction of Anterior Chamber Associated Immune Deviation. Invest Ophthalmol Vis Sci 28:1537–1542, 1987.

156. Williamson JSP, Streilein JW. Impaired induction of delayed hypersensitivity following anterior chamber inoculation of alloantigens. Reg Immunol 1:15–23, 1988.

157. Wisniewski HM, Bloom BR. Primary demyelination as a nonspecific consequence of a cell-mediated immune reaction. J Exp Med 142:346–359, 1975.

158. Wong GHW, Bartlett PF, Clark-Lewis I, Battye F, Schrader JW. Inducible expression of H-2 and Ia antigens on brain cells. Nature 310:688–691, 1984.

159. Wright KE, Buchmeier MJ: Antiviral antibodies attenuate T-cell-mediated immunopathology following acute lymphocytic choriomeningitis virus infection. J Virol 65:3001–3006, 1991.

160. Yamada S, DePasquale M, Patlak C, Cserr HF. Albumin outflow into deep cervical lymph from different regions of rabbit brain. Am J Physiol 240 (Renal Fluid Electrolyte Physiol 9): F329–F336, 1981.

161. Yoshikawa T, Streilein JW. Tumor necrosis factor-alpha and ultraviolet B light have similar effects on contact hypersensitivity in mice. Reg Immunol 3:140–145, 1991.

4

Cervical Lymphatics, the Blood-Brain Barrier, and the Immunoreactivity of the Brain

HELEN F. CSERR
PAUL M. KNOPF

Helen F. Cserr
In Memorium

Helen F. Cserr died of a brain tumor in August 1994.
We dedicate this review to her memory.

During her career, Helen contributed significantly to the understanding of brain fluid volume regulation and the blood-brain barrier. While some subsequent editing of the review has introduced minor changes in the text for clarification, the review was written before she became ill. In particular, the sections on cervical lymphatics, the blood-brain barrier, and tissue-specific features contributing to the immunoreactivity of the brain, represent to a large extent Helen's personal perspective on the significance of connections between the central nervous system and immune system and on the regulation of this interaction.

Historical Survey

The brain has been characterized immunologically as a site of limited reactivity. This concept, termed *immune privilege,* developed from classical transplantation studies showing that tissue or tumor allografts generally survive better in the brain than in more conventional sites (as reviewed in 2,9,57). Immune rejection of such allografts is usually a cell-mediated immune reaction. Mechanisms of humoral immunity in the normal brain and their relation to the concept of immune privilege were usually not addressed.

The biological significance of immune privilege in the brain and the eye seems clear. As expressed by Leslie Brent (9), "it may be supposed that it is beneficial to the organism not to turn the anterior chamber or the cornea of the eye, or the brain, into an inflammatory battlefield, for the immunological response is sometimes more damaging than the antigen insult that provoked it."

While there may be agreement as to the benefits of immune privilege, mechanisms contributing to this immune state have been a subject of debate. Classical explanations emphasized isolation of the brain from the immune system (2,32). The absence of conventional lymphatics within the brain was believed to interfere with the afferent arm of the immune response to antigen within the tissue, due to the perceived lack of drainage of immunogenic signals to regional nodes. The presence of the blood-brain barrier was thought to block the efferent arm by preventing entrance of effector cells and molecules of the immune system into the brain. According to this view, immune privilege is a state of passive nonreactivity resulting from isolation of the brain from the immune system.

Results of more recent studies are incompatible with this view: both afferent and efferent connections between the brain and the draining lymph nodes and spleen are evident. The afferent connection includes outflow of antigenic signals from brain tissue into surrounding cerebrospinal fluid (CSF), via perivascular (or Virchow-Robin) spaces, followed by subsequent passage from CSF to both cervical lymphatics and spleen (as reviewed in 6). The efferent connection, while less well characterized, includes passage of activated T cells (26,55), and possibly also B cells (16), from the cerebral vasculature into the normal brain. These results demand a new explanation for immune privilege which incorporates active communication between the brain and secondary lymphoid organs, via outflow to the cervical lymphatics and spleen, plus lymphocyte passage into the brain across the vascular endothelium.

Immunoreactivity of the normal brain has been studied in our laboratory, using a rat model with normal blood-brain barrier permeability (12,17,24). Other laboratories have studied the eye, following antigen administration into the anterior chamber (28,44,50). Antigens administered into either site elicit a sterotypic immune response. Delayed hypersensitivity (DH) is markedly suppressed (23,44), which presumably contributes to the ability to allografts to survive for prolonged periods within the brain or eye. Humoral immunity, on the other hand, is stimulated (24,59) or, in the case of brain, enhanced compared to immunization at peripheral sites (21). Antibody responses will not be inflammatory, since concentrations of complement components are very low in normal rat CSF (16) and antibody isotypes in mice immunized in the anterior chamber of the eye with soluble proteins are biased to complement nonfixing IgG subclasses (59). Moreover, the presence of decay-accelerating factor in the eye actively protects ocular tissue from complement-mediated lysis (31). These results confirm the presence of functional afferent and efferent connections between the brain or eye and the immune system. Furthermore, they suggest that the phenomenon of immune privilege may be understood in terms of selective expression of a distinctive spectrum of non-inflammatory, immune effectors within the tissue (17,45,46).

Regional specialization of immune mechanisms is well recognized. Two "regions" of the immune system are the mucosa-associated lymphoid tissues (MALT) and bronchial-associated lymphoid tissues (BALT). Streilein extended this concept of regional specialization in immune responses to include the nervous system (45,46). Furthermore, he and Taylor have proposed that the distinctive regional immune system serving the nervous system—the brain, the eye, and peripheral nerves—be called the *neural-ocular immune system* (see Chapter 3 of this monograph). No longer can the normal nervous system be viewed as isolated and beyond the purview of the immune system. Rather, it emerges as an example of a general principle of regional immunity.

This current characterization of the immunoreactivity of the nervous system remains consistent with the classical view of immune privilege as a noninflammatory state. It differs, however, in that *(1)* limited immunoreactivity of the nervous system is viewed as an active rather than a passive state, *(2)* the roles of cervical lymphatics and the blood-brain barrier are redefined as mediating and regulating interactions with the immune system, and *(3)* the relations of humoral immunity to the concept of immune privilege is addressed (17).

Our interests in the immunoreactivity of the brain developed from experiments by Cserr and colleagues on turnover of brain interstitial fluid (ISF) and its outflow to cervical lymph (7,15). Despite the absence of typical lymphatic channels in brain tissue, a significant fraction (14–47%) of protein injected into the brain could be collected from cervical lymphatics of common laboratory animals (7,61). On the basis of this finding, we began to explore connections between the brain and the immune system in a rat model with normal brain-barrier permeability. In this chapter we first review features of brain fluid dynamics, cervical lymphatics, and the blood-brain barrier essential to an understanding of interactions between the brain and immune system. We then address the issue of immunoreactivity of the normal brain. Emphasis will be on tissues and fluids of the brain, the topic of this chapter, with discussion of the eye as appropriate. The recognition that mechanisms of immunity extend to normal brain demands a critical reevaluation of the basic tenets of neuroimmunology in health and disease.

Cervical Lymphatics and Afferent Connections from the Brain to the Draining Nodes and Spleen

Turnover of Brain Interstitial Fluid (ISF)

Comparison with Extracerebral Tissues

Individual neurons and glial cells within the brain are surrounded by a thin film of ISF. In most other tissues, ISF is produced from plasma by the process of filtration across the semipermeable capillary endothelium. It is then cleared from the interstitium either by filtration back into capillaries or by drainage with escaped proteins and cells into lymphatics. The situation in the brain can be expected to differ. The blood-brain barrier restricts filtration between plasma and cerebral ISF; the brain and spinal cord are surrounded by another extracellular fluid, the CSF; and, as emphasized above, there are no conventional lymphatics. Some connection between the brain and lymphatics has long been recognized, involving outflow of CSF along certain cranial nerves and spinal nerve roots (as reviewed in 62). However, this connection was felt to be quantitatively insignificant (32).

Perivascular Spaces and Outflow of ISF from the Brain to CSF

Modern studies are consistent with a model of ISF turnover in normal brain based on secretion of ISF by cerebral vascular endothelium, or blood-brain barrier, coupled with drainage of ISF into surrounding CSF (18,40). Relevant characteristics of the blood-brain–CSF system are illustrated in Fig. 4-1. Cerebral ISF is separated from plasma by

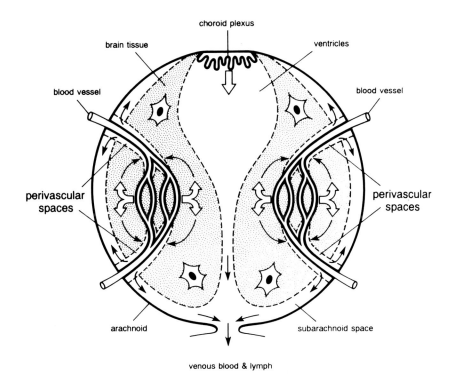

Fig. 4-1. Schematic diagram illustrating a model of interstitial fluid (ISF) turnover in the brain based on secretion of cerebral ISF by the blood-brain barrier (open arrows) and bulk flow of ISF from the brain to cerebrospinal fluid (CSF) via perivascular spaces (curved arrows). CSF is secreted by the choroid plexus (open arrow) and drains with ISF from the subarachnoid space to venous blood and to the lymph. Perivascular spaces extend along arteries and veins penetrating into the nervous tissue, down to the point at which arterioles and venules merge with capillaries.

the blood-brain barrier, whereas it is connected to CSF by specialized extracellular channels (as reviewed in 6). These channels consist principally of perivascular spaces, or Virchow-Robin spaces, which surround blood vessels as they penetrate into the brain. This vast network of perivascular channels provides a preferential pathway for outflow of ISF from the brain into surrounding CSF, as first suggested over a century ago by His (27). According to the model, secretion of ISF by the cerebral capillary endothelium through coupled transport of solutes and water generates a driving force for bulk flow of ISF from the brain to CSF, and ISF drains from the tissue.

The rate of ISF outflow from the normal brain has been estimated based on analysis of the kinetics of tracer outflow, following microinfusion of radiolabeled extracellular markers (albumin, polyethylene glycols) into brain tissue (14,15). Values $(ml \cdot g \ brain^{-1} \cdot min^{-1})$ range between 0.18 and 0.29 for different regions of rat brain (caudate nucleus, internal capsule, midbrain) (51) and between 0.10 and 0.15 for corresponding regions of rabbit brain (61). In the next section, we discuss the significance of this continuous outflow from various regions of the brain with respect to brain immunity.

Drainage of ISF and CSF into Blood and Lymph

Pathways of fluid outflow from the subarachnoid space to blood and lymph are illustrated in Fig. 4-2. From the cranial subarachnoid space, ISF and CSF can either drain into dural sinus blood, via arachnoid villi, or escape to extracranial tissue spaces, via prolongations of the subarachnoid space along certain cranial nerves. These include the olfactory, optic, trigeminal, and acoustic nerves (as reviewed in 6). The primary outflow pathway in common laboratory animals is along arachnoid sheaths of the olfactory nerves, through the cribriform plate, to nasal submucosa (8,58). Outflow from the spinal subarachnoid space also appears to involve drainage both into venous blood, via arachnoid granulations (56), and into tissue spaces outside the spinal column, by passage along spinal nerve root ganglia (10).

Substances draining from the cranial subarachnoid space via the olfactory pathway can be cleared from nasal submucosa by passage into terminal lymphatics or into blood capillaries. Proteins and other large molecular weight substances preferentially enter lymphatics and can be recovered in high concentration, relative to blood plasma, from deep cervical lymph collected from the jugular lymph trunks (8,61). Lymphocytes, macrophages (35), and erythrocytes (35,36,62) injected into brain follow the same pathway. In contrast, smaller molecular weight substances (5,000 daltons or less) only appear in low concentration in lymph, being lost to the blood due to a greater ability to penetrate the permeable vascular endothelium in the nasal submucosa and lymph nodes (8).

Quantitation of the connection to deep cervical lymph, using radioiodinated albumin as tracer, indicates that the magnitude of outflow to lymph is much larger (Table 4-1),

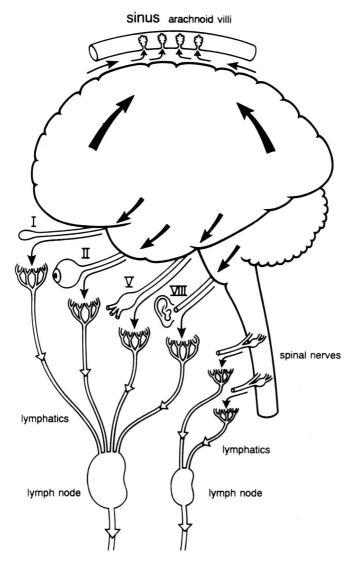

Fig. 4-2. Schematic diagram illustrating outflow pathways from the cranial and spinal subarachnoid space across the arachnoid villi to dural sinus blood or along certain cranial nerves and spinal nerve roots to lymphatics. I, olfactory nerve; II, optic; V, trigeminal; VIII, acoustic.

and the time course of passage through lymph is more prolonged than previously appreciated (61). A significant fraction of radiolabeled albumin cleared from widely dispersed regions of brain or intracranial CSF can be recovered from deep cervical lymph in common laboratory animals (61). It is important to emphasize that these values are minimal estimates of total outflow through lymph, due to the prolonged time required for passage through lymph (>26 hours), as compared to the experimental

Table 4-1 Recovery of Radioiodinated Albumin in Deep Cervical Lymph Following Injection into Brain or CSF[a], Where Recovery in Lymph is Given as a Percent of Total Outflow from the Central Nervous System

Species	Injection Site	Duration of Lymph Collection (hr)	Recovery in Lymph (percent)
Rabbit	Caudate nucleus	25	47
Rabbit	Internal capsule	25	22
Rabbit	Midbrain	25	18
Rabbit	CSF	6	30
Cat	CSF	8	14
Sheep	CSF	26	32

[a]Values from the literature compiled in ref. 61.

duration of lymph collection (6–26 hours). Following injection into brain tissue, radiolabeled protein begins to appear in lymph in about an hour. The concentration then increases slowly over time, reaching a maximum value some 15–20 hours later (61). This provides a prolonged period of antigenic exposure to the draining nodes. A similar delay in the time required to reach peak protein concentrations in lymph is seen after CSF-tracer injection, although with a shorter duration, (after 3–4 hours in the rabbit, somewhat later in the cat, and after 8–12 hours in the sheep, as reviewed in 6).

The Blood-Brain Barrier

The concept of a blood-brain barrier arose around the turn of the century based on studies showing that intravital dyes and neuroactive compounds, which pass from blood into most tissues, fail to penetrate into the brain (as reviewed in 4). Studies with protein tracers, which can be visualized by electron microscopy, localized the vascular barrier to the cerebral capillary endothelium (11). In extracerebral tissues, these tracers cross the capillary wall by passing through the narrow intercellular cleft or "pore" between adjoining endothelial cells. In the brain, this cleft is "zippered up" by bands of elaborate tight junctions, and the passage of tracers across the endothelium is blocked. The unusual tightness of these occluding junctions explains the marked impermeability of the blood-brain barrier.

The term *barrier* is probably misleading as applied to cerebral capillaries, in that it implies a physical obstacle between plasma and tissue interstitial fluid. Permeability properties of cerebral endothelium are governed both by those of the endothelial cell and of the cleft. As with cell membranes generally, lipid-soluble compounds such as blood gases and anesthetics penetrate rapidly across vascular endothelium, while passage of water-soluble molecules is highly selective. Some water-soluble molecules, including albumin and antibodies, are largely excluded. Others, including monosaccharides, amino acids, and K^+, penetrate by carrier-mediated mechanisms (as reviewed in 4,19). Furthermore, cerebral endothelia are reactive (1) and may respond to chemical or physical stimuli by modulating barrier permeability through changes in either endothelial transport (38) or junctional permeability (37,42). Clearly, the blood-brain barrier is not simply a physical barrier, but a dynamic interface between blood and the central nervous system (CNS).

The chemical composition of the extracellular fluid—or microenvironment—of the brain is more closely controlled than that of blood and general extracellular fluid. This homeostatic control extends to numerous substances, including inorganic ions, sugars, amino acids and peptide hormones. The blood-brain barrier contributes to this regulation by virtue of its selective transport and permeability properties (as reviewed in 13). In the section Immunoregulatory Molecules in the Microenvironment, we propose that the blood-brain barrier also participates in controlling immunoregulatory cells and molecules within the brain cell microenvironment.

Immunoreactivity of the Normal Brain

Overview

The immune response to tissue antigen can be considered as a circuit with afferent and efferent limbs. The *afferent limb* involves recognition of antigen from the tissue and generation of effector cells, and it includes antigen presentation and activation of lymphocytes. The *efferent limb* is concerned with the elimination of antigen by antibodies and effector cells, and it includes passage of activated lymphocytes and antibodies into the tissue via blood capillaries. Fig. 4-3 incorporates these fundamental components of an immune response with respect to the CNS and extracerebral lymphoid organs. This diagram is based on data from our laboratory, which is discussed below.

It is unlikely that the afferent limb can be completed within the tissues and fluids of the normal brain. The paucity of immunocompetent cells (32) and the limited expression of antigen-presenting major histocompatibility complex (MHC) molecules (30) reduces the probability of productive interactions between antigen and immune cells. Furthermore, brain fluids contain soluble immunoregulatory factors which selectively suppress certain immune functions (9,47,49). These findings suggest that immunogenic material must reach secondary lymphoid organs before it encounters the diversity of immunocompetent cells and chemical microenvironment required for initiation of an immune response (see Fig. 4-3A). The continual outflow from the normal brain of large molecular weight substances and mononuclear cells to blood and lymph provides for this possibility. This may be important, both for initiation of specific humoral or cell-mediated immunity against antigen draining from the brain, e.g., viral antigens, and for maintenance of self-tolerance of normal brain constituents.

PATHWAYS MEDIATING NORMAL CNS IMMUNITY

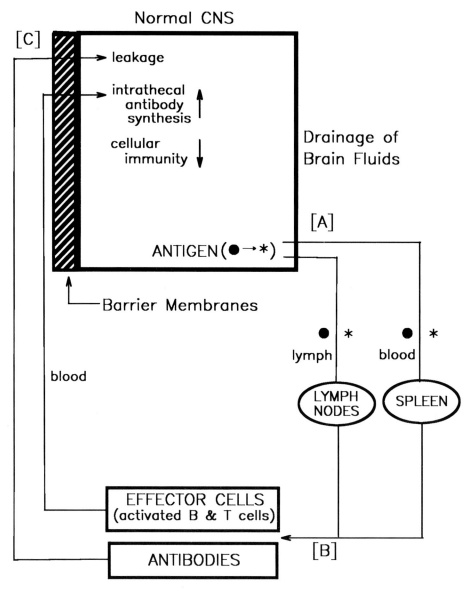

Fig. 4-3. Schematic diagram illustrating pathways leading to interaction between antigens (•) from the normal central nervous system (CNS) and extracerebral lymphoid organs (afferent arm, designated [A]). This interaction generates antigen-specific, activated effector cells and antibodies (designated [B]). The immune response loop is completed by the transbarrier movement of activated immune cells across intact brain-barrier membranes and antibody leakage across nonbarrier sites (efferent arm, designated [C]). Brain-barrier membranes consist of the cerebral endothelium, choroidal epithelium, and arachnoid. The scheme recognizes the possibility that

We have developed a rat model with normal blood-brain barrier permeability to explore the immunoreactivity of the normal brain (24). Antigen is microinfused into CSF or brain tissue, without adjuvant, through a cannula implanted 1 week previously. The 1-week recovery period ensures restoration of normal brain barrier function (12). This contrasts with the majority of other studies which have typically involved barrier disruption through acute insertion into brain tissue of needles or cannulas used to administer antigen. These other studies have also involved injection of pathogenic microorganisms (as reviewed in 24) or injection of such large volumes that immediate efflux to blood and lymph can be assumed (34).

The Systemic Response

The systemic immune response has been explored in our normal rat model using three unrelated, T-dependent protein antigens: human serum albumin (HSA), chicken oval-bumin (OV), and myelin basic protein (MBP). Microinfusion of either of the two albumins into the CNS yields a prolonged, antigen-specific serum antibody response, primarily IgG_1 and IgG_2, and antibody-secreting cells have been identified in both the cervical nodes and spleen (21,24) (see Fig. 4-3B). The nodes appear to be primary, however, based on studies showing that removal of cervical nodes markedly blunts the serum antibody response (24), whereas removal of the spleen is without effect on this response (Wu, Nolan, Cserr, and Knopf, unpublished observations).

Comparison of the magnitude of the serum antibody response in rats, following different routes of immunization, reveals that injections of albumin into CSF or brain tissue without adjuvant are far more immunogenic than injections into more conventional extracerebral sites (21,24). The immunoglobulin isotype profile is also distinctive, the ratio of $IgG_1:IgG_2$ isotypes being higher when antigen is administered via CSF rather than intramuscularly. Thus, contrary to classical interpretation of the brain as not being in communication with secondary lymphoid organs, we find that the humoral immune response to CSF-administered antigen may actually be enhanced and regulated.

MBP was used as antigen to explore the influence of CSF immunization on cell-mediated immunity. The effector T-cell response to MBP was examined using the

----

antigens in the brain are processed ($\bullet \rightarrow *$), in some way yet to be established. Immunogenic signals elicted by antigen in the CNS result in a noninflammatory response. Peripherally, this includes up-regulation of the antibody response. Within the CNS, this includes elevated antibody synthesis ($\uparrow$), and suppression of both delayed hypersensitivity and cytotoxic T-cell responses ($\downarrow$). Intrathecal antibody synthesis presumably involves activated B and T lymphocytes that have crossed intact barrier membranes from the periphery. The regulatory mechanisms responsible for such biased immune responses, involving extracerebral lymphoid organs and CNS microenvironment, are presently being investigated.

standard Lewis rat model of experimental autoimmune encephalomyelitis (EAE) (23), a neuroinflammatory disorder mediated by MBP-specific effector CD4+ T cells of the DH subset (25). Rats were initially given a single infusion of MBP into the CSF. Following subsequent encephalitogenic challenge with MBP in complete Freund's adjuvant, clinical signs of EAE were markedly suppressed in an antigen-specific manner. In addition, the number of inflammatory foci within the CNS were significantly reduced in EAE-suppressed rats as compared to controls (24a). As with the humoral response to CSF-administered albumins discussed above, CSF-administered MBP elicited suppression of DH greater than suppression elicited by systemically administered MBP (as reviewed in 23).

Synthesis of Antibodies within the Brain

Results summarized above demonstrate that the afferent connection from the brain to the immune system is intact. Numerous studies have shown that the efferent limb of the immune response to brain antigen is also intact, with respect to the passage of activated T lymphocytes into the normal brain (as reviewed in 9; 26,55). As a first step toward characterizing the efferent limb of the humoral immune response to antigen in the brain, we have examined CSF with respect to titer and isotype profile of the antibody response and with respect to complement activity (see Fig. 4-3C).

The ratio of CSF:serum titers, for antigen-specific antibody, is elevated in CSF-immunized rats. This excess antibody is present in the context of normal brain barrier permeability, as measured by serum albumin influx into CSF, and has been demonstrated using three antigens: HSA, OV, and UV-inactivated lymphocytic choriomeningitis virus (LCMV) (16,60). The mean CSF:serum ratio for anti-OV, for example, increased more than 20-fold in CSF-immunized rats as compared to those immunized intramuscularly. For HSA and OV, the CSF antibody isotype is primarily IgG (16), and the response to LCMV includes IgA (60).

Theoretically, the excess CSF antibody could be due either to receptor-mediated immunoglobulin transport from plasma to CSF or to antibody synthesis by plasma cells within the brain, i.e., the intrathecal synthesis. The possibility of receptor-mediated IgA transport was explored by analyzing the molecular form of IgA in the CSF of inactivated LCMV-immunized rats and in neuroinflammatory patients with elevated CSF IgA (60). IgA found in secretory fluids (milk, saliva, tears, etc.) is secreted across mucosal tissue membranes covalently bound to secretory component. In neither the LCMV-immunized rats nor the neuroinflammatory patients was the excess IgA in CSF associated with an increase in secretory component, showing that the secretory transport system for IgA does not extend to the brain.

Carrier-mediated transport has also been excluded as the source of the excess IgG in albumin-immunized rats (16). IgG transport in other organs is isotype specific, since it is mediated by receptors for the Fc portion of immunoglobulin. Comparison of the isotypes of anti-albumin antibodies, primarily IgG_1 and IgG_2, in serum and CSF failed to show a selective accumulation of one isotype relative to the other in CSF, a result inconsistent with carrier-mediated transport of antibody into CSF.

The conclusion that elevated CSF antibody titers in CSF-immunized rats are not associated with specific transport leaves intrathecal synthesis as the most likely source of the excess immunoglobulin both for IgA and IgG. The presence of antigen-specific plasma cells in the brain and of unique clones of antibody in CSF, as revealed by immunohistochemistry and isoelectric focusing, respectively, provides additional support for this conclusion (Cserr, Knopf, Basu, Sirulnick, Nolan, Keir, Thompson, and Hickey, unpublished observations). Intrathecal antibody synthesis has been well documented in animal models and in patients with increased brain barrier permeability or overt pathology (52,53). Our results are the first to suggest that this process also occurs in the presence of normal brain barrier permeability (see Fig. 4-3C).

The local humoral immune response within the privileged site is presumably valuable for neutralizing or opsonizing antigen. Antigen-antibody complexes formed by this process could then be cleared by cells displaying receptors for the Fc portion of IgG. These cells are located along the normal pathways of extracellular fluid outflow from the brain, including perivascular spaces, the leptomeninges, and arachnoid granulations (43).

Implications for B-cell Trafficking

What is the source of plasma cells contributing to the elevated CSF antibody response? Since activation of B cells occurs initially outside the brain, in the spleen and draining nodes, the conclusion that there is intrathecal synthesis implies passage of these activated, antigen-specific B cells from their extracerebral site of activation into the CNS. Activated T lymphocytes have the capacity to enter the brain (26). On the assumption that B-cell trafficking is similar, it may be suggested that activated B cells migrate into the brain as lymphoblasts, and those which receive the appropriate antigen-dependent cytokine stimulation remain (26,55) and differentiate to antibody-secreting cells. The concept of B-cell trafficking through the CNS under pathological conditions appears to be well accepted (53,54), although it has not been demonstrated formally using labeled B cells.

Immune Responses Elicited in the CNS Are Noninflammatory

The eye provides a convenient model for studying interactions between the immune system and normal nervous tissue since test substances can be introduced through the cornea without damaging the underlying retina. In this respect it is similar to our normal brain model. Results for both privileged sites are consistent with the view that immune responses in the normal nervous system are programmed to reduce potentially damaging inflammation (17,23,44).

Many antigens, when introduced into the anterior chamber of the eye, elicit antigen-specific systemic suppression of DH (20,44). Our finding that CSF-administered MBP suppresses the development of the neuroinflammatory disease, EAE, demonstrates the existence of similar mechanisms for the brain (23). Suppression of the inflammatory mechanisms of cell-mediated immunity is presumably a major factor contributing to the privileged status of both the anterior chamber and brain, as evidenced by the ability of allografts to survive longer in these sites. For example, following introduction of minor histoincompatible tumor cells into the anterior chamber, tumor-infiltrating cytotoxic T cells are prevented from acquiring tumor-specific cytotoxic T lymphocyte (CTL) activity at this privileged site (29). We have evidence for a similar phenomenon in the brain (Gordon, Nolan, Cserr, and Knopf, unpublished observations).

With respect to humoral immunity, soluble antigens in either the brain or anterior chamber elicit a serum antibody response (21,24,48,59) and, for the brain at least, local synthesis of antibodies within the tissue (16,60). Brain tissue will be protected from antibody-mediated inflammatory reactions associated with activation of the complement cascade, due to the low concentrations of components of the cascade within the extracellular microenvironment of the brain (16). In addition, in the case of the murine anterior chamber, the dominant isotype of serum antibody, IgG_1, does not fix complement (59).

Tissue-specific Features Contributing to the Distinctive Immunoreactivity of the Brain

The distinctive immunoreactivity of the normal brain and other privileged sites raises questions as to the mechanisms contributing to this regional specialization in immune effector mechanisms. Streilein's concept of regional specialization (see Historical Survey, above) relates the distinctive immune responses exhibited by different tissues to a number of tissue-specific features (46; Chapter 3 of this monograph). These features include a highly specialized extracellular microenvironment, tissue-specific antigen presenting cells, and unusual afferent and efferent connections from the tissue to the secondary immune organs. In the following sections, we first consider the unique immunoregulatory characteristics of the microenvironment in privileged sites. We then discuss the roles of the cervical lymphatics, spleen, and blood-brain barrier in mediating and regulating the immune response to antigen within the microenvironment of the brain.

Immunoregulatory Molecules in the Microenvironment

Recent attempts to explain the immunoreactivity of privileged sites, especially the eye, have focused on the presence or absence of immunoregulatory factors within the microenvironment. These studies have shown that the microenvironment is immunosuppressive and interferes with the expression of immunogenic inflammation and, further, that it mediates these effects by influencing both the induction and expression of immunity within the privileged site (50). It should be noted, however, that they do not address the possible role of the microenvironment in contributing to the enhanced humoral immunity characteristic of the neural-ocular immune system.

Specific examples of regulatory molecules, with extracellular concentrations unique to privileged sites, and their role in the local control of immune reactions include: *(1)* transforming growth factor β (TGF-β), which is present in the extracellular fluids of three privileged sites: CSF (47), aqueous humor (22,47), and amniotic fluid from the fetoplacental unit (49), and has been shown to endow macrophages with the capacity to induce antigen-specific suppression of DH; *(2)* an immunosuppressive protein with a molecular weight of 130,000 daltons which has been isolated from the testis, another privileged site with a blood-tissue barrier (39); and *(3)* low concentrations of complement in brain extracellular fluids that reduce the possibility of antibody-mediated inflammatory reactions (16). These results clearly identify the highly specialized microenvironment as an important factor contributing to the distinctive immunoreactivity of the normal brain and other privileged sites.

Blood Tissue Barriers and Regulation of the Microenvironment

Many privileged sites—the brain, anterior chamber of the eye, testis, and fetoplacental unit—have a blood-tissue barrier (2). The modern concept of the blood-brain barrier is that of a dynamic interface between plasma and brain extracellular fluids with selective permeability and transport characteristics (see the Blood-Brain Barrier, above). In the following section we suggest that the barrier participates in regulating the immunoreactivity of the brain by virtue of its ability to influence the concentrations of immunoregulatory cells and molecules within the brain cell microenvironment. This regulation provides a new function for the blood-tissue barrier in many privileged sites.

The blood-brain barrier may participate in the regulation of the immunoreactivity of the brain in at least two general ways: first, by selectively facilitating the transfer of some immunoregulatory cells and molecules between plasma and brain extracellular fluids, and second, by restricting the passage of others. The recent literature provides examples of both aspects of barrier function.

T lymphocytes illustrate the importance of selective passage across the barrier. Activated T lymphocytes enter the brain as part of the normal mechanisms of immune surveillance (26). Presumably this involves interactions between specific adhesion molecules on both the lymphocyte and the endothelium. In pathological situations, including the initiation of inflammation in EAE (41), the expression of receptors on the vascular endothelium is markedly increased and the flow of T lymphocytes into the tissue increases. This modulation of barrier function results in marked changes in the immunoreactivity of the inflamed nervous tissue.

Specific receptors are undoubtedly required for the passage of lymphocytes across all blood vessels, and not just the blood-brain barrier, since lymphocytes are much larger (micrometers) than the width of the narrow intercellular clefts (nanometers), or "pores", between endothelial cells. At one time, fenestrated capillaries were believed to be much more permeable than continuous endothelia, but it is now clear that the protein selectivity of both vessel types is similar (as reviewed in 1). Whether the cerebral vasculature exhibits tissue-specific lymphocyte receptors is not clear, although in vitro studies of leukocyte adhesion to cerebral endothelia are consistent with this possibility (33).

The limited permeability of the blood-brain barrier to immunoregulatory molecules contributes to the regulation of immune responses within the nervous tissue by uncoupling the compositions of plasma and brain extracellular fluids. This provides for independent control of immunoregulatory factors within the microenvironment. For example, circulating components of complement, which are synthesized in the liver, are virtually excluded from brain tissue by the vascular barrier. In contrast, substances synthesized within the brain may be maintained at elevated concentrations throughout the extracellular fluids of the privileged site.

It is important to emphasize that the ability to maintain elevated concentrations of immunoregulatory factors within the brain microenvironment extends throughout the tissue. Studies of extracellular cytokine concentrations have necessarily involved the analysis of CSF, since the thin film of ISF which surrounds individual brain cells is difficult to sample. The membranes separating CSF from the underlying nervous tissue are permeable (see Fig. 4-1), and CSF has a composition close to that of ISF with respect to ions and presumably also for larger compounds (as reviewed in 4). Thus, elevation of CSF cytokine levels, TGF-β for example, implies that concentrations of these important regulatory molecules are also elevated in tissue ISF. It also implies that continual synthesis occurs within nervous tissue (possibly by glial cells or the choroid plexus), with eventual paracrine distribution of the newly synthesized regulatory molecules throughout the neuraxis. Sites of cytokine production and their subsequent mechanisms of intracerebral distribution, both in health and disease, are just beginning to be characterized (as reviewed in 3,50). It can be anticipated that this characterization will provide a fertile area for future investigations.

Afferent Connections to the Draining Nodes and Spleen

Antigenic signals can reach the draining nodes or spleen via outflow of brain extracellular fluids to lymph or blood, respectively (Fig. 4-2). The large connection to the cervical lymphatics, measured using radiolabeled albumin, suggests a major role for this connection in mediating interactions between the brain and the immune system (Table 4-1). This view is reinforced by consideration of the kinetics of albumin passage through the nodes (61). Following microinfusion of radiolabeled albumin into brain tissue, the nodes are exposed continuously for periods in excess of a day to high albumin concentrations, relative to plasma, and for somewhat shorter periods following administration into the CSF (7,61). Similar tracer studies have failed to reveal an equivalent connection from the anterior chamber of the eye to cervical lymphatics, using lymphatic collection periods of only 6–8 hours (5). However, the fact that tumor cells injected into the anterior chamber induce a cellular immune response in the draining nodes clearly indicates that the connection is intact (29).

The relative importance of afferent connections from the nervous system and eye to the lymphatics and spleen remains to be determined. Our results suggest that the role of lymphatics is primary for induction of humoral immunity against CSF-administered albumin in the rat (as summarized in The Systemic Response, above), whereas the connection to the spleen is essential for induction of suppression of DH against antigens administered into the anterior chamber of the murine eye (as reviewed in 50). Further studies are needed to explore the relative importance of the nodes and spleen for induction of different immune effector mechanisms, with consideration given to the kinetics of the response, route of immunization, and possible species differences.

Summary and Conclusions

Recent studies provide a new view of immunoreactivity to antigens from the nervous system, which includes active and highly regulated communication with secondary lymphoid organs. The connection to the draining nodes is much larger than previously appreciated, and the blood-brain barrier, by virtue of its selective permeability properties, contributes to the control of immunoregulatory cells and molecules in the tissue microenvironment. Immune privilege is characterized as an active rather than a passive state which is associated with antigen-specific suppression of cell-mediated immunity and noninflammatory humoral immunity. The recognition that the nervous system and eye are served by a distinctive regional immune system, the neural-ocular immune system (Chapter 3 of this monograph), demands a reevaluation of the basic tenets of neuroimmunology in health and disease. We suggest the need, for example, to reconsider the tenet that antigens specific to the nervous system are not incorporated into the immune system's definition of self during ontogeny, and to reexamine the etiology of nervous system pathologies with the aim of redefining the progression from normal immunity to that associated with disease.

Acknowledgements

Financial support to both authors was provided by U.S.P.H.S. grants NS-11050 and NS-33070. P.M.K. wishes to thank the following members of the Cserr laboratory for their help in reviewing this manuscript and providing useful suggestions: Leslie Gordon, Dr. Christine Harling-Berg, Scott Nolan, and Joel Park.

References

1. Abbott NJ, Revest PA. Control of brain endothelial permeability. Cerebrovasc Brain Metab Rev 3:39–72, 1991.
2. Barker CF, Billingham RE. Immunologically privileged sites. Adv Immunol 25:1–54, 1977.
3. Benveniste EN. Inflammatory cytokines within the central nervous system: sources, function, and mechanism of action. Am J Physiol 263:C1–C16, 1992.
4. Bradbury MWB. The Concept of a Blood-Brain Barrier. Wiley, New York, 1979.
5. Bradbury MWB, Cole DF. The role of the lymphatic system in drainage of cerebrospinal fluid and aqueous humour. J Physiol 299:353–365, 1980.
6. Bradbury MWB, Cserr HF. Drainage of cerebral interstitial fluid and of cerebrospinal fluid into lymphatics. In: Experimental Biology of the Lymphatic Circulation, MG Johnston, ed. Elsevier, Amsterdam, 1985, pp 355–394.
7. Bradbury MWB, Cserr HF, Westrop RJ. Drainage of cerebral interstitial fluid into deep cervical lymph of the rabbit. Am J Physiol 240:F329–F336, 1981.
8. Bradbury MWB, Westrop RJ. Factors influencing exit of substances from cerebrospinal fluid into deep cervical lymph of the rabbit. J Physiol 339:519–534, 1983.
9. Brent L. Immunologically privileged sites. In: Pathophysiology of the Blood-Brain Barrier, BB Johansson, C Owman, H Widner, eds. Elsevier, Amsterdam, 1990, pp 383–402.
10. Brierley JB, Field EJ. The connexions of the spinal sub-arachnoid space with the lymphoid system. J Anat 82:153–166, 1948.
11. Brightman MW, Reese TS. Junctions between intimately apposed cell membranes in the vertebrate brain. J Cell Biol 40:648–677, 1969.
12. Cserr HF, Berman BJ. Iodide and thiocyanate efflux from brain following injection into rat caudate nucleus. Am J Physiol 235:F331–F337, 1978.
13. Cserr HF, Bundgaard M. Blood-brain interfaces in vertebrates: a comparative approach. Am J Physiol 246:R277–R288, 1984.
14. Cserr HF, Cooper DN, Milhorat TH. Flow of cerebral interstitial fluid as indicated by the removal of extracellular markers from rat caudate nucleus. Exp Eye Res Suppl 25:461–473, 1977.
15. Cserr HF, Cooper DN, Suri PK, Patlak CS. Efflux of radiolabeled polyethylene glycols and albumin from rat brain. Am J Physiol 240:F319–F328, 1981.
16. Cserr HF, DePasquale M, Harling-Berg CJ, Park JT, Knopf PM. Afferent and efferent arms of the humoral immune response to CSF-administered albumins in a rat model with normal blood-brain barrier permeability. J Neuroimmunol 41:195–202, 1992.
17. Cserr HF, Knopf PM. Cervical lymphatics, the blood-brain barrier and the immunoreactivity of the brain: a new view. Immunol Today 13:507–512, 1992.
18. Cserr HF, Patlak CS. Regulation of brain volume under isosmotic and anisosmotic conditions. In: Advances in Comparative and Environmental Physiology, R Gilles, EK Hoffman, L Bolis, eds. Vol 9, Springer-Verlag; Berlin, 1991, pp 61–80.
19. Davson H, Welch K, Segal MB. Physiology and Pathophysiology of the Cerebrospinal Fluid. Churchill Livingstone; New York, 1987.
20. Ferguson TA, Waldrep JC, Kaplan HJ. The immune response and the eye. II. The nature of T suppressor-cell induction in anterior chamber-associated immune deviation (ACAID). J Immunol 139:352–357, 1987.

21. Gordon LB, Knopf PM, Cserr HF. Ovalbumin is more immunogenic when introduced into brain or cerebrospinal fluid than into extracerebral sites. J Neuroimmunol 40:81–88, 1992.
22. Granstein RD, Staszewski R, Knisley TL, Zeira E, Nazareno R, Latina M, Albert DM. Aqueous humor contains transforming growth factor-beta and a small (<3500 daltons) inhibitor of thymocyte proliferation. J Immunol 144:3021–3027, 1990.
23. Harling-Berg CJ, Knopf PM, Cserr HF. Myelin basic protein infused into cerebrospinal fluid suppresses experimental autoimmune encephalomyelitis. J Neuroimmunol 35:45–51, 1991.
24. Harling-Berg C, Knopf PM, Merriam J, Cserr HF. Role of cervical lymph nodes in the systemic humoral immune response to human serum albumin microinfused into rat CSF. J Neuroimmunol 25:185–193, 1989.
24a. Harling-Berg CJ, Sobel RA, Knopf PM, Cserr HF. The role of immune cells in suppression of EAE induced by CSF-induced MBP. Society for Neuroscience: Abstracts Volume 18, Part II, Abstract #424.14 p. 1011, 1992.
25. Heber-Katz E, Acha-Orbea H. The V-region disease hypothesis: evidence from autoimmune encephalomyelitis. Immunol Today 10:164–169, 1989.
26. Hickey WF, Hsu BL, Kimura H. T-lymphocyte entry into the central nervous system. J Neurosci Res 28:254–260, 1991.
27. His W. Über ein perivasculares Kanalsystem in den nervosen Central-Organen und über dessen Beziehungen zum Lymphsystem. Z Wiss Zool 15:127–141, 1865.
28. Kaplan HJ, Stevens TR. A reconsideration of immunologic privilege within the anterior chamber of the eye. Transplantation 19:203–209, 1975.
29. Ksander BR, Streilein JW. Failure of infiltrating precursor cytotoxic T cells to acquire direct cytotoxic function in immunologically privileged sites. J Immunol 145:2057–2063, 1991.
30. Lampson L. Molecular bases of the immune response to neural antigens. Trends Neurosci 10:211–216, 1987.
31. Lass JH, Walter EI, Burris TE, Brossniklaus HE, Roat MI, Skelnik DL, Needham L, Singer M, Medof ME. Expression of two molecular forms of the complement decay-accelerating factor in the eye and lacrimal gland. Invest Opthalmol Vis Sci 31:1136–1148, 1990.
32. Leibowitz S, Hughes RAC. Immunology of the Nervous System. Edward Arnold, London, 1983, Chapt. 1, pp. 1–19.
33. Male D, Pryce G, Rahman J. Comparison of the immunological properties of rat cerebral and aortic endothelium. J Neuroimmunol 30:161–168, 1990.
34. Mims CA. Intracerebral injections and the growth of viruses in the mouse brain. Br J Exp Pathol 41:52–59, 1960.
35. Oehmichen M. Mononuclear Phagocytes in the Central Nervous System (translated by MM Clarkson). Neurology series 21. Springer-Verlag, New York, 1978, pp 65–82.
36. Oehmichen M, Wietholter H, Gruninger H, Gencic M. Destruction of intracerebrally applied red blood cells in cervical lymph nodes. Experimental investigations. Forensic Sci Int 21:43–57, 1983.
37. Olesen S-P. A calcium-dependent reversible permeability increase in microvessels in frog brain, induced by serotonin. J Physiol 361:103–113, 1985.
38. Pardridge WM. Brain metabolism: a perspective from the blood-brain barrier. Physiol Rev 63:1481–1535, 1983.
39. Pollanen P, Soder O. Uksila J. Testicular immunosuppressive protein. J Reprod Immunol 14:125–138, 1988.
40. Pullen RGL, DePasquale M, Cserr HF. Bulk flow of cerebrospinal fluid into brain in response to acute hyperosmolality. Am J Physiol 253:F538–F545, 1987.
41. Raine CS, Cannella B, Duijvestijn AM, Cross AH. Homing to central nervous system

vasculature by antigen-specific lymphocytes. II. Lymphocyte/endothelial cell adhesion during the initial stages of autoimmune demyelination. Lab Invest 63:476–489, 1990.

42. Rapoport SI, Robinson PJ. Tight-junctional modification as the basis of osmotic opening of the blood-brain barrier. In: The Neuronal Microenvironment, HF Cserr, ed. Ann N Y Acad Sci 481:250–267, 1986.

43. Siegelman J, Fleit HB, Peress NS. Characterization of immunoglobulin G-Fc receptor activity in the outflow system of the cerebrospinal fluid. Cell Tissue Res 248:599–605, 1987.

44. Streilein JW. Immune regulation and the eye: a dangerous compromise. FASEB J 1:199–208, 1987.

45. Streilein JW. Regional spheres of immunologic influence. Reg Immunol 1:1–2, 1988.

46. Streilein JW. Immunology, regional. In: Encyclopedia of Human Biology, Vol 4, R Dulbecco, ed. Academic Press, New York, 1991, pp 391–400.

47. Streilein JW, Cousins SW. Aqueous humor factors and their effect on the immune response in the anterior chamber. Curr Eye Res 9:175–182, 1990.

48. Streilein JW, Niederkorn JY, Shadduck JA. Systemic immune unresponsiveness induced in adult mice by anterior chamber presentation of minor histocompatibility antigens. J Exp Med 152:1121–1125, 1990.

49. Streilein JW, Wilbanks GA. Immune privileged fluids contain TGFβ and endow macrophages with the capacity to induce antigen-specific immune deviation. FASEB J 6:A1686, 1992.

50. Streilein JW, Wilbanks GA, Cousins SW. Immunoregulatory mechanisms of the eye. J Neuroimmunol 39:185–200, 1992.

51. Szentistvanyi I, Patlak CS, Ellis RA, Cserr HF. Drainage of interstitial fluid from different regions of rat brain. Am J Physiol 246:F835–F844, 1984.

52. Tourtellotte WW. On cerebrospinal fluid immunoglobulin-G (IgG) quotients in multiple sclerosis and other diseases: a review and a new formula to estimate the amount of IgG synthesized per day by the central nervous system. J Neurol Sci 10:279–304, 1970.

53. Tyor WR, Moench TR, Griffin DE. Characterization of the local and systemic B cell response of normal and athymic nude mice with Sindbis virus encephalitis. J Neuroimmunol 24:207–215, 1989.

54. Tyor WR, Wesselingh S, Levine B, Griffin DE. Long term intraparenchymal Ig secretion after acute viral encephalitis in mice. J Immunol 149:4016–4020, 1992.

55. Wekerle H, Linnington C, Lassmann H. Cellular immune reactivity within the CNS. Trends Neurosci 9:271–277, 1986.

56. Welch K, Pollay M. The spinal arachnoid villi of the monkeys *Cercopithecus aethiops sabaeus* and *Macara irus.* Anat Rec 145:43–48, 1963.

57. Widner H, Brundin P. Immunological aspects of grafting in the mammalian central nervous system. A review and speculative synthesis. Brain Res Rev 13:287–324, 1988.

58. Widner H, Jonsson BA, Hallstadius L, Wingardh K, Strand SE, Johansson BB. Scintigraphic method to quantify the passage from brain parenchyma to the deep cervical lymph nodes in rats. Eur J Nucl Med 13:456–461, 1987.

59. Wilbanks GA, Streilein JW. Distinctive humoral responses following anterior chamber and intravenous administration of soluble antigen. Evidence for active suppression of IgG_{2a}-secreting B-cells. Immunology 71:566–572, 1990.

60. Woo AH, Cserr HF, Knopf PM. Elevated cerebrospinal fluid IgA in humans and rats is not associated with secretory component. J Neuroimmunol 44:129–136, 1993.

61. Yamada S, DePasquale M, Patlak CS, Cserr HF. Albumin outflow into deep cervical lymph from different regions of rabbit brain. Am J Physiol 261:H1197–H1204, 1991.

62. Yoffey JM, Courtice FC. Lymphatics, Lymph and the Lymphomyeloid Complex. Academic Press, New York, 1970, Chapt. 4, pp 309–314.

III

IMMUNOLOGICALLY ACTIVE CELLS

5

Microglia and Macrophages

V. HUGH PERRY
SIAMON GORDON

Macrophages are generated in the bone marrow. They leave the bone marrow to circulate as monocytes and then take up residence in virtually all tissues of the body. At some sites they may be very long-lived cells, at others they turn over rapidly. The functions of resident tissue macrophages are not well understood, but there is evidence that they may play a role in tissue homeostasis and as the first line of defense against injury and infection (9,23). The number of resident tissue macrophages is relatively small, but after injury or infection their numbers can be rapidly augmented by recruitment of more macrophages from the circulating pool of monocytes in the blood.

There have been rapid advances in our knowledge about tissue macrophages in no small part due to the application of methods such as immunocytochemistry and in situ hybridization which allow the identification and characterization of tissue macrophages in sections. The striking differences in the phenotype of macrophages in different tissues is emerging and the effects of the local microenvironment is probably nowhere more apparent than in the central nervous system (CNS) (54).

The presence of resident macrophages in the CNS was debated for many years. The historical background to this debate on whether microglia were derived from monocytes or the neuroectoderm has been extensively reviewed elsewhere (37,54,62,67). There is now no doubt that microglia are the resident macrophages of the CNS. They and the macrophages associated with the various CNS compartments are the subject of this chapter.

Distribution and Kinetics of CNS-associated Macrophages

Ontogeny of Macrophages and Microglia

Studies on the ontogeny of microglia were greatly aided in the mid-1980s by the use of macrophage-specific (11,19) and leucocyte-specific (55) monoclonal antibodies. In the developing rodent brain, immunocytochemically labeled macrophages with a rounded or stellate form typical of other tissue macrophages are present from about the middle of the gestation period (7,8,30,55). These macrophages in the developing brain express a spectrum of leukocyte- and macrophage-restricted antigens on their surface and also express cytoplasmic antigens or have enzymatic activities associated with other tissue macrophages. As the animal matures, however, the macrophages develop an increasingly complex morphology as they differentiate to microglia. Hand in hand with this morphological differentiation the spectrum of antigens becomes increasingly restricted (65). In the developing brain there are both macrophages and cells with the morphology of microglia, depending on the region examined (7,55), but the emergence of adult distribution of microglia, morphology, and phenotypic restriction is predominantly a postnatal event. A similar sequence of morphological changes in the macrophage population is seen in developing human CNS (31).

Large numbers of macrophages are seen in the developing brain at a time when many cells, both neurons (47) and macroglia (12), are undergoing natural cell death. It has been hypothesized that the apoptotic cells provide a chemotactic signal for the entry of the macrophages into the developing nervous system, and these macrophages are seen to be phagocytosing the apoptotic cells (30,55). However, a hallmark of apoptotic cell death is that the plasma membrane remains intact as the cell degenerates and the cellular contents are not released extracellularly (6). Thus, cells about to become apoptotic must either secrete a chemotactic molecule prior to the fragmentation of the nuclear DNA, or they must induce neighboring cells to release monocyte chemoattractants. There is evidence to show that an astrocyte cell line synthesizes a monocyte chemoattractant (73). Other monocyte and macrophage chemoattractants (64) may also be released from tissues of the developing CNS. At the present time, the issues of whether apoptotic cells release monocyte chemoattractants and how macrophages might recognize these cells in the developing nervous system are unresolved. The presence of macrophages prior to the onset of large amounts of cell death certainly suggests that there are constitutive paths of entry in development that are independent of natural cell death (8). Outside the nervous system there is evidence that macrophages recognize and phagocytose senescent neutrophils in part via the vitronectin receptor (63), but other macrophage receptors (9) such as the lectin receptors or other members of the integrin family may be involved.

Distribution of Macrophages and Microglia

In the mature central nervous system the microglia are by far the largest population of macrophages, but in addition to the microglia there are macrophage populations in other compartments. We shall deal with each in turn.

Microglia

The microglia of the adult CNS are characterized by their highly specialized morphology. The cells have a small heterochromatic nucleus when stained with basic dyes. Immunocytochemistry with antibodies directed against plasma membrane components, for example, F4/80 or the complement type 3 receptor in the mouse, reveals that the cells have two or more primary processes which branch several times and have a bristled appearance (Fig. 5-1 and 5-2) (35,55). The long-branched processes mean that

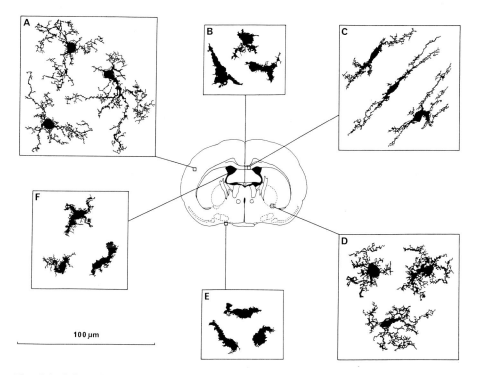

Fig. 5-1. Schematic drawing to illustrate the morphological differences in macrophages and microglia in different compartments of the CNS. A, D: Radial microglia in gray matter. Note the different appearance of microglia at these two different sites, cortex and ventral pallidum. C: Longitudinal microglia in white matter. B: Compact microglia of the subfornical organ, one of the circumventricular organs. E, F: Macrophages of the leptomeninges and choroid plexus, respectively.

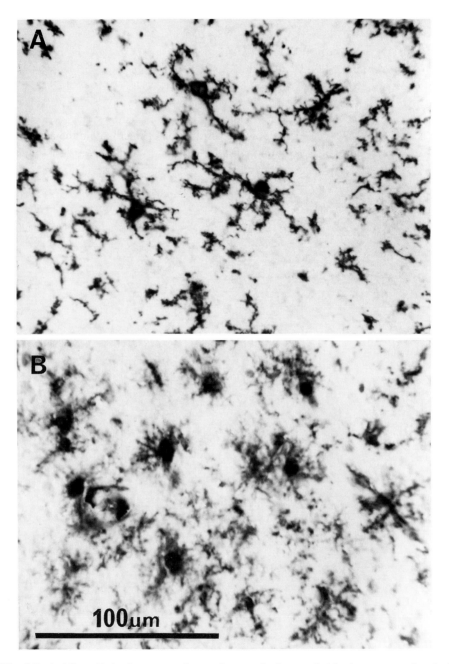

Fig. 5-2. A: Microglia in the cortex of normal mouse brain revealed by immunocytochemical detection of F4/80. B: Activated microglia in the mouse CNS.

the cell surface area of a microglial cell is much larger than that of most other tissue macrophages. Although they have a characteristic morphology, this is not constant throughout the CNS; there are subtle variations from region to region (Fig. 5-1) (35). This tells us that not only does the CNS microenvironment have an important influence on these tissue macrophages but also there are further local factors within the CNS.

Since we had suggested that natural cell death might play a role in macrophage recruitment into the developing CNS (30,55), we examined the distribution of microglia across the CNS to determine how the distribution of microglia in the adult brain might relate to the patterns of developmental cell death. The density and morphology of microglia are found to be heterogeneous with as much as a sixfold variation in density from one cytoarchitectural region to another. Regions with low density include the cerebellum and white matter, while high densities are found in the substantia nigra, ventral pallidum, and olfactory tubercle. The proportion of cells that were microglia varied from 5 to 12%. The distribution of microglia is not related to the amount of developmental cell death in that region, nor have we been able to find a correlation with the distribution of any other cell type or neurotransmitter. One interesting observation that did arise from these studies was the very large numbers of microglia present in the CNS, about 3.5 million, a comparable number to that found in the liver on a weight-for-weight basis.

The criteria for recognizing microglia at the ultrastructural level have been described (58). A striking feature of microglia in the adult CNS is their relative paucity of cellular organelles and perinuclear cytoplasm when compared to macrophages in the neonatal brain or in other tissues. The cells give the impression of being "switched off" or down-regulated, an issue we will return to again (in the subsequent section on microglia).

Perivascular Macrophages

In addition to the microglia there is a population of macrophages associated with the vasculature of the CNS (26,67). These macrophages lie within the basement membrane covering the CNS vessels and adjacent to the endothelium. They lack the highly ramified processes of the microglia. These cells are distinct from the pericytes and are indeed derived from the bone marrow, as has been shown in bone marrow chimeras (29).

Macrophages in the Choroid Plexus and Leptomeninges

Macrophages have been identified in the choroid plexus and the leptomeninges and lying on the walls of the ventricles within the cerebrospinal fluid. The macrophages most readily identified in association with the choroid plexus are the *epiplexus* or *Kolmer cells* (13). In addition to these cells, we have identified a population of macrophages that lie within the stroma of the choroid plexus where they form a regular array of branched cells akin to the Langerhans cells within the skin (41). In contrast to the large numbers of microglia, the choroid plexus macrophages number no more than a few thousand and the stromal macrophages are three times more common than the epiplexus cells. The stromal macrophages are well placed and have the phenotype to interact with cells of the peripheral immune system as is discussed below (see Macrophages of the Choroid Plexus).

The macrophages of the leptomeninges have a phenotype more typical of other non-neuronal tissue macrophages (53).

Kinetics

Macrophages in non-neuronal, non-lymphoid tissues turn over rather slowly. These populations are maintained by both local division and also by recruitment of circulating monocytes (see 36 for references). In the CNS, few microglia are labeled by systemic administration of 3H-thymidine, and this has led authors to conclude that the turnover of microglia is of no physiological significance (42,48). However, the issue as to whether microglia turn over or and whether there is influx of monocytes into the CNS in the steady state is of some interest in view of the possibility that pathogens, including HIV, might gain entry to the CNS within monocytes migrating along constitutive pathways (72). This has been termed the *Trojan Horse hypothesis* of CNS infection (50).

The combination of 3H-thymidine labeling and immunocytochemical labeling of microglia allows a rapid assay for the detection of microglia synthesizing DNA, and by varying the survival time, evidence for local division and the relative contribution of monocyte invasion can be determined (36). In the mouse CNS it has been shown that resident microglia do divide (Fig. 5-3). The labeling index for the microglia is about 0.05%, which is comparable to but slightly larger than that reported for Langerhans cells of the skin (0.01%) (39). The 3H-thymidine-labeled cells were scattered randomly throughout the CNS. In addition, this quantitative study suggested that small numbers of monocytes were entering the brain. The two processes of local division and monocyte entry contributed about equally to the turnover and maintenance of the microglia population.

The use of 3H-thymidine labeling combined with immunocytochemical detection of microglia allows the minimal amount of physiological perturbation to assess steady-state kinetics. Another approach is to use bone marrow chimeras in which the donor cells used for reconstitution of an irradiated host bear a distinct marker from the host. Given that the CNS microenvironment has a profound effect on the expression of various leucocyte antigens (see Microglia, below) the choice of polymorphic marker is of some importance. Using this approach, Hickey and Kimura (29) have shown that perivascular macrophages are more rapidly replaced by donor cells than microglia and that rare microglia are also replaced over a period of months. We have obtained evidence using male donor bone marrow into female mice that cells bearing the Y

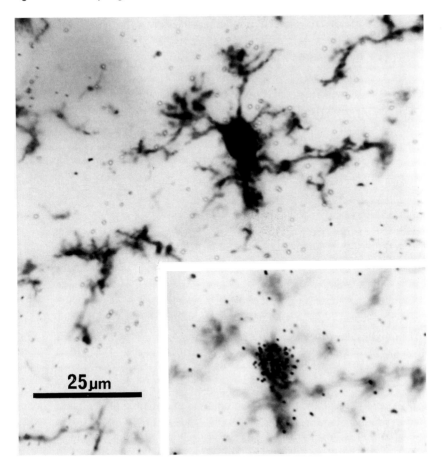

25 µm

Fig. 5-3. A microglial cell in the mature adult mouse CNS labeled with 3H-thymidine. The inset shows the silver grains over the cell nucleus.

chromosome appear in the parenchyma after several months (Perry and Gordon, unpublished results). However, at the present time, quantitative data are not available from these studies.

The turnover of macrophages in the choroid plexus has also been assayed using 3H-thymidine and immunocytochemical labeling of the macrophage population (41). The stromal macrophages in the choroid turn over faster than the microglia. By varying the survival times, it was possible to show that macrophages move from a stromal position to an epiplexus position and thence presumably to the cerebrospinal fluid since they were no longer detectable in tissue sections after 24 hours. The evidence suggests that there is a long-lived, resident stromal choroid plexus population and that these macrophages are not just cells en route to the CSF.

Thus, the macrophage populations of the CNS are not static but are in a process of continual, slow renewal, just as has been described for other tissues.

Phenotype of Macrophages Associated with the CNS

Microglia

The description above clearly indicates that microglia have a distinct morphology at both the light microscopic level and ultrastructurally. The impression is that these cells are highly differentiated and relatively quiescent cells. Further evidence that the CNS microenvironment has a powerful and possibly unique influence on macrophages comes from studies in which the expression of molecules of both known and unknown function have been examined by immunocytochemistry.

Microglia in the normal adult rodent CNS lack major histocompatibility (MHC) antigens class I and only a few cells express MHC class II, and these tend to be in white matter tracts (28,67). This lack of expression of MHC class I is particularly striking since this molecule is expressed on many macrophage populations. The absence of MHC class II on microglia is in striking contrast with that found on the macrophages of the choroid plexus and leptomeninges (41; see Macrophages of the Choroid Plexus).

In addition to the down-regulation of MHC antigens, other antigens associated with leukocytes or restricted to macrophages, for example, the leukocyte common antigen (LCA) or CD4, are either absent or only weakly expressed on microglia (52). The monoclonal antibody ED-1, which recognizes a lysosomal membrane antigen and is present on most tissue macrophages (17), is absent from microglia of the adult CNS (65). A striking feature of many lists of macrophage antigens examined on CNS tissue is the lack of some of these antigens from microglia (41,53). At the present time, there is no antigen expressed by microglia which is not expressed by other tissue macrophages.

Although progress has been made in defining cell surface antigens on microglia and, to some extent, some of the cytoplasmic antigens, it is now well known that a macrophage is not just a phagocytic cell, but that it also has the capacity to secrete an impressive spectrum of different compounds varying from small molecules, such as reactive oxygen intermediates, to larger molecules, such as growth factors (9). One clue as to the function of microglia in the normal adult brain may come from studies in which the spectrum of secretory products of microglia is discovered. Immature microglia isolated from the neonatal brain secrete interleukin-1 (IL-1) and there is evidence that they do so in vivo (20). IL-1 may promote both gliogenesis and angiogenesis (20,21).

Macrophages of the Choroid Plexus

In contrast to microglia, the macrophages of the choroid plexus and leptomeninges are much more active cells and express a much wider range of macrophage-associated antigens (53). We have examined the macrophages of the choroid plexus in some detail (41). These macrophages not only express many macrophage antigens but also express high levels of MHC class II antigen in the normal adult animal. The presence of high levels of MHC class II cells and their superficial morphological resemblance to Langerhans cells (see Macrophages in the Choroid Plexus and Leptomeninges, above) suggests that these cells may have an antigen-presenting function. This is somewhat surprising, given the location of these cells. They are situated in a region with a very high arterial perfusion rate (71) and endocytose protein from the plasma (41) and are thus in potential contact with the peripheral immune system. On the other hand, it is also possible that these cells are in contact with antigens derived from the CNS. It is known that the choroidal epithelium will take up proteins from the CSF (68) and occasional processes of the stromal macrophages are seen passing between the epithelia, thus, they may either have access to these proteins directly, or receive them from the choroidal epithelium. It is hard to image why a cell with the potential to present CNS antigens is located at such a site, but it is important to note that we do not have evidence that these cells are bona fide dendritic cells and thus able to initiate a primary immune response, an important distinction between dendritic cells and macrophages (10). On the other hand, these cells with a powerful phagocytic capacity may be positioned in such a manner as to prevent the access of CNS antigens to the peripheral immune system.

The possibility that some component of the choroid plexus is able to present antigen in an in vitro assay has been studied (46). It was shown that choroid plexus epithelium, when treated with interferon-gamma will present antigen to T-lymphocytes. However, the fact that macrophages in the stroma have high levels of MHC class II cells and that we have not been able to see this molecule on epithelium in vivo makes the macrophages the likely functional cell.

The macrophages in the choroid plexus make an interesting comparison with recent descriptions of MHC class II positive cells in the anterior chamber of the eye (44). The ciliary body in the anterior chamber is a secretory body and has a very high blood perfusion rate homologous to that of the choroid plexus. Within this structure, MHC class II–bearing cells have been identified in a network similar to that described for the choroid plexus and these cells have been described as having the phenotypic characteristics of dendritic cells, but this has not been demonstrated in functional assays.

The possible role of the macrophage or dendritic-like cells in the choroid plexus and the ciliary body requires further study to discover their possible role in immunological disorders of the brain and eye.

Blood-brain Barrier in Phenotype Regulation

Macrophages within the CNS microenvironment have a distinct morphology and phenotype. What factors might give rise to this? The obvious possibilities are the contacts they make with the different cell types of the CNS and the fact that the cells within the blood-brain barrier are isolated from plasma proteins.

Evidence for the role of plasma proteins in the control of microglia phenotype came from our studies in the rat (52). In the circumventricular organs, where plasma proteins diffuse through the fenestrated capillaries, the microglia were found to express higher levels of LCA and CD4 antigens when compared to the barely detectable levels on microglia in the parenchyma. Injury to the blood-brain barrier also resulted in increased expression of LCA and CD4 where the plasma proteins had diffused into the tissue.

Further evidence that plasma proteins may modify microglia phenotype came from studies on the sialoadhesin molecule in the mouse. Sialoadhesin is involved in macrophage–hematopoietic cell interactions, but expression of this molecule depends on the presence of a protein with a molecular weight of about 60 kilodatons present in plasma/serum (15). Microglia in the parenchyma do not express sialoadhesin, but microglia in the circumventricular organs (CVOs) express this molecule to a variable extent (51). Damage to the blood-brain barrier results in the expression of this molecule on microglia with a spatial distribution and time course consistent with the extent of the brain infiltrated by the plasma proteins.

It is as yet unclear how far it is possible to generalize from these observations and just how many and which molecules depend on exposure to serum-inducing agents for their expression to be switched on. However, from a practical point of view, the expression of a serum-induced antigen on microglia allows an assay of when the blood-brain barrier is damaged.

Microglia Activation

Microglia respond rapidly to a wide range of pathological stimuli (18,66). In pathological conditions of the CNS, typical inflammatory macrophages may appear, or under some conditions, cells referred to as *activated microglia*. These cells, when compared to the normal resident microglia, have more processes which are shorter, stouter and more arborized (Fig. 5-2). In addition, these cells may increase their level of expression of antigens that are present on the resident cells or express de novo previously down-regulated molecules. It should be noted that the term *activated* is used in a broad sense to include the responses of both resident and possibly elicited macrophages, since in the majority of experimental models of neuronal injury, the relative contributions of resident and recruited cells have not been worked out. The term *activated microglia* is used to describe responses of macrophages and microglia in both immune and nonimmune mediated injury; in the future there may be reason to distinguish between these two types.

The macrophage–microglia response to injury is discussed in the following section, but first we consider to what extent physiological conditions influence microglia phenotype.

Physiological Influences

It has been documented that microglia show increased phagocytic activity in aged brains as compared to those in juvenile animals and that there is also a small increase in the number of microglia (57,69). We have examined microglia in brains of aged rats with a panel of monoclonal antibodies to determine whether there are other phenotypic changes (56). In the brains of these aged but healthy rats, we found that there was an increase in the numbers of microglia with unusual or activated morphology, there were many microglia in white matter fiber tracts that expressed MHC class II antigen, and that the vast majority of the microglia now expressed the lysosomal membrane marker ED1, which is absent from microglia of juvenile rats (65). There was thus up-regulation of the microglia in the aged brain.

The factors that produce this up-regulation are not clear. The changes in microglia were not greater or more exaggerated in areas of the CNS where it is known that neurons have degenerated in the aging rodent brain. It is likely that many factors influence microglia activation in the aged brain. For example, neuronal degeneration, repeated subclinical infections, and exposure to environmental agents might all play a role in the up-regulation of the microglia, possibly by the production of local cytokines. These issues can all be addressed experimentally.

A second model of physiological perturbation explored in our laboratory is dehydration. There is increasing interest in the interactions between the endocrine system and the peripheral immune system (1). In a previous study, we showed that there appeared to be a highly specialized relationship between the magnocellular neurons of the hypothalamopituitary axis and microglia. In the posterior pituitary microglia represent a significant proportion of the non-neuronal population and they phagocytose the endings of magnocellular neurons (60). It has also been shown that the non-neuronal cells in the posterior pituitary and the supraoptic nucleus proliferate in response to dehydration (49). We have examined the microglial proliferative response to dehydration (36a). Although there was no change in the microglia in the brain, the microglia in the posterior pituitary underwent a dramatic, transient proliferative response. The molecules responsible for the proliferation of this highly differentiated, resident macrophage population are not known.

The systemic factors that influence microglia phenotype have not all been defined, but this may prove to be an important area of research as it becomes clear that microglia are a cornerstone of interactions between the central nervous system and the immune system.

Microglia Response to Injury

It has long been recognized that microglia respond to almost any form of CNS injury (18,62,66) and indeed, might be considered as indicators of the first signs of underlying pathology. A wide range of pathological conditions in humans and experimental animal models have been explored to define the conditions under which microglia activation occurs, how rapidly it occurs, and what molecules are expressed. We will consider some of these models but only those that involve nonimmune injury, since immune-mediated responses in the CNS are dealt with in later chapters.

Injury to non-neuronal tissues results in a stereotypic acute inflammatory response. This involves not only the local macrophages but also rapid recruitment of myelo-monocytic cells from the blood (45). These recruited cells then play a part in the removal of the debris and secrete growth factors that may play a part in the healing process. The response to CNS injury is *gliosis,* traditionally thought of as the hypertro-phy and proliferation of astrocytes. In recent years it has become clear that a major cellular element in the gliotic response is cells of the mononuclear phagocyte lineage, macrophages, and microglia. Activation of microglia in response to injury is seen as an alteration in morphology (62). These activated microglia have more processes, which are stouter than those of the resident cells, and the cell body may hypertrophy. These changes are readily appreciated when antibodies which stain the plasma membrane are used (3,16,40). In addition, the activation of microglia may be accompanied by the up-regulation of antigens already expressed on the cells (25,52) or the appearance of new antigens (24). For example, MHC class II antigen up-regulation has been identified in retrograde degeneration (67), Wallerian degeneration (33,61), excitotoxic lesions (2), and in chronic neurological disease (43). The diversity of molecules that are upregu-lated is ever increasing, but as yet, no pattern has emerged which suggests that different lesions lead to a significantly different spectrum of antigen expression.

An issue that has preoccupied experimental neuropathologists is whether the acti-vated microglia are derived from the resident microglia or from monocytes which have entered the CNS in response to the injury. There is no clear evidence to show that, at sites of neuronal degeneration accompanied by microglia activation, microglia fall into distinct categories which suggest a recruited versus resident subgrouping. In penetrat-ing wounds, it is not surprising that neutrophils and monocytes enter the CNS in the immediate proximity of the lesion and there is thus a mixture of both resident and recruited cells (32). In contrast, the evidence suggests that activated microglia around motorneurons undergoing a retrograde reaction following axotomy are largely derived from resident cells undergoing division (27). A plausible explanation for these two different responses from the mononuclear phagocyte population is that in lesions where the blood-brain barrier is breached, monocytes readily enter the CNS, but in lesions such as retrograde or Wallerian degeneration where the blood-brain barrier is not breached, the monocytes do not enter the CNS and the mononuclear phagocyte reaction is activation of the resident microglia.

However, a few experimental studies have addressed the issue of the relationship between the status of the blood-brain barrier and myelomonocytic entry into the CNS. Following neuronal cell death induced by excitatory neurotoxins (3,14) or the intra-parenchymal injection of endodotoxin (lipopolysaccharide [LPS]) (4) there is a marked mononuclear phagocyte reaction. From these studies it has emerged that the per-meability of the blood-brain barrier, as measured by the entry of exogenously delivered horseradish peroxidase (HRP), is not a major factor determining whether a monocyte will enter the CNS or not. At a time when HRP readily diffuses into the region of the cell degeneration, neither neutrophils or monocytes enter the tissue (3). In response to LPS when the blood-brain barrier is intact, it is clear that many of the cells with the morphology of activated microglia are derived from the bone marrow since irradiation prior to the injury abolishes the increase in number even when the head is shielded (4). The entry of the monocytes into the CNS parenchyma is inhibited by intravenously injected antibodies to the complement type 3 receptor (4). Circulating monocytes are able to cross the intact blood-brain barrier in response to either cell degeneration or inflammatory substances within the parenchyma. Furthermore, when a monocyte enters the adult central nervous system and the neuropil is relatively intact, the monocyte comes under the influence of the CNS microenvironment which induces the microglial phenotype. Thus, monocytes may cross the intact blood-brain barrier, as has been demonstrated for activated T-lymphocytes (70).

There is insufficient data from most experimental models of excitatory neurotoxic lesions, retrograde degeneration, and Wallerian degeneration to define the conditions under which monocyte recruitment occurs or when the response is wholly intrinsic and is a response of the resident microglia alone. There may be no hard and fast rule. A reasonable suggestion is that it is likely to depend on the degree of neuronal degeneration, the acute or chronic nature of the lesion, and the inducing agent. If microglia are able to be activated and to synthesize the majority of molecules synthesized by recruited cells, then this may be an issue of relatively little importance.

Microglia activation is associated with most neuropathologies, but the function of the cells is poorly understood. In a system with a poor capacity for regeneration and repair, the role of the macrophage is not clear. Obviously, removal of tissue debris is one function we would expect of a professional phagocyte (20). It has been shown that the macrophages associated with stab wound will produce interleukin-1, a cytokine which will stimulate astroglial proliferation and angiogenesis (20,21). The astrocyte response may be important in the re-establishment of the blood-brain barrier after such a lesion. This interaction between the astrocyte and macrophages/microglia may be of importance in determining the outcome of a particular lesion.

In contrast to the suggestion that macrophages and microglia might play a part in repair processes there is evidence emerging that macrophages and microglia may contribute directly to or exacerbate neuronal degeneration. There is evidence that HIV-infected macrophages produce substances that are neurotoxic (22,38), and since the microglia are the infected cells in the brains of patients with HIV (34), this may contribute to the neuropathology. In other conditions where large numbers of macrophages are rapidly recruited they may damage myelin (14) or secrete neurotoxic compounds (59). It is possible to speculate on the role of macrophages and microglia following many forms of CNS injury. However, at the present time their reparative or detrimental contribution remains largely unknown.

Microglia and Inflammation

The myelomonocytic response to CNS neuronal degeneration has a number of peculiarities when compared to cell degeneration in other tissues. Even when acute neuronal degeneration is provoked in the CNS by excitatory neurotoxins and neurons degenerate rapidly, there is virtually no neutrophil recruitment; the numbers of macrophages/microglia are not increased until the third day post injury (3,40). The absence of neutrophil recruitment is common to many types of neuronal degeneration (18) but has hardly been explored experimentally. The delay in monocyte recruitment is surprising given the fact that the neuronal degeneration products are present for 48 hours without recruitment.

To study this phenomenon further, we injected the potent inflammogen LPS into the CNS parenchyma (4). Low doses of this substance, which provoke a brisk inflammatory response in the dermis, will also provoke a response in the choroid plexus and ventricular compartment but not in the parenchyma. It is only at higher doses that LPS recruits monocytes to the parenchyma and this is only after a delay of 48 hours. The recruited monocytes rapidly transform to microglia. At even higher doses a unique sequence of events is seen in which a full-blown inflammatory response does not occur until about 1 week after the injection rather than in the first 24 hours (4). The unusual inflammatory response is not unique to LPS since the intraparenchymal injection of cytokines (interleukin-1 and tumour necrosis factor-alpha) and chemotaxins (interleukin-8, platelet-activating factor) at physiological doses that produce inflammation subcutaneously fails to produce this response intraparenchymally (5). We have suggested that the highly modified inflammatory response seen in the CNS may be due either to the specialized phenotype of the CNS endothelium or to the down-regulation of the microglia (4,5).

Conclusion

Microglia, the resident macrophages of the CNS, have a distinct morphology and phenotype. The CNS microenvironment appears to dramatically down-regulate these cells when compared to other tissue macrophages, including those associated with the choroid plexus and leptomeninges. This phenotype is in part regulated by the presence of the blood-brain barrier excluding plasma proteins.

Microglia readily respond to injury by changes in their morphology and phenotype. The function of these cells in response to injury is not well understood. Recent evidence suggests that properties of the CNS parenchyma play an important part in modulating the acute inflammatory response to nonimmune challenge which is quite unlike that seen in other tissues.

Microglia are a cornerstone of interactions between the CNS and the peripheral immune system and understanding factors which modulate macrophages in the CNS may be of value in both neurological and non-neurological diseases.

Acknowledgements

The work from our laboratories was supported by The Wellcome Trust, the Multiple Sclerosis Society, and the Medical Research Council.

References

1. Ader R, Felten DL, Cohen N. Psychoneuroimmunology, 2nd ed. Academic Press, San Diego, 1991.
2. Akiyama H, Itagaki S, McGeer PL. Major histocompatibility complex antigen expression on rat microglia following epidural kainic acid lesions. J Neurosci Res 20:145–157, 1988.
3. Andersson P-B, Perry VH, Gordon S. The kinetics and morphological characteristics of the macrophage-microglial response to kainic acid-induced neuronal degeneration. Neuroscience 42:201–214, 1991.
4. Andersson P-B, Perry VH, Gordon S. The acute inflammatory response to lipopolysaccharide in the CNS parenchyma differs from that of other body tissues. Neuroscience 48:169–186, 1992.
5. Andersson P-B, Perry VH, Gordon S. Intracerebral injection of proinflammatory cytokines or leukocyte chemotaxins induces minimal myelomonocytic cell recruitment to the parenchyma of the central nervous system. J Exp Med 176:255–259, 1992.
6. Arends MJ, Wyllie AH. Apoptosis—mechanisms and roles in pathology. Int Rev Exp Pathol 32:223–254, 1991.
7. Ashwell K. The distribution of microglia and cell death in the fetal rat forebrain. Dev Brain Res 58:1–12, 1991.
8. Ashwell KWS, Hollander H, Streit W, Stone J. The appearance and distribution of microglia in the developing retina of the rat. Vis. Neurosci. 2:437–488, 1989.
9. Auger MJ, Ross JA. The biology of the macrophage. In: The Natural Immune System: The Macrophage, CE Lewis, JO'D McGee, eds. IRL Press, Oxford, 1992, pp 1–74.
10. Austyn JM. Antigen-Presenting Cells. IRL Press, Oxford, 1989.
11. Austyn J, Gordon S. F4/80, a monoclonal antibody directed specifically against the mouse macrophage. Eur J Immunol 11:805–811, 1981.
12. Barres BA, Hart IK, Coles HSR, Burne JF, Voydovic JT, Richardson WD, Raff MC. Cell death and the control of cell survival in the oligodendrocyte cell lineage. Cell 70:31–46, 1992.
13. Carpenter SJ, McCarthy LE, Borison HL. Electron microscopic study of the epiplexus (Kolmer) cells of the cat choroid plexus. Z Zellforsch mikrosk Anat 110:471–486, 1970.
14. Coffey PJ, Perry VH, Rawlins JNP. An investigation into the early stages of the inflammatory response following ibotenic acid-induced neuronal degeneration. Neuroscience 35:121–132, 1990.
15. Crocker PR, Hill M, Gordon S. Regulation of a murine macrophage hemagglutinin (sheep erythrocyte receptor) by a species-restricted serum factor. Immunology 65:515–522, 1988.
16. Dickson DW, Mattiace LA, Kure K, Hutchins K, Lyman WD, Brosnan CF. Biology of disease. Microglia in human disease, with an emphasis on Acquired Immune Deficiency Syndrome. Lab Invest 64:135–156, 1991.
17. Dijkstra CD, Dopp EA, Joling P, Kraal G. The heterogeneity of mononuclear phagocytes in lymphoid organs: distinct macrophage subpopulations in the rat recognized by monoclonal antibodies ED1, ED2 and ED3. Immunology 54:589–599, 1985.
18. Duchen LW. General pathology of neurons and neuroglia. In: Greenfield's Neuropathology, 4th ed, JH Adams, JAN Corsellis, LW Duchen, eds. Arnold, London, 1984, pp 1–52.
19. Esiri MM, McGee JO'D. Monoclonal antibody to macrophages (EBM/11) labels macrophages and microglial cells in human brain. J Clin Path 39:615–621, 1986.
20. Giulian D. Ameboid microglia as effectors of inflammation in the central nervous system. J Neurosci Res 18:155–171, 1987.

21. Giulian D, Lachman LB. Interleukin-1 stimulation of astroglial proliferation after brain injury. Science 228:497–499, 1985.

22. Giulian D, Vaca K, Noonan CA. Secretion of neurotoxins by mononuclear phagocytes infected with HIV-1. Science 250:1593–1596, 1990.

23. Gordon S, Perry VH, Rabinowitz S, Chung L-P, Rosen H. Plasma membrane receptors of the mononuclear phagocyte system. J Cell Sci Suppl 9:1–26, 1988.

24. Graeber MB, Streit WJ, Kiefer R, Schoen SW, Kreutzberg GW. New expression of my-elomonocytic antigens by microglia and perivascular cells following lethal motor neuron injury. J Neuroimmunol 27:121–132, 1990.

25. Graeber MB, Streit WJ, Kreutzberg GW. Axotomy of the rat facial nerve leads to increased CR3 complement receptor expression by activated microglial cells. J Neurosci Res 21:18–24, 1988.

26. Graeber MB, Streit WJ, Kreutzberg GW. Identity of ED2-positive perivascular cells in rat brain. J Neurosci Res 22:103–106, 1989.

27. Graeber MB, Tetzlaff W, Streit WJ, Kreutzberg GW. Microglial cells but not astrocytes undergo mitosis following rat facial nerve axotomy. Neurosci Lett 85:317–321, 1988.

28. Hart DNJ, Fabre JW. Demonstration and characterization of Ia-positive dendritic cells in the interstitial connective tissues of rat heart and other tissues, but not brain. J Exp Med 153:347–361, 1981.

29. Hickey WF, Kimura H. Perivascular microglial cells of the CNS are bone-marrow derived and present antigen in vivo. Science 239:290–292, 1988.

30. Hume DA, Gordon S, Perry VH. The immunohistochemical localisation of a macrophage specific antigen in the developing mouse retina. Phagocytosis of dying neurons and differentiation of microglial cells to form a regular array in the plexiform layers. J Cell Biol 97:253–257, 1983.

31. Hutchins KD, Dickson DW, Rashbaum WK, Lyman WD. Localization of morphologically distinct microglial populations in the developing human fetal brain: implications for ontogeny. Dev Brain Res 55:95–102, 1990.

32. Imamoto K, Leblond CP. Presence of labelled monocytes, macrophages and microglia in a stab wound of the brain following an injection of bone marrow cells labeled with 3H-uridine in rats. J Comp Neurol 174:255–279, 1977.

33. Konno H, Yamamoto T, Suziki H, Saito T, Terunuma H. Wallerian degeneration induces Ia-antigen expression in the rat brain. J Neuroimmunol 25:151–159, 1989.

34. Kure K, Lyman WD, Weidenheim KM, Dickson DW. Cellular localization of an HIV-1 antigen in subacute AIDS encephalitis using an improved double-labelling immuno-histochemical method. Am J Pathol 136:1085–1092, 1990.

35. Lawson LJ, Perry VH, Dri P, Gordon S. Heterogeneity in the distribution and morphology of microglia in the normal adult mouse brain. Neuroscience 39:151–170, 1990.

36. Lawson LJ, Perry VH, Gordon S. Turnover of resident microglia in the normal adult mouse brain. Neuroscience 48:405–415, 1992.

36a. Lawson LJ, Perry VH, Gordon S. Microglial responses to physiological change: osmotic stress elevates DNA synthesis of neurohypophygeal microglia. Neuroscience 56:929–938, 1993.

37. Ling EA. The origin and nature of microglia. In: Advances in Cellular Neurobiology, Vol 2, S Federoff, L Hertz, eds., Academic Press, New York, 1981, pp 33–82.

38. Lipton SA. Models of neuronal injury in AIDS: another role for the NMDA receptor. Trends Neurosci 15:75–79, 1992.

39. Mackenzie IC. Labelling of murine epidermal Langerhans cells with 3H-thymidine. Am J Anat 144:127–136, 1975.

40. Marty S, Dusart I, Peschanski M. Glial changes following an excitotoxic lesion in the CNS-I. Microglia/macrophages. Neuroscience 45:529–539, 1991.
41. Matyszak MM, Lawson LJ, Perry VH, Gordon S. Stromal macrophages of the choroid plexus situated at an interface between the brain and peripheral immune system constitutively express MHC Class II antigen. J Neuroimmunol 40:173–182, 1992.
42. McCarthy GE, Leblond CP. Radioautographic evidence for slow astrocyte turnover and modest oligodendrocyte production in the corpus callosum of adult mice infused with 3H-thymidine. J Comp Neurol 271:589–603, 1988.
43. McGeer PL, Itagaki S, McGeer EG. Expression of the histocompatibility glycoprotein in neurological disease. Acta Neuropath 76:550–557, 1988.
44. McMenamin PG, Holthouse I, Holt PG. Class II-major histocompatibility complex (Ia) antigen-bearing cells within the iris and ciliary body of the rat eye: distribution, phenotype, ontogeny and relation to retinal microglia. Immunology 77:385–393, 1992.
45. Movat HZ. The Inflammatory Reaction. Elsevier, Amsterdam, 1985.
46. Nathanson JA, Chun LLY. Immunological function of the blood-cerebrospinal fluid barrier. Proc Natl Acad Sci USA 86:1684–1688, 1989.
47. Oppenheim RW. Cell death during development of the nervous system. Ann Rev Neurosci. 14:453–501, 1991.
48. Patterson JA. Dividing and newly produced cells in the corpus callosum of adult mouse cerebrum as detected by light microscopic autoradiography. Anat Anz 153:140–168, 1983.
49. Patterson JA, Leblond CP. Increased proliferation of neuroglial cells and endothelial cells in the supraoptic nucleus and hypophyseal neural lobe in young rats drinking hypertonic sodium chloride solution. J Comp Neurol 175:373–390, 1977.
50. Pelusso R, Haase A, Stowering L, Edwards M, Ventura P. A trojan horse mechanism for the spread of visna virus in monocytes. Virology 147:231–236, 1985.
51. Perry VH, Crocker PR, Gordon S. The blood-brain barrier regulates the expression of a macrophage sialic acid-binding receptor on microglia. J Cell Sci 101:201–207, 1992.
52. Perry VH, Gordon S. Modulation of the CD4 antigen on macrophages and microglia in rat brain. J Exp Med 166:1138–1143, 1987.
53. Perry VH, Gordon S. Resident macrophages of the central nervous system: modulation of phenotype in relation to a specialized microenvironment. In: Neuroimmune Networks: Physiology and Diseases, EJ Goetzl, NH Spector, eds. Alan R Liss, New York, 1989, pp 119–125.
54. Perry VH, Gordon S. Macrophages and the nervous system. Int. Rev. Cytol 125:203–244, 1991.
55. Perry VH, Hume DA, Gordon S. Immunohistochemical localization of macrophages and microglia in the adult and developing mouse brain. Neuroscience 15:313–326, 1985.
56. Perry VH, Matyszak MM, Fearn S. Altered antigen expression of microglia in aged rodent CNS. Glia 7:60–67, 1993.
57. Peters A, Josephson K, Vincent SL. Effects of aging on the neuroglial cells and pericytes within area 17 of the rhesus monkey cerebral cortex. Anat Rec 229:384–398, 1991.
58. Peters A, Palay SL, Webster HF. The fine structure of the nervous system: the neurons and supporting cells. WB Saunders, Philadelphia, 1976, pp 254–263.
59. Piani D, Frei K, Do KQ, Cuenod M, Fontana A. Murine brain macrophages induce NMDA receptor mediated neurotoxicity in vitro by secreting glutamate. Neurosci Lett 133:159–162, 1991.
60. Pow DV, Perry VH, Morris JF, Gordon S. Microglia in the neurohypophysis associate with

and endocytose terminal portions of neurosecretory neurons. Neuroscience 33:567–578, 1989.

61. Rao K, Lund RD. Degeneration of optic axons induces the expression of major histocompatibility antigens. Brain Res 488:332–335, 1989.

62. del Rio Hortega P. Microglia. In: Cytology and Cellular Pathology of the Nervous System, Vol 2, W Penfield, ed. Paul B Hoeber, New York, 1932, pp 482–584.

63. Savill J, Dransfield I, Hogg N, Haslett C. Vitronectin receptor-mediated phagocytosis of cells undergoing apoptosis. Nature 343:170–173, 1990.

64. Sherry B, Cerami A. Small cytokine superfamily. Curr Opin Immunol 3:56–60, 1991.

65. Sminia T, De Groot CJA, Dijkstra CD, Koetsier JC, Polman CH. Macrophages in the central nervous system of the rat. Immunobiology 174:43–50, 1987.

66. Streit WJ, Graeber MB, Kreutzberg GW. Functional plasticity of microglia: a review. Glia 1:301–307, 1988.

67. Streit WJ, Graeber MB, Kreutzberg GW. Expression of Ia antigen on perivascular and microglial cells. Exp Neurol 105:115–126, 1989.

68. Van Deurs B. Structural aspects of brain barriers with special reference to the permeability of the cerebral endothelium and choroidal epithelium. Int Rev Cytol 65:117–191, 1980.

69. Vaughan DW, Peters A. Neuroglial cells in the cerebral cortex of rats from young adulthood to old age: an electron microscopic study. J Neurocytol 3:405–429, 1974.

70. Wekerle H, Linington C, Lassmann H, Meyermann R. Cellular immune reactivity within the CNS. Trends Neurosci 9:271–277, 1986.

71. Welch K. Secretion of cerebrospinal fluid by choroid plexus of the rabbit. Am J Physiol 205:617–624, 1963.

72. Williams AE, Blakemore WF. Monocyte mediated entry of pathogens into the central nervous system. Neuropathol Appl Neurobiol 16:377–392, 1990.

73. Yoshimura T, Robinson EA, Tanaka S, Appella E, Kuratsu J-I, Leonard EJ. Purification and amino acid analysis of two human glioma-derived monocyte chemoattractants. J Exp Med 169:1449–1459, 1989.

6

Astrocytes: Normal Aspects and Response to CNS Injury

MICHAEL D. NORENBERG

Astrocytes represent the most common cellular element in the brain, outnumbering neurons by ten to one and occupying about one-third of the volume in the cerebral cortex (177). For a long time astrocytes were viewed as inert and passive cells providing physical support (scaffold), as the formers of "scar" tissue, and as the principal cell type involved in the formation of brain tumors. This view has greatly changed and it is now widely recognized that astrocytes are active and dynamic cells involved in many aspects of central nervous system (CNS) function. This chapter will review aspects of the biology of astrocytes, particularly their structure, function, and response to injury.

Historical Aspects

The concept of glia originated with Virchow (237) in 1846 when he described a *Nervenkitt*, meaning a cement or glue-like substance (hence the term *glia*), involved in holding the CNS together. In all probability, he was not describing a true cell type. It was Deiters in 1865 (54) who recognized glial cells as being distinct from neurons and who referred to them as *Sternzellen* (star cells). However, a debate persisted as to whether glia consisted of true cells rather than a network or syncytium. Camillo Golgi (87) described the perivascular astrocytic endings and also proposed that astrocytes serve a nutritive role in the CNS. The concept of heterogeneity of astrocytes was initiated by Andriezen, who in 1893, separated astrocytes into protoplasmic and fibrous types (6). In 1907 Lugaro (139) came closest to our current views regarding the function of astrocytes when he commented that they might be involved in the removal of toxic byproducts of neuronal metabolism and in the inactivation of chemical substances used as transmitting signals at nerve junctions. These views are remarkable as they were given before the enunciation of the neuron theory by Ramon y Cajal. In 1913 Ramon y Cajal (185) recognized these cells as a special class of glia and clearly established that glia were not a syncytium but rather, distinct cells.

The modern era of glial study probably began with Holgar Hyden (108), who in 1959, microdissected glial cells away from neurons. He described a reciprocal metabolic relationship between glia and neurons and was the first investigator to put forth the concept of glial-neuronal interactions. Electron microscopic studies led DeRobertis and colleagues to propose that astrocytes are involved in water and ion metabolism (81). Kuffler and colleagues, on the basis of electrophysiological data from amphibian and leech glia, established the concept of spatial buffering of potassium (126,172).

There has been a remarkable advance in our understanding of glia and their functions over the past 25 years. This has been largely due to the use of bulk fractionation (100) and cell culture (31,155). The ability to isolate these cells and study them individually (as well as in co-culture systems) has allowed investigators to more definitively examine the properties of these cells and has provided the data for our current views of glia. For a more comprehensive treatment of the history of glial cells, see the articles by Somjen (212) and Tower (227).

Morphology and Properties of Astrocytes

Astrocytes have traditionally been divided into protoplasmic and fibrous types. *Protoplasmic astrocytes* are prevalent in gray matter and have many short, irregular processes whose plasma membrane often extends outward to form a velate configuration. The extensive formation of cell processes leads to a large surface-to-volume ratio, making these cells very well suited for carrying out uptake phenomena. *Fibrous astrocytes* are found principally in the white matter and have few but long cytoplasmic processes. While these cells have many similar properties, they are biochemically and developmentally different (158).

Further classification of astrocytes was put forth by Raff (181), based on cultured astrocytes derived from the optic nerve of perinatal rats. Type 1 astrocytes, believed to represent in situ protoplasmic astrocytes, have an epithelioid appearance and stain for the glycoprotein Ran-2 but not for A2B5. Type 2 astrocytes, perhaps representing the in situ fibrous astrocytes, are smaller, process-bearing cells that stain for A2B5 as well as for tetanus toxin. Depending on culture conditions, O-2 progenitor cells with bipotential properties give rise to oligodendrocytes and type 2 astrocytes. Biochemical differences between these two types of astrocytes have been described (132). Direct evidence for the presence of these two types of astrocytes in situ, however, is not available. Moreover, current in situ data appears to be inconsistent with the concept that a progenitor cell giving rise to oligodendrocytes can also give rise to astrocytes (178).

It is now clear that astrocytes do not represent a uniform population of cells and that properties of astrocytes from one brain region may be strikingly different from those of other regions. Indeed, there are probably as many different types of astrocytes as there are types of neurons. The ability of astrocytes to take up glutamate varies between cortical astrocytes, where they are high, and astrocytes derived from the brain stem and cerebellum, where glutamate uptake is relatively low (59,94,196). Differences in their capacity to take up serotonin and catecholamines have been described (122). Not all astrocytes possess the same membrane receptors; thus receptors to dopamine are found in striatal astrocytes, whereas none are found in cortical astrocytes (99). Heterogeneity with regard to α1-adrenoreceptors occurs (189). Additionally, differences in the second messenger response of astrocytes have been described with regard to phosphoinositide hydrolysis (43,60) as well as to calcium (165). Regional differences in enzyme activity and membrane antigens have been reported (167,192). Lastly, astrocytes from different regions exert different trophic or morphogenetic influences on neurons. For instance, mesencephalic astrocytes induce dopaminergic neurons to produce extensive arborizations, whereas striatal astrocytes have minimal effects (56). Certainly, generalizations about glial properties based on studies from a single region are not tenable. For reviews dealing with aspects of astroglial heterogeneity, see articles by Hansson (93), and Wilkin and colleagues (247).

Analysis of topographical relationships provides important clues as to the function of astrocytes (Fig. 6-1). Astroglial processes cover the zone adjacent to the ependyma and pia as well as the surface of cerebral capillaries. Thus, astrocytes are located at critical interphases of the CNS with the periphery, thereby enabling them to intercept or affect the entry of various factors (metabolites, drugs, ions, infectious agents, etc.), and presumably to make appropriate responses to these factors. The close apposition of astroglial processes with the synaptic complex and nodes of Ranvier suggests a role in neurotransmission. Specialized contacts between astrocytes and neurons, oligodendrocytes, or mesenchymal elements, do not occur.

Astrocytes are interconnected to each other via gap junctions, thus creating a syncytium that allows for ionic and metabolic coupling (57,65,150,162a). This provides a means for long-distance communication and allows for functional responses extending into areas that are considerably distant from the primary site of action. Dramatic demonstration of this phenomenon is provided in studies by Smith, Cornell-Bell, and colleagues, which show glutamate-induced calcium waves in cultured astrocytes (50) as well as in astrocytes in hippocampal slices (52).

In addition to gap junctions, astrocytes are endowed with receptors to most neurotransmitters and neuropeptides (120,161), and contain appropriate second messenger systems (cyclic AMP elevations and reductions, phosphoinositide hydrolysis, calcium) which provide key intercellular communication between neurons and astrocytes. Similarly, voltage- and ligand-gated ion channels have been described which bring about

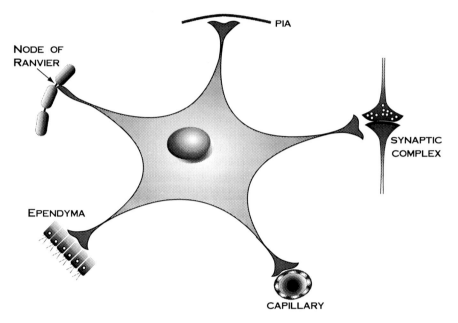

Fig. 6-1. Topographical arrangement of astrocytes with other elements of the nervous system. Note the position of astroglial processes at key interphases along the pia, ependyma, and capillaries, as well as adjacent to synaptic complexes and nodes of Ranvier.

changes in astrocytes (e.g., depolarization), providing another means for intercellular communication (14,214).

A number of biological markers have been useful in the study of astrocytes, the most common of which is glial fibrillary acidic protein (GFAP) (27,61). Other useful markers, with varying degrees of specificity, include glutamine synthetase, S-100 protein, and pyruvate carboxylase (for review see 123).

Function of Astrocytes

The precise function of atrocytes in situ remains to be defined. An enormous amount of data has been generated from cell culture studies, but their relevance to the in situ condition is not always clear. Nevertheless, there is much to indicate that astrocytes represent dynamic cells possessing a high rate of metabolic activity and pleiotropic functions responsible for the regulation of the CNS microenvironment, including ion content and extracellular neurotransmitter levels (Fig. 6-2).

Regulation of water and ion metabolism (241), the removal of excess potassium ion (242), pH regulation (42,113,125,241), and osmoregulation (241) may be among the most important of the glial functions that are required for proper neuronal activity.

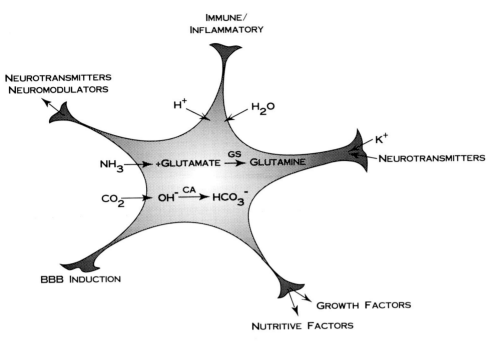

Fig. 6-2. Illustration of putative astroglial functions.

Astroglial involvement in amino acid neurotransmitter uptake, metabolism, and release (101,195) is similarly critical for neurotransmission. Through the action of glutamine synthetase, glutamate and γ-aminobutyric acid (GABA) are converted to glutamine, which is released by astrocytes and taken up by neurons. Glutamine is the principal precursor of glutamate and GABA (33). This results in the conservation and recycling of these two amino acid neurotransmitters, the so-called glutamate-glutamine cycle (17).

The astroglial involvement in glutamate metabolism has important implications in states of excitotoxicity such as stroke and trauma. It has been shown that astrocyte glutamate uptake may mitigate neuronal excitotoxicity (217), that neurons in astrocyte-poor cultures are more vulnerable to glutamate excitotoxicity (188), that astrocytes protect neurons from anoxic damage (235) and that blocking astrocytic uptake of glutamate results in neurodegeneration (186a,188a). The role of glutamine synthetase in neuroprotection against excitotoxicity has been emphasized by Oliver and colleagues (171) and by Floyd (66).

Astrocytes have also been shown to release a large number of neuroactive compounds after stimulation with neurotramsmitters, e.g., taurine release after β-adrenergic stimulation (244) and GABA release after glutamate receptor stimulation (79). Taurine, glutamate, and D-aspartate release have been documented after glial swelling (121) and following the administration of high potassium ion concentrations that result in membrane depolarization (and also probably swelling) (105,146,175,197). Potassium release following neurotransmitter stimulation has also been reported (106). A review of glial release of neuroactive compounds is provided by Martin (145).

Pyruvate carboxylase is the major anapleurotic enzyme in the brain which is involved in the net synthesis of citric acid cycle intermediates. It is found almost exclusively in astrocytes, with little or none in neurons (118,202,252). This has important implications for cooperation between astrocytes and neurons. As citric acid cycle intermediates are depleted from neurons, replenishment appears to be derived from astrocyte metabolites generated via CO_2 fixation. The release of citrate by astrocytes has been demonstrated (213), and preliminary data indicates that malate and α-ketoglutarate are also released. Synaptic endings have the capacity to take up these agents (203).

Most of the glycogen in the brain is confined to astrocytes (40,92,110). Various neurotransmitters (35,140) and potassium (34) are capable of stimulating glycogenolysis. Such breakdown of glycogen during periods of neuronal activity may provide energy subtrates to neurons (47) and may provide neuroprotection during periods of energy substrate deprivation (220). The precise metabolite that is released by glycogenolysis is not known. It is probably lactate (243), but glucose and pyruvate may also be released (198).

Detoxification appears to represent another glial function. The presence of glutamine synthetase, largely in astrocytes (168), and to some extent in oligodendrocytes (37), suggests that astrocytes are the principal site of ammonia detoxification (48,49). Carbon dioxide may be significantly metabolized via carbonic anhydrase. While chiefly present in oligodendrocytes (36,82), carbonic anhydrase has also been found in astrocytes (5,112). Additionally, pyruvate carboxylase, the principal enzyme in brain involved in CO_2 fixation (118), appears to be exclusively confined to astrocytes. Glutathione-S-transferase, which has been identified in astrocytes (2,38), may be involved in the detoxification of drugs and hormones. Astrocytes are also enriched in glutathione and are able to release it (253), which may protect neurons from free radical damage (231).

The precise role of astrocytes in blood-brain barrier (BBB) function is not known. Brain capillaries are almost totally invested by astroglial processes (248). It is clear that astrocytes exert important inductive actions during development and that they are largely responsible for the special attributes that CNS endothelial cells possess, such as the presence of tight junctions (111,215). The induction may be due to the release of a soluble factor(s) (9) or it may require cell–cell contact (222). In culture it has been shown that factors released from astrocytes increase glucose uptake (153,221), affect the polarity (15), and induce the activity of γ-glutamyltranspeptidase (53) in endothelial cells. In turn, endothelial cells exert phenotypic changes in astrocytes, resulting in stellation and increased glutamine synthetase activity (91). For reviews dealing with astrocyte–endothelial interactions, see articles by Abbott and colleagues (1), and by Goldstein (86).

Astrocytes also have a variety of neurotrophic actions (10,11,116,136,154,166), appear to support neural regeneration (78,119,183,207,208), and have been shown to promote myelin synthesis (25,29) and remyelination (70,71). They also have critical functions in guiding neuronal migration during development (184,216). Kimelberg and Norenberg provide a review of astrocytic functions (123).

Although it had been known for some time that astrocytes are capable of phagocytosis (109,130,169,226,245), the notion that astrocytes might be important in inflammatory/immune phenomena was never seriously considered until after the pioneering studies of Fontana and colleagues. In 1982 they identified interleukin-1 (IL-1) in supernatants from cultured astrocytes (68). Their subsequent demonstration of major histocompatibility complex (MHC) class II induction in astrocytes, associated with antigen-specific T-cell proliferation (67), served to further strengthen the role of astrocytes in immune phenomena.

Astrocytes produce immune mediators (Table 6-1) and in turn, respond to a number of immune factors by undergoing cell proliferation and synthesizing MHC antigens, cytokines, growth factors and adhesion molecules (Table 6-2). Thus, important interactions between astrocytes and lymphocytes, and macrophages/microglia and endothelial cells occur that may impact on immune/inflammatory phenomena (Fig. 6-3). For further details on this topic, see Chapter 11.

Reaction of Astrocytes to Injury

Astrocytes are among the first cells to respond to CNS injury. The principal responses are reactive gliosis and cell swelling. *Gliosis* represents one of the best-recognized cellular responses to CNS injury, characterized by the presence of reactive astrocytes (gemistocytic astrocytes or Nissl plump astrocytes). This change reflects largely the hypertrophy and to a lesser extent, the proliferation of astrocytes. These hypertrophic cells display a profusion of cytoplasmic processes, resulting in the laying down of a "glial scar." This response is seen following any destructive injury, be it traumatic, ischemic, degenerative, demyelinative, infectious, or immunologic. The enlarged astrocytes contain increased amounts of cytoplasmic organelles and in particular, have increased amounts of GFAP (26). These astrocytes also show increased amounts of S-100 protein (90), amyloid precursor protein (205), epidermal growth factor (EGF) receptors (164), lipocortin-1 (115), and peripheral-type benzodiazepine receptors (194). Of particular significance to inflammatory/immune phenomena is the presence of Ia antigen (69,130), IL-1 (90), and alpha-1-antichymotrypsin (124), an acute phase reactive protein. (For review of factors associated with reactive astrocytes, see 59a.)

Factors involved in the production of reactive astrocytes are beginning to be identified. These include the cytokines IL-1 (83,84), interferon-γ (IFN-γ) (251), and tumor necrosis factor (TNF) (12,199,200). Various growth factors have also been implicated, namely, EGF (131,206), platelet-derived growth factor (PDGF) (21,98), and fibroblast

Table 6-1 Immune Factors Produced by Astrocytes

Factor	Reference
MHC class I antigens to	
IFN	218,223,250
Corona virus	219
Flavivirus	137
Mouse hepatitis virus	128
MHC class II antigens to	
IFN	64,103,218,249,250
Flavivirus	137
Mouse hepatitis virus	149
Measles virus	151
Theiler's virus	187
IL-1 to	
LPS	68
Substance P	147
TNF-α to	
LPS	44,134,186
IFN	44
IL-1	22,44
Viruses	45,134,186
Phorbol esters and A23187	23,24,45,186
Substance P	147
TGF-β	
Colony-stimulating factor	4,73,95,141,232,129,170,224
Adhesion molecules (ICAM-1, LFA-3) to	
TNF, IL-1, IFN	3,75
Lymphotoxin	75
Integrins	
IFN, TNF, IL-1	3
Complement (C3, factor B)	88,133
Prostaglandin E	68,96,114,201
Apolipoprotein E	32
Leukotriene B4	97
IFN-α/β	223
α1-antichymotrypsin	124
LY-6A/E	51

Table 6-2 Effect of Immune Factors on Astrocytes

Factor	Effect	Reference
IL-1	Proliferation	83,163,176
	Production of	
	ICAM-1	3,75
	TNF-α	23,44
	IL-6	72,191
	Colony stimulating	129,224,232
	Nerve growth factor	77,78
	Integrins	3
IL-6	Proliferation	200
	Production of nerve growth factor	72
IFN-γ	Proliferation	251
	Class I antigen induction	102,249
	Class II antigens induction	64,67,180,249,234
	Production of	
	TNF (with IL-1)	44
	ICAM-1	3,75
	Integrins	3
	Complement C3	13
TNF-α	Proliferation	200
	Cell swelling	16
	Class I antigen induction	127
	Enhancement of class II antigen production by IFN and viruses	19,151,236
	Production of	
	IL-6	20,72,191
	ICAM-1	3,75,107
	Integrins	3
	NGF	77
LPS	Proliferation	117
	Production of	
	IL-1-like factor	68
	IL-6	191
TGF-β	Decreased proliferation	135,225
	Decreased stellation	225
	Reduction in glutamine synthetase activity	41
	Reduction in class II antigen expression	254

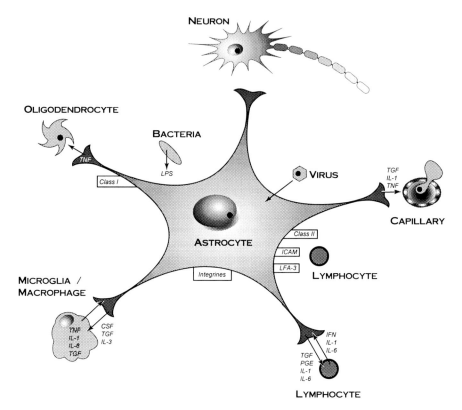

Fig. 6-3. Diagram depicts immune–inflammatory interactions between astrocytes and other cellular elements of the CNS. Important interactions among cells other than with astrocytes are not described.

growth factor (FGF) (173). Other factors include myelin basic protein (MBP) (30), cyclic adenosine monophosphate (AMP) (63), and adenosine triphosphate (ATP) (162). (For review, see 168a)

The significance of the gliotic response to CNS injury is not known. For a long time it was believed that the glial scar served as an impediment to regeneration and re-myelination. This long-held view has been seriously challenged in recent years and as discussed above, there is much evidence that these cells may have neurite- and myelin-promoting properties. It is likely that these cells may be involved in the restoration of the extracellular milieu that has been disturbed as a result of injury. For reviews of gliosis, see Kimelberg and Norenberg (123,168a).

Astrocyte swelling occurs within minutes following CNS injury and has been de-scribed in EAE (62,85). It is sometimes referred to as *cytotoxic edema.* The causes are not precisely known, but it is likely that elevated levels of potassium, glutamate, fatty acids, arachidonic acid, lactic acid, and free radicals play a role in glial swelling. This swelling leads to the production of increased intracranial pressure and consequent brain stem dysfunction. Swollen astrocytes have also been shown to release glutamate (121), which may lead to excitotoxic injury. To what extent swollen astrocytes have functional derangements remains to be defined. For a review of glial swelling, see Kimelberg and Norenberg (123,120a)

Involvement of Astrocytes in Immune Disorders

Multiple Sclerosis (MS)

The term *sclerosis* refers to the striking degree of gliosis that occurs in MS. The reactive astrocytes can be extremely large, are often binucleated, and frequently show highly atypical nuclei (182). Their role in MS is not clear. Views have varied from the inhibition of myelination to its promotion. The astrocytes may be involved in phagocytosis of myelin debris.

Class II MHC antigens have been identified on astrocytes (104,130,228,230) and their presence correlated with presence of IFN (228). Additionally, intracellular adhesion molecule-1 (ICAM-1) has been found on astrocytes (75,211) and a preliminary study has identified vascular cell adhesion molecule-1 (VCAM-1) (107).

Experimental Allergic Encephalomyelitis (EAE)

Reactive astrocytosis is a prominent histopathological feature in EAE (39,85). Astrocytes in this autoimmune demyelinative disorder have been shown to have a heightened degree of proliferation (209) and to manifest increased amounts of GFAP (7,210). Cellular edema has been described early in the disease course (62,85).

As mentioned above, astrocytes have the ability to present MBP-sensitized T cells (67). There is controversy regarding the presence of class II antigens in EAE. Some investigators have found them (218,229), while others have not (148,156). As reviewed by Benveniste (18), such failure may be due to the time at which they were looked for during the disease process, and the fact that class II antigens are more readily downregulated in astrocytes (74,76,190) as compared to microglia. Furthermore, astrocytes may be destroyed via class II MHC–restricted cytotoxicity (218).

Of considerable interest are the findings of Massa and colleagues (152), who showed that astrocytes from a susceptible rat strain (Lewis) expressed higher amounts of class II antigens in vitro after IFN or virus treatment, compared to a less susceptible strain (Brown-Norway). In keeping with this observation are studies showing that EAE-resistant and susceptible strains of rats also differ in their ability to express TNF (46). These differential responses of astrocytes suggest that these cells may indeed be playing a role in determining the outcome of this immunological condition.

AIDS

The pathogenesis of AIDS encephalopathy remains poorly understood. There is neuronal atrophy and myelin pallor, along with clusters of microglia that often contain multinucleated cells. Hypertrophic astrocytes form a prominent feature of the neuropathology of AIDS (89,174). A commonly held view focuses on the role of microglial/macrophage-released cytokines or products of HIV-1 (e.g., gp120) in having deleterious effects on various components of the CNS. Some of these cytokines may be derived from astrocytes (80) (for review, see 157,159,27a,170a).

Of interest is an interaction between astrocytes and microglia. Conditioned media of lipposaccharide (LPS)-treated astrocytes increase HIV-1 gene expression in monocytes (238) and astrocyte-derived IL-6 promotes HIV-1 replication (239). Conversely, supernatants from HIV-treated macrophages induce cultured astrocytes to release TGF (240). Clearly, a positive feedback system appears to be operative.

Related conditions seen in AIDS which have a bearing on astrocytes are progressive multifocal leukoencephalopathy (PML) and cytomegalovirus (CMV) infection. PML occurs in a setting of immunosuppression (most commonly seen now in AIDS). It is caused by an oncogenic papova virus, resulting in lytic infection of oligodendrocytes and consequent demyelination. The virus can be identified in oligodendrocytes (productive infection). Astrocytes on the other hand are transformed into bizarre-appearing cells (Alzheimer type I astrocytes). Intact virus is not present in astrocytes, although the viral genome has been identified in the astrocyte nucleus by in situ hybridization. The significance of this astroglial response is not clear, although rare reports of glial tumors occurring in PML have been described (204).

CMV infection is a frequent occurrence in AIDS patients. The virus is found chiefly in astrocytes (246), although CMV preferentially infects microglia/macrophages in culture (179). It can cause productive infection in cultured astrocytes associated with an increased production of TGF (160).

Alzheimer's Disease (AD)

Reactive gliosis is a conspicuous pathologic feature of AD and a prominent component of the neuritic plaque (55,142–144,193) which could be secondary to increased levels of IL-1 (90). IL-1 promotes amyloid precursor protein (APP) gene expression in astrocytes (28). Since astrocytes have been shown to generate IL-1 and IL-6, and since the latter cytokines appear to be involved in the generation of amyloid (233), astrocytes may contribute in a significant way to the pathology of AD. Moreover, amyloid stimulates astrocytes to produce growth factors (8). Increased levels of apolipoprotein E and cathepsin D have been identified in astrocytes (58). (For review, see 71a).

Concluding Remarks

Much data has accumulated and has transformed our view of astrocytes from one of mere passive, physically supportive cells, to that of active and dynamic partners with other cellular elements of the CNS. It is now generally accepted that astrocytes exert powerful influences on the microenvironment through the regulation of water and ion metabolism and involvement in neurotransmitter metabolism. Astrocytes also have critical functions dealing with neuronal energy metabolism, detoxification, neurotrophism, development, and the blood-brain barrier.

It has also become clear that among the repertoire of astroglial activities is involvement in immune/inflammatory phenomena, and important cooperation occurs between astrocytes and cells of the immune system. Clearly, astrocytes are immunocompetent cells that can augment, amplify, or perhaps regulate the immune response. They produce many immune/inflammatory mediators and in return are profoundly affected by these agents. Accordingly, these cells may promote a beneficial response by helping to eliminate foreign or infectious agents. On the other hand, by facilitating such responses, it may abet tissue injury. The outcome of the disease process will obviously depend on which of these two pathways dominates.

Finally, it is evident that astrocytes do not operate in a vacuum. Important interrelationships and interdependencies between astrocytes and neurons, oligodendrocytes, and endothelial cells, as well as with cells of the immune system, have been defined. A fuller insight into the operation of the CNS will require a better understanding of these cellular relationships.

Acknowledgments

This work was supported by the Department of Veterans Affairs (Merit Review and GRECC) and NIH grants DK38153 and NS30291. I am indebted to Dr. Jocelyn Bruce for her assistance in the preparation of this manuscript.

References

1. Abbott NJ, Revest PA, Romero IA. Astrocyte-endothelial interaction: physiology and pathology. Neuropathol Appl Neurobiol 18:424–433, 1992.
2. Abramovitz M, Homma H, Ishigaki S, Tansey F, Cammer W, Listowsky I. Characterization and localization of glutathione-S-transferases in rat brain and binding of hormones, neurotransmitters, and drugs. J Neurochem 50:50–57, 1988.
3. Aloisi F, Borsellino G, Samoggia P, Testa U, Chelucci C, Russo G, Peschle C, Levi G. Astrocyte cultures from human embryonic brain: characterization and modulation of surface molecules by inflammatory cytokines. J Neurosci Res 32:494–506, 1992.

4. Aloisi F, Care A, Borsellino G, Gallo P, Rosa S, Bassani A, Cabibbo A, Testa U, Levi G, Peschle C. Production of hemolymphopoietic cytokines (IL-6, IL-8, colony-stimulating factors) by normal human astrocytes in response to IL-1β and tumor necrosis factor-α. J Immunol 149:2358–2366, 1992.

5. Anderson RE, Engstrom FL, Woodbury DM. Localization of carbonic anhydrase in the cerebellum of normal and audiogenic seizure mice. Ann NY Acad Sci 429:502–504, 1984.

6. Andriezen WL. The neuroglia elements of the human brain. Br Med J 2:227–230, 1893.

7. Aquino DA, Shafit-Zagardo B, Brosnan CF, Norton WT. Expression of glial fibrillary acidic protein and neurofilament mRNA in gliosis induced by experimental autoimmune encephalomyelitis. J Neurochem 54:1398–1404, 1990.

8. Araujo DM, Cotman CW. β-amyloid stimulates glial cells in vitro to produce growth factors that accumulate in senile plaques in Alzheimer's disease. Brain Res 569:141–145, 1992.

9. Arthur FE, Shivers RR, Bowman PD. Astrocyte-mediated induction of tight junctions in brain capillary endothelium: an efficient in vitro model. Dev Brain Res 36:155–159, 1987.

10. Azmitia EC, Griffin WST, Marshak DR, Van Eldik LJ Whitaker-Azmitia PM. S-100 β and serotonin: a possible astrocytic-neuronal link to neuropathology of Alzheimer's disease. In: Neuronal-Astrocytic Interactions. Implications for Normal and Pathological CNS Function, ACH Yu, L Hertz, MD Norenberg, E Sykova, SG Waxman, eds. Elsevier, Amsterdam, 1992, pp. 459–473.

11. Banker GA. Trophic interaction between astroglial cells and hippocampal neurones in culture. Science 209:809–810, 1980.

12. Barna BP, Estes ML, Jacobs BS, Hudson S, Ransohoff RM. Human astrocytes proliferate in response to tumor necrosis factor alpha. J Neuroimmunol 30:239–243, 1990.

13. Barnum SR, Jones JL, Benveniste EN. Interferon-γ regulation of C3 gene expression in human astroglioma cells. J Neuroimmunol 38:275–282, 1992.

14. Barres BA, Chun LLY, Corey DP. Ion channels in vertebrate glia. Annu Rev Neurosci 13:441–474, 1990.

15. Beck DW, Vinters HV, Hart MN, Cancilla PA. Glial cells influence polarity of the blood-brain barrier. J Neuropathol Exp Neurol 43:219–224, 1984.

16. Bender AS, Rivera IV, Norenberg MD. Tumor necrosis factor-α induces astrocyte swelling. Trans Am Soc Neurochem 23:113, 1992.

17. Benjamin AM, Quastel JH. Locations of amino acids in brain cortex slices from the rat. Tetrodotoxin-sensitive release of amino acids. Biochem J 128:631–646, 1972.

18. Benveniste EN. Inflammatory cytokines within the central nervous system: sources, function, and mechanism of action. Am J Physiol 263:C1–16, 1992.

19. Benveniste EN, Sparacio SM, Bethea JR. Tumor necrosis factor-α enhances interferon-γ-mediated class II antigen expression on astrocytes. J Neuroimmunol 25:209–219, 1989.

20. Benveniste EN, Sparacio SM, Norris JG, Grenett HE, Fuller, GH. Induction and regulation of interleukin-6 gene expression in rat astrocytes. J Neuroimmunol 30:201–212, 1990.

21. Besnard F, Perraud F, Sensenbrenner M, Labourdette G. Platelet-derived growth factor is a mitogen for glial but not for neuronal rat brain cells in vitro. Neurosci Lett 73:287–292, 1987.

22. Bethea JR, Chung IY, Sparacio SM, Gillespie GY, Benveniste EN. Interleukin-1 β induction of tumor necrosis factor-α gene expression in human astroglioma cells. J Neuroimmunol 36:179–191, 1992.

23. Bethea JR, Gillespie GY, Benveniste EN. Interleukin-1 β induction of TNF-α gene expression: involvement of protein kinase C. J Cell Physiol 152:264–273, 1992.

24. Bethea JR, Gillespie GY, Chung IY, Benveniste EN. Tumor necrosis factor production and receptor expression by a human malignant glioma cell line, D54-MG. J Neuroimmunol 30:1–13, 1990.

25. Bhat S, Barbarese E, Pfeiffer E. Requirement for non-oligodendrocyte cells signals for enhanced myelinogenic gene expression in long term cultures or purified rat oligodendrocytes. Proc Natl Acad Sci USA 78:1283–1287, 1981.

26. Bignami A, Dahl D. The astroglial response to stabbing. Immunofluorescence studies with antibodies to astrocyte-specific protein (GFA) in mammalian and submammalian vertebrates. Neuropathol Appl Neurobiol 2:99–110, 1976.

27. Bignami AD, Dahl D, Rueger DC. Glial fibrillary acidic protein (GFA) in normal neural cells and in pathological conditions. Adv Cell Neurobiol 1:285–310, 1980.

27a. Blumberg BM, Gelbard HA, Epstein LG. HIV-1 infection of the developing nervous system: central role of astrocytes in pathogenesis. Virus Res 32:253–267, 1994.

28. Blume AJ, Vitek MP. Focusing on IL-1 promotion of β-amyloid precursor protein synthesis as an early event in Alzheimer's disease. Neurobiol Aging 10:406–408, 1989.

29. Blunt MJ, Baldwin F, Wendell-Smith CP. Gliogenesis and myelination in kitten optic nerve. Zellforsch 124:293–310, 1972.

30. Bologa L, Deugnier M, Joubert R, Bisconte J. Myelin basic protein stimulates the proliferation of astrocytes: possible explanation for multiple sclerosis plaque formation. Brain Res 346:199–203, 1985.

31. Booher J, Sesenbrenner M. Growth and cultivation of dissociated neurons and glial cells from embryonic chick, rat and human brain in flask cultures. Neurobiology 2:97–105, 1972.

32. Boyles JK, Pitas RE, Wilson E, Mahley RW, Taylor JM. Apolipoprotein E associated with astrocytic glia of the central nervous system and with nonmyelinating glia of the peripheral nervous system. J Clin Invest 76:1501–1513, 1985.

33. Bradford HF, Ward HK. Glutamine—a major substrate for nerve endings. J Neurochem 30:1453–1459, 1978.

34. Cambray Deakin M, Pearce B, Morrow C, Murphy S. Effects of extracellular potassium on glycogen stores of astrocytes in vitro. J Neurochem 51:1846–1851, 1988.

35. Cambray Deakin M, Pearce B, Morrow C, Murphy S. Effects of neurotransmitters on astrocyte glycogen stores in vitro. J Neurochem 51:1852–1857, 1988.

36. Cammer W. Carbonic anhydrase in oligodendrocytes and myelin in the central nervous system. Ann NY Acad Sci 429:494–497, 1984.

37. Cammer W. Glutamine synthetase in the central nervous system is not confined to astrocytes. J Neuroimmunol 26:173–178, 1990.

38. Cammer W, Tansey F, Abramovitz M, Ishigaki S, Listowsky I. Differential localization of glutathione-S-transferase Yp and Yb subunits in oligodendrocytes and astrocytes of rat brain. J Neurochem 52:876–883, 1989.

39. Cammer W, Tansey FA, Brosnan CF. Reactive gliosis in the brains of Lewis rats with experimental allergic encephalomyelitis. J Neuroimmunol 27:111–120, 1990.

40. Cataldo AM, Broadwell RD. Cytochemical identification of cerebral glycogen and glucose-6-phosphatase activity under normal and experimental conditions. Neurons and glia. Electron Microscop Tech 3:413–437, 1986.

41. Chao CC, Hu S, Tsang M, Weatherbee J, Molitor TW, Anderson WR, Peterson PK. Effects of transforming growth factor-β on murine astrocyte glutamine synthetase activity. Implications in neuronal injury. J Clin Invest 90:1786–1793, 1992.

42. Chesler M. The regulation and modulation of pH in the nervous system. Prog Neurobiol 34:401–427, 1990.

43. Cholewinski AJ, Hanley MR, Wilkin GP. A phosphoinositide-linked peptide response in astrocytes: evidence for regional heterogeneity. Neurochem Res 13:389–394, 1988.

44. Chung IY, Benveniste EN. Tumor necrosis factor-α production by astrocytes. Induction by lipopolysaccharide, IFN-γ and IL-1β. J Immunol 144:2999–3007, 1990.

45. Chung IY, Kwon J, Benveniste EN. Role of protein kinase C activity in tumor necrosis factor-α gene expression. Involvement at the transcriptional level. J Immunol 149:3894–3902, 1992.

46. Chung IY, Norris JG, Benveniste EN. Differential tumor necrosis factor alpha expression by astrocytes from experimental allergic encephalomyelitis-susceptible and -resistant rat strains. J Exp Med 173:801–811, 1991.

47. Coles JA, Tsacopoulos M. Ionic and possible metabolic interactions between sensory neurones and glial cells in the retina of the honeybee drone. J Exp Biol 95:75–92, 1981.

48. Cooper AJL, Lai JCK. Cerebral ammonia metabolism in normal and hyperammonemic rats. Neurochem Pathol 6:67–74, 1987.

49. Cooper AJL, Plum F. Biochemistry and physiology of brain ammonia. Physiol Rev 67:440–519, 1987.

50. Cornell-Bell FH, Finkbeiner SM, Cooper MS, Smith SJ. Glutamate induces calcium waves in cultured astrocytes: long-range glial signaling. Science 247:470–473, 1990.

51. Cray C, Keane RW, Malek TR, Levy RB. Regulation and selective expression of Ly-6A/E, a lymphocyte activation molecule, in the central nervous system. Mol Brain Res 8:9–15, 1990.

52. Dani JW, Chernjavsky A, Smith SJ. Neuronal activity triggers calcium waves in hippocampal astrocyte networks. Neuron 8:429–440, 1992.

53. Debault LE. γ-glutamyltranspeptidase induction mediated by glial foot process into endothelium contact in co-culture. Brain Res 220:432–435, 1982.

54. Deiters O. Untersuchungen über Gehirn und Rückenmark des Menschen und der Saugethiere. F. Vieweg u. Sohn, Braunschweig, 1865.

55. Delacourte A. General and dramatic glial reaction in Alzheimer brains. Neurology 40:33–37, 1990.

56. Denis-Donini S, Glowinski J, Prochiantz A. Glial heterogeneity may define the three-dimensional shape of mouse mesencephalic dopaminergic neurons. Nature (Lond) 307:641–643, 1984.

57. Dermietzel R, Hertzberg EL, Kessler JA, Spray DC. Gap junctions between cultured astrocytes: immunocytochemical, molecular, and electrophysiological analysis. J Neurosci 11:1421–1432, 1991.

58. Diedrich JF, Minnigan H, Carp RI, Whitaker JN, Race R, Frey W II, Haase AT. Neuropathological changes in scrapie and Alzheimer's disease are associated with increased expression of apolipoprotein E and cathepsin D in astrocytes. J Virol 65:4759–4768, 1991.

59. Drejer J, Meier E, Schousboe A. Novel neuron-related regulatory mechanisms for astrocytic glutamate and GABA high-affinity uptake. Neurosci Lett 37:301–306, 1883.

59a. Eddleston M, Mucke L. Molecular profile of reactive astrocytes—implications for their role in neurologic disease. Neuroscience 54:15–36, 1993.

60. El-Etr M, Cordier J, Torrens Y, Glowinski J, Premont J. Pharmacological and functional heterogeneity of astrocytes: regional differences in phospholipase C stimulation by neuromediators. J Neurochem 52:981–984, 1989.

61. Eng LF. Glial fibrillary acidic protein (GFAP): the major protein of glial intermediate filaments in differentiated astrocytes. J Neuroimmunol 8:203–214, 1985.

62. Eng LF, D'Amelio FE, Smith ME. Dissociation of GFAP intermediate filaments in EAE: observations in the lumbar spinal cord. Glia 2:308–317, 1989.

63. Fedoroff S, Mcauley WAJ, Houle JD, Devon RM. Astrocyte cell lineage. V. Similarity of astrocytes that form in the presence of dBcAMP in cultures to reactive astrocytes in vivo. J Neurosci Res 12:15–27, 1984.

64. Fierz W, Endler B, Reske K, Wekerle H, Fontana A. Astrocytes as antigen presenting cells. I. Induction of Ia expression on astrocytes by T cells via immune interferon and its effect on antigen presentation. J Immunol 134:3785–3793, 1985.

65. Fischer G, Kettenmann H. Cultured astrocytes form a syncytium after maturation. Exp Cell Res 159:273–279, 1985.

66. Floyd RA. Oxidative damage to behavior during aging. Science. 254:1597, 1991.

67. Fontana A, Fierz W, Werkele H. Astrocytes present myelin basic protein to encephalitogenic T-cell lines. Nature 307:273–276, 1984.

68. Fontana A, Kristensen F, Dubs R, Gemsa D, Weber E. Production of prostaglandin E and an interleukin-1 like factor by cultured astrocytes and C6 glioma cells. J Immunol 129:2413–2419, 1982.

69. Frank E, Pulver M, De-Tribolet N. Expression of class II major histocompatibility antigens on reactive astrocytes and endothelial cells within the gliosis surrounding metastases and abscesses. J Neuroimmunol 12:29–36, 1986.

70. Franklin RJM, Crang AJ, Blakemore WF. Transplanted type-1 astrocytes facilitate repair of demyelinating lesions by host oligodendrocytes in adult rat spinal cord. J Neurocytol 20:420–430, 1991.

71. Franklin RJM, Crang AJ, Blakemore WF. The role of astrocytes in the remyelination of glia-free areas of demyelination. Adv Neurol 59:125–133, 1993.

71a. Frederickson RCA. Astroglia in Alzheimer's disease. Neurobiol Aging 13:239–253, 1992.

72. Frei K, Malipiero UV, Leist TP, Zinkernagel RM, Schwab ME, Fontana A. On the cellular source of interleukin-6 produced in the central nervous system in viral diseases. Eur J Immunol 19:689–694, 1989.

73. Frei K, Nohava K, Malipiero UV, Schwerdel C, Fontana A. Production of macrophage colony-stimulating factor by astrocytes and brain macrophages. J Neuroimmunol 40:189–196, 1992.

74. Frohman E, Frohman T, Vayuvegula B, Gupta S, Van Den Noort S. Vasoactive intestinal polypedtide inhibits the expression of the MHC class II antigens on astrocytes. J Neurol Sci 88:339–346, 1988.

75. Frohman EM, Frohman TC, Dustin ML, Vayuvegula B, Choi B, Gupta A, Van Den Noort S, Gupta S. The induction of intracellular adhesion molecule 1 (ICAM-1) expression on human fetal astrocytes by interferon-γ, tumor necrosis factor-α, lymphotoxin, and interleukin-1: relevance to intracerebral antigen presentation. J Neuroimmunol 23:117–124, 1989.

76. Frohman EM, Vayuvegula B, Gupta S, Van Den Noort S. Norepinephrine inhibits γ interferon-induced major histocompatability class II (Ia) antigen expression on cultured astrocytes via β2-adrenergic signal transduction mechanisms. Proc Natl Acad Sci USA 85:1292–1296, 1988.

77. Gadient RA, Cron KVC, Otten U. Interleukin-1 and tumor necrosis factor-α synergistically stimulate nerve growth factor (NGF) release from cultured astrocytes. Neurosci Lett 117:335–340, 1990.

78. Gage FH, Olejniczak P, Armstrong DM. Astrocytes are important for sprouting in the septohippocampal circuit. Exp Neurol 102:2–13, 1988.

79. Gallo V, Patrizio M, Levi G. GABA release triggered by the activation of neuron-like non-NMDA receptors in cultured type 2 astrocytes is carrier mediated. Glia 4:245–255, 1991.

80. Genis P, Jett M, Bernton EW, Boyle T, Gelbard HA, Dzenko K, Keane RW, Resnick L, Mizrachi Y, Volsky DJ, Epstein LG, Gendelman, HE. Cytokines and arachidonic metabolites produced during human immunodeficiency virus (HIV)-infected macrophage-astroglia interactions: implications for the neuropathogenesis of HIV disease. J Exp Med 176:1703–1718, 1992.

81. Gerschenfeld HM, Wald F, Zadunaisky JA, DeRobertis EDP. Function of astroglia in the water-ion metabolism of the central nervous system. Neurology 9:412–425, 1959.

82. Ghandour MS, Langley OK, Vicendo G, Gombos G. Double labelling immunohistochemical techniques provides evidence of the specificity of glial cell markers. Cytochemistry 27:1634–1637, 1979.

83. Giulian D, Lachman LB. Interleukin-1 stimulation of astroglial proliferation after brain injury. Science 228:497–499, 1985.

84. Giulian D, Woodward J, Young DG, Krebs JF, Lachman LB. Interleukin-1 injected into mammalian brain stimulates astrogliosis and neovascularization. J Neurosci 8:2484, 1988.

85. Goldmuntz EA, Brosnan CF, Chiu F-C, Norton WT. Astrocytic reactivity and intermediate filament metabolism in experimental autoimmune encephalomyelitis: the effect of suppression with prazosin. Brain Res 397:16–26, 1986.

86. Goldstein GW. Endothelial cell-astrocyte interactions. A cellular model of the blood-brain barrier. Ann NY Acad Sci 529:31–39, 1988.

87. Golgi C. Opera Omnia. U. Hoepli, Milan, 1903.

88. Gordon DL, Avery VM, Adrian DL, Sadlon TA. Detection of complement protein mRNA in human astrocytes by the polymerase chain reaction. J Neurosci Methods 45:191–197, 1992.

89. Gray F, Gherardi R, Scaravilli F. The neuropathology of the acquired immune deficiency syndrome (AIDS). A review. Brain 111:245–266, 1988.

90. Griffin WS, Stanley LC, Ling C, White L, MacLeod V, Perrot LJ, White CL III, Araoz C. Brain interleukin 1 and S-100 immunoreactivity are elevated in Down syndrome and Alzheimer disease. Proc Natl Acad Sci USA 86:7611–7615, 1989.

91. Grinspan JB, Lieb M, Stern J, Rupnick M, Williams S, Pleasure D. Rat brain microvessel extracellular matrix modulates the phenotype of cultured rat type 1 astroglia. Brain Res 430:291–295, 1987.

92. Guth L, Watson PK. A correlated histochemical and quantitative study on cerebral glycogen after brain injury in the rat. Exp Neurol 22:590–602, 1968.

93. Hansson E. Astroglia from defined brain regions as studied with primary cultures. Prog Neurobiol 30:369–397, 1988.

94. Hansson E, Eriksson P, Nilsson M. Amino acid and monoamine transport in primary astroglial cultures from defined brain regions. Neurochem Res 10:1335–1341, 1985.

95. Hao C, Guilbert LJ, Fedoroff S. Production of colony-stimulating factor-1 (CSF-1) by mouse astroglia in vitro. J Neurosci Res 27:314, 1990.

96. Hartung H-P, Toyka KV. Phorbol diester TPA elicits prostaglandin release from cultured rat astrocytes. Brain Res 417:347–349, 1987.

97. Hartung HP, Heininger K, Toyka KV. Primary rat astroglial cultures can generate leukotriene B4. J Neuroimmunol 19:27, 1988.

98. Heldin C, Wasteson A, Westermark B. Partial purification and characterization of platelet

factors stimulating the multiplication of normal human glial cells. Exp Cell Res 109:429–437, 1977.

99. Henn FA, Anderson DJ, Sellstrom A. Possible relationship between glial cells, dopamine and the effects of antipsychotic drugs. Nature 266:637–638, 1977.

100. Henn FA, Hamberger A. Glial cell functions: uptake of transmitter substances. Proc Natl Acad Sci USA 68:2686–2690, 1971.

101. Hertz L. Functional interactions between neurons and astrocytes. I. Turnover and metabolism of putative amino acid transmitters. Prog Neurobiol 13:277–323, 1979.

102. Hirayama M, Yokochi T, Shimokata K, Iida M, Fujuki N. Induction of human leukocyte antigen-A, -B, -C and -DR on cultured human oligodendrocytes by β-interferon. Neurosci Lett 72:369–374, 1986.

103. Hirsch M-R, Wietzerbin J, Pierres M, Gordis C. Expression of Ia antigens by cultured astrocytes treated with γ interferon. Neurosci Lett 41:199–204, 1983.

104. Hofman FM, Vonhanwher R, Dinarello C, Mizel S, Hinton D, Merrill JE. Immunoregulatory molecules and IL-2 receptors identified in multiple sclerosis brain. J Immunol 136:3239–3245, 1986.

105. Holopainen I, Kontro P. D-aspartate release from cerebellar astrocytes: modulation of the high K-induced release by neurotransmitter amino acids. Neuroscience 36:115–120, 1990.

106. Holopainen I, Louve M, Enkvist MO, Akerman KE. ^{86}Rubidium release from cultured primary astrocytes; effects of excitatory and inhibitory amino acids. Neuroscience 30:223–229, 1989.

107. Hurwitz AA, Lyman WD, Guida MP, Calderon TM, Berman JW. Tumor necrosis factor alpha induces adhesion molecule expression on human fetal astrocytes. J Exp Med 176:1631–1636, 1992.

108. Hyden H. Quantitative assay of compounds in isolated fresh nerve cells and glial cells from control and stimulated animals. Nature (Lond) 184:433–435, 1959.

109. Iacono RF, Berria MI, Lascano EF. A triple staining procedure to evaluate phagocytic role of differentiated astrocytes. J Neurosci Methods 39:225–230, 1991.

110. Ibrahim MZM. Glycogen and its related enzymes of metabolism in the central nervous system. Adv Anat Cell Biol 52:3–89, 1975.

111. Janzer RC, Raff MC. Astrocytes induce blood-brain barrier properties in endothelial cells. Nature 325:253–257, 1987.

112. Jeffrey M, Wells GAH, Bridges AW. Carbonic anhydrase II expression in fibrous astrocytes of the sheep. J Comp Pathol 104:337–344, 1991.

113. Jendelova P, Sykova E. Role of glia in K^+ and pH homeostasis in the neonatal rat spinal cord. Glia 4:56–63, 1991.

114. Jeremy J, Murphy S, Morrow C, Pearce B, Dandona P. Phorbol ester stimulation of prostanoid synthesis by cultured astrocytes. Brain Res 419:364–368, 1987.

115. Johnson MD, Kamso-Pratt JM, Whetsell WO Jr, Pepinsky RB. Lipocortin-1 immunoreactivity in the normal human central nervous system and lesions with astrocytosis. Am J Clin Pathol 92:424–429, 1989.

116. Johnson MI, Higgins D, Ard D. Astrocytes induce dendritic development in cultured sympathetic neurons. Dev Brain Res 47:289–292, 1989.

117. Kato M, Ohno K, Takeshita K, Herz F. Stimulation of human fetal astrocyte proliferation by bacterial lipopolysaccharides and lipid A. Acta Neuropathol (Berl) 82:384–388, 1991.

118. Kaufman EE, Driscoll BF. Carbon dioxide fixation in neuronal and astroglial cells in culture. J Neurochem 58:258–262, 1992.

119. Kesslak JP, Nieto-Sampedro M, Globus J, Cotman CW. Transplants of purified astrocytes promote behavioral recovery after frontal cortex ablation. Exp Neurol 92:377–390, 1986.

120. Kimelberg HK, ed. Glial Cell Receptors. Raven Press, New York, 1988.

120a. Kimelberg HK. Current concepts of brain edema. J Neurosurg 83:1051–1059, 1995.

121. Kimelberg HK, Goderie SK, Higman S, Pang S, Waniewski RA. Swelling-induced release of glutamate, aspartate, and taurine from astrocyte cultures. J Neurosci 10:1583–1591, 1990.

122. Kimelberg HK, Katz DM. Regional differences in 5-hydroxytryptamine and catecholamine uptake in primary astrocyte cultures. J Neurochem 47:1647–1652, 1986.

123. Kimelberg HK, Norenberg MD. Astroglial responses to CNS trauma. In: The Neurobiology of Central Nervous System Trauma, SK Salzman, AI Faden, eds. Oxford University Press, New York, pp 193–208.

124. Koo EH, Abraham CR, Potter H, Cork LC, Price DL. Developmental expression of α-anti-chymotrypsin in brain may be related to astrogliosis. Neurobiol Aging 12:495–501, 1991.

125. Kraig RP, Pulsinelli WA, Plum F. Hydrogen ion buffering during complete brain ischemia. Brain Res 342:281–290, 1985.

126. Kuffler SW. Neuroglial cells: physiological properties and a potassium mediated effect of neuronal activity on the glial membrane potential. Proc R Soc Lond (Biol) 168:1–21, 1967.

127. Lavi E, Suzumura A, Murasko DM, Murray EM, Silberberg DH, Weiss SR. Tumor necrosis factor induces expression of MHC class I antigens on mouse astrocytes. J Neuroimmunol 18:245–253, 1988.

128. Lavi E, Suzumura A, Murray EM, Silberberg DH, Weiss SR. Induction of MHC class I antigens on glial cells is dependent on persistent mouse hepatitis virus infection. J Neuroimmunol 22:107–111, 1989.

129. Lee SC, Liu W, Roth P, Dickson DW, Berman JW, Brosnan LF. Macrophage colony-stimulating factor in human fetal astrocytes and microglia: differential regulation by cytokines and lipopolysaccharide, and modulation of class II MHC on microglia. J Immunol 150:594–604, 1993.

130. Lee SC, Moore GR, Golenwsky G, Raine CS. Multiple sclerosis: a role for astroglia in active demyelination suggested by class II MHC expression and ultrastructural study. J Neuropathol Exp Neurol 49:122–136, 1990.

131. Leutz A, Schachner M. Epidermal growth factor stimulates DNA-synthesis of astrocytes in primary cerebellar cultures. Cell Tiss Res 220:393–404, 1981.

132. Levi G, Patrizio M. Astrocyte heterogeneity: endogenous amino acid levels and release evoked by non-N-methyl-D-aspartate receptor agonists and by potassium-induced swelling in type-1 and type-2 astrocytes. J Neurochem 58:1943–1952, 1992.

133. Levi-Strauss M, Mallat M. Primary cultures of murine astrocytes produce C3 and factor B, two components of the alternative pathway of complement activation. J Immunol 139:2361–2366, 1987.

134. Lieberman AP, Pitha PM, Shin HS, Shin ML. Production of tumor necrosis factor and other cytokines by astrocytes stimulated with lipopolysaccharide or a neurotropic virus. Proc Natl Acad Sci USA 86:6348–6352, 1989.

135. Lindholm D, Castren E, Kiefer R, Zafra F, Thoenen H. Transforming growth factor-β1 in the rat brain: increase after injury and inhibition of astrocyte proliferation. J Cell Biol 117:395–400, 1992.

136. Lindsay RM. Adult rat brain astrocytes support survival of both NGF-dependent and NGF-insensitive neurones. Nature (Lond) 282:80–82, 1979.

137. Liu Y, King N, Kesson A, Blanden RV, Mullbacher A. Flavivirus infection up-regulates the

expression of class I and class II major histocompatibility antigens on and enhances T cell recognition of astrocytes in vitro. J Neuroimmunol 21:157–168, 1989.

138. Logan A, Frautschy SA, Gonzalez AM, Sporn MB, Baird A. Enhanced expression of transforming growth factor-β1 in the rat brain after a localized cerebral injury. Brain Res 587:216–225, 1992.

139. Lugaro E. Sulle funzioni della nevroglia. Riv Pat Nerv Ment 12:225–233, 1907.

140. Magistretti PJ, Manthorpe M, Bloom FE, Varon S. Functional receptors for vasoactive intestinal polypeptide in cultured astroglia from neonatal rat brain. Regul Peptides 6:71–80, 1983.

141. Malipiero UV, Frei K, Fontana A. Production of hemopoietic colony-stimulating factors by astrocytes. J Immunol 144:3816–3812, 1990.

142. Mancardi GL, Liwnicz BH, Mandybur TI. Fibrous astrocytes in Alzheimer's disease and senile dementia of Alzheimer type. Acta Neuropathol (Berl) 61:76–80, 1983.

143. Mandybur TI, Chuirazzi CC. Astrocytes and the plaques of Alzheimer's disease. Neurology 40:635–639, 1990.

144. Mandybur TI, Chuirazzi C, Ormsby I. The role of astrocytes in the amyloid plaques of Alzheimer's disease. J Neuropathol Exp Neurol 47:337, 1988.

145. Martin DL. Synthesis and release of neuroactive substances by glial cells. Glia 5:81–94, 1992.

146. Martin DL, Madelian V, Seligmann B, Shain W. The role of osmotic pressure and membrane potential in K$^+$-stimulated taurine release from cultured astrocytes and LRM55 cells. J Neurosci 10:571–577, 1990.

147. Martin FC, Charles AC, Sanderson, MJ, Merrill JE. Substance P stimulates IL-1 production by astrocytes via intracellular calcium. Brain Res 599:13–18, 1992.

148. Marx J. NGF and Alzheimer's: hopes and fears. Science 247:408–410, 1990.

149. Massa PT, Dorries R, Ter Meulen V. Viral particles induce Ia antigen expression on astrocytes. Nature 320:543–546, 1986.

150. Massa PT, Mugnaini E. Cell functions and intramembrane particles of astrocytes and oligodendrocytes: a freeze fracture study. Neuroscience 7:523–538, 1982.

151. Massa PT, Schimpl A, Wecker E, Ter Meulen V. Tumor necrosis factor amplifies measles virus-mediated Ia induction on astrocytes. Proc Natl Acad Sci USA 84:7242–7245, 1987.

152. Massa PT, Ter Meulen V, Fontana A. Hyperinductibility of Ia antigen on astrocytes correlates with strain-specific susceptibility to experimental autoimmune encephalomyelitis. Proc Natl Acad Sci USA 84:4219–4223, 1987.

153. Maxwell K, Berliner JA, Cancilla PA. Stimulation of glucose analogue uptake by cerebral microvessel endothelial cells by a product released by astrocytes. J Neuropathol Exp Neurol 48:69–80, 1989.

154. McCaffery CA, Raju RT, Bennett MR. Effects of cultured astroglia on the survival of neonatal rat retinal ganglion cells in vitro. Dev Biol 104:441–448, 1984.

155. McCarthy KD, De Vellis J. Preparation of separate astroglial and oligodendroglial cell cultures from rat cerebral tissue. J Cell Biol 85:890–902, 1980.

156. Merrill JE. Lymphokines, monokines, and glial cells. In: Volume Transmission in the Brain: Novel Mechanisms for Neural Transmission, K Fuxe, LF Agnati, eds. Raven Press, New York, 1991, pp 267–277.

157. Merrill JE, Chen ISY. HIV-1, macrophages, glial cells, and cytokines in AIDS nervous system disease. FASEB J 5:2391–2397, 1991.

158. Miller RH, Raff MC. Fibrous and protoplasmic astrocytes are biochemically and developmentally distinct. J Neurosci 4:585–592, 1984.

159. Morganti-Kossmann MC, Kossmann T, Brandes ME, Mergenhagen SE, Wahl SM. Auto-

crine and paracrine regulation of astrocyte function by transforming growth factor-β. J Neuroimmunol 39:163–174, 1992.

160. Morganti-Kossmann MC, Kossmann T, Wahl SM. Cytokines and neuropathology. Trends Pharmacol Sci 13:286–291, 1992.

161. Murphy S, Pearce B. Functional receptors for neurotransmitters on astroglial cells. Neuroscience 22:381–394, 1987.

162. Neary JT, Norenberg MD. Signalling by extracellular ATP: physiological and pathological considerations in neuronal-astrocytic interaction. In: Neuronal-Astrocytic Interactions: Pathological Implications, ACH Yu, L Hertz, MD Norenberg, E Sykova, SG Waxman, eds. Elsevier, Amsterdam, 1992, pp 145–151.

162a. Nedergaard M, Cooper AJL, Goldman SA. Gap junctions are required for the propagation of spreading depression. J Neurobiol 28:433–444, 1995.

163. Nieto-Sampedro M, Berman MA. Interleukin-1-like activity in rat brain: sources, targets, and effect of injury. J Neurosci Res 17:214–219, 1987.

164. Nieto-Sampedro M, Gomez-Pinilla F, Knauer DJ, Broderick JT. Epidermal growth factor receptor immunoreactivity in rat brain astrocytes. Response to injury. Neurosci Lett 91:276–282, 1988.

165. Nilsson M, Hansson E, Ronnback L. Heterogeneity among astroglial cells with respect to 5HT-evoked cytosolic Ca^{2+} responses. A microspectrofluorimetric study on single cells in primary culture. Life Sci 49:1339–1350, 1991.

166. Noble M, Fok-Seang J, Cohen J. Glia are a unique substrate for the in vitro growth of central nervous system neurons. J Neurosci 4:1892–1903, 1984.

167. Norenberg MD. The distribution of glutamine synthetase in the rat central nervous system. J Histochem Cytochem 27:756–762, 1979.

168. Norenberg MD. Immunohistochemistry of glutamine synthetase. In: Glutamine, Glutamate, and GABA in the Central Nervous System, L Hertz, E Kvamme, EG McGeer, A Schousboe, eds. Alan R. Liss, New York, 1983, pp 95–111.

168a. Norenberg MD. Reactive astrocytosis. In: The Role of Glia in Neurotoxicity, M Aschner, HK Kimelberg, eds. Boca Raton, CRC Press, 1996, 93–107.

169. Noske W, Lentzen H, Herken H. Phagocytosis and morphological development of rat astrocytes in primary cultures. Cell Mol Biol 28:235–244, 1982.

170. Ohno K, Suzumura A, Sawada M, Marunouchi T. Production of granulocyte/macrophage colony-stimulating factor by cultured astrocytes. Biochem Biophys Res Commun 169:719–724, 1990.

170a. Oldstone MBA, Vitkovic L. Role of astrocytosis in HIV-1-associated dementia. Curr Topics in Microbiol and Immunol 202:105–116, 1995.

171. Oliver CN, Starke-Reed PE, Stadtman ER, Liu GJ, Carney JM, Floyd RA. Oxidative damage to brain proteins, loss of glutamine synthetase activity, and production of free radicals during ischemia/reperfusion-induced injury to gerbil brain. Proc Natl Acad Sci USA 87:5144–5147, 1990.

172. Orkand RK, Nicholls JG, Kuffler SW. Effects of nerve impulses on the membrane potential of glial cells in the central nervous system of amphibia. J Neurophysiol 29:788–806, 1966.

173. Perraud F, Besnard F, Pettmann B, Sensenbrenner M, Labourdette G. Effects of acidic and basic fibroblastic growth factors (aFGF and bFGF) on the proliferation and the glutamine synthetase expression of rat astroblasts in culture. Glia 1:124–131, 1988.

174. Petito CK, Cho E-L, Lemann W, Navia BA, Price RW. Neuropathology of acquired immunodeficiency syndrome (AIDS): an autopsy review. J Neuropathol Exp Neurol 45:635–646, 1986.

175. Philibert RA, Rogers KL, Allen AJ, Dutton GR. Dose-dependent, K^+-stimulated efflux of endogenous taurine from primary astrocyte cultures is Ca^{2+}-dependent. J Neurochem 51:122–126, 1988.

176. Politis MJ, Lindsay JK. Exogenous interleukin regulates growth of C6 tumors in vivo. Acta Neuropathol (Berl) 77:182–185, 1988.

177. Pope A. Neuroglia: quantitative aspects. In: Dynamic Properties of Glia Cells, E Schoffeniels, G Franck, L Hertz, DB Tower, eds. Pergamon Press, London, 1978, pp 13–20.

178. Price J, Thurlow L. Cell lineage in the rat cerebral cortex: a study using retroviral-mediated gene transfer. Development 104:473–482, 1988.

179. Pulliam L. Cytomegalovirus preferentially infects a monocyte derived macrophage/microglial cell in human brain cultures: neuropathology differs between strains. J Neuropathol Exp Neurol 50:432–440, 1991.

180. Pulver M, Carrel S, Mach JP, De Tribolet N. Cultured human fetal astrocytes can be induced by interferon-γ to express HLA-DR. J Neuroimmunol 14:123–133, 1987.

181. Raff MC. Glial cell diversification in the rat optic nerve. Science 243:1450–1455, 1989.

182. Raine CS. Demyelinating diseases. In: Textbook of Neuropathology, RL Davis, DM Robertson, eds. Williams and Wilkins, Baltimore, 1991, pp 535–620.

183. Raisman G, Field PM, A quantitative investigation of the development of collateral reinnervation after partial deafferentiation of the septal nuclei. Brain Res 50:241–264, 1973.

184. Rakic P. Neuronal-glial interaction during brain development. Neuroscience 4:184–187, 1981.

185. Ramon Y Cajal S. Contribucion al conocimiento de la neuroglia del cerebro humano. Trab Lab Invest Biol 11:255–315, 1913.

186. Robbins DS, Shirazi Y, Drysdale G-E, Lieberman A, Shin HS, Shin ML. Production of cytotoxic factor for oligodendrocytes by stimulated astrocytes. J Immunol 139:2593–2597, 1987.

186a. Robinson MB, Djali S, Buchhalter JR. Inhibition of glutamate uptake with L-trans-pyrrolidine-2,4-dicarboxylate potentiates glutamate neurotoxicity in primary hippocampal cultures. J Neurochem 61:2099–2103, 1993.

187. Rodrigues M, Pierce ML, Howie EA. Immune response gene products (Ia antigens) on glial and endothelial cells in virus-induced demyelination. J Immunol 138:3438–3442, 1987.

188. Rosenberg PA, Aizenman E. Hundred-fold increase in neuronal vulnerability to glutamate toxicity in astrocyte-poor cultures of rat cerebral cortex. Neurosci Lett 103:162–168, 1989.

188a. Rothstein JD, Jin L, Dykes-Hoberg M, Kuncl RW. Chronic inhibition of glutamate uptake produces a model of slow neurotoxicity. Proc Natl Acad Sci USA 90:6591–6595, 1993.

189. Salm AK, McCarthy KD. The evidence for astrocytes as a target for central noradrenergic activity: expression of adrenergic receptors. Brain Res Bull 29:265–275, 1992.

190. Sasaki A, Levison SW, Ting JPY. Differential suppression of interferon-γ-induced Ia antigen expression on cultured rat astroglia and microglia by second messengers. J Neuroimmunol 29:213–222, 1990.

191. Sawada M, Suzumura A, Marunouchi T. TNFα induces IL-6 production by astrocytes but not by microglia. Brain Res 583:296–299, 1992.

192. Schachner M. Glial antigens and the expression of glial phenotypes. TINS 5:225–228, 1982.

193. Schecter R, Yen SC, Terry RD. Fibrous astrocytes in senile dementia of the Alzheimer type. J Neuropathol Exp Neurol 40:95–101, 1981.

194. Schoemaker H, Morelli M, Deshmukh P, Yamamura HI. [3H]Ro5-4864 benzodiazepine

binding in the kainate lesioned striatum and Huntington's diseased basal ganglia. Brain Res 248:396–401, 1982.

195. Schousboe A. Transport and metabolism of glutamate and GABA in neurons and glial cells. Int Rev Neurobiol 22:1–45, 1981.

196. Schousboe A, Divac I. Differences in glutamate uptake in astrocytes cultured from different brain regions. Brain Res 177:407–409, 1979.

197. Schousboe A, Pasantes-Morales H. Potassium-stimulated release of [3H] taurine from cultured GABAergic and glutamatergic neurons. J Neurochem 53:1309–1315, 1989.

197a. Schousboe A, Westergard N, Sonnewald U, Petersen SB, Huang R, Peng L, Hertz L. Glutamate and glutamine metabolism and compartmentation in astrocytes. Dev Neurosci 15:359–366, 1993.

198. Selak I, Skaper SD, Varon S. Pyruvate participation in the low molecular activity for CNS neurons in glia-conditioned media. J Neurosci 5:23–28, 1985.

199. Selmaj K, Shafit-Zagardo B, Aquino DA, Farooq M, Raine CS, Norton WT, Brosnan CF. Tumor necrosis factor-induced proliferation of astrocytes from mature brain is associated with down-regulation of glial fibrillary acidic protein mRNA. J Neurochem 57:823–830, 1991.

200. Selmaj KW, Farooq M, Norton WT, Raine CS, Brosnan CF. Proliferation of astrocytes in vitro in response to cytokines. A primary role for tumor necrosis factor. J Immunol 144:129–135, 1990.

201. Seregi A, Keller M, Hertting G. Are cerebral prostanoids of astroglial origin? Studies on the prostanoid forming system in developing rat brain and primary cultures of rat astrocytes. Brain Res 404:113–120, 1987.

202. Shank RP, Bennett GS, Freytag SO, Campbell GL. Pyruvate carboxylase: an astrocyte-specific enzyme implicated in the replenishment of amino acid neurotransmitter pools. Brain Res 329:364–367, 1986.

203. Shank RP, Campbell GL. α-ketoglutarate and malate uptake and metabolism by synaptosomes: further evidence for an astrocyte-to-neuron metabolic shuttle. J Neurochem 42:1153–1161, 1984.

204. Sima AAF, Finkelstein SD, McCachlan DR. Multiple malignant astrocytomas in patient with spontaneous progressive multifocal leukoencephalopathy. Ann Neurol 14:183, 1983.

205. Siman R, Card JP, Nelson RB, Davis LG. Expression of β-amyloid precursor protein in reactive astrocytes following neuronal damage. Neuron 3:275–285, 1989.

206. Simpson DL, Morrison R, De Vellis J, Herschman HR. Epidermal growth factor binding and mitogenic activity on purified populations of cells from the central nervous system. J Neurosci Res 8:453–462, 1982.

207. Smith GM, Miller RH, Silver J. Changing role of forebrain astrocytes during development, regenerative failure, and induced regeneration upon transplantation. J Comp Neurol 251:23–43, 1986.

208. Smith GM, Rutishauser U, Silver J, Miller RH. Maturation of astrocytes in vitro alters the extent and molecular basis of neurite outgrowth. Dev Biol 138:377–390, 1990.

209. Smith ME, Gibbs MA, Forno LS, Eng LF. [3H]Thymidine labeling of astrocytes in experimental autoimmune encephalomyelitis. J Neuroimmunol 15:309, 1987.

210. Smith ME, Somera FP, Eng LF. Immunocytochemical staining for glial fibrillary acidic protein and the metabolism of cytoskeletal proteins in experimental allergic encephalomyelitis. Brain Res 264:241–253, 1983.

211. Sobel RA, Mitchell ME, Fondren G. Intracellular adhesion molecule-1 (ICAM-1) in cellular immune reactions in the human central nervous system. Am J Pathol 136:1309–1316, 1990.

212. Somjen GG. Nervenkitt: Notes on the history of the concept of neuroglia. Glia 1:2–9, 1988.
213. Sonnewald U, Westergaard N, Krane J, Unsgard G, Petersen SB, Schousboe A. First direct demonstration of preferential release of citrate from astrocytes using [13C]NMR spectroscopy of cultured neurons and astrocytes. Neurosci Lett 128:235 239, 1991.
214. Sontheimer H, Black JA, Ransom BR, Waxman SG. Ion channels in spinal cord astrocytes in vitro. I. Transient expression of high levels of Na^+ and K^+ channels. J Neurophysiol 68:985–1000, 1992.
215. Stewart PA, Wiley MJ. Developing nervous tissue induces formation of blood-brain barrier characteristics in invading endothelial cells: a study using quail-chick transplantation chimeras. Dev Biol 84:183–192, 1981.
216. Stitt TN, Gasseer UE, Hatten ME. Molecular mechanisms of glial-guided neuronal migration. Ann NY Acad Sci 633:113–121, 1991.
217. Sugiyama KA, Brunori A, Mayer ML. Glial uptake of excitatory amino acids influences neuronal survival in cultures of mouse hippocampus. Neuroscience 32:779–791, 1989.
218. Sun D, Werkele H. Ia-restricted encephalitogenic T lymphocytes mediated EAE lyse autoantigen-presenting astrocytes. Nature 320:70–72, 1986.
219. Suzumura A, Lavi E, Weiss R. Coronavirus infection induces H-2 antigen expression on oligodendrocytes and astrocytes. Science 232:231–232, 1986.
220. Swanson RA, Choi DW. Glial glycogen stores affect neuronal survival during glucose deprivation in vitro. J Cereb Blood Flow Metab 13:162–169, 1993.
221. Takakura Y, Trammel AM, Kuentzel SL, Raub TJ, Davies A, Baldwin SA, Borchardt RT. Hexose uptake in primary cultures of bovine brain microvessel endothelial cells. II. Effects of conditioned media from astroglial and glioma cells. Biochim Biophys Acta 1070:11–19, 1991.
222. Tao-Cheng J-H, Nagy Z, Brightman MW. Tight junctions of brain endothelium are enhanced by astroglia. J Neurosci 7:3293–3299, 1987.
223. Tedeschi B, Barrett JN, Keane RW. Astrocytes produce interferon that enhances the expression of H-2 antigens on a subpopulation of brain cells. J Cell Biol 102:2244–2253, 1986.
224. Thery C, Stanley ER, Mallat M. Interleukin 1 and tumor necrosis factor-α stimulate the production of colony-stimulating factor 1 by murine astrocytes. J Neurochem 59:1183–1186, 1992.
225. Toru-Delbauffe D, Baghdassarian-Chalaye D, Gavaret JM, Courtin F, Pomerance M, Pierre M. Effects of transforming growth factor $\beta1$ on astroglial cells in culture. J Neurochem 54:1056–1061, 1990.
226. Toshniwal P, Tiku ML. Astrocytes can degrade myelin basic protein. Neurology 36:146–147, 1986.
227. Tower DB. A century of neuronal and neuroglial interactions, and their pathological implications: an overview. In: Neuronal-Astrocytic Interactions. Implications for Normal and Pathological CNS Function, ACH Yu, L Hertz, MD Norenberg, E Sykova, SG Waxman, eds. Elsevier, Amsterdam, 1992, pp 3–17.
228. Traugott U, Lebon P. Interferon-γ and Ia antigen are present on astrocytes in active chronic multiple sclerosis lesions. J Neurol Sci 84:257–264, 1988.
229. Traugott U, McFarlin DE, Raine CS. Experimental autoimmune encephalomyelitis (EAE) in the SJL mouse; evidence for local antigen presentation by endothelial cells and astrocytes. J Neuropathol Exp Neurol 45:354, 1986.
230. Traugott U, Scheinberg LC, Raine CS. On the presence of Ia-positive endothelial cells and astrocytes in multiple sclerosis lesions and its relevance to antigen presentation. J Neuroimmunol 8:1–14, 1985.
231. Trombetta LD, Toulon M, Jamall IS. Protective effects of glutathione on diethyldithiocarba-

mate (DDC) cytotoxicity: a possible mechanism. Toxicol Appl Pharmacol 93:154–164, 1988.

232. Tweardy DJ, Mott PL, Glazer EW. Monokine modulation of human astroglial cell production of granulocyte colony-stimulating factor and granulocyte-macrophage colony-stimulating factor. I. Effects of IL-1α and IL-β. J Immunol 144:2233–2241, 1990.

233. Vandenabeele P, Fiers W. Is amyloidogenesis during Alzheimer's disease due to an IL-1-/IL-6-mediated 'acute phase' in the brain? Immunol Today 12:217–219, 1991.

234. Vass K, Lassmann H. Intrathecal application of interferon gamma. Am J Pathol 137:789–800, 1990.

235. Vibulsreth S, Hefti F, Ginsberg MD, Dietrich WD, Busto R. Astrocytes protect cultured neurons from degeneration induced by anoxia. Brain Res 422:303–311, 1987.

236. Vidovic M, Sparacio SM, Elovitz M, Benveniste EN. Induction and regulation of class II major histocompatibility complex mRNA expression in astrocytes by interferon-γ and tumor necrosis factor-α. J Neuroimmunol 30:189–200, 1990.

237. Virchow R. Cellularpathologie in ihre Begründung auf Physiologische und Pathologische Gewebelehre, F Chance, trans. A. Hirschwald, Berlin, 1958.

238. Vitkovic L, Kalebic T, De Cunha A, Fauci S. Astrocyte-conditioned media stimulates HIV-1 expression in chronically infected promonocyte clone. J Neuroimmunol 30:153, 1990.

239. Vitkovic L, Wood GP, Major EO, Fauci AS. Human astrocytes stimulate HIV-1 expression in a chronically infected promonocyte clone via interleukin-6. AIDS Res Human Retroviruses 7:723–727, 1991.

240. Wahl SM, Allen JB, McCartney-Francis N, Morganti-Kossmann MC, Kossmann T, Ellingsworth L, Mai UE, Mergenhagen SE, Orenstein JM. Macrophage- and astrocyte-derived transforming growth factor beta as a mediator of central nervous system dysfunction in acquired immune deficiency syndrome. J Exp Med 173:981–991, 1991.

241. Walz W. Role of glial cells in the regulation of the brain ion microenvironment. Prog Neurobiol 33:309–333, 1989.

242. Walz W, Hertz L. Functional interactions between neurons and astrocytes. II. Potassium homeostasis at the cellular level. Prog Neurobiol 20:133–183, 1983.

243. Walz W, Mukerji S. Lactate production and release in cultured astrocytes. Neurosci Lett 86:296–300, 1988.

244. Waniewski RA, Martin DL, Shain W. Isoproterenol selectively releases endogenous and [14C]-labeled taurine from a single cytosolic compartment in astroglial cells. Glia 4:83–90, 1991.

245. Watabe K, Osborne D, Kim SU. Phagocytic activity of human adult astrocytes and oligodendrocytes in culture. J Neuropathol Exp Neurol 48:499–506, 1989.

246. Wiley CA, Schrier RD, Denaro FJ, Nelson JA, Lampert PW, Oldstone MB. Localization of cytomegalovirus proteins and genome during fulminant central nervous system infection in an AIDS patient. J Neuropathol Exp Neurol 45:127–139, 1986.

247. Wilkin GP, Marriott DR, Cholewinski AJ. Astrocyte heterogeneity. Trends Neurosci 13:43–46, 1990.

248. Wolff JR. The astrocyte as link between capillary and nerve cell. Triangle 9:153–164, 1970.

249. Wong GHW, Bartlett PF, Clark-Lewis I, Battye F, Schrader JW. Inducible expression of H-2 and Ia antigens on brain cells. Nature (Lond) 310:688–691, 1984.

250. Wong GHW, Bartlett PF, Clark-Lewis I, McKimm-Breschkin JL, Schrader JW. Interferon-γ induces the expression of H-2 and Ia antigens on brain cells. J Neuroimmunol 7:255, 1985.

251. Yong VW, Moumdjian R, Yong FP, Ruijs TCG, Freedman MS, Cashman N, Angel JP.

γ-interferon promotes proliferation of adult human astrocytes in vitro and reactive gliosis in the adult mouse brain in vivo. Proc Natl Acad Sci USA 88:7016–7020, 1991.

252. Yu ACH, Drejer J, Hertz L, Schousboe A. Pyruvate carboxylase activity in primary cultures of astrocytes and neurons. J Neurochem 41:1484–1487, 1983.

253. Yudkoff M, Pleasure D, Cregar L, Lin ZP, Nissim I, Stern J. Glutathione turnover in cultured astrocytes: studies with [15N]glutamate. J Neurochem 55:137–145, 1990.

254. Zuber P, Kuppner MC, De Tribolet N. Transforming factor-β2 downregulates HLA-DR antigen expression on human malignant glioma cells. Eur J Immunol 18:1623–1626, 1988.

7

Lymphocyte Entry and the Initiation of Inflammation in the Central Nervous System

WILLIAM F. HICKEY
HANS LASSMANN
ANNE H. CROSS

The human central nervous system (CNS) is susceptible to numerous inflammatory diseases including multiple sclerosis (MS), postinfectious encephalomyelitis, viral encephalitis, brain abscess, and others. All share a common feature in that the inflammation associated with them develops in an organ which exists in a relative state of immunological privilege (44,138,187,189). Investigation of the specific alterations occurring in the nervous system as it transforms from a site of relative immunological quietude to an inflammatory focus has been examined immunohistochemically, and key molecules active in the process have been defined by blocking their function with monoclonal antibodies in various in vivo or in vitro systems. However, as our knowledge of the process grows, the number of necessary participants and the intricacy of their interactions also increases.

Most studies of the mechanisms of CNS inflammation have been prompted by research on MS. This disease is believed by many investigators to involve an autoimmune attack on the brain and spinal cord initiated by CD4+ T cells specifically attacking some as of yet unidentified brain antigen (44,115,138,141,163,189). In MS research, the most widely studied animal model is experimental allergic encephalomyelitis (EAE) (3). EAE offers numerous advantages for investigators: it can be induced in a number of manipulable animal systems, and the CNS antigen being attacked has been defined to the peptide level in various rodent strains (3,87,99, 108,159,172,194). It is principally from this system that our knowledge of the specific molecular participants in the process of leukocyte entry into the nervous system parenchyma is derived. The following review will concentrate on findings relative to CNS inflammation as it progresses from the initial attachment of pathogenic leukocytes to the establishment of a defined focus of inflammation.

Types of CNS Inflammation

As noted above, leukocytes of hematogenous origin are exceptionally rare in a healthy mammalian CNS. However, they accumulate in the brain or spinal cord in response to a wide number of pathological conditions. But the type and quantity of inflammatory cells appearing in the CNS varies widely depending on the stimulus attracting them or their inherent ability to attack a CNS antigen. In areas of infarction, neutrophils appear within 12–24 hours and are themselves rapidly replaced by macrophages. In myraid bacterial infections, neutrophils and plasma cells produce either meningitis, or demarcate a zone of acute inflammation of the brain parenchyma destined to become an abscess. In tuberculous infections and the majority of acute viral encephalitides, T cells and macrophages predominate. Finally, there are a number of inflammatory CNS conditions wherein no overt tissue death or any known infectious agent is defined. Many of these conditions are believed to be autoimmune (e.g., multiple sclerosis (MS), postinfectious encephalomyelopathy); however, some are attributable to enzymatic defects (adrenoleukodystrophy) or neurodegenerative causes (amyotropic lateral sclerosis). While this is far from a complete list of conditions in which leukocytes are easily found in the normally privileged CNS, it serves to demonstrate the variety of stimuli that can induce such cells to enter. Yet all of these diseases require that leukocytes initially attach to specific adhesion molecules on CNS endothelial cells, thereby initiating their process of entry into the CNS from the circulation.

In conditions attracting neutrophils, including instances of substantial tissue death or the presence of bacteria or fungi, the blood-brain barrier (BBB) is often physically disrupted or microbial products and/or complement components attract leukocytes. In addition, changes in the CNS endothelial cells are more conducive to granulocyte attachment. Such situations are not unique to the CNS, and appear to follow the stereotypic process of the evolution of acute inflammation observed in any bodily site. In other CNS diseases such as viral infections, T cells must identify and localize the viral antigen for which they are specific in the CNS parenchyma. In these immune responses there is a foreign pathogen which is the target of the attack. T-cell mediated inflammation, as occurs in MS, postinfectious encephalomyelitis, or EAE, however, appears to be a distinct process. In such conditions there is no devitalized tissue nor microbial antigen to attack. It is the latter CNS T-cell mediated disorders which have been subjected to close scrutiny during the past decade.

General Concepts of Leukocyte Circulation

The circulation of lymphocytes through various tissues of the body had its origin decades ago in the seminal work of Gowans and Knight (63,64). These scientists established that small, nonactivated lymphocytes continually recirculated from the bloodstream into lymphoid tissues and then back to the blood via the lymph. Although such recirculation is known to play a critical role in immunological surveillance, it has required many years for the mechanisms underlying lymphocyte recirculation to begin to be elucidated.

The concept of *lymphocyte homing* was developed with the demonstration of non-random trafficking and binding of certain subsets of lymphocytes to certain lymphoid tissues. As a general rule, naive T cells were observed to migrate into lymph nodes, while memory cells preferred to enter nonlymphoid tissues at sites of their prior stimulation (102). Inflammation in an organ will itself enhance the cellular migration into that tissue and decrease the selectivity of the homing process (79). Lymphocyte homing as a physiological process is fully supported by studies demonstrating that small, recirculating lymphocytes preferentially returned to the lymphoid organ from which they were isolated (17,26). These cells would attach to the high endothelial venules (HEVs) in those organs via molecules which have subsequently been identified and characterized (15,16). It is well known that HEV-like endothelial changes occur at sites of chronic inflammation, as in granulomas, supporting the concept that the endothelial activation state is critical in establishing and maintaining leukocyte traffic through an inflammatory focus.

Early on it was noted that lymphoblasts recirculated differently than did small lymphocytes (68), which suggested that they localized selectively in celiac lymph nodes (17,26,88). In addition, differential patterns of migration have been ascribed to CD4+ vs. CD8+ lymphocytes (88). But how do lymphocytes find their antigen in the CNS?

Hematogenous cells typically have no interaction with the endothelium of parenchymal organs. At a glance, the passage of the cellular elements of the immune system through the body appears to be a random phenomenon. Yet it is now documented that leukocytes actually follow specific migratory rules that are dictated by the developmental and activation state of the circulating cell and the vascular bed through which the cell must pass (69,102). The migration of various types of leukocytes across an endothelium has been extensively characterized over the past decade (for reviews see 8,22,66,162). When interaction, binding, and transendothelial migration occur, they are extensively controlled by cell-surface glycoproteins called *adhesion molecules*. The interaction of lymphocytes and monocyte/macrophages with the endothelium, and ultimately the extravasation of the cell from the blood vessels into a target organ, are thought to occur in 3 general steps: (1) loose interaction with the endothelium, (2) firm binding to the endothelial cell, and (3) emigration from the vascular lumen and penetration of and crossing endothelial basement membrane (15,96,113,156,158). This is a carefully orchestrated process. Adhesion molecules expressed on the lymphocyte and the endothelial cells are important in this process where distinct phases of leukocyte slowing, adhesion, and emigration have been attributed to specific families of molecules. It is important to note at this point that, to date, no molecules have been identified that attract specific cells of any leukocyte group to enter the nervous system. While it remains possible that such CNS specific homing receptors or molecular addressins will be defined, our current understanding of the process indicates that the nervous system makes use of the same groups of adhesion molecules that function on leukocytes and activated endothelial cells (e.g., high endothelial venules in lymphoid organs) elsewhere in the body.

The interaction of lymphocytes with the vessel walls is orchestrated by molecules belonging to three broad classes which include *(1)* selectins (8,9,96,113), *(2)* integrins (77), and *(3)* molecules belonging to the immunoglobulin supergene family (161). The mechanism of leukocyte attachment and movement out of a vessel has been the subject of a number of reviews (15,161,162,166).

The initial step in extravasation of a lymphocyte from the vessel into the CNS parenchyma involves a slowing of the lymphocyte via rapidly made and broken interactions involving specific lectin-like molecules expressed on the endothelial cell (for a review of animal lectins see 133). When emigration is to occur, leukocytes initially make loose contact with the vascular wall via C-type lectins, or *selectin* molecules, which produce a rolling motion along the vessel wall (113). The most important members of this group of molecules are L-selectin (a.k.a., LAM-1, LECCAM-1, MEL-14), E-selectin (ELAM-1), and P-selectin (CD62), the genes for which are all tightly clustered on human chromosome 1 (8,9,69). E-selectin seems to be involved in both neutrophil and CD4$^+$ T cell adhesion; L-selectin seem to be more specifically related to T-cell homing to lymph nodes (69). Endothelial selectins can be rapidly induced; P-selectin appears within minutes, and E-selectin appears in a few hours following cytokine exposure or injury (66,69,113). The transient interaction between leukocytes and endothelial cells producing the phenomenon of leukocyte rolling along the endothelium is dictated in part by E- and P-selectins (9,15,69,93,158). However, since some circulating activated leukocytes can interact with endothelial cells that have not themselves been activated, it is probable that some lectin-like molecules are constitutively expressed and may be critical in the early phases of leukocyte passage into a noninflammed organ that does no have HEV-like endothelium.

As adhesion progresses, the leukocyte slows and sticks to the endothelial cell in a process mediated by a diverse collection of adhesion molecules, including PECAM-1, vascular cell adhesion molecule-1 (VCAM-1), very late antigen-4 (VLA-4), lymphocyte function-associated antigen-1, (LFA-1), Mac-1, and the intracellular adhesion molecules (ICAMs) (16,22,62,165). The firm adhesion of the lymphocyte to the endothelial cell predominantly involves members of the integrin and immunoglobulin (Ig)-supergene family groups of molecules (12,69,158). Composed of one α- and one β-chain, integrins are transmembrane heterodimers which can be grouped into three major classes based on the commonality of a single, unique β-chain defining each group. The VLA antigens expressed on activated and memory T cells share a common β-1 chain that has binding sites for the basement membrane components fibronectin and laminin (168). Thus, such integrins may be intimately related to the ability of a cell to migrate out of a vessel. Integrins like LFA-1 (CD11a) and Mac-1 (CD11b) share a common β2 chain (CD18). Both of these molecules have been reported to change their avidity for substrate binding when the cell on which they are expressed becomes activated (18,41), again suggesting a possible mechanism by which activation may alter cell migration capabilities.

Members of the Ig supergene family are extremely heterogeneous. This group includes such diverse elements as T-cell receptors, major histocompatibility complex (MHC) molecules, neural cell adhesion molecules (NCAMs), myelin-associated glycoprotein (MAG), the ICAMs, VCAM, and LFA-2 and -3. ICAM-1 appears to be constitutively expressed in the CNS on perivascular cells and some astrocytes, and it is readily up-regulated on endothelial cells and astrocytes in areas of experimental CNS inflammation (19,94,124,143). Likewise, ICAM-1 is detected in human brain during inflammation of various forms (160). ICAM-1 can be rapidly induced by lipopolysaccharide (LPS) or tumor necrosis factor alpha (TNF-α), and to a lesser extent by interferon gamma (IFN-γ) and interleukin-1 (IL-1) (190). Most interestingly, when CNS endothelial ICAM-1 molecules are bound by a specific antibody or by interaction with activated T cells, a transmembrane signal inducing tyrosine phosphorylation is generated in the endothelial cell, which in turn induces cytoskeletal alterations that may produce morphological changes and/or facilitate transendothelial migration of hematogenous cells (40). Less is known about other members of this group in the normal or inflamed CNS (21,95,143); however, VCAM-1 seems not to be constitutively expressed, although it probably can be rapidly induced, since it functions in experimental inflammation (6).

The question persists regarding the possible existence of a nervous system-specific addressin. *Addressins* are complex glycoproteins in the 58–80kD range which are expressed on the vascular surface of specific endothelial cells believed to confer homing properties to the sites in which they are expressed for specific subsets of lymphocytes. Addressins are currently defined by specific antibodies that react with them and block their function. The MECA-79 antigen is apparently a receptor-guiding lymphocyte homing to peripheral lymph nodes, while MECA-367 and MECA-89 direct traffic to mucosal lymph nodes (38,88). While none of these are present on normal CNS endothelial cells, they are detectable when the tissue becomes inflamed (19–21,95,124).

Once firmly attached, the cell passes through the endothelial cell, degrades the basement membrane focally, and enters the parenchyma. These later steps are not as completely defined as is the attachment phase, but they involve elaboration of appropriate basement membrane-degrading enzymes and vectorial movement out of the vessel lumen (78,120,158). The role of basement membrane-degrading enzymes might prove critical; administration of exogenous sulphated polysaccharides has proven effective in blocking the development of EAE, possibly by preventing T-cell access to the CNS by competitive inhibition of these enzymes (186).

It should be noted that these numerous analyses of the interaction of lymphocytes and monocyte/macrophages with vessel walls have been performed under a variety of in vitro and in vivo experimental settings. Such studies have used differing cell populations binding to endothelium, with different sources of endothelial cells, and under variable conditions relative to fluid movement. The available data, therefore, demonstrate a wide variation of critical molecules both for the slowing and rolling of cells on vessels and for the adhesion to vessels walls, depending upon the system studied (65,129,157). In addition to defining critical molecules for slowing, binding, and the extravasation of cells into target tissues, recent evidence also suggests that the interaction and/or mutual ligation of these adhesion molecules may initiate signal transduction by lymphocytes and endothelial cells augmenting or perpetuating their activation (77,142).

CNS Endothelial Cells

Normally, the CNS endothelium expresses low or nondetectable levels of adhesion molecules (93,94,143,158). CNS expression of adhesion molecules on the endothelium is tightly regulated (20,21,36,93,94,104). Yet in CNS inflammation, they are widely expressed and easily detected (20,21,36,90,94,106). Exposure of the endothelium to cytokines, such as IFN-γ, TNF-α, and to some extent, granulocyte-macrophage colony-stimulating factor (GM-CSF), produced by T cells and macrophages in a developing inflammatory focus, rapidly induces endothelial adhesion molecules (37,44,104, 90,94,106,112,124). Among these cytokines it appears that TNF-α plays a particularly critical role in adhesion molecule induction (103,105,111).

As noted above, activation of an endothelium results in its transformation into an HEV-like vessel. This also occurs in the CNS. At sites of inflammation in the brain, vessels with the phenotypic, molecular, and functional characteristics of HEVs have been described (20,31,32). Ultrastructurally, they are rich in organelles and often have finger-like extensions on their luminal surface not seen in resting CNS endothelia (31). It is now recognized that these activated endothelial cells play an active role in inflammatory cell adhesion (21,32,90,94,143). Activation of the endothelium can result in the expression de novo of adhesion molecules, or, alternatively, it can change the relative amount of specific adhesion molecules on the endothelial cell membrane. There is also the possibility that endothelial cell adhesion molecules may change their avidity for certain ligands without changing their relative molecular density. This latter mechanism has been demonstrated for a number of adhesion molecules of the integrin group on leukocytes (18,41); the same could also pertain to endothelial cell integrins and perhaps other molecules.

Lymphocytes do not adhere to normal, CNS-derived endothelial cells as they do to endothelia derived from most other bodily sites (104–106). Exposure of these CNS cells to cytokines like TNF-α or IFN-γ transforms them and they can readily participate in lymphocyte adhesion (104,106,135). Alternatively, activation of the lymphocytes permits them to bind to the normal CNS endothelial cells (104,135).

There has not been an extensive analysis of all known adhesion molecules relative to their presence on normal CNS endothelial cells in vivo as compared to the same type of cells in inflammatory conditions. Table 7-1 lists the adhesion molecules that CNS endothelial cells appear to have the ability to express. Favaloro (46) has performed an extensive analysis of the endothelial cell surface molecules that can be augmented or induced by exposure to thrombin, IFN-γ, and/or TNF-α. It appears that CNS endothelial cells, based on the limited data available, possess the ability to express any and all adhesion and activation-related antigens expressed by endothelial cells elsewhere in the body.

Encephalitogenic Cells

Interest in the questions surrounding lymphocyte entry into the CNS began when Gonatas and Howard demonstrated that EAE, the most widely used animal model of multiple sclerosis, was a T-cell mediated disorder (62). In both rats and mice, the pathogenic cell in EAE is the TH1 type of T lymphocyte (25,89,114,115). These T cells secrete IFN-γ, IL-2, and some TNF-α when stimulated (1,116). Moreover, such activation is required in order for the T cells to be rendered pathogenic (72,75,126,138,187). However, it is notable that not all T cells specific for CNS antigens cause clinical EAE; encephalitogenic ability appears to vary with the mouse strain from which the T cells are derived, the T-cell receptor (TcR) genes used, the cytokines produced, and the antigenic epitope for which the T cell's receptor is specific (2,10,14,27,61,123,134, 167,182,194). Thus, a constellation of parameters relative to the T cell must be correct if it is to be pathogenic in the CNS. But first the T cell must get to the target organ and recognize its antigen therein. Questions which have persisted that are relative to this

Table 7-1 Adhesion Molecules that are Enhanced or Expressed De Novo When CNS Endothelial Cells are Activated

CD54 (ICAM-1)	ICAM-2	LFA-3
CD44	CD49a/CD29 (VLA-1)	CD9
VCAM-1	HECA 452	CD31 (PECAM-1)
CD62 (P-selectin)	MECA 352	
MALA 2		
ELAM-1 (E-selectin)		

process are: Is T-cell entry into the CNS an antigen-specific process? Does lymphocyte accumulation in the CNS in conditions like EAE or MS reflect specific homing of T cells vs. specific retention of T cells?

T Lymphocytes in the CNS

Although T lymphocytes are seldom detected in the normal CNS, these cells do appear during the course of CNS inflammation in multiple sclerosis, experimental allergic encephalomyelitis, HIV-induced encephalomyelitis in humans, and simian immunodeficiency virus (SIV) infection of the CNS (71,72,92,93,127,148,151,174,183). An important question with regard to lymphocyte traffic into the CNS of diseased vs. non-diseased animals has to do with the characteristics mediating such lymphocyte entry.

Observations from the EAE model were critical in determining parameters of T-cell infiltration into the CNS. A quarter of a century ago, Werdelin and Mccluskey demonstrated that labeled, myelin antigen-specific cells localized in the CNS (185). It must be noted, however, that this study utilized as the target for homing a CNS that contained blood-brain barrier disruptions produced by various types of experimental lesions. These early studies have been subsequently confirmed and expanded by a number of investigators (30,121,171). Interestingly, all of these investigations that used radio-labeled T cells demonstrated that they not only were found in the CNS but that they were distributed widely through the body without apparent selectivity (121,171). It is important to note, however, that the pattern of distribution of activated T cells through the body is not totally independent of their antigen specificity. Cross and co-workers found that T cells specific for a myelin antigen were detectable in the CNS 24–48 hours prior to the appearance of EAE and were collected in a perivascular location (30). In contrast, cells specific for a non-self antigen, while finding their way to the CNS in lower numbers, appeared there later and were more randomly distributed through the CNS parenchyma. All the above reports have demonstrated the ability of encephalitogenic cells to localize in the CNS. But was this localization the result of selective homing or evidence of selective retention?

Over the years, numerous researchers have utilized lymph node cells from animals immunized with myelin antigens that were adoptively transferred into naive animals to produce EAE (75). One of the key observations derived from such work was that EAE would develop in animals receiving T cells only if the lymph node cells were activated prior to their injection. Activation of the cells could be achieved either by stimulation with the antigen for which the T cells were specific, or by activation via nonspecific mitogenic lectins such as phytohemagglutinin (PHA) or concanavalin-A (72,75,126, 169,184). These observations provided experimental support for a hypothesis put forth by Wekerle and collaborators that T lymphocytes in the blast stage (T lymphoblasts) could gain access into the CNS, while their resting counterparts could not (184).

In vivo studies have now shown that while T cells readily gain entry into the CNS and other organs, the entry is independent of the cell's antigen specificity, MHC restriction requirements, or the location of the antigen for which the T cell is specific (72). T cells in blast phase can be detected in the CNS within a few hours of entering the systemic circulation. While the appearance of lymphocytes in various organs seemed nonspecific and rapid following introduction of cells into the animal, if the T cells enter a target organ where their antigen is located, then the cells remain and begin the process of tissue inflammation (71,72). Whether a lymphocyte remains in the central nervous system to initiate inflammation, or exits, and/or undergoes apoptosis without inducing pathological CNS alterations, seems largely dependent upon whether that cell recognizes its antigen. While the outcome of a T cell remaining in a target organ is most likely directly related to its antigen specificity, the extravasation of the cell through the blood vessel wall into the CNS is almost certainly not antigen related. Endothelial cells permit lymphocyte transmigration into the neural parenchyma even when they are MHC incompatible with the T cell and thus unable to participate in the T cell's recognition of antigen (73,74). It appears that the most important feature in this process is the T cell's activation state, thus focusing attention on activation-related adhesion molecules. But which molecules(s) on the activated T cell mediate this transendothelial passage? Table 7-2 presents a list of the cell-surface molecules that are known to change on T cells following the cell's activation. It remains to be defined which one or combination of these molecules (assuming the critical elements have even been defined) mediate the attachment and migration of activated T cells across a resting or newly activated endothelial cell.

Having once been activated seems to induce profound and lasting changes in T cells that significantly affect their traffic through tissues. Leukocyte common antigen-(CD45) exists on hematogenous cells in many forms resulting from alternative splicing of the multiple exons contained within the gene (170). CD45R expression is charac-teristic of naive T cells; however, this molecule is rapidly down-regulated or shed

Table 7-2 Cell-Surface Antigens Changing in Concentration on the Surface of T Cells Following Activation[a]

CD2	CD3	CD4
CD5	CD6	CD8
CD28	CD31 (PECAM-1)	CD43
CD44	CD45	CD54 (ICAM-1)
VLA-4 (CD49d/CD29)	LFA-1 (CD11a/18)	LFA-2
gp39 (CD40 ligand)	ICAM-3	MHC-II (human and rat)
L-selectin	IL-2R	*fas*-ligand

[a]This is a list of the molecules currently known to alter in quantity on the T-cell membrane with stimulation. All of these have possible adhesive activities which alone or in combination could determine the adhesive-ness of a given cell for a particular vascular endothelium.

following T-cell activation, resulting in a cell with a CD45R$^-$ (CD45R0) phenotype. While a stimulated T cell will remain in the blast phase for a number of days, its CD45R0 state persists indefinitely. It has been noted that CD45R0 T cells predominate in sites of inflammation and are also the predominant T cell phenotype in MS plaques, viral encephalitis, and glioma infiltrating lymphocytes (91,128). Such "memory" cells are also known to accumulate in the lesions of EAE in experimental animals (81). It is possible that as a group, CD45R0 T cells may be more responsive to chemokine attraction, as demonstrated for CD4+ cells in a chemotaxis assay in response to the RANTES cytokine (150). Such a heightened sensitivity to subtle, attractive signals may contribute to the preferential accumulation of memory-type cells in inflammatory infiltrates, including those in the CNS.

One can envision a scenario wherein activated, cytokine-secreting T cells can pass across the CNS endothelium, resulting in endothelial cell activation. Conversely, the activation of brain endothelial cells as a result of a local CNS event including brain injury or viral infection, might also result in the expression of adhesion molecules attractive to T lymphocytes or other leukocyte classes. It seems certain that there remain to be identified other T-cell activation molecules and endothelial ligands which are important to the passage of lymphocytes into the CNS. Such critical molecules might be expected to be up-regulated on activated T cells in conditions known to permit and facilitate the traffic of these cells into the CNS. The activation-related adhesion molecule(s) responsible for the initial entry of an activated T-cell into a normal parenchymal organ would have its counter ligand molecule constitutively expressed on resting endothelial cells, including those of the CNS. In contrast to this, a number of molecules previously demonstrated on high endothelial venules, including MECA-325 and VCAM-1, have been shown to only appear in the CNS during inflammation and are considered key molecules in transendothelial cell migration (19). The expression of some of these molecules has also been noted in the CNS following HIV and SIV infection (94,143,148,149,160). They may play a critical role in attracting circulating cells to localize to that site.

Adhesion molecule pairs expressed on activated T cells and endothelium include LFA-1/ICAM-1 and VLA-4/VCAM-1. It is known that activated T cells expressing the LFA-1 molecule can bind ICAM-1 on activated endothelium (178). This interaction, gross injury, or cytokine stimulation can lead to the up-regulation of VCAM-1 on the endothelial cells. Activated T cells express the integrin VLA-4, which allows attachment to VCAM-1 on the endothelial cells facilitating the entry of the T cells into the CNS (6). Lending support to this argument is the observation that a high level of VLA-4 is expressed on activated and memory T-cell lines that can induce EAE (6,193). These data may partially explain the inability of naive T cells to enter into the CNS, based upon low VLA-4 expression.

In vivo studies of EAE in rodents, in which antibodies against cell-surface adhesion molecules expressed on either T cells or endothelial cells were administered to block disease development, have added further evidence of their importance. Yednock, et al., (193) using an antibody against the $\alpha4\beta1$ (VLA-4) integrin, were able to inhibit inflammation and clinical signs in rat EAE following the injection of encephalitogenic T cells. Baron and colleagues confirmed and expanded this observation by inhibiting EAE development in the mouse (6). Archelos and associates have demonstrated the inhibition of EAE using antibodies against ICAM-1 (4). While these studies support the notion that the disease process is blocked by stopping the entry of encephalitogenic T cells, it is not clear whether the antibodies actually function to block initial cell entry into a normal CNS parenchyma, or if they inhibit the recruitment of additional hematogenous cells to a developing inflammatory site. The latter may be the case.

In Yednock's study, a single dose of anti-VLA-4 antibody administered 2 days following T-cell injection (i.e., long after the initial T cells would have been expected to have reached the target organ) resulted in inhibition of clinical signs and inflammation in EAE (193). Also, VCAM-1, required for interaction with VLA-4 on T lymphoblasts, is not expressed on normal CNS endothelial cells; it must be induced. Likewise, ICAMs are not uniformly or constitutively present on CNS endothelial cells. It should be noted that the expression of such molecules on CNS endothelial cells can be rapidly induced following incubation with cytokines including TNF and IL-1 (104,105). Cells inducing EAE secrete TNF-α and IFN-γ. TNF and IL-1 have been demonstrated in the CSF of HIV-infected individuals (173).

The initial, rapid entry of T cells into the CNS, occurring within hours after T-lymphoblast infusion into the blood, is not blocked by either anti-VLA-4 or anti-ICAM-1 antibodies (Hickey and Yednock, unpublished observations). Thus it is possible that molecules like VCAM, ICAM, and VLA-4 play a more prominent role in the recruitment phase of EAE, during which macrophages and other T cells are recruited to the developing site of inflammation.

These observations underscore the importance of lymphocyte recruitment in the EAE model for induction of the disease. However, the adhesion molecule(s) required for initial T-cell penetration remain undefined. It is possible that poorly defined or unknown adhesion molecules may be critical for some types of T cell–endothelial cell interaction, especially those occurring in the CNS which permit EAE to develop. One recently identified, apparently unique molecule (termed *4A2*) may play a role in such a process (48,105) since blockage of this molecule with monoclonal antibodies likewise inhibits EAE development. Yet, until this and other such new antigens are more completely characterized, it is impossible to delineate the roles they might play in the development of inflammation.

B Lymphocytes in the CNS

In numerous infectious and immune-mediated processes, even those occurring in the CNS, B cells and plasma cells can frequently be demonstrated. Similar to T lymphocytes, B cells appear to have no difficulty gaining entry into different target organs.

This may also be dependent upon the activation state of the B cell, with the cell remaining in a specific site to differentiate into a plasma cell if the antigen for which it is specific is found. Interestingly, it seems that B cells are able to do this following the initial interaction of T cells with the CNS endothelium (67). Griffin et al. (67) studied the kinetics of B-cell traffic into the CNS in response to Sindbis infection and showed that the B cell entered following other cells, including TcRα/β+, CD4, and CD8 T cells and natural killer (NK) cells. One wonders if, in this viral system, the B cell is dependent upon the T cell to interact with the CNS endothelium, consequently resulting in endothelial cell activation and induction of adhesion molecules. Similar to the situation with T lymphocytes, it seems that activation of the B cell is also important for entry into organs. Activated, but not resting, B cells, can readily bind to endothelial cells via E- and P-selectins (130).

Little is known about the migratory requirements of B cells; however, it is believed that in their fully mature form, as plasma cells, their migratory potential is severely limited or absent. Recent studies of B-cell activation noted that B cells, similar to T cells, undergo a pattern of activation that results in the expression of molecules that allows the cell to bind to endothelial cells and enter into a target organ (130–132,148). Activated B cells can bind to endothelial surfaces using E- and P-selectins which can interact with CD57, CD65, and the Lewis^x and sialyl-Lewis^x antigens on the B lymphocyte. While it is an attractive hypothesis, it remains to be demonstrated that B cell–binding endothelial ligands are induced by prior T-cell antigen recognition in the region, thereby marking the path for activated B cells to follow.

Studies using rats immunized with a foreign, nonpathogenic antigen have shown that B cells and plasma cells, specific for that antigen, are found in the CNS following the placement of the antigen behind the BBB (86). These data suggest that the question of whether a B cell remains in the CNS after it has entered is partially dependent upon that cell finding its antigen. It is interesting to note in the Sindbis encephalitis model that there is a continued secretion of Ig long after the active disease has been resolved (174–176). The consequence of elevated intrathecal Ig synthesis in the CNS during viral encephalitis, MS, and EAE is not understood. It is possible that these intrathecally produced antibodies bespeak a continued pattern of B-cell entry and persistence in the CNS provoked by a low-level, continuous antigenic stimulus. So it would seem that entry of B cells into the CNS during the course of a viral infection or autoimmune event is due in part to the activation state of the cell, but similar to the T lymphocyte, the antigen specificity of the B cell or plasma cell also plays a role in determining if the B cell will remain in the CNS compartment.

Antigen-Presenting Cells (APCs)

After leukocyte entry, the next step for T cells (and possibly B cells) in the production of inflammation is the recognition of their antigen. The cells of the CNS that might serve as APCs for T cells remains an area of contention (71), and is extensively reviewed in Chapter 10. Although cogent arguments for the roles of astrocytes or endothelial cells as APCs can be formulated, it is currently felt that CNS resident members of the macrophage/monocyte family, i.e., microglia and perivascular cells, are the most important APCs in CNS inflammatory conditions. In vitro specific subsets of these CNS-resident monocytic cells serve as facile APCs, and when freshly isolated from the adult CNS, they also serve such a function (50). They express costimulatory molecules in vitro and in vivo, and can elaborate the cytokines appropriate for APC function (24,58,97,188,191,192). Perivascular cells are potentially phagocytic and can ingest and process antigen (73,85,154). Moreover, perivascular cells have been demonstrated in vivo to fill the role of APCs (73). In view of these facts and of their optimal location in the perivascular space, where they would be among the first cells to encounter the entering T cells, there is great reason to believe that they serve as the critical APC of the CNS during the initial development of inflammation.

Costimulatory Molecules

Few areas in cellular immunology have grown so rapidly in the 1990s as has research into costimulatory molecules. Numerous reviews of this area have appeared recently (34,35,80,83,89,117,153,164,188). As a group, costimulatory molecules are highly heterogeneous but have as their common denominator the ability to transduce a necessary activating signal between an antigen-specific cell and an antigen-presenting cell. However, the intercellular interaction of such molecules on cells' surfaces does not itself involve participation of the stimulating antigen. Failure of the costimulatory molecules to be engaged results in failure of stimulation, anergy, lack of cytokine production, or apoptotic death of the antigen-specific cell that did not get the co-stimulatory signal (117,152,153). While certain defined adhesion molecules and their ligands have some costimulatory functions (e.g., VLA-4/VCAM-1 [33], ICAM-1,2/LFA-1 [34,179]), it is the B7/CD28 (54,89,100) and gp39/CD40 (39,56,145) interactions which have received the most attention. The signaling between B7.1 or B7.2 on APCs and CD28 on the surface of T cells seems to be a critical part of the T cell's activation. This signal leads to IL-2 production in particular, but also induces IFN-γ, TNFα/β and GM-CSF secretion, T-cell proliferation (39,53,56), and blockage of both apoptosis and anergy (11,35,52,80,101,117,164,180). But the expression of the B7 molecules by T cells is dependent on interaction with an APC (53,54,98). Moreover, whether the T cell interacts with B7.1 vs. B7.2 during the T-cell/APC encounter may affect whether the cell becomes a Th1 vs. a Th2 type of lymphocyte (29,89,98).

The ligand for CD40, called *gp39*, is critical in the signaling between T cells and B cells, which is believed to be a Th2 type of function (39,51,145); at present its function in the appropriate activation of the Th1 type of cells known to produce EAE remains to be elucidated. It is possible that there exist other, important costimulatory molecules which remain to be identified. A novel human molecule called *4F2* (CD98) may belong to this group (55). The area of costimulatory molecule expression and function may be especially germane to neuroimmunology since antibody blockade of either B7 or gp39 inhibits the development of EAE (56,89).

Cytokines

Cytokines are soluble or cell-bound proteins which permit intercellular signaling between leukocytes or to and from parenchymal cells (23,44,125). Research into CNS inflammation has made it abundantly clear that cytokines form an important, overlapping, and intricately woven pattern for initiating and controlling immune responses in the neural parenchyma. (This topic is reviewed in Chapter 11). *Proinflammatory* cytokines such as IL-1α/β, TNF-α, IFN-γ, IL-2 and IL-6 foster the appearance and progression of inflammation, while anti-inflammatory cytokines such as IL10 and the TGFβs dampen or prevent it (7,23,114,125,147,155).

The Th1 type of T cells initiating EAE make IL-2, IFN-γ, and TNF-α (1,116); the latter two of these have potent effects on endothelial and parenchymal activation, inducing expression of MHC, costimulatory, and adhesion molecules (as above). The arrival in the CNS of activated T cells is most probably where cytokine involvement with the inflammatory cascade beings. When exposed to the products of activated T cells, microglia and perivascular cells (as a result of both exposure to T-cell derived cytokines and the act of presenting antigen to T cells) produce IL-1 and IL-6 (43). IL-1 has numerous potent proinflammatory properties among which are the ability to induce endothelial adhesion molecule expression, activate glial cells, and produce defects in the blood-brain barrier (28,37,45,97,104,106,136). IFN-γ has been long known to enhance APC function, up-regulate MHC molecule expression, and induce the expression of some adhesion molecules (95,105,138). The role of IL-6 in the establishment of CNS inflammation is more obscure, although it has been noted to be elevated during the process of EAE development in rodents (57).

TFN-α, secreted by both T cells and activated macrophages (59,97,116), appears to play a pivotal role in CNS inflammation (reviewed in 139). It also activates glial cells (59) and enhances expression of vascular adhesion molecules (as above). Anti-myelin Th1 cells must produce it in order to be encephalitogenic (134), and antibodies to TNF-α have been shown to block EAE development (110,146), thus demonstrating its central role.

In counterpoint to the proinflammatory cytokines, some cytokines appear to impede inflammation. For example, members of the TGF-β family can counteract the effects of TNF-α (147). TGF-β inhibits the secretion of many inflammatory cytokines (42,119), and its administration blocks EAE (82,137). Likewise, IL-10 administration can block EAE (144) and decrease the production of proinflammatory cytokines (47,107). Also of interest are the observations that TGF-β and IL-10 can diminish the production of nitric oxide (122,181). As can be appreciated, the interplay and balance between the known cytokines has dramatic effects on the appearance, persistence, and resolution of inflammation. It must be noted, however, that our assumptions relating the pathogenic nature of Th1 cells and the cytokines they produce to the actual production of clinical disease are based upon EAE and similar models. It remains possible that other systems wherein Th2 cells are pathogenic in the CNS will be defined.

Chemokines

Among the cytokines important to CNS inflammation are chemokines, *(chemo*attractive cyto*kines)* the role of which is just beginning to be elucidated (reviewed in 5,49,118,180). These substances are small, proinflammatory proteins, the synthesis and secretion of which can be induced in many cell types by TNF-α, IL-1 and IFN-γ (13,109,177). Chemokines produce their effects by binding to G-protein-coupled receptors on their target cells, resulting in migration toward or retention at the site of secretion (13,70,118). In the CNS, both stimulated microglial and astrocytic cells are capable of making such cytokines (140,177). The superfamily of chemokines is usually subdivided into three classes based on the location and spacing of cystine residues in the protein: *(1)* the C-X-C group includes IL-8, platelet factor 4, and interferon-V-inducible protein (IP)-10, all of which are chemoattractive for neutrophils and to some extent for monocytes; *(2)* the C-C group contains monocyte chemoattractant protein (MCP)-1a/b, macrophage inhibitory protein (MIP)-1, and regulated on activation normal T-cell expressed and secreted (RANTES) which attract T cells and monocytes; and *(3)* the C chemokines represented by lymphotactin, which influences lymphocyte traffic. MIP-1, RANTES, and MCP-1— all members of the C-C group, which attracts monocytes and T cells (and especially activated T cells)—can be detected in both rat and mouse EAE lesions (60,76). In some cases they appear even before the animal becomes ill (60). Their potential importance is underscored by studies showing that antibodies which block MCP-1 or MIP-1a inhibit clinical EAE development (84,90). There seems to be little question that they, and perhaps other members of this class of cytokines, will prove to be critically important in understanding CNS inflammation.

Conclusions

Multiple enigmas persist related to the ability to inflammatory cells to enter the CNS when needed (and unfortunately, at some less opportune times). This puzzle is somewhat less formidable if some event has occurred which would activate or induce adhesion molecule expression on the endothelium. Tissue necrosis or LPS production by some infectious agent can induce such changes. In such conditions, the endothelial cell can become HEV-like to some extent, and data exist providing clues as to the mechanisms active in attachment and migration.

The most difficult questions relate to how immunological surveillance of the CNS is achieved. This is probably the most common, almost routine, process in which the CNS participates relative to the immune system. When an individual mounts an immune response against an environmental microorganism or pathogen, it seems the T and B cells stimulated to respond to the antigen enter the CNS with alacrity. This must be a very frequent occurrence, if not a continuously ongoing process. Based upon data from the EAE system, disease occurs only if their specific antigen is localized within the brain. What molecules and cytokines and/or chemokines govern this process? There is apparently no requirement for CNS activation or endothelial changes to precede the initial event. Activated lymphocytes seem empowered in themselves to penetrate the endothelia.

It is possible, if not probable, that a number of key molecular participants in this process remain to be defined. While a specific nervous system addressin may yet be identified, it may also be the case that a common set of rules pertains to all activated cells relative to all vascular beds in all organs. Current evidence does not permit one to clearly decide where along this continuum the truth lies. In view of this dilemma, there is a continuing need for investigation to define what specific types of hematogenous cells require which adhesion molecules (or combination of adhesion molecules) to transverse the BBB. Moreover, these requirements must be defined for the various possible combinations of endothelial cells and leukocytes in both the resting and activated states. At this time, such a matrix is very incomplete.

References

1. Abbas AK, Williams ME, Burstein HJ, Chang TL, Bossu P, Lichtman AH. Activation and functions of CD4 T cell subsets. Immunol Rev 123:6–22, 1991.
2. Acha-Orbea H, Steinman L, McDevitt HO. T cell receptors in autoimmune diseases. Annu Rev Immunol 7:371–405, 1989.
3. Alvord EA Jr, Kies M, Suckling A. Experimental Allergic Encephalomyelitis: A Useful Model for Multiple Sclerosis. Alan R Liss, New York, 1984.
4. Archelos JJ, Jung S, Maurer M, Schmied M, Lassmann H, Tamatani T, Miyaska M, Toyka KV, Hartung HP. Inhibition of experimental autoimmune encephalomyelitis by an antibody to the intercellular adhesion molecule ICAM-1. Ann Neurol 34:145–154, 1993.
5. Baggiolini M, Dewald B, Moser B. Interleukin 8 and related chemotactic cytokines CXC and CC chemokines. Adv Immunol 55:97–179, 1994.
6. Baron JL, Madri JA, Ruddle NH, Hashim G, Janeway CA. Surface expression of α4 integrin by CD4 T cells is required for their entry into brain parenchyma. J Exp Med 177:57–68, 1993.
7. Bauer J, Berkenbosch F, VanDam AM, Dijkstra CD. Demonstration of interleukin 1-beta in Lewis rat brain during experimental allergic encephalomyelitis by immunohistochemistry at the light and ultrastructural level. J Neuroimmunol 48:13, 1993.
8. Bevilaqua MP. Endothelial-leukocyte adhesion molecules. Annu Rev Immunol 11:767–804, 1993.
9. Bevilacqua MP, Nelson RM. Selectins. J Clin Invest 91:379–387, 1993.

10. Blankenhorn EP, Stranford SA, Martin A-M, Hickey WF. Cloning of myelin basic protein reactive T-cells from the experimental allergic encephalomyelitis resistant rat strain, LER. J Neuroimmunol 59:173–183, 1995.

11. Boise L. CD28 costimulation can promote T cell survival by enhancing gene expression of Bcl-x. Immunity 3:87–98, 1995.

12. Boyd AW, Wawrk SO, Burns GF, Fecondo JV. Intercellular adhesion molecule 1 has a central role in cell-cell contact-mediated mechanism. Proc Natl Acad Sci USA 95:3095–3099, 1988.

13. Brown Z, Gerritesen ME, Carley MW, Strieter RM, Kunkel SL, Westwick J. Chemokine gene expression and secretion by cytokine activated human microvascular endothelial cells: different regulation of MCP-1 and IL-8 in response to IFNγ. Am J Pathol 145:913–921, 1994.

14. Burns FR, Li X, Shen N, Offner H, Chou YK, Vandenbark AA, Heber-Katz E. Both rat and mouse T cell receptors specific for the encephalitogenic determinant of myelin basic protein use similar V-alpha and V-beta even though the MHC complex and encephalitogenic determinants are different. J Exp Med 169:27–39, 1989.

15. Butcher EC. Leukocyte-endothelial cell recognition: three (or more) steps to specificity and diversity. Cell 67:1033–1036, 1991.

16. Butcher EC, Scollay RG, Weissman IL. Organ specificity of lymphocyte migration: mediation by highly selective lymphocyte interaction with organ specific determinants on high endothelial venules. Eur J Immunol 10:556–561, 1980.

17. Cahill RNP, Poskitt DC, Frost H, Trnka Z. Two distinct pools of recirculating lymphocytes: migratory characteristics of nodal and intestinal T lymphocytes. J Exp Med 145:420–428, 1977.

18. Cai T-Q, Wright SD. Energetics of leukocyte integrin activation. J Biol Chem 270:14358–14365, 1995.

19. Cannella B, Cross AH, Raine CS. Upregulation and coexpression of adhesion molecules correlate with relapsing autoimmune demyelination in the central nervous system. J Exp Med 172:1521–1524, 1990.

20. Cannella B, Cross AH, Raine CS. Adhesion related molecules in the central nervous system: upregulation correlates with inflammatory cell influx. Lab Invest 65:23–31, 1991.

21. Cannella B, Raine CS. The adhesion molecule and cytokine profile of multiple sclerosis lesions. Ann Neurol 37:424–435, 1995.

22. Carlos TM, Harlan JM. Leukocyte-endothelial cell adhesion molecules. Blood 84:2068–2101, 1994.

23. Cavallo MG, Pozzilli P, Thorpe R. Cytokines and autoimmunity. Clin Exp Immunol 91:1–7, 1994.

24. Chao CC, Hu S, Close K. Cytokine release by microglia: differential inhibition by pentoxyphyline and dexamethasone. J Infect Dis 166:847–853, 1992.

25. Chen Y, Kuchroo VK, Inobe J, Hafler DA, Weiner HL. Regulatory T cell clones induced by oral tolerance: suppression of allergic encephalomyelitis. Science 265:1237–1240, 1994.

26. Chin W, Hay JB. A comparison of lymphocyte migration through intestinal lymph nodes subcutaneous lymph nodes and chronic inflammatory sites of sheep. Gastroenterlogy 79:1231–1242, 1980.

27. Chluba J, Steeg C, Becker A, Wekerle H, Epplen JT. T cell receptor beta chain usage in myelin basic protein specific rat T lymphocytes. Eur J Immunol 19:279–285, 1989.

28. Chung IY, Benveniste EN. Tumor necrosis factor alpha production by astrocytes: induction by lipopoluysaccharide, INF-gamma and IL-1beta. J Immunol 144:2999–3007, 1990.

29. Corry DB, Linsley PS, Locksley RM. Differential effects of blocade of CD28-B7 on the development of Th1 or Th2 effector cells in experimental leishmaniasis. J Immunol 153:4142–4148, 1993.

30. Cross AH, Cannella B, Brosnan CF, Raine CS. Homing to central nervous system vasculature by antigen specific lymphocytes. I. Localization of ^{14}C-labeled cells during acute, chronic and relapsing experimental allergic encephalomyelitis. Lab Invest 63:162–170, 1990.

31. Cross AH, Girard TJ, Giacoletto KS, Evans RT, Trotter JL, Karr RW. Long term inhibition of murine experimental allergic encephalomyelitis using CTLA-4-Fc supports a role for CD28 costimulation. J Clin Invest 95:2783–2789, 1995.

32. Cross AH, Raine CS. CNS endothelial cell–polymorphonuclear cell interaction during autoimmune demyelination. Am J Pathol 139:1–8, 1991.

33. Damle NK, Aruffo A. VCAM-1 induces T cell antigen receptor dependent activation of human CD4+ T lymphocytes. Proc Natl Acad Sci USA 88:6403–6407, 1991.

34. Damle NK, Klussman K, Aruffo A. ICAM-2, a second ligand for CD11a/CD18 (LFA-1), provides a costimulatory signal for T cell receptor initiated activation of human T cells. J Immunol 148:665–671, 1992.

35. Damle NK, Klussman K, Linsley P, Aruffo A. Differential costimulatory effects of adhesion molecules B7, ICAM-1, LFA-1, LFA-3, and VCAM-1 on resting and antigen primed CD4 cells. J Immunol 148:1985–1992, 1992.

36. de Vries HE, Moor AC, Blom-Roosmalen MC, de Boer AG, Breimer DD, van Berkel TJ, Kuiper J. Lymphocyte adhesion to brain capillary endothelial cells in vitro. J Neuroimmunol 52:1–8, 1994.

37. Dore-Duffy P, Washington RA, Balabanov R. Cytokine mediated activation of cultured CNS microvessels—a system for examining antigenic modulation of CNS endothelial cells and evidence for long term expression of E-selectin. J Cereb Blood Flow Metab 14:837–846, 1994.

38. Duijvestijn A, Schreiber AB, Butcher EC. Interferon-γ regulates an antigen specific for endothelial cells involved in lymphocyte traffic. Proc Natl Acad Sci USA 83:9114–9118, 1986.

39. Durie FH, Foy TM, Noelle RJ. The role of CD40 and its ligand (gp39) in peripheral and central tolerance and its contribution to autoimmune disease. Rev Res Immunol 145:200–205, 1994.

40. Durieu-Trautmann O, Chavernot N, Cazaubon S, Strosberg AD, Couraud P-O. ICAM-1 activation induces tyrosine phosphorylation of cytoskeleton associated protein cortactin in brain microvascular endothelial cells. J Biol Chem 269:12536–12540, 1994.

41. Dustin ML, Springer TA. T cell receptor cross-linking transiently stimulates adhesiveness through LFA-1. Nature 341:619–624, 1989.

42. Espavik T, Figari IS, Shalaby MR, Lackides GA, Lewis GD, Shepard HM, Palladino MA. Inhibition of cytokine production by cyclosporin A and transforming growth factor beta. J Exp Med 166:571–576, 1987.

43. Fabry Z, Fitzsimmons K, Herlein J, Moninger T, Dobbs M, Hart MN. Production of cytokines IL-1 and Il-6 by murine brain microvessel endothelium and smooth muscle/pericytes. J Neuroimmunol 47:23–34, 1992.

44. Fabry Z, Raine CS, Hart MN. Nervous tissue as an immune compartment: the dialect of the immune response in the CNS. Immunol Today 15:218–224, 1994.

45. Fabry Z, Waldschmidt MM, Hendrickson D, Keiner J, Love L, Takei F, Hart MN. Adhesion molecules on murine brain microvascular endothelium: expression and regulation of ICAM-1 and lgp-55. J Neuroimmunol 36:1–11, 1992.

46. Favaloro EJ. Differential expression of surface antigens on activated endothelium. Immunol Cell Biol 71:571–581, 1993.

47. Fiorentino DF, Zlotnick A, Mossmann TR, Howard M, O'Garra A. IL-10 inhibits cytokines produced by macrophages. J Immunol 147:3815–3822, 1991.

48. Flaris NA, Densmore TL, Molleston MC, Hickey WF. Characterization of microglia and macrophages in the central nervous system of rats. Glia 7:34–40, 1993.

49. Flurie MB, Randolph GJ. Chemokines and tissue injury: a review. Am J Pathol 146:1287–1293, 1995.

50. Ford AL, Goodsall AL, Hickey WF, Sedgwick JD. Normal adult rat microglia separated from other CNS macrophages by flow cytometric sorting: phenotypic differences defined and direct ex vivo antigen presentation to myelin basic protein reactive CD4+ T cell compared. J Immunol 154:4309–4321, 1995.

51. Foy TM, Durie FH, Noelle RJ. The expansive role of CD40 and its ligand gp39 in immunity. Semin Immunol 6:259–267, 1994.

52. Fraser JD, Irving BA, Crabtree GR, Weiss A. Regulation of IL-2 gene enhancer activity by T cell accessory molecule CD28. Science 251:313–316, 1991.

53. Freedman AS, Freedman GJ, Rhinhart K, Nadler LM. Selective induction of B7/BB-1 on interferon-gamma stimulated monocytes: a potential mechanism for amplification of T cell activation. Cell Immunol 137:429–437, 1991.

54. Freeman GJ, Borriello F, Hodes RJ, Reiser H, Gribben GJ, Ng JW, Kim J, Goldberg JM, Hathcock K, Laszlo G, Lombard LA, Wang S, Gray GS, Nadles LM, Sharp AH. Murine B7-2, an alternative CTLA-4 counter receptor that costimulates T cell proliferation and IL-2 production. J Exp Med 178:2185–2192, 1993.

55. Freidman AW, Diaz I, Moore S, Schaller J, Fox DA. The human 4F2 antigen: evidence for cryptic and non-cryptic epitopes and a role for 4F2 in human lymphocyte activation. Cell Immunol 154:253–259, 1994.

56. Gerriste K, Noelle RJ, Aruffo A, Ledbetter J, Laman JD, Boersma WJA, Claassen E. Evidence for the role of CD40 ligand in the development of EAE and multiple sclerosis. Proc Natl Acad Sci USA 93:2499–2504, 1996.

57. Gijebels K, VanDamm J, Proost P, Put W, Carton H, Billau A. Interleukin 6 production in the CNS during experimental allergic encephalomyelitis. J Immunol 20:233–245, 1990.

58. Giulian D. Microglia and diseases of the nervous system. Curr Neurol 12:23–54, 1992.

59. Giulian D, Baker TJ, Shih L-C, Lachmann LB. Interleukin-1 of the central nervous system is produced by ameboid microglia. J Exp Med 164:594–604, 1986.

60. Godiska R, Chantry D, Dietsch GN, Gray PW. Chemokine expression in murine experimental allergic encephalomyelitis. J Neuroimmunol 58:167–175, 1995.

61. Gold DP, Offner H, Sun D, Wiley S, Vandenbark AA, Wilson DB. Analysis of T cell receptor beta chains in Lewis rats with EAE: conserved complementarity determining region 3. J Exp Med 174:1467–1477, 1991.

62. Gonatas NK, Howard JC. Inhibition of experimental allergic encephalomyelitis in rats severely depleted of T cells. Science 186:839–841, 1974.

63. Gowans JL. The recirculation of lymphocytes from blood to lymph in the rat. J Physiol 146:54–69, 1959.

64. Gowans JL, Knoght EJ. The route of recirculation of lymphocytes in the rat. Proc R Soc Lond B Biol Sci 159:257–282, 1964.

65. Granert C, Raud J, Xie X, Lindquist L, Lindbom L. Inhibition of leukocyte rolling with polysaccharide fucoidin prevents pleocytosis in experimental meningitis in the rabbit. J Clin Invest 93:929–936, 1994.

66. Granger DN, Kubes P. The microcirculation and inflammation: modulation of leukocyte-endothelial cell adhesion. J Leukoc Biol 55:662–675, 1994.
67. Griffin DE, Levine B, Tylor WR, Irani DN. The immune response in viral encephalitis. Semin Immunol 4:111–119, 1992.
68. Griscelli C, Vassalli P, McCluskey RT. The distribution of large dividing lymph node cells in syngeneic recipients after intravenous injection. J Exp Med 130:1427–1451, 1969.
69. Harlan JM, Liu DY. Adhesion: Its Role in Inflammatory Disease. WH Freeman, New York, 1992.
70. Harrison JK, Barber CM, Lynch KR. cDNA cloning of a G-protein coupled receptor expressed in rat spinal cord and brain related to chemokine receptors. Neurosci Lett 169:85–89, 1994.
71. Hickey WF. T-cell entry and antigen recognition in the central nervous system. In: Psycho-neuroimmunology, R. Ader, D. Felten, N. Cohen, ed. Academic Press, New York, pp 149–175, 1991.
72. Hickey WF, Hsu BL, Kimura H. T-lymphocyte entry into the central nervous system. J Neurosci Res 28:254–260, 1991.
73. Hickey WF, Kimura H. "Perivascular microglia" are bone marrow derived and present antigen *in vivo*. Science 239:290–292, 1988.
74. Hinrichs DJ, Wegmann KW, Dietsch GN. Transfer of EAE to bone marrow chimeras; endothelial cells are not a restricting element. J Exp Med 166:1906–1911, 1987.
75. Holda JH, Welch AM, Swanborg RH. Autoimmune effector cells I. Transfer of EAE with lymphoid cells cultured with antigen. Eur J Immunol 10:657–659, 1980.
76. Hulkower K, Brosnan CF, Aquino DA, Cammer W, Kulshresthna S, Guida MP, Rapaport DA, Berman JW. Expression of CSF-1, c-fms, and MCP-1 in the central nervous system of rats with experimental allergic encephalomyelitis. J Immunol 150:2525–2533, 1993.
77. Hynes RO. Integrins: versatility, modulation, and signaling of cell adhesion. Cell 69:11–25, 1992.
78. Ihrcke NS, Wrenshall LE, Lindman BJ, Platt JL. Role of heparin sulfate in immune system–blood vessel interactions. Immunol Today 14:500–505, 1993.
79. Issekutz TB. Effects of six different cytokines on lymphocyte adherence to microvascular endothelium and in vivo lymphocyte migration in the rat. J Immunol 144:2140–2146, 1990.
80. Jenkins MK, Johnson JG. Molecules involved in T cell costimulation. Curr Opin Immunol 5:361–367, 1993.
81. Jensen MA, Arneson BG, Toscas A, Noronha A. Preferential increase of IL-2+ CD4+ T cells and CD45RB− CD4+ T cells in the central nervous system in experimental allergic encephalomyelitis. J Neuroimmunol 38:255–261, 1992.
82. Johns L, Flanders K, Ranges G, Sriram S. Successful treatment of EAE with transforming growth factor beta-1. J Immunol 147:1792–1798, 1991.
83. June CH, Bluestone JA, Nadler LM, Thompson CB. The B7 and CD28 receptor families. Immunol Today 15:321–331, 1994.
84. Karpus WJ, Lukacs NW, McRae BL, Strieter RM, Kunkel SL, Miller SD. Prevention and treatment of PLP peptide induced EAE by anti-MIP-1a administration. J Neuroimmunol 54:171–179, 1994.
85. Kida S, Steart PV, Zhang ET, Weller RO. Perivascular cells act as scavengers in the cerebral perivascular spaces and remain distinct from pericytes, microglia and macrophages. Acta Neuropathol 86:646–652, 1993.
86. Knopf PM, Basu D, Sirulnick E, Nolan S, Cserr HM, Hickey WF. B cell traffic and intrathecal antibody synthesis in normal brain. FASEB J 8:A248, 1994.

87. Kojima K, Berger T, Lassmann H, Hinze-Selch D, Zhang Y, Gehrmann J, Reske K, Wekerle H, Linington C. Experimental autoimmune panencephalitis and uveoretinitis transferred to Lewis rats by T lymphocytes specific for the S100 beta molecule, a calcium binding protein of astroglia. J Exp Med 180:817–829, 1994.

88. Kraal G, Weissman IL, Butcher EC. Differences in *in vivo* distribution and homing of T cell subsets to mucosal *vs.* non-mucosal lymphoid organs. J Immunol 130:1097–1102, 1983.

89. Kuchroo VK, Das MP, Brown JA, Rnager AM, Zamvil SS, Sobel RA, Weiner HL, Nabavi N, Glimcher LH. B7-1 and B7-2 costimulatory molecules activate differentially the Th1/Th2 development: application of autoimmune disease. Cell 80:707–718, 1995.

90. Kuchroo VK, Martin CA, Greer JM, Ju ST, Sobel RA, Dorf ME. Cytokines and adhesion molecules contribute to the ability of myelin proteolipid protein specific T cell clones to meditate experimental allergic encephalomyelitis. J Immunol 151:4371–4379, 1993.

91. Kuppner MC, Hamou M-F, Tribolet N. Activation and adhesion molecule expression on lymphoid infiltrates in human glioblastomas. J Neuroimmunol 29:229–238, 1990.

92. Lackner AA, Dandekar S, Gardner MB. Neurobiology of simian and feline immunodeficiency virus infections. Brain Pathol 1:201–212, 1991.

93. Lassman H, Rossler K, Zimprich F, Vass K. Expression of adhesion molecules and histocompatibility antigens at the blood-brain barrier. Brain Pathol 1:115–123, 1991.

94. Lassmann H, Zimprich F, Rossler K, Vass K. Inflammation in the nervous system. Rev Neurol 147:763–781, 1991.

95. Lassmann H, Zimprich F, Vass K, Hickey WF. Microglial cells are a component of the perivascular glia limitans. J Neurosci Res 28:236–243, 1991.

96. Lawrence MB, Springer TA. Leukocytes roll on a selectins at physiologic flow rates: distinction from and prerequisite for adhesion through integrins. Cell 65:859–873, 1991.

97. Lee SC, Liu W, Roth P, Dickson DW, Brosnan CF, Berman JW. Cytokine production by human fetal microglia and astrocytes: differential induction by LPS and IL-1beta. J Immunol 150:2659–2667, 1993.

98. Lenschow DJ. Differential upregulation of the B7-1 and B7-2 costimulatory molecules following immunoglobulin receptor engagement by antigen. J Immunol 153:1990–1996, 1994.

99. Linington C, Berger T, Perry S, Weerth S, Hinze-Selch D, Zhang Y, Lu H, Lassmann H, Wekerle H. T cells specific for the myelin oligodendrocyte glycoprotein mediate an unusual autoimmune inflammatory response in the CNS. Eur J Immunol 23:1364–1369, 1993.

100. Linsley PS, Ledbetter JA. The role of CD28 receptor during T cell responses to antigen. Annu Rev Immunol 11:191–212, 1993.

101. Lucas PJ, Negishi I, Nakayama K, Fields LE, Loh DY. Naive CD28 deficient T cells can initiate but not sustain an in vitro antigen specific immune response. J Immunol 154:5757–5768, 1995.

102. Mackay CR, Marston WL, Dudler L. Naive and memory T cells show distinct pathways of lymphocyte recirculation. J Exp Med 171:801–809, 1990.

103. Mackay F, Loetscher H, Stueber D, Gehr G, Lesslauer W. Tumor necrosis factor alpha induced cell adhesion to human endothelial cells is under dominant control of one TNF receptor type, TNF-R55. J Exp Med 177:1277–1286, 1993.

104. Male D, Pryce G, Hughes C, Lantos P. Lymphocyte migration into brain modelled in vitro: control by lymphocyte activation, cytokines and antigen. Cell Immunol 127:1–11, 1990.

105. Male D, Rahman J, Linke A, Zhao W, Hickey WF. An interferon inducible molecule on brain endothelium which controls lymphocyte adherence mediated by integrins. Immunology 84:453–460, 1995.

106. Male D, Rahman G, Pryce G, Tamatani T, Miyasaka M. Lymphocyte migration into the CNS modeled in vitro: role of LFA-1, ICAM-1 and VLA-4. Immunology 81:366–374, 1994.

107. Malefet RDW, Abrahms J, Bennett B, Figdor CG, de Bries JE. Interleukin-10 inhibits cytokine synthesis by human monocytes: an autoregulatory role of IL-10 produced by monocytes. J Exp Med 174:1209–1220, 1991.

108. Mannie MD, Paterson PY, U'Pprichard DC, Fluoret G. Induction of EAE in Lewis rats with purified synthetic peptides. Proc Natl Acad Sci USA 82:5515–5519, 1985.

109. Marfang-Koka A, Devergne O, Gorgone G, Portier A, Schall TJ, Galanaud P, Emilie D. Regulation of the products of the RANTES chemokine by endothelial cells: syntergistic induction by INFg and TNFa, and inhibition by IL4 and IL13. J Immunol 154:1870–1877, 1995.

110. Martin D, Near SL, Bendele A, Russell DA. Inhibition of tumor necrosis factor is protective against neurological dysfunction after active immunization of Lewis rats with myelin basic protein. Exp Neurol 131:211–229, 1995.

111. Mattila P, Majuri M-L, Mattila PS, Renkonen R. TNF-alpha induced expression of endothelial cell adhesion molecules ICAM-1 and VCAM-1 is linked to protein kinase activation. Scand J Immunol 36:159–162, 1992.

112. McCarron RM, Wang L, Racke MK, McFarlin DE, Spatz M. Cytokine regulated adhesion between encephalitogenic T lymphocytes and cerebrovacular endothelial cells. J Neuroimmunol 43:23–30, 1993.

113. McEver RP. Selectins. Curr Opin Immunol 6:75–84, 1994.

114. Merrill JE, Kono DH, Clayton J, Ando DG, Hinton DR, Hofmann FM. Inflammatory leukocytes and cytokines in peptide induced experimental allergic encephalomyelitis in SJL/J and B10.PL mice. Proc Natl Acad Sci USA 89:574–578, 1992.

115. Miller SD, Karpus WJ. The immunopathogenesis and regulation of T cell mediated demyelinating diseases. Immunol Today 15:356–361, 1994.

116. Mossman TR, Coffman RL. Different patterns of lymphokine secretion lead to different functional properties. Annu Rev Immunol 7:145–173, 1989.

117. Mueller DL, Jenkins MK, Schwartz RH. Clonal expansion versus functional clonal inactivation: a costimulatory signalling pathway determines the outcome of T cell antigen receptor. Annu Rev Immunol 7:445–480, 1989.

118. Murphy PM. The molecular biology of leukocyte chemoattractant receptors. Annu Rev Immunol 12:593–633, 1994.

119. Musso T, Espinoza-Delgado I, Pulkki K, Gussella GL, Longo DL, Varesio L. Transforming growth factor beta downregulates IL-1 induced IL-6 production by human monocytes. Blood 76:2466–2469, 1990.

120. Naparstek Y, Cohen IR, Fuks Z, Vlodavsky I. Activated T lymphocytes produce a matrix degrading heparin sulphate endoglycosidase. Nature 310:241–244, 1984.

121. Naparstek Y, Holoshitz J, Eisenstein S, Cohen IR. Effector T lymphocyte cell lines migrate to the thymus and persist there. Nature 300:262–265, 1982.

122. Nathan C, Xie Q-W. Nitric oxide synthases: roles, tolls and controls. Cell 78:915–918, 1994.

123. Offner H, Buenafe AC, Vainiene M, Celnik B, Weinberg AD, Gold DP, Hashim G, Vandenbark AA. Where, when and how to detect biased expression of disease relevant Vβ genes in rats with EAE. J Immunol 151:506–517, 1993.

124. O'Neill JK, Butter C, Baker D, Geschemeisser SE, Kraal G, Butcher EC, Turk JL. Expression of vascular addressins and ICAM-1 by endothelial cells of the spinal cord during relapsing EAE in the Biozzi AB/H mouse. Immunology 72:520–525, 1991.

125. Owens T, Renno T, Taupin V, Krakowski M. Inflammatory cytokines in the brain: does the CNS shape the immune response? Immunol Today 15:566–571, 1994.

126. Panitch HS. Adoptive transfer of EAE with activated spleen cells: comparison of in vitro activation by concavalin A and myelin basic protein. Cell Immunol 56:163–171, 1980.

127. Pender MP, Nguyen KB, McCombe PA, Kerr JFR. Apoptosis in the nervous system in experimental allergic encephalomyelitis. J Neurol Sci 14:81–87, 1991.

128. Pitzalis C, Kingsley G, Haskard D, Panayi G. The preferential accumulation of helper-inducer T lymphocytes in inflammatory lesions: evidence for regulation by selective endothelial and homotypic adhesion. Eur J Immunol 18:1397–1404, 1988.

129. Pizcueta P, Luscinskas FW. Monoclonal antibody blockade of L-selectin inhibits mononuclear leukocyte recruitment to inflammatory sites in vivo. Am J Pathol 145:461–469, 1994.

130. Postigo AA, Marazuela M, Sanchez-Madri F, deLandazuri MO. B lymphocyte binding to E- and P-selectins is mediated through the de novo expression of carbohydrates or in vitro and in vivo activated human B cells. J Clin Invest 94:1585–1596, 1994.

131. Postigo AA, Pulido R, Campanero MR, Acevedo A, Garcia-Pardo A, Corbi AL, Sanchez-Madri F, deLandazui MO. Differential expression of LVA-4 integrin by resident and peripheral blood B lymphocytes. Acquisition of functionally active $\alpha 4\beta 1$ fibronectin receptors upon B cell activation. Eur J Immunol 21:2437–2445, 1991.

132. Postigo AA, Sanchez-Madri F, Lazarovits AI, Sanchez-Madri F, deLandazui MO. $\alpha 4\beta 1$ Integrin mediates B cell binding to fibronectin and vascular cell adhesion molecule-1. Expression and function of $\alpha 4$ integrins on human B lymphocytes. J Immunol 151:2471–2483, 1993.

133. Powell LD, Varki A. I-type lectins. J Biol chem 270:14243–14246, 1995.

134. Powell MB, Mitchell D, Lederman J, Buchmeier J, Zamvil SS, Graham M, Ruddle NH, Steinman L. Lymphotoxin and tumor necrosis factor-alpha production by MBP specific T cell clones correlates with encephalitogenicity. J Immunol 2:539–545, 1990.

135. Pryce G, Male DK, Sarkar C. Control of lymphocyte migration into brain, selective interactions of lymphocyte subpopulations with brain endothelium. Immunology 72:393–398, 1991.

136. Quaglierello VJ, Wispelwey B, Scheld WM. Recombinant human IL-1 induces meningitis and blood-brain barrier injury in the rat. J Clin Invest 87:1360–1366, 1991.

137. Racke MK, Dhib-Jalbut S, Cannella B, Albert PS, Raine CS. Prevention and treatment of chronic relapsing experimental allergic encephalomyelitis with transforming growth factor beta-1. J Immunol 146:3012–3017, 1991.

138. Raine CS. The Dale McFarlin Memorial Lecture: the immunology of multiple sclerosis. Ann Neurol 36:S61–S72, 1994.

139. Raine CS. Multiple sclerosis: TNF revisited with promise. Nature Med 1:211–214, 1995.

140. Ransohoff RM, Hamilton TA, Tani M, Stoler MH, Shick HE, Major JA, Estes ML, Thomas TM, Tuohy VK. Astrocyte expression of mRNA encoding cytokines IP-10 and JE/MCP-1 in EAE. FASEB J 7:592–600, 1993.

141. Ransohoff RM, Tuohy V, Lehmann P. The immunology of multiple sclerosis: new intricacies and new insights. Curr Opin Neurol 7:242–249, 1994.

142. Rosales C, Juliano RL. Signal transduction by cell adhesion receptors in leukocytes. J Leukoc Biol 57:189–198, 1995.

143. Rossler K, Neuchrist C, Kitz K, Scheiner O, Kraft D, Lassmann H. Expression of leucocyte adhesion molecules at the human blood-brain barrier (BBB). J Neurosci Res 31:365–374, 1992.

144. Rott W, Fleischer B, Cash E. Interleukin-10 prevents experimental allergic encephalomyelitis in rats. Eur J Immunol 24:1434–1440, 1994.

145. Roy M, Waldschmidt T, Aruffo A, Ledvbetter JA, Noelle RJ. The regulation of expression of gp39, the CD40 ligand, on normal and cloned CD4+ T cells. J Immunol 151:2497–2510, 1993.

146. Ruddle NH, Bergman CM, McGrath KM, Lingenheld EC, Grunnet ML, Padula SJ, Clark RB. An antibody to lymphotoxin and tumor necrosis factor prevents transfer of experimental allergic encephalomyelitis. J Exp Med 172:1193–1200, 1990.

147. Santambrogio L, Hochwald, G. Sexena B, Thorbecke GJ. Studies on the mechanisms by which transforming growth factor beta protects against allergic encephalomyelitis: antagonism between TGF-b and TNF. J Immunol 151:1116–1122, 1993.

148. Sasseville VG, Newman W, Brodie SJ, Hesterberg P, Pauley D, Ringler DJ. Monocyte adhesion to endothelium in simian immunodeficiency virus-induced AIDS encephalitis is mediated by vascular cell adhesion molecule 1 $\alpha4\beta1$ integrin interactions. Am J Pathol 144:27–40, 1994.

149. Sasseville VG, Newman WA, Lackner AA, Smith MO, Lausen NCG, Beall D, Ringler DJ. Elevated vascular cell adhesion molecule-1 in AIDS encephalitis induced by simian immunodeficiency virus. Am J Pathol 141:1021–1130, 1992.

150. Schall TJ, Bacon KB. Chemokines, leukocyte trafficking, and inflammation. Curr Opin Immunol 6:865–873, 1994.

151. Schmied M, Breitschopf H, Gold R, Zischler H, Rothe G, Wekerle H, Lassmann H. Apoptosis of T lymphocytes in experimental autoimmune encephalomyelitis. J Pathol 143:446–452, 1993.

152. Schwartz RH. A cell culture model for T lymphocyte clonal anergy. Science 248:1349–1356, 1990.

153. Schwartz RH. Costimulation of T lymphocytes: the role of CD28, CTLA-4 and BB/B71 in interleukin 2 production and immunotherapy. Cell 71:1065–1068, 1992.

154. Scolding NJ, Zaficek JP, Compston DAS. The pathogenesis of demyelinating disease. Prog Neurobiol 43:143–173, 1994.

155. Selmaj K. The role of cytokines in inflammatory conditions of the central nervous system. Semin Neurosci 4:221–229, 1992.

156. Shimizu Y, Newman W, Tanhka Y, Shaw S. Lymphocyte interactions with endothelial cell. Immunol Today 13:106–112, 1992.

157. Silber A, Newman W, Sasseville VG, Pauley D, Beall D, Walsh DG, Ringler DJ. Recruitment of lymphocytes during cutaneous delayed hypersensitivity in nonhuman primates is dependent on E-selectin and vascular cell adhesion molecule 1. J Clin Invest 93:1554–1563, 1994.

158. Sloan DJ, Wood MJ, Charlton HM. Leukocyte recruitment and inflammation in the CNS. TINS 15:276–280, 1992.

159. Sobel RA, Greer JM, Kuchroo VK. Minireview: autoimmune responses to myelin proteolipid protein. Neurochem Res 19:915–921, 1994.

160. Sobel R, Mitchell ME, Fondren G. Intercellular adhesion molecule-1 (ICAM-1) in cellular immune reactions in the human central nervous system. Am J Pathol 136:1309–1316, 1990.

161. Springer TA. Adhesion receptors of the immune system. Nature 346:425–434, 1990.

162. Springer TA. Traffic signals for lymphocyte recirculation and leukocyte emigration. Cell 76:301–314, 1994.

163. Steinman L, Miller A, Bernard CCA, Oksenberg JR. The epigenetics of multiple sclerosis: clues to etiology and a rationale for therapy. Annu Rev Neurosci 17:247–265, 1994.

164. Steinman RM, Young JW. Signals arising from antigen presenting cells. Curr Opin Immunol 3:361–364, 1991.

165. Stephan BJ, Butcher EC, Engelhardt B. Evidence for the involvement of ICAM-1 and VCAM-1 in lymphocyte interaction with endothelium in EAE in the CNS of the SJL/J mouse. Am J Pathol 145:189, 1994.

166. Stoolman LM. Adhesion molecules controlling lymphocyte migration. Cell 56:907–910, 1989.

167. Sun D, Klinkert WEF. Functional heterogeneity among CD4+ encephalitogenic T cells in recruitment of CD8+ T cells in experimental allergic encephalomyelitis. J Immunol 143:2867, 1989.

168. Takada Y, Huang C, Hemler ME. Fibronectin receptor structures are included within VLA family heterodimers. Nature 326:607–609, 1987.

169. Takenaka A, Minigawa H, Kaneka K, Mori R, Itoyama Y. Adoptive transfer of EAE with lectin activated spleen cells, part 2. Studies on T-cell and interleukin 2 production. J Neurol Sci 72:337–345, 1986.

170. Thomas ML. The leukocyte common antigen family. Annu Rev Immunol 7:339–369, 1989.

171. Trotter J, Steinman L. Homing of Lyt2+ and Lyt2− T cell subsets and B lymphocytes to the central nervous system of mice with acute experimental allergic encephalomyelitis. J Immunol 132:2919–2923, 1984.

172. Tuohy VK, Laursen RA, Lees MB. Acute experimental allergic encephalomyelitis in SJL/mice induced by a synthetic peptide of myelin proteolipid protein. J Neuropathol Exp Neurol 49:468–479, 1990.

173. Tyor WR, Glass JD, Griffin JW, Becker PS, McArthur JC, Bezmen L, Griffin DE. Cytokine expression in the brain during the acquired immunodeficiency syndrome. Ann Neurol 32:349–360, 1992.

174. Tyor W, Griffin DE. Virus specificity and isotype expression of intraparenchymal antibody-secreting cells during Sindbis virus encephalitis in mice. J Neuroimmunol 48:37–44, 1993.

175. Tyor WR, Moench TR, Griffin DE. Characterization of the local and systemic B cell response of normal and athymic nude mice with sindbis virus encephalitis. J Neuroimmunol 24:207–215, 1989.

176. Tyor WR, Wesselingh S, Levine B, Griffin DE. Long term intraparenchymal Ig secretion after acute encephalitis in mice. J Immunol 149:4016–4020, 1992.

177. Vanguri P, Farber JM. IFN and virus inducible expression of an immediate early geen, crg-2/IP-10, and a delayed gene, I-Aa, in astrocytes and microglia. J Immunol 152:1411–1418, 1994.

178. van Kooyk Y, van de Wiel-van Kemenade E, Weder P, Huibens JF, Figdor CG. Lymphocyte function-associated antigen 1 dominates very late antigen 4 in binding of activated T cells to endothelium. J Exp Med 177:185–190, 1993.

179. VanSeventer GA, Shimizu Y, Hogan KJ, Shaw S. The LFA-1 ligand ICAM-1 provides an important costimulatory signal for T cell receptor mediated activation of resting T cells. J Immunol 122:4579–4587, 1990.

180. Verweij CL, Geerts M, Aarden LA. Activation of IL-2 gene transcription via the T cell surface molecule CD28 is mediated through an NF-κB like response element. J Biol Chem 266:14179–14183, 1991.

181. Vodovoltz Y, Bogdan C, Paik J, Xie Q-W, Nathan C. Mechanisms of suppression of macrophage nitric oxide release by transforming growth factor beta. J Exp Med 178:605–613, 1993.

182. Wall M, Southwood S, Sidney J, Oseroff C, del Guercio MF, Lamont A, Colon SM,

Arrhenius T, Gaeta FCA, Sette A. High affinity for class II molecules as a necessary but not sufficient characteristic of encephalitogenic determinants. Int Immunol 4:773–777, 1992.

183. Weidenheim K, Epsyteyn I, Lyman WD. Immunocytochemical identification of T-cells in HIV encephalitis: implications for pathogenesis of CNS disease. Mod Pathol 6:167–204, 1993.

184. Wekerle H, Linington H, Lassman H, Meyermann R. Cellular immune reactivity within the CNS. Trends Neurosci 9:271–276, 1986.

185. Werdelin O, McCluskey RT. The nature and specificity of mononuclear cells in experimental autoimmune inflammations and the mechanisms leading to their accumulation. J Exp Med 133:1242–1263, 1971.

186. Willenborg DP, Parish CR. Inhibition of allergic encephalomyelitis in rats by treatment with sulfated polysaccharides. J Immunol 140:3401–3405, 188.

187. Williams KC, Hickey WF. Migration of hematogenous cells through the central nervous system. Curr Top Microbiol Immunol 202:221–245, 1995.

188. Williams KC, Ulvestad E, Antel JP. B7-BB1 antigen expression on adult human microglia studies in vitro and in situ. Eur J Immunol 24:3031–3037, 1994.

189. Williams KC, Ulvestadt E, Hickey WF. The immunology of multiple sclerosis. Clin Neurosci 2:229–245, 1995.

190. Wong D, Dorovini-Zis K. Upregulation of intracellular adhesion molecule-1 (ICAM-1) expression in primary cultures of human brain microvessel endothelial cells by cytokines and lipopolysaccharide. J Neuroimmunol 39:11–22, 1992.

191. Woodroofe MN, Sarna GS, Wadna M, Hayes GM, Loughlin AJ, Tinker A, Cuzner ML. Detection of interleukin-1 and interleukin-6 in adult rat brain following mechanical injury by in vivo microdialysis: evidence for microglia in cytokine production. J Immunol 33:227–236, 1992.

192. Yao J, Keri JE, Taffs RE, Colton CA. Characterization of IL-1 production by microglia in culture. Brain Res 591:88–93, 1992.

193. Yednock TA, Cannon C, Fritz LC, Sanchez-Madri F, Steinman L, Karin N. Prevention of experimental autoimmune encephalomyelitis by antibodies against $\alpha 4 \beta 1$ integrin. Nature 356:63–66, 1992.

194. Zamvil SS, Steinman L. The T lymphocyte in experimental allergic encephalomyelitis. Annu Rev Immunol 8:579–621, 1990.

8

Innervation of Lymphoid Organs and Neurotransmitter–Lymphocyte Interactions

DENISE L. BELLINGER
SUZANNE Y. FELTEN
DIANNE LORTON
DAVID L. FELTEN

The central nervous system (CNS) signals cells of the immune system via two major communication routes: neuroendocrine mediators, and neurotransmitters released from nerve fibers that innervate primary and secondary lymphoid organs. Hormonal signaling of lymphocyte and macrophage functions has been reported for releasing factors, anterior and posterior pituitary hormones, and hormones produced by target organs. CNS signaling mediated by the release of hormones depends on blood-borne access to the hypophyseal portal system and then the general circulation of these substances through the lymphoid organs (anterior pituitary hormones, target organ hormones). Neurotransmitter influences on immunocytes via receptors for these neurotransmitters have been reported for acetylcholine (ACh), catecholamines (CAs), and neuropeptides. CA innervation of primary and secondary lymphoid organs is the most extensively examined. Neurotransmitter signaling as a link between the brain and the immune system depends on the availability of the neurotransmitter released from nerve fibers that directly innervate primary and secondary lymphoid organs.

Establishing neurotransmission with cells of the immune system as targets requires that four criteria be met: *(1)* demonstration of the neurotransmitter and its metabolic machinery in nerves that course in close proximity to cells of the immune system, or that permit sufficient diffusion of the neurotransmitter to cells with the capacity to respond; *(2)* release and availability of the neurotransmitter in concentrations that will allow appropriate signaling via receptors on target cells; *(3)* the presence of specific receptors that bind the ligand on cells of the immune system and are linked to second messengers, changes in ion channels in the cell membrane, or other intracellular processes; and *(4)* a pharmacologically predictable functional impact of the neurotransmit-

226

ter on cells of the immune system such that reproducible effects on immune function are seen following manipulation of the nerve terminal or administration of specific agonist and antagonist pharmacologic agents (reviewed in 154,155). These criteria should be fulfilled for each neurotransmitter in specific compartments of lymphoid organs in all species examined under defined physiological conditions. The criteria for neurotransmission have been best satisfied for noradrenergic (NA) innervation of cells of the immune system.

NA, as well as peptidergic, nerves that distribute to lymphoid organs also may have non-lymphoid cell targets, such as vascular smooth muscle and endothelial cells, lymphatic vessels, and reticular cells that provide the supportive framework of the organ. Innervation of these targets may influence immune function indirectly by altering vascular permeability, chemotaxis, cellular migration, and release of factors from these targets that effect lymphocyte function.

In this chapter, we will describe NA, cholinergic, and peptidergic innervation of lymphoid organs, largely from rodents, and the extent to which the criteria for neurotransmission have been fulfilled for these neurotransmitters. Further, we will discuss the relationship of NA and peptidergic innervation of lymphoid organs during development, maturation, and aging, and examine changes that occur in the organization of lymphoid compartments and the regulation of immunocompetence. Nerves present in lymphoid organs are responsive to, and may contribute to, developmental, plastic, and age-associated changes in the immune system. Lastly, we will explore the possible implications of neural signaling through direct innervation of the immune system in autoimmunity.

Neurochemically Identified Nerves in Primary and Secondary Lymphoid Organs—Criteria for Neurotransmission

NA Sympathetic Nerves in Lymphoid Organs

NA innervation of lymphoid organs (reviewed in 36,37,154,163,308) is best demonstrated using two techniques: *(1)* fluorescence histochemistry for CAs, which permits the localization of CA-containing nerves; and *(2)* double-label immunocytochemistry (ICC) using anti-sera against tyrosine hydroxylase (TH), the rate-limiting enzyme in the synthesis of norepinephrine (NE), and anti-sera against specific surface markers on cells of the immune system. Fluorescence histochemistry for CAs is a tool that is most powerful when coupled with neurochemical assessment of CAs and their metabolites. Using these methods, NA innervation has been demonstrated in both primary and secondary lymphoid organs including lymphoid tissue associated with the respiratory and gastrointestinal systems. (reviewed in 37,152,163,308).

Bone Marrow

In young adult rodents, NA sympathetic innervation distributing to long bones courses along branches of the appropriate spinal nerve supplying that region of the body. These nerves then form small nerve bundles that delve into the bone through the nutrient foramena, along with the vasculature. Within the marrow, fine, varicose NA nerves form dense plexuses along the vasculature (37,163). From these vascular plexuses, occasional nerve fibers branch into the surrounding parenchyma among hemopoietic cells in the marrow. ICC localization of TH-positive[+] nerve cells in bone marrow has recently been worked out in our laboratory (196) and reveals TH nerve fibers (Fig. 8-1) with a distribution similar to that described with fluorescence histochemistry. Nerve plexuses along the vasculature in the bone marrow contain TH[+] fibers that extend into the surrounding parenchyma. Once released from these nerve terminals, NE can diffuse through the bone marrow to interact with adrenergic receptors present on vascular endothelial and smooth muscle cells and on a variety of bone marrow cells.

The presence of NA nerves adjacent to the vasculature suggests that NE may have vasomotor activity, controlling blood flow and volume within the bone marrow. Stimulation of sympathetic nerves that innervate bone marrow causes a release of reticulocytes (125,559). Stimulation of the posterior hypothalamus (149) may activate descending sympathetic innervation to produce this effect. It is not clear whether the release of reticulocytes is due to a direct action of NE on these cells or to an indirect action of NE on the vasculature. NE also mobilizes fat from the bone marrow (535).

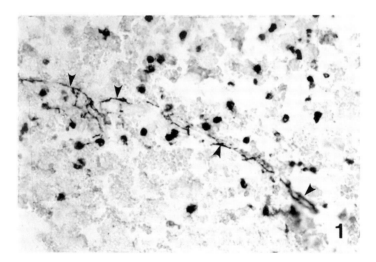

Fig. 8-1. TH[+] nerves (arrowheads) surround a blood vessel in the bone marrow of the rat femur. Single-label ICC for TH; ×110. (Courtesy of Kim Gibson-Berry, Department of Neurobiology and Anatomy, University of Rochester School of Medicine.)

Thymus

NA sympathetic innervation of the thymus originates from postganglionic cell bodies in the upper paravertebral ganglia of the sympathetic chain, primarily the superior cervical (SCG) and stellate ganglia (75,366,532). NA innervation of the thymus is well characterized in the rodent thymus (34,45,75,153,157,164,366,478,571,572; reviewed in 153,163). NA fibers enter the thymus adjacent to large blood vessels as dense vascular plexuses, and travel in the capsule and interlobular septa, or continue with the vasculature into the cortex (Fig. 8-2). From these plexuses, NA nerves appear to course along very fine septa into the cortical region, in close proximity to thymocytes (less than 1 μm). Cortical fibers often reside in close proximity to cells with yellow auto-fluorescence (CAF) a macrophage-like cell in the cortex. In the capsule and septa, NA nerve fibers, as well as peptidergic nerves, course adjacent to mast cells. At the corticomedullary junction, NA nerves are present along the medullary venous sinuses, which are continuous with the system of innervated vessels in the septa. NA fibers extend from these sinuses into the adjacent cortical region, and occasionally into the medullary parenchyma. Neurochemical analysis of CAs in the thymus indicates that virtually all of the CA-containing nerves are NA.

Without the presence of any diffusion barrier, it is likely that NE released from NA nerves can interact with thymocytes, particularly because extensive diffusion of NE from sympathetic postganglionic nerves is well documented in other peripheral target organs. The functional significance of NA innervation of the thymus is not clear. Experimental studies by Singh and colleagues (492,493,495,496,498,499) suggest that

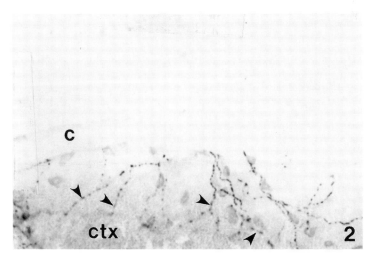

Fig. 8-2. TH+ nerves (arrowheads) travel from the capsule (c) into the cortex (ctx) of the rat thymus. Single-label ICC for TH; ×215.

NE exerts an effect on the maturation of thymocytes, since it inhibits proliferation and promotes differentiation of thymocytes in vitro. This effect is mediated through the activation of β-adrenergic receptors via adenosine 3'-5'-cyclic monophosphate (cAMP) as a second messenger (reviewed in 154,308).

Spleen

Innervation of the spleen has been studied more widely than innervation of any other lymphoid organ. Both fluorescence histochemical localization of CAs and ICC staining for localization of TH or NE demonstrate robust NA sympathetic innervation of the spleen in a variety of species, including humans (285), dog (117), cat (167,169), beluga whale (447), mouse (45,88,435,571), rat (7–9,29,33,38,165,166,170; reviewed in 6,36,37,154,158,164,227,308), African lungfish (3), dogfish (3), cod (370,574), and cane toad (369).

NA nerves that distribute to the rat spleen derive from postganglionic cell bodies mainly in the superior mesenteric–celiac ganglionic complex (SMCG) (38,152,365), and to a lesser extent, the sympathetic trunk (365) that sends fibers through the SMCG. NA nerves enter the spleen as a dense plexus associated with the splenic artery and its branches beneath the capsule of the spleen. NA fibers from this subcapsular plexus plunge into the depths of the spleen along the trabeculae and its associated vasculature. NA plexuses follow the central arterioles and their branches into the white pulp of the spleen (Fig. 8-3). NA nerve fibers exit this vascular plexus and travel into the surrounding periarteriolar lymphatic sheaths (PALS), regions composed primarily of T-lymphocytes. The extent to which these NA fibers actually branch from vascular plexuses into the parenchyma needs to be further verified.

In transgenic mice that over express nerve growth factor (NGF) in the skin and other epithelial structures, the marginal zone is hyperinnervated compared with control mice (86). Further, concanavalin A (Con A)-induced proliferation is suppressed in splenocytes from NGF transgenic mice suggesting that NGF-induced sympathetic hyperinnervation of the spleen has functional consequences on immune response (86).

.60Ackerman et al. (5,6,9) found that NA nerve fibers enter the parenchymal lymphoid component of the 1-day-old rat spleen and form neuroeffector junctions with lymphocytes and macrophages at a time before smooth muscle even exists along the vasculature and before NA fibers along the vasculature can be found. NA nerves are also present along the marginal sinus and in the marginal zone along blood vessels, in nerve bundles, or as free fibers that course adjacent to B-lymphocytes and macrophages. Occasionally, NA fibers are found in the follicles among B-lymphocytes, but this is seen more frequently in neonatal development. In the red pulp, NA fibers are found along the trabeculae and venous sinuses that drain splenic blood. A few fibers can be seen exiting these plexuses to course through the parenchyma of the red pulp.

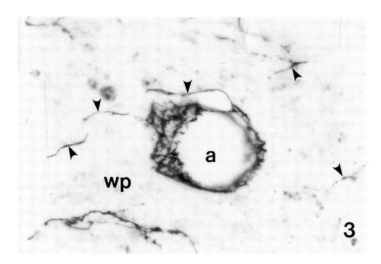

Fig. 8-3. TH$^+$ nerves form a dense plexus around the central arteriole (a) of the rat splenic white pulp (wp). TH$^+$ nerve fibers (arrowheads) extend from this plexus into the surrounding PALS. Single-label ICC for TH; ×215.

ICC studies for the localization of TH confirm and extend observations with fluorescence histochemistry (8,9,29,165). Spleen sections stained with antibodies directed against TH and antibodies directed against surface antigens specific for different populations of immunocytes reveal the anatomical relationship of TH$^+$ nerves with specific populations of cells of the immune system. In the PALS, TH$^+$ nerves (Fig. 8-4) reside in close proximity to T-lymphocytes of both the T-helper and T-cytotoxic/suppressor subsets. TH$^+$ nerves also course along the marginal sinus adjacent to ED3$^+$ macrophages, and in the marginal zone in close association with ED3$^+$ macrophages (Fig. 8-5) and immunoglobulin (Ig)M$^+$ B-lymphocytes (Fig. 8-6). Only an occasional TH$^+$ nerve fiber is present among IgM$^+$ B-lymphocytes in the follicle.

Electron microscopic (EM) examination of ICC sections stained for TH (165) have revealed TH$^+$ nerve terminals adjacent to smooth muscle cells of the central arteriole (Fig. 8-7). Like typical sympathetic synapses in other non-lymphoid target organs, TH$^+$ terminals are separated from these smooth muscle cells by a basement membrane and often by additional cell processes. These neuroeffector junctions are in the range of 150 nm or more. Surprisingly, TH$^+$ nerve terminals are also found in direct contact with lymphocytes in the PALS (Fig. 8-8), at sites distant from the central arterioles. These terminals possess long, smooth zones of contact with lymphocyte plasma membranes, separated by as little as 6 nm. In many cases, the TH$^+$ terminals indent along the lymphocyte membrane. Similar close appositions are present at the marginal sinus and in the marginal zone between TH$^+$ nerve terminals and lymphocytes and macro-

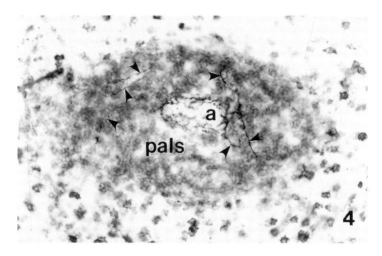

Fig. 8-4. Linear varicose TH⁺ nerves surround the central arteriole in the white pulp of the rat spleen. TH⁺ fibers (arrowheads) exit this plexus and run adjacent to OX19⁺ T-lymphocytes (cell membrane staining of spherically shaped cells) in the periarteriolar lymphatic sheath (pals). Double-label ICC for TH and OX19 (a pan T lymphocyte marker); ×110.

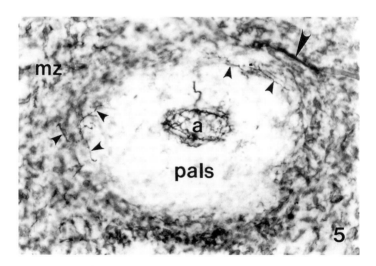

Fig. 8-5. Linear TH⁺ nerves (small arrowheads) are present at the site of the marginal sinus and in the marginal zone (mz) adjacent to ED3⁺ macrophages (stellate-shaped cellular staining) as individual profiles and in a large TH⁺ nerve bundle (large arrowhead). TH⁺ nerves also surround the central arteriole (a) and in the adjacent periarteriolar lymphatic sheath (pals). Double-label ICC for TH and ED3 (a marker for macrophages in the inner and outer marginal zone); ×110.

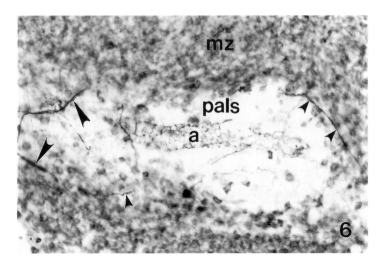

Fig. 8-6. TH[+] nerves reside in bundles (large arrowheads) or as free fibers (small arrowheads) among IgM[+] B-lymphocytes (cell membrane staining reveals spherically shaped cells) in the marginal zone (mz). Double-label ICC for TH and IgM. a, central arteriole; pals, periarteriolar lymphatic sheath; ×110.

phages. No postsynaptic specializations are apparent. However, such CNS-type synaptic specialization is rarely found at any peripheral sympathetic neuroeffector junctions with any target cells. These TH[+] profiles are not present in spleens denervated either by 6-hydroxydopamine (6-OHDA, a neurotoxin that destroys nerve terminals) or by ganglionectomy, or in ICC-stained tissue sections incubated with goat anti-rabbit IgG (the secondary antibody) alone.

Lymph Nodes

Fluorescence histochemical and ICC staining for NA sympathetic innervation of lymph nodes in rats (200) and several strains of mice (7,8,30,37,154,159) reveal dense plexuses of NA nerves along blood vessels at the hilus, the presumed point of entry of NA nerves. In lymph nodes, NA nerves travel in a subcapsular plexus or continue in vascular plexuses through the medullary cords. NA fibers distribute adjacent to many lymphoid cell types and to both vascular and lymphatic channels in the medulla. These fibers continue with small vessels that course from the medulla into the paracortical regions, which are rich in T-lymphocytes. Single NA profiles exit these plexuses and travel in the paracortical parenchyma. NA fibers that contribute to subcapsular plexuses also course along small vessels into the cortex and give off individual fibers that project into the cortical parenchyma. Linear fibers that enter into T-lymphocyte com-

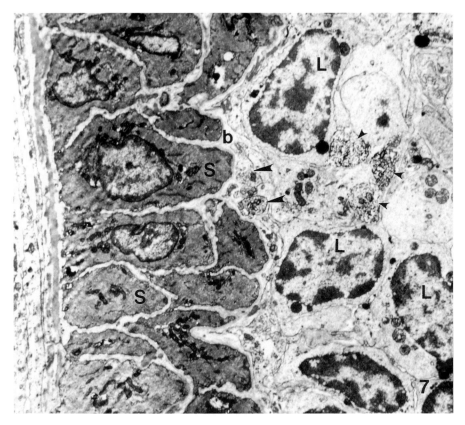

Fig. 8-7. TH$^+$ nerve terminals directly contact the basement membrane (b) of smooth muscle (s) of the central arteriole (large arrowheads), as well as lymphocytes (L) (small arrowheads) in the periarteriolar lymphatic sheath of the rat spleen. Single-label ICC for TH with TEM; ×6,860.

partments of the cortex and paracortex do not travel into the adjacent nodular regions and germinal centers where B-lymphocytes predominate. Dopamine β-hydroxylase$^+$ (an enzyme that converts the precursor, dopamine, to NE) nerve fibers have also been demonstrated in lymph nodes from rats, guinea-pigs, mice, cats, pigs, and humans (172).

In NGF transgenic mice where NGF is over expressed by the skin, peripheral lymph nodes that drain the skin are more densely innervated compared to peripheral lymph nodes from control mice, and compared to mesenteric lymph nodes from transgenic and control mice (86). NGF concentration in peripheral lymph nodes is also elevated thirteen-fold. These findings suggest that NGF provides trophic influence on sympathetic nerves in this genetic mouse model.

At the ultrastructural level, Novotny and colleagues (375,376) have described axonal profiles with synaptic vesicles, presumed to be NA, in close proximity to vascular

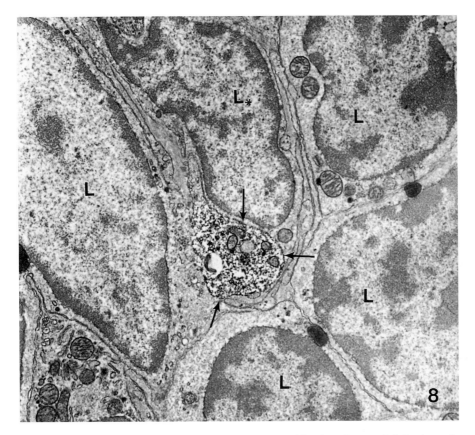

Fig. 8-8. TH$^+$ nerve terminal (arrows) in direct contact with a lymphocyte (L*) in the periarteriolar lymphatic sheath in the rat spleen. Single-label ICC for TH with TEM. L, lymphocyte; ×10,600.

smooth muscle, reticular cells, plasma cells, and lymphocytes. They report at least three different vesicle populations and suggest that these populations result from colocalization of peptides. NA nerves also travel along lymphatic vessels (13) forming a loose network in the adventitia of the lymph vessel, where they are proposed to regulate vessel contraction.

The origin of NA innervation of lymph nodes has not been thoroughly investigated. Removal of the SCG decreases NA innervation of the cervical nodes in the rat (200). It is presumed that since lymph nodes are regional structures draining the areas with which they are associated, their innervation must also be regional.

The compartmentalization of NA nerves in lymph nodes displays many similarities with NA innervation of the spleen, suggesting a common functional role in both organs (see Table 8-1) (reviewed in 154). A role for NE in antigen processing, i.e., antigen

Table 8-1 Noradrenergic Innvervation of Functional Compartments of Secondary Lymphoid Organs

Compartments with NA Innvervation	Functional Significance of Compartment
Spleen	
Marginal zone (macrophages/B-lymphocytes)	Site of lymphocyte entry
Marginal zone (macrophages/B-lymphocytes)	Site of antigen capture
PALS (T-lymphocytes)	Site of antigen presentation/lymphocyte activation
Parafollicular/marginal zone (macrophages/ B-lymphocytes)	Site of antigen presentation/lymphocyte activation
Outer marginal zone	Site of lymphocyte egress
Lymph node	
Corticomedullary junction	Site of lymphocyte entry
Subcapsular sinus	Site of antigen capture
Paracortex	Site of antigen presentation/lymphocyte activation
Medullary cords	Site of antigen presentation/lymphocyte activation
Medullary sinuses	Site of lymphocyte egress

capture and antigen presentation, is supported by studies showing reduced primary antibody responses in spleen and lymph nodes following sympathetic denervation (308). Egress of activated lymphocytes into the circulation from spleen and lymph nodes occurs following the infusion of CAs (37,138,154), suggesting an additional role for NE at these secondary lymphoid organs in lymphocyte trafficking.

Gut-Associated Lymphoid Tissue (GALT) and other Lymphoid Tissue

The more diffuse accumulations of lymphoid tissue in the mucosa of the gastrointestinal and respiratory systems make interpretation of innervation more difficult. It is not clear whether the nerve fibers that are present signal lymphoid components, or whether other non-lymphoid components with the lymphoid elements come into proximity of nerve profile by chance. In some regions of the gut, lymphoid tissue forms discrete compartments, including tonsils, Peyer's patches, and appendix, that are integral and large and clearly important compartments of the gut-associated immune system. If one assumes that innervation is present, transmitter is released and binds to the appropriate receptor on target cells, and the target cell is altered intracellularly by this ligand-receptor interaction, then classic criteria for neurotransmission are met. In vitro studies show that transient exposure of lymphocytes or other immunocytes to a variety of neurotransmitters can result in profound functional alterations (reviewed in 41). It does not matter if the association with the target cell is transient; this may be the case for some cells in other lymphoid organs as well, such as the spleen and thymus. It is likely that the presence of the target cell is the result of a previous interaction of receptors with transmitter substances, such as vasoactive intestinal polypeptide (VIP), that determines the migration of the cell to that location, as shown in the elegant studies by Ottaway (385,386,390,392). He has demonstrated that the expression of VIP receptors on murine T-lymphocytes mediates cell homing to Peyer's patches and mesenteric lymph nodes. Very high concentrations of VIP in mesenteric lymph nodes in the rat that are not seen in spleen, thymus, or lymph nodes from other sites in the body support his findings (39).

Sympathetic NA innervation has also been described in the human palatine tonsils (577), the rabbit appendix (161), the sacculus rotundus and Peyer's patches of the rabbit (250), and the bursa of Fabricius of the chicken (239). Even though the bursa of Fabricius is considered a primary lymphoid organ in birds, it is associated with, and anatomically similar to, other GALT.

In the tonsil (577), NA nerves distribute in dense perivascular plexuses, particularly along the arteries. Individual fluorescent profiles enter parafollicular regions of the tonsil, but no fibers travel into the epithelium or the lymphoid nodules. In the rabbit appendix (161), NA nerves enter lymphoid tissue with the vasculature and muscularis interna. NA fibers travel longitudinally inside the muscularis interna for short distances until they reach a zone between lymphoid nodules. These NA plexuses turn radially to course perpendicular to the long axis of the lumen and continue toward the lumen between the large lymphoid nodules. Like the tonsil, no fibers enter the lymphoid nodule. NA nerves traverse through interdomal zones of T-lymphocytes between lymphoid nodules at the entrance to the lamina propria. NA fibers then enter the lamina propria, traveling along small blood vessels and arborizing into the surrounding parenchyma to end among lymphocytes, enterochromaffin cells (some of which may contain serotonin), and other accessory cells. They also form delicate arborizations in the subepithelial region adjacent to plasma cells.

The general pattern of NA innervation in the sacculus rotundus and Peyer's patches (250) is similar to that in the appendix. However, the enterochromaffin cells that are juxtaposed with NA terminals are more abundant in the appendix. A similar pattern of innervation is present in the bursa of Fabricius. NA nerves form perivascular plexuses in the perimuscular connective tissue, muscle, and mucosa, often in close proximity to autofluorescent cells. Fine, linear fibers travel between the lymphoid nodules, but do not enter the nodules. NA fibers are also not found in the epithelium.

Peptidergic Nerves in Lymphoid Organs

More recently, we and others have begun to explore the presence and role of peptide-containing nerves in lymphoid organs (reviewed in 41,163). Identification of peptidergic nerves in lymphoid organs has been determined by ICC with antibodies directed against the neuropeptide of interest. Thus far, there is substantial evidence for nerves containing neuropeptide Y (NPY), substance P (SP), calcitonin gene-related peptide (CGRP), VIP, somatostatin (SOM), and opiate peptides in lymphoid organs.

These neuropeptides are sometimes colocalized with classical amines (i.e., NPY with NE) or with other neuropeptide transmitters (i.e., SP and CGRP).

Additionally, there is recent evidence to suggest that in vivo administration of some cytokines, or activation of the immune system, can reveal nerve fibers that contain peptides (i.e., corticotropin-releasing factor [CRF], SP, and CGRP) in lymphoid organs that are not visualized with ICC staining in these organs from vehicle-treated animals (135; D. L. Bellinger, unpublished observations).

Bone Marrow

The identification of neurotransmitter-specific nerves innervating the bone marrow, other than NA sympathetic nerves, is not clearly established. Using general histological staining methods (such as silver stains and methylene blue) and EM (82,83,125,305), nerve bundles are found that supply the periosteum and enter the interior of the bone via the nutrient foramena to the medulla. These medullary bundles, consisting of both myelinated and unmyelinated nerve fibers, then distribute in a fashion similar to the branching of the nutrient artery. Some of these fibers enter the parenchyma to course among blood-forming cells in the marrow. Clearly some, but not all, of these nerves are NA (125), since sympathectomy results in the degeneration of some of these fibers (262,524).

The localization of peptidergic nerves with ICC in the bone marrow has been hampered by the difficulty preserving antigenicity with standard decalcification methods used in the tissue preparation of bone. Recently, we have overcome this problem with staining for PGP 9.5 (a general neuronal marker), TH, and NPY (196). NPY[+] profiles have a distribution similar to that of NA nerves, traveling adjacent to the vasculature and in the parenchyma among hemopoietic and lymphopoietic cells in the marrow (Fig. 8-9).

PGP 9.5 staining (Fig. 8-10) reveals a greater density of nerve profiles associated with the vasculature and in the marrow parenchyma than is seen with TH- or NPY-staining, indicating the presence of non-NA sympathetic nerve fibers. In support of these findings, Bjurholm et al. (51) report SP[+] and CGRP[+] nerves in the bone marrow. The pattern of distribution of these two types of nerves is similar, although CGRP[+] fibers are more numerous. Varicose, winding fibers are present among hemopoietic cells of the bone marrow and generally do not course along the vasculature. Long, non-varicose fibers course along the bone trabeculae and in close relation to blood vessels in the marrow.

Thymus

In the mammalian thymus, nerve fibers stained with ICC for NPY, tachykinins (TKs) (SP, neurokinin A and B, collectively), SP, CGRP, and VIP are present (36,41, 76,157,172,315,561). NPY[+] nerves (41,561) provide the most extensive inner-

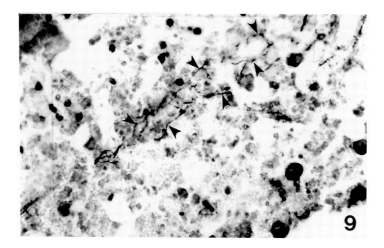

Fig. 8-9. NPY⁺ nerves (arrowheads) form a dense plexus around a blood vessel in the bone marrow of the rat femur. Single-label ICC for NPY; ×215.

vation of the thymus to date. The distribution of NPY⁺ nerves overlaps with the NA innervation of the thymus. NPY⁺ fibers travel in bundles that enter the thymus through the capsule or with surface arteries that extend along the thymic capsule and traverse the interlobular septa. From these plexuses, NPY⁺ nerves (Fig. 8-11) extend into superficial and deep cortical regions to arborize among thymocytes and other support

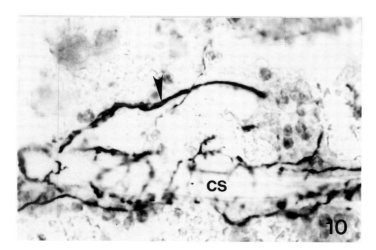

Fig. 8-10. PGP 9.5⁺ nerves distribute as individual fibers or as nerve bundles (large arrowheads) along the central sinus (cs) and in the surrounding parenchyma of the bone marrow of the rat femur. Single-label ICC for PGP 9.5 (a general marker for nerve fibers); ×215. (Courtesy of Kim Gibson-Berry, Department of Neurobiology and Anatomy, University of Rochester School of Medicine.)

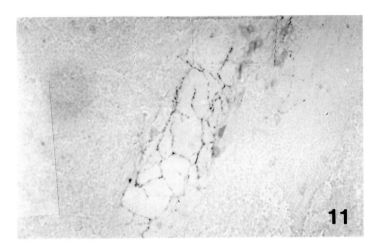

Fig. 8-11. NPY+ nerves course along a blood vessel in the cortex of the rat thymus. Single-label ICC for NPY; bar = μm.

ive cells of the thymus. The densest innervation occurs at the corticomedullary junction. NPY+ profiles are also found in the medulla along the vasculature adjacent to the corticomedullary junction.

The thymus also receives innervation from numerous SP- and CGRP-containing nerve fibers (36,41,76,172,561). SP+ and CGRP+ nerves enter the thymus along the capsule and travel along the interlobular septa, where they frequently reside adjacent to mast cells (Fig. 8-12). An occasional nerve fiber exits from the interlobular septa to

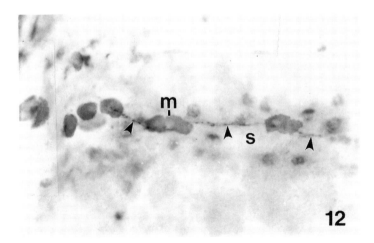

Fig. 8-12. CGRP+ nerve fibers (arrowheads) traverse adjacent to mast cells (m) in an interlobular septum (s) of the rat thymus. Single-label ICC for CGRP; ×215.

pass among immature thymocytes in the parenchyma of the cortex or to enter the medulla (Fig. 8-13). SP$^+$ and CGRP$^+$ fibers also course along blood vessels, particularly those of the corticomedullary boundary, and are found in close association with the large number of mast cells also present along these vessels. Treatment with capsaicin, a neurotoxin specific for SP$^+$ nerve terminals when administered in low concentrations, depletes SP in the thymus (194), indicating that SP resides in neural compartments. The distribution of CGRP$^+$ nerves in the thymus closely overlaps the distribution of SP$^+$ staining. However, based on neurochemical measurements of SP and CGRP using radioimmunoassay following capsaicin treatment, these two peptides do not appear to be colocalized in the thymus (193).

We have also found VIP$^+$ nerve fibers are present in the thymus (41,157). VIP$^+$ nerves have a different pattern of innervation than SP and CGRP. Most VIP$^+$ fibers are present in the capsule and interlobular septa, often residing close to mast cells (Fig. 8-14). Some VIP$^+$ nerves are also seen along blood vessels at the corticomedullary junction and perivascular mast cells, and as free fibers in the capsule, cortex, and medulla (Fig. 8-15). This association of peptide-containing nerves with mast cells is similar to that described in mucosa of the gut (516) and may be a source of neuropeptide signals for regulation of mast cell secretion.

A recent report by Weihe et al. (561) describing the distribution of TK$^+$, CGRP$^+$, and NPY$^+$ fibers in the rat thymus, supports our earlier findings. Most of these fibers form perivascular plexuses and come in close proximity to mast cells, with TK and CGRP displaying similar distribution patterns. These investigators suggest that TK and CGRP serve a sensory function, and that NPY may colocalize with sympathetic fibers of the vasculature. However, until appropriate tracing studies are done, the identity of

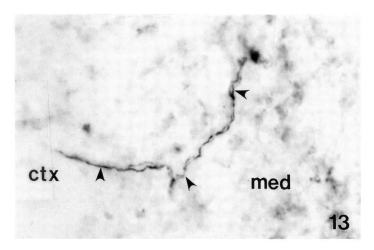

Fig. 8-13. SP$^+$ nerves (arrowheads) travel among thymocytes at the corticomedullary junction of the rat thymus. Single-label ICC for SP. ctx, cortex; med, medulla; ×215.

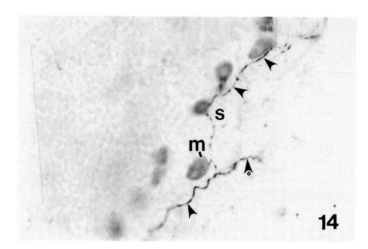

Fig. 8-14. VIP+ nerves (arrowheads) are present in close proximity to mast cells (m) in the interlobular septum (s) of the rat thymus. An occasional VIP+ fiber (open circle-arrowhead) exits this plexus into the adjacent thymic cortex. Single-label ICC for VIP; ×215.

TK+ and CGRP+ nerves as primary sensory afferents must be viewed with caution and considered unsubstantiated.

Myelinated fibers travel in nerve bundles in the capsule and septa of the murine and human thymus. While they have not been demonstrated in the parenchyma of the thymus, the finding of SP+ and CGRP+ nerves in the parenchyma, some of which possibly derive from dorsal root ganglia, may indicate sensory innervation. ICC staining for oxytocin, vasopressin, and associated neurophysins is present in epithelial cells,

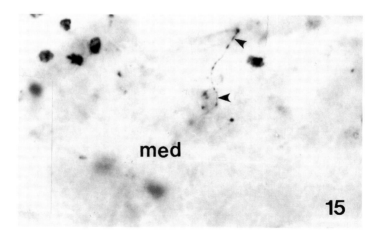

Fig. 8-15. VIP+ varicose profile (arrowheads) in the rat thymic medulla (med). Single-label ICC for VIP; ×215.

nurse cells, and other non-neural elements in the human thymus (106,190,191,335) but has not been reported in nerves. Recently, we have found CRF-containing nerves in the thymus and spleen 12 and 24 hours after intraperitoneal injection of human recombinant IL-2 into Fischer 344 rats (D. L. Bellinger, unpublished observations).

Spleen

Early observations from our laboratories using immunofluorescent techniques reported the presence of immunoreactive profiles for NPY, Met-enkephalin, cholecystokinin (CCK), and neurotensin (NT) along the central arteriole of the white pulp and its smaller branches, with only sparse fibers of most of these peptides entering the parenchyma (157). Lundberg et al. (321) reported NPY, SP, and VIP innervation of the splenic vasculature on which the nerves produce vascular and volume control. These investigators did not further describe the distribution of these nerves in specific compartments of the spleen. Using light microscopic ICC methods, we demonstrated NPY+, SP+, and CGRP+ nerves along the vasculature and in lymphoid compartments of the spleen (41,314,316,384,446–448). The distribution of NPY+ nerves (41,384,446,448) parallel NA innervation of the spleen. NPY+ nerves travel along the capsular, trabecular, and venous systems, and along the arterial systems, including prominent innervation of the central arterioles in the white pulp. NPY+ nerves (Fig. 8-16) arborize into the surrounding PALS away from the central arteriolar plexuses; these fibers end among T-lymphocytes. Additional NPY+ fibers extend along the marginal sinus and are scattered in the marginal zone, where they branch among

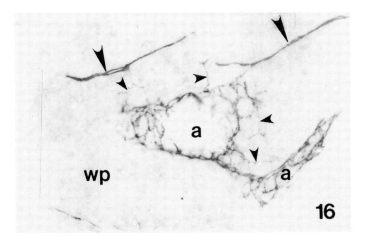

Fig. 8-16. NPY+ staining demonstrates a dense plexus of NPY+ nerves surrounding the central arteriole (a) of the rat spleen. Additional NPY+ nerves (small arrowheads) exit this plexus to travel among T lymphocytes in the PALS. Large NPY+ nerve bundles (large arrowheads) also occur in the white pulp (wp) of the spleen. Single-label ICC for NPY; ×215.

B-lymphocytes and macrophages. Ultrastructural analysis of ICC-stained spleen sections revealed direct contacts between NPY$^+$ terminals and lymphocytes, similar to those seen for TH$^+$ terminals (384,446).

Romano and colleague (446) have shown that destruction of sympathetic NA nerves with 6-OHDA depletes NPY and eliminates NPY$^+$ profiles in ICC-stained sections. By differential staining of consecutive tissue sections, they showed direct colocalization of TH and NPY in some nerve fibers in the rat spleen. Studies of the bovine splenic nerve (182) demonstrated NE and NPY colocalized in large, dense core vesicles with enkephalins. Immunofluorescence staining also supports colocalization of these neurotransmitters in some nerves along the large blood vessels near their entry into the bovine spleen. NE and NPY colocalize in vascular and trabecular nerves of spleens from cats (321) and pigs (322), where NPY is believed to mediate vasoconstriction and possibly play a neuromodulatory role, enhancing the action of NE on the vasculature. A report by Schultzberg and colleagues (470) described IL-1-containing nerve fibers in the spleen, perhaps colocalized in sympathetic NA nerves.

Fried and colleagues (182) reported the presence of SP-, SOM-, and VIP-immunoreactive nerve profiles in the bovine splenic nerve that are not colocalized with NE. VIP also was described along the vasculature in the cat spleen (321). Infusion of VIP results in vasodilation and increased splenic volume, suggesting that VIP may exert at least some of its effects directly on the vasculature. Similarly, we found a sparse VIP innervation of the splenic vasculature (41,157) and adjacent PALS, and relatively low VIP concentration in the rat spleen (31). VIP$^+$ nerves course along the venous sinuses and trabeculae, in the red pulp, in the marginal zone, and along the central artery and in the adjacent PALS (Fig. 8-17). The sparcity of VIP-

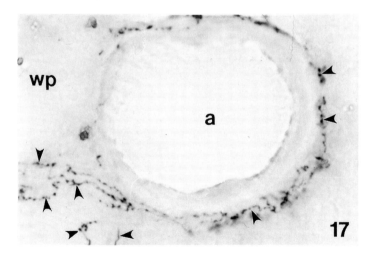

Fig. 8-17. VIP$^+$ fibers (arrowheads) are present around the central arteriole (a) and in the adjacent periarteriolar lymphatic sheath of the rat splenic white pulp (wp). Single-label ICC for VIP; ×215.

immunoreactive fibers in the spleen is supported by the findings of Chevendra and Weaver (100) indicating that less than 1% of the mesenteric neurons that innervate the spleen is immunoreactive for VIP. VIP-immunoreactivity is also present in cells of the immune system, suggesting an additional source of VIP in the spleen (reviewed in 39).

SP$^+$ and CGRP$^+$ nerves (36,41,314,316) also appear to have overlapping distributions in the rat spleen, but a distribution distinct from that of TH$^+$, NPY$^+$, or VIP$^+$ nerve fibers. Overall, the spleen is more densely innervated by CGRP$^+$ profiles. SP$^+$ (Fig. 8-18) and CGRP$^+$ (Fig. 8-19) nerves travel along the large venous sinuses and extend from these sinuses along the trabeculae. Numerous linear SP$^+$ and CGRP$^+$ nerves extend from the venous plexuses and trabeculae into the surrounding red pulp. SP$^+$ and CGRP$^+$ long, linear profiles occasionally travel through the marginal zone (Fig. 8-20), and to a lesser extent, the PALS (Fig. 8-21). SP$^+$ fibers are sometimes present adjacent to large arteries near the hilus of the spleen, which is presumably their site of entry into the spleen. Lundberg et al. (32) also have described SP$^+$ fibers in the splenic nerve and around the arteries and arterioles in the cat spleen, but do not further describe fibers in other splenic compartments. Infusion of SP reduces perfusion pressure but also reduces splenic volume as a result of capsule contraction. Whether SP$^+$ and CGRP$^+$ nerves in the spleen represent sensory innervation is not clear. Very few myelinated fibers are reported in the splenic nerve (22,168), and none are thus far described within the spleen itself. Tracing studies reveal very few labeled cells in sensory ganglia (38,365). In a careful tracing study by Baron and Jänig (22) only 5% of the fibers in the splenic nerve of the cat are sensory. Anterograde tracing of primary sensory afferents from throacic dorsal root ganglia (T7-T12) also indicates the existence of sensory nerve fibers that contain SP and CGRP in the guinea-pig spleen (132). Physiological evidence of reflexes between the spleen and kidney indicates that some fibers are able to evoke reflex responses (reviewed in 163).

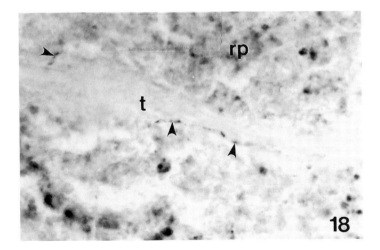

Fig. 8-18. SP$^+$ fibers (arrowheads) travel along the trabeculae (t) in the red pulp (rp) of the rat spleen. Single-label ICC for SP; ×215.

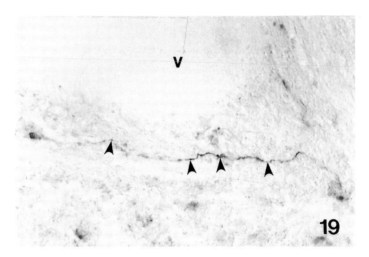

Fig. 8-19. CGRP$^+$ nerves (arrowheads) traverse the venous sinus (v) in the red pulp of the rat spleen. Single-label ICC for CGRP; ×215.

An early report by Felten et al. (157) indicates Met-enkephalin-containing nerves in the rodent spleen. Nohr et al. (372) have recently demonstrated proenkephalin opioid peptides in the porcine and bovine splenic nerves, but were unable to find them in splenic nerves from rats, mice, hamsters, and guinea-pigs. This study confirms earlier work by Fried and co-workers (182) who reported enkephalin-immunoreactive nerves in bovine spleen. In addition, Fried et al. (182) have provided evidence that enkephalin is coexpressed with NE and NPY in the splenic nerve. Nohr et al. (372) did not confirm the findings by Felten et al. (157) of enkephalin-containing nerves in the rat spleen.

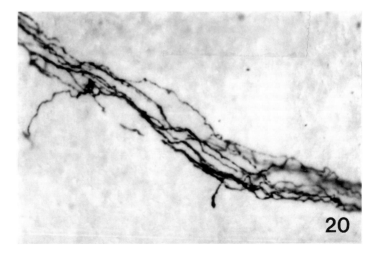

Fig. 8-20. A CGRP$^+$ nerve bundle runs through the inner marginal zone of the rat splenic white pulp. Single-label ICC for CGRP; ×215.

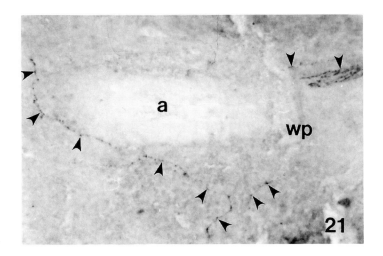

Fig. 8-21. SP⁺ nerves (arrowheads) are distributed along the central arteriole (a) and proceed into the adjacent periarteriolar lymphatic sheath in the white pulp (wp) of the rat spleen. Single-label ICC for SP; ×215.

This discrepancy may be due to the use of antibodies with different specificities, or to rat strain differences. Enkephalin-containing nerves form a dense plexus along blood vessels in the spleen suggesting a functional role of opioid peptides in modulating vascular effector functions similar to that described for NPY and NE (372). In the PALS, numerous peri- and paravascular proenkephalin-immunoreactive fibers course in close apposition to lymphocytes and reticular cells. Proenkephalin-immunoreactive fibers also reside in the red pulp.

Lymph Nodes

Immunoreactivity for NPY, VIP, SP, CGRP, peptide histidine isoleucine (PHI), dynorphin A, and CCK in nerves has been described in lymph nodes in a variety of mammalian species (41,163,172,286,424,449) including rat, mouse, guinea-pig, cat, pig, and human. VIP⁺ nerve fibers are found along the vasculature in internodal regions of the cortex, with meager innervation of surrounding parenchyma, and along medullary cords (Fig. 8-22) (172,424). VIP and PHI staining overlap in their distribution and may be colocalized. These fibers generally are found in association with the vasculature. Based on radioimmunoassay for VIP, VIP⁺ nerves may be much more abundant in mesenteric lymph nodes than in popliteal lymph nodes (31). Dynorphin A⁺ and CCK⁺ profiles travel in the medulla of lymph nodes from the guinea-pig (286). Retrograde tracing studies in Wistar rats indicate separate NPY- and proenkephalin-containing neurons in the SCG project to the submaxillary lymph nodes (449).

Studies from our laboratories demonstrated NPY-, SP-, and CGRP-immunoreactive nerve fibers in mesenteric, popliteal, and inguinal lymph nodes of the rat (41,163). The

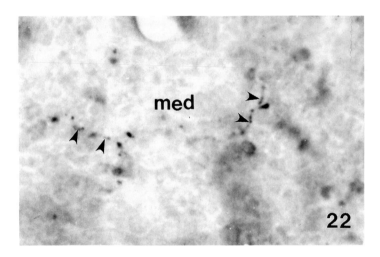

Fig. 8-22. VIP+ nerves (arrowheads) traversing the medulla (med) of the rat mesenteric lymph node. Single-label ICC for VIP; ×215.

distribution of NPY+ nerves again appears to overlap NA innervation. NPY+ nerves (Fig. 8-23) course along blood vessels in the hilus, medullary, and interfollicular regions of lymph nodes. Some NPY+ fibers are present as linear profiles in the parenchyma in paracortical and cortical regions, where they end among fields of lymphocytes. SP+ and CGRP+ nerves (Fig. 8-24) closely overlap in their distribution in lymph nodes and are found in the hilus, beneath the capsule, at the corticomedullary junction, in medullary regions, and in internodal regions of the lymph nodes. These

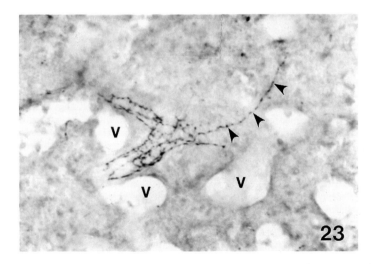

Fig. 8-23. NPY+ nerve fibers associated with a vascular plexus in the medullary cords near the hilus of a rat mesenteric lymph node. Some linear fibers (arrowheads) radiate into the cords from this plexus. Single-label ICC for NPY. v, venous sinus; ×215.

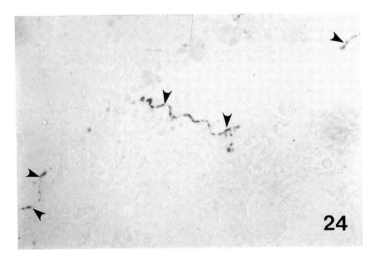

Fig. 8-24. CGRP$^+$ nerves (arrowheads) run through the cortex of a rat mesenteric lymph node. Single-label ICC for CGRP; ×215.

nerve fibers course along the vasculature or branch into the parenchyma among lymphocytes and accessory cells.

GALT

Direct demonstration of peptidergic nerves innervating lymphoid components of the gut is incomplete (reviewed in 515). Early studies using silver stains of the bursa of Fabricius indicate nerves within the nodules (110,238). These are not likely to be NA nerves, since fluorescence histochemistry fails to reveal NA nerves in lymphoid nodules. An ultrastructural study of Peyer's patches from the Syrian hamster demonstrated nonmyelinated nerve bundles traversing the lymphoid follicles (420). Within the lymphoid nodule, free nerve fibers containing snyaptic vesicle aggregates reside within 20 nm of reticular cells and lymphocytes. Similar direct contacts were reported between catecholaminergic nerve terminals and plasma cells in the lacrimal gland of the pigeon (552) and between nonmyelinated nerve endings and small lymphocytes in the jugular body, a lymphomyeloid organ, of the leopard frog (583). A variety of peptidergic nerves reside in the lamina propria (109,131,426), which contains large numbers of lymphocytes, plasma cells, mast cells, and macrophages, including SP-, SOM-, VIP-, CCK-, and CGRP-containing nerves.

VIP$^+$ nerve fibers are present in murine (392) and cat (236) Peyer's patches, coursing predominantly along small caliber blood vessels. In the human colon, SP$^+$ nerves are closely apposed to both T$_4$-cells and IgA-bearing B-cells (565). SOM-immunoreactive nerves have also been described in the Peyer's patches from cats (147). SOM$^+$ nerves and SOM$^+$ cell bodies of enteric neurons are present in the tela submucosa very close to the Peyer's patches. SOM$^+$ (147) and VIP$^+$ (392,236) fibers course along the margin of the follicle and few fibers are found in the follicle. With EM analysis, very close contacts of SOM-immunoreactive nerves with lymphocytes and plasma cells (gap junction of 20–200 nm) with no Schwann cell sheath interposed have been observed (147).

The mast cell is one cell type that has received a great deal of attention as a potential target for neural signals in the gut and elsewhere. Numerous investigators have reported nerve fibers in close contact with mast cells. With ICC, Stead et al. (516) demonstrated close associations between SP$^+$ and CGRP$^+$ nerve fibers and mast cells in the lamina propria of the jejunum intestinal mucosa. Skofitsch and co-workers (502) reported SP$^+$ nerve terminals in contact with mast cells in the rat diaphragm and mesentery. Functional studies indicate that SP can induce release of histamine from mast cells (502). VIP-, CGRP-, SP-, and SOM-containing nerves have also been described in the rat mesentery where there is a close anatomical relationship with serotonin$^+$ mast cells (116). It should be noted that similar associations between SP$^+$, CGRP$^+$, and VIP$^+$ nerves and mast cells are also reported in the rodent thymus (41,315).

Cholinergic Innervation of Lymphoid Organs

A variety of techniques can be used to demonstrate the presence of cholinergic innervation. With antibodies directed against choline acetyltransferase ChAT), an enzyme necessary for the synthesis of ACh, ICC has been used successfully to demonstrate cholinergic neurons and their projections in the CNS, since other techniques used in conjunction with this method such as measurements of ACh content and ChAT activity can confirm the existence of cholinergic innervation in these sites. In the past, acetylcholinesterase (AChE) staining has been the method of choice for revealing putative cholinergic innervation in many peripheral organs. In lymphoid organs, however, interpretation of AChE staining is greatly complicated because many cellular elements stain positively for AChE, including thymocyte and lymphocyte membranes, reticular cells, dendritic cells, and smooth muscle of the vascular and connective tissue. Furthermore, non-cholinergic nerves, including NA nerve fibers, appear to contain AChE. Thus, given the inherent problems with anatomical staining methods for cholinergic nerves, accurate neurochemical measurements of ACh and measurements of ChAT activity are necessary to even propose the existence of any putative cholinergic nerves in lymphoid organs. For most lymphoid organs, a thorough examination of putative cholinergic innervation is not available.

Bone Marrow

Few studies have examined the possibility of cholinergic innervation of bone marrow. DePace and Webber (125) described AChE$^+$ staining in blood vessel walls of the bone marrow and interpreted these as AChE$^+$ nerve fibers that are sensory in function, although no further experimental evidence is given to support either the cholinergic nature of AChE$^+$ nerve fibers or any sensory function. They reported such nerve fibers within the parenchyma, but found no nerve endings, suggesting that these fibers pass through the area without specific association with hemopoietic cells.

Thymus

Several lines of evidence have been cited to infer cholinergic innervation in the thymus. Studies have been performed using retrograde tracing with horseradish peroxidase (HRP) injected into the mouse and rat thymus to determine the cells of origin of the nerve fibers. They describe labeled neurons in three areas of the brain stem (the retrofacial nucleus, nucleus ambiguus, and the dorsal medullary tegmentum adjacent to the dorsal motor nucleus of the vagus) and three areas of the spinal cord (C2-C4 lateral ventral horn, C2-C4 medial ventral horn, and a group of large motoneurons in the medial ventral horn from the decussation of the pyramids through the C1 segment). Later, work by Bulloch and Pomerantz (75) combined gross anatomical observations with AChE staining to identify AChE$^+$ nerves in the thymus. They reported that the mouse thymus receives AChE$^+$ nerves from the vagus nerve, the phrenic nerve, and the recurrent laryngeal nerve. They further reported that the latter two sources, along with fibers from the sympathetic chain, provide innervation in the subcapsular region, but the investigators have not provided experimental evidence to substantiate this contention. In similar studies in the 1-day-old chick, using retrograde tracing from the thymus, positively-labeled neurons were found in the cervical spinal cord and in the IX and X nerve nuclei of the brain stem (71). More recently, a double-labeling retrograde tracing study by Tollefson and Bullock (532) reported that tracers injected into the thymus and the esophagus adjacent to the thymus label separate cell populations in both the spinal cord and brain stem. However, as many as 30% of cells in the nucleus ambiguus and 20% of cells in the nucleus retrofacial and spinal cord are labeled with both tracers. Double-labeling of these cells was interpreted to indicate that either the tracer diffused directly onto adjacent tissue or into the lymphatics, or that collaterals of vagus nerve fibers innervate these areas.

Nance and co-workers (366) carefully reinvestigated innervation of the thymus by using injections of HRP conjugated to wheat germ agglutinin (WGA-HRP) into the thymus, but using small injection volumes followed by application of wound sealants to eliminate diffusion of the dye from the thymus. They confirmed Bullock and co-workers (74,75) findings of sympathetic innervation, but were unable to verify any labeled cells in the spinal cord and brain stem. Control injections into the esophagus and the longus colli muscles produced extensive labeling of nucleus ambiguus and the cervical spinal cord, respectively. They have suggested the CNS-derived innervation from the dorsal motor nucleus of the vagus to the thymus (532) is an artifact caused by the diffusion of tracer from the thymus onto these adjacent structures. The problem of the diffusion of tracer from peripherally innervated organs is not a new one. Early reports of direct CNS innervation of the pancreas (293) have later been shown to result from diffusion from the organ (181). In fact, the gradual diffusion of the label from an injected organ can produce even denser CNS labeling than direct injection of the tracer into the peritoneum, possibly because slowly diffusing tracers escape phagocytosis by macrophages. In our laboratory, we were unable to show anterograde tracing from the brain stem to the thymus (D. L. Bellinger, unpublished results) using either WGA-HRP or fluorogold, although these labels were transported in an anterograde fashion to the esophagus.

The second line of evidence for cholinergic innervation of the thymus comes from AChE staining. There are many reports in the literature of AChE[+] nerve fibers distributing to the thymus (71,72,75,146). It has been inferred that these nerves derive from branches of the vagus nerve on its course through the diaphragm to innervate other visceral organs. However, AChE staining is not diminished by experimental vagotomy in the rat (366), suggesting that even if some nerve fibers from the vagus do supply the thymus, they most likely are not AChE[+] and are therefore not likely to be cholinergic, or that the AChE component is so minute that vagotomy has little effect on AChE staining. We have performed AChE staining in the thymus and indeed, at both the light and ultrastructural level, there are nerve profiles that are positively stained for AChE, particularly around the vasculature (30,35). Despite this staining, we are not sure that these nerve profiles are cholinergic, since non-cholinergic nerve fibers can also stain for AChE. Clearly, at least some of the AChE is colocalized within NA nerves, because treatment with 6-OHDA, which produces chemical sympathectomy, also diminishes AChE staining in neural profiles in these same sites of the thymus. In our AChE-stained sections of the thymus, the AChE[+] cellular element, which comprises most of the AChE staining, is the more prominent feature. These cellular elements include thymocyte membranes and endoplasmic reticulum of epithelial reticular cells. Similar staining is reported in the human thymus (533). The presence of such large amounts of AChE may be important for neurotransmission with neuropeptides. Besides hydrolyzing ACh, AChE has also been shown to hydrolyze and inactivate SP (103) and perhaps other peptides (104,129,245). Therefore, the presence of AChE[+]-stained profiles, even if they are shown to be nerves, is not evidence for cholinergic innervation.

An alternative to staining for AChE is to use ICC for ChAT. There are no convincing data indicating cholinergic innervation of the thymus using this technique. Fatani and colleagues (146) reported a rather modest density of stained profiles that were presumed to be nerves largely associated with the vasculature, with only a few fibers extending into the parenchyma. They did not report extensive subcapsular plexuses, and contrary to studies using AChE staining that report staining early in ontogeny, these ChAT[+] profiles were not seen until day 17–18 of gestation. If these are nerve fibers, the discrepancy could result from differential expression of genes that code for these two enzymes that are turned on at different time periods during development. Interpretation of ChAT staining with ICC must be done with utmost caution. The enzyme appears to be processed post-translationally, is notoriously unreliable for demonstrating even the most robust peripheral cholinergic nerve fibers, and is problematic for false-positive staining. In a collaborative study between our laboratory and Robert Hamill we have measured ChAT activity and total acetyltransferase activity in lymphoid organs (34,35). In the rat thymus, only a very low level of total activity is measurable, less than the $2 \times$ background activity which is needed to claim that activity is present. This low level of ChAT activity is not consistent with a large cholinergic nerve supply, and it is substantially below the levels detected in other peripheral organs, such as the heart, salivary glands, and penile corpora, that are known to be innervated by parasympathetic cholinergic nerve fibers.

The third line of evidence cited in support of cholinergic innervation of lymphoid organs, the presence of muscarinic receptors on lymphocytes (205,210,338,519), is the best established component of a possible cholinergic link for cells of the immune system. Of course, the presence of muscarinic receptors on cells of the immune system does not provide any clues about a possible ligand, if one exists. Mismatches between localization of presynaptic neurotransmitters and receptors on the responding cells are commonplace both centrally and peripherally. This is not to say that thymocytes that possess muscarinic receptors will never be in a microenvironment where there is ligand to bind to muscarinic receptors. It is possible that muscarinic receptors will become activated on cells that migrate from the thymus into a site (e.g., skin, gut, or lung) where cholinergic nerves are present and can secrete the ligand, ACh. It is also possible that the endogenous ligand for muscarinic receptors on cells of the immune system is a peptide and not yet identified. In summary, at the present time the evidence for cholinergic innervation of the thymus is weak. If cholinergic innervation is present, it is probably minimal when contrasted with innervation of the thymus and with cholinergic innervation of other target tissues.

Spleen

In the spleen, histochemical staining of AChE has been demonstrated by numerous investigators (35,169,285,435). These studies describe the largest compartment of AChE staining to be in cellular elements. These authors are generally cautious in their statements of AChE staining in nerve profiles in the spleen. Kudoh et al. (138) reported AChE[+] nerve fibers associated with trabecular arteries, presuming them to be cholinergic, a contention unsubstantiated by other evidence. We found extensive AChE staining associated with lymphoid and reticular elements of the spleen (35), some of which resemble nerve-like profiles but are not nerves; this supports findings in the earlier literature (169,285,435). In addition, we found AChE staining in nerve-like profiles; however, vagotomy did not alter this staining pattern. Instead, surgical removal of the SMCG totally eliminated all neural and non-neural AChE staining. Chemical sympathectomy with 6-OHDA eliminated some, but not all, of the AChE staining. Collectively, these studies indicate that the majority of AChE staining in the rat spleen is non-neural, and that AChE staining present in nerves derives from sympathetic NA nerves as well as from non-NA non-vagal nerves. The presence of AChE staining in non-neural cellular elements of the spleen may function in detoxification of bacterial toxins (20) or hydrolysis of peptides (103,104,129,245).

Lymph Nodes

There are a few preliminary reports of AChE staining in nerve profiles that innervate lymph nodes (32), but no definitive evidence that these nerves are cholinergic. Clearly, there are non-NA nerve fibers in lymph nodes as seen with EM (375,376) and ICC studies (172). The possibility that some of these fibers are cholinergic remains to be demonstrated.

GALT

Two types of AChE staining have been reported in GALT (161,239,577): AChE staining in nerve-like fibers in the lamina propria and between lymphoid nodules of the rabbit appendix, and lymphoid nodules of the human tonsil. There is no evidence that these nerves represent cholinergic fibers. Rather, it is likely that AChE colocalizes with NA nerve fibers in these zones. This colocalization is probably the case for nerve-like AChE$^+$ staining in the rabbit appendix (161). It is probable that at least some of the AChE staining in GALT is cholinergic, since parasympathetic ganglia are present within the enteric nervous system. However, no definitive studies have demonstrated that AChE$^+$ nerve fibers associated with lymphoid tissue in the gut are truly cholinergic. In addition, there is a more diffuse non-neural staining associated with the lymphoid nodules. In the rabbit appendix (161), this staining forms a dense network surrounding the B-lymphocytes deep within the nodules and at the crown of the domes. Similar staining is seen in the germinal centers in the tonsil (577).

Release and Availability of Neurotransmitter for Interaction with Target Cells

The second criterion for neurotransmission, release and availability, is the most difficult criterion to fulfill (reviewed in 154,155). Because of inherent technical problems with direct measurement of neurotransmitter release from stimulated nerves that distribute to lymphoid organs, much of the evidence for neurotransmitter release has come from studies that indirectly measure this phenomenon. Release and availability of NE have been most convincingly demonstrated in the spleen. Early studies of CAs used the spleen as a rich source of both NE and its associated enzymes. Stimulation of the splenic nerve (550), which is composed almost exclusively of NA postganglionic, sympathetic fibers, released NE into the microenvironment of the spleen that is subsequently drained by splenic venous blood. Indirect evidence for release of NE from neural compartments comes from the use of pharmacologic agents that have direct effects on NA nerve fibers. Chemical sympathectomy with 6-OHDA depletes splenic NE concentration by greater than 95% (317,572). After inhibition of TH with alpha-methyl-para-tyrosine, NE levels decline with time, revealing a turnover time of 8–16 hours in the spleen of young adult rats (6,36). NE released from sympathetic nerve terminals diffuses through the local environment in a paracrine fashion (65) and can act at a considerable distance from the site of release (520).

The diverse compartmentalization of NA nerve fibers suggests that the concentration of NE will vary in the local microenvironment, depending on the exact spatial relationship of the target cell to the sites of release from the NA nerve terminals. Pharmacologic methods described above do not provide information about the concentration of NE in a particular microenvironment of specific compartments of the spleen. Direct measurements of NE in splenic microenvironments have not been attainable by such techniques as in vivo microdialysis, since the effects of tissue injury and inflammation cannot be easily controlled in the spleen. Superimposed on paracrine-like effects is the presence of direct junctional appositions between nerve fibers and lymphocytes and macrophages described above. These synapse-like contacts may provide the transmitter in an even higher concentration for a more immediate effect than is available at a distance. Signaling from the target cell to the nerve terminal via these direct contacts may, in turn, modulate release of NE, perhaps via IL-1 or other cytokines or by the release of extraneuronal NE (or epinephrine) that has been taken up by macrophages (508), and subsequently released upon appropriate stimulation. Bergquist et al. (43) has reported that T- and B-lymphocytes can synthesize NE, suggesting that NE released from these cells also may modulate sympathetic outflow and/or lymphocyte activity.

Neurotransmitter release and availability have been shown to be even more complex by studies suggesting that uptake of other biogenic amines from the circulation and local microenvironment into NA nerve terminals may occur in the spleen. After uptake of these amines (NE and epinephrine, which are secreted by the adrenal medulla [42] and serotonin, which is released from platelets [107]) into NA nerve terminals, they can be released upon nerve stimulation. Additionally, cytokines have been shown modulate neurotransmitter expression in cultured sympathetic neurons (20,128,267,480), and release of CAs from sympathetic nerves (235,456,506). Colocalization of NE in sympathetic nerves with other neurotransmitters, such as NPY, provides the potential for simultaneous release and availability, possibly under the influence of the axonal firing frequency of the specific nerve fiber. Colocalization of neuropeptides with CAs or with each other adds another level of complexity to fulfilling the criterion of release and availability, since some of the neurotransmitter content may be derived from hormonal sources, and the efficacy of one neurotransmitter may be augmented or inhibited by the presence of another neurotransmitter. As an example, NPY has been shown to augment to vasoconstrictive effects of NE in vascular nerve beds (321).

Presence of Receptors on Cells of the Immune System

Adrenergic Receptors

NE released from activated sympathetic nerve fibers will influence cells of the immune system that possess adrenergic receptors. By direct receptor–ligand binding techniques, β-adrenergic receptors, mainly of the β_2 subclass, have been demonstrated on lymphocytes, macrophages, granulocytes, and bone marrow stem cells (4,48,64,115, 183,211,252,291,319,423,497,573; reviewed in 215,216). These receptors display high affinity, are saturable, and are displacable binding sites, which are important characteristics of true receptors. Moreover, β-adrenergic receptors are linked intracellularly to the GTP-binding protein, Gs, of the adenylate cyclase complex, and ligand-receptor interaction leads to a rise in cAMP as a second messenger. Therefore, NE feeds into a signal transduction pathway stimulated by a host of other bioactive molecules, including cytokines known to be involved in immunoregulation. α-Adrenergic receptors have not been demonstrated on murine or rat lymphocytes; however, there are reports of α-adrenergic receptors on human and guinea-pig lymphocytes (203,346,530). Activated rodent macrophages express α_2- and β-adrenergic receptors (4,66). α_1-adrenergic receptors stimulate phosphatidylinositol turnover and a rise in intracellular calcium, while α_2-adrenergic receptors are linked to the G_i subunit of the adenylate cyclase complex. As discussed later in this chapter, pharmacologic studies have demonstrated that α- and β-adrenergic agents can affect the number, or functions, of immunocytes, suggesting the presence of α- and β-adrenergic receptors on cells of the immune system. While they have been difficult to identify by direct receptor-binding studies, pharmacologic studies indicate that α-adrenergic receptors are present, at least on a small subset(s) of cells within unfractionated lymphoid populations (461,464,509,510) (see Table 8-2).

β-adrenergic receptor density varies among lymphocyte populations. Murine splenic B-lymphocytes generally express twice the number of β-adrenergic receptors as that expressed by murine T-cells (115,183). Higher β-adrenergic receptor expression in B-cells may result from a sparse NA innervation of B-cell compartments in the spleen, or it may simply reflect heterogeneity within these two lymphocyte populations. Among human T-lymphocyte subsets, suppressor T-cells possess the highest β-adrenergic receptor density, cytotoxic T-cells (CTLs) have an intermediate density, and helper T-cells express the lowest number (268,546). Resting Th_1-cells, but not resting Th_2-cells, express β-adrenergic receptors and accumulate cAMP in response to β_2-adrenergic agonists (466). In lymphocytes from young adult rodents, intracellular cAMP concentrations generated by receptor-ligand interactions correlate with receptor density.

The presence of NE and other CAs can regulate the density of adrenoreceptors' expression on immunocytes in young adult animals, the presence or absence of the ligand leading to down- or up-regulation, respectively (1,2,358). Regulation of receptor

Table 8-2 Adrenergic Stimulation and Subsequent Inhibition of Cytotoxic T-Lymphocyte (CTL) Responses

Agonist[a]	Selectivity	CTL Reponse (% increase)[b]	Antagonist (0.1 μM)[c]	Reduction of Agonist Response (%)[d]
Norepinephrine	alpha > beta	40–250	Propranolol (beta)	42–45
			Phentolamine (alpha)	25–31
			Both	75–85
Epinephrine	beta > alpha	45–350	Propranolol	30–40
			Phentolamine	25–31
			Both	36–47
			Timolol (beta) (1 μM)	82
Isoproterenol	beta	25–120		
Dobutamine	beta$_1$	No change		
Terbutaline	beta$_2$	50–500	Propranolol	48–54
			Timolol	94
Methoxamine	alpha	±0–80		

[a]Adrenergic compounds in the nM to μM range were added to mixed lymphocyte cultures (C3H spleen + LN responder cells, irradiated BALB/c stimulators) in 24-well plates or upright 25 cm^2 flasks. After 4–5 days of culture, cells were harvested and CTL activity was assessed against P815 targets in a standard 4-h ^{51}Cr-release assay. Multiple effector:target ratios were tested and CTL activity expressed as lytic units per 10^6 cells (or per culture).

[b]Results are expressed as percent increase (e.g., 50% increase = 150% of control) or decrease of lytic units compared to control cells to which diluent was added. Results are based on 3–11 experiments with each compound.

[c]In a second set of experiments, blockers were added at the initiation of the culture.

[d]Results are expressed as percent reduction of agonist-induced potentiation of the CTL response (e.g., 100% reduction indicates that the response was suppressed to background levels [no agonist added]).

[d]Ranges of values indicate results of 2–4 experiments.

expression on lymphocytes and other cells of the immune systems is likely to have functional implications. A lymphocyte adjacent to a NA nerve terminal in the splenic white pulp (with a relatively low density of receptors) may have its receptors saturated and may be most sensitive to a change in CA levels during a decrease in sympathetic nerve activity. On the other hand, a lymphocyte distant to the nearest nerve terminal may seldom see enough CAs to saturate receptors, resulting in up-regulation of adrenergic receptors, and may respond best to increased NE released during sympathetic nerve activation. Location-based regulation of lymphocyte β-adrenergic receptor expression in vivo has not yet been demonstrated, but it is suggested by the greater density of β-adrenoreceptors on B-lymphocytes as compared with T-lymphocytes (183,192,350), which may be predicted based on the compartmentalization of NA nerves in the spleen.

β-adrenergic receptor density may be altered by activation of lymphocytes by antigen or mitogen. Expression of β-adrenergic receptors in splenocytes is reduced after immunization with sheep red blood cells (183), but is increased in draining lymph node cells after contact sensitization with picryl chloride (326). Depending on the number of immunizations, alloimmunization increase, decrease, or do not alter β-adrenergic receptor density on B-cells, and do not change β-adrenergic receptor density on T-cells (192). These changes in receptor number correlate with changes in cAMP production. It is likely that changes in neurotransmitter availability during an immune response (123,124), alter β-adrenergic receptor expression, thereby regulating lymphocyte responsiveness to CAs at the level of the target cell. Alternatively, there is evidence that it is the state of activation of the specific signal transduction pathways that dictates β-adrenergic receptor number and sensitivity of target cells (427,567).

Peptidergic Receptors

VIP

Peptidergic receptors that act through known intracellular second messenger mechanisms are present on cells of the immune system. A variety of human and rodent lymphoid cell lines have been used to demonstrate specific binding sites for VIP. VIP receptors are closely associated with G_s-adenylate cyclase complex (112), and functional responses resulting from the interaction of VIP with these receptors are generally mediated via cAMP-dependent protein kinase (27,378). Some functional responses induced by VIP appear not to use this intracellular pathway (59,243,414,445; reviewed in 39). VIP binding sites have been characterized in Molt-4b (27,380), SUPT-1 (442), and Jurkat (171) T-cell lines, and Raji (444), Dakiki (379), Nalm6 (379), U266 (171), and SKW 6.4 (99) B-cell lines. VIP receptors in most of these cell lines have selectivity and/or a molecular weight comparable to that encountered in normal tissue preparations (reviewed in 39,441).

Receptors for VIP have been found on human peripheral blood mononuclear cells (79,118,209,389,443,570), but there is controversy as to which subpopulations of cells express these receptors. Wiik et al. (570) have reported binding on monocytes and in T-cell-depleted populations, but not in T-cell-enriched fractions. This is in contrast to other studies showing that the predominant VIP binding occurs in lymphocyte-enriched fractions (118,79,443). Further fractionation of mononuclear cells by Calvo et al. (79) has suggested that VIP binding sites are present on B-lymphocytes and/or cells of the (killer/natural killer) K/NK system. O'Dorisio and colleagues (378) have been unable to demonstrate VIP receptors or VIP-induced stimulation of adenylate cyclase in suspensions of human blood monocytes, neutrophils, and erythrocytes. Guerrero et al. (209) have reported both high- and low-affinity VIP binding sites in circulating human mononuclear leukocytes. On the contrary, Danek et al. (118) and Ottaway et al. (389) have demonstrated only a single class of VIP receptors in human monocyte-depleted, lymphocyte-enriched cell suspensions. In the study by Ottaway et al. (389), VIP binds to human blood lymphocytes with CD8$^+$ (32%), CD4$^+$ (23%), and/or CD2$^+$ phenotypes (391,443).

Rodent lymphocytes from primary and secondary lymphoid tissue possess a single class of high-affinity receptors for VIP (52,80,390,563). Regional differences occur in binding capabilities of specific subsets of T- and B-lymphocytes, but T-cells generally have a much greater binding capacity for VIP than do non-T-cells. The density of VIP binding sites on T-cells from mesenteric and superior cervical lymph nodes, spleen and Peyer's patches appears to be similar (about 2,600 sites per cell). Thymocytes have few VIP binding sites (150 sites per cell), suggesting that expression of these receptors occurs as T-cells differentiate and mature. Recently, VIP receptors have been reported in murine peritoneal (81), rat peritoneal (476), and alveolar (237) macrophages. In the avian bursa Fabricius and thymus, Lacey et al. (289) have demonstrated high- and low-affinity VIP receptors.

With northern blot analysis, Ishihara and colleagues (242) have reported no VIP receptor mRNA expression in spleen, and weak expression in thymus. However, using a cloned cDNA probe that codes for VIP receptor protein isolated in rat lung, Gomariz and co-workers (204) have demonstrated VIP receptor mRNA and VIP receptor protein expression in rat thymocytes, splenocytes, and lymph node cells with reverse transcription polymerase chain reaction (RT-PCR). In mesenteric lymph nodes from dogs, VIP receptors are located in the internodular and T-cell regions, in the medullary cords, and germinal centers (424).

NPY

NPY acts on three subclasses of NPY receptors, referred to as NPY Y_1, Y_2, and Y_3 receptors (reviewed in 207). The receptors for NPY that cause vasoconstriction and elevated systemic blood pressure, are mainly the Y_1 type. The Y_1 receptor requires the N-terminus of NPY for binding. The Y_2 is mainly prejunctional and is activated by C-terminal fragments of NPY. Both of these receptors recognize the homologous peptide YY. In contrast, the NPY Y_3 receptor does not recognize peptide YY. None of the three receptor types recognized N-terminal NPY fragments. Two types of NPY receptors have been reported in murine peritoneal macrophages: one is a high-affinity (K_d = 2.7 ± 0.4 nM) and a low binding capacity (38.0 ± 3.5 fmol/10^6 cells) receptor, and the other type is a low-affinity K_d = 64.2 ± 7.1 nM) and a high binding capacity (420.5 ± 65.0 fmol/10^6 cells) receptor (121). Peptide YY was eight-fold less potent in binding with these receptors. Whether specific populations of lymphocytes or other immunocytes possess specific subtypes of NPY receptors have not yet been determined.

Substance P

Receptors for SP are present on human (408) and murine (513,514) lymphocytes, the IM-9, 5F5, and 4810 human B-lymphoblast cell lines (399,407), human fibroblasts (255,256), rat peritoneal mast cells (421), rat alveolar macrophages (237), and guinea-pig macrophages (222). Cells isolated from murine Peyer's patches possess a greater number of SP binding sites than cells from the spleen (513). The expression of SP binding sites in murine lymphocytes does not appear to be strictly dependent on a specific stage of the cell cycle (419). SP receptors are coupled with the phosphotidyl inositol pathway, activation of protein kinase C, and calcium mobilization (219, 412,558). Most of these cell types possess NK-type SP receptors. SP receptors on lymphocytes and most inflammatory cells appear to be different from those on mast cells. The carboxy–terminal end of the SP molecule is important in ligand binding on lymphocytes (406), while the amino acid–terminal end is necessary for release of inflammatory mediators from mast cells (201).

Parnet and colleagues (396) have shown that preincubation of IM-9 cells with micromolar concentrations of SP decreases the number of receptors per cell but does not influence the affinity of SP binding. Alternatively, pretreatment of IM-9 cells with testosterone, but not estradiol or progesterone, results in approximately a ten-fold decrease in the affinity for radiolabeled-SP. The significance of steroid treatment on SP receptor affinity is not clear.

SOM

SOM receptors are not as well characterized as those for VIP and SP, but they are present on human peripheral blood (HPB) monocytes and lymphocytes (47), murine T- and B-lymphocytes in Peyer's patches and spleen (472,516), the Jurkat human leukemic T-cell line (509), the U266 human IgE-producing cell line (509), and basophils (202).

There are at least five SOM receptor subtypes with differing affinities for SOM-14, SOM-28, and SOM analogs (reviewed in 85). There is controversy over whether cells of the immune system express some or all SOM receptor subtypes (reviewed in 85). Bathena et al. (47) was the first to report SOM receptors on human mononuclear leukocytes. They found low-affinity receptors on resting monocytes and lymphocytes (450–500 and 220–250 sites/cells, respectively). With a binding assay, Hiruma et al. (232) subsequently have found SOM binding sites on more than 95% of normal mitogen-activated human peripheral lymphocytes. These activated lymphocytes express a single class of low affinity receptors with a K_d of 10^{-8} nM. Approximately 50% of murine B- and T-lymphocytes from Peyer's patches and 30% of the lymphocytes from spleen express SOM receptors (473). In Peyer's patches, these receptors are not differentially expressed on T-cell subsets, but in spleen approximately 30% of pan T- and T-helper cells, 52% of T-suppressor cells and the majority of IgA$^+$ B-lymphocytes bear SOM binding sites (473). High- and/or low-affinity SOM receptors also have been reported in (1) Jurkat, a human T-leukemic cell line; (2) U266, a human IgE-secreting myeloma; (3) MT-2, a human T-leukemic cell line; (4) MOLT-4b, a human T-cell line; (5) Isk, an Epstein-Barr virus-transformed B-cell line; and (6) MOPC-315, a murine IgA-secreting plasmacytoma cell line (232,363,438,474,509). In contrast to the observations by Sreedharan et al. (509), Nakamura and co-workers (363) did not find

SOM receptors on the Jurkat cell line. Collectively, these studies suggest that SOM receptors are expressed in both lymphoid and monocyte cells. The greater proportion of SOM receptor[+] cells in Peyer's patches may be related to continuous antigenic stimulation, and the two subtypes of SOM receptors in the cell lines may result from malignant transformation. Monocytes/macrophages, basophils and eosinophils also possess SOM receptors (47,202).

With in vitro receptor autoradiography, SOM receptors have been reported in human GALT (palatine tonsils, ileal Peyer's patches, vermiform appendix, and colonic solitary lymphatic follicles [437]), but not in canine mesenteric lymph nodes (424). In GALT, the distribution of SOM receptors was confined to germinal centers, the luminal aspect of the follicles expressing a greater density of receptors than the serosal aspect. This observation suggests that SOM receptor expression may be related to the proliferative state of lymphoid cells, and that the activity of SOM may be greater in the activated state. Since germinal centers are sites of intensive B-cell lymphoblast proliferation, SOM may modulate B-cell maturation and differentiation.

Binding of SOM with its receptor in many tissues is reported to be linked to G proteins, and to suppress cAMP production (reviewed in 545). SOM inhibits adenylate cyclase by a membrane receptor coupled to the activation of adenylate cyclase-inhibiting G-protein complex. Inhibition of adenylate cyclase activity does not appear to occur in lymphocytes and leukaemic cells at physiological concentrations, but does occur with high concentrations of SOM (415). Conversely, the SOM analogue, RC-102-2H, does decrease cAMP production in spleen lymphocytes (403). GTP can reduce agonist binding to SOM receptors by uncoupling GTP-binding proteins from the receptors (134,334,433).

CGRP

Specific binding sites for CGRP have been reported on rodent T-lymphocytes from spleen and lymph nodes (345,364,424), B- lymphocytes (345), macrophages (549), and murine thymocytes (73). Functional studies indicate that rat lymphocytes express only one class of CGRP receptors (type I) (345), while murine lymph node cells and the murine 70Z/3 pre-B-cell line express two classes of CGRP binding sites (345,538). CGRP binding sites in T- and B-lymphocytes are linked to G proteins and adenylate cyclase (101,231,345,538). CGRP binding sites in macrophages may be directly coupled to multiple signaling systems to regulate macrophage functions, including protein kinase C and cAMP (549).

CGRP binding sites also have been reported on several cell lines, including the murine 70Z/3 pre-B-cell line (343,344). Receptors on cells of the 70Z/3 pre B-cell line have both high- and low-affinity binding states (344). These cells also appear to express a peptidase (distinct from neutral endopeptidase) that can inactivate CGRP (343). Findings by McGillis et al. (343) indicate that the peptidase that is capable of inactivating CGRP is a cysteine peptidase. Treatment of these cells with the mitogen, lipopolysaccharide (LPS), resulted in a four-fold increase in the density of CGRP receptors, with no changes in receptor affinity (343). CGRP binding sites also are present on 3-1 cells, another murine B-cell line, but these sites have low affinity for binding CGRP, and remain unchanged after treatment with LPS (343). Combined treatment with LPS and CGRP also inhibits the induction of sIg by LPS on these cells (344). McGillis et al. (343) did not find CGRP receptors on Jurkat cells, a human T-cell line, the IM-9 human B-lymphoblast cell line, the M12 murine B-cell line, the X16c murine IgM$^+$, IgD$^+$, B-cell line, the A20 murine B-cell line, the 38c-13 murine IgM-secreting B-cell line, and the WEHI 231 murine B-cell line.

Opioid Receptors

Functional evidence for opioid receptors on human T-lymphocytes was first reported by Wybran et al. (576), after which numerous reports have appeared. At present, a clear functional role has not yet emerged for the opioid peptides (reviewed in 488), a result of the heterogeneity of the opioid peptides and the opioid receptors. Numerous bioactive derivatives of opiate metabolism may be present in the in vivo microenvironment. Also, the heterogeneity of the cell types that possess opioid receptor complicates functional studies. Structural similarities between opiate peptides does not lead to predictable functional immune responses in many cases. Although α-, γ-, and β-endorphins and Met-enkephalin have identical NH$_2$-terminals, they have differential immunologic effects in vitro. Additionally, the effects of opioid peptides are not always blocked by naloxone or other classical opioid receptor blockers, again suggesting heterogeneity of opioid receptors on cells of the immune system.

Classical receptors (where ligands displace naloxone and morphine) are present on mouse splenocytes (91,253), HPB lymphocytes and platelets (347), human polymorphonuclear leukocytes (144), human granulocytes (311), and human monocytes (311). Jurkat cells (16), HPB lymphocytes (504), and EL4 thymoma cells (471) possess non-classical opiate receptors where opiate peptides cannot displace naloxone and morphine. The second messenger system coupled with opiate receptors is dependent upon the specific opioid peptide, type of receptor on the target cell, and type of immunocyte (reviewed in 90).

Investigators are beginning to use pharmacological and molecular means to identify the lymphocyte/macrophage opioid receptor types. Pharmacological studies (reviewed later in this chapter) suggest that all three of the major opioid receptor types (μ, δ, and κ) are expressed by at least some populations of cells of the immune system. However, most investigators have found that these binding sites are different from the classical receptors present in mammalian brain (reviewed in 488). For example, in IL-1- or PHA-induced activation of thymocytes, the binding characteristics of morphine are different from classical opioid receptors in brain in that they display little stereoselectivity, have relatively low-affinity and high-capacity, are resistant to trypsin, and are strongly inhibited by millimolar concentrations of Mg^{2+}, Ca^{2+}, and Cl^- after ligand-receptor binding (452). Multiple types of low- and high-affinity opioid receptors on cells of the immune system whose expression of one receptor type may be regulated by the other, further add to the complexity of the system.

Probably best characterized of the three opioid receptor types for its effects on immune functions are μ-opioid receptors. μ-Opioid receptor agonists generally suppress *(1)* respiratory burst activity by peripheral blood mononuclear cells (417); *(2)* granulocyte chemotaxis (333); *(3)* T-cell-dependent antibody production (528); and *(4)* macrophage colony formation by bone marrow stem cells (454). These compounds enhance mitogen-induced lymphocyte proliferation (49,56,429).

Non-opioid-mediated effects of β-endorphin may be due to COOH-terminal binding to an as yet unidentified receptor. Gilmore and Weiner (198) have shown that β-endorphin enhancement of Con A-stimulated proliferation of murine spleen cells requires the COOH-terminal of the peptide and that the NH_2-terminal potentiated this enhancement. Findings by Van den Bergh et al. (541) provide evidence for multiple opioid receptors on lymphocyte populations. They have shown that enhancement of Con A-stimulated proliferation of rat lymphocytes occurs only if the cells are pretreated with β-endorphin and then washed to remove the peptide. Along with an enhancement of proliferation, IL-2 production and IL-2 receptor expression is elevated. These effects are not blocked by naloxone. When β-endorphin is present continuously in the culture, no effect of the peptide on proliferation is detectable. An inhibitory effect of α- and β-endorphin is observed if each of these compounds is added after the β-endorphin pretreatment. This inhibition is opioid receptor-mediated. Collectively, these experiments suggest the presence of both opioid and non-opioid receptors on cells that participate in the Con A proliferative response. More recently, they have shown that the C-terminal moiety of opioid peptides enhances T-cell proliferation, whereas this stimulatory effect can be prevented by peptides that possess the N-terminal enkephalin sequence (543).

A few studies have used pharmacological means to identify the lymphocyte/macrophage opioid receptor types that bind β-endorphin. Taub et al. (528) have assessed alkaloid compounds with selective activity for δ-, μ-, or κ-opioid receptors. In vitro antibody production by murine splenocytes is reduced in the presence of the κ-agonists, U-50,488H and U-69,593 at concentrations as low as 10^{-10} M. This inhibitory effect is stereoselective. At high concentrations (10^{-6} and 10^{-7} M, respectively), the μ-selective agonists, morphine and Tyr-D-Ala-Gly-*N*-Me-Phe-Gly-ol (DAMGE), are also inhibitory. The δ-agonist has no effect up to 10^{-5} M. Both μ- and κ-mediated effects are inhibited by naltrexone or naloxone. This data provides strong evidence for the presence of classical μ- and κ-opioid receptors on the surface of murine splenocytes. In addition, opiate alkaloid-selective, opioid peptide insensitive $μ_3$-opioid receptors have been demonstrated in three murine macrophage cell lines (J774.2, RAW 264.7, and BAC1.2F5) (330).

Gaveriaux et al. (189) have identified opioid receptor transcripts in HPB lymphocytes, murine splenocytes, and a variety of human and murine cell lines. In HPB mononuclear cells and monocyte preparations, μ receptors are present but δ are undetectable. Human cell lines have low but significant levels of δ-opioid receptor transcripts in T-, B-, or monocyte cell lines, while only μ receptors are found in B-cell lines. In murine cells, transcripts for the δ-opioid receptor are present in splenocytes and in some T- and B-cell lines, but μ-opioid receptors are not expressed by these cells. Chuang et al. (102) have demonstrated mRNA encoding the κ-opioid receptor in human and monkey lymphocytes.

Collectively, these studies indicate that the criteria for the presence of bona fide opiate receptors have not been adequately fulfilled in many systems, although the recent development of more selective opiate agonist and antagonist has begun to better define opiate receptor expression on cells of the immune system. Further work is required to elucidate more detailed characteristics of specific opioid receptors and their functions on cells of the immune system. It will be important to fulfill the classical criteria for receptors, including stereospecificity, saturability, and displacability, on each cell type at each phase of development and activation. For a more exhaustive discussion of this topic, consult Blalock in chapter 14.

Functional Impact of Innervation on the Immune System

A large body of literature indicates that both CAs and neuropeptides can influence the functional capabilities of the immune system. Neurotransmitters can influence immune function at several hierarchical levels of complexity (155). The most basic interactions occur at the level of individual cellular responses, including neurotransmitter influences on such activities as proliferation, differentiation, expression of specific receptors, synthesis and secretion of specific cellular proteins, cell adhesion, and cellular migration or trafficking.

At the second level of complexity, neurotransmitters can influence the collective interaction of cells of the immune system, including primary and secondary antibody responses, cytotoxic T-lymphocyte activity, NK cell activity, lymphocyte-activated killing (LAK), and delayed-type hypersensitivity (DTH) responses. The third level in this hierarchical scheme is the impact of neurotransmitter signaling on the reactivity of the total capacity of the immunological response of the host to immune challenge by bacteria, virus, tumor cell, alloantigen, autoimmune or other antigens, or to autoimmunity. Important host factors to this overall immune responsiveness are age, gender, genetic factors, previous experiences, physiological capacity, and behavioral status of the host.

At the highest level of complexity are neurotransmitter influences that might provide an assessment of the host's health status, or the ability to respond immunologically to a wide range of potential challenges under certain physiological conditions. While this level of neurotransmitter–immune interactions has received the most widespread public attention, it is currently the least understood. At each level of interaction, neuro-transmitter modulation of immune function must take into account an increasingly complex set of variables, making it impossible to extrapolate data from any one category to the next level without direct experimental testing.

NA Modulation of the Immune System

An abundant literature supports a modulatory role for NE on the immune system. Studies examining CA-induced modulation of B-lymphocyte proliferation and differentiation indicate a complex interaction between adrenergic receptor stimulation and lymphocyte activation. The effects of β-adrenergic agents on B-cell proliferation and differentiation are dependent on the stimulus used for induction (280,303). Co-incubation of NE or isoproteronol (5×10^{-6}——10^{-5} M) and mitogen, enhances LPS-induced proliferation and differentiation of unfractionated splenocytes. An effect that is blocked by propranolol (β-blocker), but not by phentolamine (α-blocker), indicating a β-adrenergic receptor mechanism (280). In contrast, NE added 2 hours or more after incubation of splenocytes with LPS has no effect on B-cell proliferation (280). Similarly, NE enhances proliferation of splenocytes stimulated by Klebsiella pneumoniae, another polyclonal B-cell mitogen. However, other agents that elevate cAMP inhibit LPS-stimulated proliferation, suggesting a divergent intracellular pathway after elevation of cAMP, since the rise in cAMP does not predict the directional change induced by CA interaction with adrenergic receptors on B-cells. T-cells and adherent cells were not involved in NE-induced enhancement of LPS-stimulated B-cell proliferation (280). NE activation of β-adrenergic receptors reduces B-cell proliferation stimulated with antibody to Ig mμ-chain (303). Anti-IgM induces B-cell proliferation through different intracellular mechanisms than those used by LPS. Likewise, the signal pathway induced in B-cells after interaction with Th-cells that recognize antigen expressed in conjunction with a class II major histocompatibility complex determinant on the B-cell differs from that induced by LPS or anti-IgM (95,275). Lower cAMP concentrations are necessary to inhibit B-cell activation induced by anti-IgM compared with Th-cells (263). These data suggest that the directional change induced by CAs is in part determined by the mode of B-cell activation and the subsequent intracellular signaling pathway. Further, cAMP modulates these pathways differently.

Several laboratories have reported reduced mitogen-induced T-cell proliferation with β-adrenergic stimulation as well as other agents that increase cAMP (87,211,252,257). Anti-CD3-stimulated proliferation of T-cells and enriched CD4$^+$, CD8$^+$, and CD45$^+$ RO$^+$ (memory) T-lymphocytes is inhibited by 10^{-5} M isoproteronol and prostaglandin E$_2$ (23). NE added in bone marrow cultures decreases the number of granulocyte-macrophage colony forming units, an effect that is blocked by prazosin (328). Only a modest reduction in IL-2 production suggests altered generation of other cytokines. While inhibition of proliferation correlates with increased intracellular cAMP, the equimolar concentrations of cAMP induced by isoproteronol and prostaglandin E_2 did not induce similar levels of inhibition, indicating that some other factor(s) help to determine the degree of inhibition.

CAs can also influence lytic activity, an effector function of NK cells and cytotoxic T-lymphocytes (CTLs). Katz et al. (261) have reported that isoproteronol and other cAMP-inducers inhibit NK cell activity when added directly to target and effectors in a ^{51}Cr release assay (261). Other reports indicate more complex effects of CAs. Hellstrand and co-workers (229) have found that epinephrine at 10^{-6} and 10^{-8} M inhibits and potentiates, respectively, NK cell lysis. These effects are prevented by propranolol. The effects of epinephrine were mediated through interaction with β-adrenergic receptors in NK cells, since similar effects of epinephrine are seen when NK cells are incubated in epinephrine, washed to remove the agonist and then incubated with target cells. Lysis of specific target cells by mature CTLs also is inhibited when isoproteronol is added to the ^{51}Cr-release assay (518). A more recent study (525) demonstrating that cAMP-enhancing agents prevent exocytosis of granules from cloned CTLs is consistent with these findings.

Agents that elevate intracellular cAMP also diminish neutrophil phagocytosis, and lysosomal enzyme release in neutrophils (585). Isoproteronol and prostaglandin E_2, in low concentrations, inhibit the respiratory burst of neutrophils associated with degranulation (368). This effect occurs only when neutrophil activation occurs through an increase in intracellular calcium. Isoproteronol also reduces the concentration of neutrophil leukotriene B_4, a calcium-dependent metabolite of arachidonic acid (368). It has been suggested that CAs may also act by inhibiting the rise in intracellular calcium in neutrophils. Furthermore, β-adrenergic receptor stimulation or dibutyryl cAMP decreases the maximal rate of superoxide production and increases the rate of termination of superoxide production (195). CAs also may alter neutrophil movement and chemotaxis. When rabbit peritoneal neutrophils are incubated with epinephrine or isoproteronol, spontaneous motility and chemotaxis are inhibited (440), an effect that is prevented by propranolol indicating that the response was β-adrenergic receptor mediated. Similarly, chemotaxis of human neutrophils also is inhibited by β-adrenergic stimulation (224). Their finding that forskolin, which induced a greater increase in cAMP than isoproteronol, had no effect of leukotriene B_4-induced chemotaxis, indicates that elevating intracellular cAMP does not mediate the change in responsiveness of neutrophils to all chemoattractants.

CAs can modulate inflammatory responses through interaction with adrenergic receptors on granulocytes. In one of the earliest reports of adrenergic effects on immunocytes, Lichtenstein and Margolis (304) have shown that isoproteronol, epinephrine, and dibutyryl cAMP inhibit antigen-stimulated release of histamine from sensitized basophils, in proportion to their ability to elevate intracellular cAMP. These findings indicate a role for CAs in IgE-mediated immediate-type hypersensitivity. Similarly, several reports have shown that cAMP-inducers inhibit release of inflammatory mediators in a number of other cell types, including histamine release from peripheral blood leukocytes (60), and histamine release and slow-reacting substance of anaphylaxis (SRS-A) from the lung (19,244). The order of potency for this inhibitory action of adrenergic agents (isoproteronol > epinephrine > NE > phenylephrine) (60), and the ability of propranolol to block the adrenergic-induce inhibition of inflammatory mediator released suggests involvement of β-adrenergic receptors in these cells. While β-adrenergic receptors have been demonstrated on eosinophils, stimulating these receptors have no effect on either superoxide anion generation or the release of eosinophil peroxidase (581). Idazoxan (α-antagonist) and propranolol (β-antagonist) can inhibit hydrogen peroxide and superoxide secretion, although the timing of the inhibition is different (486). Idazoxan, but not propranolol, also can reduce nitrite accumulation in macrophages (486). For many functional parameters tested in macrophages, α-agonists and β-agonists have opposite effects. Further, endogenous NE is released following LPS stimulation of macrophages that can regulate LPS-induced TNF production in an autocrine fashion (508). Incubation of human monocytes with epinephrine, NE, or phenylephrine (an α-adrenergic agonist) increases synthesis of complement components (292).

Cytokine production and immunocyte responsiveness to cytokines can be altered by the sympathetic nervous system. Adding epinephrine or isoproteronol to normal HPB monocytes or the THP-1 monocyte cell line reduces LPS-induced TNF-β production (479). β-receptor blockade prevented the epinephrine-induced inhibition. In contrast, preincubation of THP-1 cells with isoproteronol for 24 hours before adding LPS enhances TNF-β production. In activated murine macrophages, stimulation of α_2-adrenergic receptors increases LPS-induced TNF-α production and gene expression (290), while β-adrenergic receptor activation decreases it (508). Collectively, these findings indicate that both α-adrenergic and β-adrenergic receptor stimulation may influence cytokine production in accessory cells, and that the timing of β-adrenergic receptor activation in relation to a primary activating signal (i.e., LPS) may be critical in determining the direction of change in the response to CAs.

NE reduces chemiluminescent oxidative burst in a murine macrophage cell line (J774) acutely stimulated with zymosan in the presence of IFN-γ (534). NE downregulates TNF secretion by LPS-stimulated macrophages (234), and suppresses the killing of virus-infected cells and tumor cells by macrophages activated with IFN-γ (240,278). Isoproterenol increases intracellular cAMP in macrophages and suppresses their capacity to phagocytize aggregated γ-globulin (278). IL-2 induced-LAK cell activity is enhanced by phenylephrine, an α-agonist (26). Finally, β-adrenergic receptor activation synergized the IL-4-induced increase in CD23 expression, the low-affinity IgE receptor, on human promonocytic cell line U937 (401), suggesting that the cytokine microenvironment may be important in determining the outcome of β-adrenergic receptor activation.

Melmon and co-workers (348) have demonstrated that adding cAMP-elevating agents to splenocytes from mice immunized with sheep red blood cells 15 minutes before performing the plaque assay resulted in fewer plaques formed. Sanders and

Munson (262–266) also have assess catecholaminergic effects on the generation of anti-sheep red blood cell antibodies in an in vitro system in which three cell types are involved in the responses: *(1)* antigen-presenting cells (macrophages, dendritic cells), *(2)* Th-cells, and *(3)* antibody-forming B-cells. Antibody response is enhanced on the peak day of culture (day 5) when NE (10^{-6}–10^{-5} M) is added at the beginning of culture. This enhancing effect is blocked by propranolol when added within 6 hours of culture initiation, and is mimicked with terbutaline, a β_2-agonist. β-adrenergic receptor blockade with propranolol unmasks an NE-mediated enhancement of the primary antibody response that is mediated via activation of α_1-adrenergic receptors (464). The α_2-agonist, clonidine, causes a 50% reduction in the plaque-forming cell response at day 5. This effect is due to events occurring within 2 hours of clonidine addition. Both α-receptor mediated responses are inhibited by phentolamine. In the presence of phenylephrine (α-agonist), but not isoproteronolol (β-agonist), antigen-specific proliferation by in vivo-primed lymph node cells is reduced in vitro. This inhibitory effect is greatest at suboptimal doses of antigen, and is completely blocked by α-adrenergic receptor blockade. The target cell(s) that mediate(s) these α-adrenergic receptor effects is not clear from these studies. Since α-adrenergic receptor expression in mouse T-lymphocytes has not been demonstrated with radioligand binding studies, it is possible that α-agonists act on receptors expressed by antigen-presenting cells.

Recently, Sanders and Powell-Oliver (465) have extended these findings using trinitrophenyl (TNP)-specific B-cells to serve the dual role of antigen-presentation and antibody formation. In this in vitro model, a keyhole limpet hemocyanin (KLH)-specific Th_2-cell line was used as the source of cytokines necessary for B-cell differentiation to antibody-secreting cells. With this system, terbutaline increases the number of IgM anti-TNP-secreting cells, and the amount of anti-TNP antibodies secreted by these cells. The increase in the number of anti-TNP-secreting cells is due to an increase in the number of anti-TNP B-cell precursors, but not from an increase in the clonal proliferation of B-cells that have already been induced to differentiate. No change in B-cell MHC class II expression or IgG_1 anti-TNP antibodies indicate that lymphokine secretion by the Th_2-cell line is not affected by β-adrenergic receptor stimulation. These findings suggest that β_2-adrenergic agonists induce a larger proportion of B-cells to become capable of producing antibody.

From these studies it is possible to make some generalizations regarding CA interactions with cells of the immune system. In vitro effects of adrenergic agents on immune responses requiring multiple cellular interactions are dependent on the cell type(s) involved in the response, subtype of adrenergic receptor activated, the immune stimulus, and the timing of receptor activation with respect to the immune stimulus. In general, in vitro studies indicate that if a β-adrenergic receptor agonist is present during the activation phase of the response, then enhancement may occur, depending on the immune stimulus. If β-adrenergic receptor stimulation occurs late in the immune response, then inhibition of the effector function is a possible outcome. Furthermore, these in vitro studies support a synergistic, regulatory, or modulatory role for CAs, since they do not initiate or completely suppress a response on their own at any single step in the immune response, and they are most effective when cells are activated by mitogen, antigen, or cytokines.

In vivo approaches that examine CA-immune system interactions are necessary to demonstrate physiological relevance of in vitro phenomena and to understand the full range of the interactions in an intact animal. These studies add a level of complexity that is not present in vitro, since CAs can exert an effect on immune response through multiple interactions with a variety of cell types, and may alter a wide variety of functions such as antigen presentation, lymphocyte proliferation, differentiation, expression of specific receptors, lymphokine production, cell trafficking, and vascular changes.

Several laboratories have examined the effects of chemical sympathectomy with 6-OHDA or surgical sympathectomy on subsequent immunization. Chemical sympathectomy with 6-OHDA in newborn animals produces a long-lasting depletion of NE, particularly in lymphoid organs. However, it also depletes NE and dopamine in CNS catecholaminergic neurons. Denervation centrally can also modulate neuroendocrine and autonomic outflow back to lymphoid structures and may alter the development of the immune system. In young adult animals, 6-OHDA causes an acute depletion of NE, since nerve terminals are destroyed and not the cell bodies of origin. NE depletion of lymphoid organs, such as the spleen, can also be achieved by surgical removal of the ganglion of origin. Generally, adult animals that are chemically sympathectomized as neonates, or young adult animals that are surgically denervated, have enhanced antibody responses (46,574). In contrast, in animals that are chemically sympathectomized as adults, antibody responses to T-dependent antigens, delayed-type hypersensitivity, and interleukin-2 (IL-2) production are reduced (217,260,308,326), while antibody responses to T-independent antigen are enhanced (351). These results have not yet been fully explained on the individual cellular level, but they suggest that there may be a dichotomy of responsiveness to CAs by T- and B-cells. There probably is an effect of NE on early events, such as antigen recognition, processing, or presentation, and removal of NE fibers from a mature immune system that results in strikingly different effects than removal of those same fibers at birth.

Following chemical sympathectomy in non-immunized adult mice, in vivo cellular proliferation in spleen, lymph node, and bone marrow is transiently enhanced (324,327). LPS-stimulated lymph node cells from chemically sympathectomized mice show enhanced proliferation in vitro and an increase in the number of B-cells expressing Ig mμ-chain (sIgM$^+$) (327). These cells also display a striking isotype shift from IgM to IgG, compared with vehicle controls. Conversely, in chemically sympathectomized mice, Con A-induced proliferation of lymph node and spleen cells is reduced, corresponding to a reduction in Thy-1$^+$, CD4$^+$, and CD8$^+$ T-cells in lymph nodes. Con A-stimulated IFN-γ production is increased, while IL-2 production is not altered. These data reveal clear-cut differences in the responsiveness of B-cells and T-cells from lymph nodes to NE depletion following administration with 6-OHDA. In the spleen, Con A and LPS responsiveness is reduced after sympathectomy, as well as IL-2 and IFN-γ production, without changes in splenic T-cell and B-cell populations. Collectively, these findings indicate that sympathetic influences on immune functions may be enhancing or inhibiting, and are organ-specific.

Antibody and cell-mediated responses are also altered in chemically sympathectomized animals. Antibody responses to T-dependent antigens are reduced in spleen and lymph nodes from adult rodents treated with 6-OHDA before immunization (309,326). However, animals that are sympathectomized neonatally, and adult animals in which the splenic nerve is cut surgically, exhibit enhanced antibody production (47,572). Miles et al. (351) have reported that chemical sympathectomy in young adult rodents enhances antibody response to a T-independent antigen, but has no effect on a T-dependent antibody response. Brenner et al. (62) have shown that chemical sympathectomy before i.v. injection of the alveolar carcinoma line 1 significantly increases the number of pulmonary metastases, but there is no correlation of denervation with alterations in either NK cell cytotoxicity or priming mice with lethally irradiated line 1 cells.

In Fischer 344 rats, chemical sympathectomy with 6-OHDA modestly elevates antibody production to KLH in young adult rats, but markedly enhances antibody production in old rats, suggesting that age may play a role in the functional consequences of chemical sympathectomy (325). Other studies from our laboratories (284) have examined the effect of chemical sympathectomy on cytokine production in two strains of mice that differ in their response to a variety of pathogens and in the dominant types of cytokines produced in response to immunization. Chemical sympathectomy significantly increases KLH-stimulated in vitro proliferation and IL-2 and IL-4 production in splenocytes from both mouse strains following immunization with KLH. However, serum titers of IgM, IgG, IgG_1, and IgG_{2a} are enhanced in sympathectomized C57Bl/6J mice, the Th_1-predominant strain, but only a small increase in IgG_1 occurs in sympathectomized BALB/c mice, the Th_2-predominant strain. These findings suggest that sympathectomy cannot further potentiate antibody production in a strain already shifted towards Th_2-cytokine production. Therefore, Th subtype predominance may determine the functional consequences of sympathectomy.

Chemical sympathectomy in adult mice that is performed before or after the initial sensitization reduces DTH (326). In these animals, in vitro generation of CTLs specific for the contact sensitizing agent also is reduced, likely the result of reduced IL-2 production necessary for maturation of the CTL response. Chemical sympathectomy also lowers CTL responses to alloantigen in vitro and in vivo (154,223). Collectively, these finding suggest that the sympathetic nervous system potentiates cell-mediated immune responses. Enhancement of phagocytosis by macrophages occurs in adult animals injected with 6-OHDA, 3 and 1 days before sacrifice, an effect that is only partially blocked by the NE uptake blocker, desipramine (323). Chelmicka-Schorr et al. (97) have shown that chemical sympathectomy in neonatal mice and rats augments TNF-α secretion by peritoneal macrophage (two-fold increase) in adult rodents, while isoproteronol inhibits this release in a dose-dependent manner.

Chemical sympathectomy also influences lymphocyte migratory patterns. After injection of ^{51}Cr-labeled lymphocytes from non-treated mice into sympathectomized animals, radiolabeled lymphocytes migrate with greater frequency to lymph nodes, but not to spleen. In contrast, ^{51}Cr-labeled lymphocytes from sympathectomized animals injected into control mice, have reduced migration to lymph nodes (324). CAs may alter the microenvironment of lymphoid organs, and/or influence the expression of adhesion molecules on lymphoid cells and endothelial cells. Chemical sympathectomy increases the number of peripheral blood leukocytes (including granulocytes, platelets, and bone marrow granulocyte-macrophage-colony forming units), and induces granulocytic hyperplasia in the spleen after syngeneic bone marrow transplantation in mice (328). The effects of sympathetic outflow are mediated via an α-adrenergic mechanism.

Peripheral infusion of CAs can modulate efflux of leukocytes from the spleen (113,186,354), and lymphocyte responsiveness to immunization in vivo (122). In mice, the timing of epinephrine administration (4 μg i.p.) relative to immunization determines the effect on the subsequent immune response (122). Injections of epinephrine 6 hours before primary or secondary challenge with sheep red blood cells, changes the kinetics of the IgM and IgG antibody response in the spleen, shifting it one day earlier compared with control mice. If it is administered 2–4 days before immunization, infusion of epinephrine inhibits the primary response at all time points examined.

In humans, a single epinephrine injection induces transient increases in the number of circulating blood lymphocytes and monocytes and decreases proliferative responsiveness to T-cell mitogens (113,186). These functional alterations are accompanied by reduced $T_4{}^+$-cells (CD4$^+$, T-helper cells) and increased HNK-1$^+$ cells (NK/killer cells), indicative of cellular redistribution (114). Five minutes after intracardiac injection of either NE or the β-adrenergic agonist isoproteronol, lymphocyte, and granulocyte release from the guinea-pig spleen occurs (136). These effects are mediated by both α-adrenergic and β-adrenergic receptors. Ernstrom and Soder (138) also have demonstrated that plaque-forming cell release from guinea-pig spleen after secondary immunization with sheep red blood cells is enhanced and sustained after intracardial administration of epinephrine. Using sustained release pellets containing NE or epinephrine, Felsner et al. (150) have found that 24 hours after pellet implantation, plasma NE concentration increases of about ten-fold reduce peripheral blood lymphocyte proliferation to Con A in vitro by approiimately 50%, while epinephrine had no effect. Concomitant administration of propranolol with NE reduces T-cell proliferation in vitro by 80%–90%, an effect that is blocked by administration of phentolamine. This decrease occurs without changes in CD5$^+$ (pan) T-cell number, suggesting that α-adrenergic receptor stimulation inhibits markedly the ability of T-cells to proliferate to Con A. Spleen cells treated with epinephrine in vitro (10^{-5} M for 1 hour) enhances the antibody response in normal recipients, but epinephrine-treated recipients receiving control cells showed no effect compared with control recipients, suggesting that epinephrine acted directly on lymphocytes to alter antibody responses. These studies indicate that adrenergic suppression of peripheral blood T-cell reactivity in the rat can be due to activation of peripheral α_2-adrenergic receptors (151).

Neuropeptidergic Modulation of Immune Function

VIP

VIP immunomodulation has recently been reviewed by Bellinger and colleagues (39). VIP reduces mitogen-induced proliferation of T-lymphocytes from murine Peyer's patches and spleen (59,282,283,349,390,511,512,578). An inhibitory effect of VIP has also been observed in the rabbit (418). In contrast, VIP modulation of mitogen-stimulated proliferation in HPB lymphocytes, and in cell lines, has not been consistent (reviewed in 39). VIP also appears to inhibit antigen-induced lymphocyte proliferation (282,283,349). Reduced proliferative responses probably are in part mediated by a VIP-induced reduction in IL-2 production by activated lymphocytes (187,388,387,521). In unfractionated murine splenocytes and purified CD4+ T-cell cultures stimulated with antibodies directed against CD3, VIP suppresses IL-2 and IL-4, but not IFN-γ, in a dose-dependent fashion (187,521). VIP also suppresses IL-2 production, with no effect on IL-5 or IFN-γ release, in granuloma and splenic T-cells from mice infected with *Schistosoma mansoni* (a model for delayed hypersensitivity) stimulated with Con A or soluble egg antigen (SEA) in vitro (349). In murine schistosomiasis, VIP evokes IL-5 release from activated T-cells that are not undergoing immediate T-cell receptor stimulation (339). These investigators suggest that VIP may signal preactivated T-cells to secrete IL-5 that then regulates eosinophil maturation at the site of the granulomatous lesions.

VIP effects on antibody production are isotype-specific and tissue-specific (511,512). VIP (10^{-8} M) increases the IgA response in mesenteric lymph nodes (20%) and spleen (30%), but suppresses IgA synthesis in cells from Peyer's patches (60%). IgM synthesis in Peyer's patches is increased by VIP (80%), but is not affected by 10^{-8} M VIP in spleen and mesenteric lymph nodes. IgG synthesis is not altered in these lymphoid organs by VIP. VIP effects on Ig synthesis are thought to be T-cell-mediated and involve the generation of cAMP. Differences in organ responses may be related to differences in local T-cell subpopulations in these organs. In contrast to the findings of Stanisz and colleagues (511), Neil et al. (367) have found no effect of VIP on Ig production by splenic and liver granuloma cell preparations from *Schistosoma mansoni*-infected mice incubated with VIP for 4 hours. The differences in the outcomes of these studies may result from differences in antigen used to activate B-cells, or may reflect the length of time that the cells are cultured in the presence of VIP.

Several studies by Kimata et al. have demonstrated VIP modulation of antibody production in human tonsillar mononuclear cells (272,273), several B-cell lines (243), and fetal B-cells (270). VIP elevates Ig production and proliferation in several lymphoblastoid B-cell lines, including IgA, IgM, and IgG production in GM-1056, CBL, and

IM-9 B-cell lines, respectively. VIP stimulatory effects on these cell lines occur without cAMP generation. In human mononuclear cells obtained by tonsillectomies for chronic tonsillitis from non-atopic children, VIP inhibits IL-4-stimulated IgE, IgG_2, and IgG_4 production (272). Both T-cells and monocytes are required for this VIP effect. (Atopy is an inherited sensitivity to naturally occurring allergens that is characterized by continuous elevation in IgE antibodies.) VIP elevates IgG_4 and IgE production in $sIgG_4^-$ and $sIgE^-$ B-cells, respectively, indicating IL-4 induces isotype switching. In cultures of mononuclear cells from human atopic tonsils, VIP suppresses both spontaneous IgE and IgG_4 production (273). In unfractionated small resting B-cells stimulated with anti-CD40 monoclonal antibodies, VIP induces IgA_1 and IgA_2 production (271). VIP can induce isotype switching in anti-CD40-stimulated tonsillar B-cells, since it stimulates IgA_1 and IgA_2 production in $sIgA_1^-$ and $sIgA_2^-$ B-cells (271). IgA_1, IgA_2, and IgM production are induced by VIP in $sIgM^+$ and $sIgM^-$, $CD19^+$ fetal B-cells ($sIgA^-$) after stimulation with anti-CD40 monoclonal antibodies. In IgM^- B-cells, the effects of VIP are enhanced by IL-7. Collectively, these studies show selective modulation of different antibody classes and subclasses by VIP that involve isotype switching. Further, the effects of VIP on antibody production require the presence of both T-cells and monocytes in B-cell cultures.

The effects of VIP on NK cell activity are variable depending on the source of NK cells, activational state, the target cells, whether cells are pre-incubated with VIP before, but not during the assay, or whether VIP is present throughout the assay period (co-incubation), assay incubation time, and concentration of VIP. VIP produces a potent inhibition of NK cell activity in HPB lymphocytes to K-562 target cells when continually present in a 4-hour cytotoxicity assay (130,445,501). This effect is not blocked by adenylate cyclase inhibitors (445). In contrast, when HPB lymphocyte cultures are pre-incubated in VIP for 30–60 minutes and washed before the assay, VIP-enhanced cytotoxicity of cells against the target occurs (445), an effect that requires cAMP accumulation in NK cells. The enhancing effect of pre-incubating NK cells with VIP results from an increased interaction of target cells with effector cells, and not from an increase in lytic efficiency.

Van Tol et al. (547,548) have reported that pre-incubation with VIP stimulates cytotoxicity of HPB mononuclear cells, and lamina propria mononuclear cells from normal mucosa, against CaCo-2 human colon cancer cells. Contrary to the findings of Rola-Pheszczynski et al. (445), they report no change in NK cell activity in these lymphocyte cultures against K562 target cells. Ginsburg and co-workers (199) have found a decrease in NK cell activity without a decrease in NK cell number in patients with inflammatory bowel disease, a condition associated with the loss of VIP-containing nerves in the gut (276,277).

Several studies document VIP modulation of the regional distribution and trafficking of lymphocytes, particularly in GALT. The migration of T-lymphocytes into GALT (385,392) and mesenteric lymph nodes (355,356) is altered through binding with VIP receptors. Preincubation of rat T-lymphocytes from Peyer's patches with VIP in concentrations that down-regulate VIP receptors on T-lymphocytes prevents homing of these lymphocytes to Peyer's patches following adoptive transfer into a syngeneic host. Further, VIP alters the composition of the lymphocyte pool in lymph flow through the popliteal lymph nodes (357), particularly increasing the egress of CD4$^+$ T-cells, consistent with decreased homing of CD4$^+$ VIP-treated cells to GALT (382,391). Bondesson and colleagues (58) have demonstrated that VIP at concentrations ranging from 10^{-7}–10^{-9} inhibits, and at 10^{-12}–10^{-14} M stimulates, mononuclear leukocyte migration.

Continuous infusion of VIP into the superior mesenteric artery of the rat significantly reduces lymphocyte migration through intestinal (especially T-helper cells) and mesenteric lymph (particular T-suppressor cells) without changing lymph flow (382). In VIP-infused rats, there is a decrease in pan T-cells, T-helper cells, and IgA-containing cells in the lamina propria. No change in the hemodynamics of the intestines occurs after VIP infusion suggesting a direct effect on lymphocytes.

Johnson et al. (254) have found that VIP stimulates in vitro chemotaxis of T-lymphocytes from both CD4$^+$ and CD8$^+$ subsets (as well as monocytes, but not neutrophils). These chemotactic effects are more potent on unstimulated cells compared with anti-CD3-activated cells that results in reduced VIP receptor expression. Pre-incubation of unstimulated T-cells with VIP increases cell adhesion to intercellular and vascular adhesion molecule (ICAM and VCAM, respectively) integrins, and significantly increases unstimulated T-cell adhesion to fibronectin, an extracellular matrix protein. VIP also enhances the aggregation of Raji cells, a response dependent on cAMP generation and lymphocyte function-associated adhesive protein (LFA)-1 and ICAM-1 (444). Litwin et al. (307) also have reported that VIP inhibits rat alveolar macrophage phagocytosis and chemotaxis in vitro.

Several studies document VIP involvement in inflammatory responses. VIP protects lung tissue from injury caused by HCl (174), xanthine/xanthine oxide (44), and toxic oxygen metabolites (287). Some effects of VIP on inflammation are indirect, stimulating vasodilatation of vascular beds during local inflammatory responses (175,410), and acting on endothelial cells to change plasma extravasation, and cell adhesion molecule expression (reviewed in 458). Still VIP does exert direct effects on accessory cells that mediate inflammation. VIP inhibits superoxide anion (O_2^-) formation in N-formyl-methione-leucine-phenylalanine (fMLP)-activated inflammatory cells (peripheral blood neutrophils) and mononuclear cells from healthy human subjects (287). A similar effect of VIP on superoxide anion (O_2^-) occurs in the human monoblast cell line, U937, peripheral eosinophils, and alveolar macrophages obtained by bronchoalveolar lavage (287). Respiratory bursts in human monocytes after activation by zymozan are suppressed by VIP through a cAMP-mediated mechanism. In contrast, pre-incubation with VIP for 2 minutes primed respiratory bursts in human neutrophils induced by either phorbol myristate acetate or fMLP, an effect that does not appear to be mediated through binding of VIP with VIP receptors (414).

VIP is moderately inhibitory for antigen-induced release of histamine from guinea-pig lung (540), and for peptidoleukotriene release from platelet-activating factor-stimulated rat lung tissue (127). This is not the case for VIP modulation of antigen-induced histamine in rat peritoneal mast cells, and in human skin where VIP has been shown to evoke histamine release in a non-cytolytic manner (105,173,481).

Neuropeptide Y

There is some evidence that NPY modulates inflammatory responses. Incubation of NPY with rat peritoneal mast cells (206,359,485) or human cutaneous mast cells (133) results in histamine release. In rat peritoneal mast cells this histamine response is not receptor-mediated but does involve activation of G proteins (359). In anesthetized rats, NPY causes a biphasic blood pressure response; however, in conscious rats, NPY decreases blood pressure. The depressor effects of NPY can be abolished by pretreatment with a histamine H_1 receptor blocker, suggesting that NPY induces the release of histamine that causes the subsequent decrease in blood pressure. Intradermal injection of NPY induces a flare response in humans, suggesting a similar role of NPY in vivo.

NPY causes no change in spontaneous lymphoproliferation (251) and a decrease in the mitogen-stimulated T-cell proliferative response (505). NK activity against K-562 target cells, and NK-enriched large granular lymphocytes against LAV-infected 8Ef/LAV target cells, are significantly suppressed by NPY (10^{-9}–10^{-12} M) (362). This finding is consistent with data by Chelmicka-Schorr and co-workers (434) demonstrating that chemical sympathectomy increases NK cell activity. Irwin et al. (241) have shown that chronic activation of sympathetic nervous system causes an elevation in NPY that correlates with a reduction in NK cell activity. Interpretation of these in vivo studies, however, is complicated by the loss or co-release of CAs (or other neuropeptides), respectively.

De La Fuente et al. (121) have demonstrated that incubation of resting murine peritoneal macrophages with NPY and peptide YY at concentrations from 10^{-12} M–10^{-8} M stimulates adherence of macrophages to substrate, chemotaxis, ingestion of inert particles and foreign cells, and production of superoxide anion. A dose response is seen, with a maximal stimulation of macrophage function at 10^{-10} M. These macrophage responses to NPY are receptor-mediated, and cause a significant increase in intracellular protein kinase C, but no change in intracellular cAMP. Hafstrom and colleagues (212) have shown that NPY can prime polymorphonuclear oxidative metabolism. In this study, NPY is not able to prime fMLP-induced rises in cytosolic calcium, but it does cause a direct and dose-related increase in cytosolic calcium concentrations. NPY also is not able to prime polymorphonuclear aggregation or directly induce oxidative metabolism, aggregation, or chemotaxis.

Substance P

Both, neurally-derived SP and SOM play a prominent role in local inflammatory responses. Typically, small nonmyelinated sensory nerve fibers, which contain SP, SOM, CGRP, and several other peptidergic neurotransmitters, are found in close proximity to mast cells in a variety of tissues, including respiratory airways, joint synovium, kidney, vas deferens, thymus, and gastrointestinal tract (50,61,315,502,515). Foreman and co-workers (175,176) have provided evidence that NT can prevent SP-induced release of histamine by competing for SP receptors on target cells, and that SOM can block release of SP from peripheral nerve endings.

During inflammatory responses, neuropeptides from sensory nerves are released and modulate both acute hypersensitivity and delayed-type immune responses. SP dilates vascular beds (310,322), and stimulates mast cells and basophils to release histamine and other mediators, such as leukotrienes (175,177,201,306,410). Morphological support for this action of SP comes from a study by Oura et al. (393). They report a decrease in SP-immunoreactive nerves, vasodilation, and degranulation of mast cells 10 minutes after topical application of a corticosteroid cream onto the back skin of rats. They suggest that corticosteroids cause release of SP, which in turn, stimulates blood vessels to dilate, and mast cells to release histamine and other inflammatory mediators.

The role of SP in inflammation also is indicated by its ability to stimulate chemotaxis of monocyte/macrophages, mast cells, fibroblasts, and polymorphonuclear cells (89,256,397,455). These effects of SP can be blocked by D-amino acid analogs of SP but not by antagonists of the chemotactic peptide fMLP, suggesting SP specificity. However, SP can prime the fMLP-induced rise in cytosolic calcium (212). SP-induced chemotaxis may in part be indirect by inducing endothelial-leukocyte adhesion molecule (ELAM)-1 on endothelial cells (341), and by stimulating mast cells to release TNF-α (which increases expression of ELAM-1 in the microvascular endothelium) or leukotriene B$_4$ (247,248,555). In contrast, using in vitro cultures of human T-lymphocytes and endothelial cultures from human umbilical vein, Smart and co-workers (503) did not find an effect of SP on T-lymphocyte adhesion to vascular endothelium or on surface adhesion receptor expression. Proliferation of connective tissue cells (smooth muscle cells, fibroblasts, and endothelial cells) in the proximity of an inflammatory site may be regulated by SP (371,405). Both neurokinin A and SP stimulate proliferation (10^{-7} to 10^{-4} M) and chemotaxis (10^{-10} M maximal) of human HFL1 and IMR-90 fibroblasts (220). These findings suggest a role for SP in the activation of mesenchymal cells that could contribute to the structural abnormalities observed in the airways of asthmatic patients.

A role for SP in inflammatory diseases also has been suggested by many investigators. Increases in SP in the site of disease has been demonstrated with many inflammatory-mediated diseases, including rheumatoid arthritis, Crohn's disease, asthma, and ulcerative colitis (11,295). In animals treated with *Clostridium difficile,* they have found that the SP antagonist, CP-96,345, completely inhibits the acute inflammatory enterocolitis that results from toxin A produced by this pathogen (425). In contrast, the SP antagonist has no effect on cholera toxin that causes a noninflammatory secretory diarrhea (425). Similarly, in *Trichinella spiralis*-infected mice, Agro and Stanisz (12) have demonstrated a rise in SP concentration in the jejunum and serum that parallels the course of the infection, and administration of anti-SP antibodies lowers lymphocyte responsiveness to SP, both systemically and locally, and blocks the intestinal inflammation.

Topical application of SP in doses ranging from 10^{-6}–10^{-9} M onto human nasal mucosa can enhance the expression of mRNA for IL-1β, IL-3, IL-4, IL-5, IL-6, TNF-α, and IFN-γ (383), particular in allergic patients. The cell types that are activated by SP to increase cytokine mRNA expression were not examined. Ansel and co-workers (15) have found that SP stimulates TNF-α gene expression and TNF-α secretion in a dose-dependent manner in a murine mast cell line, CFTL 12, and in isolated murine peritoneal mast cells. SP can modulate macrophage functions, including enhancing phagocytosis by mouse macrophages and human polymorphonuclear cells (24), inducing the oxidative burst and thromboxane generation from guinea-pig peritoneal macrophages (221), promoting chemotaxis of macrophages into sites of inflammation (222), stimulating cytokine production (IL-1, IL-6, and TNF-α) by monocyte/macrophages (274,294,318), and down-regulating membrane-associated enzymes and the release of inflammatory products derived from the lipoxygenase and cyclooxygenase pathways (222). Conversely, in human fibroblasts SP stimulates the arachidonic pathway (255). Stimulation of inflammatory cytokine production by macrophages also may play a role in fever induction, the production of acute phase proteins, and late-stage differentiation of B-lymphocytes into antibody-producing cells resulting in SP-induced enhancement of murine Ig synthesis (345).

In the activation of human neutrophils by SP, the *N*-terminal peptide of SP enhances phagocytosis (24,481) and the C-terminal peptides induce the respiratory burst (477,481). Eosinophils from chronic granulomas isolated from the liver of mice infected with *Schistosomiasis mansoni* express and release both SP and SOM. This finding indicates that these neuropeptides come from multiple sources. Regardless of the source once they are released they are available to modulate the activity of local eosinophils, macrophages, and lymphocytes involved in the inflammatory response to the parasite (564). SP and other TKs substantially increase IFN-γ production from spleen or granuloma inflammatory cells primed in vitro by suboptimal stimulatory concentrations of egg antigen or mitogen, while optimal doses are much less effective (53). This SP-induced IFN-γ secretion is blocked by antagonists specific for NK$_1$ receptors. Animals treated in vivo with an NK$_1$ receptor antagonist produce smaller granulomas. Conversely, SOM inhibits SEA-induced IFN-γ production. SP increases polyclonal and SEA-specific, IgG$_{2a}$ secretion from spleen cells challenged with SEA, while IgG$_{2a}$ production in splenocytes exposed to SOM is inhibited (55). Granuloma cells constitutively express IgG$_{2a}$, and this antibody is not affected by SP or SOM. If mice are treated with an SOM agonist in vivo, granulomas produce little or no IgG$_{2a}$. They have concluded from these studies, that in the spleen SP and SOM are important for IgG$_{2a}$ class switching, while cells in the granulomas are mostly activated B-cells that have completed the switch recombination.

SP potentiates in vitro IgA antibody production in murine lymphocytes from spleen and Peyer's patches by 70% and 300%, respectively (511). SP may exert this effect through the release of IL-6. Using subclones of the CD5$^+$ CH12 B-lymphoma cell line that secrete either IgM or IgA, SP potentiates LPS-stimulated antibody response by 172% and 45%, respectively (398). In purified splenic B-cell cultures, SP enhances LPS-triggered IgM and IgG production 500% and 572% (399). These SP-dependent increases are blocked by SP antagonists. SP-induced enhancement of antibody production does not result from an increase in B-cell proliferation. Instead, SP increases the number of B-cells secreting antibodies. SP also can synergize IL-6-induced differentiation of, and IgG production by, B-cells from Peyer's patch (400). Pascual and co-workers (400) believe that SP can drive the differentiation of co-stimulated B-cells by direct stimulation, or indirectly by activation of macrophages or Th$_2$-cells through the release of cytokines. SP injected into benzylpenicilloyl (BPO)-KLH sensitized mice at the time of peak antibody responses strongly inhibits IgE production within 48 hours, and BPO-specific memory IgE response in vitro (94). This effect of SP involves the carboxy terminal of the SP molecule, and involves IFN-γ (94). In human mononuclear cell cultures from tonsils, SP inhibited spontaneous IgG$_4$ production without affecting production of other isotypes or other IgG subclasses (273).

SP, at nanomolar concentrations, promotes unstimulated and mitogen-induced proliferation of murine, human lymphocytes, and human lymphocyte cell lines (406,512,526). SP-induced proliferation of the Molt-4 T-cell line could not be inhibited by other neuropeptides like CCK, VIP, or SOM, that inhibit proliferative responses in this cell line and in human and murine T-lymphocytes (526). This effect may result from a SP-induced increase in IL-2 production in activated lymphocytes (77,432) through an increased stability of the IL-2 mRNA (78). SP also enhances hematopoiesis in bone marrow cultures, an effect that is mediated by increased IL-3 and granulocyte-macrophage colony-stimulating factor production by bone marrow mononuclear cells and involves release of IL-1 and IL-6 (430,431). T-cells play a minimal role in this response.

SOM

Generally, SOM exerts inhibitory effects, opposite to those of SP. In most studies, SOM causes a concentration-dependent suppression of the spontaneous and lectin-induced proliferative responses of lymphocytes and cell lines (reviewed in 85,545). At low concentrations (10 pM-1 nM), SOM inhibits proliferation, including *(1)* spontaneous proliferation of murine splenocytes (402); *(2)* mitogen-stimulated proliferation of murine lymphocytes (10,511,514); *(3)* mitogen-stimulated human T-lymphocytes and the Molt-4b human lymphoblasts (142,331,409); *(4)* IgA secreting plasmacytoma MOPC-315 cell proliferation (474); *(5)* Con A-stimulated rat thymocytes (337); and *(6)* colony-stimulating activity of murine splenocytes (529). In several reports, SOM has a biphasic proliferation response on lymphocytes, where at low concentrations SOM suppresses, and at above 0.1 μM SOM stimulates proliferation (251,374,402,409, 418,474). Van Hagen et al. (546) has postulated that low numbers of high-affinity receptors, and high numbers of low-affinity receptors could explain inhibitory and stimulatory effects on lymphocyte proliferation, respectively. Alternatively, they suggest that direct and indirect effects of SOM may be antagonistic.

In vitro polyclonal IgA and IgM production by lymphocytes from murine Peyer's patch, spleen, and mesenteric lymph nodes are reduced in the presence of 10^{-7} M or lower concentrations of SOM (514). This effect is higher on IgA (20%–50%) than on IgM (10%–30%) synthesis. Since all three Ig-producing B-cell isotypes in Peyer's patches bind SOM in a similar fashion, the inhibition of Ig production by SOM is not explainable based on binding to distinct subsets of B-lymphocytes. In unstimulated and mitogen-stimulated human peripheral blood lymphocytes, SOM suppresses IgA, IgG, and IgM production, with the highest percentage inhibition in IgG and IgA synthesis (142). Schistosome-infected mice treated with octreotide show complete inhibition of IgG_{2a} production from pulmonary granulomas and reduction of hepatic granuloma size, and IFN-γ production is reduced (53,55). Similarly, spontaneous production of IgE and IgG_4 in mononuclear cells from atopic patients is inhibited by SOM (273). The IgE response is not affected by antisera to either IFN-α and IFN-γ, or indomethacin, similar to findings in mononuclear cells from non-atopic patients (272). Further, SOM promotes isotype switching induced by IL-4 plus anti-CD40 monoclonal antibody in a T-cell- and monocyte-dependent fashion (273). These effects of SOM require the presence of monocytes and T-lymphocytes present with B-lymphocytes. Therefore, SOM, as well as SP, appears to mediate isotype-specific and organ-specific regulation of B-cell differentiation in vitro, suggesting that in vivo they may act as neurophysiological regulators to influence tissue-specific synthesis of a particular isotype. Further, SOM-induced decrease in IgE production, suggests that SOM may act to down-regulate allergic or immediate hypersensitivity responses.

SOM and the analogue BIM 23014c administered to mice inhibit in vitro NK cell activity of splenocytes and Peyer's patch lymphocytes (10). This effect is greater in lymphocytes from Peyer's patches compared with splenocytes, and may be related to differences in SOM receptor expression and/or state of activation of the lymphocytes. A similar effect of SOM on NK activity of human peripheral lymphocytes has been reported (500). This effect of SOM is not due to a decrease response of NK cells to IL-2. Kroc et al. (282,283) has reported a suppressive effect of SOM on mixed lymphocyte reaction. SOM did not alter the cytotoxic response against K-562 and CaCo-2 colon carcinoma target cells (531). The effects of SOM on the production of cytotoxic cytokines also have been examined. SOM enhances lymphotoxin-induced and TNF-induced destruction of mitomycin-C-treated murine L929 cells (580). They suggest that SOM promotes cell injury by preventing repair mechanisms of the affected cells. SOM also enhances lymphotoxin and TNF secretion (at concentrations ranging from 10–100 nM) (580), and IFN-γ (at concentrations higher than 1 μM) (579) from peripheral mononuclear cells. SOM (10 nM) suppresses IFN-γ production stimulated by the T-cell mitogen staphylococcal enterotoxin A (360), by schistosome-induced granulomas (562), and by mitogen-stimulated splenic T-lymphocytes (54).

SOM is an important signal molecule in immediate hypersensitivity through its modulation of leukocyte and monocyte chemotaxis (455), neutrophil phagocytosis (24), macrophage effector functions (222), and release of histamine and leukotrienes by basophils and mast cells (202,482). Karalis et al. (259) have reported that glucocorticoid suppression of inflammation may in part be mediated by stimulation of SOM (in parallel with other local inflammatory mediators like SP, corticotropin releasing factor and TNF-α), which in turn inhibits leukocyte chemotaxis into the inflamed site. In micromolar concentrations, SOM stimulates chemotaxis of monocytes, but pretreatment with nanomolar concentrations of SOM (or IL-1, or SP) inhibits the chemotactic response of monocytes to growth hormone (568). Similarly, octreotide, a SOM analogue, antagonizes growth hormone-induced or prolactin-induced activation of neutrophils for enhanced respiratory bursts, and growth hormone-induced or prolactin-induced stimulation of neutrophil migration (569). SP and SOM exert opposing effects on human neutrophils. SP is restricted in its capacity to activate human neutrophil: SP does not provoke aggregation, superoxide anion generation, or rises in intracellular free calcium, but it does provoke directed migration. In contrast, SOM does not elicit neutrophil activation, but significantly inhibits SP-induced neutrophil activation (279). SOM exerts a biphasic pattern of histamine release, with low concentrations suppressing the release and high concentrations enhancing it. Concentrations of SOM in the nM–pM range suppress the anti-human myeloma IgE-induced histamine and leukotriene release by human basophils, mouse bone marrow-derived mast cells, and rat leukemia basophils (202,436), while SOM, at μM concentrations, enhance histamine release by mast cells (529) and white blood cells from patients with allergic hyperreactivity (126). Hypereosinophilia in rats can be suppressed by administration of SOM analogues (140,141), possibly by increasing the formation of human leukocyte migration inhibiting factor (403).

SOM inhibits the IFN-γ-induced tumoricidal capacity of macrophages (413) at concentrations 1 nM–10 μM, an effect that is reversed by the addition of SP. They suggest that high concentrations of SOM are required to elicit this effect on macrophages, which then causes an increase in protease activity in the culture medium and subsequent rapid degradation of the peptide. An SOM anologue, octreotide, but not SOM-14, enhances chemotaxis in patients with acromegaly (457). Octreotide also enhances phagocytic activity of monocytes from patients with cirrhosis of the liver (249).

CGRP

The principal activity CGRP in immediate hypersensitivity reactions is vasodilatation. CGRP induces protracted vasodilatation when administered extra-vascularly (reviewed in 61), to mimic release from nerves. When CGRP and SP are administered together into human skin, the response is transient, and is dependent on protease-mediated degradation of CGRP by mast cells that are stimulated by SP. Release of histamine from mast cells is not required for this effect. CGRP and SP can release serotonin from cerebrovascular mast cells (439). CGRP augments SP-induced increase in microvascular permeability, manifested by a greater cutaneous flare and wheal, but has no effect on vascular permeability in the absence of SP. CGRP causes migration of guinea-pig and human airway epithelial cells in primary culture through stimulation of specific CGRP receptors, suggesting a role for this peptide in regulating airway epithelial migration and repair (467). In human lungs, CGRP was more potent than SP in stimulating bronchoconstriction in vitro (395), but in vivo studies regarding CGRP function in the lungs are inconclusive. CGRP inhibits the enzymatic degradation of SP, thereby enhancing the activity of this peptide when both are present in the microenvironment. Like SP-immunoreactive nerves, nerves that contain CGRP also reside near subepithelial mast cells (516). CGRP can evoke release of histamine from rat connective tissue mast cells in vitro (411); however, unlike SP this activation is not mediated through activation of CGRP receptors on these cells. CGRP inhibits the release of leukotrienes from lung tissue challenged with the phospholipid platelet-activating factor (127). CGRP also exhibits chemotactic activity for hematopoietic cells (179), increases neutrophil infiltration after injection of IL-1 in vivo (70), and enhances neutrophil adhesion to vascular endothelial cells in vitro (522). Findings by Davies et al. (119) suggest that neutral endopeptidase (CD10), which is expressed in lymphoid progenitor cells and a subpopulation of mature B-cells, can generate a fragment of CGRP that is chemotactic for eosinophils.

CGRP is detected at low concentrations in nasal lavage of allergic and normal control subjects (553), and the concentration of CGRP in the lavage fluid is elevated 1.5–4.0-fold from 15–24 hours after local challenge with antigen selected for known sensitivity. Similarly, infusion of IL-2 intravenously, or intraperitoneally, combined with LAK cells to treat metastatic carcinoma results in a marked increase in intraperitoneal concentrations of SP or CGRP, respectively. IL-2 injection also caused edema, and serosal effusions, possibly mediated by the rise in neuropeptide concentrations in the peritoneal cavity. An increase of CGRP release (as well as SP and VIP) from peripheral nerve endings of small nonmyelinated sensory axons has been suggested in certain skin diseases (145,554), and in rheumatoid arthritis (269). Plasma CGRP levels also are elevated after injection of endotoxin, and in patients with septic shock (reviewed in 557).

CGRP can inhibit the proliferative response of mouse splenocytes, thymocytes, lymph node cells, and human T-cells to mitogens (59,73,557,539). In the murine Th_1-cell clones, 5.9 and 5.5, CGRP inhibits mitogen-induced IL-2 mRNA and IL-2 production, as well as mRNA for TNF-α and IFN-γ (556). These cytokine-induced effects of CGRP are reversible by adding a CGRP antagonist selective for $CGRP_1$ receptors to the cultures, and are at least in part mediated by an increase in cAMP. Conversely, CGRP causes an elevation in cAMP, has no effect on mitogen-induced proliferation of rat splenocytes (536). CGRP also inhibits murine NK cell activity (537). CGRP stimulates IL-6 production in pituitary cells and in a bone marrow-derived preadipocyte-like cell line (469,527). In fibroblasts, CGRP enhances IL-1β- or TNF-α-induced bio-synthesis of IL-6 by a non-transformed fibroblast cell line (Swiss 3T3), an effect that is in part mediated by stabilization of IL-6 mRNA (460).

CGRP also effects some macrophage functions. CGRP stimulates Na/H-exchangers in rat peritoneal macrophages through a protein kinase C-dependent mechanism (549), inhibits antigen-presenting activity by suppression of class II MHC molecules, de-creases IL-1 production (373,394), inhibits H_2O_2 production in IFN-γ-stimulated mac-rophages (373), and suppresses antigen presentation by epidermal Langerhans cells (233).

Opioid Peptides

Considerable evidence now indicates that opioids can play a major role in immune activation and effector processes. Early studies have indicated that endogenous opioid peptides modulate immune responses, including opioid peptide-mediated alterations in antibody production (228,311), mitogen-stimulated proliferation of lymphocytes (342,422,575), expression of surface receptors on T-lymphocytes (E-rosette, IL-2, and Ia receptors) (352,576), production of lymphokines (interferon and T-lymphocyte che-motactic factor (66,67,332), NK (143,266,340,484), and cytotoxic T-cell activity (93), and a number of phagocytic functions (178,422,488,489).

Several studies have reported that β-endorphin augments Con A-stimulated prolif-eration of spleen cells, and PHA-stimulated proliferation of human lymphocytes through a non-opioid receptor-mediated mechanism (197,198,342,541). Hemmick and Bidlack (230) have shown that prostaglandin E_1-induced suppression is partially blocked by β-endorphin. This effect is not blocked by naloxone, and the reduced proliferation induced by two other compounds that increase adenosine cAMP is not affected by β-endorphin. Zaitsev et al. (582) have found that Met-enkephalin modula-tion of blast-transformation in murine splenocytes depends on the stimulus used to induce proliferation. Con A-induced proliferation is suppressed, and *Staphylococcus enterotoxin A*-induced proliferation is enhanced by Met-enkephalin. Both of these effects are blocked by naloxone indicating an opioid-mediated mechanism; however, the affinity of these receptors for ligand ($K_d < 10^{-10}$ M) is greater in these cells than in other tissues of the body. Activation of splenocytes increases the density of opioid receptors on these cells. Further, the amplitude of the proliferative response is depen-dent on the animals sensitivity to painful stimuli (i.e., higher proliferative responses in mice with a higher threshold for pain).

Opioid peptides also modulate thymocyte and bone marrow cell development and maturation (213,453,454). IL-1 activation of thymocytes results in a dramatic increase in the specific binding of morphine (453), and administration of morphine or β-endor-phin inhibits IL-1-induced proliferation of thymocytes (452,453). Forty-eight hours after subcutaneous implantation of a time-release pellet of morphine induces rapid and profound thymic atrophy (18,68,69,475) with a 30% loss in thymic cellularity, and a decrease in CD4$^+$/CD8$^+$ thymocytes (68,69). Adrenalectomy prevents the morphine-induced loss in thymic atrophy (18). Fuchs and Pruett (184) have shown that morphine induces an increased rate of apoptosis in thymocytes in vivo but not in vitro. This in vivo effect of morphine can be blocked by an opiate or by a glucocorticoid antagonist, indicating that other types of receptors play a role in the process. Recently, Hagi et al. (213) have shown that in mixed cell culture, β-endorphin acts in concert with IL-1 to potentiate LPS-induced macrophage-colony stimulating factor-dependent macrophage differentiation from immature bone marrow precursor cells.

Opioid peptides also alter antibody response. α-Endorphin and Met-enkephalin, but not β-endorphin or γ-endorphin diminish primary antibody production by murine splenocytes after immunization with sheep red blood cells (253), and with ovalbumin (228). In vitro T-cell dependent antibody responses are also inhibited after administration of the κ-opioid agonist U50,488H or U69,593 (528). This immunosuppression is reversible by pretreatment with either naloxone or naltrexone or by the κ-selective antagonist, norbinaltorphimine. In a subsequent study, they showed that short-term treatment of either T-cells or macrophages with the κ-opioid agonist, U50,488H results in significant inhibition of in vitro antibody responses (208). Inhibition of both T-cell and macrophage activity is blockable by naloxone. These findings indicate that resting T-cells and macrophage express κ-opioid receptors and responsive to opioid signaling before activation by antigen. The α-endorphin-mediated suppression is antagonized by naloxone and β-endorphin. Similarly, Radulovic et al. (428) show that the selective κ-opioid receptor agonist MR2034 exerts a pronounced suppression of plaque-forming cell response following i.p. administration in the rat, an effect they attribute to direct action on plasma cell activity. Rowland and co-workers (450,451) have found that modulation of in vitro primary antibody response by Met-enkephalin depends on the dose of antigen used to stimulate the immune system. For example, when an optimal dose of antigen is used to induce the maximal immune response, the addition of Met-enkephalin to the culture medium suppresses the response. When the immune response is suppressed by supraoptimal doses of antigen, Met-enkephalin enhances the immune response. Lastly, Met-enkephalin has no detectable effect in regions of the antigen dose-response curve where there is insufficient antigen to induce strong immune signals.

Using suboptimal doses of LPS to induce IL-1 production by bone marrow-deprived macrophages β-endorphin enhances cytokine production (17). This effect is inhibited by naloxone, although naloxone itself also inhibited IL-1 production. β-endorphin and Met-enkephalin enhances Con A-induced production of IFN-γ, and stimulates NK cell activity in vitro (67,172,332). Singh et al. (490,491) have demonstrated that Met-enkephalin and a potent Met-enkephalin analogue, 82/205, can biphasically modulate malarial antigens-induced production of colony-stimulating factors by macrophages, and Con A-induced elaboration of phagocytosis-promoting lymphokines (IFN-γ and IL-4) by murine spleen cells, in vitro. The enhancing effect appears to be mediated via μ-receptors, while the suppressive effect is mediated through δ-receptors. Production of a T-lymphocyte chemotactic factor by Con A-stimulated human peripheral blood mononuclear cells is inhibited by β-endorphin (66). In the presence of β-endorphin, Met-enkephalin, and Leu-enkephalin increased migration of human T-lymphocytes has been demonstrated in vitro (226). Recently, Iuvone and co-workers (246) have demonstrated that pretreatment with morphine, or with a selective μ-agonist or a selective κ-agonist, inhibit the induction of nitric oxide synthase in LPS-stimulated J774 macrophages.

Van Den Bergh and colleagues (544) have examined the effects of opioid peptides on in vitro cultures of purified CD4$^+$ T-cells stimulated with Con A (or immobilized anti-CD3 antibodies) in the presence or absence of macrophages. The presence of α-endorphin and β-endorphin (dose range from 10^{-12}–10^{-10} M), but not Met-enkephalin, stimulates IL-2, IL-4, IL-6, and IFN-γ production. IL-1 secretion is not altered by these opioid peptides in their culture system. The effect occurs when either Con A or immobilized anti-CD3 antibodies are used to stimulate the CD4$^+$ T-cells. Cytokine production induced by these opioid peptides does not require the presence of macrophages. Several findings by this group of investigators indicate that the endorphin-mediated cytokine production does not result from activation of classical opioid receptors: *(1)* the opioid receptor agonist, Met-enkephalin does not enhance cytokine production; *(2)* the opioid receptor antagonist naloxone does not prevent the stimulatory effects of α-endorphin and β-endorphin; *(3)* naloxone in fact stimulates IL-2 and IL-4 production by itself indicating that there are classical opioid receptors on CD4+ T-cells; and *(4)* incubation of CD4$^+$ T-cells with these endorphins does not alter intracellular cAMP concentrations. Interestingly, these opioid peptides do not stimulate the expression of IL-2 or IL-4 receptors on CD4$^+$ T-cells in the culture system. Further, they have shown that β-endorphin-stimulated IL-4 production by CD4$^+$ T-cells, and IL-1 and IL-6 secretion by splenic macrophages enhances Ia expression on murine B-cells (542).

Opioid peptides modulate a variety of phagocytic and inflammatory functions in macrophages and granulocytes. Enkephalins stimulate neutrophil superoxide anion production and neutrophil migration (482,487). Neutrophil activation by Met-enkephalin and Leu-enkephalin is enhanced by an inhibitor of neutral endopeptidase 24.11 activity (487). This peptidase, known as CD10 or common acute lymphoblastic leukemia antigen, is expressed on normal lymphoid progenitors, neutrophils, and acute lymphoblastic leukemia cells. CD10 may be an important regulator of enkephalin activity in these cells. Activation of classical opioid receptors by Met-enkephalin stimulates and inhibits H_2O_2 release from macrophages from Dark August and Albino Oxford male rats, respectively, indicating that the effects of opioid peptides are strain-dependent (428). Stefano and colleagues (329,517) have demonstrated that HPB monocytes possess δ$_2$-receptors that stimulate, and μ$_3$-receptors that inhibit cytokine-induced activation and chemotactic activity of granulocytes by cytokines.

Foster and Moore (180) have found that dynorphin-A and its related opioid peptides increase the tumoricidal activity of murine peritoneal macrophages activated with IFN and LPS. After treatment with IFN and LPS, tumorcidal responses in peritoneal macrophages become more responsive to opioid peptides (214). U50,488H, the κ-selective agonist, suppresses the production of IL-1, IL-6, and TNF-α by resting peritoneal macrophages (14). This suppression is reversible by pretreatment with naloxone and, by the κ-receptor antagonist, norbinaltorphimine. Similarly, in the PD388D1 macrophage cell line, nanomolar concentrations of U50,488H inhibit LPS-induced IL-1 and TNF-α production (but not IL-6), an effect that is reversible by naloxone, and norbinaltorphimine (28). Examination of IL-1 mRNA concentrations in these macrophages indicates that the opioid peptide-mediated effects on cytokine production occurs at the level of transcription. In contrast, cytokine production by the macrophage-like cell line, RAW 264.7 is not altered by activation of κ-opioid receptors (28). Murine peritoneal macrophage phagocytic activity also is inhibited by μ-, κ-, and δ-opioid agonists (523).

Stimulation of NK cytotoxicity in vitro by Leu-enkephalin and Met-enkephalin was first reported by Faith et al. (143). Administration of Leu-enkephalin, intraperitoneally, suppresses splenic NK cell activity in a naloxone-reversible manner 12 hours after injection, and enhances NK cell activity in a naloxone-irreversible manner 24 and 48 hours after treatment (185). Acute morphine exposure in vivo suppresses splenic NK activity (483) and mitogen-induced proliferation (25). Similar findings have been reported for acute in vivo modulation of these immune parameters by Met-enkephalin (336). There is convincing evidence to indicate that these in vivo effects of opioid peptides are mediated via interaction with receptors in the periaqueductal gray of the mesencephalon (560) to modulate sympathetic outflow (92). Gatti et al. (188) have data that indicate that both ACTH and β-endorphin can effectively counteract the in vitro cortisol-induced inhibition of human NK cell activity and potentiate spontaneous and lymphokine-inducible cytotoxicity.

In in vitro work using cocultures of the U1 monocyte cell line and human brain cells, morphine amplifies LPS-induced HIV-1 expression in brain (416). This effect is dose-dependent with the maximal activity at 10^{-12} M morphine, and is blocked by naloxone and by the selective μ-selective opioid receptor antagonist, β-funaltrexamine. The bell-shaped characteristics of the dose-response suggest that in addition to high affinity μ-opioid receptors that are stimulatory, there also may be low-affinity sites, possibly δ- or κ-opioid receptors, that down-regulate HIV-1 expression.

Development of NA Nerves in Lymphoid Organs

Bone Marrow

Very few developmental studies examining the innervation of bone marrow have been undertaken (83,84,353). In the Wistar rat (84) and the New Zealand rabbit (353), innervation of the bone marrow is first apparent during late fetal life. Miller and McCuskey (353) reported that NA fibers are present prior to the onset of hemopoietic activity, suggesting a role for NA innervation in the subsequent development of hema-topoiesis.

Thymus

The development of NA nerves into the thymus is largely a postnatal event (5; re-viewed in 6,37). NA sympathetic nerves are present in the rodent thymus by embryonic day 17–18, just prior to birth (full term is 20–21 days) (72,494). At birth, NA nerves are sparse. The intensity of fluorescence in CA histochemistry is dull compared with that seen in the adult thymus, suggesting a low concentration of NE in nerve terminals. Most of the NA nerves travel in nerve bundles in the capsule and along the interlobular septa, with a few nerve fibers exiting into the adjacent thymic cortex. At the cor-ticomedullary junction, relatively dense plexuses of fine fibers run adjacent to some of the small-to-medium-sized arteries, with an occasional fluorescent profile extending into the surrounding parenchyma.

By postnatal day 7, the thymus increases in size and becomes further subdivided into lobules by connective tissue septa. A greater density of NA nerves is present in all compartments of the thymus, compared with innervation at birth, but the thymus is still incompletely innervated, compared with that seen in young adult rodents. Individual nerve fibers extend from arteriolar plexuses in the interlobular septa, arborizing among thymocytes and CAF cells in the adjacent thymic cortex, especially near the cor-ticomedullary boundary where CAF cells are most abundant. Large venous sinuses also are innervated by NA nerves at postnatal day 7.

By postnatal day 14, the density and intensity of NA innervation of the capsular/septal system and vasculature approach the extent of NA innervation described in thymuses from young adult animals. Occasionally, single linear fluorescent profiles extend from arteriolar plexuses into the deep cortex, especially along the zone of the CAF cells at the corticomedullary junction. NA fibers also are present along the venous sinuses. The concentration of NE in the 14-day-old thymus approaches adult thymic NE levels. From 14 to 56 days of age, NA innervation of septal and cortical arteries, sinuses, capsule, and interlobular septa keeps pace with thymic growth. During this period of development, CAF cells form a concentrated zone of cells at the corticomedullary junction. As this zone of CAF cells forms, NA innervation becomes more robust.

Spleen

NA innervation of the rat spleen develops principally in the postnatal period (5,7–9,156,158; reviewed in 6,37). In newborn rats, sparse plexuses of NA nerves enter the spleen at the hilus in bundles traveling with the splenic artery and its branches. The most striking finding in neonatal rat spleens is the virtual lack of TH[+] nerve fibers associated with the central arteriole. Instead, TH[+] nerves encircle the outer border of the PALS, several cell layers distant from the central arteriole, among T- and B-lym-phocytes (Figs. 8-25, 8-26). These fibers persist at the adult stage along the marginal

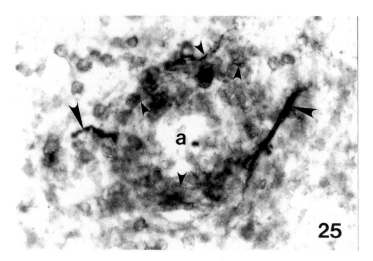

Fig. 8-25. One-day-old rat spleen stained for TH⁺ nerves and OX19⁺ T lymphocytes. TH⁺ nerves fibers in nerve bundles (large arrowheads) or as free fibers (small arrowheads) contact the outer limit of the region delineated by OX19⁺ T-lymphocytes. Occasional TH⁺ fibers enter this compartment but do not contact the cental arteriole (a). Double-label ICC TH and OX19; ×215.

sinus. At the ultrastructural level, TH⁺ nerve terminals directly contact lymphocytes similar to those observed in the PALS of adult rats. Direct appositions also occur between TH⁺ nerve terminals and reticular-like cells, a cell type mainly seen in the PALS of the neonatal rat spleen. Despite the low density of NA nerves, splenic NE concentration is approximately 25% of adult values.

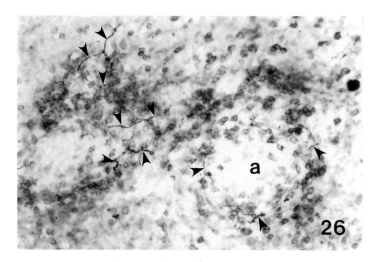

Fig. 8-26. One-day-old rat spleen stained for TH⁺ nerves and IgM⁺ T-lymphocytes. TH⁺ nerve fibers (arrowheads) proceed among IgM⁺ B-lymphocytes in the external portion of the periarteriolar lymphatic sheath. Double-label ICC for TH and IgM. a, central arteriole; ×110.

By postnatal day 7, the white pulp consists of the central PALS, the peripheral PALS, the marginal sinus, and the marginal zone. T-lymphocytes are present throughout the PALS, intermixed with B-lymphocytes in the periphery. The marginal zone contains B-lymphocytes and ED3$^+$ macrophages. The density and the intensity of TH staining in nerves throughout the white pulp is greater than at any other age examined. The central arterioles are surrounded by dense TH$^+$ nerve plexuses. TH$^+$ profiles exit from these vascular plexuses into the PALS among T- and B-lymphocytes (Figs. 8-27, 8-28). TH$^+$ nerves arborize extensively among B-lymphocytes in the outer PALS and inner marginal zone. At the inner edge of the marginal zone, ED3$^+$ macrophages reside adjacent to bundles of TH$^+$ nerves (Fig. 8-29) that traverse the marginal sinus.

NA innervation resembles the adult pattern by postnatal day 14. ED3$^+$ macrophages and T- and B-lymphocytes reorganize to form adult-like white pulps. Concomitant with this cellular rearrangement, NA nerves also redistribute to the inner PALS, forming dense, tangled plexuses of fibers along the central arteriole and adjacent regions of the PALS (Fig. 8-30). TH$^+$ nerve fibers are also present in the parafollicular zone and in the marginal sinus. From the marginal sinus, TH$^+$ fibers arborize among ED3$^+$ macrophages (Fig. 8-30) and B-lymphocytes in the inner marginal zone. Splenic NE concentration progressively increases, approaching young adult levels at day 14.

By 28 days of age, the relative size of each splenic compartment shifts. The inner PALS develops a thin and elongated appearance. The follicles and marginal zones greatly increase in size. NA nerves accomodate the changes in the organization of the white pulp. TH$^+$ nerves are localized in the inner one-third of the PALS, which is

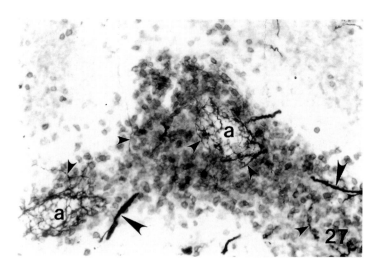

Fig. 8-27. Ten-day-old rat spleen stained for TH$^+$ nerves and OX19$^+$ T-lymphocytes. TH$^+$ nerve fibers (small arrowheads) travel throughout the inner PALS formed by OX19$^+$ T-lymphocytes. Additional bundles (large arrowheads) in long, linear arrays encircle this region, at the site of the marginal sinus. Double-label ICC for TH and OX19. a, central arteriole; ×215.

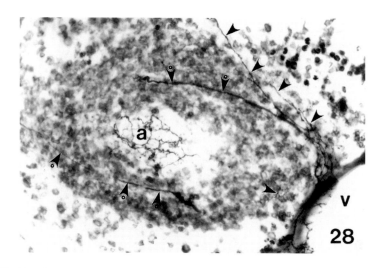

Fig. 8-28. Ten-day-old rat spleen stained for TH⁺ nerves and IgM⁺ T-lymphocytes. TH⁺ nerve fibers are present along the venous sinus (v), and exit from this compartment into the white pulp of the spleen. Long, linear profiles of TH⁺ nerves (open circle-arrowheads) separate lightly stained IgM⁺ cell of the PALS from the darkly stained IgM⁺ cells of the marginal zone. Additional TH⁺ fibers form a dense plexus within the periarteriolar lymphatic sheath arborizing among B lymphocytes within the outer portion of the this region and adjacent to branches of the central arteriole (a). Double-label ICC for TH and IgM; ×215.

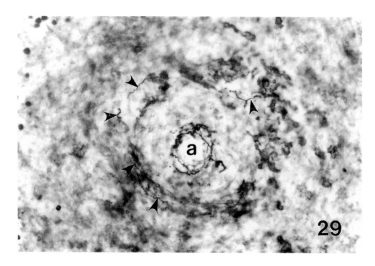

Fig. 8.29. Ten-day-old rat spleen stained for TH⁺ nerves and ED3⁺ macrophages. TH⁺ nerve fibers form a dense plexus throughout the inner portion of the periarteriolar lymphatic sheath devoid of ED3⁺ cells. Additional TH⁺ fibers (small arrowheads) run among ED3⁺ macrophages at the site of the marginal sinus. Large TH⁺ nerve bundles (large arrowheads) also traverse this region. Double-label ICC for TH and ED3; ×215.

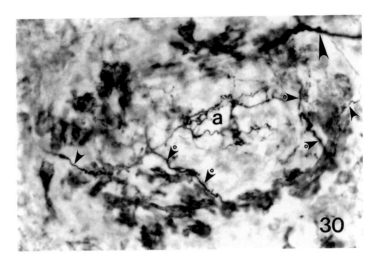

Fig. 8-30. Fourteen-day-old rat spleen stained for TH$^+$ nerves and ED3$^+$ macrophages. TH$^+$ nerves (open circle-arrowheads) arborize within the thickened rim of ED3$^+$ cells along the marginal sinus. Additional ED3$^+$ cells are present in the marginal zone among individual TH$^+$ nerve fibers (small arrowheads) and TH$^+$ nerve bundles (large arrowheads). The typical plexus of TH$^+$ nerve fibers is found associated with the central arteriole (a) and adjacent to the periarteriolar lymphatic sheath. Double-label ICC for TH and ED3; $\times$215.

similar to the distribution in the adult spleen. NA nerve fibers remain in the marginal zone among the thickening rim of ED3$^+$ macrophages, and the outer portion of this zone receives additional fibers from NA plexuses that course along the venous sinuses and trabeculae. TH$^+$ nerves also reside in the parafollicular zone, with some fibers occasionally extending from this zone into the follicle itself. By 28 days of age, the most prominent change in NA innervation is the marked increase in density of TH$^+$ nerves along the venous sinuses and trabeculae. Relatively few fibers extend from the venous sinuses and trabeculae into the surrounding red pulp. Throughout young adulthood, all compartments of the spleen increase in size and are accompanied by parallel growth of NA innervation.

Estimates of NE turnover in the developing spleen reveal enhanced NE metabolism throughout development, which parallels increases in NE concentration and in density of NA nerve fibers. NE turnover is relatively low at birth, increases from birth to postnatal day 7, reaches a second plateau from day 14 to 56, then gradually increases to adult values. The density of β-adrenergic receptors on splenocytes from developing spleens parallels the pattern of NE turnover. Splenocytes from 1- to 10-day-old rats display a B$_{max}$ of 400–500 sites/cell, whereas splenocytes from 14- to 90-day old rats contain adult levels of 800–1,000 sites/cell. This shift in receptor expression may reflect a change in spleen cell populations or the development of immunocompetent cells approaching a state where they are more capable of responding to NE released from NA nerves.

The presence of NA nerves in developing compartments of the thymus and spleen throughout development suggests a role for NE in the development of immunocompetence. The presence of β-adrenergic receptors on developing cells of the immune system supports this hypothesis. In the thymus, NE released from NA nerves is available for interaction with thymocytes and supportive cells. NE may modulate thymic stem cell migration into the thymus possibly through direct interaction with thymocytes to induce chemotaxis and migration, or indirectly through the regulation of blood flow. Increasing concentrations of NE in the developing thymus may subsequently promote maturation and emigration of mature thymocytes for the seeding of secondary lymphoid organs. In the spleen, NE may play a role in the formation and maturation of splenic compartments through selective migration of specific populations of cells into the spleen, modulation of proliferation and maturation of lymphocytes, and activation of specific cell functions at critical time points during the splenic development. Conversely, lymphoid and non-lymphoid cells that reside near nerve fibers in the marginal sinus may provide signals that influence the growth and maturation of NA nerves and the release of NE from those nerves.

Aging and Innervation of Lymphoid Organs

Bone Marrow

In preliminary studies, we have examined bone marrow from 3- and 21-month-old F344 rats with fluorescence histochemistry for CAs (D. L. Bellinger, unpublished observations). NA innervation of bone marrow from 3-month-old rats is similar to that described above. We found no remarkable differences in the density or pattern of NA innervation of bone marrow from rats at 21 months of age compared with their young adult counterparts.

Thymus

In humans and in experimental animals, the maximum size of the thymus is attained at sexual maturation and then begins to atrophy shortly after puberty, continuing to degenerate with normal aging (34,469). Before the onset of thymic involution, a decline in thymic hormone secretion has also been reported (218). Clearly, the neuroendocrine system plays a role in this process. It is not clear what role, if any, direct sympathetic innervation of the thymus has on thymic involution. In a longitudinal study examining NA innervation of the thymus with fluorescence histochemistry for localization of CAs, we have found that, between 8 and 27 months of age, as the thymus progressively atrophies, the density of NA nerve fibers in all compartments of the thymus progressively increases (34), probably reflecting the maintenance of intact innervation in the face of marked cortical involution. NA innervation is especially dense in the cortical and paracortical regions of the aging thymus, forming more extensive plexuses of sympathetic fibers than has been described anywhere else in the body, with the possible exception of the vas deferens. Dense tangles of NA nerves course along the vasculature and as free profiles through the parenchyma of the cortex and paracortex. These fibers generally form longitudinal arrays oriented parallel to the long axis of the thymic surface.

The number of CAF cells in the thymus also increase with age (34), making the boundary between the cortex and medullary much more distinct than at younger ages. These cells are often present as single cells or in clusters among dense tangles of NA fibers. The density of NA nerve fibers in the medulla is not as markedly altered with advancing age, also making the boundary between the medulla and the cortex more distinct. We suggest that the increase in density of NA innervation of the thymus with age results from the preservation of the full complement of NA nerves in the face of a progressively diminishing volume of thymic tissue.

Neurochemical measurement on NE is consistent with this hypothesis (34). Thymic NE content expressed per whole thymus reveals relatively stable NE levels from 3 to 27 months of age. These findings indicate that, with advancing age, NA nerves in the thymus accommodate to the collapsing thymic cortex. As the thymic parenchyma recedes, the remaining nerves fibers become packed into a smaller volume of tissue, resulting in an increased NE concentration in the microenvironment of age-resistant thymocytes. Whether these target cells are capable of responding to enhanced NE availability has not been examined; this would depend on the continued presence of adrenergic receptors on these cells and on the ability of the ligand-receptor interaction to initiate an appropriate second messenger response with functional consequences for the target cells.

Spleen

The mature pattern of NA innervation of specific compartments of the spleen (Fig. 8-31) persists through approximately 17 months of age in F344 rats (6,29,33,162). From 17 to 27 months of age, (Fig. 8-32), NA innervation shows a progressive diminution in all compartments of the spleen (6,29,33,162). At 27 months of age, the total NE content is diminished by approximately 50%, and the density of fluorescent profiles, evaluated morphometrically, is reduced by more than 80% in the parenchyma and around the central arteriolar system (33). However, all compartments show at least a 60% reduction in the density of nerve profiles. We have some evidence to indicate that the discrepancy in the NE content, compared with the decline in the density of NA nerve profiles, is likely the result of altered NE metabolism in, and enhanced ability for uptake of NE into, age-resistant nerve terminals persisting in the splenic white pulp.

Double-labeled ICC for TH and specific cellular markers on immunocytes further demonstrates a gradual decline in the density of T-lymphocytes in the PALS (Figs.

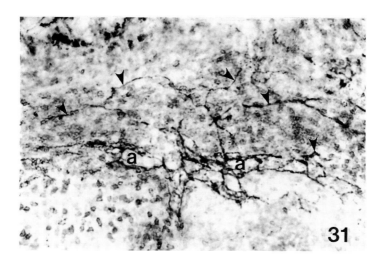

Fig. 8-31. TH$^+$ nerves (arrowheads) course along the central arteriole (a) and arborize into the surrounding periarteriolar lymphatic sheath among OX19$^+$ T-lymphocytes in spleens from 3-month-old rats. Double-label ICC for TH; ×215.

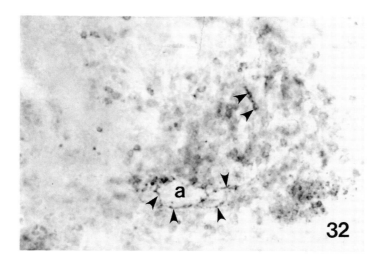

Fig. 8-32. The density of TH$^+$ nerves (arrowheads) along the central arteriole (a) and among OX19$^+$ T-lymphocytes in the surrounding PALS of the rat splenic white pulp is diminished at 21 months of age. Additionally, the fewer OX19$^+$ cells are present in the PALS of spleens from 21-month-old rats. Double-label ICC for TH and OX19; ×110.

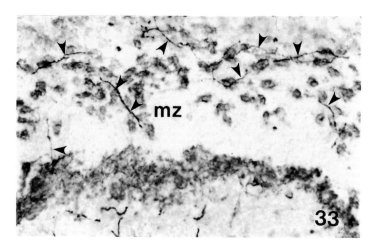

Fig. 8-33. TH+ nerves (arrowheads) distribute among ED3+ macrophages in the inner and outer marginal zone of the rat spleen at 3 months of age. Double-label ICC for TH and ED3; ×215.

8-31, 8-32) and in ED3+ macrophages in the marginal zone (Figs. 8-33, 8-34). This decline begins just prior to, and progresses in parallel with, the loss of NA innervation (29). The density of NA nerves in the aged spleen displays a high-to-low gradient with respect to the distance from the hilar region of the spleen (i.e., higher density nearer the hilus). The density of T-lymphocytes in the PALS and ED3+ macrophages in the marginal zone displays a similar pattern of loss that closely overlaps the loss of NA

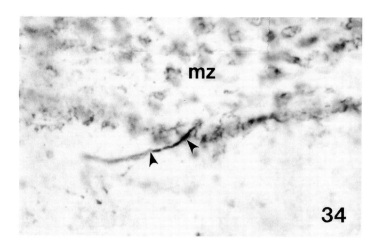

Fig. 8-34. The density of TH+ nerves (arrowheads) that proceed from the marginal sinus and into the marginal zone (mz) of the rat spleen is diminished at 21 month of age. Concomitant with this decline in NA innervation, the density of ED3+ macrophages in the inner and outer marginal zone also declines. Double-label ICC for TH and ED3; ×215.

innervation. Cell loss in these compartments occurs to the greatest extent most distal to the hilar region and proceeds toward the hilus with advancing age. In contrast, the density of IgM$^+$ B-lymphocytes is not altered in the follicle or marginal zone in spleens from aged F344 rats.

We have some preliminary data to suggest that the extent and time course of age-related decline in splenic NA innervation is dependent upon the continued exposure of the adult rat to environmental antigens. Pilot data suggest that splenic NA denervation is accelerated in rats raised under vivarium conditions as compared with rats raised in barrier facilities (pathogen-free). A similar decline in NPY innervation which overlaps the distribution of NA nerves and parallels the loss of T-lymphocytes and ED3$^+$ macrophages occurs with age. In contrast, SP innervation does not appear to change with the normal aging process, based on both ICC staining and direct measurement of splenic SP. These findings support the hypothesis that NPY, but not SP, is colocalized in NA sympathetic nerves that distribute to the spleen.

A loss in NA innervation of the spleen can result from *(1)* an inability of NA nerve terminals to synthesize enough NE to form observable fluorophore (or enough TH for immunostaining, since this decline in NA nerve fibers in the spleen is also observed with ICC staining for TH); or *(2)* an absence of the terminals. Administration of α-methylNE, a compound that is taken up by the high-affinity carrier into NA terminals and persists because it cannot be catabolized by monoamine oxidase, is able to restore fluorescence in only a few nerve profiles in 27-month-old rat spleens as compared with untreated and vehicle-treated controls, but not to the level of 3-month-old rats (40). These findings support an actual retraction and loss of NA fibers in the aging spleen; however, these findings could also be attributed to a deficit in the high-affinity uptake system in the aging spleen.

We have developed a perfused spleen model to examine the high-affinity uptake, release, and metabolism of [^{3}H]-NE in spleen slices, coupled with fluorescence histo-chemistry for CAs to quantitate NA innervation in alternate slices (36,37,40). In preliminary studies using this technique with spleen slices from 3- and 21-month-old rats, we have found that total uptake of [^{3}H]-NE in old rats is significantly less than uptake in young rats, but that the efficiency of uptake of [^{3}H]-NE per nerve terminal is greatly enhanced in old rats. Kinetic analysis of the data suggests an increase in NE uptake in the aging spleen, probably as a compensatory mechanism resulting from the decline in NE concentration, and/or loss of NA nerve terminals that occurs with aging. We have not yet examined the effect of age on synthesis of NE in spleens from young and old rats. It is likely that synthesis in age-resistant terminals in the spleen also is enhanced, and may account for the higher splenic NE content compared with the density of nerve terminals. Increased circulating NE reported to occur with aging (39,281,290,338), which might be available for uptake into age-resistant terminals, also contributes to this process.

Radioligand binding studies (6) show an increase in the density of β-adrenergic receptors in splenocytes with age, which is consistent with up-regulation in response to declining splenic NE concentration. No differences in receptor affinity occur with age. De Blasi and co-workers (120) reported that aged rats respond to restraint stress (as a mechanism to increase NE availability) more slowly and with diminished down-regulation of lymphocyte β-adrenergic receptor density in response to agonist avail-ability. However, the fact that restraint stress also increases circulating glucocorticoid levels, which have also been shown to modulate β-adrenoreceptor expression, and that old rats may have exaggerated responses to stressors as compared with young rats, makes this study difficult to interpret at a mechanistic level. Measurements of β-adren-ergic receptors over time, following administration of exogenous adrenergic agonists, has not been performed to test this hypothesis throughout the age span.

Expression of β-adrenoceptors may not be an accurate indicator of the ability of cells to respond to NA stimulation, especially in lymphocytes from aged subjects. Based on several studies examining β-adrenergic receptor coupling with adenylate cyclase (148,381), lymphocyte responsiveness to NA stimulation may be impaired, despite the greater number of receptors. These studies indicate an age-related, intrinsic defect in the activation of the adenylate cyclase system following β-adrenergic receptor stimula-tion, resulting from an inability of the receptor to activate adenylate cyclase and/or alter the catalytic capacity of adenylate cyclase. Similar findings have been reported in non-lymphoid organs that receive sympathetic innervation, such as rat myocardium and lung (288,377,468).

Extensive investigations of immune reactivity in aging (reviewed in 264,265) have demonstrated a decline in normal immune functions, primarily those involving T-cell–mediated responses (summarized in Table 8-3), that parallels the decline in the peripheral NA system. Age-related immunologic dysfunction is associated with an increased incidence of autoimmune and immune-complex diseases, certain types of cancer, and viral and fungal infections. Impairment of immune capacity with age is likely to result from a combination of both age-related changes in immune cells and alterations in their microenvironment. That the normal aging process is associated with both a decline in immunocompetence and in NA innervation of secondary lymphoid organs makes it tempting to hypothesize a causal relationship. Conversely, NA denervation may be compensatory rather than causal to immune dysfunction. The finding that the direction of change in immune responses following acute chemical sympathectomy with 6-OHDA is often similar to that of immune responses measured in aged rodents supports the possibility that NA nerve fiber loss plays at least a partial causal role in the loss of immune competence with age. NA innervation of the murine spleen remains fully intact but becomes more dense, in the white pulp following lymphocyte depletion using hydrocor-tisone or cyclophosphamide in young adults (88), suggesting that NA denervation may not be compensatory to the loss of T-lymphocytes in the white pulp of the spleen with age. Whether or not a compensatory loss of NA nerve fibers occurs with chronic depletion of T-lymphocytes remains to be demonstrated. However, in SCID mice, with the absence of both T- and B-lymphocytes, NA innervation of the small white pulp remains intact over several months (S. Y. Felten, unpublished observations).

Table 8-3 Effect of Aging and Acute Chemical Sympathectomy on Immune Responsiveness

Immune Response	Age-Related Changes	Sympathectomy-Induced Changes
T-cell–mediated responses		
Delayed-type hypersensitivity	Decreased	Decreased
Cytotoxic T-lymphocyte activity	Decreased	Decreased
Con A-induced proliferation	Decreased	Decreased
IL-2 receptors	Decreased	ND[a]
B cell–mediated responses		
LPS-induced proliferation	Mixed	Mixed
Ig secretion in response to polyclonal B-cell differentiation	Increased	Increased
Response to antigen stimulation		
Primary antibody response (T-dependent)	Decreased	Decreased
Secondary antibody response (T-dependent)	Mixed	Decreased[b]
Primary antibody response (T-independent)	Mixed	Increased
IL-2 production	Decreased	Decreased
Lymph node cellular proliferation	Increased	Increased
Response to autologous antigen	Increased	Increased
Tumoricidal activity		
NK-cell activity	Mixed	Increased
Resistance to tumor challenge	Decreased	Increased

ND, not determined.

[a]Sympathectomy prior to boosting.

[b]From Ackerman KD, Bellinger, DL, Felten SY, Felten DL. Ontogeny and senescence of noradrenergic innervation of the rodent thymus and spleen. In: Psychoneuroimmunology II, 2nd ed., R Ader, DL Felten, N Cohen, eds. Academic Press, New York, 1991, pp. 71–125, with permission. See Ackerman KD, Bellinger DL, Felten SY, Felten DL, 1991 for a review of the effects of aging and acute sympathectomy on immune responsiveness.

Lymph Nodes

We have examined cervical, mesenteric, and popliteal lymph nodes from several strains of aged mice, including C3H, C57B1/6, New Zealand white and black (NZW), (NZB), NZB × NZW F1, and in aged F344 rats with fluorescence histochemistry for CAs. NA innervation in all compartments of lymph nodes was diminished in all lymph nodes examined (30,37). The time course of decline varied depending on the strain, and correlated with the expected life span of the animals.

NA Sympathetic Innervation and Autoimmunity

Studies in animal models of autoimmunity (including adjuvant-induced experimental arthritis (AA) [rheumatoid arthritis], New Zealand mice strains [hemolytic anemia and lupus-like syndrome], and experimental allergic encephalomyelitis [EAE; multiple sclerosis]), as well as clinical studies, suggest a role for neural signaling in the development and progression of autoimmune disorders (30,36,37,96,98,108,111,160,295,297, 299–302,312,566). The expression of EAE was attenuated following lesions in the anterior hypothalamus prior to immunization (566). Direct involvement of the sympathetic nervous system in the expression of autoimmune disease is suggested by the work of Chelmicka-Shorr and co-workers (96,98) and by studies from our laboratories (160,312). Chemical sympathectomy in Lewis rats exacerbates EAE (96), while administration of isoproterenol, an adrenergic agonist, to susceptible rats is protective against the development of EAE (98). Clinical and animals studies also point toward involvement of the nervous system in the inflammation and joint destruction in rheumatoid arthritic patients, and in rats with AA. Neonatal treatment with capsaicin, a neurotoxin that destroys small nonmyelinated fibers, including SP-containing fibers, reduces the severity of joint injury in arthritic rats (295,298,299). NE- and SP-containing nerves in the joint can mediate the extent of inflammation and subsequent destruction of affected joints in laboratory animals with AA, and in arthritic patients (258,551).

Recent studies from our laboratory have examined the role of NA and SP innervation of secondary lymphoid organs, without manipulation of the innervation of the joint tissue, in the development and progression of AA in young adult Lewis rats (36,160,312,313). Selective denervation of NA nerves in draining popliteal and inguinal lymph nodes by local application of 6-OHDA prior to challenge with Freund's complete adjuvant into the hind footpad exacerbates the subsequent inflammatory responses and joint destruction following adjuvant-induced arthritis. By contrast, selective denervation of SP-containing nerves in draining popliteal and inguinal lymph nodes by local application of capsaicin 1 day after immunization delays the onset and attenuates the severity of arthritis.

Summary and Conclusions

NA and peptidergic nerve fibers have been demonstrated in both primary and secondary lymphoid organs among cells of the immune system. We and others have demonstrated that these nerves can transmit signals to the immune system that are capable of altering immune functions and reactivity. Further, we have shown that dynamic changes occur in sympathetic innervation throughout the lifespan of an individual, with possible functional implications for the development and senescence of the immune system and for disease processes such as autoimmune disorders. Collectively, these findings indicate that the development of disease states, including autoimmune disorders, depends on highly complex interactions between the nervous and immune systems at multiple sites (i.e., at all effector tissues, at the site of antigen presentation and processing, and at the CNS). The mechanisms of action, routes of communication between these sites, and the neural and immune mediators that determine the overall health status of an individual await further investigation. However, the detailed investigation of neurotransmitters, such as NE in nerves in the spleen and lymph nodes offers several clues. Innervation of primary and secondary lymphoid organs can play an important role in health and illness, and under conditions of marginal functioning of the immune system, neural signaling may be a particularly important factor. Future research to elucidate pathways for neural–immune interactions and to identify neural and immune mediators and their mechanisms of action in models of aging, disease, and autoimmunity may ultimately lead to unique pharmacological approaches to the maintenance of immune-system homeostasis and host defense-mechanism throughout the life span of an individual, and to intervention in autoimmune disorders, such as rheumatoid arthritis.

Acknowledgments

We thank Kim Gibson-Berry for use of her micrographs, Dorothy Herrera and Jennifer Loughlin for excellent photographic work, and John Housel, Charley Richardson, and Angela Tong for expert technical assistance. This work was supported by grants R37 NIMH MH42076, P50 NIMH MH40381, R01 NIH NS25223, R29 NIMH MH47783, and the Lucille Markey Charitable Trust Award.

References

1. Aarons RD, Nies AS, Gall J, Hegstrand LF. Elevation of beta-adrenergic receptor density in human lymphocytes after propranolol administration. J Clin Invest 65:949–957, 1980.
2. Aarons RD, Nies AS, Gerber JG, Molinoff PB. Decreased beta adrenergic receptor density on human lymphocytes after chronic treatment with agonists. J Pharmacol Exp Ther 224:1–6, 1982.
3. Abrahamsson T, Holmgren S, Nilsson S, Pettersson K. Adrenergic and cholinergic effects on the heart, the lung and the spleen of the African lungfish, *Protopterus aethiopicus*. Acta Physiol Scand 107:141–147, 1979.
4. Abrass CK, O'Connor SW, Scarpace PJ, Abrass IB. Characterization of the β-adrenergic receptor of the rat peritoneal macrophage. J Immunol 135:1338–1341, 1985.
5. Ackerman KD. Noradrenergic sympathetic neurotransmission in the adult and neonatal rat spleen. Ph.D. thesis, University of Rochester, Rochester N.Y..
6. Ackerman KD, Bellinger DL, Felten SY, Felten DL. Ontogeny and senescence of noradrenergic innervation of the rodent thymus and spleen. In Psychoneuroimmunology, 2nd ed, R Ader, DL Felten, N Cohen eds. Academic Press, New York, 1991, 71–125.
7. Ackerman KD, Felten SY, Bellinger DL, Felten DL. Noradrenergic sympathetic innervation of the spleen: III. Development of innervation in the rat spleen. J Neurosci Res 18:49–54, 1987.
8. Ackerman KD, Felten SY, Bellinger DL, Livnat S, Felten DL. Noradrenergic sympathetic innervation of spleen and lymph nodes in relation to specific cellular compartments. Prog Immunol 6:588–600, 1987.

9. Ackerman KD, Felten SY, Dijkstra CD, Livnat S, Felten DL. Parallel development of noradrenergic innervation and cellular compartmentation in the rat spleen. Exp Neurol 103:239–255, 1989.

10. Agro A, Padol I, Stanisz AM. Immunomodulatory activity of the somatostatin analogue BIM 23014c: effects on murine lymphocyte proliferation and natural killer activity. Regul Peptides 32:129–139, 1991.

11. Agro A, Stanisz AM. Are lymphocytes the main target for neuromodulation by substance P in rheumatoid arthritis? Seminar Arthritis Rheum 21:252–258, 1992.

12. Agro A, Stanisz AM. Inhibition of murine intestinal inflammation by anti-substance P antibody. Reg Immunol 5:120–126, 1993.

13. Alessandrini C, Gerli R, Sacchi G, Ibba L, Pucci AM, Fruschelli C. Cholinergic and adrenergic innervation of mesenteric lymph vessels in guinea pig. Lymphology 14:1–6, 1981.

14. Alicea C, Belkowski S, Einstein TK, Adler MW, Rogers TJ. Inhibition of primary murine macrophage cytokine production in vitro following treatment with the κ-opioid agonist U50,488H. J Neuroimmunol 64:83–90, 1996.

15. Ansel JC, Brown JR, Payan DG, Brown MA. Substance P selectively activates TNF-α gene expression in murine mast cells. J Immunol 150:4478–4485, 1993.

16. Ansiello CM, Roda LG. Leu-enkephalin binding to cultured human T lymphocytes. Cell Biol Int Rep 8:353–362, 1984.

17. Apte RN, Oppenheim JJ, Durum SK. β-endorphin regulates interleukin 1 production and release by murine bone marrow macrophages. Int Immunol 1:465–470, 1989.

18. Arora PK, Rfide E, Petitto J, Waggie K, Skolnick P. Morphine-induced immune alteration in vivo. Cell Immunol 126:343–353, 1990.

19. Assem ESK, Schild HO. Inhibition by sypathomimetic amines of histamine release induced by antigen in passively sensitized human lung. Nature 224:1028–1029, 1969.

20. Ballantyne, B. The reticuloendothelial localization of splenic esterases. J Reticuloendothel 5:399–411, 1968.

21. Barbany G, Friedman WJ, Persson H. Lymphocyte-mediated regulation of neurotransmitter gene expression in rat sympathetic ganglia. J Neuroimmunol 32:97–104, 1991.

22. Baron R, Jänig W. Sympathetic and afferent neurons projecting in the splenic nerve of the cat. Neurosci Lett 94:109–113, 1988.

23. Bartik MM, Brooks WH, Roszman TL. Modulation of T cell proliferation by stimulation of the β-adrenergic receptor: lack of correlation between inhibition of T cell proliferation and cAMP accumulation. Cell Immunol 148:408–421, 1993.

24. Bar-Shavit Z, Goldman R, Stabinsky Y, Gottleib F, Fridkin M, Teichberg V, Blumberg S. Enhancement of phagocytosis—a newly found activity of substance P residing in its N-terminal tetrapeptide sequence. Biochem Biophys Res Commun 94:1445–1451, 1980.

25. Bayer BM, Daussin A, Hernandez M, Irwin L. Morphine inhibition of lymphocyte activity is mediated by an opioid dependent mechanism. Neuropharmacol 29:369–374, 1990.

26. Beckner SK, Farrar WL. Potentiation of lymphokine-activated killer cells differentiation and lymphocyte proliferation by stimulation of protein kinase C or inhibition of adenylate cyclase. J Immunol 140:208–214, 1988.

27. Beed EA, O'Dorisio MS, O'Dorisio TM, Gaginella TS. Demonstration of a functional receptor for vasoactive intestinal polypeptide on Molt 4b lymphoblasts. Regul Pept 6:1–12, 1983.

28. Belkowski SM, Alicea C, Einstein TK, Adler MW, Rogers TJ. Inhibition of interleukin-1 and tumor necrosis factor-α synthesis following treatment of macrophages with the kappa opioid agonist U50,488H. J Pharmacol Exp Ther 273:1491–1496, 1995.

29. Bellinger DL, Ackerman KD, Felten SY, Felten DL. Loss of noradrenergic nerves and lymphoid cells in the aged rat spleen. Exp Neurol 116:295–311, 1991.

30. Bellinger DL, Ackerman KD, Felten SY, Lorton D, Felten DL. Noradrenergic sympathetic innervation of thymus, spleen and lymph nodes: aspects of development, aging and plasticity in neural-immune interactions. In: Interactions Between the Neuroendocrine and Immune Systems, G Nistico, ed. Pythogora Press, Rome, 1989, pp 35–66.

31. Bellinger DL, Earnest DJ, Gallagher M, Felten DL. Presence and availability of VIP in primary and secondary lymphoid organs. Soc Neurosci Abstr 18:1009, 1992.

32. Bellinger DL, Felten SY, Coleman PD, Yeh P, Felten DL. Noradrenergic innervation and acetylcholinesterase activity of lymph nodes in young adult and aging mice. Soc Neurosci Abstr 11:663, 1985.

33. Bellinger DL, Felten SY, Collier TJ, Felten DL. Noradrenergic sympathetic innervation of the spleen: IV. Morphometric analysis in adult and aged F344 rats. N Neurosci Res 18:55–63, 1987.

34. Bellinger DL, Felten SY, Felten DL. Maintenance of noradrenergic sympathetic innervation in the involuted thymus of the aged Fischer 344 rat. Brain Behav Immunol 2:133–150, 1988.

35. Bellinger DL, Felten SY, Felten DL. The origin of acetylcholinesterase-positive nerve fibers in the spleen of young adult rats. Soc Neurosci Abstr 14:956, 1988.

36. Bellinger DL, Felten SY, Felten DL. Neural-immune interactions: neurotransmitter signaling of cells of the immune system. Annu Rev Psychiatry 11:127–144, 1991.

37. Bellinger DL, Felten SY, Felten DL. Noradrenergic sympathetic innervation of lymphoid organs during development, aging, and autoimmunity. In Aging of the Autonomic Nervous System, F Amenta, ed. CRC Press, Boca Raton, FL, 1993:243–284.

38. Bellinger DL, Felten SY, Lorton D, Felten DL. Origin of noradrenergic innervation of the spleen in rats. Brain Behav Immunol 3:291–311, 1989.

39. Bellinger DL, Lorton D, Brouxhon S, Felten SY, Felten DL. The significance of vasoactive intestinal polypeptide (VIP) in immunomodulation. Adv Neuroimmunol 6:5–27, 1996.

40. Bellinger DL, Lorton D, Felten SY, Felten DL. Age-related alteration in norepinephrine uptake in the rat spleen. Soc Neurosci Abstr 16:1210, 1990.

41. Bellinger DL, Lorton D, Romano T, Olschowka JA, Felten SY, Felten DL. Neuropeptide innervation of lymphoid organs. Ann NY Acad Sci 594:17–33, 1990.

42. Berecek KH, Brody MJ. Evidence for a neurotransmitter role for epinephrine derived from the adrenal medulla. Am J Physiol 242:H593–H601, 1982.

43. Bergquist J, Tarkowski A, Ekman R, Ewing A. Discovery of endogenous catecholamines in lymphocytes and evidence for catecholamine regulation of lymphocyte function via an autocrine loop. Proc Natl Acad USA 91:12912–12916, 1994.

44. Berisha H, Foda HD, Sakakibara H, Trotz M, Pakbaz H, Said SI. Vasoactive intestinal peptide prevents lung injury due to xanthine/xanthine oxidase. Am J Physiol 259:L151–L155, 1990.

45. Besedovsky HO, del Rey AE, Sorkin E, Burri R, Honegger CG, Schlumpf M, Lichtensteiger W. T lymphocytes affect the development of sympathetic innervation of mouse spleen. Brain Behav Immunol 1:185–193, 1987.

46. Besedovsky HO, del Rey A, Sorkin E, Da Prada M, Keller HH. Immunoregulation mediated by the sympathetic nervous system. Cell Immunol 48:346–355, 1979.

47. Bhathena SJ, Louie J, Schechter GP, Redman RS, Wahl L, Recant L. Identification of human mononuclear leukocytes bearing receptors for somatostatin and glucagon. Diabetes 30:127–131, 1981.

48. Bidart JM, Motte Ph, Assicot M, Bohuon C, Bellett D. Catechol-O-methyltransferase

activity and aminergic binding sites distribution in human peripheral blood lymphocyte subpopulations. Clin Immunol Immunopathol. 26:1–9, 1983.

49. Bidlack JM, Hemmick LM. Morphine enhancement of mitogen-induced T-cell proliferation. In: The International Narcotics Research Conference (INRC) '89, F Quirion, K Jhamandas, C Gianoulakis, eds. Alan R. Liss, New York, 1990, 405–408.

50. Bienenstock J, Tomioka M, Matsuda H, Stead RH, Quinonez G, Simon GT, Coughlin MD, Denburg JA. The role of mast cells in inflammatory processes: evidence for nerve-mast cell interactions. Int Arch Allergy Appl Immunol 82:238–243, 1987.

51. Bjurholm A, Kreicbergs A, Broden E, Schultzberg M. Substance P- and CGRP-immunoreactive nerves in bone. Peptides 9:165–171, 1989.

52. Blum AM, Mathew R, Cook GA, Metwall A, Felman R, Weinstock JV. Murine mucosal T cells have VIP receptors functionally distinct from those on intestinal epithelial cells. J Neuroimmunol 39:101–108, 1992.

53. Blum AM, Metwall A, Cook G, Mathew RC, Elliott D, Weinstock JV. Substance P modulates antigen-induced, IFN-γ production in murine *Schistosomiasis mansoni.* J Immunol 151:225–233, 1993.

54. Blum AM, Metwali A, Matthew RC, Cook G, Elliot D, Weinstock JV. Granuloma T lymphocytes in murine *Schistosomiasis mansoni* have somatostatin receptors and respond to somatostatin with decreased IFN-gamma secretion. J Immunol 149:3621–3626, 1992.

55. Blum AM, Metwali A, Mathew RC, Elliot D, Weinstock JV. Substance P and somatostatin can modulate the amount of IgG$_{2a}$ secreted in response to schistosome egg antigens in murine *Schistosomiasis mansoni.* J Immunol 151:6694–7004, 1993.

56. Bocchini G, Bonanno G, Canevari A. Influence of morphine on human peripheral blood T-lymphocytes. Drug Alcohol Depend 11:233–237, 1983.

57. Bond RA, Charlton KG, Clark DE. Evidence for a receptor to clonidine distinct from alpha$_2$ sites. Federation Proc 44:1248, 1985.

58. Bondesson L, Norolind K, Liden S, Gafvelin G, Theodorsson E, Mutt V. Dual effects of vasoactive intestinal peptide (VIP) on leucocyte migration. Acta Physiol Scand 141:477–481, 1991.

59. Boudard R, Bastide M. Inhibition of mouse T-cell proliferation by CGRP and VIP: effects of these neuropeptides on IL-2 production and cAMP synthesis. J Neurosci Res 29:29–41, 1991.

60. Bourne HR, Lichtenstein LM, Melmon K, Henney CS, Weinstein Y, Shearer GM. Modulation of inflammation and immunity by cyclic AMP. Science 184:19–28, 1974.

61. Brain S, Williams TJ. Substance P regulates the vasodilator activity of calcitonin gene-related peptide. Nature 335:73–75, 1988.

62. Brenner GJ, Felten SY, Felten DL, Moynihan JA. Sympathetic nervous system modulation of tumor metastases and host defense mechanisms. J Neuroimmunol 37:191–202, 1992.

63. Brimijoin S, Hammond P, Rakonczay Z. Two-site immunoassay for acetylcholinesterase in brain, nerve, and muscle. J Neurochem 49:555–562, 1987.

64. Brodde OE, Engel G, Hoyer D, Block KD, Weber F. The beta-adrenergic receptor in human lymphocytes—subclassification by the use of a new radio-ligand (±)[125 Iodo]cyano-pindolol. Life Sci 29:2189–2198, 1981.

65. Brown GL, Gillespie JS. The output of sympathetic transmitter from the spleen of the cat. J Physiol 138:81–102, 1957.

66. Brown SL, Van Epps DE. Suppression of T lymphocyte chemotactic factor production by the opioid peptides β-endorphin and met-enkephalin. J Immunol 134:3384–3390, 1985.

67. Brown SL, Van Epps DE. Opioid peptides modulate production of interferon gamma by human mononuclear cells. Cell Immunol 103:19–26, 1986.

68. Bryant HU, Bernton EW, Holaday JW. Immunosuppressive effects of chronic morphine treatment in mice. Life Sci 41:1731–1738, 1987.

69. Bryant HU, Bernton EW, Holaday JW. Morphine-induced immunosuppression: involvement of glucocorticoids and prolactin. Natl Inst Drug Abuse Res Monogr Ser 90:323, 1988.

70. Buckley TL, Brain SD, Collins PD, and Williams TJ. Inflammatory edema induced by interactions between IL-1 and the neuropeptide calcitonin gene-related peptide. J Immunol 146:3424–3430, 1991.

71. Bulloch KA. A comparative study of the autonomic nervous system innervation of the thymus in the mouse and chicken. Int J Neurosci 40:129–140, 1988.

72. Bulloch K, Cullen MR, Schwartz RH, Longo DL. Development of innervation within syngeneic thymus tissue transplanted under the kidney capsule of the nude mouse: a light and ultrastructural microscope study. J Neurosci Res 18:16–27, 1987.

73. Bulloch K, McEwen BS, Diwa A, Radojcic T, Hausman J, Baird S. The role of calcitonin gene-related peptide in the mouse thymus revisited. Ann NY Acad Sci 741:129–136, 1994.

74. Bulloch K, Moore RY. Innervation of the thymus gland by brain stem and spinal cord in mouse and rat. Am J Anat 162:157–166, 1981.

75. Bulloch K, Pomerantz W. Autonomic nervous system innervation of thymic related lymphoid tissue in wild-type and nude mice. J Comp Neurol 228:57–68, 1984.

76. Bulloch K, Radojcic T, Yu R, Hausman J, Lenhard L, Baird S. The distribution and function of calcitonin gene-related peptide in the mouse thymus and spleen. Prog Neuroendocrinol 4:186–194, 1991.

77. Calvo CF, Chavanel G, Senik A. Substance P enhances IL-2 expression in activated human T cells. J Immunol 148:3505–3512, 1992.

78. Calvo CF. Substance P stabilizes interleukin-2 mRNA in activated Jurkat cells. J Neuroimmunol 51:85–91, 1994.

79. Calvo JR, Guerrero JM, Molinero P, Blasco R, Goberna R. Interaction of vasoactive intestinal peptide (VIP) with human peripheral blood lymphocytes: specific binding and cyclic AMP production. Gen Pharmac 17:185–189, 1986a.

80. Calvo JR, Molinero P, Jiminez J, Goderna R, Guerrero JM. Interaction of vasoactive intestinal peptide (VIP) with rat lymphoid cells. Peptides 7:177–1181, 1986b.

81. Calvo JR, Montilla ML, Guerrero JM, Segura JJ. Expression of VIP receptors in mouse peritoneal macrophages: functional and molecular characterization. J Neuroimmunol 50:85–93, 1994.

82. Calvo W. The innervation of the bone marrow in laboratory animals. Am J Anat 123:315–328, 1968.

83. Calvo W, Forteza-Vila J. On the development of bone marrow innervation in new-born rats as studied with silver impregnation and electron microscopy. Am J Anat 126:355–359, 1969.

84. Calvo W, Haas RJ. Die Histogenese des Knochemarks der Ratte. Z Zellforsch 95:377–395, 1969.

85. Campbell RM, Scanes CG. Endocrine peptides 'moonlighting' as immune modulators: roles for somatostatin and GH releasing factor. J Endocrinol 147:383–396, 1995.

86. Carlson SL, Albers KM, Beiting DJ, Parish M, Conner JM, Davis BM. NGF modulates sympathetic innervation of lymphoid tissues. J Neurosci 15:5892–5899, 1995.

87. Carlson SL, Brooks WH, Roszman TL. Neurotransmitter-lymphocyte interactions: dual receptor modulation of lymphocyte proliferation and cAMP production. J Neuroimmunol 24:155–162, 1989.

88. Carlson SL, Felten DL, Livnat S, Felten SY. Noradrenergic sympathetic innervation of the spleen: V. Acute drug-induced depletion of lymphocytes in the target fields of innervation results in redistribution of noradrenergic fibers but maintenance of compartmentation. J Neurosci Res 18:64–69, 1987.

89. Carolan, EJ, Casale TB. Effects of neuropeptides on neutrophil migration through noncellular and endothelial barriers. J Allergy Clin Immunol 92:589–598, 1993.

90. Carr D, Blalock JE. Neuropeptide hormones and receptors common to both the immune and neuroendocrine systems: a bidirectional pathway of intersystem communication. In: Psychoneuroimmunology, 2nd ed, R Ader, N Cohen, DL Felten, eds. Academic Press, New York, 1991, pp 573–588.

91. Carr DJ, Bubein JK, Woods WT, Blalock JE. Opioid receptors on murine splenocytes: possible coupling to K^+ channels. Ann NY Acad Sci 540:694–697, 1988.

92. Carr DJJ, Gebhardt BM, Paul D. Alpha adrenergic and mu-2 opioid receptors are involved in morphine-induced suppression of splenocyte natural killer activity. J Pharmacol Exp Ther 264:1179–1186, 1993.

93. Carr DJJ, Klimpel GR. Enhancement of the generation of cytotoxic T cells by endogenous opiates. J Neuroimmunol 12:75–87, 1986.

94. Carucci JA, Herrick CA, Durkin HG. Neuropeptide-mediated regulation of hapten-specific IgE responses in mice. II. Mechanisms of substance P-mediated isotype-specific suppression of BPO-specific IgE antibody-forming cell responses induced in vitro. J Neuroimmunol 49:89–95, 1994.

95. Chartash EK, Imai A, Gershengorn MC, Crow MK, Friedman SM. Direct human T helper cell-mediated B cell activation is not mediated by inositol lipid hydrolysis. J Immunol 140:1974–1981, 1988.

96. Chelmicka-Schorr E, Checinski M, Arnason BGW. Chemical sympathectomy augments the severity of experimental allergic encephalomyelitis. J Neuroimmunol 17:347–350, 1988.

97. Chelmicka-Schorr E, Kwasniewski MN, Czlonkowska A. Sympathetic nervous system modulates macrophage function. Int J Immunopharmac 14:841–846, 1992.

98. Chelmicka-Schorr E, Kwasniewski MN, Thomas BE, Arnason BGW. The β-adrenergic agonist isoproterenol suppresses experimental allergic encephalomyelitis in Lewis rats. J Neuroimmunol 25:203–207, 1989.

99. Cheng PP-J, Sreedharan SP, Kishiyama JL, Goetzl EJ. The SKW 6.4 line of human B lymphocytes specifically binds and response to vasoactive intestinal peptide. Immunology 79:64–68, 1993.

100. Chevendra V, Weaver LC. Distribution of neuropeptide Y, vasoactive intestinal peptide and somatostatin in populations of postganglionic neurons innervating the rat kidney, spleen and intestine. Neuroscience 50:727–743, 1992.

101. Chiba T, Yamaguchi A, Yamatani T, Nakamura A, Morishita T, Inui T, Fukase M, Noda T, Fujita T. Calcitonin gene-related peptide receptor antagonist to human CGRP-(8-37). Am J Physiol 256:E331–E335, 1989.

102. Chuang LF, Chuang TK, Killam KF Jr, Qui Q, Wang XR, Lin J-J, Kung H-F, Sheng W, Chao C, Yu L, Chuang RY. Expression of kappa opioid receptors in human and monkey lymphocytes. Biochem Biophys Commun 209:1003–1010, 1995.

103. Chubb IW, Hodgson AJ, White GH. Acetylcholinesterase hydrolyzes substance P. Neuroscience 5:2065–2072, 1980.

104. Chubb IW, Ranieri R, White GH, Hodgson AJ. The enkephalins are amongst the peptides hydrolyzed by purified acetylcholinesterase. Neuroscience 10:1369–1377, 1983.

105. Church MK, El-Lati S, Caulfield JP. Neuropeptide-induced secretion from human skin mast cells. Int Arch Allergy Appl Immunol 94:310–318, 1991.

106. Clements JA, Funder JW. Arginine vasopressin (AVP) and AVP-like immunoreactivity in peripheral tissues. Endocr Rev 7:449–460, 1986.
107. Cohen RA. Platelet-induced neurogenic coronary contractions due to accumulation of the false neurotransmitter, 5-hydroxytryptamine. J Clin Invest 75:286–292, 1985.
108. Colpaert FC, Donnerer J, Lembeck F. Effects of capsaicin on inflammation and on the substance P content of nervous tissue in rats with adjuvant arthritis. Life Sci 32:1827–1834, 1983.
109. Cooke HJ. Neurobiology of the intestinal mucosa. Gastroenterology 90:1057–1081, 1986.
110. Cordier A. L'innervation de la bourse de fabricius durant l'embryogenese et la vie adulte. Acta Anat 73:38–47, 1969.
111. Costa MC, Sutter P, Gybel J. Adjuvant-induced arthritis in rats: a possible animal model of chronic pain. Pain 10:173, 1985.
112. Couvineau A, Amiranoff B, Laburthe M. Solubilization of the liver vasoactive peptide receptor. Hydrodynamic characterization of evidence for an association with a functional GTP regulatory protein. J Biol Chem 261:14482–14489, 1986.
113. Crary B, Hauser SL, Borysenko M, Kutz I, Hoban C, Ault KA, Weiner HL, Benson H. Decreased mitogen responsiveness of mononuclear cells from peripheral blood after epinephrine administration in humans. J Immunol 130:694–597, 1983.
114. Crary B, Hauser SL, Borysenko M, Kutz I, Hoban C, Ault KA, Weiner HL, Benson H. Epinephrine-induced changes in the distribution of lymphocyte subsets in peripheral blood of humans. J Immunol 131:1178–1181, 1983a.
115. Cremashi GA, Fisher P, Boege F. β-adrenoceptor distribution in murine lymphoid cell lines. Immunopharmacology 22:195–206, 1991.
116. Crivellato E, Damiani D, Mallardi F, Travan L. Suggestive evidence for a microanatomical relationship between mast cells and nerve fibers containing substance P, calcitonin gene-related peptide, vasoactive intestinal polypeptide, and somatostatin in the rat mesentery. Acta Anat 141:127–131, 1991.
117. Dahlström AB, Zetterström BEM. Noradrenaline stores in nerve terminals of the spleen: changes during hemorrhagic shock. Science 147:1583–1585, 1965.
118. Danek A, O'Dorisio MS, O'Dorisio TM, George JM. Specific binding sites for vasoactive intestinal polypeptide on nonadherent peripheral blood lymphocytes. J Immunol 131:1173–1177, 1983.
119. Davies D, Medeiros MS, Keen J, Truner AJ, Haynes LW. Endopeptidase-24.11 cleaves a chemotactic factor from alpha-calcitonin gene-related peptide. Biochem Pharmacol 43:1753–1756, 1992.
120. DeBlasi A, Lipartiti M, Algeri S, Sacchetti G, Costantini C, Fratelli M, Cotecchia S. Stress induced desensitization of lymphocyte β-adrenoceptors in young and aged rats. Pharmacol Biochem Behav 24:991–998, 1986.
121. De La Fuente M, Bernaez I, Del Rio M, Hernanz A. Stimulation of murine peritoneal macrophage functions by neuropeptide Y and peptide YY. Involvement of protein kinase C. Immunology 80:259–265, 1993.
122. Depelchin A, Letesson JJ. Adrenaline influence on the immune response. I. Accelerating or suppressor effects according to the time of application. Immunol Lett 3:199–205, 1981.
123. del Rey AE, Besedovsky HO, Sorkin E, Da Prada M, Arrenbrechts S. Immunoregulation mediated by the sympathetic nervous system. Cell Immunol 63:329–334, 1981.
124. del Rey AE, Besedovsky HO, Sorkin E, Da Prada M, Bondiolotti GP. Sympathetic immunoregulation: difference between high- and low-responder animals. Am J Physiol 242:R30–R33, 1982.

125. DePace DM, Webber RH. Electrostimulation and morphologic study of the nerves to the bone marrow of the albino rat. Acta Anat 93:1–18, 1975.

126. Diel F, Bethge N, Opree W. Histamine secretion in leukocyte incubates of patients with allergic hyperreactivity induced by somatostatin-14 and somatostatin-18. Agents Actions 13:216–218, 1983.

127. Di Marzo V, Tippins JR, Morris HR. The effect of vasoactive intestinal peptide and calcitonin gene-related peptide on peptidoleukotriene release from platelet activating factor stimulated rat lungs and ionophore stimulated guinea-pig lungs. Biochem Int 13:933–942, 1986.

128. Ding M, Hart RP, Jonakait GM. Tumor necrosis factor-α induces substance P in sympathetic ganglia through sequential induction of interleukin-1 and leukemia inhibitory factor. J Neurobiol 28:445–454, 1995.

129. Dowton M, Boelen M. Acetylcholinesterase converts Met5-enkephalin-containing peptides to Met5-enkephalin. Neurosci Lett 94:151–155, 1988.

130. Drew P, Shearman D. Vasoactive intestinal peptide: a neurotransmitter which reduces human NK cell activity and increases Ig synthesis. Aust J Exp Biol Med Sci 63:313–318, 1985.

131. Ekblad E, Winther C, Ekman R, Hakanson R, Sundler F. Projections of peptide-containing neurons in rat small intestine. Neuroscience 20:169–188, 1987.

132. Elfvin L-G, Aldskogius H, Johansson J. Splenic primary sensory afferents in the guinea pig demonstrated with anterogradely transported wheat-germ agglutinin conjugated to horseradish peroxidase. Cell Tissue Res 269:229–234, 1992.

133. Emadi-Khiav B, Bousli M, Bronner C, Landry Y. Human and rat cutaneous mast cells: involvement of a G protein in the response to peptidergic stimuli. Eur J Pharmacol 272:97–102, 1994.

134. Enjalbert A, Rasolon-Janahary R, Moyse E, Kordon C, Epelbaum J. GTP sensitivity of [^{125}I]Tyr^{11}-SRIF binding in rat adenohypophysis and cerebral cortex. Endocrinology 113:822–824, 1983.

135. Enzmann V, Drossler K. Immunohistochemical detection of substance P and vasoactive intestinal peptide fibres in the auricular lymph nodes of sensitized guinea-pigs and mice. Acta Histochem Jena 96:15–18, 1994.

136. Ernström U, Sandberg G. Effects of alpha- and beta-receptor stimulation on the release of lymphocytes and granulocytes from the spleen. Scan J Haematol 11:275–286, 1973.

137. Ernström U, Sandberg G. Stimulation of lymphocyte release from the spleen by theophylline and isoproterenol. Acta Physiol Scand 90:202–209, 1974.

138. Ernström U, Söder O. Influence of adrenaline on the dissemination of antibody-producing cells from the spleen. Clin Exp Immunol 21:131–140, 1975.

139. Esler M, Skews H, Leonard P, Jackman G, Bobik A, Korner P. Age dependence of noradrenaline kinetics in normal subjects. Clin Sci 60:217–219, 1981.

140. Etienne A, Soulard C, Thonier F, Braquet P. Modulation by drugs of eosinophil recruitment induced by immune challenge in the rat. Possible roles of interleukin 5 and platelet-activating factor. Int Arch Allergy Appl Immunol 88:216–221, 1989.

141. Etienne A, Soulard C, Thonier F, Braquet P. Modulation of eosinophil recruitment in the rat by the platelet-activating factor (PAF) antagonist, BN 52021, the somatostatin analog, BIM 23014, and by cyclosporin A. Prostaglandins 37:345–351, 1989.

142. Fais S, Annibale B, Boirivant M, Santoro A, Pallone F, Delle Fave G. Effects of somatostatin on human intestinal lamina propria lymphocytes. J Neuroimmunol 31:211–219, 1991.

143. Faith RE, Liang HJ, Murgo AJ, Plotnikoff NP. Neuroimmunomodulation with enkephalins:

enhancement of human natural killer (NK) cell activity in vitro. Clin Immunol Immunopathol 31:412–418, 1984.

144. Falke NE, Fischer EG. Opiate receptor mediated internalization of 125-I-β-End in human polymorphonuclear leukocytes. Cell Biol Int Rep 19:429–435, 1986.

145. Farber EM, Nickollof BJ, Recht B, Fraki JE. Stress, symmetry and psoriasis. J Am Acad Dermatol 14:305–311, 1986.

146. Fatani JA, Qayyum MA, Mehta L, Singh U. Parasympathetic innervation of the thymus: a histochemical and immunocytochemical study. J Anat 147:115–119, 1986.

147. Feher E, Fodor M, Burnstock G. Distribution of somatostatin-immunoreactive nerve fibres in Peyer's patches. Gut 33:1195–1198, 1992.

148. Feldman RD, Limbird LE, Nadeau J, Robertson D, Wood AJJ. Alterations in leukocyte β-receptor affinity with aging. A potential explanation for altered β-adrenergic sensitivity in the elderly. N Engl J Med 310:815–819, 1984.

149. Feldman S, Rachmilewitz EA, Izak G. The effect of central nervous system stimulation on erythropoiesis in rat with chronically implanted electrodes. J Lab Clin Med 67:713–725, 1966.

150. Felsner P, Hofer D, Rinner I, Mangge H, Gruber M, Korsatko W, Schauenstein K. Continuous in vivo treatment with catecholamines suppresses in vitro reactivity of rat peripheral blood T-lymphocytes via α-mediated mechanisms. J Neuroimmunol 37:47–57, 1992.

151. Felsner P, Hofer D, Rinner I, Porta S, Korsatko W, Schauenstein K. Adrenergic suppression of peripheral blood T cell reactivity in the rat is due to activation of peripheral α_2-receptors. J Neuroimmunol 57:27–34, 1995.

152. Felten DL, Bellinger DL, Ackerman KD, Felten SY. Denervation of splenic sympathetic fibers in the young adult rat. Soc Neurosci Abstr 12:1064, 1986.

153. Felten DL, Felten SY. Innervation of the thymus. In: Thymus Update, MD Kendall, MA Ritter, eds. Harwood Academic Publishers, London, 1989, pp 73–88.

154. Felten DL, Felten SY, Bellinger DL, Carlson SL, Ackerman KD, Madden KS, Olschowka JA, Livnat S. Noradrenergic sympathetic neural interactions with the immune system: structure and function. Immunol Rev 100:225–260, 1987.

155. Felten DL, Felten SY, Bellinger DL, Madden KS. Fundamental aspects of neural-immune signaling. Psychother Psychosom 60:46–56, 1993.

156. Felten DL, Felten SY, Carlson SL, Bellinger DL, Ackerman KD, Romano TA, Livnat S. Development, aging, and plasticity of noradrenergic sympathetic innervation of secondary lymphoid organs: Implications for neural-immune interactions. In: Progress in Catecholamine Research Part A: Basic Aspects and Peripheral Mechanisms, A Dahlstrom, RM Belmaker, M Sandler, eds. Alan R. Liss, New York, 1988, pp 517–524.

157. Felten DL, Felten SY, Carlson SL, Olschowka JA, Livnat S. Noradrenergic and peptidergic innervation of lymphoid tissue. J Immunol 135:755s–765s, 1985.

158. Felten DL, Felten SY, Madden KS, Ackerman KD, Bellinger DL. Development, maturation, and senescence of sympathetic innervation of secondary immune organs. In: Development, Maturation, and Senescence of Neuroendocrine Systems, MP Schreibman, CG Scanes, eds. Academic Press, San Diego, 1989, pp 381–396.

159. Felten DL, Livnat S, Felten SY, Carlson SL, Bellinger DL, Yeh P. Sympathetic innervation of lymph nodes in mice. Brain Res Bull 13:693–699, 1984.

160. Felten DL, Lorton D, Bellinger DL, Duclos M, Felten SY. Substance P (SP) denervation of lymph nodes attenuates the expression of adjuvant induced arthritis. Soc Neurosci Abstr 16:1210, 1990.

161. Felten DL, Overhage JM, Felten SY, Schmedtje JF. Noradrenergic sympathetic innervation

of lymphoid tissue in the rabbit appendix: further evidence for a link between the nervous and immune systems. Brain Res Bull 7:595–612, 1981.

162. Felten SY, Bellinger DL, Collier TJ, Coleman PD, Felten DL. Decreased sympathetic innervation of spleen in aged Fischer 344 rats. Neurobiol Aging 8:159–165, 1987.

163. Felten SY, Felten DL. The innervation of lymphoid tissue. In: Psychoneuroimmunology, 2nd ed, R Ader, DL Felten, N Cohen, eds. Academic Press, New York, 1991, pp 27–69.

164. Felten SY, Felten DL, Bellinger DL, Carlson SL, Ackerman KD, Madden KS, Olschowka JA, Livnat S. Noradrenergic sympathetic innervation of lymphoid organs. Prog Allergy 43:14–36, 1988.

165. Felten SY, Olschowka JA. Noradrenergic sympathetic innervation of the spleen: II. Tyrosine hydroxylase (TH)-positive nerve terminals form synaptic-like contacts on lymphocytes in the splenic white pulp. J Neurosci Res 18:37–48, 1987.

166. Felten SY, Olschowka JA, Ackerman KD, Felten DL. Catecholaminergic innervation of the spleen: Are lymphocytes targets of noradrenergic nerves? In: Progress in Catecholamine Research, Part A: Basic Aspects and Peripheral Mechanisms. A Dahlström, RH Belmaker, M Sandler, eds. Alan R. Liss, New York, 1988, pp 525–531.

167. Fillenz M. Innervation of blood vessels of lung and spleen. In: Sympathetic Electric Activation and Innervation of Blood Vessels, B Karger, ed. Cambridge, London, 1966, pp 56–59.

168. Fillenz M. Innervation of the cat spleen. Proc Physiol Soc 25–26:2P–3P, 1966.

169. Fillenz M. The innervation of the cat spleen. Proc R Soc Lond 174:459–468, 1970.

170. Fillenz M, Pollard RM. Quantitative differences between sympathetic nerve terminals. Brain Res 109:443–454, 1976.

171. Finch R, Sreedharan SP, Goetzl EJ. High affinity receptors for vasoactive intestinal peptide on human myeloma cells. J Immunol 142:1977–1981, 1989.

172. Fink T, Weihe E. Multiple neuropeptides in nerves supplying mammalian lymph nodes: messenger candidates for sensory and autonomic neuroimmunomodulation? Neurosci Lett 90:39–44, 1988.

173. Fjellner B, Hagermark O. Studies on pruritogenic and histamine-releasing effects of some putative peptide neurotransmitters. Act Dermatovener (Stockholm) 61:245–250, 1981.

174. Foda HD, Iwanaga T, Liu LW, Said SI. Vasoactive intestinal peptide protects against HCl-induced pulmonary edema in rats. Ann NY Acad Sci 527:633–636, 1988.

175. Foreman JC, Jordan CC. Histamine release and vascular changes induced by neuropeptides. Agents Actions 13:105–111, 1983.

176. Foreman JC, Jordan CC, Piotrowski W. Interaction of neurotensin with the substance P receptor mediating histamine release from rat mast cells and the flare in human skin. Br J Pharmacol 77:531–539, 1982.

177. Foreman JC, Piotrowski W. Peptides and histamine release. J Allergy Clin Immunol 74:127–131, 1984.

178. Foris G, Medgyesi E. Gyimesi E, Hauck E. Met-enkephalin induced alterations of macrophage functions. Mol Immunol 21:747–750, 1984.

179. Foster CA, Mandak B, Kromer E, Rot A. Calcitonin gene-related peptide is chemotactic for human T lymphocytes. Ann NY Acad Sci USA 657:397–404, 1992.

180. Foster JS, Moore RN. Dynorphin and related opioid peptides enhance tumoricidal activity mediated by murine peritoneal macrophages. J Leukocyte Biol 42:171–174, 1987.

181. Fox EA, Powley TL. Tracer diffusion has exaggerated CNS maps of direct preganglionic innervation of pancreas. J Autonom Nerv Syst 15:55–69, 1986.

182. Fried G, Terenius L, Brodin E, Efendic S, Dockray G, Fahrenkrug J, Goldstein M, Hökfelt T. Neuropeptide Y, enkephalin and noradrenaline coexist in sympathetic neurons inner-

vating the bovine spleen. Biochemical and immunohistochemical evidence. Cell Tissue Res 243:495–508, 1986.

183. Fuchs BA, Albright JW, Albright JF. β-Adrenergic receptors on murine lymphocytes: density varies with cell maturity and lymphocyte subtype and is decreased after antigen administration. Cell Immunol 114:231–245, 1988.

184. Fuchs BA, Pruett SB. Morphine induces apoptosis in murine thymocytes in vivo but not in vitro: involvement of both opiate and glucocorticoid receptors. J Pharmacol Exp Ther 266:417–423, 1993.

185. Gabrilovac J, Antica M, Osmak M. In vivo bidirectional regulation of mouse natural killer (NK) cell cytotoxic activities by Leu-enkephalin: reversibility by naloxone. Life Sci 50:29–37, 1992.

186. Gader AMA. The effects of beta adrenergic blockage on the response of leukocyte counts to intravenous epinephrine in man. Scand J Haematol 13:11–16, 1974.

187. Ganea D, Sun L. Vasoactive intestinal peptide downregulates the expression of IL-2 but not of IFNγ from stimulated murine T lymphocytes. J Neuroimmunol 47:147–158, 1993.

188. Gatti G, Gabriella R, Masera G, Pallavicini L, Sartori ML, Staurenghi A. Orlandi F, Angeli A. Interplay in vitro between ACTH, β-endorphin and glucocorticoids in the modulation of spontaneous and lymphokine-inducible human natural killer (NK) cell activity. Brain Behav Immun 7:16–28, 1993.

189. Gaveriaux C, Peluso J, Simonin F, Laforet J, Kieffer B. Identification of κ- and δ-opioid receptor transcripts in immune cells. FEBS Lett 369:272–276, 1995.

190. Geenen V, Legros J-J, Franchimont P, Baudrihaye M, Defresne MP, Boniver J. The neuro-endocrine thymus: coexistence of oxytocin and neurophysin in the human thymus. Science 232:508–510, 1986.

191. Geenen V, Legros J-J, Franchimont P, Defresne MP, Boniver J, Ivell R, Richter D. The thymus as a neuroendocrine organ: synthesis of vasopressin and oxytocin in human thymic epithelium. Ann NY Acad Sci 496:56–66, 1987.

192. Genaro AM, Borda E. Alloimmunization-induced changes in β-adrenoceptor expression and cAMP on B lymphocytes. Immunopharmacology 18:63–70, 1989.

193. Geppetti P, Frilli S, Renzi D, Santicioli P, Maggi CA, Theodorsson E, Fanciullacci M. Distribution of calcitonin gene-related peptide-like immunoreactivity in various rat tissues: correlation with substance P and other tachykinins and sensitivity to capsaicin. Regul Pept 23:289–298, 1988.

194. Geppetti P, Maggi CA, Zecchi-Orlandini S, Santicioli P, Meli A, Frilli S, Spillantini MG, Amenta F. Substance P-like immunoreactivity in capsaicin-sensitive structures of the rat thymus. Regul Pept 18:321–329, 197.

195. Gibson-Berry KL, Whitin JC, Cohen HJ. Modulation of the respiratory burst in human neutrophils by isoproteronol and dibutyryl cyclic AMP. J Neuroimmunol 43:59–68, 1993.

196. Gibson-Berry KL, Richardson C, Felten SY, Felten DL. Immunocytochemical and neuro-chemical analyses of sympathetic nerves in rat bone marrow. Soc Neurosci Abstr 19:944, 1993.

197. Gilman SC, Schwartz JM, Milner RJ, Bloom FE, Feldman JD. β-endorphin enhances lymphocyte proliferative responses. Proc Natl Acad Sci USA 79:4226–4230, 1982.

198. Gilmore W, Weiner LP. The opioid specificity of beta-endorphin enhancement of murine lymphocyte proliferation. Immunopharmacol 17:19–30, 1989.

199. Ginsburg CH, Dambrauskas JT, Ault KA, Falchuk ZM. Impaired natural killer cell activity in patients with inflammatory bowel disease: evidence for a qualitative defect. Gastroenterology 85:846–851, 1983.

200. Giron LT, Crutcher KA, Davis JN. Lymph nodes—a possible site for sympathetic neuronal regulation of immune responses. Ann Neurol 8:520–525, 1980.

201. Goetzl EJ, Chernov T, Renold F, Payan DG. Neuropeptide regulation of the expression of immediate hypersensitivity. J Immunol 135:802S–805S, 1985.

202. Goetzl EJ, Payan DG. Inhibition by somatostatin of the release of mediators from human basophils and rat leukemic basophils. J Immunol 133:3255–3259, 1984.

203. Goin JC, Sterin-Borda L, Borda ES, Finiasz M, Fernandez J, de Bracco MME. Active alpha$_2$ and beta adrenoceptors in lymphocytes from patients with chronic lymphocytic leukemia. Int J Can 49:178–181, 1991.

204. Gomariz RP, Leceta J, Garrido E, Garrido T, Delgado M. Vasoactive intestinal peptide (VIP) mRNA expression in rat T and B lymphocytes. Regul Pept 50:177–184, 1994.

205. Gordon MA, Cohen JJ, Wilson IB. Muscarinic cholinergic receptors in murine lymphocytes: demonstration by direct binding. Proc Natl Acad Sci USA 75:2902–2904, 1978.

206. Grundemar L, Hakanson R. Neuropeptide Y, peptide YY and C-terminal fragments release histamine from rat peritoneal mast cells. Br J Pharmacol 104:776–778, 1991.

207. Grundemar L, Sheikh SP, Wahlestedt. Characterization of receptor types for neuropeptide Y and related peptides. In: The Biology of Neuropeptide Y and Related Peptides, WF Colmers, C Wahlestedt, eds. Humana Press, Totowa, 1993, pp 197–216.

208. Guan L, Townsend R, Eisenstein TK, Adler MW, Rogers TJ. Both T cells and macrophages are targets of κ-opioid-induced immunosuppression. Brain Behav Immun 8:229–240, 1994.

209. Guerrero JM, Prieto JC, Elorza FL, Ramirez R, Goberna R. Interaction of vasoactive intestinal peptide with human blood mononuclear cells. Mol Cell Endocrinol 21:151–160, 1981.

210. Hadden JW. Cyclic nucleotides in lymphocyte proliferation and differentiation. In: Immunopharmacology, JW Hadden, RG Coffey, F Spreafico, eds. Plenum Press, New York, 1977, pp 1–28.

211. Hadden JW, Hadden EM, Middleton E Jr. Lymphocyte blast transformation. I. Demonstration of adrenergic receptors in human peripheral lymphocytes. Cell Immunol 1:583–595, 1970.

212. Hafstrom I, Ringertz B, Lundeberg T, Palmblad J. The effect of endothelin, neuropeptide Y, calcitonin gene-related peptide and substance. P Acta Physiol Scand 148:341–346, 1993.

213. Hagi K, Inaba K, Sakuta H, Muramatsu S. Enhancement of murine bone marrow macrophage differentiation by β-endorphin. Blood 86:1316–321, 1995.

214. Hagi K, Uno K, Inaba K, Muramatsu S. Augmenting effect of opioid peptides on murine macrophage activation. J Neuroimmunol 50:71–76, 1994.

215. Hall NR, Goldstein AL. Neurotransmitters and the immune system. In Psychoneuroimmunology, R Ader, ed. Academic Press, New York, 1981, pp 521–544.

216. Hall NR, Goldstein AL. Neurotransmitters and host defense. In: Neural Modulation of Immunity, R Guillemin, M Cohn, T Melnechuk, eds. Raven Press, New York, 1985, pp 143–154.

217. Hall NR, McClure JE, Hu S-K, Tare NS, Seals CM, Goldstein AL. Effects of 6-hydroxydopamine upon primary and secondary thymus dependent immune responses. Immunopharmacology 5:39–48, 1982.

218. Hall NRS, O'Grady MP, Farah JR Jr. Thymic hormones and immune function: mediation via neuroendocrine circuits. In: Psychoneuroimmunology, 2nd ed, R Ader, N Cohen, DL Felten, eds. Academic Press, New York, 1991, pp 515–528.

219. Hanley MR, Lee CM, Jones LM, Michel RH. Similar effects of substance P and related

peptides on salivation and on phosphatidylinositol turnover in rat salivary glands. Mol Pharmacol 18:78–83, 1980.

220. Harrison NK, Dawes KE, Kwon OJ, Barnes PJ, Laurent GJ, Chung KF. Effects of neuropeptides on human lung fibroblast proliferation and chemotaxis. Am J Physiol 268:L278–L283, 1995.

221. Hartung HP, Toyka KV. Activation of macrophages by substance P: induction of oxidative burst and thromboxane release. Eur J Pharmacol 89:301–305, 1983.

223. Hatfield SM, Petersen BH, DiMicco JA. Beta adrenoceptor modulation of the generation of murine cytotoxic T lymphocytes in vitro. J Pharmacol Exp Ther 239:460–466, 1986.

224. Harvath L, Robbins JD, Russell AA, Seamon KB. cAMP and human neutrophil chemotaxis. Elevation of cAMP differentially affects chemotactic responsiveness. J Immunol 146:224–232, 1991.

225. Hazum E, Chang K-J, Cuatrecasas P. Specific nonopiate receptors for β-endorphin. Science 205:1033–1035, 1979.

226. Heagy W, Laurance M, Cohen E, Finberg R. Neurohormones regulate T cell function. J Exp Med 171:1625–1633, 1990.

227. Hedfors E, Holm G, Ivansen M, Wahren J. Physiological variation of blood lymphocyte reactivity: T-cell subsets, immunoglobulin production, and mixed-lymphocyte reactivity. Clin Immunol Immunopathol 27:9–14, 1983.

228. Heijnen CJ, Bevers C, Kavelaars A, Ballieux RE. Effect of alpha-endorphin on the antigen-induced primary antibody response of human blood B cells in vitro. J Immunol 136:213–216, 1986.

229. Hellstrand K, Hermodsson S, Strannegard O. Evidence for a β-adrenoceptor-mediated regulation of human natural killer cells. J Immunol 134:4095–4099, 1985.

230. Hemmick LM, Bidlack JM. β-Endorphin stimulates rat T lymphocyte proliferation. J Neuroimmunol 29:239–248, 1990.

231. Hirata Y, Takagi Y, Takata S, Fukuda Y, Yoshimi H, Fujita T. Calcitonin gene-related peptide receptors in cultured vascular smooth muscle and endothelial cells. Biochem Biophys Res Commun 151:1113–1121, 1988.

232. Hiruma K, Koike T, Nakamura H, Sumida T, Maeda T, Tomioka H, Yoshida S, Fujita T. Somatostatin receptors on human lymphocytes and leukemia cells. Immunology 71:480–485, 1990.

233. Hosoi J, Murphy GF, Egan CL, Lerner EA, Grabbe S, Asahina A, Granstein RD. Regulation of Langerhans cell function by nerves containing calcitonin gene-related peptide. Nature 363:159–162, 1989.

234. Hu X, Goldmuntz EA, Brosnana CF. The effect of norepinephrine on endotoxic-mediated macrophage phagocytosis following peripheral activation. J Neuroimmunol 31:35–42, 1991.

235. Hurst S, Collins S. IL-1β modulation of NE release from rat myenteric nerves. Am J Physiol 264:G30–G35, 1993.

236. Ichikawa S, Sreedharan SP, Goetzl EJ, Owen RL. Immunohistochemical localization of peptidergic nerve fibers and neuropeptide receptors in Peyer's patches of the cat ileum. Regul Pept 54:385–395, 1994.

237. Ichikawa S, Sreedharan SP, Owen RL, Goetzl EJ. Immunochemical localization of type 1 VIP receptor and NK-1-type substance P receptor in rat lung. Am J Physiol 268:L584–L588, 1995.

238. Inoue K. Innervation of the bursa of Fabricius in the domestic fowl. Kaibogaku Zasshi 46:403–415, 1971.

239. Inoue K. Distribution of adrenergic and cholinergic nerve cells and fibers in the bursa of fabricius of chicken. Okajimas Folia Anat Jpn 50:317–325, 1973.

240. Irimajiri N, Bloom ET, Makinodan T. Suppression of murine natural killer cell activity by adherent cells from aging mice. Mech Ageing Dev 31:155–162, 1985.

241. Irwin M, Brown M, Patterson T, Hauger R, Mascovich A, Grant I. Neuropeptide Y and natural killer cell activity: findings in depression and Alzheimer caregiver stress. FASEB J 5:3100–3107, 1991.

242. Ishihara T, Sigemoto R, Mori K, Takahashi K, Nagata S. Functional expression and tissue distribution of a novel receptor for vasoactive intestinal polypeptide. Neuron 8:811–819, 1992.

243. Ishioka C, Yoshida A, Kimata H, Midawa H. Vasoactive intestinal peptide stimulates immunoglobulin production and growth of human B cells. Clin Exp Immunol 87:504–508, 1992.

244. Ishizaka T, Ishizaka K, Orange RP, Austen KF. Pharmacologic inhibition of the antigen-induced release of histamine and slow reacting substance of anaphylaxis (SRS-A) from monkey lung tissues mediated by human IgE. J Immunol 106:1267–1273, 1971.

245. Ismael Z, Millar TJ, Small DH, Chubb IW. Acetylcholinesterase generates enkephalin-like immunoreactivity when it degrades the soluble proteins (chromogranins) from adrenal chromaffin granules. Brain Res 376:230–238, 1986.

246. Iuvone T, Capasso A, D'Acquisto F, Camuccio R. Opioids inhibit the induction of nitric oxide synthase in F774 macrophages. Biochem Biophys Res Commun 212:975–980, 1995.

247. Iwamoto I, Tomoe S, Tomioka H, Yoshida S. Substance P-induced granulocyte infiltration in mouse skin: the mast cell-dependent granulocyte infiltration by the N-terminal peptide is enhanced by the activation of vascular endothelial cells by the C-terminal peptide. Clin Exp Immunol 87:203–207, 1992.

248. Iwamoto I, Tomoe S, Tomioka H, Yoshida S. Leukotriene B4 mediates substance P-induced granulocyte infiltration into mouse skin. J Immunol 151:2116–2123, 1993.

249. Jenkins SA, Baxter JN, Day DW, Al-Sumidaie AM, Leinster SJ, Shields R. The effects of somatostatin and SMS 201-995 on experimentally-induced pancreatitis and endotoxaemia in rats, and on monocyte activity in patients with cirrhosis and portal hypertension. Klin Wochenschr 64:100–106, 1986.

250. Jesseph JM, Felten DL. Noradrenergic innervation of the gut-associated lymphoid tissues (GALT) in the rabbit. Anat Rec 208:81A, 1984.

251. Johansson O, Sandberg G. Effect of neuropeptides beta-MSH, neurotensin, NPY, PHI, somatostatin and substance P on proliferation of lymphocytes in vitro. Acta Physiol Scand 137:107–111, 1989.

252. Johnson DL, Ashmore RC, Gordon MA. Effects of beta-adrenergic agents on the murine lymphocyte response to mitogen stimulation. J Immunopharmacol 3:205–219, 1981.

253. Johnson HM, Smith EM, Torres BA, Blalock JE. Regulation of the in vitro antibody response by neuroendocrine hormones. Proc Natl Acad Sci USA 79:4171–4174, 1982.

254. Johnston JA, Taub DD, Lloyd AR, Conlon K, Oppenheim JJ, Kevlin DJ. Human T lymphocyte chemotaxis and adhesion induced by vasoactive intestinal peptide. J Immunol 153:1762–1768, 1994.

255. Kahler CM, Herold M, Wiedermann CJ. Substance P: a competence factor for human fibroblast proliferation that induces the release of growth-regulatory arachidonic acid metabolites. J Cell Physiol 155:579–587, 1993a.

256. Kahler CM, Sitte BA, Reinisch N, Wiedermann CJ. Stimulation of the chemotactic migration of human fibroblasts by substance P. Eur J Pharmacol 249:281–286, 1993.

257. Kammer GM, Boehm CA, Rudolph SA, Schultz LA. Mobility of the human T lymphocyte surface molecules CD3, CD4, and CD8: regulation by a cAMP-dependent pathway. Proc Natl Acad Sci USA 85:792–796, 1988.

258. Kaplan R, Robinson CA, Scavulli JF, Vaughan JH. Propranolol and the treatment of rheumatoid arthritis. Arthritis Rheum 23:253–255, 1980.

259. Karalis K, Mastorakos G, Sano H, Wilder RL, Chrousos GP. Somatostatin may participate in the antiinflammatory actions of glucocorticoids. Endocrinology 136:4133–4138, 1995.

260. Kasahara K, Tanaka S, Ito R, Hamashima Y. Suppression of the primary immune response by chemical sympathectomy. Res Commun Chem Pathol Pharmacol 16:687–694, 1977.

261. Katz P, Zaytoun AM, Fauci AS. Mechanisms of human cell-mediated cytotoxicity. I. Modulation of natural killer cell activity by cyclic nucleotides. J Immunol 129:287–296, 1982.

262. Kawahara G, Osada N. Studies on the innervation of bone marrow with special reference to the intramedullary fibers in the dog and goat. Arch Histol Jpn 24:471–487, 1962.

263. Kawakami K, Parker DC. Antigen and helper T lymphocytes activate B lymphocytes by distinct signaling pathways. Eur J Immunol 23:77–84, 1993.

264. Kay MMB. Immunological aspects of aging. In: Aging Immunity and Arthritic Disease, MMB Kay, J Galpin, T Makinodan, eds. Raven Press, New York, 1980, pp 33–78.

265. Kay MMB, Makinodan T. Relationship between aging and the immune system. Prog Allergy 29:134–181, 1981.

266. Kay N, Allen J, Morley JE. Endorphins stimulate normal human peripheral blood lymphocyte natural killer activity. Life Sci 35:53–59, 1984.

267. Kessler JA, Freidin MM, Kalberg C, Chandross KJ. Cytokines regulate substance P expression in sympathetic neurons. Regul Pept 46:70–75, 1993.

268. Khan MM, Sansoni P, Silverman ED, Engleman EG. Beta-adrenergic receptors on human suppressor, helper, and cytolytic lymphocytes. Biochem Pharmacol 35:1137–1142, 1986.

269. Kidd BL, Mapp PI, Gibson SJ, Polak JM, O'Higgins FO. Buckland-Wright JC, Blake DR. A neurogenic mechanism for symmetrical arthritis. Lancet 2:1128–1130, 1989.

270. Kimata H, Fujimoto M. Induction of IgA$_1$ and IgA$_2$ production in immature human fetal B cells and pre-B cells by vasoactive intestinal peptide. Blood 85:2098–2104, 1995.

271. Kimata H, Fujimoto M. Vasoactive intestinal peptide specifically induces human IgA$_1$ and IgA$_2$ production. Eur J Immunol 24:2262–2265, 1994.

272. Kimata H, Yoshida A, Fujimoto M, Mikawa H. Differential effect of vasoactive intestinal peptide, somatostatin, and substance P on human IgE and IgG subclass production. Cell Immunol 144:429–442, 1992.

273. Kimata H, Yoshida A, Fujimoto M, Mikawa H. Effect of vasoactive intestinal peptide, somatostatin, and substance P on spontaneous IgE and IgG$_4$ production in atopic patients. J Immunol 150:4630–4640, 1993.

274. Kimball ES, Persico FJ, Vaught JL. Substance P, neurokinin A, and neurokinin B induce generation of IL-1-like activity in P388D1 cells: possible relevance to arthritis disease. J Immunol 141:3564–3569, 1988.

275. Klaus SJ, Parker DC. Inducible cell contact signals regulate early activation gene expression during B-T lymphocyte collaboration. J Immunol 149:1867–1875, 1992.

276. Koch TR, Carney JA, Go VLW. Distribution and quantitation of gut neuropeptides in normal intestine and inflammatory bowel disease. Dig Dis Sci 32:369–376, 1987.

277. Koch TR, Carney JA, Go VLW, Szurszewski JH. Altered inhibitory innervation of circular smooth muscle in Crohn's colitis: association with decreased vasoactive intestinal polypeptide levels. Gastroenterology 98:1437–1444, 1990.

278. Koff WC, Dunegan MA. Neuroendocrine hormones suppress macrophage-mediated lysis of herpes simplex virus-infected cells. J Immunol 136:705–709, 1986.

279. Kolasinski SL, Haines KA, Siegel EL, Cronstein BN, Abramson SB. Neuropeptides and inflammation. A somatostatin analog as a selective antagonist of neutrophil activation of substance P. Arthritis Rheum 35:369–375, 1992.

280. Kouassi E, Li YS, Boukhris W, Millet I, Revillard J-P. Opposite effects of the catecholamines dopamine and norepinephrine on murine polyclonal B-cell activation. Immunopharmacology 16:125–137, 1988.

281. Krall JF, Connelly M, Weisbart R, Tuck ML. Age-related elevation of plasma catecholamine concentration and reduced responsiveness of lymphocyte adenylate cyclase. J Clin Endocrinol Metab 52:863–867, 1981.

282. Kroc C, Gores A, Go V. Gastrointestinal regulatory peptides modulate mouse lymphocyte functions under serum free conditions in vitro. Immunol Invest 15:103–111, 1986.

283. Kroc C, Gores A, Go V. Gastrointestinal regulatory peptides modulate in vitro immune reactions of mouse lymphocytes. Clin Immunol Immunopathol 39:308–318, 1986.

284. Kruszewska B, Felten SY, Moynihan JA. Alterations in cytokine and antibody production following chemical sympathectomy in two strains of mice. J Immunol 155:4613–4620, 1995.

285. Kudoh G, Hoshi K, Murakami T. Fluorescence microscopic and enzyme histochemical studies of the innervation of the human spleen. Arch Histol Jpn 42:169–180, 1979.

286. Kurkowski R, Kummer W, Heym C. Substance P-immunoreactive nerve fibers in tracheobronchial lymph nodes of the guinea pig: origin, ultrastructure and coexistence with other peptides. Peptides 11:13–20, 1990.

287. Kurosawa M, Ishizuka T. Inhibitory effects of vasoactive intestinal peptide on superoxide anion formation by N-formyl-methionyl-leucyl-phenylalanine-activated inflammatory cells in vitro. Int Arch Allergy Appl Immunol 100:28–34, 1993.

288. Kusiak JW, Pitha J. Decreased response with age of the cardiac catecholamine sensitive adenylate cyclase system. Life Sci 33:1679–1686, 1983.

289. Lacey CB, Elde RP, Seybold VS. Localization of vasoactive intestinal peptide binding sites in the thymus and bursa of fabricius of the chick. Peptides 12:383–391, 1991.

290. Lake CR, Zeigler MG, Coleman MD, Kopin IJ. Age related norepinephrine levels are similar in normotensive and hypertensive subjects. N Engl J Med 296:208–209, 1977.

291. Landmann R, Burgisser E, West M, Buhler FR. Beta adrenergic receptors are different in subpopulations of human circulating lymphocytes. J Recept Res 4:37–50, 1985.

292. Lappin D, Whaley K. Adrenergic receptors on monocytes modulate complement component synthesis. Clin Exp Immunol 47:606–612, 1982.

293. Laughton W, Powley TL. Four central nervous system sites project to the pancreas. Soc Neurosci Abstr 5:46, 1979.

294. Laurenzi MA, Persson MAA, Dalsgaard CJ, Haegerstrand A. The neuropeptide substance P stimulates production of interleukin 1 in human blood monocytes: activated cells are preferentially influenced by the neuropeptide. Scand J Immunol 31:529–533, 1990.

295. Levine JD, Clark R, Devor M, Helms C, Moskowitz MA, Basbaum AI. Intraneuronal substance P contributes to the severity of experimental arthritis. Science 226:547–549, 1984.

296. Levine JD, Coderre TJ, Helms C, Basbaum AI. β_2-adrenergic mechanisms in experimental arthritis. Proc Natl Acad Sci USA 85:4553–4556, 1988.

297. Levine JD, Collier DH, Basbaum AI, Moskowitz MA, Helms CA. Hypothesis: the nervous system may contribute to the pathophysiology of rheumatoid arthritis. J Rheumatol 12:406–411, 1985.

298. Levine JD, Dardick SJ, Basbaum AI, Scipio E. Reflex neurogenic inflammation. I. Contribution of the peripheral nervous system to spatially remote inflammatory responses that follow injury. J Neurosci 5:1380–1386, 1985.

299. Levine JD, Dardick SJ, Roizen MF, Helms C, Basbaum AL. Contribution of sensory afferents and sympathetic efferents to joint injury in experimental arthritis. J Neurosci 6:3423–3429, 1986.

300. Levine JD, Fye K, Heller P, Basbaum AI, Whiting-O'Keefe Q. Clinical response to regional intravenous guanethidine in patients with rheumatoid arthritis. J Rheumatol 13:1040–1043, 1986.

301. Levine JD, Moskowitz MA, Basbaum AI. The contribution of neurogenic inflammation in experimental arthritis. J Immunol 135:843s–847s, 1985.

302. Levine JD, Taiwo YO, Collins SD, Tam JK. Noradrenaline hyperalgesia is mediated through interaction with sympathetic postganglionic neurone terminals rather than activation of primary afferent nociceptors. Nature 323:158–160, 1986.

303. Li YS, Kouassi E, Revillard JP. Differential regulation of mouse B-cell activation of β-adrenoceptor stimulation depending on type of mitogens. Immunology 69:367–372, 1990.

304. Lichtenstein LM, Margolis S. Histamine release in vitro: inhibition by catecholamines and methylxanthenes. Science 161:902–903, 1968.

305. Lichtman MA. The ultrastructure of the hemopoietic environment of the marrow: a review. Exp Hematol 9:391–410, 1981.

306. Lilly CM, Hall AE, Rodger IW, Kobzik L, Haley KJ, Drazen JM. Substance P-induced histamine release in tracheally perfused guinea-pig lungs. J Appl Physiol 78:1234–1241, 1995.

307. Litwin DK, Wilson AK, Said SI. Vasoactive intestinal polypeptide (VIP) inhibits rat alveolar macrophage phagocytosis and chemotaxis in vitro. Regul Pept 40:63–74, 1992.

308. Livnat S, Felten SY, Carlson SL, Bellinger DL, Felten DL. Involvement of peripheral and central catecholamine systems in neural-immune interactions. J Neuroimmunol 10:5–30, 1985.

309. Livnat S, Madden KS, Felten DL, Felten SY. Regulation of the immune system by sympathetic neural mechanisms. Prog Neuro-Psychopharmacol Biol Psychiatry 11:145–152, 1987.

310. Lofstrom B, Pernow B, Wahren J. Vasodilating action of substance P in human forearm. Acta Physiol Scand 63:311–315, 1985.

311. Lopker A, Abood LG, Hoss W, Lionetti FJ. Stereoselective muscarinic acetylcholine and opiate receptors in human phagocytic leukocytes. Biochem Pharmacol 29:1361–1365, 1980.

312. Lorton D, Bellinger DL, Duclos M, Felten SY, Felten DL. Sympathectomy of lymph nodes exacerbates the expression of experimental arthritis. Soc Neurosci Abstr 16:1210, 1990.

313. Lorton D, Bellinger DL, Duclos M, Felten SY, Felten DL. Application of 6-hydroxydopamine into the fatpads surrounding the draining lymph nodes exacerbates adjuvant-induced arthritis. J Neuroimmunol 64:103–113, 1996.

314. Lorton D, Bellinger DL, Felten SY, Felten DL. Substance P (SP) and calcitonin gene-related peptide (CGRP) innervation of the rat spleen. Soc Neurosci Abstr 15:714, 1989.

315. Lorton D, Bellinger DL, Felten SY, Felten DL. Substance P innervation of the rat thymus. Peptides 11:1269–1275, 1990.

316. Lorton D, Bellinger DL, Felten SY, Felten DL. Substance P innervation of spleen in rats: nerve fibers associate with lymphocytes and macrophages in specific compartments of the spleen. Brain Behav Immun 5:29–40, 1991.

317. Lorton D, Hewitt D, Bellinger DL, Felten SY, Felten DL. Noradrenergic reinnervation of the rat spleen following chemical sympathectomy with 6-hydroxydopamine: pattern and time course of reinnervation. Brain Behav Immunol 4:198–222, 1990.

318. Lotz M, Vaughan JH, Carson DA. Effect of neuropeptides on production of inflammatory cytokines by human monocytes. Science 241:1218–1221, 1988.

319. Loveland BE, Jarrott B, McKenzie IFC. The detection of beta adrenoceptors on murine lymphocytes. Int J Immunopharmacol 3:45–55, 1981.

320. Lundberg JM, Rudehill A, Sollevi A, Theodorsson-Norhein E, Hamberger B. Frequency- and reserpine-dependent chemical coding of sympathetic transmission: differential release of noradrenaline and neuropeptide Y from pig spleen. Neurosci Lett 63:96–100, 1986.

321. Lundberg JM, Änggård A, Pernow J, Hökfelt T. Neuropeptide Y-, substance P- and VIP-immunoreactive nerves in cat spleen in relation to autonomic vascular and volume control. Cell Tissue Res 239:9–18, 1985.

322. Lundberg JM, Saria A, Brodin E, Rosell S, Folkars K. A substance P antagonist inhibits vagally-induced increase in vascular permeability and bronchial smooth muscle contraction in the guinea pig. Proc Natl Acad Sci USA 80:1120–1124, 1983.

323. Lyte M, Ernst S, Driemeyer J, Baissa B. Strain-specific enhancement of splenic T cell mitogenesis and macrophage phagocytosis following peripheral axotomy. J Neuroimmunol 31:1–8, 1991.

324. Madden KS, Felten SY, Felten DL, Hardy CA, Livnat S. Sympathetic nervous system modulation of the immune system. II. Induction of lymphocyte proliferation and migration in vivo by chemical sympathectomy. J Neuroimmunol 49:67–75, 1994.

325. Madden KS, Felten SY, Felten DL, Bellinger DL. Sympathetic nervous system—Immune system interactions in young and old Fischer 344 rats. Ann NY Acad Sci 771:523–533, 1995.

326. Madden KS, Felten SY, Felten DL, Livnat S. Sympathetic neural modulation of the immune system. I. Depression of T cell immunity in vivo and in vitro following chemical sympathectomy. Brain Behav Immunol 3:7–89, 1989.

327. Madden KS, Moynihan JA, Brenner GJ, Felten SY, Felten DL. Sympathetic nervous system modulation of the immune system. III. Alterations in T and B cell proliferation and differentiation in vitro following chemical sympathectomy. J Neuroimmunol 49:77–87, 1994.

328. Maestroni GJ, Conti A. Noradrenergic modulation of lymphohematopoiesis. Int J Immunopharmacol 16:117–122, 1994.

329. Makman MH, Bilfinger TV, Stefano GB. Human granulocytes contain an opiate alkaloid-selective receptor mediating inhibition of cytokine-induced activation and chemotaxis. J Immunol 154:1323–1330, 1995.

330. Makman MH, Dvorkin B, Stefano GB. Murine macrophage cell lines contain μ_3-opiate receptors. Eur J Pharmacol 273:R5–R6, 1995.

331. Malec P, Zeman K, Markiewicz K, Tchorzewski H, Nowak Z, Baj Z. Short-term somatostatin infusion affects T lymphocyte responsiveness in humans. Immunopharmacology 17:45–49, 1989.

332. Mandler RN, Biddison WE, Mandler R, Serrate SA. β-endorphin augments the cytolytic activity and interferon production of natural killer cells. J Immunol 136:934–939, 1986.

333. Marcoli M, Ricevuti G, Mazzone A, Bekkering M, Lecchini S, Frigo GM. Opioid-induced modification of granulocyte function. Int J Immunopharmacol 10:425–433, 1988.

334. Marie JC, Cotroneo P, de Chasseval R, Rosselin G. Solubization of somatostatin receptors

in hamster pancreatic beta cells. Characterization as a glycoprotein interacting with a GTP-binding protein. Eur J Biochem 186:181–188, 1989.

335. Markwick AJ, Lolait SJ, Funder JW. Immunoreactive arginine vasopressin in the rat thymus. Endocrinology 119:1690–1696, 1986.

336. Marotti T, Rabatic S, Gabrilovac J. A characterization of the in vivo immunomodulation by Met-enkephalin in mice. Int J Immunopharmac 15:919–926, 1993.

337. Mascardo RN, Barton RW, Sherline P. Somatostatin has an antiproliferative effect on concancavalin-activated rat thymocytes. Clin Immunol Immunopathol 33:131–138, 1984.

338. Maslinski W, Kullberg M, Nordström O, Bartfai T. Muscarinic receptors and receptor-mediated actions on rat thymocytes. J Neuroimmunol 17:265–274, 1988.

339. Mathew RC, Cook GA, Blum AM, Metwall A, Felman R, Weinstock JV. Vasoactive intestinal peptide stimulates T lymphocytes to release IL-5 in murine *Schistosomiasis mansoni* infection. J Immunol 148:3572–3577, 1992.

340. Mathews PM, Froelich CJ, Sibbitt WL Jr, Bankhurst AD. Enhancement of natural cytotoxicity by β-endorphin. J Immunol 130:1658–1662, 1983.

341. Matis WL, Lavker RM, Murphy GF. Substance P induces expression of an endothelial-leukocyte adhesion molecule by microvascular endothelium. J Invest Dermatol 94:492–495, 1990.

342. McCain HW, Lamster IB, Bozzone JM, Grbic JT. β-endorphin modulates human immune activity via non-opiate receptor mechanisms. Life Sci 31:1619–1624, 1982.

343. McGillis JP, Humphreys S, Rangnekar V, Ciallella J. Modulation of B lymphocyte differentiation by calcitonin gene-related peptide (CGRP). II. Inhibition of LPS-induced κ light chain expression by CGRP. Cell Immunol 150:405–416, 1993.

344. McGillis JP, Humphreys S, Rangnekar V, Ciallella J. Modulation of B lymphocyte differentiation by calcitonin gene-related peptide (CGRP). I. Characterization of high-affinity CGRP receptors on murine 70Z/3 cells. Cell Immunol 150:391–404, 1993.

345. McGillis JP, Humphreys S, Reid S. Characterization of functional calcitonin gene-related peptide receptors on rat thymocytes. J Immunol 147:3482–3489, 1991.

346. McPherson GA, Summers RJ. Characteristics and localization of ^{3}H-clonidine binding in membranes prepared from guinea-pig spleen. Clin Exp Pharmacol Physiol 9:77–87, 1982.

347. Mehrishi JN, Mills IH. Opiate receptors on lymphocytes and platelets in man. Clin Immunol Immunopathol 27:240–249, 1983.

348. Melmon KL, Bourne HR, Weinstein Y, Shearer GM, Kram J, Bauminger S. Hemolytic plaque formation by leukocytes in vitro—control by vasoactive hormones. J Clin Invest 53:13–21, 1974.

349. Metwall A, Blum A, Mathew R, Sandor M, Lynch RG, Weinstock JV. Modulation of T lymphocyte proliferation in mice infected with *Schistosome mansoni*: VIP suppresses mitogen- and antigen-induced T cell proliferation possibly by inhibiting IL-2 production. Cell Immunol 149:11–23, 1993.

350. Miles K, Atweh S, Otten G, Arnason BGW, Chelmicka-Schorr E. Beta-adrenergic receptors on splenic lymphocytes from axotomized mice. Int J Immunopharmacol 6:171–177, 1984.

351. Miles K, Quintáns J, Chelmicka-Schorr E, Arnason BGW. The sympathetic nervous system modulates antibody response to thymus-independent antigens. J Neuroimmunol 1:101–105, 1981.

352. Miller GC, Murgo AJ, Plotnikoff NP. Enkephalins: enhancement of active T cell rosettes from normal volunteers. Clin Immunol Immunopathol 31:132–137, 1984.

353. Miller ML, McCuskey RS. Innervation of bone marrow in the rabbit. Scand J Haematol 10:17–23, 1973.

354. Modin A, Pernow J, Lundberg JM. Comparison of the acute influence of neuropeptide Y and sympathetic stimulation on the composition of blood cells in the splenic vein in vivo. Regul Peptides 47:159–169, 1993.

355. Moore TC. Modification of lymphocyte traffic by vasoactive neurotransmitter substances. Immunology 52:511–518, 1984.

356. Moore TC, Lachmann PJ. Cyclic AMP reduces and cyclic GMP increases the traffic of lymphocytes through peripheral lymph nodes of sheep in vivo. Immunology 47:423–428, 1982.

357. Moore TC, Spruck CH, Said SI. 1998. Depression of lymphocyte traffic in sheep by vasoactive intestinal peptide (VIP). Immunology 64:475–478, 1988.

358. Motulsky HJ, Cunningham EMS, DeBlasi A, Insel PA. Desensitization and redistribution of β-adrenergic receptors on human mononuclear leukocytes. Am J Physiol 250:E583–E590, 1986.

359. Mousli M, Trifilieff A, Pelton JT, Gies J-P, Landry Y. Structural requirements for neuropeptide in mast cell and G protein activation. Eur J Pharmacol 289:125–133, 1995.

360. Muscettola M, Grasso G. Somatostatin and vasoactive intestinal peptide interferon gamma production by human peripheral blood mononuclear cells. Immunobiology 180:419–430, 1990.

361. Myers AC, Undem BJ, Weinreich D. Influence of antigen on membrane properties of guinea-pig bronchial ganglion neurons. J Appl Physiol 71:970–976, 1991.

362. Nair MP, Schwartz SA, Wu K, Kronfol Z. Effect of neuropeptide Y on natural killer activity of normal human lymphocytes. Brain Behav Immun 7:70–78, 1993.

363. Nakamura H, Koike T, Hiruma K, Sato T, Tomioka H, Yoshida S. Identification of lymphoid cell lines bearing receptors for somatostatin. Immunology 62:655–658, 1987.

364. Nakamuta H, Fukada Y, Koida M, Fujii N, Otaka S, Funakoshi S, Yajima H, Mitsuyasu N, Orlowski RC. Binding sites of calcitonin gene-related peptide (CGRP): abundant occurrence in visceral organs. Jpn J Pharmacol 42:175–180, 1986.

365. Nance DM, Burns J. Innvervation of the spleen in the rat: evidence for absence of afferent innervation. Brain Behav Immun 3:281–290, 1989.

366. Nance DM, Hopkins DA, Bieger D. Re-investigation of the innervation of the thymus gland in mice and rats. Brain Behav Immun 1:134–147, 1987.

367. Neil GA, Blum A, Weinstock JV. Substance P but not vasoactive intestinal peptide modulates immunoglobulin secretion in murine schistosomiasis. Cell Immunol 135:394–401, 1991.

368. Nielson CP. β-Adrenergic modulation of the polymorphonuclear leukocyte respiratory burst is dependent upon the mechanism of cell activation. J Immunol 139:2392–2397, 1987.

369. Nilsson S. Sympathetic innervation of the spleen of the cane toad, *Bufo marinus*. Comp Biochem Physiol 61C:133–139, 1978.

370. Nilsson S, Grove DJ. Adrenergic and cholinergic innervation of the spleen of the cod: *Gadus morhua*. Eur J Pharmacol 28:135–143, 1974.

371. Nilsson J, Von Euler AM, Dalsgaard CJ. Stimulation of connective tissue cell growth by substance and substance K. Nature London 315:61–63, 1985.

372. Nohr D, Michel S, Fink T, Weihe E. Pro-enkephalin opioid peptides are abundant in porcine and bovine splenic nerves, but absent from nerves of rat, mouse, hamster, and guinea-pig spleen. Cell Tissue Res 281:215–219, 1995.

373. Nong Y, Titus RG, Ribeiro JMC, Remold HG. Peptides encoded by the calcitonin gene inhibit macrophages function. J Immunol 143:45–49, 1989.

374. Nordlind K, Mutt V. Influence of beta-endorphin, somatostatin, substance P, and vasoactive intestinal peptide on the proliferative response of human peripheral blood T lymphocytes to mercuric chloride. Int Archs Allergy Appl Immunol 80:326–328, 1986.

375. Novotny GEK. Ultrastructural analysis of lymph node innervation in the rat. Acta Anat 133:57–61, 1988.

376. Novotny GEK, Kliche KO. Innervation of lymph nodes: a combined silver impregnation and electron-microscopic study. Acta Anat 127:243–248, 1986.

377. O'Connor SW, Scarpace PJ, Abrass IB. Age-associated decrease in the catalytic unit activity of rat myocardial adenylate cyclase. Mech Ageing Dev 21:357–363, 1983.

378. O'Dorisio MS, Hermina NS, O'Dorisio TM, Balcerzak SP. Vasoactive intestinal polypeptide modulation of lymphocyte adenylate cyclase. J Immunol 127:2551–2554, 1981a.

379. O'Dorisio MS, Shannon BT, Fleshman DJ, Campolito LB. Identification of high affinity receptors for vasoactive intestinal peptide on human lymphocytes of B cell lineage. J Immunol 142:3533–3536, 1989.

380. O'Dorisio MS, Wood C, Wenger G, Vasalo L. Cyclic AMP-dependent protein kinase in MOLT-4B lymphoblasts: identification by photoaffinity labeling and activation in intact cells by VIP and PHI. J Immunol 134:4078–4085, 1985.

381. O'Hara N, Daul AE, Fesel R, Siekmann U, Brodde O-E. Different mechanisms underlying reduced β_2-adrenoceptor responsiveness in lymphocytes from neonates and old subjects. Mech Ageing Dev 31:115–122, 1985.

382. Ohkubo N, Miura S, Serizawa H, Yan HJ, Kimura H, Imaeda H, Tashiro H, Tsuchiya M. In vivo effect of chronic administration of vasoactive intestinal peptide on gut-associated lymphoid tissues in rats. Regul Pept 50:127–135, 1994.

383. Okamoto Y, Shirotori K, Kudo K, Ishikawa K, Ito E, Togawa K, Saito I. Cytokine expression after the topical administration of substance P to human nasal mucosa. The role of substance P in nasal allergy. J Immunol 151:4391–4398, 1993.

384. Olschowka JA, Felten SY, Bellinger DL, Lorton D, Felten DL. NPY-positive nerve terminals contact lymphocytes in the periarteriolar lymphatic sheath of the rat splenic white pulp. Soc Neurosci Abstr 14:1280, 1988.

385. Ottaway CA. In vitro alteration of receptors for vasoactive intestinal peptide changes the in vivo localization of mouse T cells. J Exp Med 160:1054–1069, 1984.

386. Ottaway CA. Evidence for local neuromodulation of T cell migration in vivo. Adv Exp Med 186:637–645, 1985.

387. Ottaway CA. Vasoactive intestinal peptide as a modulator of lymphocyte and immune functions. Ann NY Acad Sci 527:486–500, 1988.

388. Ottaway CA. Vasoactive intestinal peptide and immune function. In: Psychoneuroimmunology, 2nd ed, R Ader, DL Felten, N Cohen, eds. Academic Press, New York, 1991, pp 225–262.

389. Ottaway CA, Bernaerts C, Chan B, Greenberg GR. Specific binding of vasoactive intestinal peptide to human circulating mononuclear cells. Can J Physiol Pharmacol 61:664–671, 1983.

390. Ottaway CA, Greenberg GR. Interaction of vasoactive intestinal peptide with mouse lymphocytes: Specific binding and the modulation of mitogen responses. J Immunol 132:417–423, 1984.

391. Ottaway CA, Lay T, Greenberg G. High affinity specific binding of vasoactive intestinal peptide to human circulating T cells, B cells and large granular lymphocytes. J Neuroimmunol 29:149–155, 1990.

392. Ottaway CA, Lewis DL, Asa SL. Vasoactive intestinal peptide-containing nerves in Peyer's patches. Brain Behav Immun 1:148–158, 1987.

393. Oura H, Takeda K, Daikoku S. Blood vessels and immunoreactive substance P-containing nerve fibers in rat skin treated topically with clobetasol propionate, a corticosteroid. J Dermatol 19:355–341, 1992.

394. Owan I, Ibaraki K. The role of calcitonin gene-related peptide (CGRP) in macrophages: the presence of functional receptors and effects on proliferation and differentiation into osteoclast-like cells. Bone Mineral 24:151–164, 1994.

395. Palmer JBD, Cuss FMC, Mulderry PK, Ghatei MA, Springall DR, Cadieux A, Bloom SR, Polak JM, Barnes PJ. Calcitonin gene-related peptide is localized to human airway nerves and potently constricts human airway smooth muscle. Br J Pharmacol 91:95–101, 1987.

396. Parnet P, Payan DG, Kerdelhue B, Mitsuhashi M. Neuroendocrine interaction on lympho-cytes: testosterone-induced modulation of the lymphocyte substance P receptor. J Neuro-immunol 28:185–188, 1990.

397. Partsch G, Matucci-Cerinic M. Effect of substance P and somatostatin on migration of polymorphonuclear (PMN) cells in vitro. Inflammation 16:539–547, 1992.

398. Pascual DW, McGhee JR, Kiyono H, Bost KL. Neuroimmune modulation of lymphocyte function. I. Substance P enhances immunoglobulin synthesis in LPS activated murine splenic B cell cultures. Int Immunol 3:1223–1229, 1991a.

399. Pascual DW, Xu-Amano J, Kiyono H, McGhee JR, Bost KL. Substance P acts directly upon cloned B lymphoma cells to enhance IgA and IgM production. J Immunol 146:2130–2136, 1991b.

400. Pascual DW, Beagley KW, Kiyono H, McGhee JR. Substance P promotes Peyer's patch and splenic B cell differentiation. In: Advances in Mucosal Immunol, J Mestechky, ed. Plenum Press, New York, 1995, pp 55–59.

401. Paul-Eugene N, Dugas B, Gordon J, Kolb JP, Cairns JA, Paubert-Braquet M, Mencia-Huerta JM, Braquet P. β_2-adrenoceptor stimulation augments the IL-4-induced CD23 expression and release and the expression of differentiation markers (CD14, CD18) by the human monocyte cell line. Clin Exp Allergy 23:317–325, 1993.

402. Pawlikowski M, Stepien H, Kunert-Radek J, Schally AV. Effect of somatostatin on the proliferation of mouse spleen lymphocytes in vitro. Biochem Biophys Res Commun 129:52–55, 1985.

403. Pawlikowski M, Stepien H, Kunert-Radek J, Zelazowski P, Schally AV. Immunomodula-tory action of somatostatin. Ann NY Acad Sci 496:233–239, 1987.

404. Pawlikowski M, Zelazowski P, Stepien HQ, Schally HV. Somatostatin and its analog enhance the formation of human leukocyte migration inhibiting factor: further evidence of immunomodulatory action of somatostatin. Peptides 8:951–952, 1987.

405. Payan DG. Receptor-mediated mitogenic effects of substance P on cultured smooth muscle cells. Biochem Biophysical Res Commun 130:104–109, 1985.

406. Payan DG, Brewster DR, Goetzl EJ. Specific stimulation of human T lymphocytes by substance P. J Immunol 131:1613–1615, 1983.

407. Payan DG, Brewster DR, Goetzl EJ. Stereospecific receptors for substance P on cultured human IM-9 lymphoblasts. J Immunol 133:3260–3265, 1984.

408. Payan DG, Brewster DR, Missirian-Bastian A, Goetzl EJ. Substance P recognition by a subset of human T lymphocytes. J Clin Invest 74:1532–1539, 1984.

409. Payan DG, Hess CA, Goetzl EJ. Inhibition by somatostatin of the proliferation of T-lym-phocytes and Molt-4 lymphoblasts. Cell Immunol 84:433–438, 1984.

410. Payan DG, Levine JD, Goetzl EJ. Modulation of immunity and hypersensitivity by sensory neuropeptides. J Immunol 132:1601–1604, 1984.

411. Payan DG, McGillis JP, Goetzl EJ. Neurommunology In: Advances in Immunology, FJ Dixon, KF Austen, L Hood, JW Uhr, eds. Academic Press, New York, 1986a, pp 299–323.

412. Payan DG, McGillis JP, Organist ML. Characterization of the lymphocyte substance P receptor. J Biol Chem 261:14321–14329, 1986.

413. Peck R. Neuropeptides modulating macrophage function. Ann NY Acad Sci 496:264–270, 1987.

414. Pedrera C, Lucas M, Bellido J, Lopez-Gonzalez MA. Receptor-independent mechanisms are involved in the priming of neutrophil's oxidase by vasoactive intestinal peptide. Regul Pept 54:505–511, 1994.

415. Perachi M, Bamonti-Catena F, Bareggi B. Effect of high doses of somatostatin on adenylate cyclase activity in peripheral mononuclear leukocytes from normal subjects and from acute leukemia patients. Experientia 44:613–615, 1988.

416. Peterson PK, Gekker G, Hu S, Anderson WR, Kravitz F, Portoghese PS, Balfour HH Jr, Chao CC. Morphine amplifies HIV-1 expression in chronically infected promonocytes cocultured with human brain cells. J Neuroimmunol 50:167–175, 1994.

417. Peterson PK, Sharp B, Bekker G, Brummitt C, Keane WF. Opioid-mediated suppression of culture peripheral blood mononuclear cell respiratory burst activity. J Immunol 138:3907–3912, 1987.

418. Peuriere S, Susini C, Alvinerie M, Vaysse N, Escoula L. Interactions between neuropeptides and dexamethasone on the mitogenic response of rabbit spleen lymphocytes. Peptides 12:645–651, 1991.

419. Pezzati P, Agro A, Dazin P, Payan DG, Stanisz AM. The apparent lack of cell cycle dependency for substance P binding to murine lymphocytes. Ann NY Acad Sci 650:226–229, 1992.

420. Pfoch M, Unsicker K. Electron microscopic study on the innervation of Peyer's patches of Syrian hamster. Z Zellforsch 123:425–429, 1972.

421. Piotrowski W, Mead M, Foreman JC. Action of the SP2-11 and SP3-11 fragments of substance P on rat peritoneal mast cells. Agents Actions 20:178–180, 1987.

422. Plotnikoff NP, Miller GC. Enkephalins as immunomodulators. Int J Immunopharmacol 5:437–441, 1983.

423. Pochet R, Delespesse G, Gausset PW, Collet H. Distribution of beta-adrenergic receptors on human lymphocyte subpopulations. Clin Exp Immunol 38:578–584, 1979.

424. Popper P, Mantyh CR, Vigna SR, Magioos JE, Mantyh PW. The localization of sensory nerve fibers and receptor binding sites for sensory neuropeptides in canine mesenteric lymph nodes. Peptides 9:257–267, 1988.

425. Pothoulakis C, Castagliuolo I, LaMont T, Jaffer A, O'Keane JC, Snider RM, Leeman SE. CP-96,345, a substance P antagonist, inhibits rat intestinal responses to *Clostridium difficile* toxin A but not cholera toxin. Proc Natl Acad Sci USA 91:947–951, 1994.

426. Probert L, de Mey J, Polak JM. Distinct subpopulations of enteric p-type neurones contain substance P and vasoactive intestinal polypeptide. Nature 294:470–471, 1981.

427. Radojcic T, Baird S, Darko D, Smith D, Bulloch K. Changes in β-adrenergic receptor distribution on immunocytes during differentiation: an analysis of T cells and macrophages. J Neurosci Res 30:328–335, 1991.

428. Radulovic J, Miljevic C, Djergovic D, Vujic V, Antic J, von Horsten S, Jankovic BD. Opioid receptor-mediated suppression of humoral immune response in vivo and in vitro: involvement of κ opioid receptors. J Neuroimmunol 57:55–62, 1995.

429. Radulescu RT, DeCosta BR, Jacobson AE, Rice KC, Blalock JE, Carr DJJ. Biochemical and functional characterization of a mu-opioid receptor binding site on cells of the immune system. Prog Neuroendocrinimmunol 4:166–179, 1991.

430. Raneshwar P, Ganea D, Gascon P. In vitro stimulatory effect of substance P on hematopoiesis. Blood 81:391–398, 1993.

431. Rameshwar P, Ganea D, Gascon P. Induction of IL-3 and granulocyte-macrophage colony-stimulating factor by substance P in bone marrow cells is partially mediated through the release of IL-1 and IL-6. J Immunol 152:4044–4054, 1994.

432. Rameshwar P, Gascon P, Ganea D. Immunoregulatory effects of neuropeptides. Stimulation of interleukin-2 production by substance P. J Neuroimmunol 37:65–74, 1992.

433. Raynor K, Reisine T. Analogs of somatostatin selectively label distinct subtypes of somatostatin receptors in rat brain. J Pharmacol Exp Ther 251:510–517, 1989.

434. Reder A, Checinski M, Chelmicka-Schorr E. The effect of chemical sympathectomy on natural killer cells in mice. Brain Behav Immun 3:110–118, 1989.

435. Reilly FD, McCuskey PA, Miller ML, McCuskey RS, Meineke HA. Innervation of the periarteriolar lymphatic sheath of the spleen. Tissue and Cell 11:121–126, 1979.

436. Renold F, Chernov T, Lee J, Payan DG, Furuichi K, Goetzl EJ. Somatostatin (SOM 14) modulation of mediator release by mouse bone marrow-derived mast cells (BMMC), rat serosal mast cells (SMC), and rat basophilic leukemia cells (RBL-2H3). Federation Proc 44:1917, 1985.

437. Reubi JC, Horisberger U, Waser B, Gebber JO, Laissue J. Preferential location of somatostatin receptors in germinal centres of human gut lymphoid tissue. Gastroenterology 103:1207–1214, 1992.

438. Reubi JC, Kvols LK, Krenning EP, Lamberts SWJ. Distribution of somatostatin receptors in normal and tumor tissue. Metabolism 39:78–81, 1990.

439. Reynier-Rebuffel A-M, Mathiau P, Callebert J, Dimitriadou V, Farjaudon N, Kacem K, Launay J-M, Seylaz J, Aubineau P. Substance P, calcitonin gene-related peptide, and capsaicin release serotonin from cerebrovascular mast cells. Am J Physiol 267:R1421–R1429, 1994.

440. Rivkin I, Rosenblatt J, Becker EL. The role of cyclic AMP in the chemotactic responsiveness and spontaneous motility of rabbit peritoneal neutrophil. The inhibition of neutrophil movement and the elevation of cyclic AMP levels by catecholamines, prostaglandins, theophylline, and cholera toxin. J Immunol 115:1126–1134, 1975.

441. Robberecht P, Cauvin A, Gourlet P, Christophe J. Heterogeneity of VIP receptors. Arch Int Pharmacodyn 303:51–66, 1990.

442. Robberecht P, De Neef P, Gourlet P, Cauvin A, Coy DH, Christophe J. Pharmacological characterization of the novel helodermin/VIP receptor present in Human SUP-T1 lymphoma cell membranes. Regul Pept 26:117–126, 1989.

443. Roberts AI, Panja A, Brolin RE, Ebert EC. Human intraepithelial lymphocytes. Immunomodulation and receptor binding of vasoactive intestinal peptide. Dig Dis Sci 36:341–346, 1991.

444. Robichon A, Sreedharan SP, Yang J, Shames RS, Gronroos EC, Cheng PP-J, Goetzl EJ. Induction of aggregation of Raji human B-lymphoblastic cells by vasoactive intestinal peptide. Immunology 79:574–579, 1993.

445. Rola-Pleszczynski M, Bulduc D, St. Pierre A. The effects of VIP on human NK cell function. J Immunol 135:2659–2673, 1985.

446. Romano TA, Felten SY, Felten DL, Olschowka JA. Neuropeptide-Y innervation of the rat spleen: another potential immunomodulatory neuropeptide. Brain Behav Immun 5:116–131, 1991.

447. Romano T, Felten SY, Olschowka JA, Felten DL. Noradrenergic and peptidergic innervation of lymphoid organs in the beluga, *Delphinapterus leucas:* an anatomical link between the nervous and immune systems. J Morphol 221:243–259, 1994.

448. Romano TA, Olschowka JA, Felten SY, Felten DL. Neuropeptide-Y involvement in neural-immune interactions in the rat spleen. Soc Neurosci Abstr 15:714, 1989.

449. Romeo HE, Fink T, Yanaihara N, Weihe E. Distribution and relative proportions of neuropeptide Y- and proenkephalin-containing noradrenergic neurones in rat superior cervical ganglion: separate projections to submaxillary lymph nodes. Peptides 15:1479–1487, 1994.

450. Rowland RRR, Chukwuocha RU, Tokuda S. Modulation of the in vitro murine immune response by met-enkephalin. Brain Behav Immun 1:342–348, 1987.

451. Rowland RRR, Tokuda S. Dual immunomodulation by met-enkephalin. Brain Behav Immun 3:171–174, 1989.

452. Roy S, Ge B-L, Loh HH, Lee N. Characterization of [^{3}H]morphine binding to interleukin-1-activated thymocytes. J Pharmacol Exp Ther 263:451–456, 1992.

453. Roy S, Ge B-L, Ramakrishnan S, Lee NM, Loh HH. ^{3}H-Morphine binding to thymocytes is enhanced by IL-1 stimulation. FEBS Lett 287:93–96, 1991a.

454. Roy S, Ramakrishnan S, Loh HH, Lee NM. Chronic morphine treatment selectively suppresses macrophage colony formation in bone marrow. Eur J Pharmacol 195:359–363, 1991b.

456. Ruhl A, Berezin I, Collins SM. Involvement of eicosanoids and macrophage-like cells in cytokine-mediated changes in rat myenteric nerves. Gastroenterology 109:1852–1862, 1995.

457. Sacerdote P, Bianchi M, Panerai AE. Human monocyte chemotactic activity of calcitonin and somatostatin related peptides: Modulation by chronic peptide treatment. J Clin Endocrinol Metab 70:141–148, 1990.

458. Said SI. Vasoactive intestinal peptide in the lung. Ann NY Acad Sci 527:450–464, 1988.

459. Sakagami Y, Girasole G, Yu X-P, Boswell HS, Manolagas SC. Stimulation of interleukin-6 production by either calcitonin gene-related peptide or parathyroid hormone in two phenotypically distinct bone marrow-derived murine stromal cell lines. J Bone Mineral Res 8:811–816, 1993.

460. Sakuta H, Inaba K, Muramatsu S. Calcitonin gene-related peptide enhances cytokine-induced IL-6 production by fibroblasts. Cell Immunol 165:20–25, 1995.

461. Sanders VM, Munson AE. Beta adrenoceptor mediation of the enhancing effect of norepinephrine on the murine primary antibody response in vitro. J Pharmacol Exp Ther 230:183–192, 1984.

462. Sanders VM, Munson AE. Kinetics of the enhancing effect produced by norepinephrine and terbutaline on the murine primary antibody response in vitro. J Pharmacol Exp Ther 231:527–531, 1984.

463. Sanders VM, Munson AE. Norepinephrine and the antibody response. Pharmacol Rev 37:229–248, 1985.

464. Sanders VM, Munson AE. Role of alpha adrenoceptor activation in modulating the murine primary antibody response in vitro. J Pharmacol Exp Ther 232:395–400, 1985.

465. Sanders VM, Powell-Oliver FE. β_2-adrenoceptor stimulation increases the number of antigen specific precursor B lymphocytes that differentiate into IgM-secreting cells without affecting burst size. J Immunol 148:1822–1828, 1992.

466. Sanders VM, Street NE, Fuchs BA. Differential expression of the β-adrenoceptor by subsets of T-helper lymphocytes. FASEB J 8:A114, 1994.

467. Sanghavi JN, Rabe KR, Kim JS, Magnussen H, Leff AR, White SR. Migration of human and guinea-pig airway epithelial cells in response to calcitonin gene-related peptide. Am J Respir Cell Mole Biol 11:183–187, 1994.

468. Scarpace PJ, Abrass IB. Decreased beta-adrenergic agonist affinity and adenylate cyclase activity in senescent rat lung. J Gerontol 38:143–147, 1983.

469. Scatchard G. The attractions of protein for small molecules and ions. Ann NY Acad Sci 51:660–672, 1949.
470. Schultzberg M, Svenson SB, Unden A, Bartfai T. Interleukin-1-like immunoreactivity in peripheral tissues. J Neurosci Res 18:184–189, 1987.
471. Schweigerer L, Schmidt W, Teschemacher H, Gramsch C. β-Endorphin: surface binding and internalization in thymoma cells. Proc Natl Acad Sci USA 82:5751–5755, 1985.
472. Scicchitano R, Biennenstock J, Stanisz AM. In vivo immunomodulation by the neuropeptide substance P. Immunology 63:733–735, 1988.
473. Scicchitano R, Dazin P, Bienenstock J, Payan DG, Stanisz AM. Distribution of somatostatin receptors on murine spleen and Peyer's patch T and B lymphocytes. Brain Behav Immun 1:173–183, 1987.
474. Scicchitano R, Dazin P, Bienenstock J, Payan DG, Stanisz AM. The murine IgA-secreting plasmacytoma mopc-315 expresses somatostatin receptors. Am Assoc Immunologists 937–941, 1988.
475. Sei Y, Yoshimoto K, McTintyre T, Skolnick P, Arora PK. Morphine-induced hypoplasia is glucocorticoid dependent. J Immunol 146:194–198, 1991.
476. Segura JJ, Guerrero JM, Goberna R, Calvo JR. Characterization of functional receptors for vasoactive intestinal peptide (VIP) in rat peritoneal macrophages. Regul Pept 35:133–143, 1991.
477. Serra MC, Bazzoni F, Bianca VD, Greskowiak M, Rossi R. Activation of human neutrophils by substance P. Effect on oxidative metabolism, exocytosis, cytosolic Ca^{2+} concentration and inositol phosphate formation. J Immunol 141:2118–2124, 1988.
478. Sergeeva VE. Histotopography of catecholamines in the mammalian thymus. Bull Exp Bio Med 77:456–458, 1974.
479. Severn A, Rapson NT, Hunter CA, Liew FY. Regulation of tumor necrosis factor production by adrenaline and β-adrenergic agonists. J Immunol 148:3441–3445, 1992.
480. Shadlack AM, Hart RP, Carlson CD, Jonakait GM. Interleukin-1 induces substance P in sympathetic ganglia through the induction of leukemia inhibitory factor (LIF). J Neuroscience 13:2601–2609, 1993.
481. Shanahan F, Denburg JA, Fox J, Bienenstock J, Befus D. Mast cell heterogeneity: effects of neuroenteric peptides on histamine release. J Immunol 135:1331–1337, 1985.
482. Sharp BM, Tsukayama DT, Gekker G, Keane WF, Peterson PK. β-Endorphin stimulates human polymorphonuclear leukocyte superoxide production via a stereoselective opiate receptor. J Pharmacol Exp Ther 242:579–582, 1987.
483. Shavit Y, Depaulis A, Martin RC, Terman GW, Pechnick RN, Zane CJ, Gale RP, Liebeskind JC. Involvement of brain opiate receptors in the immune-suppressive effect of morphine. Proc Natl Acad Sci USA 83:7114–7117, 1986.
484. Shavit Y, Lewis JW, Terman GW, Gale RP, Liebeskind JC. Opioid peptides mediate the suppressive effect of stress on natural killer cell cytotoxicity. Science 223:188–190, 1984.
485. Shen GH, Grundemar L, Zukowska-Grojec Z, Hakanson R, and Wahlestedt C. C-terminal neuropeptide Y fragments are mast cell-dependent vasodepressor agents. Eur J Pharmacol 204:249–256, 1991.
486. Shen HM, Sha LX, Kennedy JL, Ou DW. Adrenergic receptors regulate macrophage secretion. Int J Immunopharmacol 16:905–910, 1994.
487. Shipp MA, Stefano GB, D'Adamio L, Switzer SN, Howard FD, Sinisterra J, Scharrer B, Rheinerz EL. Downregulation of enkephalin-mediated inflammatory responses by CD10/neutral endopeptidase 24.11. Nature London 347:394–396, 1990.
488. Sibinga NES, Goldstein A. Opioid peptides and opioid receptors in cells of the immune system. Annu Rev Immunol 6:219–249, 1988.

489. Simpkins CO, Dickey CA, Fink MP. Human neutrophil migration is enhanced by beta-endorphin. Life Sci 34:2251–2255, 1984.
490. Singh PP, Singh S, Dhawan VC, Haq W, Mathur KB, Dutta GP, Srimal RC, Dhawan BN. Enkephalins-modulation of *Plasmodium cynomolgi* antigens-induced colony-stimulating factors elaboration by macrophages. J Biol Regul Domest Agents 5:133–137, 1991.
491. Singh PP, Singh S, Dhawan VC, Haq W, Mathur KB, Dutta GP, Srimal RC, Dhawan BN. Lymphokines production by concanavalin A-stimulated mouse splenocytes: modulation by Met-enkephalin and a related peptide. Immunopharmacology 27:245–251, 1994.
492. Singh U. Effect of catecholamines on lymphopoiesis in fetal mouse thymic explants. J Anat 129:279–292, 1979.
493. Singh U. Effect of catecholamines on lymphopoiesis in fetal mouse thymic explants. Eur J Immunol 14:757–759, 1979.
494. Singh U. Sympathetic innervation of fetal mouse thymus. Eur J Immunol 14:757–759, 1984.
495. Singh U. Effect of sympathectomy on the maturation of fetal thymocytes grown within the anterior eye chambers in mice. Adv Exp Biol Med 186:349–356, 1985.
496. Singh U. Lymphopoiesis in the nude fetal mouse thymus following sympathectomy. Cell Immunol 93:222–228, 1985.
497. Singh U, Millson S, Smith PA, Owen JJT. Identification of β adrenoceptors during thymocyte ontogeny in mice. Eur J Immunol 9:31–35, 1979.
498. Singh U, Owen JJT. Studies on the effect of various agents on the maturation of thymus stem cells. Eur J Immunol 5:286–288, 1975.
499. Singh U, Owen JJT. Studies on the maturation of thymus stem cells. The effects of catecholamines, histamine, and peptide hormones on the expression of T alloantigens. Eur J Immunol 6:59–62, 1976.
500. Sirianni MC, Annibale B, Fais S, Delle Fave G. Inhibitory effect of somatostatin-14 and some analogues on human natural killer cell activity. Peptides 15:1033–1036, 1994.
501. Sirianni MC, Annibale B, Tagliaferri F, Fais S, De Luca S, Pallone F, Delle Fave G, Aiuti F. Modulation of human natural killer activity by vasoactive intestinal peptide (VIP) family. VIP, glucagon, and GHRF specifically inhibit NK activity. Regul Pept 38:79–87, 1992.
502. Skofitsch G, Savitt JM, Jacobowitz DM. Suggestive evidence for a functional unit between mast cells and substance P fibers in the rat diaphragm and mesentery. Histochemistry 82:5–8, 1985.
503. Smart BA, Rao KMK, Cohen HJ. Substance P and adrenocorticotropic hormone do not affect T-lymphocyte adhesion to vascular endothelium or surface expression adhesion receptors. Int J Immunpharmac 16:137–149, 1994.
504. Smolen AJ. Postnatal development of ganglionic neurons in the absence of preganglionic input: morphological observations on synapse formation. Dev Brain Res 1:49–58, 1981.
505. Soder O, Hellstrand PM. Neuropeptide regulation of human thymocyte, guinea-pig T lymphocyte and rat B lymphocyte mitogenesis. Int Arch Allergy Appl Immunol 84:205–211, 1987.
506. Soliven B, Albert J. Tumor necrosis factor modulates the inactivation of catecholamine secretion in cultured neurons. J Neurochem 58:1073–1078, 1992.
507. Spengler RN, Allen RM, Remick DG, Strieter RM, Kunkel SL. Stimulation of alpha-adrenergic receptor augments the production of macrophage-derived tumor necrosis factor. J Immunol 145:1430–1434, 1990.
508. Splengler RN, Chensue SW, Giacherio DA, Blenk N, Kundel SL. Endogenous norepinephrine regulates tumor necrosis factor-alpha production from macrophages in vitro. J Immunol 152:3024–3031, 1994.

509. Sreedharan SP, Kodama KT, Peterson KE, Goetzl EJ. Distinct subsets of somatostatin receptors on cultured human lymphocytes. J Biol Chem 264:949–952, 1989.

510. Staehelin M, Muller P, Portenier M, Harris AW. Beta adrenergic receptors and adenylate cyclase activity in murine lymphoid cell lines. J Cyc Nucl Prot Phosphoryl Res 10:55–64, 1985.

511. Stanisz AM, Befus D, Bienenstock J. Differential effects of vasoactive intestinal peptide, substance P, and somatostatin on immunoglobulin synthesis and proliferation by lymphocytes from Peyer's patches, mesenteric lymph nodes, and spleen. J Immunol 136:152–156, 1986.

512. Stanisz AM, Scicchitano R, Bienenstock J. The role of vasoactive intestinal peptide and other neuropeptides in the regulation of the immune response in vitro and in vivo. Ann NY Acad Sci USA 527:478–485, 1988.

513. Stanisz AM, Scicchitano R, Dazin P, Bienenstock J, Payan DG. Distribution of substance P receptors on murine spleen and Peyer's patch T and B cells. J Immunol 139:749–754, 1987.

514. Stanisz AM, Scicchitano R, Payan DG, Bienenstock J. In vitro studies of immunoregulation of substance P and somatostatin. Ann NY Acad Sci 496:217–225, 1987.

515. Stead RH, Bienenstock J, Stanisz AM. Neuropeptide regulation of mucosal immunity. Immunol Rev 100:333–359, 1987.

516. Stead RH, Tomioka M, Quinonez G, Simon G, Felten SY, Bienenstock J. Intestinal mucosal mast cells in normal and nematode-infected rat intestines are in intimate contact with peptidergic nerves. Proc Natl Acad Sci USA 84:2975–2979, 1987.

517. Stefano GB, Melchiorri P, Negri L, Hughes TK Jr, Scharrer B. [D-Ala^2]deltorphin I binding and pharmacological evidence for a special subtype of δ opioid receptor on human and invertebrate immune cells. Proc Natl Acad Sci USA 89:9316–9320, 1992.

518. Strom TB, Carpenter CB, Garovoy MR, Austen KF, Merrill JP, Kaliner M. The modulating influence of cyclic nucleotides upon lymphocyte-mediated cytotoxicity. J Exp Med 138:381–393, 1973.

519. Strom TB, Lundin AP, Carpenter CB. The role of cyclic nucleotides in lymphocyte activation and function. Prog Clin Immunol 3:115–153, 1977.

520. Su C, Bevan JA. The release of ^{3}H-norepinephrine in arterial strips studied by the technique of superfusion and transmural stimulation. J Pharmacol Exp Ther 172:62–68, 1970.

521. Sun L, Ganea D. Vasoactive intestinal peptide inhibits interleukin (IL)-2 and IL-4 production through different molecular mechanisms in T cells activated via the T cell receptor/CD3 complex. J Neuroimmunol 48:59–70, 1993.

522. Sung CP, Arleth AJ, Aiyar N, Bhatnager PK, Lysko PG, Feuerstein G. CGRP stimulates the adhesion of leukocytes to vascular endothelial cells. Peptides 13:429–434, 1992.

523. Szabo I, Rojavin M, Bussiere JL, Eisenstein TK, Adler MW, Rogers TJ. Suppression of peritoneal macrophage phagocytosis of *Candida albicans* by opioids. J Pharmacol Exp Ther 267:703–706, 1993.

524. Takase B, Nomura S. Studies on the innervation of the bone marrow. J Comp Neurol 108:421–443, 1957.

525. Takayama H, Trenn G, Sitkovsky MV. Locus of inhibitory action of cAMP-dependent protein kinase in the antigen receptor-triggered cytotoxic T lymphocyte activation pathway. J Biol Chem 263:2330–2336, 1988.

526. Tang SC, Braunsteiner, Wiedermann CJ. Regulation of human T lymphoblast growth by sensory neuropeptides: augmentation of cholecystokinin-induced inhibition of Molt-4 proliferation by somatostatin and vasoactive intestinal peptide in vitro. Immunol Lett 34:237–242, 1992.

527. Tatsuno I, Somogyvari-Vigh A, Mizuno K, Gottschall PE, Hidaka H, Arimura A. Neuropeptide regulation of interleukin-6 production from the pituitary: stimulation by pituitary adenylate cyclase activating polypeptide and calcitonin gene-related peptide. Endocrinology 129:1797–1804, 1991.

528. Taub DD, Eisenstein TK, Gellar EB, Adler MW, Rogers TJ. Immunomodulatory activity of mμ- and kappa-selective opioid agonists. Proc Natl Acad Sci USA 88:360–364, 1991.

529. Theoharides TC, Douglas WW. Mast cell histamine secretion in response to somatostatin analogues: structural considerations. Eur J Pharmacol 73:131–136, 1981.

530. Titinchi S, Clark B. Alpha$_2$-adrenoceptors in human lymphocyte: direct characterisation by [^{3}H]yohimbine binding. Biochem Biophys Res Commun 121:1–7, 1984.

531. Tol AF, Verspaget HW, Lamers CB. Neuropeptide regulation of cell-mediated cytotoxicity against human tumor cells. Neuropeptides 16:25–32, 1990.

532. Tollefson L, Bulloch K. Dual-label retrograde transport: CNS innervation of the mouse thymus distinct from other mediastinum viscera. J Neurosci Res 25:20–28, 1990.

533. Topilko A, Caillou B. Fine structural localization of acetylcholinesterase activity in rat submandibular gland. J Histochem Cytochem 33:439–445, 1985.

534. Tosk JM, Grim JR, Kinback KM, Sale EJ, Bozzetti LP, Will AD. Modulation of chemiluminescence in a murine macrophage cell line by neuroendocrine hormones. Int J Immunopharmac 15:615–620, 1993.

535. Tran MA, Dang TL, Lafontan MS, Montastruc P. Adrenergic neurohumoral influences of FFA release from bone marrow adipose tissue. J Pharmacologie 16:171–179, 1985.

536. Umeda Y. Inhibition of immune responses by calcitonin gene-related peptide. Ann NY Acad Sci 657:552–554, 1992.

537. Umeda Y, Arisawa M. Inhibition of natural killer activity by calcitonin gene-related peptide. Immunopharmacol Immunotoxicol 11:309–320, 1989.

538. Umeda Y, Arisawa M. Characterization of the calcitonin gene-related peptide receptor in mouse T lymphocytes. Neuropeptides 14:237–242, 1990.

539. Umeda Y, Takamiya M, Yoshizaki H, Arisawa M. Inhibition of mitogen-stimulated T lymphocyte proliferation by calcitonin gene-related peptide. Biochem Biophys Res Commun 154:227–235, 1988.

540. Undem BJ, Dick EC, Buckner CK. Inhibition by vasoactive intestinal peptide of antigen-induced histamine release from guinea-pig minced lung. Eur J Pharmacol 88:247–249, 1983.

541. Van Den Bergh P, Rozing J, Nagelkerken L. Two opposing modes of action of β-endorphin on lymphocyte function. Immunology 72:537–543, 1991.

542. Van Den Bergh P, Rozing J, Nagelkerken L. β-Endorphin stimulates Ia expression on mouse B cells by inducing interleukin-4 secretion by CD4$^+$ T cells. Cell Immunol 149:180–192, 1993.

543. Van Den Bergh P, Rozing J, Nagelkerken L. Identification of two moieties of β-endorphin with opposing effects on rat T-cell proliferation. Immunology 79:18–23, 1993.

544. Van Den Bergh P, Rozing J, Nagelkerken L. Role of opioid peptides in the regulation of cytokine production by murine CD4$^+$ T cells. Cell Immunol 154:109–122, 1994.

545. Van Hagen PM, Krenning EP, Kwekkeboom DJ, Reubi JC, Anker-Lugtenburg PJ, Lowenberg B, Lamberts SWJ. Somatostatin and the immune and haematopoetic system: a review. Eur J Clin Invest 24:91–99, 1994.

546. Van Tits LJH, Michel MC, Grosse-Wilde H, Happel M, Eigler FW. Catecholamines increase lymphocyte β$_2$-adrenergic receptors via a β$_2$-adrenergic, spleen-dependent process. Am J Physiol 258:E191–E202, 1990.

547. van Tol EAF, Verspaget HW, Hansen BE, Lamers CBHW. Neuroenteric peptides affect

natural killer activity by intestinal lamina propria mononuclear cells. J Neuroimmunol 42:139–146, 1993.

548. van Tol EAF, Verspaget HW, Pena AS, Jansen JBMJ, Aparicio-Pages N, Lamers CBHW. Modulatory effects of VIP and related peptides from the gastrointestinal tract on cell mediated cytotoxicity against tumour cells in vitro. Immunol Invest 20:257–267, 1991.

549. Vignery A, Wang F, Ganz MB. Macrophages express functional receptors for calcitonin gene-related peptide. J Cell Physiol 149:301–306, 1991.

550. von Euler US. The presence of a substance with sympathin E properties in spleen extracts. Acta Physiol Scand 11:168, 1946.

551. Vyden JK, Groseth-Dittrich MF, Callis G, Lars MM, Weinberger H. The effect of propranolol on peripheral hemodynamics in rheumatoid arthritis. Arthritis Rheum 14:420, 1971.

552. Walcott B, McLean JR. Catecholamine-containing neurons and lymphoid cells in a lacrimal gland of the pigeon. Brain Res 328:129–137, 1985.

553. Walker KB, Serwonska MH, Valone FH, Harkonen WS, Frick OL, Scriven KH, Ratnoff WD, Browning JG, Payan DG, Goetzl EJ. Distinctive patterns of release of neuroendocrine peptides after nasal challenge of allergic subjects with ryegrass antigen. J Clin Immunol 8:108–113, 1988.

554. Wallengren J, Moller H, Ekman R. Occurrence of substance P, vasoactive intestinal peptide, and calcitonin gene-related peptide in dermographism and cold urticaria. Arch Dermatol 279:512–515, 1987.

555. Walsh LJ, Trinchieri G, Waldorf HA, Whitaker D, Murphy GF. Human dermal mast cells contain and release tumor necrosis factor a which induces endothelial leukocyte adhesion molecule 1. Proc Natl Acad Sci USA 88:4220–4224, 1991.

556. Wang F, Millet I, Bottomly K, Vignery A. Calcitonin gene-related peptide inhibits interleukin 2 production by murine T lymphocytes. J Biol Chem 267:21052–21057, 1992.

557. Wang X, Fiscus RR, Tang Z, Yany L, Wu J, Fan S, Mathews HL. CGRP in the serum of endotoxin-treated rats suppresses lymphoproliferation. Brain Behav Immun 8:282–292, 1994.

558. Watson SP, Downes DP. Substance P induced hydrolysis of inositol phospholipids in guinea-pig ileum and rat hypothalamus. Eur J Pharmacol 93:245–253, 1983.

559. Webber RH, DeFelice R, Ferguson RJ, Powell JP. Bone marrow response to stimulation of the sympathetic trunks in rats. Acta Anat 77:92–97, 1970.

560. Weber RJ, Pert A. The periaqueductal gray matter mediates opiate-induced immunosuppression. Science Wash DC 245:188–190, 1989.

561. Weihe E, Müller S, Fink T, Zentel HJ. Tachykinins, calcitonin gene-related peptide and neuropeptide Y in nerves of the mammalian thymus: interactions with mast cells in autonomic and sensory neuroimmunomodulation. Neurosci Lett 100:77–82, 1989.

562. Weinstock JV. Neuropeptides and the regulation of granulomatous inflammation. Clin Immunol Immunopathol 64:17–22, 1992.

563. Weinstock JV, Blum AM, Khetarpal S. Granulomas in murine *Schistosomiasis mansoni* contain vasoactive intestinal peptide-responsive lymphocytes. Cell Immunol 134:458–472, 1991.

564. Weinstock JV, Blum A, Walder J, Walder R. Eosinophils from granulomas in murine *Schistosomiasis mansoni* produce substance P. Immunology 71:52–56, 1988.

565. Weisz-Carrington P, Nagomoto N, Farraj M, Buschmann R, Rypins EB, Stanisz A. Analysis of SP/VIP fiber association with T_4 and T_8 lymphocytes in normal human colon. In: Advances in Mucosal Immunology, J Mestechky, ed. Plenum Press, New York, 1995, pp 559–561.

566. Wertian E, Ovadia H, Ferran S, Abramsky O. Prevention of allergic experimental encephalomyelitis by anterior hypothalamic lesions in rats. Neurology 35:1468–1470, 1985.

567. Westly HJ, Kelley KW. Down regulation of glucocorticoid and β-adrenergic receptors on lectin-stimulated splenocytes. Proc Soc Exp Biol Med 185:211–218, 1987.
568. Wiedermann CJ, Reinisch, Braunsteiner H. Stimulation of monocyte chemotaxis by human growth hormone and its deactivation by somatostatin. Blood 82:954–960, 1993.
569. Wiedermann CJ, Reinisch, Niedermuhlbichler M, Braunsteiner H. Inhibition of recombinant human growth hormone-induced and prolactin-induced activation of neutrophils by octreotide. Naunyn-Schmiedeberg's Arch Pharmacol 347:347–341, 1993a.
570. Wiik P, Opstad PK, Boyum A. Binding of vasoactive intestinal polypeptide (VIP) by human blood monocytes: demonstration of specific binding sites. Regul Pept 12:145–153, 1985.
571. Williams JM, Felten DL. Sympathetic innervation of murine thymus and spleen: a comparative histofluorescence study. Anat Rec 199:531–542, 1981.
572. Williams JM, Peterson RG, Shea PA, Schmedtje JF, Bauer DC, Felton DL. Sympathetic innervation of murine thymus and spleen: evidence for a functional link between the nervous and immune systems. Brain Res Bull 6:83–94, 1981.
573. Williams LT, Snyderman R, Lefkowitz RJ. Identification of β-adrenergic receptors in human lymphocytes by (−)[³H]-alprenolol binding. J Clin Invest 57:149–155, 1976.
574. Winberg M, Holmgren S, Nilsson S. Effects of denervation of 6-hydroxydopamine on the activity of choline acetyltransferase in the spleen of the cod, *Gadus morhua*. Comp Biochem Physiol 69C:141–143, 1981.
575. Wybran J. Enkephalins as molecules of lymphocyte activation and modifiers of the biological response. In: Enkephalins and Endorphins, NP Plotnikoff, RE Faith, AJ Murgo, RA Good, eds. Plenum Press, New York, 1986, pp 253–282.
576. Wybran J, Appelboom T, Famaey J-P, Govaerts A. Suggestive evidence for receptors for morphine and methionine-enkephalin on normal blood T lymphocytes. J Immunol 123:1068–1070, 1979.
577. Yamashita T, Kumazawa H, Kozuki K, Amano H, Tomoda K, Kumazawa T. Autonomic nervous system in human palatine tonsil. Acta Otolaryngol 416:63–71, 1984.
578. Yiangou Y, Serrano R, Pena J, Festenstein H. Effects of prepro-vasoactive intestinal peptide-derived peptides on the murine immune response. J Neuroimmunol 29:65–72, 1990.
579. Yousefi S, Ghazinouri A, Vaziri N, Tilles J, Carandang G, Cesario T. The effect of somatostatin on the production of human interferons by mononuclear cells. PSEBM 194:114–118, 1990.
580. Yousefi S, Varizi N, Carandang G, Le W, Yamamoto R, Granger G, Ocariz J, Cesario T. The paradoxical effects of somatostatin on the bioactivity and the production of cytotoxins derived from human peripheral blood mononuclear cells. Br J Cancer 64:243–246, 1991.
581. Yukawa T, Ukena D, Kroegel C, Chanez P, Dent G. Beta₂-adrenergic receptors on eosinophils. Am Rev Respir Dis 141:1446–1452, 1990.
582. Zaitsev SV, Khegia LA, Kim BB, Gavrilova EM, Yanovsky OG, Zakharova LA. Involvement of opioid receptors in Met-enkephalin modulation of blast-transformation of mouse splenocytes. Immunol Lett 32:27–30, 1992.
583. Zapata A, Villena A, Cooper EL. Direct contacts between nerve endings and lymphoid cells in the jugular body of *Rana pipiens*. Experientia 38:623–624, 1982.
584. Ziegler MG, Lake CR, Kopin IJ. Plasma noradrenaline increases with age. Nature (Lond) 261:333–335, 1976.
585. Zurier RB, Weissman G, Hoffstein S, Kammerman S, Tai HH. Mechanisms of lysosomal enzyme release from human leukocytes: II. Effects of cAMP and cGMP, autonomic agonists, and agents which affect microtubule function. J Clin Invest 53:297–309, 1974.

IV

CELLULAR AND HUMORAL IMMUNE RESPONSES IN THE NERVOUS SYSTEM

9

Autoantigens of the Nervous System

LOU ANN BARNETT
ROBERT S. FUJINAMI

Many diseases of the nervous system have been thought to be autoimmune in nature because of the extreme immune response measured in patients and the pathological pattern that ensues. This measurable immune response can be in the form of antibody or T cells. Several proteins have emerged as prominent autoantigens in these diseases. In most cases the autoantigens characterized have several elements in common. For example, many are highly abundant proteins, such as the myelin proteins (e.g., myelin basic protein and proteolipid protein). Another common factor of autoantigens of the nervous system is the extreme conservation of many of the proteins among various species, reflecting an evolutionary pressure to maintain a specific functional structure. Lastly, many of the identified autoantigens have physiological importance in the normal nervous system. Clearly, an immune response directed at an essential protein could easily culminate in disease.

In normal immunologic homeostasis, unresponsiveness to self antigens is intact, whereas in autoimmune disease, reactivity to self has been abolished or modulated. Several mechanisms have been postulated to account for the lack of tolerance. Epidemiological and clinical studies have linked viral infection with the development of autoimmune disease. The mechanism of molecular mimicry could explain some of these observations. Molecular mimicry suggests that there are shared sequences between host proteins and viral proteins. These homologous sequences are sufficiently different to elicit an immune response initially directed at the virus, but ultimately directed at self. In this way, tolerance to self is broken.

Early studies by Fujinami and Oldstone (45) involved computer-aided analysis to identify sequences in hepatitis B virus polymerase that were homologous to myelin

333

basic protein (MBP). Antibodies made to peptides of this viral sequence were reactive with MBP. Rabbits immunized with this peptide also had mononuclear cells reactive to viral peptide and MBP. Lastly, pathological examination of the rabbits immunized with this viral peptide showed lesions similar to those seen in experimental allergic encephalomyelitis (EAE; described later). This study was the first to identify autoreactivity that resulted from immunization with a viral peptide, and it supports molecular mimicry as a mechanism for autoimmune disease. Many subsequent studies have used molecular mimicry as a means to correlate microbial proteins and autoantigens, and these have led to a more thorough characterization of both. These studies have been recently reviewed (10).

This chapter will focus on some of the recognized autoantigens of the nervous system. Various proteins have been thoroughly characterized biochemically, whereas a few have only been identified. The following discussion is not meant to be conclusive, as other nervous system antigens are probably also involved.

Peripheral Nervous System

Myelin P2

Myelin P2 is a 14.8 kDa basic protein which is found primarily in the peripheral nervous system (PNS), with lesser amounts found in the spinal cord, brainstem, and cerebrum (179). Myelin in the PNS is produced by Schwann cells, which initially wrap the axon in a loose manner, with compaction of the myelin occurring later. Because of the variability in the relative abundance of P2 between species (less than 1% in rodents, but 5–12% in human, bovine, and rabbit [54] and in the tissue distribution of myelin P2, its part in actively maintaining the myelin lamellae structure is unlikely. P2 is highly expressed during myelination, suggesting a supportive role in that process.

Like MBP (described later), P2 is an extrinsic membrane protein localized with a cytoplasmic orientation (189). The myelin P2 is produced by free polysomes in rabbit spinal cord with the P2 mRNA localized to the perikaryon of the cell (52). Gillespie et al. (52) have postulated that P2 requires a receptor molecule for membrane binding, as P2 does not bind freely to membranes in translation reactions in vitro.

Myelin P2 is the only myelin protein whose three-dimensional structure has been elucidated. The structure of the P2 protein has been resolved using X-ray crystallography and it consists of a flattened barrel shape (72). The protein is at least 70% β-sheet structure, sequentially ordered with extensive hydrophilic pairing between the sheets. The β-sheets constituting the barrel surround a hydrophobic pocket in which a fatty acid molecule may reside. P2 has been determined to bind oleic acid, retinoic acid, and retinol (189), although a natural ligand has not been determined.

The DNA sequence of the myelin P2 gene has been determined for various species, including rabbit (115), mouse (116), and human (62). The deduced amino acid sequence reveals a high degree of intraspecies homology for myelin P2. Narayanan et al. (116) have determined the genomic organization of mouse myelin P2. The mouse gene contains 4 exons and 3 introns, covering approximately 3 kb in size. There are two transcriptional start sites found by primer extension analysis which suggest that two P2 mRNAs may be produced.

By the proposed structure and amino acid analysis of myelin P2, it has been determined that P2 belongs to a family of cytoplasmic binding proteins which include the retinol- and retinoic acid–binding proteins (26,36). These proteins function to solubilize and transport fatty acids. Myelin P2 may have a similar function, although this has not been confirmed.

P2 has been identified as an autoantigen in relationship to its involvement in experimental allergic neuritis (EAN), which is considered to be a relevant animal model of Guillian-Barré syndrome (GBS). As in studies of EAE, this disease of the PNS, EAN, was initially induced by injection of homogenized nerve or purified PNS myelin (195). The disease was considered autoimmune because T cells from diseased animals could transfer EAN to naive recipients (144). In addition, immunosuppressive corticosteroids prevented or reduced EAN (120). Later, studies identified P2 as one of the autoantigens in the PNS that induced EAN (73), the other being PO glycoprotein (discussed later).

Clinical symptoms of EAN are weight loss, ataxia, paralysis, and death in affected animals. Pathogenic findings in diseased animals are inflammatory cell infiltrates of peripheral nerves, accompanied by edema and increased endoneurial fluid pressure. In studies by Rosen et al. (143), myelin injury has been found to occur prior to cellular infiltration. The inflammatory cells are mainly Ia+, with the T-cell phenotype of T helper cells predominating early, and T suppressor/cytotoxic cells found in later stages of EAN. After recovery from EAN, a refractory time for reinduction of disease is observed, which is antigen-specific to P2 (29). Strigard et al. (170) found that antibodies to the CD5 receptor abrogated this refractory stage, resulting in disease relapse and implicating cells bearing this receptor in the recovery from EAN.

The disease-inducing or neuritogic regions for the autoantigen P2 have been identified. This region in the rat corresponds to amino acids 53-78 (188), with the minimum peptide size of 61-70 (122). Low doses of this peptide in adjuvant administered to rats resulted in pure demyelination, whereas higher doses of the peptide resulted in edema and inflammation associated with demyelination. Axonal degeneration was found in close proximity with macrophages (61). A CD4+, Ia+ T-cell line reactive to $P2_{53-78}$ was found to transfer EAN to naive recipient rats, with animals developing disease on days 7–8 post transfer (145).

Interestingly, by using computer-aided searches of amino acid sequences, the neuritogenic region of P2 has been found to share significant homology with the influenza A NS2 protein (71). This influenza region has been found to be mitogenic for lymphocytes from some GBS patients, and may explain the outbreak of GBS associated with swine flu vaccination. In this case, molecular mimicry between a virus and a myelin protein may serve as an explanation for immune-mediated PNS injury.

Myelin-Associated Glycoprotein

Myelin-associated glycoprotein (MAG) is a glycoprotein produced by myelin-forming oligodendrocytes and Schwann cells. Although MAG is located in the CNS and PNS myelin, it is found in higher abundance in the PNS. MAG is located in the periaxonal membranes of the developing myelin, but it is completely absent from the compact myelin (reviewed in 134).

The genes for rat (82), human (167), and mouse (32) MAG have been cloned and sequenced. The rodent gene for MAG covers 16 kb and contains 13 exons (82). There are two isoforms of MAG, early and late, that differ in the carboxy (cytoplasmic) region of the protein (82,181). These isoforms are produced by alternative splicing (of exon 12) of the mRNA encoding them and are found in active myelination (early) and adult myelin (late) (181). Regulation of MAG gene expression is developmentally controlled with predominant expression postnatally (133).

MAG is similar in structure to another myelin glycoprotein, PO glycoprotein (28 kDa), but it is much larger at 100 kDa in size (135). Both are members of the immunoglobulin (Ig) gene superfamily (152). MAG contains a cytoplasmic domain, transmembrane domain, and 5 extracellular immunoglobulin-like domains (Fig. 9-1). These extracellular domains are heavily glycosylated (30% carbohydrate), with sulfation of some of these oligosaccharides occurring (105). These glycosylated/sulfated epitopes share immunological epitopes with natural killer (NK) cells. This homology has been determined by reactivity with antibodies specific for the HNK-1/L2 determinant found on NK cells (80). In addition, the terminal extracellular domain contains a Arg-Gly-Asp (RGD) binding site found on integrin-like receptors. Other posttranslational modifications of MAG include acylation of the transmembrane region and phosphorylation of the cytoplasmic tail of this protein (35,124). The phosphorylation sites of MAG produced in the PNS and CNS are different, and studies are underway to identify the kinases responsible for specific phosphorylation (35).

MAG is implicated in two neurological disorders, multiple sclerosis (MS) and peripheral neuropathy. The role of MAG in the pathogenesis of multiple sclerosis is unclear. In studies of acute plaques in MS by Itoyama et al. (69), MAG was found to be one of the earliest myelin proteins lost at the lesion margin. Several investigators have found a small but significant MAG antibody response in the cerebrospinal fluid (CSF) of multiple sclerosis patients versus controls (114). These studies have been extended to identify B cells producing antibodies against MAG in the CSF of MS patients (8). In addition, Link et al. (96) have identified T cells that produce interferon-γ (IFN-γ) in response to MAG. When compared to blood and bone marrow, a higher proportion of B

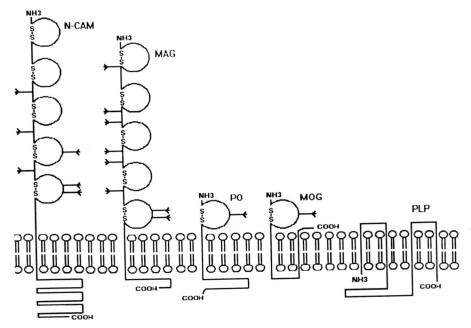

Fig. 9-1. Proposed membrane orientation of myelin proteins MAG, PO, MOG, and PLP (49,82,84,89). N-CAM is shown as a reference. Glycosylation sites are marked (Ψ), as are disulfide bonds.

and T cells specific for MAG were found in the CSF, indicating a sequestering of MAG-reactive cells in the CNS.

MAG has been implicated as an autoantigen in peripheral neuropathy. Studies of patients with peripheral neuropathy demonstrated that 50% had IgM antibodies to MAG (reviewed in 134). In animal studies, endoneurial injection of anti-MAG antibody produced conduction block in feline sciatic nerve which lasted longer and showed more demyelination than that produced by injection of control antibody (180). The B cells which produce the anti-MAG antibody have been found to express the CD5 molecule, a cell-surface marker which is implicated in autoimmune disease (86). Evidence is suggestive that anti-MAG antibodies participate in the pathogenesis of peripheral neuropathy, but more studies are required to determine their disease-inducing potential.

PO Glycoprotein

PO glycoprotein is produced by Schwann cells in the PNS, but none is found in CNS myelin (68). This 28 kDa protein is the most abundant protein in PNS myelin, comprising 50% of the total protein. In contrast to proteolipid protein (PLP), which is the most abundant CNS protein, PO glycoprotein is glycosylated (37). Additional post-translational modifications of this protein include acylation, phosphorylation, and sulfation (105,202). PO glycoprotein has been suggested to assume the role of MBP and PLP in the PNS (108a).

The amino acid sequences for rat, bovine, and mouse PO glycoprotein have been determined by direct protein sequencing or deduced from the nucleic acid sequence of PO cDNAs (89,90,151). The genomic organization of rodent PO includes 6 exons separated by 5 introns and encompasses 7 kb (90). Exon I encodes the amino-terminal signal sequence and 5' untranslated regions. The extracellular domain of PO glycoprotein is encoded by exons II and III. This region of the protein is glycosylated and hydrophobic. The transmembrane region of the protein is coded in exon IV. Cytoplasmic portions of the molecule are encoded in exons V and VI. This intracellular domain is quite basic and may function in a similar manner to MBP in binding acidic lipids.

It was determined by sequence analysis that PO belongs to the immunoglobulin superfamily of molecules (90). The extracellular domain is very similar in amino acid sequence to a variable domain of immunoglobulin (Fig. 9-1). This family of adhesion glycoproteins includes MAG and neural cell adhesion molecules (NCAM). These molecules function in either adhesion or recognition.

Although PO glycoprotein has not been well characterized as a recognition molecule, its role in adhesion is well documented. Filbin et al. (39) transfected Chinese hamster ovary cells with the gene encoding PO glycoprotein. Such transfected cells in suspension culture adhered to each other, resulting in large aggregates of cells. These results support the hypothesis that PO integral membrane protein acts extracellularly by homophilic interactions between opposing myelin membranes in the developing compact myelin (39). In studies by Schneider-Schaulies et al. (155), PO glycoprotein was expressed in CV-1 cells using a recombinant vaccinia virus encoding the gene for PO. In vitro homophilic interactions between the recombinant integral protein in CV-1 cells and a bacterially expressed outer immunoglobulin-like domain of PO were observed. In addition, the recombinant extracellular domain of PO interacted with neurons, resulting in neuronal outgrowth. This study suggests that PO glycoprotein may function not only in the compaction of myelin, but in the initial contact between axon and Schwann cells.

PO glycoprotein has been linked with the diseases of polyneuropathy and monoclonal IgM gammopathy by the presence of antibodies to PO in the sera of patients with these disorders (13). Since antibodies to MAG were also found in monoclonal IgM gammopathy, it is believed that the shared HNK-1 epitope between MAG, PO glycoprotein, and NCAM (80) is recognized by antibodies in these peripheral neuropathy patients. The role of such antibodies in the development of neuropathy is currently under study.

PO glycoprotein is one of the peripheral nervous system antigens responsible for the development of EAN (19,112), which is an animal model for GBS (see Myelin P2). Two T-cell epitopes have been identified in PO. The first epitope is contained in amino acid sequences 56-71 (found in the extracellular domain) and the second in 180-199 (located in the cytoplasmic domain) (94). T-cell lines stimulated with peptides to these regions are capable of transferring EAN. However, draining lymph node cells form rats immunized with purified PO or PNS myelin respond only to peptide 180-199 (94). These results suggest that region 180-199 is immunodominant in the rat immune response to PO.

Molecular mimicry between PO glycoprotein and viral proteins has been suggested as a mechanism for GBS. Homologous amino acid sequences have been identified between PO and several viruses, including Epstein-Barr virus, cytomegalovirus, and varicella zoster virus (2). All of these viruses have been associated clinically with the development of GBS. Viral peptides corresponding to these shared sequences were unable to induce EAN (2). Therefore, the significance of homologies between viruses and GBS has yet to be determined.

Acetylcholine Receptor

The identification and characterization of the acetylcholine receptor (AChR) has been facilitated because of two natural phenomenon. First, the AChR is found in abundance in the electric organs of electric fish, allowing a source for purification. Second, the AChR also binds with high affinity to neurotoxins found in snake venoms, permitting its purification. Numerous excellent reviews are available on the biochemical characterization of the AChR (20,48,171,172).

The AChR is a transmitter-gated cation channel located on the target muscle at the neuromuscular junction. In response to a nerve impulse, acetylcholine is released from the nerve terminal in vesicles that fuse with the plasma membrane of the muscle. After binding with the AChR, the ion channels in the muscle cell membrane open, allowing positive ions to pass through (mostly Na^+ and K^+) and resulting in an altered membrane potential which allows signal transmission.

The AChR been extensively characterized at the molecular level. The receptor is a glycoprotein consisting of 5 subunits, α, β, γ (or ϵ), and δ in the stoichiometry $\alpha 2\beta\gamma\delta$ (5,137). Developmental regulation of the AChR results in an embryonic form ($\alpha 2\beta\gamma\delta$) expressed prior to innervation, and an adult form ($\alpha 2\beta\epsilon\delta$) that is expressed after innervation.

Orientation of the subunits within the plasma membrane has been hypothesized in several models (23,40,60). One model proposes that each subunit consists of an extracellular, membrane, and cytoplasmic domain (40). The four hydrophobic regions (MI–IV) make up the membrane spanning domains (Fig. 9-2). An amphipathic membrane

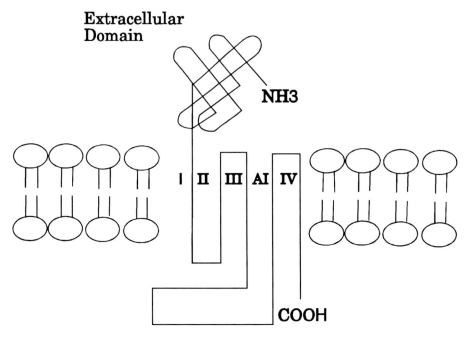

Fig. 9-2. Proposed membrane orientation of alpha subunit of acetylcholine receptor (40). Extracellular domain is indicated, as are membrane domains I, II, III, AI, and IV.

domain designated *AI* is thought to form the interface between the hydrophobic domains and the pore that forms an ion channel. This model is supported by proteolysis experiments which have identified the extracellular N-terminal and cytoplasmic regions (5,197).

Assembly of the subunits into a functional receptor occurs in several phases. Initially, the subunits are glycosylated in the endoplasmic reticulum. At this time, it is proposed that membrane regions MI, MII, and MIII are stably inserted into the membrane, with the cytoplasmic tail and MIV free-floating in the membrane. Subunit assembly presumably occurs during passage through the Golgi to the cell surface. The amphipathic helix A is thought to enter the membrane only after all subunits have combined (40). These subunits are encoded by four different genes.

The AChR has been implicated as an autoantigen in the study of myasthenia gravis (MG). This disease is manifested by muscle weakness and has been attributed to the presence of AChR antibodies in patients (91,139). Antibodies from MG patients can transfer myasthenic symptoms to laboratory animals (168,178). Rather than block function of the receptor, these antibodies result in accelerated degradation of the AChR. The mechanism of this destruction is unknown, although complement-mediated lysis or antibody cross-linking of adjacent receptors has been postulated (101,178). Several noteworthy reviews on the immunological aspects of the AChR are available (101, 142,192).

Central Nervous System

Myelin Basic Protein (MBP)

MBP is an abundant protein found in the myelin sheath of the CNS and PNS myelin, at amounts of 30% and 15%, respectively (reviewed in 88). MBP is associated with the cytoplasmic side of the oligodendrocyte membrane (123). The protein is highly cationic and interacts with the negative phospholipids in the myelin membrane. This membrane interaction may result in compaction of the CNS myelin by adjoining opposing membrane structures (88).

The family of rodent MBPs is comprised of several isoforms with molecular weights of 21.5, 18.5, 17, and 14 kDa (9). Human MBP has similar isoforms of sizes 21.5, 20.2, 18.5, and 17.2 kDa (74). These isoforms are generated by alternative splicing of the MBP mRNA transcript (30). Isoform expression is developmentally regulated, with MBP protein produced at the same time or earlier than PLP, although PLP mRNA is expressed earlier than MBP mRNA (79,212). The different isoforms of MBP are produced within the same oligodendrocyte. MBP mRNA is translated on free ribosomes which apparently enter the oligodendrocyte processes to produce MBP at the site of utilization (25). The isoforms are postulated to have different functions, as their expression is tightly regulated (9).

Rodent MBP is encoded by a single gene which contains 7 exons that encompass a 30-kb region of DNA (30,177). Alternative splicing of the mRNA of exons 2 and 6 generates the different isotypes of MBP. Functional roles or differences between the different isoforms of MBP are currently under investigation.

There are two mutant murine stains that are deficient in MBP expression, both of which express the deficiency in an autosomal recessive fashion. In the *shiverer* mutant, a large portion of the MBP gene is deleted (140,141). This deletion results in hypomyelination of oligodendrocytes and the *shiverer* phenotype, which includes hindquarter tremors, tonic seizures, and premature death. The *myelin-deficient (mld)* mutant also lacks MBP but is produced by a different genetic mechanism. In the *mld* mutant, a large portion of the MBP gene is duplicated and invertly placed upstream from the functional MBP gene (127). Antisense mRNA from this inverted duplicate portion of the MBP gene is thought to either interfere with transcription or repress the MBP gene. These two mutant strains have been partially or fully corrected in transgenic mice containing the wild-type MBP gene (77,128,138).

MBP is an autoantigen because of its well-documented role in EAE, an animal model of multiple sclerosis (158). EAE is induced in laboratory animals by injecting spinal cord homogenates in complete Freund's adjuvant. Clinical signs of EAE include paralysis of hind quarters to forelimbs and incontinence. This disease has been defined as autoimmune because it is transferable into naive animals by class II-restricted, CD4+ T cells isolated from animals with EAE (reviewed in 43,211). Two autoantigens found in the spinal cord that will induce EAE are MBP and PLP

(42,186,206). These antigens have been extensively studied as to their role in this autoimmune disease.

The encephalitogenic, or disease-producing, epitopes of MBP, have been defined in numerous laboratory animals, although for this discussion, we will focus on the murine model (Table 9-1). When peptides corresponding to these regions are used for immunization, animals exhibit clinical signs of EAE. The size of peptide used is important, presumably because of enhanced binding of the peptide to class II molecules. For example, acetylated peptide M1-11 (M1-11ac) has been found to induce disease in H-2^u mice (209). Larger peptides, such as M1-16ac, are less encephaltogenic than shorter forms of the peptide. Therefore, binding of peptide to class II molecule is one important aspect of this autoimmune response.

Another important point that has been observed is the gene usage of the variable (V) region of the T-cell receptor (TcR). A limited heterogeneity of Vβ and Vα usage has been observed in T cells responsive to MBP (Table 9-1) (1,187,208). Although early studies of TcR-β gene usage in the rat model of EAE found a predominant Vβ8.2 usage (18,22), recent studies indicate the TcR usage to be more heterogeneous (173). Encephalitogenic T cells in the H-2^u mouse are predominantly Vβ8.2+ (1,187,208), whereas in the H-2^s mouse, 50% of encephalitogenic T cells are Vβ17a+ (148). This limited heterogeneity has made the TcR the focus for immunomodulation (discussed later).

Proteolipid Protein (PLP)

PLP is an extrinsic membrane protein of high abundance in the CNS and comprises 50% of the total protein in CNS myelin. PLP has also been found in PNS Schwann cells (mRNA and protein), although its function in the PNS is uncertain (reviewed in

Table 9-1 Encephalitogenic Epitopes of MBP and PLP in the Mouse

Haplotype	Disease-Inducing Epitope	H-2 Restriction	Comments	References
H-2^u	MBP1-11ac	IA^u	Dominant epitope in H-2$^{(uxs)}$ F1 mice	209
	MBP34-47	IE^u		210
H-2^s	MBP89-101	IA^s		150
	MBP89-100	IA^s		148
	MBP17-27			44
H-2^u	PLP43-64			200
H-2^s	PLP178-191	IA^s		56
	PLP139-151	IA^s	Codominant epitopes in H-2$^{(sxq)}$ F1 mice	185
H-2^q	PLP 103-116			184

87,110). Hydropathy profiles reveal that the PLP has very strong hydrophobic domains, as do other membrane proteins. The overall charge of this protein, like MBP, is basic, with a isoelectric point of greater than 9. Covalent binding of fatty acids adds to the hydrophobicity of the protein. Purification of PLP requires a chloroform-methanol extraction of CNS tissues because of the extreme hydrophobic nature of the protein. A water-soluble form of PLP is produced upon gradual addition of water to the chloroform-methanol extract (reviewed in 87).

PLP is a 25-kDa protein that exists in multiple forms, including DM-20, which has a 5-kDa deletion from PLP protein (3). The deletion arises via alternative splicing of its mRNA. This observation was confirmed by direct sequencing of a cDNA of DM-20 (118). Other forms of PLP include a higher molecular weight form of PLP which arises from aggregation and low molecular weight forms that may correspond to carboxy- and amino-terminal regions of PLP. Primary sequence data indicate that PLP is highly conserved between species (79,98,118).

The gene encoding PLP has been determined in human and mouse species (32,67,98). Remarkable conservation is observed at the nucleotide level. The PLP gene encompasses nearly 17 kb of DNA, containing 7 exons. Exon 1 is separated from the other 6 exons by approximately 7 kb, and it encodes only the initial methionine and first amino acid of PLP. The other 6 exons encode protein domains which are mostly hydrophobic regions with polar segments contained in exons 4 and 5. Exon 3 contains a proposed extracellular β-sheet structure, much of which is deleted in the DM-20 isoform (118). Several models for the orientation of PLP in membranes have been proposed, based on biochemical analysis and antibody-binding studies (32,66,84,169). One of these models by Laursen et al. (84) is depicted in Fig. 9-1. It has been suggested that PLP may form a membrane ion channel (87).

Early developmental expression of PLP and DM-20 mRNA has been observed in rats at 1 day postnatally (75). Coculture of oligodendrocytes and neurons resulted in increased PLP (and MBP) mRNA production which suggests that a factor or axonal contact is important in PLP expression (100). Although mRNA expression of PLP is early, PLP protein does not appear until later in the developing human CNS (79). DM-20 is expressed earlier than PLP and may be a marker for immature oligodendrocytes (79,191).

As with MBP, there are mice strains which have a mutation in the gene for PLP. The *jimpy* mouse has a lethal sex-linked mutation in PLP (28), resulting in death by 30 days. The PLP gene in the *jimpy* mouse has a point mutation in the splice site of intron 4. This mutation results in aberrant splicing of the mRNA transcript, which results in a shortened PLP mRNA (99,117). Myelin loss is observed, with degeneration of oligodendrocytes and the appearance of immature oligodendrocytes. Another mutant strain, the *rumpshaker,* is myelin deficient but has a normal murine life span and normal oligodendrocytes (59). The *rumpshaker* mutation has been defined by a single amino acid substitution at residue 186 (Ile to Thr), which is found in a transmembrane domain of PLP (154). In addition to these specific PLP mutant strains, the expression of PLP is abnormally low in the *twitcher* (galactosylceramidase defect), *shiverer* (MBP defect), and *myelin-deficient* (*shiverer* allele) mice (109,166), suggesting the important regulatory relationships among the myelin proteins.

As described above, the role of PLP as an autoantigen comes from the study of its role in the induction of EAE. PLP and MBP have been identified as the major autoantigens found in CNS myelin. There are similarities and differences found when comparing MBP- vs. PLP-induced EAE. Active EAE can be induced by PLP (186) or synthetic peptides (56,184,185,200) of PLP that vary with species or H-2 haplotype of the mice (Table 9-1). PLP-induced EAE can be passively transferred with T cells isolated from mice immunized with PLP (190). These T-cell lines must be restimulated in vitro with PLP in order to efficiently transfer disease. The PLP-cell lines responsible for transfer of EAE are similar to their MBP counterparts with a L3T4 (CD4+) phenotype and class II restriction (190). Active and passive PLP-induced EAE results in a relapsing form of EAE (186).

However, in vitro proliferation studies have found PLP to be the predominant encephalitogen in spinal cord homogenate-induced disease, since T cells from SJL mice immunized with spinal cord proliferated selectively to $PLP_{139-151}$ versus whole MBP or the encephalitogenic peptide MBP_{87-99} (199). Encephalitogenic T-cell lines isolated from mice immunized with spinal cord homogenate were specific for PLP and were able to transfer the relapsing form of EAE (199).

The TCR usage in MBP-induced EAE is restricted, whereas in PLP-induced EAE no such restriction has been observed. T-cell clones derived from H-2s mice immunized with PLP peptide 139-151 were determined to have varying TcR-β genes (81). In studies by Sobel and Kuchroo (165), CNS-cell infiltrates were evaluated in active and passive EAE for the types of cells present. The T cells in these lesions were heterogeneous in TcR-β usage, with expression of Vβ2, 3, 4, 6, 7, and 14. When T-cell clones of one Vβ type were used for transfer of disease, the infiltrates were heterogeneous, implying recruitment of other cells in these lesions.

As with other major myelin proteins, PLP has been associated with the pathogenesis of MS. Peripheral and CSF T cells from most MS patients produce IFN-γ in response to PLP (175,182), with higher numbers of positive cells found in the CSF relative to the periphery. B cells producing antibody to PLP were also found in the CSF and blood in these patients, with higher comparative numbers in the CSF (175). In another study, PLP-specific T-cell lines could be obtained from some MS patients (182). The actual role of this measurable anti-PLP immune response in the pathogenesis of MS has yet to be determined.

Myelin Oligodendrocyte Glycoprotein (MOG)

MOG is found exclusively in the CNS on the extracellular surface of myelin and oligodendrocytes (16,93). Quantitatively, MOG is classified as a minor myelin protein

(85,95). The function of MOG is unknown. During myelination, oligodendroglia expression of MOG lags behind MBP (104,157), therefore MOG may be involved in myelin sheath completion and maintenance. Scolding et al. (157) have proposed MOG as a surface marker for oligodendrocyte maturation.

This 25-kDa protein contains 2 structural domains: an amino-terminal cysteine-rich domain, followed by a domain containing tandem leucine-rich repeats. This associates MOG with a group of proteins known as the *CR-LR family* (cysteine-rich, leucine-rich repeats) (108). The spacing of the N-terminal cysteines of MOG are a primary requirement of the V-set subfamily member of the immunoglobulin superfamily (49). V- and C-set subfamilies of the immunoglobulin superfamily are defined in part by the spacing between cysteine residues that compromise a domain. However, MOG is a unique member of this family in that two transmembrane domains are predicted (Fig. 9-1).

The gene encoding human MOG has been determined to be embedded within one of the introns of the neurofibromatosis type 1 gene (193). The gene covers at least 2.7 kb of genomic DNA and contains no introns in its coding region (107). The 5' noncoding region contains one intron.

MOG may play an important role in autoimmunity as a target of antibody-mediated demyelination. Antibodies to MOG have been shown in vitro to either directly induce demyelination of brain cell cultures (in a complement-dependent manner) (64) or to induce macrophages to phagocytize oligodendrocytes (156). Treatment with monoclonal antibody to MOG augmented EAE in rats and mice (93,153). This experiment serves as a good model for evaluating the influence of antibody of a T-cell mediated disease. Other studies by Yamada et al. (203) have determined augmentation of EAE with antibody to galactocerebroside, emphasizing the importance of antibody in CNS autoimmune disease.

MOG may play an important role as an autoantigen in MS. MOG-reactive T cells were found in the periphery and CSF of patients with MS, but rarely in controls (174). B cells producing antibodies to MOG were detected in MS patients as well. Importantly, in these studies there were more MOG-reactive cells in the CSF than in the blood, suggesting sequestering of the cells to the CNS. In addition, MOG-reactive cells were found only rarely in normal controls, unlike MBP-reactive cells, which are found in both MS patients and normal populations (125).

Purkinje Cell Antigens Associated with Paraneoplastic Neurological Syndromes

Paraneoplastic syndromes have been defined as nonmetastatic complications of systemic cancer or "remote effects of cancer" (reviewed in 129). The etiology of paraneoplastic syndromes is unknown, however antibodies reactive with neuronal proteins have been found in the sera and CSF of affected individuals (55,70). These antibodies are also specific for the patient's tumor (47). Based on the presence of these antibodies, paraneoplastic neurological syndromes are thought to be autoimmune, with the tumor eliciting an immune response directed at neuronal tissue. Three major types of antibodies have been characterized, each associated with different tumors and neurological symptoms.

Type I, or *anti-Yo* antibody is found in association with paraneoplastic cerebellar degeneration (PCD), with adenocarcinomas of the ovary, fallopian tube, uterus, and breast (7,55,70). Pathologically, brains of affected individuals have extensive loss of Purkinje cells, with variable loss of other cerebellar neuronal cells (14,15). Anti-Yo antibodies stain the cytoplasm of Purkinje cells (4), and in Western-blot analysis of cerebellar Purkinje cell lysates, they identify antigens of 34 and 62 kDa (27). Three Purkinje cell antigens recognized in this type I staining have been characterized at the molecular level.

A cDNA corresponding to CDR-34 was isolated from a cerebellar expression library (34). Further characterization of CDR-34 indicated that this antigen was uniquely expressed in Purkinje cells of the cerebellum (46). Patients with PCD also contained this antigen in their tumors (34). The structure of CDR-34 contains tandemly repeated, hexapeptide units (Leu-Leu-Glu-Asp-Val-Asp) (34). The gene for CDR-34 is a single-exon gene that covers 1.4 kb of DNA. The CDR-34 gene maps to the X chromosome in humans and mice (21).

The CDR-62 protein has also been characterized at the cDNA level. Fathallah-Shaykh et al. (38) screened an expression library made from a HeLa tumor cell line with anti-Yo antibody. Positive clones expressing protein reactive with anti-Yo did not react with normal sera. Protein sequence deduced from the DNA sequence of CDR-62 revealed a leucine-zipper motif at amino acid residues 171-192, a motif that is present in DNA-binding proteins. In addition, CDR-62 bound strongly to DNA (38), which suggests that CDR-62 functions in regulating gene expression. CDR-62 has been mapped to chromosome 16 and localized to interval 16p12-16p13.1 (58).

Another antigen termed *PCD-AA* (paraneoplastic cerebellar degeneration–associated autoantigen) has been identified (146,147). This 52-kDa antigen, in addition to being present in the cytoplasm of Purkinje cells, was also found in the cytoplasm of brain stem and cerebrum neurons. Sakai et al. (146) identified a cDNA encoding a 52-kDa protein recognized by antibodies of a PCD patient with uterine cancer. This antigen was not unique to the nervous system, for gene expression was also found in the intestine. The PCD-AA shares similarities with CDR-34 in being hydrophilic and acidic. Although there was no significant homology at the nucleic acid or amino acid level between CDR-34 and the 52-kDa antigen, there was significant homology between CDR-62 and PCD-AA at the C terminus of these proteins (38,146).

Type IIa, or *anti-Hu* antibody is found associated with small-cell carcinoma of the lung, along with a spectrum of paraneoplastic neurological syndromes such as cerebellar degeneration, encephalomyelitis, limbic or brain stem encephalotides, and dorsal sensory neuronopathy (14). These patients may have one or more of these syndromes during the course of the disease. Type IIa antibodies are reactive with the nucleus and cytoplasm of all CNS and PNS neurons. Antigens of 35 to 42 kDa are labeled by anti-Hu antibody in Western blots (6).

A protein associated with the type IIa pattern of staining has been characterized at the DNA level. Using the anti-Hu antibody to screen a cerebellar cDNA library, Szabo et al. (176) cloned a neuronal antigen (HuD). HuD mRNA was expressed exclusively in the brain. Significant homology between HuD and the *Drosophila* proteins Elav (51% identity) and Sex-lethal (42% identity) was found by comparing the predicted amino acid primary sequence of HuD (176). These *Drosophila* proteins have RNA-binding domains and function in sex determination and development of the brain, possibly through control of RNA-splicing. Szabo and colleagues suggested that HuD may also function as an RNA-binding protein in the control of RNA-processing in neurons.

Type IIb, or *anti-Ri* antibody is found exclusively in patients with carcinoma of the breast, with syndromes of opsoclonus, and ataxia (17). The staining pattern of type IIb antibody is similar to that of type IIa, with nuclear and cytoplasmic staining of most neurons (17). Antigens detected by type IIb antibody are of approximately 55 and 70 to 80 kDa in Western blots (97). To date, genes corresponding to these antigens have not been characterized.

S Antigen (Arrestin)

Soluble antigen (S antigen) was originally identified because of its role in the development of experimental autoimmune uveoretinitis (EAU). Later it was discovered that S antigen was identical to arrestin, the 48-kDa protein important in the regulation of light transmittance into nerve impulses (126). This complex reaction begins with the photo-excited rhodopsin binding to the α-subunit of transducin as it catalyzes the binding of guanosine 5'-triphosphate (GTP) (214). GTP-bound transducin then separates from rhodopsin and activates cGMP phosphodiesterase. Quenching of this reaction occurs when arrestin, in the presence of ATP, inactivates the phosphodiesterase (201).

Arrestin is one of the most abundant proteins in rod photoreceptors. The genes for mouse, human, and bovine arrestin have been cloned and sequenced (159,183,205). The N terminal–conserved region of arrestin has been found to contain homologous regions to α-transducin, which includes regions thought to bind GTP and rhodopsin (159,183,205). Predictions of arrestin's secondary structure indicate predominantly β-sheet conformation (159).

EAU is induced in laboratory animals by the immunization of S antigen in complete Freund's adjuvant (194). EAU acts as a model for autoimmune disease of the eye involving the retina and pineal gland (76). The disease is class II restricted, CD4$^+$ T-cell mediated (113). Inflammatory cell infiltrates are found in the anterior vitreous chamber. Pathological examination indicates complete destruction of the retinal layer of photoreceptor cells (194). In addition to S antigen, a retinol-binding protein, interphotoreceptor retinoid-binding protein (IRBP), is also capable of inducing EAU (15a).

Several epitopes of S antigen can induce uveitis. To date, six of these have been identified: peptide M (303-314), peptide N (286–297), peptide 3 (221-240), and peptide K sequences 241-260, 333-352, and 352-364 (33,106,160,162). Using anti–S antigen monoclonal antibodies, B-cell immunodominant regions of arrestin were localized to the C-terminal region, which is distal to peptide M found in the N-terminal region (78).

Interestingly, the uveitogenic sites in S antigen were adjacent to sites that are responsible for T-cell proliferation. In studies by Gregerson et al. (57) peptides corresponding to the proliferative epitopes were unable to induce EAU when injected into rats. However, a T-cell line repeatedly stimulated with peptide to this site was able to transfer EAU transiently. Although the reason for the separation of proliferative and disease-inducing sites is unknown, it has been hypothesized that there is an interaction between the two types of cells. A similar segregation of proliferation and disease-inducing epitopes has been found in rat studies of EAE (102).

Shared sequences have been found between viral and bacterial peptides and arrestin. These homologous epitopes may elicit an immune reaction directed to self as proposed in the mechanism of molecular mimicry. Singh et al. (163) identified an amino acid sequence in yeast histone H3 that shares homology with peptide M. This sequence, 106-121, contained five consecutive amino acids identical to those in peptide M. When the yeast histone peptide or native yeast histone was injected into rats, clinical EAU was observed. These studies argue in favor of a molecular mimicry model of uveitis.

In other studies, several viral proteins, including hepatitis B virus DNA polymerase, gag-pol polyprotein of Baboon endogenous virus, and gag-pol polyprotein of AKV murine leukemia virus, were found to contain homologous sequences to S-antigen peptide M (161). Peptides corresponding to these viral sequences induced EAU in rats. When rats and a monkey were immunized with peptide M, a proliferative response to the viral peptides was found. Singh et al. suggested that as little as three shared consecutive amino acids were sufficient to induce an immunological cross-reactivity and they hypothesize that viral infection could lead to an autoimmune reaction (161).

Astrocyte 43-kDa Antigen (HIV)

A common manifestation of infection with HIV is AIDS dementia complex (ADC), a neurological condition with manifestations of cognitive, motor, and behavioral disorders (reviewed in 131). The pathology of ADC includes white matter leukoencephalopathy, with demyelination or reactive astrocytosis with ares of demyelination. The virus infects microglial or macrophage cells located in the brain, but it spares astrocytes and rarely infects neuronal cells (130). These findings suggest that the pathogenesis of ADC is not totally attributable to direct infection by virus but may be linked to immunological dysfunction.

The HIV glycoprotein 41 (gp41) has been shown to contain an immunodominant epitope within the transmembrane domain. Most HIV patients produce antibodies to the region of amino acids 598 through 609 (53). In studies by Yamada et al. (204), monoclonal antibodies were produced to a synthetic peptide corresponding to this region. Upon characterization, these antibodies were found to react with a subpopulation of astrocytes. The astrocyte antigen was determined by immunoblotting to be a 43-kDa antigen. In immunohistochemical studies of mouse and human brain sections, the number of positive-staining cells increased in the pathological states of murine EAE and human cerebral infarction. The positive astrocytes were morphologically similar to reactive astrocytes. The peptide $gp41_{598-690}$ blocked reactivity of spinal fluid antibodies from AIDS patients with reactive astrocytes, further supporting its relevance in this disease. Further studies are currently in progress to characterize this 43-kDa astrocyte antigen.

Conclusions

Identification of autoantigens and characterization of the immune response directed toward them in autoimmune disease is the first step in developing strategies for prevention and treatment. Most of the examples of prevention and treatment to be followed are found in studies of EAE. This has proven to be an excellent model to manipulate, as most of the components involved have been thoroughly characterized. Many of the techniques used for therapeutic approaches focus on one or more of the trimolecular complex of the class II MHC molecule, the TcR, and peptide.

Oral Tolerance

Prevention of autoimmune disease has been accomplished by the oral administration of autoantigens including MBP (12,63), collagen (213), and S antigen (119). In the rat model of EAE, oral feeding of MBP resulted in the prevention of EAE (12,63). In studies by Lider et al. (92), this prevention could be transferred by CD8+ T cells that acted through the release of transforming growth factor β (TGF-β, 111). Diminished disease was observed when oral MBP was given after immunization, suggesting a means for treatment. In separate studies of oral tolerance in the rat model of EAE by Whitacre et al. (198), no immunoregulatory cells were found, and anergy as a mechanism of nonresponsiveness was proposed. Clinical trials determining the effects of oral tolerance on patients with MS have begun (196).

Antigen and Peptide Inhibition

One approach to the prevention or treatment of autoimmune disease is that of antigen or peptide inhibition. This method depends on either competitive inhibition of peptide binding in the TcR–MHC class II complex or on functional inactivation or tolerization of the effector T cell. Qin et al. (132) found that neonatal rats immunized with MBP or peptides were totally resistant to EAE, probably via the mechanism of deletion of the effector T cells. In these studies, antigen immunization was made in incomplete Freund's adjuvant, which was not disease inducing. Tolerance to M1-11ac was induced in studies by Clayton et al. (24) by injection of peptide M1-11ac into neonatal mice. This tolerance was specific for M1-11ac and not for whole MBP, which suggests additional encephalitogenic epitope(s) in MBP. In recent studies by Gaur et al. (50), intraperitoneal injection of encephalitogenic peptides of MBP in incomplete Freund's adjuvant resulted in peptide-specific tolerance of effector T cells with almost complete prevention of EAE in mice. In addition, peptide immunization at the onset of clinical signs of EAE decreased the severity of disease and blocked its progression.

Antagonist inhibition of encephalitogenic peptide binding to class II molecules has been successful in preventing EAE. Synthetic peptide analogs of M1-11ac have been found to be capable of preventing and treating peptide-induced disease (164). Non-self peptides that bound to class II were effective at inhibiting M1-11ac-induced EAE in the H-2^u mouse (149), and PLP 139-151-induced EAE in the H-2^s mouse (83).

TcR Peptide Therapy

TcR analysis of EAE in the mouse (H-2^u) and rat has determined a restricted usage of TcR variable genes when EAE is induced with MBP or MBP peptides (1,187,208). These findings have prompted investigators to focus on this region of the TcR in formulating means of preventing EAE. These treatments include TcR-peptide vaccination (65) or administering antibody specific for these TcR-V regions (207). These methods have worked with some success in the animal models of EAE, however TcR usage in MS populations appears to be more heterogeneous (51).

Recent studies by Oksenberg et al. (121) have determined TcR rearrangements in MS brain plaques. Five common sequence motifs in Vβ5.2 were identified in HLA-matched individuals. One of these motifs was found in a Vβ5.2 T-cell clone from a MS patient that had been characterized as cytotoxic in vitro (103). Rat encephalitogenic T cells isolated from rats with EAE also contained this motif. These common motifs will be the attention of future investigations designed to treat and/or prevent MS.

Cytokine Inhibition

As described above, CD8$^+$ T cells have been determined to transfer the protection observed in orally tolerized rats by secreting the cytokine TGF-β. Antibodies directed at this cytokine are successful in removing this protective effect (111). Other studies by Racke et al. (136) have used TGF-β1 in successful prevention and treatment of relapsing EAE. This cytokine may therefore be an important cytokine for future consideration in the treatment of autoimmune disease. Another cytokine, IL-10, may also be important in the regulation of EAE. The effector cell of EAE has been found to be of the TH1 phenotype, which is known to be suppressed by IL-10. This cytokine is produced by TH2 CD4+ T cells (41). It has yet to be determined if IL-10 has any effects on EAE or other autoimmune disease.

Vaccination

Our studies have focused on the effects viral infection may have on the development of autoimmune disease. Vaccinia virus constructs have been developed that encode the disease-inducing region of MBP. Mice vaccinated with recombinant virus are protected against the induction of EAE in an antigen-specific manner (11). This model has the benefit of evaluating peptides presented by either the class I or class II pathway. Class I presentation of MBP has not been verified in autoimmune disease, although it may occur in the oral tolerance model of prevention of EAE, in which CD8+ T cells transfer protection. Future studies will determine if such recombinant virus are capable of treatment of disease.

Acknowledgments

The authors wish to thank Drs. John Greenlee and Yoshiaka Wada for helpful discussions, and Jewelyn Jenson for manuscript preparation.

References

1. Acha-Orbea H, Mitchell DJ, Timmermann L, Wraith DC, Tausch GS, Waldor MK, Zamvil SS, McDevitt HO, Steinman L. Limited heterogeneity of T cell receptors from lymphocytes mediating autoimmune encephalomyelitis allows specific immune intervention. Cell 54:263–273, 1988.
2. Adelmann M, Linington C. Molecular mimicry and the autoimmune response to the peripheral nerve myelin PO glycoprotein. Neurochem Res 17:887–891, 1992.
3. Agrawal HC, Burton RM, Fishman AM, Mitchell RF, Prensky AL. Partial characterization of new myelin protein component. J Neurochem 19:2083–2089, 1972.
4. Altermatt HJ, Rodriguez M, Scheithauer BW, Lennon VA. Paraneoplastic anti-Purkinje and type I anti-neuronal nuclear autoantibodies bind selectively to central, peripheral, and autonomic nervous system cells. Lab Invest 65:412–420, 1991.
5. Anderson DJ, Blobel G. *In vitro* synthesis, glycosylation and membrane insertion of the four subunits of Torpedo acteylcholine receptor. Proc Natl Acad Sci USA 78:5598–5602, 1981.
6. Anderson NE, Rosenblum MK, Graus F, Wiley RG, Posner JB. Autoantibodies in paraneoplastic syndromes associated with small-cell lung cancer. Neurology 38:1391–1398, 1988.

7. Anderson NE, Rosenblum MK, Posner JB. Paraneoplastic cerebellar degeneration: clinical-immunological correlations. Ann Neurol 24:559–567, 1988.

8. Baig S, Olsson T, Yu-Ping J, Hojeberg B, Cruz M, Link H. Multiple sclerosis: cells secreting antibodies against myelin-associated glycoprotein are present in cerebrospinal fluid. Scand J Immunol 33:73–79, 1991.

9. Barbarese E, Carson JH, Braun PE. Accumulation of the four myelin basic proteins in mouse brain during development. J Neurochem 31:779–782, 1978.

10. Barnett LA, Fujinami RS. Molecular mimicry: a mechanism for autoimmune injury. FASEB J 6:840–844, 1992.

11. Barnett LA, Whitton JL, Wang L-Y, Fujinami RS. Virus encoding an encephalitogenic peptide protects mice from experimental allergic encephalomyelitis. J Neuroimmunol 64:163–173, 1996.

12. Bitar DM, Whitacre CC. Suppression of experimental autoimmune encephalomyelitis by the oral administration of myelin basic protein. Cell Immunol 112:364–370, 1988.

13. Bollensen E, Steck AJ, Schachner M. Reactivity with the peripheral myelin glycoprotein PO in serum from patients with monoclonal IgM gammopathy and polyneuropathy. Neurology 38:1266–1270, 1988.

14. Brain L, Wilkinson M. Subacute cerebellar degeneration associated with neoplasms. Brain 88:465–478, 1965.

15. Brain WR, Daniel PM, Greenfield JG. Subacute cortical cerebellar degeneration and its relation to carcinoma. J Neurol Neurosurg Psychiatry 14:59–75, 1951.

15a. Broekhuyse RM, Winkens HJ, Kuhlmann ED. Induction of experimental autoimmune uveoretinitis and pinealitis by IRBP. Comparison to uveoretinitis by S-antigen and opsin. Curr Eye Res 5:231–240, 1986.

16. Brunner C, Lassmann H, Waehneldt TV, Matthieu JM, Linington C. Differential ultrastructural localization of myelin basic protein, myelin/oligodendroglial glycoprotein, and 2′,3′-cyclic nucleotide 3′-phosphodiesterase in the CNS of adult rats. J Neurochem 52:296–304, 1989.

17. Budde-Steffen C, Anderson NE, Rosenblum MK, Graus F, Ford D, Synek BJL, Wray SH, Posner JB. An antineuronal autoantibody in paraneoplastic opsoclonus. Ann Neurol 23:528–531, 1988.

18. Burns FR, Li XB, Shen N, Offner H, Chou YK, Vandenbark AA, Heber-Katz E. Both rat and mouse T cell receptors specific for the encephalitogenic determinant of myelin basic protein use similar V α and V β chain genes even though the major histocompatibility complex and encephalitogenic determinants being recognized are different. J Exp Med 169:27–39, 1989.

19. Carlo DJ, Karkhanis YD, Bailey PJ, Wisniewski HM, Brostoff SW. Experimental allergic neuritis: evidence for the involvement of the P0 and P2 proteins. Brain Res 88:580–584, 1975.

20. Changeux JP. The acetylcholine receptor: its molecular biology and biotechnological prospects. BioEssays 10:48–54, 1989.

21. Chen YT, Rettig WJ, Yenamandra AK, Kozak CA, Chaganti RS, Posner JB, Old LJ. Cerebellar degeneration-related antigen: a highly conserved neuroectodermal marker mapped to chromosomes X in human and mouse. Proc Natl Acad Sci USA 87:3077–3081, 1990.

22. Chluba J, Steeg C, Becker A, Wekerle H, Epplen JT. T cell receptor β chain usage in myelin basic protein-specific rat T lymphocytes. Eur J Immunol 19:279–284, 1989.

23. Claudio T, Ballivet M, Patrick J, Heinemann S. Nucleotide and deduced amino acid sequences of Torpedo californica acetylcholine receptor alpha subunit. Proc Natl Acad Sci USA 80:1111–1115, 1983.

24. Clayton JP, Gammon GM, Ando DG, Kono DH, Hood L, Sercarz EE. Peptide-specific prevention of experimental allergic encephalomyelitis. Neonatal tolerance induced to the dominant T cell determinant of myelin basic protein. J Exp Med 169:1681–1691, 1989.

25. Coleman DR, Kreibich G, Frey AB, Sabatini DD. Synthesis and incorporation of myelin polypeptides into CNS myelin. J Cell Biol 95:598–608.

26. Crabb JW, Saari JC. N-terminal sequence homology among retinoid-binding proteins from bovine retina. FEBS Lett 130:15–18, 1981.

27. Cunningham J, Graus F, Anderson N, Posner JB. Partial characterization of the Purkinje cell antigens in paraneoplastic cerebellar degeneration. Neurology 36:1163–1168, 1986.

28. Dautigny A, Mattei MG, Morello D, Alliel PM, Pahm-Dinh D, Amar L. Arnaud D, Simon D, Mattei JF, Guenet JL, Jolles P, Avner P. The structural gene coding for myelin-associated proteolipid protein is mutated in *jimpy* mice. Nature 321:867–869, 1986.

29. Day MJ, Tse A, Mason DW. The refractory phase of experimental allergic encephalomyelitis in the Lewis rat is antigen specific in its induction but not in its effect. J Neuroimmunol 34:197–203, 1991.

30. de Ferra F, Engh H, Hudson L, Kamholz J, Puckett C, Molineaux S, Lazzarini RA. Alternative splicing accounts for the four forms of myelin basic protein. Cell 43:721–727, 1985.

31. D'Eustachio P, Colman DR, Salzer JL. Chromosomal location of the mouse gene that encoded the myelin-associated glycoproteins. J Neurochem 50:589–593, 1988.

32. Diehl HJ, Schaich M, Budzinski RM, Stoffel W. Individual exons encode the integral membrane domains of human myelin proteolipid protein. Proc Natl Acad Sci USA 83:9807–9811, 1986.

33. Donoso LA, Merryman CF, Sery TW, Shinohara T, Dietzschold B, Smith A, Kalsow CM. S-antigen: characterization of a pathogenic epitope which mediates experimental autoimmune uveitis and pinealitis in Lewis rats. Curr Eye Res 6:1151–1159, 1987.

34. Dropcho EJ, Chen YT, Posner JB, Old LJ. Cloning of a brain protein identified by autoantibodies from a patient with paraneoplastic cerebellar degeneration. Proc Natl Acad Sci USA 84:4552–4556, 1987.

35. Edwards AM, Braun PE, Bell JC. Phosphorylation of myelin-associated glycoprotein *in vivo* and *in vitro* occurs only in the cytoplasmic domain of the large isoform. J Neurochem 52:317–320, 1989.

36. Eriksson U, Sundelin J, Rask L, Peterson PA. The NH2-terminal amino acid sequence of cellular retinoic-acid binding protein from rat testis. FEBS Lett 135:70–72, 1981.

37. Everly JL, Brady RO, Quarles RH. Evidence that the major protein in rat sciatic nerve myelin is a glycoprotein. J Neurochem 21:329–334, 1973.

38. Fathallah-Shaykh H, Wolf S, Wong E, Posner JB, Furneaux HM. Cloning of a leucine-zipper protein recognized by the sera of patients with antibody-associated paraneoplastic cerebellar degeneration. Proc Natl Acad Sci USA 88:3451–3454, 1991.

39. Filbin MT, Walsh FS, Trapp DB, Pizzey JA, Tennekoon GI. Role of myelin PO protein as a homophilic adhesion molecule. Nature 344:871–872, 1990.

40. Finer-Moore J, Stroud RM. Amphipathic analysis and possible formation of the ion channel in an acetylcholine receptor. Proc Natl Acad Sci USA 81:155–159, 1984.

41. Fiorentino DF, Bond MW, Mosmann TR. Two types of mouse T helper cell. IV. Th2 clones secrete a factor that inhibits cytokine production by Th1 clones. J Exp Med 170:2081–2095, 1989.

42. Fritz RB, Chou CHJ, McFarlin DE. Relapsing murine experimental allergic encephalomyelitis induced by myelin basic protein. J Immunol 130:1024–1026, 1983.

43. Fritz RB, McFarlin DE. Encephalitogenic epitopes of myelin basic protein. Chem Immunol 46:101–125, 1989.
44. Fritz RB, Skeen MJ, Chou CHJ, Zamvil SS. Localization of an encephalitogenic epitope for the SJL mouse in the N-terminal region of myelin basic protein. J Neuroimmunol 26:239–243, 1990.
45. Fujinami RS, Oldstone MBA. Amino acid homology between the encephalitogenic site of myelin basic protein and virus: mechanism for autoimmunity. Science 230:1043–1045, 1985.
46. Furneaux HM, Dropcho EJ, Barbut D, Chen YT, Rosenblum MK, Old LJ, Posner JB. Characterization of a cDNA encoding a 34-kDa Purkinje neuron protein recognized by sera from patients with paraneoplastic cerebellar degeneration. Proc Natl Acad Sci USA 86:2873–2877, 1989.
47. Furneaux HM, Rosenblum MK, Dalmau J, Wong E, Woodruff P, Graus F, Posner JB. Selective expression of Purkinje-cell antigens in tumor tissue from patients with paraneoplastic cerebellar degeneration. N Engl J Med 322:1844–1851, 1990.
48. Galzi JL, Revah F, Bessis A, Changeux JP. Functional architecture of the nicotinic acetylcholine receptor: from electric organ to brain. Annu Rev Pharmacol 31:37–72, 1991.
49. Gardinier MV, Amiguet P, Linington C, Matthieu JM. Myelin/oligodendrocyte glycoprotein is a unique member of the immunoglobulin superfamily. J Neurosci Res 33:177–187, 1992.
50. Gaur A, Wiers B, Liu A, Rothbard J, Fathman CG. Amelioration of autoimmune encephalomyelitis by myelin basic protein synthetic peptide-induced anergy. Science 258:1491–1494, 1992.
51. Giegerich G, Pette M, Meinl E, Epplen JT, Wekerle H, Hinkkanen A. Diversity of T cell receptor α and β chain genes expressed by human T cells specific for similar myelin basic protein peptide/major histocompatibility complexes. Eur J Immunol 22:753–758, 1992.
52. Gillespie CS, Trapp BD, Colman DR, Brophy PJ. Distribution of myelin basic protein and P2 mRNAs in rabbit spinal cord oligodendrocytes. J Neurochem 54:1556–1561, 1990.
53. Gnann JWJ, Schwimmbeck PL, Nelson JA, Truax B, Oldstone MBA. Diagnosis of AIDS by using a 12-amino acid peptide representing an immunodominant epitope of the human immunodeficiency virus. J Infect Dis 156:261–267, 1987.
54. Greenfield S, Brostoff S, Eylar EH, Morell P. Protein composition of myelin of the peripheral nervous system. J Neurochem 20:1207–1216, 1973.
55. Greenlee JE, Brashear HR. Antibodies to cerebellar Purkinje cells in patients with paraneoplastic cerebellar degeneration and ovarian carcinoma. Ann Neurol 14:609–613, 1983.
56. Greer JM, Kuchroo VK, Sobel RA, Lees MB. Identification and characterization of a second encephalitogenic determinant of myelin proteolipid protein (residues 178-191) for SJL mice. J Immunol 149:783–788, 1992.
57. Gregerson DS, Fling SP, Obritsch WF, Merryman CF, Donoso LA. Identification of T cell recognition sites in S-antigen: dissociation of proliferative and pathogenic sites. Cell Immunol 123:427–440, 1989.
58. Gress T, Baldini A, Rocchi M, Furneaux H, Posner JB, Siniscalco M. In situ mapping of the gene coding for a leucine zipper DNA binding protein (CDR62) to 16p12-16p13.1. Genomics 13:1340–1342, 1992.
59. Griffiths IR, Scott I, McCulloch MC, Barrie JA, McPhilemy K, Cattanach BM. *Rump-shaker* mouse: a new X-linked mutation affecting myelination: evidence for a defect in PLP expression. J Neurocytol 19:273–283, 1990.

60. Guy HR. A structural model of the acetylcholine receptor channel based on partition energy and helix packing calculations. Biophys J 45:249–261.

61. Hahn AF, Feasby TE, Wilkie L, Lovgren D. P2-peptide induced experimental allergic neuritis: a model to study axonal degeneration. Acta Neuropathol (Berl) 82:60–65, 1991.

62. Hayasaka K, Nanao K, Tahara M, Sato W, Takada G, Miura M, Uyemura K. Isolation and sequence determination of cDNA encoding P2 protein of human peripheral myelin. Biochem Biophys Res Commun 181:204–207, 1991.

63. Higgins PJ, Weiner HL. Suppression of experimental autoimmune encephalomyelitis by oral administration of myelin basic protein and its fragments. J Immunol 140:440–445, 1988.

64. Honegger P, Matthieu JM, Lassmann H. Demyelination in brain cell aggregate cultures, induced by a monoclonal antibody against the myelin/oligodendrocyte glycoprotein (MOG). Schweiz Arch Neurol Psychiatr 140:10–13, 1989.

65. Howell MD, Winters ST, Olee T, Powell HC, Carlo DJ, Brostoff SW. Vaccination against experimental allergic encephalomyelitis with T cell receptor peptides. Science 246:668–670, 1989.

66. Hudson LD, Friedrich VL Jr, Behar T, Dubois-Dalcq M, Lazzarini RA. The initial events in myelin synthesis: orientation of proteolipid protein in the plasma membrane of cultured oligodendrocytes. J Cell Biol 109:717–727, 1989.

67. Ikenaka K, Furuichi T, Iwasaki Y, Moriguchi A, Okano H, Mikoshiba K. Myelin proteolipid protein gene structure and its regulation of expression in normal and *jimpy* mutant mice. J Mol Biol 199:587–596, 1988.

68. Ishaque A, Roomi MW, Szymanska I, Kowalski S, Eylar EH. The PO glycoprotein of peripheral nerve myelin. Can J Biochem 58:913–921, 1980.

69. Itoyama Y, Sternberger NH, Webster HF, Quarles RH, Cohen SR, Richardson EP. Immunocytochemical observations on the distribution of myelin-associated glycoprotein and myelin basic protein in multiple sclerosis lesions. Ann Neurol 7:167–177, 1980.

70. Jaeckle KA, Graus F, Houghton A, Cardon-Cardo C, Nielsen SL, Posner JB. Autoimmune response of patients with paraneoplastic cerebellar degeneration to a Purkinje cell cytoplasmic protein antigen. Ann Neurol 18:592–600, 1985.

71. Jahnke U, Fischer EH, Alvord EC, Jr. Sequence homology between certain viral proteins and proteins related to encephalomyelitis and neuritis. Science 229:282–284, 1985.

72. Jones TA, Bergfors T, Sedzik J, Unge T. The three-dimensional structure of P2 myelin protein. EMBO J 7:1597–1604, 1988.

73. Kadlubowski M, Hughes RAC. Identification of the neuritogen for experimental allergic neuritis. Nature 277:140–141, 1979.

74. Kamholz J, Toffenetti J, Lazzarini RA. Organization and expression of the human myelin basic protein gene. J Neurosci Res 21:62–70, 1988.

75. Kanfer J, Parently M, Goujet-Zalc D, Monge M, Bernier L, Campagnoni AT, Dautigny A, Zalc B. Developmental expression of myelin proteolipid, basic protein, and 2′,3′-cyclic nucleotide 3′-phosphodiesterase transcripts in different rat brain region. J Mol Neurosci 1:39–46, 1989.

76. Kaslow CM, Wacker WB. Pineal gland involvement in retina-induced experimental allergic uveitis. Invest Ophthalmol Vis Sci 17:774–783, 1978.

77. Kimura MK, Sato M, Akatsuka A, Nozawa-Kimura S, Takahashi R, Yokoyama M, Normura T, Katsuki M. Restoration of myelin formation by a single type of myelin basic protein in transgenic *shiverer* mice. Proc Natl Acad Sci USA 86:5661–5665, 1989.

78. Knospe V, Gregerson DS, Donoso LA. Identification of the main immunogenic region of

retinal S-antigen: subordinate influence of MHC, IGH, species or strain differences on the specificity of the antibody response. Autoimmunity 4:153–169, 1989.

79. Kronquist KE, Crandall BF, Macklin WB, Campagnoni AT. Expression of myelin proteins in the developing human spinal cord: cloning and sequencing of human proteolipid protein cDNA. J Neurosci Res 18:395–401, 1987.

80. Kruse F, Mailhammer R, Wernecke H, Faissner A, Sommer I, Goridis C, Schachner M. Neural cell adhesion molecules and myelin-associated glycoprotein share a common carbohydrate moiety recognized by monoclonal antibodies L2 and HNK-1. Nature 311:153–155, 1984.

81. Kuchroo VK, Sobel RA, Laning JC, Martin CA, Greenfield E, Dorf ME, Lees MB. Experimental allergic encephalomyelitis mediated by cloned T cells specific for a synthetic peptide of myelin proteolipid protein. Fine specificity and T cell receptor V β usage. J Immunol 148:3776–3782, 1992.

82. Lai C, Brow MA, Nave KA, Noronha AB, Quarles RH, Bloom FE, Milner RJ, Sutcliffe JG. Two forms of 1B236/myelin-associated glycoprotein, a cell adhesion molecule for postnatal neural development, are produced by alternative splicing. Proc Natl Acad Sci USA 84:4337–4341, 1987.

83. Lamont AG, Sette A, Fujinami R, Colon SM, Miles C, Grey HM. Inhibition of experimental autoimmune encephalomyelitis induction in SJL/J mice by using a peptide with high affinity for IAs molecules. J Immunol 145:1687–1693, 1990.

84. Laursen RA, Samiullah M, Lees MB. The structure of bovine brain myelin proteolipid and its organization in myelin. Proc Natl Acad Sci USA 81:2912–2916, 1984.

85. Lebar R, Lubetzki C, Vincent C, Lombrail P, Boutry JM. The M2 autoantigen of central nervous system myelin, a glycoprotein present in oligodendrocyte membrane. Clin Exp Immunol 66:423–434, 1986.

86. Lee KW, Inghirami G, Spatz L, Knowles DM, Latov N. The B-cells that express anti-MAG antibodies in neuropathy and non-malignant IgM monoclonal gammopathy belong to the CD5 subpopulation. J Neuroimmunol 31:83–88, 1991.

87. Lees MB, Bizzozero OA. Structure and acylation of proteolipid protein. In: Myelin: Biology and Chemistry. RE Martenson, ed. CRC Press, Boca Raton, 1992, pp 237–255.

88. Lees MB, Brostoff SW. Proteins of myelin. In: Myelin, P Morell, ed. Plenum Press, New York, 1984, pp 197–224.

89. Lemke G, Axel R. Isolation and sequence of a cDNA encoding the major structural protein of peripheral myelin. Cell 40:501–508, 1985.

90. Lemke G, Lamar E, Patterson J. Isolation and analysis of the gene encoding peripheral myelin protein zero. Neuron 1:73–83, 1988.

91. Lennon VA, Lambert EH, Myasthenia gravis induced by monoclonal antibodies to acetylcholine receptors. Nature 285:238–240, 1980.

92. Lider O, Santos LM, Lee CS, Higgins PJ, Weiner HL. Suppression of experimental autoimmune encephalomyelitis by oral administration of myelin basic protein. II. Suppression of disease and *in vitro* immune responses is mediated by antigen-specific CD8+ T lymphocytes. J Immunol 142:748–752, 1989.

93. Linington C, Bradl M, Lassmann H, Brunner C, Vass K. Augmentation of demyelination in rat acute allergic encephalomyelitis by circulating mouse monoclonal antibodies directed against a myelin/oligodendrocyte glycoprotein. Am J Pathol 130:443–454, 1988.

94. Linington C, Lassmann H, Ozawa K, Kosin S, Mongan L. Cell adhesion molecules of the immunoglobulin supergene family as tissue-specific autoantigens: induction of experimental allergic neuritis (EAN) by PO protein-specific T cell lines. Eur J Immunol 22:1813–1817, 1992.

95. Linington C, Webb M, Woodhams PL. A novel myelin-associated glycoprotein defined by a mouse monoclonal antibody. J Neuroimmunol 6:387–396, 1984.

96. Link H, Sun JB, Wang Z, Xu Z, Love A, Fredrikson S, Olsson T. Virus-reactive and autoreactive T cells are accumulated in cerebrospinal fluid in multiple sclerosis. J Neuroimmunol 38:63–73, 1992.

97. Luque FA, Furneaux HM, Ferziger R, Rosenblum MK, Wray SH, Schold SC Jr, Glantz MJ, Jaeckle KA, Biran H, Lesser M. Anti-Ri: an antibody associated with paraneoplastic opsoclonus and breast cancer. Ann Neurol 29:241–251, 1991.

98. Macklin WB, Campagnoni DW, Deininger PL, Gardinier MV. Structure and expression of the mouse myelin proteolipid protein gene. J Neurosci Res 18:383–394, 1987.

99. Macklin WB, Gardinier MV, King KD, Kampf K. An AG to GG transition at a splice site in the myelin proteolipid protein gene in *jimpy* mice results in the removal of an exon. FEBS Lett 223:417–421, 1987.

100. Macklin WB, Weill CL, Deininger PL. Expression of myelin proteolipid and basic protein mRNAs in cultured cells. J Neurosci Res 16:203–217, 1986.

101. Manfredi AA, Protti MP, Bellone M, Moiola L, Conti-Tronconi BM. Molecular anatomy of an autoantigen: T and B epitopes on the nicotinc acetylcholine receptor in myasthenia gravis. J Lab Clin Med 120:13–21, 1992.

102. Mannie MD, Paterson PY, U'Prichard DC, Flouret G. Encephalitogenic and proliferative responses of Lewis rat lymphocytes distinguished by position 75- and 80-substituted peptides of myelin basic protein. J Immunol 142:2608–2616, 1989.

103. Martin R, Howell MD, Jaraquemada D, Flerlage M, Richert J, Brostoff S, Long EO, McFarlin DE, McFarland HF. A myelin basic protein peptide is recognized by cytotoxic T cells in the context of four HLA-DR types associated with multiple sclerosis. J Exp Med 173:19–24, 1991.

104. Matthieu JM, Amiguet P. Myelin/oligodendrocyte glycoprotein expression during development in normal and *myelin-deficient* mice. Dev Neurosci 12:293–302, 1990.

105. Matthieu JM, Quarles RH, Poduslo J, Brady RO. 35S-sulfate incorporation into myelin glycoproteins. I. Central nervous system. Biochim Biophys Acta 392:159–166, 1975.

106. Merryman CF, Donoso LA, Zhang XM, Heber-Katz E, Gregerson DS. Characterization of a new, potent, immunopathogenic epitope in S-antigen that elicits T cells expressing V β 8 and V α 2-like genes. J Immunol 146:75–80, 1991.

107. Mikol DD, Alexakos MJ, Bayley CA, Lemons RS, Le Beau MM, Stefansson K. Structure and chromosomal localization of the gene for the oligodendrocyte-myelin glycoprotein. J Cell Biol 111:2673–2679, 1990.

108. Mikol DD, Gulcher JR, Stefansson K. The oligodendrocyte-myelin glycoprotein belongs to a distinct family of proteins and contains the HNK-1 carbohydrate. J Cell Biol 110:471–479, 1990.

108a. Mikoshiba K, Aruga J, Ikenada K, Okano H. Shiverer and allelic mutant MLD mice. In: Myelin: Biology and Chemistry, R Martenson, ed. CRC Press, Boca Raton, 1992, pp 723–744.

109. Mikoshiba K, Fujishiro M, Kohsaka S, Okano H, Takamatsu K, Tsukada Y. Disorders in myelination in the twitcher mutant: immunohistochemical and biochemical studies. Neurochem Res 10:1129–1141, 1985.

110. Mikoshiba K, Okano H, Tamura T, Ikenaka K. Structure and function of myelin protein genes. Annu Rev Neurosci 14:201–217, 1991.

111. Miller A, Lider O, Roberts AB, Sporn MB, Weiner HL. Suppressor T cells generated by oral tolerization to myelin basic protein suppress both *in vitro* and *in vivo* immune

responses by the release of transforming growth factor β after antigen-specific triggering. Proc Natl Acad Sci USA 89:421–425, 1992.

112. Milner P, Lovelidge CA, Taylor WA, Hughes RAC. PO myelin protein produces experimental allergic neuritis in Lewis rats. J Neurol Sci 79:275–285, 1987.

113. Mochizuki M, Kuwabara T, McAllister C, Nussenblatt RB, Gery I. Adoptive transfer of experimental autoimmune uveoretinitis in rats. Invest Ophthalmol Vis Sci 26:1–9, 1985.

114. Moller JR, Johnson D, Brady RO, Tourtellotte WW, Quarles RH. Antibodies to myelin-associated glycoprotein (MAG) in the cerebrospinal fluid of multiple sclerosis patients. J Neuroimmunol 22:55–61, 1989.

115. Narayanan V, Barbosa E, Reed R, Tennekoon G. Characterization of a cloned cDNA encoding rabbit myelin P2 protein. J Biol Chem 263:8332–8337, 1988.

116. Narayanan V, Kaestner KH, Tennekoon GI. Structure of the mouse myelin P2 protein gene. J Neurochem 57:75–80, 1991.

117. Nave KA, Bloom FE, Milner RJ. A single nucleotide difference in the gene for myelin proteolipid protein defines the *jimpy* mutation in mouse. J Neurochem 49:1873–1877, 1987.

118. Nave KA, Lai C, Bloom FE, Milner RJ. Splice site selection in the proteolipid protein (PLP) gene transcript and primary structure of the DM-20 protein of central nervous system myelin. Proc Natl Acad Sci USA 84:5665–5669, 1987.

119. Nussenblatt RB, Caspi RR, Mahdi R, Chan CC, Roberge F, Lider O. Weiner HL. Inhibition of S-antigen induced experimental autoimmune uveoretinitis by oral induction of tolerance with S-antigen. J Immunol 144:1689–1695, 1990.

120. Ohno R, Hamaguchi K, Nomura K, Sowa K, Tanaka H, Negishi T, Yamashita T. Immune responses in experimental allergic neuritis treated with corticosteroids. Acta Neurol Scand 77:468–473, 1988.

121. Oksenberg JR, Panzara MA, Begovich AB, Mitchell D, Erlich HA, Murray RS, Shimonkevitz R, Sherritt M, Rothbard J, Bernard CCA, Steinman L. Selection for T-cell receptor Vβ-Dβ-Jβ gene rearrangements with specificity for a myelin basic protein peptide in brain lesions of multiple sclerosis. Nature 362:36–70, 1993.

122. Olee T, Powell HC, Brostoff SW. Minimum length requirement for a T-cell epitope for experimental allergic neuritis. J Neuroimmunol 27:187–190, 1990.

123. Omlin FX, Webster HD, Palkovits CG, Cohen SR. Immunocytochemical localization of basic protein in major dense line regions of central and peripheral myelin. J Cell Biol 95:242–248, 1982.

124. Pedraza L, Owens GC, Green LAD, Salzer JL. The myelin-associated glycoproteins: membrane disposition, evidence of a novel disulfide linkage between immunoglobulin-like domains, and posttranslational palmitylation. J Cell Biol 111:2651–2661, 1990.

125. Pette M, Fujita K, Wilkinson D, Altmann DM, Trowsdale J, Giegerich G, Hinkkanan A, Epplen JT, Kappos L, Wekerle H. Myelin autoreactivity in multiple sclerosis: recognition of myelin basic protein in the context of HLA-DR2 products by T lymphocytes of multiple-sclerosis patients and healthy donors. Proc Natl Acad Sci USA 87:7968–7972, 1990.

126. Pfister C, Chabre M, Plouet J, Tuyen VV, deKozak Y, Faure JP, Kuhn H. Retinal S antigen identified as the 48K protein regulating light-dependent phosphodiesterase in rods. Science 228:891–893, 1985.

127. Popko B, Puckett C, Hood LE. A novel mutation in *myelin-deficient* mice results in unstable myelin basic protein gene transcripts. Neuron 1:221–225, 1988.

128. Popko B, Puckett C, Lai E, Shine HD, Readhead C, Takahashi N, Hunt SW, Sidman RL, Hood L. Myelin deficient mice: expression of myelin basic protein and generation of mice with varying levels of myelin. Cell 48:713–721, 1987.

129. Posner JB, Furneaux HM. Paraneoplastic syndromes. Res Publ Assoc Res Nerv Ment Dis 68:187–219, 1990.
130. Price RW, Brew B, Sidtis J, Rosenblum M, Scheck AC, Cleary P. The brain in AIDS: central nervous system and HIV-1 infection and AIDS dementia complex. Science 239:586–592, 1988.
131. Price RW, Sidtis J, Rosenblum M. The AIDS dementia complex: some current questions. Ann Neurol 23(suppl):S27–S33, 1988.
132. Qin Y, Sun D, Goto M, Meyermann R, Wekerle H. Resistance to experimental autoimmune encephalomyelitis induced by neonatal tolerization to myelin basic protein: clonal elimination vs. regulation of autoaggressive lymphocytes. Eur J Immunol 19:373–380, 1989.
133. Quarles RH. Myelin-associated glycoprotein in development and disease. Dev Neurosci 6:285–303, 1984.
134. Quarles RH. Myelin-associated glycoprotein in demyelinating disorders. Crit Rev Neurobiol 5:1–28, 1989.
135. Quarles RH, Barbarash HR, Figlewiez DA, McIntyre LJ. Purification and partial characterization of the myelin-associated glycoprotein from adult rat brain. Biochim Biophys Acta 757:140–143, 1983.
136. Racke MK, Dhib-Jalbut S, Cannella B, Albert PS, Raine CS, McFarlin DE. Prevention and treatment of chronic relapsing experimental allergic encephalomyelitis by transforming growth factor-β1. J Immunol 146:3012–3017, 1991.
137. Raftery MA, Hunkapiller MW, Strader CD, Hood LE. Acetylcholine receptor: complex of homologous subunits. Science 208:1454–1457, 1980.
138. Readhead C, Popko B, Takahashi N, Shine RA, Saavedra RL, Sidman RL, Hood LE. Expression of a myelin basic protein gene in transgenic *shiverer* mice: correction of the dysmyelination phenotype. Cell 48:703–712, 1987.
139. Richman DP, Gomez MC, Berman PW, Burres SA, Fitch FW, Arnason BGW. Monoclonal anti-acetylcholine receptor antibodies can cause experimental myasthenia. Nature 286:738–739, 1980.
140. Roach A, Boylan K, Horvath S, Prusiner SB, Hood LE. Characterization of cloned cDNA representing rat myelin basic protein: absence of expression in *shiverer* mutant mice. Cell 34:799–806, 1983.
141. Roach A, Takahashi N, Pravtcheva D, Ruddle F, Hood L. Chromosomal mapping of mouse myelin basic protein gene and structure and transcription of the partially deleted gene in *shiverer* mutant mice. Cell 42:149–155, 1985.
142. Rose JW, McFarlin DE. Myasthenia gravis. In: Immunological Diseases, M Samter, ed. Little, Brown and Company, Boston, 1988, pp 1851–1875.
143. Rosen JL, Brown MJ, Rostami A. Evolution of the cellular response in P2-induced experimental allergic neuritis. Pathobiology 60:108–112, 1992.
144. Rostami A, Burns JB, Brown MJ, Rosen J, Zweiman B, Lisak RP, Pleasure DE. Transfer of experimental allergic neuritis with P2-reactive T-cell lines. Cell Immunol 91:354–361, 1985.
145. Rostami A, Gregorian SK. Peptide 53-78 of myelin P2 protein is a T cell epitope for the induction of experimental autoimmune neuritis. Cell Immunol 132:433–441, 1991.
146. Sakai K, Mitchell DJ, Tsukamoto T, Steinman L. Isolation of a complementary DNA clone encoding an autoantigen recognized by an anti-neuronal cell antibody from a patient with paraneoplastic cerebellar degeneration. Ann Neurol 28:692–698, 1990.
147. Sakai K, Negami T, Yoshioka A, Hirose G. The expression of a cerebellar degeneration-associated neural antigen in human tumor line cells. Neurology 42:361–366, 1992.
148. Sakai K, Sinha AA, Mitchell DJ, Zamvil SS, Rothbard JB, McDevitt HO, Steinman L.

Involvement of distinct murine T-cell receptors in the autoimmune encephalitogenic response to nested epitopes of myelin basic protein. Proc Natl Acad Sci USA 85:8608–8612, 1988.

149. Sakai K, Zamvil SS, Mitchell DJ, Hodgkinson S, Rothbard JB, Steinman L. Prevention of experimental encephalomyelitis with peptides that block interaction of T cells with major histocompatibility complex proteins. Proc Natl Acad Sci USA 86:9470–9474, 1989.

150. Sakai K, Zamvil SS, Mitchell DJ, Lim M, Rothbard JB, Steinman L. Characterization of a major encephalitogenic T cell epitope in SJL/J mice with synthetic oligopeptides of myelin basic protein. J Neuroimmunol 19:21–32, 1988.

151. Sakamoto Y, Kitamura K, Yoshimura K, Nishijima T, Uyemura K. Complete amino acid sequence of PO protein in bovine peripheral nerve myelin. J Biol Chem 262:4208–4214, 1987.

152. Salzer JI, Holmes WP, Colman DR. The amino acid sequences of the myelin-associated glycoproteins: homology to the immunoglobulin gene superfamily. J Cell Biol 104:957–965, 1987.

153. Schluesener HJ, Sobel RA, Linington C, Weiner HL. A monoclonal antibody against a myelin oligodendrocyte glycoprotein induces relapses and demyelination in central nervous system autoimmune disease. J Immunol 139:4016–4021, 1987.

154. Schneider A, Montague P, Griffiths I, Fanarraga M, Kennedy P, Brophy P, Nave KA. Uncoupling of hypomyelination and glial cell death by a mutation in the proteolipid protein gene. Nature 358:758–761, 1992.

155. Schneider-Schaulies J, von Brunn A, Schachner M. Recombinant peripheral myelin protein Po confers both adhesion and neurite outgrowth-promoting properties. J Neurosci Res 27:286–297, 1990.

156. Scolding NJ, Compston DA. Oligodendrocyte-macrophage interactions *in vitro* triggered by specific antibodies. Immunology 72:127–132, 1991.

157. Scolding NJ, Frith S, Linington C, Morgan BP, Campbell AK, Compston DA. Myelin-oligodendrocyte glycoprotein (MOG) is a surface marker of oligodendrocyte maturation. J Neuroimmunol 22:169–176, 1989.

158. Shaw CM, Alvord EC Jr. Experimental allergic encephalomyelitis: a useful model for multiple sclerosis. Alan R. Liss, New York, 1984, pp 61–64.

159. Shinohara T, Dietzschold B, Craft CM, Wistow G, Early JJ, Donoso LA, Horwitz J, Tao R. Primary and secondary structure of bovine retinal S antigen (48-kDa protein). Proc Natl Acad Sci USA 84:6975–6979, 1987.

160. Singh VK, Donoso LA, Yamaki K, Shinohara T. Uveitopathogenic sites in bovine S-antigen. Autoimmunity 3:177–187, 1989.

161. Singh VK, Kalra HK, Yamaki K, Abe T, Donoso LA, Shinohara T. Molecular mimicry between a uveitopathogenic site of S-antigen and viral peptides. Induction of experimental autoimmune uveitis in Lewis rats. J Immunol 144:1282–1287, 1990.

162. Singh VK, Nussenblatt RB, Donoso LA, Yamaki K, Chan CC, Shinohara T. Identification of a uveitopathogenic and lymphocyte proliferation site in bovine S-antigen. Cell Immunol 115:413–419, 1988.

163. Singh VK, Yamaki K, Donoso LA, Shinohara T. Molecular mimicry. Yeats histone H3-induced experimental autoimmune uveitis. J Immunol 142:1512–1517, 1989.

164. Smilek DE, Wraith DC, Hodgkinson S, Dwivedy S, Steinman L, McDevitt HO. A single amino acid change in a myelin basic protein peptide confers the capacity to prevent rather than induce experimental autoimmune encephalomyelitis. Proc Natl Acad Sci USA 88:9633–9637, 1991.

165. Sobel RA, Kuchroo VK. The immunopathology of acute experimental allergic encepha-

lomyelitis induced with myelin proteolipid protein. T cell receptors in inflammatory lesions. J Immunol 149:1444–1451, 1992.

166. Sorg BJA, Smith MM, Campagnoni AT. Developmental expression of the myelin proteolipid protein and basic protein mRNAs in normal and dysmyelinating mutant mice. J Neurochem 49:1146–1154, 1987.

167. Spagnol G, Williams M, Srinivasan J, Golier J, Bauer D, Lebo RV, Latov N. Molecular cloning of human myelin-associated glycoprotein. J Neurosci Res 24:137–142, 1989.

168. Stanley EF, Drachman DB. Effect of myasthenic immunoglobulin on acetylcholine receptor of intact mammalian neuromuscular junction. Science 200:1285–1286, 1978.

169. Stoffel W, Hillen G, Giersiefen H. Structure and molecular arrangement of proteolipid protein of central nervous system myelin. Proc Natl Acad Sci USA 81:5012–5016, 1984.

170. Strigard K, Larsson P, Holmdahl R, Klareskog L, Olsson T. *In vivo* monoclonal antibody treatment with Ox19 (anti-rat CD5) causes disease relapse and terminates P2-induced immunospecific tolerance in experimental allergic neuritis. J Neuroimmunol 23:11–18, 1989.

171. Stroud RM, Finer-Moore J. Acetylcholine receptor structure, function, and evolution. Annu Rev Cell Biol 1:317–351, 1985.

172. Stroud RM, McCarthy MP, Shuster M. Nicotinic acetylcholine receptor superfamily of ligand-gated ion channels. Biochemistry 29:11009–11023, 1990.

173. Sun D, Le J, Coleclough C. Diverse T cell receptor β chain usage by rat encephalitogenic T cells reactive to residues 68-88 of myelin basic protein. Eur J Immunol 23:494–498, 1993.

174. Sun J, Link H, Olsson T, Xiao BG, Andersson G, Ekre HP, Linington C, Diener P. T and B cell responses to myelin-oligodendrocyte glycoprotein in multiple sclerosis. J Immunol 146:1490–1495, 1991.

175. Sun JB, Olsson T, Wang WZ, Xiao BG, Kostulas V, Fredrikson S, Ekre HP, Link H. Autoreactive T and B cells responding to myelin proteolipid protein in multiple sclerosis and controls. Eur J Immunol 21:1461–1468, 1991.

176. Szabo A, Dalmau J, Manley G, Rosenfeld M, Wong E, Henson J, Posner JB, Furneaux HM. HuD, a paraneoplastic encephalomyelitis antigen, contains RNA-binding domains and is homologous to Elav and Sex-lethal. Cell 67:325–333, 1991.

177. Takahashi N, Roach A, Teplow DB, Prusmer S, Hood L. Cloning and characterization of the myelin basic protein gene from mouse. One gene can encode both 14 kD and 18.5 kD MBPS by alternate use of exons. Cell 42:139–148, 1985.

178. Toyka KV, Drachman DB, Pestronk A, Kao I. Myasthenia gravis: passive transfer from man to mouse. Science 190:397–399, 1975.

179. Trapp BD, Itoyama Y, MacIntosh TD, Quarles RH. P2 protein in oligodendrocytes and myelin of the rabbit central nervous system. J Neurochem 40:47–54, 1983.

180. Trojaborg W, Galassi G, Hays AP, Lovelace RE, Alkaitis M, Latov N. Electrophysiologic study of experimental demyelination induced by serum of patients with IgM M proteins and neuropathy. Neurology 39:1581–1586, 1989.

181. Tropak MB, Johnson PW, Dunn RJ, Roder JC. Differential splicing of MAG transcripts during CNS and PNS development. Mol Brain Res 4:143–155, 1988.

182. Trotter JL, Hickey WF, van der Veen RC, Sulze L. Peripheral blood mononuclear cells from multiple sclerosis patients recognize myelin proteolipid protein and selected peptides. J Neuroimmunol 33:55–62, 1991.

183. Tsuda M, Syed M, Bugra K, Whelan JP, McGinnis JF, Shinohara T. Structural analysis of mouse S-antigen. Gene 73:11–20, 1988.

184. Tuohy VK, Lu Z, Sobel RA, Laursen RA, Lees MB. A synthetic peptide from myelin

proteolipid protein induces experimental allergic encephalomyelitis. J Immunol 141: 1126–1130, 1988.

185. Tuohy VK, Lu Z, Sobel RA, Laursen RA, Lees MB. Identification of an encephalitogenic determinant of myelin proteolipid protein for SJL mice. J Immunol 142:1523–1527, 1989.

186. Tuohy VK, Sobel RA, Lees MB. Myelin proteolipid protein-induced experimental allergic encephalomyelitis: variations of disease expression in different strains of mice. J Immunol 140:1868–1873, 1988.

187. Urban JL, Kumar V, Kono DH, Gomez C, Horvath SJ, Clayton J, Ando DG, Sercarz EE, Hood L. Restricted use of T cell receptor V genes in murine autoimmune encephalomyelitis raises possibilities for antibody therapy. Cell 54:577–592, 1988.

188. Uyemura K, Suzuki M, Kitamura K, Horie K, Ogawa Y, Matsuyama H, Nozaki S, Muramatsu I. Neuritogenic determinant of bovine P2 protein in peripheral nerve myelin. J Neurochem 395:895–898, 1982.

189. Uyemura K, Yoshimura K, Suzuki M, Kitamura K. Lipid binding activities of the P2 protein in peripheral nerve myelin. Neurochem Res 9:1509–1514, 1984.

190. van der Veen RC, Trotter JL, Hickey WF, Kapp JA. The development and characterization of encephalitogenic cloned T cells specific for myelin proteolipid protein. J Neuroimmunol 26:139–145, 1990.

191. Van Dorsselaer A, Nebhi R, Sorokine O, Schindler P, Luu B. The DM-20 proteolipid is a major protein of the brain. It is synthesized in the fetus earlier than the major myelin proteolipid (PLP). C R Acad Sci III 305:555–560, 1987.

192. Vincent A. Autoimmunity to acetylcholine receptors in myasthenia gravis. Biochem Soc Trans 19:180–183, 1991.

193. Viskochil D, Cawthon R, O'Connell P, Xu GF, Stevens J, Culver M, Carey J, White R. The gene encoding the oligodendrocyte-myelin glycoprotein is embedded within the neurofibromatosis type 1 gene. Mol Cell Biol 11:906–912, 1991.

194. Wacker WB, Donoso LA, Kalsow CM, Yankeelov JA, Jr, Organisciak DT. Experimental allergic uveitis. Isolation, characterization, and localization of a soluble uveitopathogenic antigen from bovine retina. J Immunol 119:1949–1958, 1977.

195. Waksman BH, Adams RD. Allergic neuritis: an experimental disease of rabbits induced by the injection of peripheral nervous tissue and adjuvants. J Exp Med 102:213–235, 1955.

196. Weiner HL, Mackin GA, Matsui M, Orav EJ, Khoury SJ, Dawson DM, Hafler DA. Double-blind pilot trial of oral tolerization with myelin antigens in multiple sclerosis. Science 259:1321–1324, 1993.

197. Wennogle LP, Changeux JP. Transmembrane orientation of proteins present in acetylcholine receptor rich membranes from *Torpedo marmorata* studied by selective proteolysis. Eur J Biochem 106:381–393, 1980.

198. Whitacre CC, Gienapp IE, Orosz CG, Bitar DM. Oral tolerance in experimental autoimmune encephalomyelitis. III. Evidence for clonal anergy. J Immunol 147:2155–2163, 1991.

199. Whitham RH, Bourdette DN, Hashim GA, Herndon RM, Ilg RC, Vandenbark AA, Offner H. Lymphocytes from SJL/J mice immunized with spinal cord respond selectively to a peptide of proteolipid protein and transfer relapsing demyelinating experimental autoimmune encephalomyelitis. J Immunol 146:101–107, 1991.

200. Whitham RH, Jones RE, Hashim GA, Hoy CM, Wand RY, Vandenbark AA, Offner H. Location of a new encephalitogenic epitope (residues 43 to 64) in proteolipid protein that induces relapsing experimental autoimmune encephalomyelitis in PL/J and (SJL x PL)F1 mice. J Immunol 147:3803–3808, 1991.

201. Wilden U, Hall SW, Kuhn H. Phosphodiesterase activation by photoexcited rhodopsin is quenched when rhodopsin is phosphorylated and binds the intrinsic 48-kDa protein of rod outer segments. Proc Natl Acad Sci USA 83:1174–1178, 1986.
202. Wood JG, Dawson RM. A major myelin glycoprotein of sciatic nerve. J Neurochem 21:717–719, 1973.
203. Yamada M, Zurbriggen A, Fujinami RS. Monoclonal antibody to Theiler's murine encephalomyelitis virus defines a determinant on myelin and oligodendrocytes, and augments demyelination in experimental allergic encephalomyelitis. J Exp Med 171:1893–1907, 1990.
204. Yamada M, Zurbriggen A, Oldstone MBA, Fujinami RS. Common immunologic determinant between human immunodeficiency virus type I gp41 and astrocytes. J Virol 65:1370–1376, 1991.
205. Yamaki K, Tsuda M, Shinohara T. The sequence of human retinal S-antigen reveals similarities with alpha-transducin. FEBS Lett 234:39–43, 1988.
206. Yasuda T, Tsumita T, Nagai Y, Mitsuzawa E, Ohtani S. Experimental allergic encephalomyelitis in mice. I. Induction of EAE with mouse spinal cord homogenate and myelin basic protein. Jpn J Exp Med 45:423–427, 1975.
207. Zaller DM, Osman G, Kanagawa O, Hood L. Prevention and treatment of murine experimental allergic encephalomyelitis with T cell receptor V β-specific antibodies. J Exp Med 171:1943–1955, 1990.
208. Zamvil SS, Mitchell DJ, Lee NE, Moore AC, Waldor MK, Sakai K, Rothbard JB, McDevitt HO, Steinman L, Acha-Orbea H. Predominant expression of a T cell receptor V β gene subfamily in autoimmune encephalomyelitis. J Exp Med 167:1586–1596, 1988 [erratum in J Exp Med 168:455, 1988].
209. Zamvil SS, Mitchell DJ, Moore AC, Kitamura K, Steinman L, Rothbard JB. T-cell epitope of the autoantigen myelin basic protein that induces encephalomyelitis. Nature 324:258–260, 1986.
210. Zamvil SS, Mitchell DJ, Powell MB, Sakai K, Rothbard JB, Steinman L. Multiple discrete encephalitogenic epitopes of the autoantigen myelin basic protein include a determinant for I-E class II-restricted T cells. J Exp Med 168:1181–1186, 1988.
211. Zamvil SS, Steinman L. The T lymphocyte in experimental allergic encephalomyelitis. Annu Rev Immunol 8:579–621, 1990.
212. Zeller NK, Hunkeler MJ, Campagnoni AT, Sprague J, Lazzarini RA. Characterization of mouse myelin basic protein messenger RNAs with a myelin basic protein cDNA clone. Proc Natl Acad Sci USA 81:18–22, 1984.
213. Zhang ZJ, Lee CSY, Lider O, Weiner HL. Suppression of adjuvant arthritis in lewis rats b oral administration of type II collagen. J Immunol 145:2489–2493, 1990.
214. Zuckerman R, Cheasty JE. A 48 kDa protein arrests cGMP phosphodiesterase activation in retinal rod disk membranes. FEBS Lett 207:35–41, 1986.

10

Antigen Presentation in the Central Nervous System

JONATHON D. SEDGWICK
WILLIAM F. HICKEY

Inflammatory diseases of the central nervous system (CNS) have always presented a complex puzzle to physicians and scientists who strive to understand them. The CNS is isolated behind the blood-brain barrier (BBB), a structural and functional obstacle to the entry of cells, macromolecules, and even simple substances like ions. In the healthy CNS it is possible to detect only very rare cellular elements of the immune system, thus suggesting that the brain, spinal cord, and, to a lesser extent, the peripheral nervous system (PNS) are immunologically privileged. Nevertheless, a wide spectrum of inflammatory disorders can and do develop therein. For infectious conditions such as meningitis and abscess, or during the cellular response to devitalized tissue, the brain appears to respond in a manner quite similar to all parenchymal organs. However, there are a spectrum of illnesses in which the pathogenesis is unclear. Among these are multiple sclerosis (MS), postinfectious encephalomyelitis, certain viral infections, and experimental allergic encephalomyelitis (EAE, an animal model of MS). These are believed to involve T cells as the major effector arm of the immune system.

One of the central problems when considering such diseases is that T cells, which are normally excluded from the CNS, must find their way to the appropriate site and mount an immunospecific attack against their chosen antigen. While in some viral infections and in EAE the antigens are fairly well defined, in others they are totally unknown. To complicate the issue is the elaborate mechanism by which T cells must recognize their antigen (see Chapter 2). T cells of both the CD4+ and CD8+ groups require that their antigen be processed into small peptides, associated with a macromolecule encoded in the major histocompatibility complex (MHC), and expressed on the surface of a certain type of cell in sufficient density in order to stimulate or activate the T cells' effector

364

functions (242). Such cells, whose function it is to provide the appropriate stimulatory signals to T cells, are referred to as *antigen presenting cells* (APCs). In the EAE and lymphocytic choriomeningitis virus (LCMV) models of CNS inflammation—and thus presumably in human diseases as well—the pathogenic T lymphocytes must be MHC compatible with the host or disease will not develop (30,31,75,77,80,144). Here there has historically been a problem.

In the normal CNS, MHC molecules are virtually undetectable, yet these cell-surface elements are the *sine qua non* of antigen recognition for pathogenic T lymphocytes. While it is easily demonstrated that MHC expression is readily apparent in the inflamed nervous system, this presents one with a type of "chicken and egg" problem: how can T cells recognize their antigen and thus cause inflammation when the MHC molecules needed for antigen recognition become detectible only after inflammation has started? Obviously, there must be "sufficient" MHC expression somewhere in the nervous system, and some resident cell therein has processed and is ready to present MHC-bound peptide. When the problem is viewed in this way, it is easy to understand why many of the studies attempting to unravel the pathogenesis of T-cell mediated CNS disease have sought to define cells which express MHC molecules, and delineate the conditions and factors which make them do so. Thus, the debate begins. For more than a decade various factions have championed the role of their favorite cell as the APC of the CNS. The purpose of this review is to weigh the evidence supporting or refuting the claim of specific CNS cell types to that role.

General Concepts of Antigen Presentation

The usual concept of an antigen presentation is that embodied in the image of a "professional," MHC class II–positive cell, such as a dendritic cell or a B lymphocyte (158), interacting with and "presenting" appropriately processed, MHC-bound peptide to a CD4+ T lymphocyte. The latter cell then proliferates, secretes cytokines, and thereby gains its effector functions. Yet, this is a relatively narrow interpretation.

It was clear from early studies that antigen requires some form of intracellular proteolytic processing in order to be recognized by MHC class II–restricted (CD4+) T cells (242; see also Chapter 2). This concept was also extended to MHC class I–restricted CD8+ T-cell responses when, in a series of studies in the mid to late 1980s, it was demonstrated that cytotoxic T lymphocytes (CTL) specific for *intracellular* proteins (viral nucleocapsid protein, for example) could nevertheless kill an infected (or transfected) target cell. Like CD4+ T cells, CD8+ T cells also recognize short peptides, but for CD8+ cells the antigenic peptides derived from the intracellular proteins were presented by MHC class I molecules on the cell surface (233). Therefore, all cells expressing MHC class I or II molecules can qualify as antigen-presenting cells. Importantly, since *most* cells are MHC class I positive, T lymphocytes specific for a viral antigen can recognize and kill MHC class II–negative, virus-infected cells, thereby eliminating viral infections from virtually any tissue. In the CNS this is vitally important since a number of cells unable to express MHC class II (neurons and oligo-dendrocytes, for example) can express MHC class I under some circumstances.

Undoubtedly, the minimum requirement necessary for effective antigen presentation is the existence of cell surface molecules that can bind antigenic peptides in such a way that T cells can recognize them. In almost every case, this role is filled by MHC molecules. Yet, recent evidence suggests that a minor population of T cells (T-cell receptor (TcR)+ CD4− CD8−) specific for some microbial antigens may recognize their antigen in the context of non-MHC, CD1 antigens (178). Notwithstanding such rare exceptions, overwhelming evidence supports the essential role of MHC class I or II molecules in presentation of antigen to the vast majority of T lymphocytes.

With regard to the full activation of an effector cell, the act of MHC-restricted antigen presentation by an APC to a T cell is an incomplete process. This interaction is often a low-affinity one, and for T-cell activation or killing of target cells by activated CD8+ CTL to occur, the TcR-peptide-MHC interaction must be stabilized by antigen–nonspecific molecular interactions between the T-cell and the APC membranes. The first such molecules to be considered are the CD4 and CD8 coreceptors on the T cell, which bind to the APC's MHC class II and class I molecules, respectively (44). It has been estimated that in the case of MHC class II–restricted T cells, the CD4 molecule may potentiate antigen recognition by 100 times (88). Even these two MHC-associated binding events (i.e., TcR-peptide-MHC binding plus CD4/CD8–MHC interaction) are in themselves not sufficient to activate T cells. Additional interactions between cell-surface adhesion or costimulatory molecules are needed to augment the strength of binding or provide other second signals, thus allowing T-cell effector functions to proceed (reviewed in 115,214).

Many studies have concentrated on the roles of adhesion molecules in terms of their costimulatory abilities for CD4+ cells—that is, the capacity of molecular interactions between the T-cell and APC surfaces to increase levels of T-cell proliferation and/or cytokine secretion. There is no doubt that some similar processes are involved in the binding of CD8+ CTL to their target, as illustrated by the inhibition of cell lysis by a variety of adhesion molecule–specific antibodies (215).

Transfection studies have shown the importance in T-cell activation of interactions between APC-expressed intercellular adhesion molecule (ICAM)-1 (4) and leukocyte function–associated molecule (LFA)-3 (159) and the T-cell molecules, LFA-1 and CD2, respectively. ICAM-1 also binds to T cell CD43 (174). Another molecule, ICAM-2, which is constitutively expressed on endothelial cells, also binds LFA-1 and has been shown to participate in T-cell activation (115). A molecule on T cells termed *CD28* (132), or its homologue, *CTLA-4* (115), binds to a family of molecules that include B7-1, B7-2(B70), and B7-3 (6,50,51,70) found on activated B cells and other professional APC such as dendritic cells (DC) (227). There is substantial evidence for the role of CD28/CTLA-4-B7 interactions in the activation of both CD4+ and CD8+

T lymphocytes, including the observation that binding of the CD28 molecule on CD4+ T cells can prevent anergy induction (66). More recently, similar, T-cell empowering interactions between CD40 and its ligand gp[39] have been defined (35,48).

Vascular cell adhesion molecule (VCAM)-1 present on cytokine-activated vascular endothelial cells (21) and heat-stable antigen (HSA) (113), which is found on a range of potential APCs, also have demonstrable costimulatory roles in the T-cell activation process as evidenced by the ability of antibodies to these molecules or their receptors to inhibit T-cell activation. The counter receptor on T cells for VCAM-1 is VLA-4, while that for HSA is currently unknown.

It was originally believed that the costimulatory signals necessary for T-cell activation to occur were provided solely by cytokines released by the APC. While this is not totally correct, as noted above, cytokines including interleukin (IL)-1 and IL-6 do participate in the T-cell activation process. They serve to increase the T cell's production of IL-2 or IL-4 or the T cell's responsiveness to such cytokines (111,244), or they may enhance the efficiency of the APC's function (98). In the latter case, IL-1 has been shown to have an enhancing effect on antigen presentation by dendritic cells which, while being the most potent type of APC, do not themselves produce that factor (158). Conversely, cells such as macrophages, which can produce a variety of cytokines (including IL-1 and IL-6), are not necessarily very effective APC, at least in terms of primary T-cell activation (85). Thus, the ability of a given cell to secrete cytokines known to increase T-cell responsiveness by whatever mechanism does not necessarily correlate with its ability to interact with and stimulate T lymphocytes.

It is difficult to generalize about the conditions necessary for successful T-cell activation. For example, unprimed/naive CD4+ T cells are particularly rigorous in their activation requirements. Both in vitro (17,158) and in vivo (190) dendritic cells (and B-cell blasts in vitro) are the APCs that most efficiently stimulate these T cells. Once the CD4+ T cell is primed, a greater range of cell types can act as APCs, at least for proliferation and cytokine secretion (158); this is certainly germane to the consideration of antigen presentation in parenchymal, nonlymphoid target organs like the CNS. CD8+ T cells, on the other hand, appear less discriminating in their activation requirements (18,101), although it has been argued that their CTL effector functions are best elicited by leukocyte dendritic cells (86,122). It may be advantageous for CD8+ T cells to be activated by a broader range of cells than CD4+ T lymphocytes, given their role in killing virus-infected cells which might lack the set of costimulatory molecules necessary for a successful interaction with CD4+ T cells.

A final question particularly relevant to antigen presentation in the CNS concerns the level of MHC molecule expression required to permit antigen recognition. Studies using an MHC class II–restricted T-cell hybridoma specific for a hen egg lysozyme peptide (27) and an MHC class I–restricted influenza viral peptide-specific CTL line (14) indicate that as few as 200 T-cell receptor-MHC-peptide interactions are sufficient to activate the T-cell hybridoma or induce target lysis by the CTL. At high antigen concentration (which could conceivably be attained for some autoantigens within the confines of the CNS), around 10% (and up to 40%) of the APC or target cell-surface MHC class I or II molecules of a particular haplotype can be occupied by peptide. Taken to its logical conclusion, this means that a cell expressing 2,000 or less MHC molecules capable of binding a particular peptide could activate or be killed by specific T lymphocytes. Under most circumstances, even the sensitive technique of flow cytometry requires 3000–4000 molecules on the cell surface before the cell can be detected as being positive, and most immunohistological methods are far less sensitive than this. Given the artificial nature of the studies alluded to above, in particular the use of highly sensitive readouts (T-cell hybridomas, for example, and readily lysed target cells), it is likely that the in vivo system is not always that sensitive. Yet, the fact remains that the expression of relatively few MHC molecules may be sufficient to qualify a given CNS cell to act as an APC.

Thus, the ability of a cell to function as an APC entails more than the mere expression of MHC molecules. The requirements are necessarily complex. The neuroimmunology literature is crowded with reports of CNS cells expressing MHC (usually class II) molecules in situ, with the inevitable conclusion that the cell is likely to be important in T-cell activation. Obviously, the matter is more intricate. Little is known about the in vivo APC potential of most of the cells of the CNS. The following overview attempts to address these issues by critically assessing the literature on the APC function of the cells illustrated in Fig. 10-1.

Vascular Endothelial Cells and Smooth Muscle Cells/Pericytes

These two anatomically related, but quite distinct, cell populations will be considered together. Their identities have been inextricably linked as a result of a small number of recent studies on brain microvessel smooth muscle cells/pericytes (SM/P) by Hart and Fabry (38–40,69).

While very few leukocytes can be detected within the healthy CNS, there is ample evidence that the organ is effectively patrolled by the immune system (reviewed in 200). Moreover, the development of an inflammatory immune response (EAE) to self antigens present within the CNS, following the transfer of antigen-specific CD4+ T cells to normal, healthy animals, clearly indicates T-cell recognition of CNS-associated antigen *in spite of* the sequestration of the antigen behind an intact blood-brain barrier. Recognition of viral antigen in the CNS by transferred virus-specific CD4+ (183) and CD8+ (31) T cells can also be demonstrated.

Examination of Fig. 10-1 suggests that a logical site for antigen recognition in the CNS would be the vascular endothelial cell (EC), given its direct contact with leukocytes in the blood. Moreover, the paucity of T cells in the CNS might suggest that the EC is the only place where sufficient T cell–antigen–MHC interaction could occur.

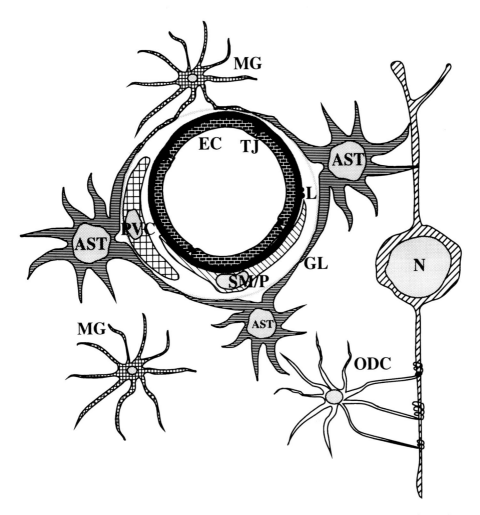

Fig. 10-1. Potential antigen-presenting cells of the CNS. Brain macrophages in localities such as the meninges and choroid plexus are not included (see text). The anatomical locality of the different cell types is approximate but essentially as found in vivo. The glia limitans (GL) is mostly formed by astrocyte (AST) endfeet with some contribution from microglia (MG) processes. Perivascular cells (PVC) abut the GL. Smooth muscle cells/pericytes (SM/P) are associated with the endothelial cell (EC) basal lamina (BL). There are tight junctions (TJ) between individual EC. Axons and dendrites of the neuron (N) are wrapped by layers of myelin formed by oligodendrocytes (ODC).

However, the observation that *activated* T cells of any specificity can cross the intact BBB and enter CNS (75,121,250) shows that antigen recognition at the EC surface is not necessary. This is not to say that it does not occur, and at least for CD8+ MHC class I–restricted anti-viral CTL, there is some in vivo evidence for direct T cell–EC interactions (30,32; see below). There is little doubt that T cell–endothelium interactions are very important in the pathogenesis of T-cell-mediated diseases such as EAE (199) and MS (156). Whether this involves MHC class II–restricted antigen presentation by EC or SM/P, or merely "bystander" damage by T cells following initial interaction with other cells in the vicinity of vessels (astrocytes, perivascular cells, some microglia; see below), is less clear (200).

CNS Vascular Endothelial Cells and Smooth Muscle Cells/Pericytes as APC in vivo

One notes with caution that much of the evidence that CNS endothelial cells express MHC class II molecules come from light microscopic studies. In many cases they do not (and cannot) exclude the possibility that associated cells are actually the MHC+ ones. In locations where endothelial MHC class II expression is patchy, it is possible that perivascular macrophages are responsible for the positivity which appears localized to the endothelium (218; see below). On the other hand, extensive continuous MHC class II expression around vessels may signal involvement of SM/P (69), and ultrastructural analyses have been performed in some cases to confirm EC MHC expression.

MHC class II expression on CNS EC may be species dependent. Early studies investigating MHC class I and II expression on normal rat (67,68,248), mouse (166,229), and human (19,20,71) CNS tissue using polyclonal and monoclonal antibodies (MAb), invariably noted the absence (or at least paucity of) MHC class II expression both in the parenchyma as well as on the ECs. The endothelium was, however, frequently noted to be MHC class I positive. Guinea pig EC are apparently different with respect to MHC expression. Sobel et al. in 1984 (209) and subsequently others (251) demonstrated that a small proportion of vessels in the normal guinea pig CNS express MHC class II, and that the frequency of positive EC increases substantially during the early stages of EAE development when inflammation is minimal. By light and electron microscopy (EM), MHC class II molecule expression was detected both on the luminal face of the EC as well as in the cytoplasm (209,212). It was also reported (211) that in [resistant (strain 2) x susceptible (strain 13)]F$_1$ guinea pigs, MHC class II expression of the susceptible haplotype was enhanced on vasculature during EAE development while the resistant haplotype was not. This was not related to an intrinsic inability of strain 2 guinea pig EC to express MHC class II in vivo, so the relationship of this effect to disease susceptibility is uncertain.

In most other species, MHC class II expression on EC is irregular even after CNS inflammation develops. Studies of rats with EAE (142,143,145,246), two of these at the EM level, failed to detect any MHC class II+ EC. However, the type of stimulus in vivo may be important since focal endothelial MHC class II expression can be detected in the CNS of rats with graft-versus-host-disease (GvHD), an overwhelming, systemic immunological condition (76). It has also been reported that intravenous administration of interferon (IFN)-γ to rats (216,217) induced MHC class II expression on large-vessel but not capillary EC in the CNS. It is interesting to note that most in vitro studies of EC use this cytokine. Despite the above reports, some detailed studies in rats with analysis done at both light and electron microscope levels (245), have failed to detect MHC class II molecules on vessels of any size.

In mice and humans, MHC class II expression on EC in the CNS has been reported in both normal and inflammatory situations, but in most cases the studies do not confirm the locality of expressing cells by EM. In normal human CNS, more recent work (104,173,197) has confirmed earlier observations that CNS EC are rarely MHC class II positive. In cases when some staining of the vasculature was observed, it tended to be discontinuous (104) (possibly due to associated cells) or related to perivascular elements rather than to EC (173). Examination of postmortem MS brain (236,238), biopsy material from herpes simplex virus (HSV) encephalitis (210) and EAE-diseased mice (194,235), all report some EC MHC class II expression. However, it is difficult to determine whether the staining is actually localized to EC in these cases. Subsequent studies in mice in systems other than EAE have produced conflicting data. Two studies of intraventricular allogeneic neural tissue transplantation (97,169) report vascular MHC class II expression of both host and donor CNS, although the point is raised that associated cells other than the EC may be responsible. Indeed, the intermittent nature of MHC class II expression on the vasculature (e.g., see 169) closely resembles MHC expression by perivascular macrophages. Following Sindbis virus infection in mice, MHC class II+ EC were rarely observed (241). This is in contrast to MHC expression by EC in mice infected with Theiler's virus which was confirmed by electronmicroscopy (189).

In summary, endothelial cell MHC class II expression in vivo is inconsistent, potentially species related, possibly directly related to the presence of certain cytokines in adequate quantity, and not necessarily related to the development of inflammatory responses. This relatively uncertain conclusion is mirrored by the essentially indirect nature of the evidence suggesting MHC class II–restricted interactions between CD4+ T cells and EC or SM/P in vivo.

Studies in irradiation bone marrow chimeric rats and in *SCID* mice have demonstrated that MHC compatibility between EC and SM/P and encephalitogenic T cells is *not* required for EAE development. EAE can be generated following transfer of encephalitogenic T cells in which the only MHC-compatible APC present in the CNS are macrophage-like perivascular cells (PVC) (77,80) and other such bone marrow–derived monocytic cells in the choroid plexus and meninges (79). Similarly, it has been shown more recently that SCID mice reconstituted with rat or allogeneic mouse fetal liver cells and later injected with encephalitogenic T cells that are MHC compatible with the donor hematopoietic cells develop EAE (91). Thus, MHC compatibility between T cells and all irradiation-resistant cells not replaced from the bone marrow but normally resident in the adult CNS—including EC, astrocytes (AST), SM/P, oligodendroglia, neurons, and even most parenchymal microglia (MG)—is not essential for inflammation and disease to develop. Such bone marrow–transfer studies do not prove that potentially important interactions between T cells and irradiation-resistant CNS cells cannot occur. There is some evidence that they do, and that they could be very relevant to disease susceptibility. Studies using irradiation bone marrow chimeras between H-2-identical susceptible and resistant mouse strains (100,119) have provided evidence that some cellular element not of bone marrow origin played a critical role in governing EAE susceptibility. Subsequent experiments (120) in which CNS tissue from one mouse strain was transplanted into the anterior eye chamber of the other and EAE induced in the host animal clearly showed that inflammation of the *donated* CNS tissue depended on the susceptibility of the host. Such evidence could indicate that vascularization of the graft by susceptible or resistant EC is a critical parameter. Unquestionably, other host cells would also enter the allografts, but it appears from earlier work that susceptibility is not related to bone marrow–derived elements (120). In a recent study (165), irradiation bone marrow chimeric mice and encephalitogenic T-cell lines were constructed in which the injected T cells were MHC compatible *only* with irradiation-resistant elements in the animal and not with bone marrow–derived, irradiation-sensitive cells. These mice did develop EAE, although the severity was less and onset significantly delayed compared with those mice in which the injected encephalitogenic T cells were MHC compatible with irradiation-sensitive, bone marrow–derived cells. Thus, cells other than those from the marrow can present autoantigen to T cells within the CNS, but they appear to do so in a relatively inefficient way, and the role of EC and SM/P specifically is still not known.

While evidence is lacking for direct CD4+ T cell–MHC class II+ EC and SM/P interactions in vivo, this is not the case for cytolytic CD8+ T cell-MHC class I+ EC interactions. Intracerebral infection of mice with LCMV causes fatal disease (264). In normal mice, the disease is initiated by virus-specific CD8+ CTLs. A series of experiments in virus-infected, irradiation bone marrow chimeric mice have demonstrated that disease only develops when virus-specific effector cells are transferred into recipients in which there is MHC compatibility between radiation-resistant cells of the host and the donor T cells (30–32). Where MHC compatibility resides only between donor effector T cells and bone marrow–derived cells in the recipient, disease is less virulent. This result is completely opposite to that found with EAE-inducing CD4+ T cells.

It has been recognized for many years that CNS vascular EC, like EC in all tissues, constitutively express MHC class I molecules and it is highly likely (although actually unproven) that the principle APC in this disease model is infected endothelial cells presenting viral peptides to the CD8+ CTL. The concurrent BBB dysfunction appearing early in the disease (5,31), while consistent with targeting of the vasculature by effector CTLs, is not in fact proof of direct interactions since loss of BBB integrity is also an early feature of EAE development in which (MHC-restricted) EC–CD4+ T-cell interactions do not necessarily have to occur.

Undoubtedly, the most important function of CNS endothelium is to regulate traffic of leukocytes into the CNS. Like vascular EC in other tissues, the ECs in the CNS express a range of cell adhesion molecules which subserve this role. The importance of nonspecific adhesion interactions in the development of CNS inflammation was elegantly demonstrated in a study showing that MBP-specific CD4+ T-cell clones, which were *unable* to cause EAE after transfer to naive host mice, expressed low constitutive levels of the β1 integrin, α4β1(VLA-4). Encephalitogenic clones, on the other hand, were strongly VLA+ (8). EAE can also be prevented in rats by administration of MAb specific for α4 integrin (261). These important and dominant effects are independent of MHC expression by the EC, although presumably, localized T cell–dependent, cytokine-mediated up-regulation of MHC expression on EC in situ is unlikely to occur until successful interactions between the EC and effector T cell not involving antigen recognition have already taken place.

CNS Vascular Endothelial Cells and Smooth Muscle Cells/Pericytes as APC in vitro

Studies in the late 1970s and early '80s established that in vitro–cultured EC derived from the umbilical vein were not only capable of expressing MHC class II in response to treatment by the T-cell cytokine IFN-γ but could also act as APC for proliferative T-cell responses (84,176). The early reports of MHC class II expression on CNS EC in diseases like MS (see above) stimulated an interest in the potential of CNS EC to process and present antigen to T lymphocytes in vitro in a manner similar to umbilical vein EC. The ensuing results from an ever-increasing number of such studies are sometimes difficult to interpret, given the potential of small numbers of nonendothelial contaminating cells (SM/P, for example) to alter the outcome of the experiments. However, a consensus view is beginning to emerge.

Investigations of MHC-expressing ability and APC function of brain endothelial and SM/P in vitro have employed adult rather than fetal or neonatal tissue. This is undoubtedly beneficial with respect to the extrapolation of in vitro–derived data to the in vivo situation. In all species thus examined (mouse [152], rat [130], guinea pig [251], bovine [15], human [155]), brain vascular EC in culture constitutively express MHC class I and, with the exception of guinea pig EC, are essentially MHC class II negative. That is, in vitro MHC expression mimics that seen in vivo. Constitutive MHC class II expression on guinea pig EC in vitro is in itself atypical however, since expression is predominantly cytoplasmic (251); this mode of MHC expression could be immunologically irrelevant, at least in terms of CD4+ T cell interactions. Unlike mouse EC, a proportion (up to 30%) of mouse SM/P spontaneously express MHC class II molecules in vitro (39,69).

Enhanced MHC expression in vitro can be achieved in a variety of ways; predictably, IFN-γ is the most potent modulator, at least for MHC class II expression. The studies in the five species listed record the induction or enhancement of MHC expression following treatment of the EC or SM/P cultures with recombinant IFN-γ or culture supernatants containing this cytokine. Male and colleagues (129) have formally examined the response of brain EC vs. aortic EC to IFN-γ and have found similar constitutive and inducible levels of MHC class I to this stimulus. MHC class II could be induced on both cell types, although levels of expression were two- to three-fold higher on brain EC after cytokine treatment. There exists considerable disparity between rat and mouse CNS endothelia in terms of the effects of monokines on MHC levels. Tumor necrosis factor (TNF) alone up-regulates MHC class I on rat EC and synergizes with IFN-γ in the up-regulation of MHC class II molecules. Interestingly, IL-1 has little effect in this species (127). In mice, both IL-1 and TNF synergistically *inhibit* the MHC class II–inducing effects of IFN-γ (228)! No simple explanations for these differences are apparent.

Stimulated by earlier work of Massa and colleagues (135,140) describing the differences in levels of MHC class II inducible on cultured astrocytes derived from different strains of mice and rats, strain variability in the levels of MHC class II expressed on brain EC in vitro following treatment with IFN-γ has also been described. Significantly, in both rats (128) and mice (89), *more* MHC class II is induced on brain EC derived from strains that are susceptible to EAE than is found on EC from EAE-resistant strains. In mice, this phenomenon occurs even when MHC-identical mice (with differing EAE susceptibility) are used. The possible relevance of these findings to disease susceptibility will be discussed later.

Viral infection is known to alter endothelial MHC class I expression and may influence the ability of CTL to recognize and kill infected cells. Infection of mouse brain EC in vitro by neurotropic murine hepatitis (corona) virus (92) and LCMV (56) resulted in enhanced MHC class I expression in both cases. This affect was thought to be due to a direct viral effect rather than to cytokine production. No (or minimal) MHC class II on EC has been reported to be mediated by a virus.

Can MHC-expressing brain EC and SM/P process and present antigen to T cells in vitro? The answer is most probably yes, but it is unclear to what extent antigen presentation by endothelia can support *proliferative* T-cell responses. The type of responding T cell, the antigen used, and the animal species from which the EC are derived all seem to be important variables.

In 1985 McCarron and colleagues (152) were the first to report the ability of mouse CNS EC to present myelin basic protein (MBP) to MBP-primed T lymphocytes. T cells in these studies were purified from the draining lymph nodes of previously immunized animals. T-cell proliferation was only observed when the EC were pretreated with IFN-γ-containing supernatants to induce MHC class II and T-cell proliferation could be blocked by anti-MHC class II MAb. They went on to demonstrate that EC isolated from mice with EAE (the EC of which already expressed some MHC class II) could directly act as APC without further IFN-γ pretreatment (154). As in many studies, the central question here remains whether significant "other" types of cells were present in the endothelial cell cultures used.

Examination of EC from mice and other species followed in 1989/1990 with very different results emerging. First, in two independent studies (179,186) using rat brain EC and short- or long-term T-cell lines specific for MBP or ovalbumin (OVA), virtually no T-cell proliferation could be obtained whether or not the EC were pretreated with IFN-γ to induce MHC class II expression. Interestingly, both of these studies as well as another contemperaneous one (201) reported antigen-specific, MHC class II–restricted, T-cell mediated cytolytic damage to the EC monolayers. That is, the EC were clearly processing and presenting antigen (OVA and MBP) to T cells, and the latter were then killing the EC—but they were not proliferating! The same studies also showed that preactivated T lymphoblasts could damage EC in an antigen-nonspecific manner. Mouse brain EC have now also been shown to be susceptible to lysis by MBP and purified protein derivative (PPD)–specific T cells in vitro (153).

Again, results from studies in guinea pigs are different. A 1989 report (252) showed that MBP-reactive but *not* OVA- or PPD-reactive T cells would proliferate in the presence of EC and antigen. However, responses were not particularly vigorous even with MBP-reactive T cells where the stimulation indices were highest. The counts were merely two- to threefold above background levels, and a tenfold increase in the number of EC (purportedly the APCs in the system) with T cells and antigens held constant, resulted in only a doubling of the T-cell response. T cells in these studies (252), like those by McCarron in mice, were purified from the draining lymph nodes of immunized animals. It was argued that the lack of response to OVA and PPD could reflect inefficient processing of these antigens by EC, but this is questionable in view of the ability of EC from mice and rats to process and present these antigens (see above). Using a different type of reaction, T cells primed in vivo by an injection of allogeneic macrophages also responded in vitro in a secondary mixed leukocyte-type reaction (MLR) when allogeneic EC were added to the primed T cells. There was no evidence that EC themselves could stimulate unprimed (naive) T cells.

Finally, an important study by Fabry and colleagues in 1990 (39) showed that flow cytometrically purified mouse brain EC did *not* support the proliferation of CD4+ T-cell clones specific for OVA or keyhole limpet hemocyanin. However, SM/P could be, and in all respects were, vastly superior APC for these T-cell responses. Levels of MHC class II inducible by IFN-γ were also considerably higher on SM/P than on EC. SM/P apparently also stimulate the proliferation of normal (unprimed) *syngeneic* CD4+, but not CD8+ T cells in vitro. This is an unusual result suggesting that SM/P are presenting an antigen (via their own surface MHC class II) to which T cells in the same strain are not tolerant. The kinetics of the response suggests a primary rather than secondary stimulation, but there was no evidence that SM/P could stimulate a primary allogeneic T-cell response (40).

Possible explanations for the differences between EC and SM/P as APCs include *(a)* lack of antigen processing by the EC, and *(b)* insufficient levels of MHC class II on the EC. Both possibilities are effectively excluded by a recent report (38) in which the same authors have demonstrated that mouse EC can indeed support the proliferation of OVA- or rabbit Ig–specific CD4+ TH2 cells producing IL-4 but not IL-2. SM/P, in contrast, appear to present antigen to, and support the proliferation and cytokine secretion (IL-2) of, TH1-type T cells.

The data on SM/P provides a number of explanations for the differences observed with EC in different laboratories. First, where T-cell proliferation was observed, possibly minor contamination of the EC preparations by SM/P provided the APC function. This is not the most likely explanation since in the studies using rat EC, one group (186) went to some lengths to remove contaminating pericytes and astrocytes, while the other did not (179). Yet neither group observed T-cell proliferation in response to EC APC. Another possibility relates to the type of T cells used to test the APC properties of EC. In the rat studies and in the original report by Fabry et al. (39), in vitro propagated T-cell lines or clones were used, all of which were of the TH1 type. On the other hand, where T-cell proliferation was observed (152,252), T cells isolated directly from the draining lymph nodes of immunized animals were used, and these preparations presumably contain at least some TH2 T cells. It would be of interest to determine the cytokine secretion pattern of bulk antigen-primed T cells stimulated in the presence of endothelial cells as APCs. The third explanation is that a small number of B cells, macrophages, or dendritic cells that might contaminate some T-cell populations, while insufficient to stimulate the T cells alone, may be empowered to do so in the presence of EC-secreted factors, such as IL-1, which are known to enhance DC function (98). It should also be emphasized that guinea pig ECs do appear different to those in other species as evidenced in the in vivo and constitutive in vitro MHC class II expression and so it may transpire that brain EC in this species also exhibit functional properties different to those from rats and mice.

There are few studies on MHC class I–restricted interactions between EC or SM/P and CD8+ T cells in vitro. The report that LCMV-infected mouse EC are indeed a lysable target of virus-specific CTL in vitro (56) is consistent with the hypothesis that CD8+ CTL-mediated immunopathology in LCMV-infected mice is due to killing of infected ECs.

What the in vitro results tell us about possible interactions between EC-SM/P and T cells in vivo is difficult to decipher, particularly since the evidence for in situ MHC expression (especially MHC class II) on EC or SM/P is limited, except in guinea pigs. Levels of MHC expression detectable by T cells are much lower than that detected by most immunohistochemical staining techniques, so no strict conclusions can be drawn until definitive experiments targeting MHC expression only to EC or SM/P have been performed. The comparisons made by Fabry of EC and SM/P are also relevant here, as the conclusion one must draw is that TH1 cells (all encephalitogenic T cells fall into this category) are unlikely to be further activated by brain EC, although they potentially may be by SM/P. In theory, however, there is nothing preventing T cells of this type from directly damaging EC in an MHC-restricted or nonrestricted fashion. In the end, one must conclude that endothelial cells are probably not functioning as typical APCs, and the role of SM/P as APCs appears promising but is in need of further study.

Astrocytes

While the appearance of MHC class II molecules on a variety of nonlymphoid cells was reported in the late 1970s and early '80s (103,133,257), it was only umbilical cord endothelial cells that had been analyzed for their ability to process and present antigen to induce T-cell proliferation (84). Thus, the study published in 1984 by Fontana, Fierz, and Wekerle (46) was highly significant in demonstrating that astrocytes could stimulate a CD4+ T-cell line specific for MBP to proliferate in vitro. Astrocytes were not only nonlymphoid, they were unique to the CNS itself. This was an exciting and important observation which set in motion a cascade of events that dramatically altered many concepts in neuroimmunology.

Astrocytes as APC in vivo

The 1984 report by Fontana and colleagues (46) served as a catalyst for the investigation of astrocytic MHC molecule expression in situ, particularly in situations where an inflammatory response had been initiated, such as in EAE or MS. While it was apparent from earlier studies on normal brain tissue that astrocytes were not MHC positive—or at least that expression was at a level undetectable by immunohistological techniques (e.g., 68)—it was reasonable to assume that if these cells were involved in antigen presentation in the CNS, then they should express MHC antigen after T-cell infiltration.

A number of early studies in rats with EAE (78,143,145,246) and in human brain biopsies (104) failed to demonstrate significant expression of MHC class I or II molecules on astrocytes. These cells, when isolated from mice inoculated intracranially with the JHM-A59 coronavirus, were MHC class I+ but MHC class II− (224). Nevertheless, a number of studies emerging around the same time reported the presence of MHC class II on astrocytes, particularly in MS brain tissue (234,236,238). In mice with EAE (194,235) and Theiler's virus–induced demyelination (189) and in tumor-infiltrated human CNS (49), MHC class II+ astrocytes were also found. The reasons for the discrepancy in these reports is not clear. A possibility is the lack of definitive double labeling procedures to ensure that it was astrocytes that were MHC+, although this criticism cannot be leveled at the study by Frank et al. (49). Species differences could also be an explanation. Moreover, it was unclear to what extent exogenous factors (e.g., viral infection, other diseases in the host-patient) other than T-cell-mediated CNS inflammation might be influencing MHC expression by astrocytes.

More recently, there is data both for and against the presence of MHC expression on astrocytes—and in these cases dual labeling is used to confirm the cell's lineage. A number of studies failed to detect MHC class II+ astrocytes in MS (72) and Alzheimer's disease brain tissue (87,221). Interestingly, in both these conditions it was the MG that were the predominant MHC-expressing population (73). Ransohoff and Estes

(181), on the other hand, describe quite extensive MHC class I and some MHC class II expression by astrocytes at the edge of MS lesions (as shown some years before by Traugott and Raine, 236). It was a significant observation since it employed fresh tissue obtained by stereotactic biopsy, rather than postmortem material. In progressive multifocal leukoencephalopathy (PML, JC virus infection of oligodendrocytes), astrocytes express MHC class I but are MHC class II negative (1). Later studies in experimental animals have supported the earlier observations of astrocytic MHC class II negativity in EAE in two different susceptible mouse strains (157), after IFN-γ infusion in rats (217,245), and following virus-induced encephalitis in mice and rats (28,241,249).

As noted above, MHC molecules are not the only ones required for effective antigen presentation. The essential role of costimulatory and adhesion molecules in this process would imply that the detection of such surface molecules is important in vivo as well as in vitro. Unfortunately, very few studies have addressed this issue, at least for astrocytes. In experimental animals, where it is possible to obtain absolutely normal CNS tissue, it is the vascular endothelium rather than cells within the parenchyma that express the highest levels of molecules such as ICAM-1 (13,253), although there is some evidence of glial cell ICAM-1 expression in the normal mouse CNS (13). In pathologically normal (peritumoral) tissue from the human CNS, ICAM-1 and some LFA-3+ cells, thought to be astrocytes, have been reported (191). Yet, the incidental induction of these molecule in a brain containing a neoplasm is difficult to allow for. It is probably safe to assume that astrocytes in situ do express some relevant adhesion molecules under normal situations, but their identity and functional relevance is not known. Astrocyte expression of B7 or CD40 has not been reported.

The irradiation bone marrow chimera experiments mentioned above were equally relevant here in showing that T cell–astrocyte interactions are nonessential in the development of some CNS immune responses. But it must be remembered that this result does not mean that such interactions do not or cannot occur. The definitive study to determine whether astrocytes, as the *only* element in the CNS MHC-compatible with pathogenic T cells, could function as APCs and permit disease to develop, has not been performed. In essence, therefore, there is no evidence available that clearly indicates that astrocyte–T cell interactions *do* occur in vivo; nor is there evidence to show that they do not!

Astrocytes as APC in vitro

To assess the astrocyte's antigen-presenting abilities in vitro, cells have been derived from a variety of sources including the newborn CNS of rats and mice, and both fetal and adult human CNS tissue. There is some species-related variation regarding the MHC expression by astrocytes after culture. The almost universal finding in rodent-derived astrocytes from newborn animals is that MHC class I expression rapidly and spontaneously appears during cell culture. MHC class II expression remains undetectable. In the years 1983–1985, a number of studies (33,83,258) demonstrated that while most glial cells isolated from the neonatal CNS and cultured in vitro were MHC class II negative, some of them, including astrocytes, could be induced to express MHC class II by treatment with IFN-γ. For typical flow cytometric profiles, see Sedgwick et al.'s study (202). Human astrocytes are clearly different. In each case, culture of such cells derived from fetal (3,109,151,180) or freshly resected CNS tissue (65,262) shows that, like rodent astrocytes, MHC class I is induced spontaneously. However, in many cases so is MHC class II (at least on a proportion of the cells), and without the addition of IFN-γ. As expected, human astrocytes also respond to IFN-γ by greatly increased surface MHC expression above that occurring spontaneously. When sought, such MHC expression was not evident by immunohistological staining in the tissue from which the astrocytes were derived (65,180). Thus, there is a clear disparity between what is seen in vivo and what develops under tissue culture conditions. The reasons for the differences between human and rodent astrocytes (in terms of MHC class II expression) is unclear.

In 1986 Massa and colleagues (136) demonstrated for the first time that a neurotropic form of murine hepatitis (corona) viral particles could induce MHC class II expression on rat astrocytes when added to these cells in culture. Virus–cell contact appeared necessary, thus the role of a soluble factor was discounted. Subsequent studies showed that this was not a unique feature of this particular virus; measles virus on rat astrocytes (138) and flavivirus on mouse astrocytes (114) mediated similar MHC class II–inducing effects. There is also a single report (81) of human T-cell lymphotropic virus (HTLV)-1 infection inducing MHC class II expression on human astrocytes in vitro.

There are some unusual features of astrocytic MHC class II induction by virus in vitro. First, the mechanism by which this occurs is clearly independent of IFN-γ (139), but little more is known. Second, there is no similar effect on cells of macrophage/microglia lineage (136,139). Even when the astrocytic MHC class II-inducing effect of virus is minimal (as was observed in one study [102]) it is only the astrocytes, and not macrophage/microglial cells, which are in any way induced to express MHC class II by the virus alone. Third, viral infection can readily and reproducibly induce or up-regulate astrocytic MHC class I expression in vitro, but this might be attributed to cytokines (including type-1 IFN [102,163] and other unidentified factors [223,224]) released from these infected glial cells. It should be noted that type-1 IFN is not a specific MHC class I–inducing substance for astrocytes. The point of these various studies is that astrocytes do appear unusual in their propensity to express MHC class II following viral infection. This could be attributed to the differences that exist between astrocytes and other cells within the CNS in terms of MHC class II regulation at the transcriptional level (137). Whatever the explanation, it is possible that the spontaneous appearance of MHC class II on human astrocytes in vitro reflects the presence of viral infection that is revealed in the dysregulated environment of tissue culture.

There are a number of accounts of rat and mouse strain variability in levels of expression of MHC class II on AST after stimulus in vitro. The original studies reporting higher levels of IFN-γ-inducible class II expression on astrocytes derived from EAE and coronavirus-susceptible mouse and rat strains (compared with resistant strains) (135,140) have been confirmed by others. Two studies in the rat (25,202) found that after IFN-γ treatment in vitro, more astrocytes from an EAE-susceptible strain (Lewis) expressed MHC class II, and at higher levels, than did similar cells from EAE-resistant strains (PVG, Brown Norway, and Wistar). This was the case with type-1 astrocytes. Expression of MHC class II on type-2 astrocytes (which are also MHC inducible by IFN-γ [12]) did not vary between strains (25). In another system (11), astrocytes from SJL/J mice susceptible to Theiler's virus–induced demyelinating disease expressed more MHC class II after IFN-γ treatment in vitro than did disease-resistant BALB/c mouse astrocytes. These independent studies have mostly used the same mouse and rat strains. Subsequent studies have not reproduced the correlation between EAE susceptibility and astrocytic MHC class II inducibility. One report using cells from EAE-resistant BALB/c mice (7) found that astrocytes that had been in vitro for an extended period expressed MHC class II after the addition of IFN-γ; in contrast, astrocytes that had just reached confluence in tissue culture did not. The astrocytes used in all other studies cited above were probably of the latter variety. In another report (10), astrocytes from MHC-identical mouse strains which varied relative to their susceptibility to EAE (i.e., SJL and B10.S) were tested for MHC class II induction in response to activated T-cell supernatants (presumably containing IFN-γ). At higher supernatant concentrations no differences were observed, while at low levels the cells from EAE-resistant mice expressed *more* MHC class II. Nevertheless, astrocytes from the susceptible strain were superior stimulators of alloreactive CD4+ T-cell clones in vitro.

In view of the variability in these findings, one is hard pressed to assign a clear in vivo correlate to them. Notwithstanding this, distinct strain differences in inducible levels of MHC class II expression on astrocytes in vitro obviously exist and explanations for the phenomenon at the level of gene regulation are of clear interest.

Finally, expression of costimulatory and adhesion molecules by astrocytes in vitro has received only limited attention, and all studies with human (54), mouse (198), and rat (102) astrocytes report the constitutive expression of ICAM-1 (and ICAM-2 in one study [198]). Levels of expression are augmented in the presence of IFN-γ or type-1 IFN. The expression and regulation of ICAM-1 looks very similar to that seen with MHC class I.

What APC functions do astrocytes display in vitro? As noted above, they were originally shown to present soluble protein antigen (MBP) to specific CD4+ T-cell lines, leading to the proliferation of the responding T lymphocyte (46). In that study they were not pretreated with IFN-γ to induce MHC class II, although it was shown that anti-MHC class II MAb can block MBP–T-cell proliferation induced by these ostensibly class II− cells (41). It is possible either that the T cells produced small amounts of IFN-γ, which induced enough MHC class II expression on the astrocytes to initiate the antigen presenting process, or that the astrocytes in vitro expressed very low levels of MHC class II that were sufficient to lead to T-cell activation but undetectable by normal techniques, including flow cytometry. The final possibility that the astrocyte cultures contained a tiny, but effective, population of nonastrocytic APCs also cannot be excluded.

Many other studies on the APC role of astrocytes followed, and to date there have been well over 60 reports on the in vitro function of astrocytes specifically related to their potential as CNS APCs. To the extent that it is unclear how many of these studies relate to the in vivo situation (see above), an analysis of all of them is unwarranted, particularly as many of them report similar features of astrocyte function. However, there are a number of studies of significant theoretical interest which deserve analysis.

The range of antigens that have been used in in vitro antigen presentation experiments with astrocytes is not restricted to self antigen such as MBP (41,46) but includes viral antigens (e.g., MHV-JHM [164] and Theiler's [11]). The T-cell responses in all these cases are secondary since the T cells with which the astrocytes interact have previously been activated by interaction with "professional" APC—first in the lymphoid tissue in the animal from which the T cells were derived, and subsequently on a number of occasions in vitro. Similarly, astrocytes can also present alloantigen to *previously stimulated* alloreactive CD4+ T cells in a secondary MLR in which the astrocytes serve as the stimulators of the reaction (202). It should also be mentioned that there is some evidence that, by analogy with Müller's cells in the retina (187), astrocytes suppress the response of T cells to other potential APCs such as microglial cells (147). The mechanism underlying the curious effect is unclear, but it could be important, particularly if the observation that minimal T-cell proliferation occurs once T cells enter the CNS (170) turns out to be a consistent phenomenon in other experimental systems.

The situation is far less clear in terms of the astrocyte's ability to act as an APC in primary T-cell responses. Before the introduction of T-cell receptor transgenic mice, in which there exists a very high frequency of T cells specific for a single antigen in an unimmunized mouse, the only way of investigating primary T-cell responses was via the detection of responses to allogeneic APCs, since the frequency of alloresponsive T cells in a normal T-cell population is high. The requirements for this "primary" response to be successful do indeed appear to match those of a T cell responding to a defined protein antigen (17,158). There have been only a limited number of studies along these lines and the results are confusing, at least when results from mice and rats are compared. A study utilizing murine astrocytes (45) indicated that a mixture of CD4+ and CD8+ T cells could be induced to proliferate if allogeneic astrocytes were pretreated and they were cultured in the presence of Con-A supernatants or IL-2 and IFN-γ. It was assumed that it was the CD4+ T cells that responded to allogeneic MHC class II+ astrocytes. In rats, highly purified CD4+ T cells showed no evidence of activation (either by proliferation or IL-2 secretion) following coculture with allogeneic, IFN-γ-pretreated, MHC class II+ astrocytes (202). However, in the latter studies it was also shown that CD8+ T cells could be primed by the constitutively MHC class I+ allogeneic astrocytes, and that this priming was particularly effective in the presence of exogenous IL-2 (predominantly a CD4+ T-cell cytokine). It is conceivable, therefore, that the difference between the mouse and rat studies lies at the level of the purity of the responding T-cell population and that it is CD8+ T cells rather than CD4+ T cells which react well to alloantigens on astrocytes in primary responses.

The degree of activation of the astrocyte may itself be important. The studies using rat astrocytes have now been repeated, but this time the astrocytes were pretreated with a combination of TNF-α and IFN-γ (J. Sedgwick, unpublished observations). While this treatment did not substantially increase astrocytic MHC class II expression, there was clear and specific priming of the responding allogeneic CD4+ T cells, but only when IL-2 was added to the cultures. In other words, the astrocyte appeared to impart some signal to the T cells, resulting in the expression of IL-2 receptors; however, that signal was not in itself a sufficient stimulus to induce the T cells to produce IL-2 themselves. Overall, therefore, it is likely that if astrocytes act at all as APCs in terms of CD4+ T-cell activation, it would be in the context of perpetuating a response that was initiated by another APC. Given the general dependence of CD8+ T cells on other sources of IL-2 (CD4+ T cells in particular), direct CNS priming of this population by astrocytes would also seem unlikely.

The other major facet of antigen presentation, the presence of MHC-peptide complexes on the astrocyte membrane rendering the astrocyte a target for CTLs, has been demonstrated. There are many reports that alloreactive (45,93,102,163,207) and viral antigen–specific (163) MHC class I–restricted CD8+ CTLs can lyse astrocytic targets; MHC class II+ astrocytes can also be the target for MBP-specific, MHC class II–restricted CD4+ CTLs (222). Astrocytes may also be lysed by CD4+ T-cell blasts in an MHC-nonrestricted fashion (193), although they are resistant to natural killer (NK) cell lysis (116). Within this group of studies, one (207) is particularly interesting in that it demonstrates that astrocytes can be killed in an MHC class I–restricted fashion by CD8+ CTL, even when the MHC class I expression on the astrocyte was undetectable by immunohistochemical staining. This is a clear demonstration that the apparent absence (by immunohistochemistry or even flow cytometry) of MHC expression on cells within the CNS does not preclude the cells from interacting with T cells whose sensitivity for detection of antigen is very high.

It is very difficult to define the relevance of the above investigations to actual antigen presentation by astrocytes in vivo. One major reason is that most in vitro investigations are conducted with astrocytes derived from the developing (fetal or early postnatal) CNS; in vivo correlates are almost all in relation to the mature, adult CNS. The astrocytes' populations may be functionally quite different in terms of APC function and MHC expression. Moreover, clearly there is something profoundly different about MHC regulation of the astrocyte after it is removed from the CNS. Astrocytes appear to be capable of expressing MHC antigens and responding to factors such as IFN-γ, but apparently only in vitro. There are now a variety of studies demonstrating that some substances likely to be present in the CNS, but not usually present in vitro, are potent inhibitors of astrocytic MHC class I and II expression or their induction by IFN-γ. These include norepinephrine (55,108) and glutamate (108). Addition of cortical neurons to astrocyte cultures has a similar effect (231), although neuron–astrocyte contact is required for this in vitro suppression. Whether MHC inhibition in this latter case is due to gangliosides (which also prevent astrocytic MHC expression if added in vitro [134]) remains to be determined. Significantly, microglial and macrophage MHC expression is not negatively affected by these treatments. If such suppressive actions are indeed occurring within the CNS, it is unlikely that under most circumstances astrocytes could express significant levels of MHC class I and II in situ. Thus, it could be argued that immune interactions are not a significant feature of this cell's functional repertoire. However, the fact that MHC expression occurs sometimes, particularly after some virus infections—and particularly with respect to MHC class I expression—implies that the suppressive environment can be overcome and that it is possible that astrocytes may present antigen to T cells, especially viral antigens to CD8+ T cells.

Macrophages and Microglia

The fact that the astrocyte was the first CNS cell to be used in studies of antigen presentation, and not cells of hematopoietic derivation such as microglia (MG) or macrophages resulted in the latter being virtually ignored in the first half of the 1980s. As we now know, the predominant MHC-expressing population in the normal or inflamed CNS is cells of macrophage/MG lineage, although the evidence that the bulk of these cells are truly effective APC is lacking. First, however, it may be useful to briefly define, with reference to Fig. 10-1, the different populations of cells we will analyse in this section. A more detailed analysis of the origins and localization of MG and macrophages in the CNS can be found in Chapter 5.

Microglia

This term is usually reserved for cells exhibiting a branching, ramified morphology which reside throughout the CNS parenchyma, within the confines of the glia limitans. They constitutively express the CD11b (Mac-1) and CD45 (leukocyte common antigen) molecules (148) and are the resident "macrophage" of the CNS. Foot processes of a minority of these cells which are close to vessels may contribute to the glia limitans (106). The latter could, in principle, be termed *perivascular MG* but are distinct from the perivascular cell (PVC). Most microglia stay of host type in irradiation bone marrow chimeras (144), that is, they are irradiation resistant and turnover is minimal, at least in the noninflamed CNS (79).

Perivascular Cells (PVC)

In normal CNS tissue these cells, also called *perivascular macrophages,* are localized within the perivascular space, outside the endothelial basement membrane, interposed between that structure and the layer of astrocytic and microglial foot processes defining the edge of the CNS parenchyma proper (60,61,77,79). Like MG, they are CD11b+, and in rats they also stain positively with the ED2 monoclonal antibody (29) which additionally labels some cells in the meninges but does not stain parenchymal MG (177). PVC are repopulated from the bone marrow, being replaced approximately every 3–4 months. Thus, in irradiation bone marrow chimeras, a progressively increasing proportion of the PVC becomes of donor type (77,79).

Other CNS Macrophages

The other main populations of macrophages are found within the meninges and in the choroid plexus. In rats, these stain with a number of monoclonal antibodies known to label macrophages, including ED1 (CD68-like) (22,208). Those within the meninges at least, are highly irradiation sensitive and are rapidly replaced by marrow-derived cells in irradiation chimeras (79). It is likely that the early studies by Ting et al. in mice (230) showing that brain MHC class II+ cells have a bone marrow origin, revealed the existence of PVC and meningeal macrophages.

Microglia as APC in vivo

As mentioned above, confirmed reports of MHC-expressing microglia in vivo were relatively rare in the early 1980s since the predominant search was for MHC class II+ astrocytes. In all likelihood, at least some of the MHC-expressing cells present in normal or inflamed tissue that were originally designated as oligos or astrocytes were actually MG. Similarly, cells designated as MHC class II+ macrophages in MS lesions (37,237) probably included a major MG component. In the CNS of rats with EAE, Hickey in 1985 (78) had made the observation that exceptionally few of the MHC class II+ cells were astrocytes, while MHC+ cells were numerous. In 1986 Matsumoto (145) and Vass (246) made clear reference to the presence of large numbers of MHC class II+ cells with a dendritic morphology that were neither endothelial nor astrocytic. While most of these MHC class II+ cells were probably MG, the studies could not exclude the possibility that some of the "MG" were inflammatory macrophages that had entered the parenchyme from the blood and adopted a dendritic or ramified appearance. The propensity of microglia (as distinguished from inflammatory macrophages) to up-regulate MHC class II and CD4 in vivo was soon unequivocally demonstrated in rats with graft-versus-host disease (GvHD) (76). Since there was only a very low level of inflammation into the CNS of these rats, most of which were T cells rather than blood-derived monocytes, the microglia became identified as the MHC-expressing population. The first clear statement regarding the potential antigen-presenting role of MG in human CNS tissue came from Cuzner and colleagues who demonstrated in two studies that MG, rather than astrocytes, were the main cell type expressing MHC class II in human MS tissue (73,259).

These initial reports on microglial MHC expression have been confirmed in numerous studies over recent years. These studies include the demonstration that some expression of MHC class II on MG occurs in normal human CNS tissue, usually in white matter, and that levels of MHC class II expression increase with the age of the tissue donor (149,197). Injection of IFN-γ either intravenously (217) or directly into the rodent CNS (205,245,247) has established that it is predominantly MG and to a very minor extent, astrocytes and endothelial cells, but not oligos or neurons, that respond to this cytokine by up-regulation of MHC class I and II. Inflammation after viral infection (1,28,241,249) is also associated with MG MHC class II expression. Two other in vivo experimental approaches demonstrating immunological activation of MG are worthy of further discussion.

Neuronal Damage and Microglial Cell MHC Expression

A number of studies emerged in 1988 which illustrated the highly reactive nature of MG. Two groups (2,125) demonstrated that a nonimmunological, noninflammatory nerve injury resulted in the up-regulation of MHC class II on MG in the vicinity of the damaged neuron. CD45 expression on MG was also increased. Almost simultaneously, using a different system, Rao and Lund (1982) reported MHC class I and II expression in the superior colliculus of the rat following contralateral optic nerve transection. Subsequently, it has been discovered in a number of variations on the theme that damage of axons—leading to either Wallerian degeneration within the CNS or to the reaction or death of a neuron—can rapidly induce MG reaction, including MHC and CD4 molecule expression. These systems are depicted in Fig. 10-2. The concept of neuronal injury or death producing MG responses is potentially important, and could explain MG reactivity observed in Alzheimer brain (87,118).

Parenchymal MG cells are evidently very sensitive to the health of the neurons and axons in their immediate vicinity (57,58,63,64,95,160,218–220,232). If the neuron becomes reactive, if it dies, or if its axon is damaged, the MG cells become activated in such a way that MHC class I and II and CD4 molecules (at least in the rat) become expressed on their surface, and in some systems the MG cells synthesize IL-6 and TGF-β (95). In short, they become activated *potential* APCs. Other glial cells in the vicinity do not appear to be either so rapidly or extensively affected.

As noted in Fig. 10-2, many permutations of this theme have been examined, and all lead to the same conclusions: neuroaxonal pertubation leads to MG activation and a

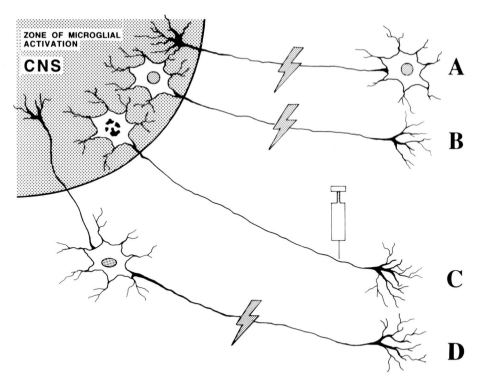

Fig. 10-2. Various model systems in which axonal or neuronal damage induces microglial activation. In these situation, the type of damage varies; however, the microglial reaction is always detected in the CNS parenchyma, as depicted. *A* demonstrates the transection of the optic nerve in which the neurons of the retina are separated from the terminal projections of the axons to the superior colliculus, where the reaction occurs. *B* depicts the transection of the facial nerve; microglial reaction occurs in the facial nerve nucleus around the reactive motor neurons. *C* is a system in which toxic ricin is injected into the facial nerve and transported in a retrograde manner to induce the death of the CN VII motor neurons. Microglia surrounding them become reactive and phagocytic. *D* illustrates the effect of sciatic nerve damage. In this paradigm both motor axons (with their neurons in the anterior spinal cord) and sensory axons of neurons in the dorsal root ganglia are severed; however, the reactive microglia appear around the *undamaged* projections from these neurons into the CNS parenchyma.

change in the baseline predisposition of that area of the CNS to inflammation (57,58, 63,64,95,99,160,218–220,232). Since none of these systems involve direct trauma to the area in which the MG become activated, it raises numerous questions about the nature of the relationship existing between these cells and the neurons. Little is known about the mechanisms that are active, except that it appears to be steroid sensitive (94).

Axonal injury systems involve transection of the optic nerve, the seventh cranial nerve (CN VII), or sectioning a peripheral nerve (57,58,63,64,99,160,218). More elaborately, an intraneural injection of a toxin which is transported to the nerve cell body in the CNS causing neuronal death stimulates MG cells (219,220). In all cases where such manipulations have been followed by the induction of EAE, the site in which the MG have been activated exhibits a new or enhanced susceptibility to EAE inflammation (99,160). Such observations lend support to the contention that it is MG which function most optimally as APC in the nervous system, although there are alternative explanations, and these are considered below.

Irradiation Bone Marrow Chimeras and Microglia

Irradiation bone marrow chimeras have seen extensive use in the field of immunology for analysis of the lineage and function of specific subtypes of leukocytes. More recently, this technique has been used to probe the origins and in vivo functions of cells normally resident in the CNS or entering it during disease. Parenchymal MG are largely irradiation resistant (79,144), and in studies involving the isolation of MG from the CNS of adult chimeric rats, little exchange of MG to the donor bone marrow type is seen even 12 months after transplantation (203,204). This has subsequently been shown to be true in mice by employing a system which did not involve irradiation (see Chapter 5). The EAE induction studies alluded to above wherein disease could only be induced in rats in which the encephalitogenic T cells were MHC compatible with APCs derived from the donor bone marrow provide the strongest available evidence that some macrophages and/or perivascular cells are effective APCs. In these systems, astrocytes, endothelial cells, oligos and neurons, *as well as most parenchymal MG* are unnecessary for disease development. However, in the interpretation of these experiments, the same limitations that were discussed for astrocytes and endothelial cells apply to MG; complex and pathogenic interactions might occur, but are not required in the development of EAE.

   With this background in mind, evidence can be evaluated for the in vivo role of MG as APCs. The first point, which could be derived from the nerve damage models, is that the expression of MHC class II on microglia is almost certainly no more than an indicator of MG activation, not a signature of a totally functional APC. Activated T cells in rats and humans also express MHC class II, but their primary role is certainly not currently believed to be as an APC! There are some clues about the potential of MG to participate in T-cell-mediated immune responses in vivo. Needless to say, the results are indirect and contradictory.

   First, in a number of studies (99,124,172), EAE was induced in rats *after* nerve injury had caused increased MHC class I and II expression on the MG in the vicinity of the damaged neurons or neural tracts (but actually a centimeter or more from the actual site of injury). Thus, it is possible that the activated, MHC+ MG do present antigen more efficiently/effectively and thereby precipitate inflammatory foci (58,99,160). A more prosaic explanation is that enhanced MHC expression by MG is unrelated to

T-cell localization, reflecting some other effect of neuronal or axonal injury, for example, an alteration in vascular permeability. One way of assessing this latter notion is to create chimeras, as done previously (77,80), in which most MG are not MHC compatible with the encephalitogenic T cells. If the same effects are observed, then it could not be due to (MHC-restricted) T-cell activation by MG. An alternative and completely opposite role to that normally considered for ramified MG expressing MHC molecules is as suppressors of T-cell responses. Again, the evidence permitting this idea is indirect. Voorthuis et al. (247) reported that while intraventricular administration of IFN-γ induced high levels of MHC class II on MG, the ability to induce EAE in these rats was completely prevented. If IFN-γ was administered intravenously, EAE severity was not affected either in a positive or negative way. In another study (203), constitutive MHC class expression on MG isolated from the normal rat CNS was examined; in general, MG from EAE-resistant rats (the BN strain in particular) exhibited greater constitutive MHC expression than MG from EAE-susceptible strains. It is noteworthy that after EAE is induced in resistant (BN strain) and susceptible (Lew strain) rats, MG MHC class II expression is about the same in the CNS parenchyma of both (146). Such studies, however, do not directly implicate MG as being inhibitory to T cells. What they do indicate is that MHC expression by MG alone cannot be taken as an indicator that an immune response will necessarily proceed or be enhanced. It is possible that the opposite may be the case.

It is interesting to consider why MG, but not astrocytes, can so readily express MHC class II in vivo. It seems to be an innate function. Emerging evidence from in vitro studies (using glia derived from neonatal rodents) indicate that MHC expression, particularly MHC class II, is differentially regulated in the two cell types, at least in response to the cytokine IFN-γ. Thus, reagents which increase intracellular cAMP and protein kinase C block IFN-γ-induced MHC class II on astrocytes but not on MG (196). As reviewed in the astrocyte section above, similarly differential affects are seen after addition of norepinephrine, glutamate, neurons, and gangliosides; moreover, the block to astrocytic MHC expression appears to be at the transcriptional level (55,108,134,231). Whether similar mechanisms preventing MHC expression by astrocytes but not MG exist in vivo in the adult mammal is not known.

Microglia as APC in vitro

Interest in the antigen processing and presenting capabilities of MG stemmed from observations regarding the propensity of these cells to express MHC molecules in situ. This is in contrast to astrocytes, for which the first observations were made from in vitro cultured cells. The available data is accordingly biased, so that relatively few studies address the APC properties of isolated MG, while many in vivo observations are available. As was the case for astrocytes, in vitro studies that have used "MG" derived from the rodent neonatal CNS or human fetal CNS are difficult to reconcile with immunological events occurring in the adult CNS. It has been argued that the cells so frequently employed in vitro are MG precursors that pass through a series of differentiation steps and develop into a fully ramified adult MG (see 175 and Chapter 5). There is no direct evidence that this occurs, nor is there proof that the functions exhibited by "immature MG" bear any relationship to the adult cell. The only evidence available shows that some (a small proportion) of adult MG are derived from hematopoietic precursors entering from the blood (79). This has also been noted in mice when sex-mismatched marrow was given, or where the marrow cells were derived from a mouse expressing a bacteriophage γ transgene (23). It is notable in the latter study that approximately the same number of labeled MG were found in those recipient mice that had received bone marrow as neonates 3 months earlier, as was found when injection of bone marrow was delayed until the mice were 3 months old. Thus, there was no evidence that seeding of MG precursors occurred at a greater rate in the newborn at the time when MG differentiation is thought to occur (175). It is possible that seeding of the CNS by microglia or their progenitors has already occurred before birth (see 175, and Chapter 5). Phenotypically and morphologically, such early "MG" are very different from the cells found in adult tissue; they are more like a typical lymphoid tissue macrophage (24,175,208). However, it is also apparent that adult MG activated in situ can express the ED1 antigen in rats, (62)—a marker of macrophage activation—or up-regulate CD45 and CD4 (203,204). These are some of the markers normally associated with "immature MG." Importantly, it should be noted that there is no proof that the cells obtained from culture of neonatal CNS and called *MG* are actually parenchymal microglia. As noted above, there is a wide variety of other macrophage-like cells in the CNS, all of which have a somewhat similar phenotype to MG (e.g., CD11b expression).

Two early studies using primary mixed glial cultures derived from neonatal mice (258) and rats (33), and other subsequent reports (25,195,255), observed some constitutive MHC class I expression on MG, as well as IFN-γ/Con-A supernatant-induced expression of MHC class II on these same cells. One study using human fetal tissue found a high basal level of MHC class II on MG (and astrocytes) which was augmented by IFN-γ (109). It is possible that this constitutive MHC class II expression represents a developmental stage of these cells only, since a much smaller proportion of MG and astrocytes isolated in culture from adult human tissue express MHC class II spontaneously (65).

Guilian and colleagues (59), and Frei and colleagues (52,53) were among the first to devise methods to separate MG from other glial cells in culture. Using purified microglia, Frei demonstrated that MG from neonatal brain share many of the properties with macrophages, including phagocytic ability, expression of IgG-Fc receptors, nonspecific esterase activity, and stimulation of growth by IL-3 and granulocyte-macrophage colony-stimulating factor (GM-CSF). Also, the cells were induced to express MHC class II by treatment with IFN-γ, and after this, could process and present protein antigen to CD4+ T cells. Microglia were also shown to produce the cytokines IL-1 and

TNF-α, which (potentially) could enhance their APC properties (59,131). These studies reinforced the then emerging belief (based on in vivo observations) that MG were the important APC of the CNS.

Relatively few other studies have followed. Rat neonatal MG, after treatment with IFN-γ, were shown to act as APC for MBP-specific CD4+ T-cell lines (147). Mouse neonatal MG derived in the presence of GM-CSF exhibited good APC function for a range of protein- and alloantigen-specific CD4+ Th1 and Th2 T-cell lines (42). Interestingly, cells cultured in M-CSF with or without IFN-γ, were less potent APC. It is believed that surface IL-1 induced by GM-CSF may be responsible for the increase in activity. Finally, a single study has examined the ability of neonatal mouse MG to prime allogeneic CD4+ and CD8+ T cells (162). The results are similar to those reported for rat astrocytes (202) in that both MG and astrocytes are good stimulators of naive CD8+ T cells. CD4+ T cells did not respond to allogeneic MG, but there was also no evidence that the MG expressed MHC class II. The difference between the astrocytes and MG studies is that there appeared to be no requirement for CD4+ T-cell help (IL-2) to obtain a strong response from allogeneic CD8+ T cells. This could indicate a real difference between the two types of APC. Alternatively, it could represent a species difference as, depending on the strain combinations used, mouse CD8+ T cells can exhibit quite strong proliferation to allogeneic macrophage stimulators in the absence of exogenous IL-2 (213). Finally, it would have been useful to see the extent of CD8+ T-cell proliferation to MG in the presence of anti-CD4 MAb and to know how pure the T-cell subpopulations were. In some studies, the presence of even a small, contaminating population of CD4+ T cells has been known to provide sufficient IL-2 to help CD8+ T cells to proliferate.

In recent years, a number of studies from Antel and colleagues have investigated the immunological function of MG derived from human CNS material surgically resected from epilepsy patients. The cells were cultured for some weeks prior to use and probably were already highly activated on isolation in view of their constitutive MHC class II expression and long-term viability in vitro (254). It was also reported that these MG have a low basal level of the B7/BB-1 costimulatory molecule which increased with addition of IFN-γ (255). Like astrocytes, the MG in culture were lysed by activated but antigen nonspecific CD4+ T cells. Whether these MG can act as targets of specific CTL (requiring "MHC-restricted" recognition of peptide antigens) is not known. The MG were reported to act as APCs for proliferative secondary (254) and primary (256) T-cell responses, the latter involving stimulation of allogeneic CD4+ T cells. The result, with unprimed T cells in particular, is an unusual result, given that their activation is normally achieved only by a small number of cell types, including DC and B-cell blasts (see beginning of chapter). No strict comparison between cultured MG and cells of this type have been reported, so it is possible that the microglia can stimulate T cells, but in relative terms, are poor at this. This is the experience when normal macrophages are compared with DC or B-cell blasts (98,158). One additional uncertainty is the effect of extended culture on the APC function of MG, and given the very limited APC abilities of astrocytes in vivo, for example, which are revealed only after extended culture, some degree of caution in extrapolating these finding to the situation in vivo is warranted.

MG have also been isolated from the adult rat and human CNS by a rosetting technique, which utilizes the expression of Fc receptors by MG (and macrophages generally [74]). The cultured cells respond to IFN-γ, IL-1, and TNF-α by up-regulating Fc receptor levels, and MHC expression is increased after IFN-γ treatment (117,260). One problem with this approach is that cells other than true MG (e.g., PVC, and macrophages of the meninges and choroid) are also likely to be isolated when Fc receptor expression is used as the isolating criterion.

Two alternative approaches have been adopted to analyze the function of adult microglia in vitro. The first (203,204) utilizes flow cytometry to separate adult MG from other CNS macrophages based on their relatively low levels of CD45 expression as compared with other bone marrow–derived cells in the CNS. Studies have concentrated on the phenotype of MG isolated directly ex vivo; Fig. 10-3 illustrates the typical profiles of such MG isolated from the normal and graft-versus-host disease rat CNS in which microglial activation occurs (76). All CD45^{low} cells (MG) are CD11b/c+ and up-regulate MHC class II after GvHD induction. In the normal CNS, class II expression is mostly confined to CD45^{high} cells, which includes both T cells and non-MG brain macrophages. Using fluorescence-activated cell sorter (FACS) separation of cells and purifying them into their constituent populations has permitted in vitro examination of the specific APC effectiveness of freshly isolated microglia and other resident macrophage cells from the CNS (47). Most interestingly, the freshly isolated microglial cells (from the normal CNS), although they could present antigen to resting, previously stimulated MBP-reactive CD4+ T cells, resulted in relatively low levels of T-cell proliferation and IL-2 production. One reason might be that freshly isolated cells might express only low levels of the needed MHC or costimulatory molecules. However, other cells isolated from the CNS and belonging to the greater macrophage–monocyte family did function very well as APCs. It is possible that these represent PVCs or meningeal resident monocytes.

The second approach adopted by Rieske and colleagues (184) has utilized the microglial cell-activating properties of nerve transection in adult rats (see above). Explants from the facial nucleus were cultured, and outgrowth of both ramified cells and macrophage-like cells was observed. Both expressed MHC class I and II molecules as they do in vivo after this treatment, and there was substantial proliferation observed. The APC functions of the cells have not been examined.

Perivascular Cells

These cells are defined entirely on the basis of in vivo studies. They have never been studied in vitro as there is no clear way of separating them from other CNS macro-

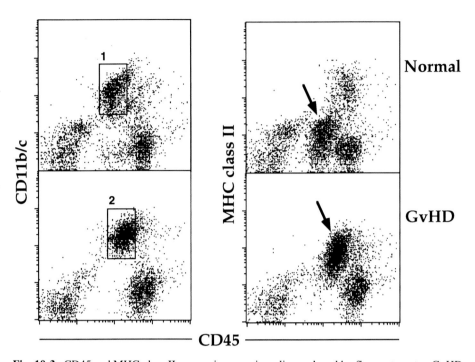

Fig. 10-3. CD45 and MHC class II expression on microglia, analyzed by flow cytometry. GvHD was induced in lightly irradiated F1 rats by intravenous injection of parent splenocytes. Ten days after cell injection, PBS-perfused CNS was removed from normal or GvHD rats and cells isolated (47) and stained for CD45 vs. CD11b/c and CD45 vs. MHC class II. Note that most microglia (CD45^{low} CD11b/c$^+$, population 1) in the normal CNS are MHC class II$^-$ (arrow) while microglia in GvHD (population 2) are MHC class II$+$ (arrow). Note also the increased CD45 expression (x-axis) of activated microglia where population 2 is shifted to the right relative to population 1.

phages or MG. Paradoxically, however, they are the only type of CNS cell where a reasonably strong case can be made that they do indeed act as APC in vivo, at least for MBP-reactive T cells in the induction of EAE (77).

Other than the original description of PVC by del rio Hortega in 1932 (26), delineation of this cell type is just evolving (16,77,79,141,142,218,246). All studies using normal rat CNS tissue note that they are sparse, MHC class II+ cells in close apposition to small vessels. In the rat irradiation bone marrow chimeric EAE experiments alluded to above (77), researchers report that the only cell type expressing the donor MHC in the CNS of the chimeras was an infrequent population of cells in close apposition to vessels. These were identified as the PVCs (105,185). This population of cells stained with an antibody recognizing donor bone marrow MHC but not host cells is illustrated in Fig. 10-4. This cell type is almost certainly the same as that detected previously in normal rats. It was surmized that this population was responsible for

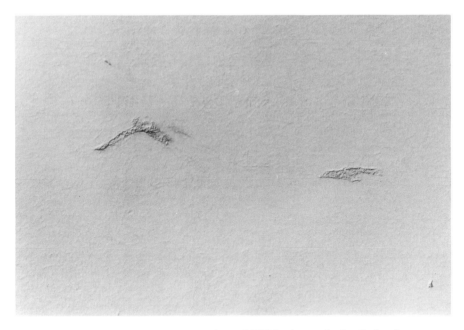

Fig. 10-4. Perivascular cells express the donor MHC haplotype in irradiation bone marrow chimeras indicating bone-marrow origin. This photomicrograph depicts two perivascular cells adjacent to a venule in the CNS parenchyma. These cells are interposed between the glial foot processes and the basement membrane of the endothelial cells. Immunohistochemical staining for the RT1.B^1 molecule, interference optics; $\times 325$.

MBP presentation to the encephalitogenic T cells. Studies in irradiation bone marrow chimeras (79,105,144,185; see Chapter 5) have shown that more than just perivascular cells are replaced by the transplanted marrow. This includes macrophage and monocytic cells in the meninges, subarachnoid space, and choroid plexus. It remains possible that some of these latter cell types may also act as APC in the induction of EAE and the perivascular cell is not exclusive in this APC role.

MHC class II+ cells in a perivascular location have also been identified in normal human CNS tissue, although in prior studies they were identified as endothelial cells or pericytes (104,173). In view of the recent studies on the APC properties of SM/P, this is a distinct possibility. Subsequent work with human tissue has clearly identified MHC class II+ macrophage-like cells in the Virchow-Robin space (36) and around capillaries; in the latter case, the cells localized between the endothelial cell basal lamina and the glia limitans, but distinct from pericytes (61). It has also been shown using CNS tissue from human bone marrow transplant recipients where the recipient was female and donor bone marrow was male that some PVC bore the Y chromosome indicating the hematopoietic derivation of the cells (243). As in rats, few cells in the parenchyma were of the donor type.

Other CNS Macrophages

It has been known for some time (79,105,185,208) that macrophages are present in a variety of sites in the CNS, other than in a perivascular location (PVC) and within the parenchyma. Constitutive expression of MHC class II by these cells is an indicator (although possibly an irrelevant one!) of potential APC function, and it has recently been shown (150) that stromal macrophages of the choroid plexus in rodents are MHC class II+. The nonmicroglial macrophages isolated directly from the normal CNS by flow cytometry which show potent T-cell activating properties (47) would include these other CNS macrophages, so it is likely that they do function as APCs in vivo as well.

Choroid Plexus Epithelial Cells (CPEC)

There is a single report on the antigen-presenting properties of these cells (167). CPEC derived from adult mice were exhaustively purified, allegedly to >99.9% purity. The cells were MHC class II negative, both in vivo and in vitro, but responded to IFN-γ treatment in vitro by up-regulation of MHC class II. The absence of constitutive MHC class II expression supports claims about the purity of the cell population, given that choroid macrophages in situ in rats and mice normally express this molecule (150). A CD4+ OVA-specific T-cell clone formed aggregates with MHC class II+ CPEC and proliferated in the presence of specific antigen and the appropriate MHC-compatible CPEC. T-cell proliferation was inhibited by appropriate monoclonal antibodies to the Ia restriction element on the CPEC. Also demonstrated was the uptake of small (100 nm) particles by the CPEC following intraventricular injection, which suggests that these cells could, in principle, gather antigen (including viral particles) from the CSF and process and present it to T cells. Thus, the choroid plexus which contains macrophages as well as epithelial cells with interfaces impinging on the CSF and, via fenestrated capillaries, with cells in blood, is another potential site at which T cells in the periphery may interact with CNS-associated antigens. It must be noted in passing, however, that in most T-cell mediated CNS diseases, with the notable exception of that associated with LCMV infection, the choroid plexus itself is rarely the site of significant inflammation.

Oligodendrocytes

The interest in oligodendroglial cells *(oligos)* obviously stems from the role of these cells in myelination of axons within the CNS and in the group of inflammatory, demyelinating diseases (e.g., multiple sclerosis) that result from the interruption of the normal myelination process or destruction of myelin that has already been layed down. Mechanisms of demyelination could potentially include stripping of myelin sheaths from axons as a direct result of anti-myelin antibody-directed macrophage phago-cytosis. Alternatively, myelin destruction may be secondary to oligo damage or lysis mediated by direct viral infection or immunologically mediated events, including cyto-kine secretion (TNF, for example) by T cells or macrophages, or direct MHC-restricted T-cell-mediated lysis. The latter mechanism, of course, would require the expression of MHC class I or II molecules on the cell surface. In principle, such a scenario could involve T cells specific for either an oligo or myelin (self) antigen or viral antigen expressed on the surface of the oligo. Unfortunately, there is debate about the oligo's ability to present antigen. After more than a decade of investigation into this matter, evidence is ultimately emerging that the APC potential of these cells is probably limited to MHC class I–restricted interactions.

Oligodendrocytes as APC in vivo

It can be taken for granted, at least with respect to MHC class II expression and bearing in mind the limitations in the sensitivity of the assays used, that in the many studies of normal and inflamed CNS cited above in which astrocytes and endothelial were found to be class II negative, oligos were also probably negative. Moreover, of the relatively few reports in which MHC expression by oligos has been specifically sought in vivo, a minority detect MHC expression on this cell type. In the normal human CNS, they are negative for both MHC class I and II (65,104). Oligos in two types of noninflammatory CNS diseases (Alzheimer's [221] and PML [1]) were MHC class II negative, despite the expression of significant levels of these molecules on MG. However, in PML (1), JC virus-infected oligos did stain positively for $\beta 2$ microglobulin, the necessary com-olecule for full class I expression; yet, since the staining appeared to be predominantly intracellular, its significance for actual surface MHC class I expression remains ques-tionable. In rodents and humans alike, it is likely that oligos do not express MHC class II, even during inflammatory conditions. For example, in EAE (143) and CNS herpes simplex virus infection in the rat (249), no MHC expression on oligos was observed—again, despite substantial induction on MG. Direct injection of IFN-γ into the CNS of newborn mice and recovery of neural cells 2 days later resulted in the expression of MHC class I but not class II by oligos (258). Similarly, in mice infected with a neurotropic form of coronavirus (224), this type of cell expressed MHC class I but not class II in situ.

Two reports of MHC class II expression on oligos in vivo must be considered. First, one early study reported the presence of MHC class II+ cells in the white matter of the normal mouse CNS (229). These cells were assumed to be oligos, but it is more likely, given our current knowledge, that the cells were ramified MG. The second study by Rodriguez et al. (189) in which mice infected by Theiler's virus were examined for CNS MHC expression, has already been mentioned above in the context of the expres-sion of MHC class II on both endothelial and astrocytes. This was a careful, ultrastructural study that is more convincing than others. However, the alleged MHC class II expression by oligos seems unusual for two reasons: first, the molecule appeared to be expressed cytoplasmically rather than on the surface; and second, serial section staining (at the light microscope level) showing that a proportion (25%) of MHC class II+ cells coincided with those staining positively for galactocerebroside (Gal-C), must be viewed with caution as it is known that some anti-Gal-C antibodies also bind macrophages in addition to oligos (24)!

Finally, two independent transgenic mouse studies (240,263) deserve mention. Both described the production of transgenic mice in which murine MHC class I was overexpressed in oligos. In both cases, the mice were hypomyelinated, apparently due to the MHC class I molecule (somehow) interfering with the ability of the cell to effectively myelinate axons. There was also an overall reduction in the number of oligos present in these mice. No CNS inflammation was evident. The other point of significance was that MHC class I was not expressed on the cell surface, but appeared to accumulate in the cytoplasm of these cells. While these are artificial systems and it is unclear whether the accumulation of other, non-MHC proteins within the oligodendroglia would lead to a similar phenotype, the results indicate that there is at least a reluctance of oligos to express MHC molecules in vivo. It would be of some interest if it could be demonstrated that they have an unusual propensity to accumulate MHC molecules intracellularly. It is of note that in the studies by Rodriguez et al. (189) and Achim et al. (1), MHC class II and β2 microglobulin expression, respectively, were apparently again cytoplasmic.

On the basis of current evidence, the only conclusion one can reach is that oligos are unlikely to participate in MHC class II–restricted (CD4+ T-cell) interactions in vivo. In contrast, interaction between oligos and CD8+ T cells may occur, and there is good evidence that in vivo they can express MHC class I. This tends to occur in the context of viral infection. Thus, immune-mediated lysis of oligos is a real possibility, and studies of oligos in vitro strongly support these general conclusions.

Oligodendrocytes as APC in vitro

Mouse and rat oligodendrocytes are prepared from the CNS or optic nerve of newborn pups up to the age of 1 week. In vitro culture times vary from a few days to a week or longer before the cells are used for experimental purposes. This could explain some of the minor differences in MHC expression reported by different laboratories.

All studies emerging in the years 1983 to 1985 (33,83,112,258) found that rat and mouse oligos in culture were constitutively MHC class I and class II negative, and it was only MHC class I that could be induced in response to treatment with activated T-cell supernatants or IFN-γ. Thus, these cells were clearly different from astrocytes. In general, the results of these early studies have stood the test of time, except for the later observation (135) that rat oligos will, like astrocytes, spontaneously express MHC class

I—particularly after extended culture periods. Culture conditions such as the concentration of serum may be important. Oligos remain MHC class I negative in the presence of TNF (107,239), unlike astrocytes, although in the case of the latter cell type, TNF is probably enhancing an already existing basal level MHC class I expression (138; see above). The combination of TNF and IFN-γ has no synergistic effect on MHC class I expression above IFN-γ treatment alone (239). Apart from IFN-γ, only one other factor produced by coronavirus-infected glia in vitro has been reported to induce MHC class I expression on oligos (223). This is thought not to be type-1 IFN and is probably produced by infected astrocytes. Little is known about the propensity of oligos to express adhesion and costimulatory molecules in vivo or in vitro. In a single study, mouse oligos in culture exhibited no ICAM-1 expression in response to IFN-γ treatment; this is in contrast to astrocytes that did (198).

Of the few studies with human oligos, all involve cells isolated from adult postmortem material. While one report (96) describes a high percentage of spontaneously MHC class II+ oligos (Gal-C+ cells) in culture, this is probably artifactual in view of a number of other studies demonstrating (as in rodents) constitutive (65) or IFN-γ-inducible (82) MHC class I expression, but no detectable MHC class II expression with or without IFN-γ treatment.

There appears to be a clear developmental stage at which oligodendroglial precursors lose the ability to express MHC class II molecules. Oligos and type-2 astrocytes in vitro have a common precursor, the O-2A+ progenitor cell. Interestingly, it was noted by Calder et al. (12) that this cell lineage as well as type-1 and type-2 rat astrocytes, but not oligos, expressed MHC class II in response to IFN-γ. As described by others, oligos, as well as all other cell lineages, up-regulated MHC class I in response to IFN-γ. Thus, something happens between the O-2A+ progenitor stage and development into a fully differentiated oligo that renders the mature oligo incapable of expressing MHC class II. A timely and important study by Massa et al. (137) has demonstrated that it is differences in MHC class I gene regulation between astrocytes and oligos that underly the dissimilar levels of MHC class I expression on these cell types. By using cells from newborn mice cultured for 8–10 days, it was demonstrated that astrocytes that spontaneously display MHC class I in vitro showed constitutive MHC class I regulatory element (CRE) region I binding activity as well as interferon consensus sequence (ICS) binding activity. Oligos that remained MHC class I negative in culture did not express these activities. However, both cell types (but not neurons; see below) responded to IFN-γ treatment by induction of ICS-binding activity: the activity was minimal in the case of oligos and further enhanced in astrocytes. Thus, these findings are entirely consistent with the actual expression of MHC class I seen both in vivo and in vitro.

There are very few studies on the functional interaction between T cells and oligos. Nevertheless, those that do exist confirm in a functional sense the absence of MHC class II on the cell's surface. A study by Takiguchi and Frelinger (226) showed that IFN-γ-treated astrocytes but not oligos could present antigen to, and activate, CD4+

T-cell hybridomas. The latter cell type provides a highly sensitive detection mechanism for T-cell-APC interactions. This is solid, albeit indirect, evidence for oligo class II negativity. In contrast, oligos are lysed specifically by CD8+ alloreactive T cells in vitro, which is consistent with their MHC class I expression (192). Oligos also appear to be sensitive to lysis by preactivated CD4+ T cells acting in a fashion that is not MHC restricted—so called bystander killing (193). The mechanism of lysis is unclear in this system as it does not involve simple secretion of factors like TNF. This sort of experimental result, also noted above in the context of T-cell–endothelial interactions (201), highlights the possibility that MHC class II− cells may be susceptible to damage by CD4+ T cells. Such a mechanism could explain the development of EAE, for example, in irradiation bone marrow chimeric animals where many potential target tissues (such as the vasculature) are MHC incompatible with the encephalitogenic T cells responsible for the disease (77,80).

Perhaps ironically, the role of oligos as an APC within the CNS is probably less complex and more clearly defined than any other cell so far reviewed. There seems to be general agreement that this cell type cannot express any MHC class II (confirmed at the functional level), but that they can up-regulate MHC class I, both in vivo and in vitro, and thus be specifically recognized and killed by CD8+ CTL. Some evidence exists for the latter process in mice infected with neurotropic coronavirus (MHV-4) wherein a combination of viral tropism for oligos and development of anti-viral CTL (43) may be in part responsible for the extensive demyelination that occurs in this condition. However, reports of viral persistence in oligos should also be noted (188), as they may indicate that levels of MHC class I up-regulation in vivo are not always sufficient for T cell recognition to occur.

Neurons

Neurons, the major signal-transducing cell type in the central and peripheral nervous system, appear to have little role in presentation of antigen to T cells. Of all the cells in the nervous system, it is the neuron which is the least able to express MHC molecules. Emerging evidence would indeed suggest that normal neurons (as distinct from those infected by certain viruses or those otherwise damaged) are probably unable to respond even to MHC-inducing cytokines like IFN-γ (see below). In this sense, by definition, the neuron has little potential as an APC. However, the few reports of in vivo MHC expression in nontransformed, virus-infected neurons are of interest, and some in vitro studies on T-cell interactions with transformed neurons have been particularly enlightening.

Neurons as APC in vivo

Neurons in the CNS of rodents injected with IFN-γ remain MHC negative (161,205,217,245,247). In one study where neurons were found to be MHC class I positive after intracranial IFN-γ injection (258), it was possible the glial fibrillary acidic protein (GFAP)− Gal-C− A2B5+ phenotype was O2-A progenitor cells rather than neurons, as suggested. There are, on the other hand, reports (both direct and indirect) of MHC expression on neurons in vivo following infection; but where this has been described, expression is usually limited to MHC class I. Some neurons in herpes simplex virus (HSV) encephalitis-affected human CNS tissue were reported as being MHC class I and II positive (210). This was not confirmed at the EM level, the presence of MHC class II being particularly unusual. In contrast, HSV infection of rat CNS neurons results in MG but not neuronal MHC expression (249). In a recent study (206) it was shown that CD8+ T-cell depletion of mice resulted in a substantial increase in HSV-mediated destruction of peripheral nerve neurons, implying first, that under normal circumstances, CD8+ (MHC class I–restricted) T-cell responses control the infection and second, that the infected neurons express MHC class I. The latter was not formally demonstrated but was implied. While these results are of significant interest in relation to possible neuron–T-cell interactions in vivo, it cannot, of course, be ruled out that CD8+ T cells mediate their protection of infected neurons by inducing an anti-viral state in the cells, for example, via secretion of IFN-γ. In a similar vein, Maehlen et al. (123) described increased persistence of measles virus in rat CNS neurons in animals depleted of CD8+ T cells. The interpretations and limitations of this study are essentially the same as those mentioned above. Moreover, a definitive demonstration of persistently infected neurons (as opposed to glial elements, for example) was not made in the latter study. There exists one report of elevated MHC class I gene expression in scrapie-infected guinea-pig CNS (34). β2 microglobulin protein was demonstrated in neurons. Notably, no evidence of *surface* MHC class I expression on neurons was provided, so the relevance for T-cell interactions is unclear.

A well-studied model of neuronal virus infection–immune system interaction is that of LCMV infection in mice. This virus is eventually cleared from the CNS, and from infected neurons specifically, but without apparent neuronal destruction (171). Importantly, since the mice can be shown to harbor LCMV-specific CTL, and since it is likely that CD8+ T-cell blasts (75) will enter the CNS, these investigations could be construed as providing clear *functional* evidence for the lack of effective T-cell–neuron interactions. While this might be in part due to the absence of MHC class I on the infected neuron, there could be additional factors which prevent T cells and neurons interacting as revealed in some in vitro studies (see below). Viral clearance from neurons in this system and in others (110) could involve antibody (9) or possibly the effect of cytokines such as IFN-γ, without the necessity of cell elimination.

Evidence from studies of neural allograft rejection also lend support to the idea that neurons are less visible to the immune system since they are spared, while other glial elements are destroyed following transplantation (169). It is only after sustained secondary rejection processes are initiated that neurons are affected, and this may be due to nonspecific bystander events, rather than specific cytolysis.

In summary, there is some in vivo evidence (albeit indirect) that certain viruses, perhaps those with substantial transactivating potential like HSV, may dysregulate neurons (peripheral nerve neurons at least; see below), resulting in MHC class I expression that is detectable by virus-specific CTL. There is no indication that this occurs following LCMV infection of mouse CNS neurons, and there is a paucity of in vivo evidence that "normal" neurons can express MHC class I and II molecules, even in the presence of an inflammatory infiltrate or injected inflammatory cytokines.

To date, the most compelling example of MHC class I expression by neurons comes from the work of Neumann et al. (168). In this exacting study it was shown that neurons that were rendered electrically quiet by axonal damage did indeed synthesize and express MHC class I molecules following exposure to IFN-γ. It seems that the critical regulatory step for the neuron is at the level of expression of β2 microglobulin, which is apparently tightly controlled (168). Thus, the ability of neurons to interact with T cells seems to exist, but the parameters governing it are still obscure.

Neurons as APC in vitro

Before analyzing the few published studies on T cell–neuron interactions in vitro, the analysis by Massa et al. (137) of MHC regulation in neural cell cultures deserves mention. IFN-γ treatment of normal, nontransformed neurons derived from normal fetal or 8-day-old mice did not result in induction of MHC class I promoter activity or induction of interferon consensus sequence binding activity, as occurred with both astrocytes and oligos. Thus, of all neural cells, neurons are unique in their resistance to MHC class I up-regulation, as noted in the study above (168).

Transformed neurons are clearly different in that MHC class I is often present constitutively at low level and can be substantially up-regulated in response to IFN-γ treatment. One report (90) showed that an LCMV-infected transformed mouse CNS neuronal cell line was not susceptible to lysis by specific CTL. However, treatment of the cells with IFN-γ to increase MHC class I, or transfection with a construct which resulted in surface MHC class I expression, led to lysis of virus-infected cells. This clearly demonstrated that resistance to lysis was related to the lack of MHC class I expression on the cell surface. Examination of the data in this study indicates that other factors may be involved in resistance to lysis by CTL since neurons expressing very high levels of MHC class I were less susceptible to lysis than fibroblasts expressing lower MHC levels. The defect may lie in the capacity of T cells to form stable conjugates with neurons due to the latter's lack of costimulatory or adhesion molecules. Alternatively, there may exist an innate resistance of neurons to T-cell-mediated lysis.

In this context, it has been reported (126) that MHC class I+ human neuroblastomas are resistant to alloreactive CTL, but this resistance could be reversed by non-specifically binding effector T cells to the neurons with lectins like phytohemagglutinin (PHA). A related study (93) using nontransformed fetal mouse CNS neurons and peripheral nervous system neurons from newborn mice demonstrated that the latter cell type was susceptible to alloreactive CTL lysis, while CNS neurons were not. Direct addition of isolated lytic granules to CNS neurons had no affect, while PNS neurons and astrocytes were destroyed. Additionally, agglutination of neurons and CTL with PHA, while not resulting in neuronal lysis in this study (there was no MHC class I expression in these nontransformed neurons), did increase the levels of lytic serine esterase secretion by the CTL. The conclusion from these studies is that the absence of MHC class I is but only one factor that renders these cells particularly poor APCs and a poor target for CTL.

Questions, Conflicts, and Conclusions

Tables 10-1 and 10-2 summarize current knowledge on the MHC expression and antigen-presenting role of each cell in the CNS. Importantly, the in vivo information is not only from models like EAE but also from viral infections and, in the case of the human CNS, from naturally occurring neurodegenerative diseases, viral infections, and autoimmunity. The in vitro analysis is also broad ranging, encompassing the response of these CNS cells to a range of stimuli but particularly cytokines and a number of different viruses. The following broad picture has emerged.

In vivo, there is a relatively consistent response of all these cell types to a widely divergent set of stimuli. That is, the APC does not vary, depending on the system. For example, astrocytes in *all* species and circumstances *can* express MHC class II, but normally, they do not. In contrast, MG *always* up-regulate MHC class I and II. This does not mean, of course, that MG are efficient APC (see below).

Across species, there are only minor differences in MHC expression (with the exception of MHC class II expression by guinea pig EC). Human CNS cells both in vivo and in vitro seem to be more reactive than their laboratory animal counterparts. Constitutive MHC expression, particularly MHC class II, is usually greater in human tissue. It should also be remembered that tissue from animals is usually removed for analysis immediately after death. This is rarely the case with human tissue. Therefore, in some cases apparent constitutive MHC expression in the human CNS could be due to the disease causing death or to agonal or postmortem changes.

It seems likely that in vitro studies of MHC expression and antigen presentation by long-term cultured CNS cells may not be very relevant to the in vivo situation. Both tables reflect the substantial differences between the two environments, and this is probably most evident with astrocytes and to some extent EC—at least in terms of MHC class II–restricted responses. It is difficult to draw any firm conclusions from the studies with both astrocytes and EC reporting increased MHC class II–inducibility in vitro in response to IFN-γ in cells derived from rats and mice susceptible to EAE and some types of viral encephalomyelitis. Altered conditions may give opposite results. Moreover, the apparent influence of exogenous substances (which are found in the CNS but not normally in vitro) on astrocytic MHC expression is an important consideration that could also be relevant to EC.

Table 10-1 MHC Expression of CNS Cells In vivo and In vitro

Cell Type	In vivo			In vitro		
	MHC Class I	MHC Class II	Comments	MCH Class I	MHC Class II	Comments
Neurons	- → -(+?)	- → -	?Transactivation by virus but mostly negative	- → +	- → -	Electrically silent neurons may express MHC class I
Oligodendrocytes	- → +	- → -	Consistent results	-(+ → ++	- → -	Constitutive MHC class I reported
Astrocytes	- → +	- → -(+)	Species variable but usually negative	++ → +++	-(+) → ++	Human adult AST constitutively MHC class II+
Microglia (MG)	+/- → +++	-(+) → +++	Constitutive MHC class II, strain variable	++ → +++	- → +++	Data from newborn MG; adult MG data not available
Perivascular cells	++ → ?++	+ → ?++	Postinflammation data not clear	—	—	No data available
Other CNS macrophages	+++ → +++	#PL → ?++	Postinflammation data not clear	—	—	No data available
Endothelial cells	+++ → +++	-(+) → -(++)	Constitutive MHC class II, species variable	+++ → ++	-(+) → ++	Only guinea pig constitutively MHC class II+
Smooth muscle cells/perigiles	+/- → ?	- → ?	Postinflammation data not clear	?+ → ?++	+ → ++	Mouse data only

This information refers to normal (nontransformed) cells and is cumulative data derived from immunohistochemical, immunofluorescent, flow cytometric, or functional analyses. → indicates before (normal CNS in vivo) and after activation or stimulation associated with infection, autoimmunity, or cytokine treatment in vivo or in vitro (usually IFN-γ). Note that MG respond similarly in some noninflammatory disorders, Alzheimer's disease, for example. −, negative. +/−, weak. +, ++, +++, positive but only in some species or animal strains. ?, clear data not available.

Table 10-2 Antigen-Presenting Capacity of CNS Cells In vivo and In vitro

	In vivo		In vitro	
Cell Type	MHC Class I Restricted	MHC Class II Restricted	MHC Class I Restricted	MHC Class II Restricted
Neurons	Possibly with some viral infections, otherwise no	No	No	No
Oligodendrocytes	[a]Possible	No	Yes	No
Astrocytes	[a]Possible	[a,b]Possible	Yes	Yes
Microglia	[a]Possible	[c]Yes	Not tested	Not tested
Perivascular cells	[a]Possible	[c]Yes	Not tested	Not tested
Other CNS macrophages	[a]Possible	[c]Yes	Not tested	Not tested
Endothelial cells	[d]Yes	[e]Species dependent	Yes	[f]Yes
Smooth muscle cells/ pericytes	[a]Possible	[a]Possible	Not tested	[g]Yes

This information refers to normal (nontransformed) cells. MHC class I restricted indicates that the CNS cell type can be a MHC-restricted target for CD8[+] CTL and/or can present alloantigen to naive CD8[+] T cells inducing proliferation. MHC class II restricted indicates the capacity of the different cell types to present protein or alloantigen to primed CD4[+] T cells inducing proliferation or cytokine secretion in the responding T cell and, in some cases, acting as an MHC-restricted target for cytolytic CD4[+] T cells.

[a]On the basis of MHC expression, antigen presentation to CD4[+] or CD8[+] T cells is *possible* although there is no direct evidence for it actually occurring.

[b]Probably is not a significant APC in view of the limited potential for MHC class II expression in vivo.

[c]Evidence from irradiation bone marrow chimera experiments (77). The APC in these experiments could be PVC or other brain macrophages, but not MG.

[d]LCMV-infected EC are almost certainly the target of specific CTL, although this has not been proven formally.

[e]In all species except the guinea pig, EC are probably not a significant APC in view of the limited potential for MHC class II expression in vivo.

[f]Th2 responses > Th1.

[g]Th1 responses > Th2.

MG, unlike astrocytes, readily express MHC molecules in vivo, but there is no evidence to implicate these cells as the APCs of the CNS. Most telling is the increased MHC expression by MG in situations that are essentially nonimmunological (e.g., nerve transection), which indicates that MG express MHC molecules in response to a variety of activation signals unrelated to immune responses. This may place the MG in a state where antigen presentation is possible, but there is no guarantee that the resultant T-cell–MG interaction will lead to T-cell activation (see below).

For CD4+ MHC class II–restricted responses, the irradiation bone marrow chimera studies clearly indicate that populations like PVC and meningeal and choroid macrophages (the experiments cannot distinguish between these) are very effective at presenting antigen (to encephalitogenic cells in vivo). It is very likely that it is these CNS cells which are also responsible for presenting antigen on a routine basis to patrolling

CD4+ T-cell blasts. In the one chimera study where cells of this type were MHC incompatible with injected CD4+ encephalitogenic T cells while resident CNS cells (EC, astrocytes, MG, and so on) were the MHC-compatible elements, EAE was induced but the disease was weak and delayed (165). Thus, the latter cell types are also CNS APCs for CD4+ T cells but appear to be less effective, or possibly they provide negative, anergizing signals to the T cells rather than positive, activating ones. (Note that it is almost certain that resident MG in this latter chimera study would have become MHC class II+ but still disease induction was poor.) In terms of CD8+ MHC class I–restricted responses, it is likely, with the exception of neurons, that all CNS cells, EC in particular, can act as APC.

Unequivocal experiments for testing the APC role of each CNS resident cell are not easy to design. Using cells isolated from neonatal tissue which have been grown for extended periods in vitro may teach us very little about the situation in vivo. The simpler approach to this problem is to isolate and purify cells directly ex vivo and test for T-cell responses to these potential APC. In vivo studies require specific targeting of T cells to each cell type, which can be achieved in transgenic animals by expressing a specific MHC in a given cell. Targeting antigen is probably less useful as there is no guarantee that some of it will not be picked up, processed, and presented secondarily within the CNS by cells other than the one to which it was targeted. To date, studies in transgenic mice (e.g., using GFAP or MBP promoters) have not yielded any data which address the question of antigen presentation by astrocytes or oligos, respectively. The approach clearly has merit however.

Thus, the resolution of the identity of the APC in the CNS is still wanting. With the increasing availability of highly specific cell isolation methods, novel in vivo systems, and transgenic and knock-out technology, however, the answer may be rapidly approaching.

References

1. Achim CL, Wiley CA. Expression of major histocompatibility complex antigens in the brains of patients with progressive multifocal leukoencephalopathy. J Neuropathol Exp Neurol 51:257, 1992.
2. Akiyama H, Itagaki S, McGeer PL. Major histocompatibility complex antigen expression on rat microglia following epidural kainic acid lesions. J Neurosci Res 20:147, 1988.
3. Aloisi F, Borsellino G, Samoggia P, Testa U, Chelucci C, Russo G, Peschle C, Levi G. Astrocyte cultures from human embryonic brain: characterization and modulation of surface molecules by inflammatory cytokines. J Neurosci Res 32:494, 1992.
4. Altmann DM, Hogg N, Trowsdale J, Wilkinson D. Cotransfection of ICAM-1 and HLA-DR reconstitutes human antigen-presenting cell function in mouse L cells. Nature 343:512, 1989.
5. Andersen IH, Marker O, Thomsen AR. Breakdown of blood-brain barrier function in the murine lymphocytic choriomeningitis virus infection mediated by virus-specific CD8+ T cells. J Neuroimmunol 31:155, 1991.

6. Azuma M, Ito D, Yagita H, Okumura K, Phillips JH, Lanier LL, Somoza C. B70 antigen is a second ligand for CTLA-4 and CD28. Nature 366:76, 1993.
7. Barish ME, Raissdana SS. Induction of class II major histocompatibility complex antigens on a population of astrocytes from a mouse strain (BALB/c) resistant to experimental allergic encephalomyelitis. Brain Res 510:329, 1990.
8. Baron JL, Madri JA, Ruddle NH, Hashim G, Janneway CAJ. Surface expression of alpha 4 integrin by CD4 T cells is required for their entry into brain parenchyma. J Exp Med 177:57, 1993.
9. Barrett PN, Koschel K, Carter M, ter Meulen V. Effect of measles virus antibodies on a measles SSPE virus persistently infected C6 rat glioma cell line. J Gen Virol 66:1411, 1985.
10. Birnbaum G, Kotilinek L. Immunologic differences in murine glial cells and their association with susceptibility to experimental allergic encephalomyelitis. J Neuroimmunol 26:119, 1990.
11. Borrow P, Nash AA. Susceptibility to Theiler's virus-induced demyelinating disease correlates with astrocyte class II induction and antigen presentation. Immunology 76:133, 1992.
12. Calder VL, Wolswijk G, Noble M. The differentiation of O-2A progenitor cells into oligodendrocytes is associated with a loss of inducibility of Ia antigens. Eur J Immunol 18:1195, 1988.
13. Cannella B, Cross AH, Raine CS. Upregulation and coexpression of adhesion molecules correlates with relapsing autoimmune demyelination in the central nervous system. J Exp Med 172:1521, 1990.
14. Christinck ER, Luscher MA, Barber BH, Williams DB. Peptide binding to class I MHC on living cells and quantitation of complexes required for CTL lysis. Nature 352:67, 1991.
15. Coutinho GC, Durieu TO, Strosberg AD, Couraud PO. Catecholamines stimulate the IFN-gamma-induced class II MHC expression on bovine brain capillary endothelial cells. J Immunol 147:2525, 1991.
16. Craggs RI, Webster HD. Ia antigens in the normal rat nervous system and in lesions of experimental allergic encephalomyelitis. Acta Neuropathol (Berl) 68:263, 1985.
17. Croft M, Duncan DD, Swain SL. Response of naive antigen-specific CD4+ T cells *in vitro:* Characteristics and antigen-presenting cell requirements. J Exp Med 176:1431, 1992.
18. Czitrom AA, Sunshine GH, Reme T, Ceredig R, Glassebrook AL, Kelso A, MacDonald HR. Stimulator cell requirements for allospecific T cell subsets: specialized cells are required to activate helper but not cytolytic T lymphocyte precursors. J Immunol 130:546, 1983.
19. Daar AS, Fuggle SV, Fabre JW, Ting A, Morris PJ. The detailed distribution of HLA-A, B, C antigens in normal human organs. Transplantation 38:287, 1984.
20. Daar AS, Fuggle SV, Fabre JW, Ting A, Morris PJ. The detailed distribution of MHC Class II antigens in normal human organs. Transplantation 38:293, 1984.
21. Damle NK, Aruffo A. Vascular cell adhesion molecule 1 induces T-cell receptor-dependent activation of CD4+ T lymphocytes. Proc Natl Acad Sci USA 88:6403, 1991.
22. Damoiseaux JGMC, Dopp EA, Calame W, Chao D, Macpherson GG, Dijkstra CD. Rat macrophage lysosomal membrane antigen recognized by monoclonal antibody ED1. Immunology 83:140, 1994.
23. de Groot CJ, Huppes W, Sminia T, Kraal G, Dijkstra CD. Determination of the origin and nature of brain macrophages and microglial cells in mouse central nervous system, using non-radioactive *in situ* hybridization techniques. Glia 6:301, 1992.
24. de Groot CJ, Sminia T, Dijkstra CD. Isolation and characterization of brain macrophages

from the central nervous system of newborn and adult rats and of rats with experimental allergic encephalomyelitis. Immunobiology 179:314, 1989.

25. de Groot CJ, Sminia T, Dijkstra CD, Van der Pal RH, Lopes-Cardozo M. Interferon-gamma induced IA antigen expression on cultured neuroglial cells and brain macrophages from rat spinal cord and cerebrum. Int J Neurosci 59:53, 1991.

26. del rio Hortega P. In: Cytology and Cellular Pathology of the Nervous System, W Penfield, ed. Hoeber, New York, 1932, p 481.

27. Demotz S, Grey HM, Sette A. The minimal number of class II MHC-antigen complexes needed for T cell activation. Science 249:1028, 1990.

28. Deschl U, Stitz L, Herzog S, Frese K, Rott R. Determination of immune cells and expression of major histocompatibility complex class II antigen in encephalitic lesions of experimental Borna disease. Acta Neuropathol (Berl) 81:41, 1990.

29. Dijkstra CD, Dopp EA, Joling P, Kraal G. The heterogeneity of mononuclear phagocytes in lymphoid organs: distinct macrophage subpopulations in the rat recognized by monoclonal antibodies ED1, ED2 and ED3. Immunology 54:589, 1985.

30. Doherty PC, Allan JE. Role of the major histocompatibility complex in targeting effector T cells into a site of virus infection. Eur J Immunol 16:1237, 1986.

31. Doherty PC, Allan JE, Lynch F, Ceredig R. Dissection of an inflammatory process induced by CD8+ T cells. Immunol Today 11:55, 1990.

32. Doherty PC, Ceredig R, Allan JE. Immunogenetic analysis of cellular interactions governing the recruitment of T lymphocytes and monocytes in lymphocytic choriomeningitis virus-induced immunopathology. Clin Immunol Immunopathol 47:19, 1988.

33. DuBois JH, Hammond-Tooke GD, Cuzner ML. Expression of major histocompatibility complex antigens in neonate rat primary mixed glial cultures. J Neuroimmunol 9:363, 1985.

34. Duguid J, Trzepacz C. Major histocompatibility complex genes have an increased brain expression after scrapie infection. Proc Natl Acad Sci USA 90:114, 1993.

35. Durie FH, Foy TM, Noelle RJ. The role of CD40 and its ligand (gp39) in peripheral and central tolerance and its contribution to autoimmune disease. Res Immunol 145:200, 1994.

36. Esiri MM, Gay D. Immunological and neuropathological significance of the Virchow-Robin space. J Neurol Sci 100:3, 1990.

37. Esiri MM, Reading MC. Macrophage populations associated with multiple sclerosis plaques. Neuropathol Appl Neurobiol 13:451, 1987.

38. Fabry Z, Sandor M, Gajewski TF, Herlein JA, Waldschmidt MM, Lynch RG, Hart MN. Differential activation of Th1 and Th2 CD4+ cells by murine brain microvessel endothelial cells and smooth muscle/pericytes. J Immunol 151:38, 1993.

39. Fabry Z, Waldschmidt MM, Moore SA, Hart MN. Antigen presentation by brain microvessel smooth muscle and endothelium. J Neuroimmunol 28:63, 1990.

40. Fabry Z, Waldschmidt MM, Van Dyk L, Moore SA, Hart MN. Activation of CD4+ lymphocytes by syngeneic brain microvascular smooth muscle cells. J Immunol 145:1099, 1990.

41. Fierz W, Endler B, Reske K, Wekerle H, Fontana A. Astrocytes as antigen-presenting cells. I. Induction of Ia antigen expression on astrocytes by T cells via immune interferon and its effect on antigen presentation. J Immunol 134:3785, 1985.

42. Fischer HG, Nitzgen B, Germann T, Degitz K, Daubener W, Hadding U. Differentiation driven by granulocyte-macrophage colony-stimulating factor endows microglia with interferon-gamma-independent antigen presentation function. J Neuroimmunol 42:87, 1993.

43. Fleming JO, Wang FI, Trousdale MD, Hinton DR, Stohlman SA. Immunopathogenesis of demyelination induced by MHV-4. Adv Exp Med Biol 276:565, 1990.
44. Fleury SG, Croteau G, Sékaly R-P. CD4 and CD8 recognition of class II and class I molecules of the major histocompatibility complex. Semin Immunol 3:177, 1991.
45. Fontana A, Erb P, Pircher H, Zinkernagel R, Weber E, Fierz W. Astrocytes as antigen-presenting cells. Part II; Unlike H-2K-dependent cytotoxic T cells, H-2Ia-restricted T cells are only stimulated in the presence of interferon-γ. J Neuroimmunol 12:15, 1986.
46. Fontana A, Fierz W, Wekerle H. Astrocytes present myelin basic protein to encephalitogenic T-cell lines. Nature 307:273, 1984.
47. Ford AL, Goodsall AL, Hickey WF, Sedgwick JD. Normal adult ramified microglia separated from other central nervous system macrophages by flow cytometric sorting. Phenotypic differences defined and direct ex vivo antigen presentation to myelin basic protein-reactive CD4+ T cells compared. J Immunol 154:4309, 1995.
48. Foy TM, Durie FH, Noelle RJ. The expansive role of CD40 and its ligand, gp39, in immunity. Semin Immunol 6:259, 1994.
49. Frank E, Pulver M, de Tribolet N. Expression of class II major histocompatibility antigens on reactive astrocytes and endothelial cells within the gliosis surrounding metastases and abscesses. J Neuroimmunol 12:29, 1986.
50. Freeman GJ, Borriello F, Hodes RJ, Reiser H, Hathcock KS, Laszlo G, McKnight AJ, Kim J, Du L, Lombard DB, Gray GS, Nadler LM, Sharpe AH. Uncovering of functional alternative CTLA-4 counter-receptor in B7-deficient mice. Science 262:907, 1993.
51. Freeman GJ, Gribben JG, Boussiotis VA, Ng JW, Restivo VA, Lombard LA, Gray GS, Nadler LM. Cloning of B7-2: a CTLA-4 counter-receptor that costimulates human T cell proliferation. Science 262:909, 1993.
52. Frei K, Bodmer S, Schwerdel C, Fontana A. Astrocyte-derived interleukin 3 as a growth factor for microglia cells and peritoneal macrophages. J Immunol 137:3521, 1986.
53. Frei K, Siepl C, Groscurth P, Bodmer S, Schwerdel C, Fontana A. Antigen presentation and tumor cytotoxicity by interferon-γ-treated microglial cells. Eur J Immunol 17:1271, 1987.
54. Frohman EM, Frohman TC, Dustin ML, Vayuvegula B, Choi B, Gupta A, van den Noort S, Gupta S. The induction of intercellular adhesion molecule 1 (ICAM-1) expression on human fetal astrocytes by interferon-gamma, tumor necrosis factor alpha, lymphotoxin, and interleukin-1: relevance to intracerebral antigen presentation. J Neuroimmunol 23:117, 1989.
55. Frohman EM, Vayuvegula B, Gupta S, van den Noort S. Norepinephrine inhibits gamma-interferon-induced major histocompatibility class II (Ia) antigen expression on cultured astrocytes via beta-2-adrenergic signal transduction mechanisms. Proc Natl Acad Sci USA 85:1292, 1988.
56. Gairin JE, Joly E, Oldstone MB. Persistent infection with lymphocytic choriomeningitis virus enhances expression of MHC class I glycoprotein on cultured mouse brain endothelial cells. J Immunol 146:3953, 1991.
57. Gehrmann J, Gold R, Linington C, Lannes-Vieira J, Wekerle H, Kreutzberg GW. Microglial involvement in experimental autoimmune inflammation of the central and peripheral nervous system. Glia 7:50, 1993.
58. Gehrmann J, Monaco S, Kreutzberg GW. Spinal cord microglia and DRG satellite cells respond rapidly to transection of the rat sciatic nerve. Restor Neurol Neurosci 2:181, 1991.
59. Giulian D, Baker TJ, Shih L-CN, Lachman LB. Interleukin 1 of the central nervous system is produced by ameboid microglia. J Exp Med 164:594, 1986.
60. Graeber MB, Streit WJ. Perivascular cells defined. Trends Neurosci 13:366, 1990.

61. Graeber MB, Streit WJ, Buringer D, Sparks DL, Kreutzberg GW. Ultrastructural location of major histocompatibility complex (MHC) class II positive perivascular cells in histologically normal human brain. J Neuropathol Exp Neurol 51:303, 1992.

62. Graeber MB, Streit WJ, Kiefer R, Schoen SW, Kreutzberg GW. New expression of myelomonocytic antigens by microglia and perivascular cells following lethal motor neuron injury. J Neuroimmunol 27:121, 1990.

63. Graeber MB, Streit WJ, Kreutzberg GW. Axotomy of the rat facial nerve leads to increased CR3 complement receptor expression by activated microglial cells. J Neurosci Res 21:18, 1988.

64. Graeber MB, Tetzlaff W, Streit WJ, Kreutzberg GW. Microglial cells but not astrocytes undergo mitosis following rat facial nerve axotomy. Neurosci Lett 85:317, 1988.

65. Grenier Y, Ruijs TC, Robitaille Y, Olivier A, Antel JP. Immunohistochemical studies of adult human glial cells. J Neuroimmunol 21:103, 1989.

66. Harding FA, McArthur JG, Gross JA, Raulet DH, Allison JP. CD28-mediated signalling costimulates murine T cells and prevents induction of anergy in T-cell clones. Nature 356:607, 1992.

67. Hart DN, Fabre JW. Quantitative studies on the tissue distribution of Ia and SD antigens in the DA and Lewis rat strains. Transplantation 27:110, 1979.

68. Hart DN, Fabre JW. Demonstration and characterization of Ia-positive dendritic cells in the interstitial connective tissues of rat heart and other tissues, but not brain. J Exp Med 154:347, 1981.

69. Hart MN, Waldschmidt MM, Hanley HJ, Moore SA, Kemp JD, Schelper RL. Brain microvascular smooth muscle expresses class II antigens. J Immunol 138:2960, 1987.

70. Hathcock KS, Laszlo G, Dickler HB, Bradshaw J, Linsley P, Hodes RJ. Identification of an alternative CTLA-4 ligand costimulatory for T cell activation. Science 262:905, 1993.

71. Hauser SL, Bhan AK, Gilles FH, Hoban CJ, Reinherz EL, Schlossman SF, Weiner HL. Immunohistochemical staining of human brain with monoclonal antibodies that identify lymphocytes, monocytes, and the Ia antigen. J Neuroimmunol 5:197, 1983.

72. Hayashi T, Morimoto C, Burks JS, Kerr C, Hauser SL. Dual-label immunocytochemistry of the active multiple sclerosis lesion: major histocompatibility complex and activation antigens. Ann Neurol 24:523, 1988.

73. Hayes GM, Woodroofe MN, Cuzner ML. Microglia are the major cell type expressing MHC class II in human white matter. J Neurol Sci 80:25, 1987.

74. Hayes GM, Woodroofe MN, Cuzner ML. Characterization of microglia isolated from adult human and rat brain. J Neuroimmunol 19:177, 1988.

75. Hickey WF, Hsu BL, Kimura H. T-lymphocyte entry into the central nervous system. J Neurosci Res 28:254, 1991.

76. Hickey WF, Kimura, H. Graft-vs.-host disease elicits expression of class I and class II histocompatibility antigens and the presence of scattered T lymphocytes in rat central nervous system. Proc Natl Acad Sci USA. 84:2082, 1987.

77. Hickey WF, Kimura H. Perivascular microglial cells of the CNS are bone marrow-derived and present antigen *in vivo*. Science 239:290, 1988.

78. Hickey WF, Osborn JP, Kirby WM. Expression of Ia molecules by astrocytes during acute experimental allergic encephalomyelitis in the Lewis rat. Cell Immunol 91:528, 1985.

79. Hickey WF, Vass K, Lassmann H. Bone marrow-derived elements in the central nervous system: an immunohistochemical and ultrastructural survey of rat chimeras. J Neuropathol Exp Neurol 51:246, 1992.

80. Hinrichs DJ, Wegmann KW, Dietsch GN. Transfer of experimental allergic encepha-

lomyelitis to bone marrow chimeras. Endothelial cells are not a restricting element. J Exp Med 166:1906, 1987.

81. Hirayama M, Miyadai T, Yokochi T, Sato K, Kubota T, Iida M, Fujiki N. Infection of human T-lymphotropic virus type I to astrocytes in vitro with induction of the class II major histocompatibility complex. Neurosci Lett 92:34, 1988.

82. Hirayama M, Yokochi T, Shimokata K, Iida M, Fujiki N. Induction of human leukocyte antigen-A,B,C and -DR on cultured human oligodendrocytes and astrocytes by human gamma-interferon. Neurosci Lett 72:369, 1986.

83. Nirsch MR, Wietzerbin J, Pierres M, Goridis C. Expression of Ia antigens by cultured astrocytes treated with gama interferon. Neurosci Lett 41:199, 1983.

84. Hirschberg H, Braathen LR, Thorsby E. Antigen presentation by vascular endothelial cells and epidermal Langerhan cells: the role of HLA-DR. Immunol Rev 66:57, 1982.

85. Inaba K, Steinman RM. Resting and sensitized T lymphocytes exhibit distinct stimulatory (antigen-presenting cell) requirements for growth and lymphokine release. J Exp Med 160:1717, 1984.

86. Inaba, K, Young JW, Steinman RM. Direct activation of CD8+ cytotoxic T lymphocytes by dendritic cells. J Exp Med 166:182, 1987.

87. Itagaki S, McGeer PL, Akiyama H. Presence of T-cytotoxic suppressor and leucocyte common antigen positive cells in Alzheimer's disease brain tissue. Neurosci Lett 91:259, 1988.

88. Janeway CAJ. The co-receptor function of CD4. Semin Immunol 3:153, 1991.

89. Jemison LA, Williams SK, Lublin FD, Knobler RL, Korngold R. Interferon-γ-inducible endothelial cell class II major histocompatibility complex expression correlates with strain- and site-specific susceptibility to experimental allergic encephalomyelitis. J Neuroimmunol 47:15, 1993.

90. Joly E, Mucke L, Oldstone MB. Viral persistence in neurons explained by lack of major histocompatibility class I expression. Science 253:1283, 1991.

91. Jones RE, Bourdette DN, Whitham RH, Offner H, Vandenbark AA. Induction of experimental autoimmune encephalomyelitis in severe combined immunodeficient mice reconstituted with allogeneic or xenogeneic hematopoietic cells. J Immunol 150:4620, 1993.

92. Joseph J, Knobler RL, Lublin FD, Hart MN. Differential modulation of MHC class I antigen expression on mouse brain endothelial cells by MHC-4 infection. J Neuroimmunol 22:241, 1989.

93. Keane RW, Tallent MW, Podack ER. Resistance and susceptibility of neural cells to lysis by cytotoxic lymphocytes and by cytolytic granules. Transplantation 54:520, 1992.

94. Kiefer R, Kreutzberg GW. Effects of dexamethasone on microglial activation in vivo: selective downregulation of major histocompatibility complex class II expression in regenerating facial nucleus. J Neuroimmunol 34:99, 1991.

95. Kiefer R, Lindholm D, Kreutzberg GW. Interleukin-6 and transforming growth factor-beta 1 mRNAs are induced in rat facial nucleus following motoneuron axotomy. Eur J Neurosci 5:775, 1993.

96. Kim SU, Moretto G, Shin DH. Expression of Ia antigens on the surface of human oligodendrocytes and astrocytes in culture. J Neuroimmunol 10:141, 1985.

97. Kohsaka S, Shinozaki T, Nakano Y, Takei K, Toya S, Tsukada Y. Expression of Ia antigen on vascular endothelial cells in mouse cerebral tissue grafted into the third ventricle of rat brain. Brain Res 484:340, 1989.

98. Koide SL, Inaba K, Steinman RM. Interleukin 1 enhances T-dependent immune responses by amplifying the function of dendritic cells. J Exp Med 165:515, 1987.

99. Konno H, Yamamoto T, Suzuki H, Yamamoto H, Iwasaki Y, Ohara Y, Terunuma H, Harata

N. Targeting of adoptively transferred experimental allergic encephalitis lesion at the sites of wallerian degeneration. Acta Neuropathol (Berl) 80:521, 1990.

100. Korngold R, Feldman A, Rorke LB, Lublin FD, Doherty PC. Acute experimental allergic encephalomyelitis in radiation bone marrow chimeras between high and low susceptible strains of mice. Immunogenetics 24:309, 1986.

101. Kosaka H, Surh CD, Sprent J. Stimulation of mature unprimed CD8+ T cells by semi-professional antigen-presenting cells *in vivo*. J Exp Med 176:1291, 1992.

102. Kraus E, Schneider-Schaulies S, Miyasaka M, Tamatani T, Sedgwick J. Augmentation of major histocompatibility complex class I and ICAM-1 expression on glial cells following measles virus infection: evidence for the role of type-1 interferon. Eur J Immunol 22:175, 1992.

103. Lampert IA, Suitters AJ, Chisholm PM. Expression of Ia antigen on epidermal keratinocytes in graft-versus host disease. Nature 293:149, 1981.

104. Lampson LA, Hickey WF. Monoclonal antibody analysis of MHC expression in human brain biopsies: tissue ranging from "histologically normal" to that showing different levels of glial tumor involvement. J Immunol 136:4054, 1986.

105. Lassmann H, Schmied M, Vass K, Hickey WF. Bone marrow derived elements and resident microglia in brain inflammation. Glia 7:19, 1993.

106. Lassmann H, Zimprich F, Vass K, Hickey WF. Microglial cells are a component of the perivascular glia limitans. J Neurosci Res 28:236, 1991.

107. Lavi E, Suzumura A, Murasko DM, Murray EM, Silberberg DH, Weiss SR. Tumor necrosis factor induces expression of MHC class I antigens on mouse astrocytes. J Neuroimmunol 18:245, 1988.

108. Lee SC, Collins M, Vanguri P, Shin ML. Glutamate differentially inhibits the expression of class II MHC antigens on astrocytes and microglia. J Immunol 148:3391, 1992.

109. Lee SC, Liu W, Brosnan CF, Dickson DW. Characterization of primary human fetal dissociated central nervous system cultures with an emphasis on microglia. Lab Invest 67:465, 1992.

110. Levine B, Hardwick JM, Trapp BD, Crawford TO, Bollinger RC, Griffin DE. Antibody-mediated clearance of alphavirus infection from neurons. Science 254:856, 1991.

111. Lichtman AH, Chin J, Schmidt JA, Abbas AK. Role of interleukin 1 in the activation of T lymphocytes. Proc Natl Acad Sci USA 85:9699, 1988.

112. Lisak RP, Hirayama M, Kuchmy D, Rosenzweig A, Kim SU, Pleasure DE, Silberberg DH. Cultured human and rat oligodendrocytes and rat Schwann cells do not have immune response gene associated antigen (Ia) on their surface. Brain Res 289:285, 1983.

113. Liu Y, Jones B, Aruffo A, Sullivan KM, Linsley PS, Janeway CAJ. The heat-stable antigen is a co-stimulatory molecule for T cell growth. J Exp Med 175:437, 1992.

114. Liu Y, King N, Kesson A, Blanden RV, Müllbacher A. Flavivirus infection up-regulates the expression of class I and class II major histocompatibility antigens on and enhances T cell recognition of astrocytes *in vitro*. J Neuroimmunol 21:157, 1989.

115. Liu Y, Linsley PS. Costimulation of T-cell growth. Curr Opin Immunol 4:265, 1992.

116. Liu Y, Mullbacher A. Astrocytes are not susceptible to lysis by natural killer cells. J Neuroimmunol 19:101, 1988.

117. Loughlin AJ, Woodroofe MN, Cuzner ML. Regulation of Fc receptor and major histocompatibility complex antigen expression on isolated rat microglia by tumour necrosis factor, interleukin-1 and lipopolysaccharide: effects on interferon-gamma induced activation. Immunology 75:170, 1992.

118. Luber NJ, Rogers J. Immune system associated antigens expressed by cells of the human central nervous system. Neurosci Lett 94:17, 1988.

119. Lublin FD, Knobler RL, Doherty PC, Korngold R. Relapsing experimental allergic encephalomyelitis in radiation bone marrow chimeras between high and low susceptible strains of mice. Clin Exp Immunol 66:491, 1986.

120. Lublin FD, Knobler RL, Marini J, Goldowitz D. Brain transplantation in genetic analysis of experimental allergic encephalomyelitis. Ann NY Acad Sci 540:252, 1988.

121. Ludowyk PA, Willenborg DO, Parish CR. Selective localisation of neuro-specific T lymphocytes in the central nervous system. J Neuroimmunol 37:237, 1992.

122. Macatonia SE, Taylor PM, Knight SC, Askonas BA. Primary stimulation by dendritic cells induces antiviral proliferative and cytotoxic T cell responses *in vitro*. J Exp Med 169:1255, 1989.

123. Maehlen J, Olsson T, Love A, Klareskog L, Norrby E, Kristensson K. Persistence of measles virus in rat brain neurons is promoted by depletion of CD8+ cells. J Neuroimmunol 21:149, 1989.

124. Maehlen J, Olsson T, Zachau A, Klareskog L, Kristensson K. Local enhancement of major histocompatibility complex (MHC) class I and II expression and cell infiltration in experimental allergic encephalomyelitis around axotomized motor neurons. J Neuroimmunol 23:125, 1989.

125. Maehlen J, Schroder HD, Klareskog L, Olsson T, Kristensson K. Axotomy induces MHC class I antigen expression on rat nerve cells. Neurosci Lett 92:8, 1988.

126. Main EK, Monos DS, Lampson LA. IFN-treated neuroblastoma cell lines remain resistant to T cell-mediated allo-killing, and susceptible to non-MHC-restricted cytotoxicity. J Immunol 141:2943, 1988.

127. Male D, Pryce G. Synergy between interferons and monokines in MHC induction on brain endothelium. Immunol Lett 17:267, 1988.

128. Male D, Pryce G. Induction of Ia molecules on brain endothelium is related to susceptibility to experimental allergic encephalomyelitis. J Neuroimmunol 21:87, 1989.

129. Male D, Pryce G, Rahman J. Comparison of the immunological properties of rat cerebral and aortic endothelium. J Neuroimmunol 30:161, 1990.

130. Male DK, Pryce G, Hughes CC. Antigen presentation in brain: MHC induction on brain endothelium and astrocytes compared. Immunology 60:453, 1987.

131. Malipiero UV, Frei K, Fontana A. Production of hemopoietic colony-stimulating factors by astrocytes. J Immunol 144:3816, 1990.

132. Martin PJ, Ledbetter JA, Morishita Y, June CH, Beatty PG, Hansen JA. A 44 kilodalton cell surface homodimer regulates interleukin 2 production by activated human T lymphocytes. J Immunol 136:3282, 1986.

133. Mason DW, Dallman M, Barclay AN. Graft-versus-host disease induces expression of Ia antigen in rat epidermal cells and gut epithelium. Nature 293:150, 1981.

134. Massa PT. Specific suppression of major histocompatibility complex class I and class II genes in astrocytes by brain-enriched gangliosides. J Exp Med 178:1357, 1993.

135. Massa PT, Brinkmann R, ter Meulen V. Inducibility of Ia antigen on astrocytes by murine coronavirus JHM is rat strain dependent. J Exp Med 166:259, 1987.

136. Massa PT, Dorries R, ter Meulen V. Viral particles induce Ia antigen expression on astrocytes. Nature 320:543, 1986.

137. Massa PT, Ozato K, McFarlin DE. Cell type-specific regulation of major histocompatibility complex (MHC) class I gene expression in astrocytes, oligodendrocytes and neurons. Glia 8:201, 1993.

138. Massa PT, Schimpl A, Wecker E, ter Meulen V. Tumor necrosis factor amplifies measles virus-mediated Ia induction on astrocytes. Proc Natl Acad Sci USA 84:7242, 1987.

139. Massa PT, ter Meulen V. Analysis of Ia induction on Lewis rat astrocytes in vitro by virus particles and bacterial adjuvants. J Neuroimmunol 13:259, 1987.

140. Massa PT, ter Meulen V, Fontana A. Hyperinducibility of Ia antigen on astrocytes correlates with strain-specific susceptibility to experimental autoimmune encephalomyelitis. Proc Natl Acad Sci USA. 84:4219, 1987.

141. Mato M, Aikawa E, Mato TK, Kurihara K. Tridimensional observation of fluorescent granular perithelial (FGP) cells in rat cerebral blood vessels. Anat Rec 215:413, 1986.

142. Mato M, Ookawara S, Saito-Taki T. Serological determinants of fluorescent granular perithelial cells along small cerebral blood vessels in rodent. Acta Neuropathol (Berl) 72:117, 1986.

143. Matsumoto Y, Fujiwara M. In situ detection of class I and II major histocompatibility complex antigens in the rat central nervous system during experimental allergic encephalomyelitis. An immunohistochemical study. J Neuroimmunol 12:265, 1986.

144. Matsumoto Y, Fujiwara M. Absence of donor-type major histocompatibility complex class I antigen-bearing microglia in the rat central nervous system of radiation bone marrow chimeras. J Neuroimmunol 17:71, 1987.

145. Matsumoto Y, Hara N, Tanaka R, Fujiwara M. Immunohistochemical analysis of the rat central nervous system during experimental allergic encephalomyelitis, with special reference to Ia-positive cells with dendritic morphology. J Immunol 136:3668, 1986.

146. Matsumoto Y, Kawai K, Fujiwara M. In situ Ia expression on brain cells in the rat: autoimmune encephalomyelitis-resistant strain (BN) and susceptible strain (Lewis) compared. Immunology 66:621, 1989.

147. Matsumoto Y, Ohmori K, Fujiwara M. Immune regulation by brain cells in the central nervous system: microglia but not astrocytes present myelin basic protein to encephalitogenic T cells under in vivo-mimicking conditions. Immunology 76:209, 1992.

148. Matsumoto Y, Watabe K, Ikura F. Immunohistochemical study on neuroglia identified by the monoclonal antibody against a macrophage differentiation antigen (Mac-1). J Neuroimmunol 9:379, 1985.

149. Mattiace LA, Davies P, Dickson DW. Detection of HLA-DR on microglia in the human brain is a function of both clinical and technical factors. Am J Pathol 136:1101, 1990.

150. Matyszak MK, Lawson LJ, Perry VH, Gordon S. Stromal macrophages of the choroid plexus situated at an interface between the brain and peripheral immune system constitutively express major histocompatibility class II antigens. J Neuroimmunol 40:173, 1992.

151. Mauerhoff T, Pujol BR, Mirakian R, Bottazzo GF. Differential expression and regulation of major histocompatibility complex (MHC) products in neural and glial cells of the human fetal brain. J Neuroimmunol 18:271, 1988.

152. McCarron RM, Kempski O, Spatz M, McFarlin DE. Presentation of myelin basic protein by murine cerebral vascular endothelial cells. J Immunol 134:3100, 1985.

153. McCarron RM, Racke M, Spatz M, McFarlin DE. Cerebral vascular endothelial cells are effective targets for in vitro lysis by encephalitogenic T lymphocytes. J Immunol 147:503, 1991.

154. McCarron RM, Spatz M, Kempski O, Hogan RN, Muehl L, McFarlin DE. Interaction between myelin basic protein-sensitized T lymphocytes and murine cerebral vascular endothelial cells. J Immunol 137:3428, 1986.

155. McCarron RM, Wang L, Cowan EP, Spatz M. Class II MHC antigen expression by cultured human cerebral vascular endothelial cells. Brain Res 566:325, 1991.

156. McDonald WI, Barnes D. Lessons from magnetic resonance imaging in multiple sclerosis. Trends Neurosci 12:376, 1989.

157. Merrill JE, Kono DH, Clayton J, Ando DG, Hinton DR, Hofman FM. Inflammatory

leukocytes and cytokines in the peptide-induced disease of experimental allergic encephalomyelitis in SJL and B10.PL mice. Proc Natl Acad Sci USA 89:574, 1992.

158. Metlay JP, Pure E, Steinman RM. Control of the immune response at the level of antigen-presenting cells: a comparison of the function of dendritic cells and B lymphocytes. Adv Immunol 47:45, 1989.

159. Moingeon P, Chang H, Wallner BP, Stebbins C, Frey AZ, Reinherz EL. CD2-mediated adhesion facilitates T lymphocyte antigen recognition function. Nature 339:312, 1989.

160. Molleston MC, Thomas ML, Hickey WF. Novel major histocompatibility complex expression by microglia and site-specific experimental allergic encephalomyelitis lesions in the rat central nervous system after optic nerve transection. Adv Neurol 59:337, 1993.

161. Momburg F, Koch N, Moller P, Moldenhauer G, Butcher GW, Hammerling GJ. Differential expression of Ia and Ia-associated invariant chain in mouse tissues after in vivo treatment with IFN-gamma. J Immunol 136:940, 1986.

162. Moore SC, McCormack JM, Armendariz E, Gatewood J, Walker WS. Phenotypes and alloantigen-presenting activity of individual clones of microglia derived from the mouse brain. J Neuroimmunol 41:203, 1992.

163. Morris A, Tomkins PT, Maudsley DJ, Blackman M. Infection of cultured murine brain cells by Semliki Forest virus: effects of interferon-αβ on viral replication, viral antigen display, major histocompatibility complex antigen display and lysis by cytotoxic T lymphocytes. J Gen Virol 68:99, 1987.

164. Mößner R, Sedgwick J, Flory E, Körner H, Wege H, ter Meulen V. Astrocytes as antigen presenting cells for primary and secondary T cell responses. Effect of astrocyte infection by murine hepatitis virus. Adv Exp Med Biol 276:647, 1991.

165. Myers KJ, Dougherty JP, Ron Y. In vivo antigen presentation by both brain parenchymal cells and hematopoietically derived cells during the induction of experimental autoimmune encephalomyelitis. J Immunol 151:2252, 1993.

166. Natali PG, De Martino C, Pellegrino MA, Ferrone S. Analysis of the expression of I-Ak-like antigens in murine fetal and adult tissues with the monoclonal antibody 10-2.16. Scand J Immunol 13:541, 1981.

167. Nathanson JA, Chun LL. Immunological function of the blood-cerebrospinal fluid barrier. Proc Natl Acad Sci USA. 86:1684, 1989.

168. Neumann H, Cavalie A, Jenne DE, Wekerle H. Induction of MHC class I genes in neurons. Science 269:549, 1995.

169. Nicholas MK, Antel JP, Stefansson K, Arnason BG. Rejection of fetal neocortical neural transplants by H-2 incompatible mice. J Immunol 139:2275, 1987.

170. Ohmori K, Hong Y, Fujiwara M, Matsumoto Y. In situ demonstration of proliferating cells in the rat central nervous system during experimental autoimmune encephalomyelitis. Evidence suggesting that most infiltrating cells do not proliferate in the target organ. Lab Invest 66:54, 1992.

171. Oldstone MB, Blount P, Southern PJ, Lampert PW. Cytoimmunotherapy for persistent virus infection reveals a unique clearance pattern from the central nervous system. Nature 321:239, 1986.

172. Olsson T, Diener P, Ljungdahl A, Hojeberg B, van der Meide P, Kristensson K. Facial nerve transection causes expansion of myelin autoreactive T cells in regional lymph nodes and T cells homing to the facial nucleus. Autoimmunity 13:117, 1992.

173. Pardridge WM, Yang J, Buciak J, Tourtellotte WW. Human brain microvascular DR-antigen. J Neurosci Res 23:337, 1989.

174. Park JK, Rosenstein YJ, O'Donnell R, Bierer BE, Rosen FS, Burakoff SJ. Enhancement of

T cell activation by the CD43 molecule whose expression is defective in Wiskott-Aldrich syndrome. Nature 350:706, 1991.

175. Perry VH, Gordon S. Macrophages and microglia in the nervous system. Trends Neurosci 11:273, 1988.

176. Pober JS, Gimbrone MAJ, Cotran RS, Reiss CS, Burakoff SJ, Fiers W, Ault KA. Ia expression by vascular endothelium is inducible by activated T cells and by human γ interferon. J Exp Med 157:1339, 1983.

177. Polman CH, Dijkstra CD, Sminia T, Koetsier JC. Immunohistological analysis of macrophages in the central nervous system of lewis rats and acute experimental allergic encephalomyelitis. J Neuroimmunol 11:215, 1986.

178. Porcelli S, Morita CT, Brenner MB. CD1b restricts the response of human CD4-CD8- T lymphocytes to a microbial antigen. Nature 360:593, 1992.

179. Pryce G, Male D, Sedgwick J. Antigen presentation in brain: brain endothelial cells are poor stimulators of T-cell proliferation. Immunology 66:207, 1989.

180. Pulver M, Carrel S, Mach JP, de Tribolet N. Cultured human fetal astrocytes can be induced by interferon-gamma to express HLA-DR. J Neuroimmunol 14:123, 1987.

181. Ransohoff RM, Estes ML. Astrocyte expression of major histocompatibility complex gene products in multiple sclerosis brain tissue obtained by stereotactic biopsy. Arch Neurol 48:1244, 1991.

182. Rao K, Lund RD. Degeneration of optic axons induces the expression of major histocompatibility antigens. Brain Res 488:332, 1989.

183. Richt JA, Stitz L, Wekerle H, Rott R. Borna disease, a progressive meningoencephalomyelitis as a model for CD4 T cell-mediated immunopathology in the brain. J Exp Med 170:1045, 1989.

184. Rieske E, Graeber MB, Tetzlaff W, Czlonkowska A, Streit WJ, Kreutzberg GW. Microglia and microglia-derived brain macrophages in culture: generation from axotomized rat facial nuclei, identification and characterization in vitro. Brain Res 492:1, 1989.

185. Rinner WA, Bauer J, Schmidts M, Lassmann H, Hickey WF. Resident microglia and hematogenous macrophages as phagocytes in adoptively transferred experimental autoimmune encephalomyelitis—an investigation using rat radiation bone marrow chimeras. Glia 14:257, 1995.

186. Risau W, Engelhardt B, Wekerle H. Immune function of the blood-brain barrier: incomplete presentation of protein (auto-)antigens by rat brain microvascular endothelium in vitro. J Cell Biol 110:1757, 1990.

187. Roberge FG, Caspi RR, Nussenblatt RB. Glial retinal Muller cells produce IL-1 activity and have a dual effect on autoimmune T helper lymphocytes. Antigen presentation manifested after removal of suppressive activity. J Immunol 140:2193, 1988.

188. Rodriguez M, Leibowitz JL, Lampert PW. Persistent infection of oligodendrocytes in Theiler's virus-induced encephalomyelitis. Ann Neurol 13:426, 1983.

189. Rodriguez M, Pierce ML, Howie EA. Immune response gene products (Ia antigens) on glial and endothelial cells in virus-induced demyelination. J Immunol 138:3438, 1987.

190. Ronchese F, Hausmann B. B lymphocytes *in vivo* fail to prime naive T cells but can stimulate antigen-experienced T lymphocytes. J Exp Med 177:679, 1993.

191. Rössler K, Neuchrist C, Kitz K, Scheiner O, Kraft D, Lassmann H. Expression of leucocyte adhesion molecules at the human blood-brain barrier (BBB). J Neurosci Res 31:365, 1992.

192. Ruijs TC, Freedman MS, Grenier YG, Olivier A, Antel JP. Human oligodendrocytes are susceptible to cytolysis by major histocompatibility complex class I-restricted lymphocytes. J Neuroimmunol 27:89, 1990.

193. Ruijs TC, Louste K, Brown EA, Antel JP. Lysis of human glial cells by major histocompatibility complex-unrestricted CD4+ cytotoxic lymphocytes. J Neuroimmunol. 42:105, 1993.

194. Sakai K, Tabira T, Endoh M, Steinman L. Ia expression in chronic relapsing experimental allergic encephalomyelitis induced by long-term cultured T cell lines in mice. Lab Invest 54:345, 1986.

195. Sasaki A, Levison SW, Ting JP. Comparison and quantitation of Ia antigen expression on cultured macroglia and ameboid microglia from Lewis rat cerebral cortex: analyses and implications. J Neuroimmunol 25:63, 1989.

196. Sasaki A, Levison SW, Ting JP. Differential suppression of interferon-gamma-induced Ia antigen expression on cultured rat astroglia and microglia by second messengers. J Neuroimmunol 29:213, 1990.

197. Sasaki A, Nakazato Y. The identity of cells expressing MHC class II antigens in normal and pathological human brain. Neuropathol Appl Neurobiol 18:13, 1992.

198. Satoh J, Kim SU, Kastrukoff LF, Takei F. Expression and induction of intercellular adhesion molecules (ICAMs) and major histocompatibility complex (MHC) antigens on cultured murine oligodendrocytes and astrocytes. J Neurosci Res 29:1, 1991.

199. Sedgwick J, Brostoff S, Mason D. Experimental allergic encephalomyelitis in the absence of a classical delayed-type hypersensitivity reaction. Severe paralytic disease correlates with the presence of interleukin 2 receptor-positive cells infiltrating the central nervous system. J Exp Med 165:1058, 1987.

200. Sedgwick JD, Dörries R. The immune system response to viral infection of the CNS. Semin Neurosci 3:93, 1991.

201. Sedgwick JD, Hughes CC, Male DK, MacPhee IA, ter Meulen V. Antigen-specific damage to brain vascular endothelial cells mediated by encephalitogenic and nonencephalitogenic CD4+ cell lines in vitro. J Immunol 145:2474, 1990.

202. Sedgwick JD, Mößner R, Schwender S, and ter Meulen V. MHC-expressing non-hematopoietic astroglial cells prime only CD8+ T lymphocytes: astroglial cells as perpetuators but not initiators of CD4+ T cell responses in the central nervous system. J Exp Med 173:1235, 1991.

203. Sedgwick JD, Schwender S, Gregersen R, Dörries R, ter Meulen V. Resident macrophages (ramified microglia) of the BN-strain rat central nervous system are constitutively MHC class II-positive. J Exp Med 177:1145, 1993.

204. Sedgwick JD, Schwender S, Imrich H, Dörries R, Butcher GW, ter Meulen V. Isolation and direct characterization of resident microglial cells from the normal and inflamed central nervous system. Proc Natl Acad Sci USA 88:7438, 1991.

205. Sethna MP, Lampson LA. Immune modulation within the brain: recruitment of inflammatory cells and increased major histocompatibility antigen expression following intracerebral injection of interferon-gamma. J Neuroimmunol 34:121, 1991.

206. Simmons A, Tscharke DC. Anti-CD8 impairs clearance of herpes simplex virus from the nervous system: implications for the fate of virally infected neurons. J Exp Med 175:1337, 1992.

207. Skias DD, Kim DK, Reder AT, Antel JP, Lancki DW, Fitch FW. Susceptibility of astrocytes to class I MHC antigen-specific cytotoxicity. J Immunol 138:3254, 1987.

208. Sminia T, de Groot CJ, Dijkstra CD, Koetsier JC, Polman CH. Macrophages in the central nervous system of the rat. Immunobiology 174:43, 1987.

209. Sobel RA, Blanchette BW, Bhan AK, Colvin RB. The immunopathology of experimental allergic encephalomyelitis. II. Endothelial cell Ia increases prior to inflammatory cell infiltration. J Immunol 132:2402, 1984.

210. Sobel RA, Collins AB, Colvin RB, Bhan AK. The in situ cellular immune response in acute herpes simplex encephalitis. Am J Pathol 125:332, 1986.

211. Sobel RA, Colvin RB. The immunopathology of experimental allergic encephalomyelitis (EAE). III. Differential in situ expression of strain 13 Ia on endothelial and inflammatory cells of (strain 2 × strain 13)F1 guinea pigs with EAE. J Immunol 134:2333, 1985.

212. Sobel RA, Natale JM, Schneeberger EE. The immunopathology of acute experimental allergic encephalomyelitis. IV. An ultrastructural immunocytochemical study of class II major histocompatibility complex molecule (Ia) expression. J Neuropathol Exp Neurol 46:239, 1987.

213. Sprent J, Schaefer M. Antigen-presenting cells for unprimed T cells. Immunol Today 10:17, 1989.

214. Springer TA. Adhesion receptors of the immune system. Nature 346:425, 1990.

215. Springer TA, Dustin ML, Kishimoto TK, Marlin SD. The lymphocyte function-associated LFA-1, CD2 and LFA-3 molecules: cell adhesion receptors of the immune system. Annu Rev Immunol 5:223, 1987.

216. Steiniger B, Falk P, Van der Meide PH. Interferon-gamma in vivo. Induction and loss of class II MHC antigens and immature myelomonocytic cells in rat organs. Eur J Immunol 18:661, 1988.

217. Steiniger B, van der Meide PH. Rat ependyma and microglia cells express class II MHC antigens after intravenous infusion of recombinant gamma interferon. J Neuroimmunol 19:111, 1988.

218. Streit WJ, Graeber MB. Heterogeneity of microglial and perivascular cell populations: insights gained from the facial nucleus paradigm. Glia 7:68, 1993.

219. Streit WJ, Graeber MB, Kreutzberg GW. Expression of Ia antigen on perivascular and microglial cells after sublethal and lethal motor neuron injury. Exp Neurol 105:115, 1989.

220. Streit WJ, Kreutzberg GW. Response of endogenous glial cells to motor neuron degeneration induced by toxic ricin. J Comp Neurol 268:248, 1988.

221. Styren SD, Civin WH, Rogers J. Molecular, cellular, and pathologic characterization of HLA-DR immunoreactivity in normal elderly and Alzheimer's disease brain. Exp Neurol 110:93, 1990.

222. Sun D, Wekerle H. Ia-restricted encephalitogenic T lymphocytes mediating EAE lyse autoantigen-presenting astrocytes. Nature 320:70, 1986.

223. Suzumura A, Lavi E, Bhat S, Murasko D, Weiss SR, Silberberg DH. Induction of glial cell MHC antigen expression in neurotropic coronavirus infections. Characterization of the H-2-inducing soluble factor elaborated by infected brain cells. J Immunol 140:2068, 1988.

224. Suzumura A, Lavi E, Weiss SR, Silberberg DH. Coronavirus infection induces H-2 antigen expression on oligodendrocytes and astrocytes. Science 232:991, 1986.

225. Suzumura A, Mezitis SG, Gonatas NK, Silberberg DH. MHC antigen expression on bulk isolated macrophage-microglia from newborn mouse brain: induction of Ia antigen expression by gamma-interferon. J Neuroimmunol 15:263, 1987.

226. Takiguchi M, Frelinger JA. Induction of antigen presentation ability in purified cultures of astroglia by interferon-gamma. J Mol Cell Immunol 2:269, 1986.

227. Tan R, Teh SJ, Ledbetter JA, Linsley PS, Teh HS. B7 costimulates proliferation of CD4-8+ T lymphocytes but is not required for the deletion of immature CD4+8+ thymocytes. J Immunol 149:3217, 1992.

228. Tanaka M, McCarron RM. The inhibitory effect of tumor necrosis factor and interleukin-1 on Ia induction by interferon-gamma on endothelial cells from murine central nervous system microvessels. J Neuroimmunol 27:209, 1990.

229. Ting JP, Shigekawa BL, Linthicum DS, Weiner LP, Frelinger JA. Expression and synthesis of murine immune response-associated (Ia) antigens by brain cells. Proc Natl Acad Sci USA 78:3170, 1981.

230. Ting JP-Y, Nixon DF, Weiner LP, Frelinger JA. Brain Ia antigens have a bone marrow origin. Immunogenetics 17:295, 1983.

231. Tontsch U, Rott O. Cortical neurons selectively inhibit MHC class II induction in astrocytes but not in microglial cells. Int Immunol 5:249, 1993.

232. Töpper R, Gehrmann J, Schwarz M, Block F, Noth J, Kreutzberg GW. Remote microglial activation in the quinolinic acid model of Huntington's disease. Exp Neurol 123:271, 1993.

233. Townsend A, Bodmer H. Antigen recognition by class I-restricted T lymphocytes. Annu Rev Immunol 7:601, 1989.

234. Traugott U. Multiple sclerosis: relevance of class I and class II MHC-expressing cells to lesion development. J Neuroimmunol 16:283, 1987.

235. Traugott U, McFarlin DE, Raine CS. Immunopathology of the lesion in chronic relapsing experimental autoimmune encephalomyelitis in the mouse. Cell Immunol 99:395, 1986.

236. Traugott U, Raine CS. Multiple sclerosis. Evidence for antigen presentation in situ by endothelial cells and astrocytes. J Neurol Sci 69:365, 1985.

237. Traugott U, Reinherz EL, Raine CS. Multiple sclerosis. Distribution of T cells, T cell subsets and Ia-positive macrophages in lesions of different ages. J Neuroimmunol 4:201, 1983.

238. Traugott U, Scheinberg LC, Raine CS. On the presence of Ia-positive endothelial cells and astrocytes in multiple sclerosis lesions and its relevance to antigen presentation. J Neuroimmunol 8:1, 1985.

239. Turnley AM, Miller JF, Bartlett PF. Regulation of MHC molecules on MBP positive oligodendrocytes in mice by IFN-gamma and TNF-alpha. Neurosci Lett 123:45, 1991.

240. Turnley AM, Morahan G, Okano H, Bernard O, Mikoshiba K, Allison J, Bartlett PF, Miller JF. Dysmyelination in transgenic mice resulting from expression of class I histocompatibility molecules in oligodendrocytes. nature 353:566, 1991.

241. Tyor WR, Stoll G, Griffin DE. The characterization of Ia expression during Sindbis virus encephalitis in normal and athymic nude mice. J Neuropathol Exp Neurol 49:21, 1990.

242. Unanue ER. Antigen presenting function of the macrophage. Annu Rev Immunol 2:395, 1984.

243. Unger ER, Sung JH, Manivel JC, Chenggis ML, Blazer BR, Krivit W. Male donor-derived cells in the brains of female sex-mismatched bone marrow transplant recipients: a Y-chromosome specific in situ hybridization study. J Neuropathol Exp Neurol 52:460, 1993.

244. Van Snick J. Interleukin-6: an overview. Annu Rev Immunol 8:253, 1990.

245. Vass K, Lassmann H. Intrathecal application of interferon gamma. Progressive appearance of MHC antigens within the rat nervous system. Am J Pathol 137:789, 1990.

246. Vass K, Lassmann H, Wekerle H, Wisniewski HM. The distribution of Ia antigen in the lesions of rat acute experimental allergic encephalomyelitis. Acta Neuropathol (Berl) 70:149, 1986.

247. Voorthuis JAC, Uitdehaag BMJ, de Groot CJA, Goede PH, van der Meide PH, Dijkstra CD. Suppression of experimental allergic encephalomyelitis by intraventricular administration of interferon-gamma in Lewis rats. Clin Exp Immunol 81:183, 1990.

248. Weinberg WC, Deamant FD, Iannaccone PM. Patterns of expression of class I antigens in the tissues of congenic strains of rat. Hybridoma 4:27, 1985.

249. Weinstein DL, Walker DG, Akiyama H, McGeer PL. Herpes simplex virus type I infection

of the CNS induces major histocompatibility complex antigen expression on rat microglia. J Neurosci Res 26:55, 1990.

250. Wekerle HC, Linington H, Lassmann H, Meyermann R. Cellular immune reactivity within the CNS. Trends Neurosci 9:271, 1986.

251. Wilcox CE, Baker D, Butter C, Willoughby, DA, Turk JL. Differential expression of guinea pig class II major histocompatibility complex antigens on vascular endothelial cells in vitro and in experimental allergic encephalomyelitis. Cell Immunol 120:82, 1989.

252. Wilcox CE, Healey DG, Baker D, Willoughby DA, Turk JL. Presentation of myelin basic protein by normal guinea-pig brain endothelial cells and its relevance to experimental allergic encephalomyelitis. Immunology 67:435, 1989.

253. Wilcox CE, Ward AM, Evans A, Baker D, Rothlein R, Turk JL. Endothelial cell expression of the intercellular adhesion molecule-1 (ICAM-1) in the central nervous system of guinea pigs during acute and chronic relapsing experimental allergic encephalomyelitis. J Neuroimmunol 30:43, 1990.

254. Williams K, Bar-Or A, Ulvestad E, Olivier A, Antel JP, Yong VW. Biology of adult human microglia in culture: comparisons with peripheral blood monocytes and astrocytes. J Neuropathol Exp Neurol 51:538, 1992.

255. Williams K, Ulvestad E, Antel JP. B7/BB-1 antigen expression on adult human microglia studied in vitro and in situ. Eur J Immunol 24:3031, 1994.

256. Williams K, Ulvestad E, Cragg L, Blain M, Antel JP. Induction of primary T cell responses by human glial cells. J Neurosci Res 36:382, 1993.

257. Wiman K, Curman B, Forsum U, Klareskog L, Malmnäs-Tjernlund U, Rask L, Trägårdh, L, Petersen PA. Occurrence of Ia antigens on tissues of non-lymphoid origin. Nature 276:711, 1978.

258. Wong GH, Bartlett PF, Clark LI, Battye F, Schrader JW. Inducible expression of H-2 and Ia antigens on brain cells. Nature 310:688, 1984.

259. Woodroofe MN, Bellamy AS, Feldmann M, Davison AN, Cuzner ML. Immunocytochemical characterisation of the immune reaction in the central nervous system in multiple sclerosis. Possible role for microglia in lesion growth. J Neurol Sci 74:135, 1986.

260. Woodroofe MN, Hayes GM, Cuzner ML. Fc receptor density, MHC antigen expression and superoxide production are increased in interferon-gamma-treated microglia isolated from adult rat brain. Immunology 68:421, 1989.

261. Yednock TA, Cannon C, Fritz LC. Sanchez-Madrid F, Steinman L, Karin N. Prevention of experimental autoimmune encephalomyelitis by antibodies against α4β1 integrin. Nature 356:63, 1992.

262. Yong VW, Yong FP, Ruijs TC, Antel JP, Kim SU. Expression and modulation of HLA-DR on cultured human adult astrocytes. J Neuropathol Exp Neurol 50:16, 1991.

263. Yoshioka T, Feigenbaum L, Jay G. Transgenic mouse model for central nervous system demyelination. Mol Cell Biol 11:5479, 1996.

264. Zinkernagel RM, Doherty PC. MHC-restricted cytotoxic T cells: studies on the biological role of polymorphic major transplantation antigens determining T-cell restriction-specificity, function and responsiveness. Adv Immunol 27:51, 1979.

11

Cytokine Expression in the Nervous System

ETTY N. BENVENISTE

This chapter on cytokines in the central nervous system (CNS) will emphasize the expression and action of a select group of cytokines, namely those implicated in inflammatory and immune responses within the CNS. These cytokines include interleukin-1 (IL-1), interferon gamma (IFN-γ), interleukin-6 (IL-6), tumor necrosis factor alpha and beta (TNF-α/TNF-β), transforming growth factor beta (TGF-β) and the colony stimulating factors (CSFs). Specifically, the emphasis will be on the ability of glial cells to both produce and respond to such cytokines.

The chapter begins with the historical background and the reasons why cytokine expression in the CNS was initially investigated. Next comes a brief overview of the "traditional" (i.e., immunological) functions of the above cytokines. Finally, the main part of this chapter concerns how glial cells both respond to, and synthesize, cytokines, and how these changes in gene expression and function may contribute to various neurologic disease states such as multiple sclerosis (MS), experimental allergic encephalomyelitis (EAE), and AIDS dementia complex (ADC). Where applicable, information about the intracellular signaling pathways and molecular mechanisms by which genes are expressed in glial cells will be discussed.

Historical Background

The CNS is generally regarded as an immunologically privileged site for several reasons: 1) the CNS is devoid for the most part of a lymphatic system that captures potential antigens, and 2) the CNS is protected from circulating blood by the blood-

419

brain barrier (BBB), a specialized vasculature consisting of endothelial cells with tight junctions, which is impermeable to many soluble substances, including immunoglobulins and growth factors, and which acts to restrict the migration of lymphoid cells into the CNS. Additionally, cells of the CNS (neurons, astrocytes, oligodendrocytes, microglia) constitutively express very low levels of class I and II major histocompatibility complex (MHC) antigens, which play a fundamental role in the induction and regulation of immune responses (10,192). Injury and pathological events within the CNS often result in a breakdown of the BBB, which permits cells of the peripheral immune system access to this site. During human diseases such as viral encephalitis (113), MS (64,134), and ADC (119), and animal models of CNS disease such as EAE (139), inflammatory infiltrates composed of varying ratios of activated T cells, B cells, and macrophages are found in the brain.

Studies were initially directed towards investigating whether factors from immune cells were contributing to astrocytic activation or astrogliosis. Astrogliosis is the result of astrocyte proliferation, hypertrophy, and the increased synthesis of glial fibrillary acidic protein (GFAP), an astrocyte-specific protein (20). The astrogliotic process eventually produces dense glial scars in the CNS. Astrogliosis is often associated with inflammatory infiltrates in the CNS, and is one of the characteristic hallmarks of the diseases MS and ADC. Because of the close proximity of astrocytes and activated lymphocytes in the CNS, the question arose as to whether lymphocytes might contribute to the process of astrogliosis.

Fontana et al. (38,43) tested this hypothesis by examining the ability of lymphocytes to produce glial-stimulating factors in vitro, specifically looking for soluble products that might modulate astrocyte proliferation. Supernatants from rat lymphocytes stimulated with the mitogen concanavalin A or sensitized rat lymphocytes challenged with antigen in vitro were collected and tested for glial-stimulating activity. Indeed, they found that these supernatants enhanced both RNA synthesis and DNA synthesis in rat astrocyte cultures (39). This factor, named *glial-stimulating factor,* was produced by both activated T and B lymphocytes. A factor with similar activity was also derived from mitogen-activated human T lymphocytes (43). Merrill et al. (110) later demonstrated that both rat astrocytes and oligodendrocytes could respond by increased proliferation to supernatants from activated human T cells. The supernatants tested were derived from a T-lymphoblast line (MO) which was infected with the retrovirus human T-cell lymphotropic virus (HTLV)-II; human T lymphocytes transformed by HTLV-II; and human T lymphocytes activated by the mitogen phytohemagglutinin. Additionally, the MO cell line also produced factors which enhanced maturation of oligodendrocytes as assessed by the increased expression of myelin basic protein (12). The above studies indicated that lymphoid cells activated by three different mechanisms: 1) nonspecifically by mitogen; 2) in an antigen-specific fashion; and 3) by viral transformation, were all capable of secreting factors which stimulated the growth of glial cells.

In light of the fact that soluble factors from activated lymphoid cells could enhance the growth of glial cells, investigators were interested in determining whether the reverse could occur, i.e., whether glial cells might secrete soluble products that would affect lymphoid cells and/or monocytes/macrophages. Fontana et al. (41,42) discovered that cultured murine astrocytes, upon stimulation with lipopolysaccharide (LPS), secreted significant amounts of prostaglandin and an IL-1-like factor, and that human glioblastoma cell lines constitutively secreted an IL-1-like molecule.

These early studies provided evidence that glial cells and lymphocytes could communicate via soluble mediators. By necessity, these studies were performed using crude cell-derived supernatants, or partially purified proteins. The use of these materials to detect a specific biological effect was complicated by the fact that numerous cytokines were present in these preparations and exerted synergistic or inhibitory effects, thereby masking or altering the activity of the cytokine in question. The availability of recombinant purified cytokines has greatly facilitated the study of cytokine influences on glial cell function. Additionally, the use of specific neutralizing antibodies against individual cytokines and highly specific bioassays, enzyme-linked immunoadsorbent assays (ELISA), and radioimmunoassays (RIA) for cytokines has allowed for the precise determination of cytokine activity in glial cell supernatants and permits the definitive assignment of cytokine production with a particular glial cell.

Cytokines

Cytokines play a major role in the initiation, propagation, regulation, and suppression of immune and inflammatory responses. In this section, the characteristics of the cytokines most relevant to inflammatory and immune responses within the CNS will be described. For more detailed information on cytokine function, see numerous referenced review articles.

Although cytokines comprise a diverse group of proteins, they share a number of general properties. Cytokines are low molecular weight (MW) proteins that are produced during the effector phases of immunity and serve to mediate and regulate immune and inflammatory responses. Most cells do not constitutively produce cytokines, instead, an activation event results in cytokine gene transcription. Cytokines in general are secreted, but they can also be expressed on the cell surface. An individual cytokine can be produced by many different cell types and have multiple effects on different cell types. Cytokines have also been shown to have redundant functions, i.e., several cytokines can mediate a common event. Thus, the cytokine system displays pleiotropism and redundancy. Cytokines can have synergistic or antagonistic effects, and they can induce or inhibit the synthesis of other cytokines, resulting in complex "cytokine cascades" for immune and inflammatory responses. Cytokines generally act locally and initiate their action by binding to specific cell-surface receptors on target cells; these receptors generally show high affinities for their ligands, with dissociation constants in the range of 10^{-10}–10^{-12} M. These low dissociation constants suggest that very small amounts of a cytokine need to be produced to elicit a biological response. The ultimate response of a particular cell to a particular cytokine is determined by the level of expression of the cytokine receptor, the signal transduction pathways of the target cell that are activated by that cytokine, and the microenvironment of the target cell.

Interleukin-1

IL-1 is a 17,000 dalton cytokine produced predominantly by activated macrophages, although other cell types, such as endothelial cells, B cells, keratinocytes, microglia, and astrocytes, can also secrete IL-1 upon stimulation (for review see 3,36). IL-1 is a cytokine responsible for mediating a variety of processes in the host response to microbial and inflammatory diseases. IL-1 is expressed in two major forms, IL-1α and IL-1β, which are the products of two different genes. Although these two forms of IL-1 have less than 30% homology between their amino acid sequences, they both bind to identical receptors and have similar biologic activities. Both forms of IL-1 lack signal peptide sequences characteristic of many secretory proteins, suggesting that IL-1 may function as a cell-associated protein or that IL-1 follows a novel secretory process. IL-1 is the major costimulator for T helper–cell activation via the augmentation of both IL-2 and IL-2 receptor expression. These effects allow antigen-stimulated T helper cells to rapidly proliferate and expand in number. IL-1, in cooperation with other cytokines, can also enhance the growth and differentiation of B cells. IL-1 is a principal participant in inflammatory reactions through its induction of other inflammatory metabolites such as prostaglandin, collagenase, and phospholipase A2. IL-1 acts on endothelial cells to promote leukocyte adhesion and induces the production of various cytokines such as IL-6, TNF-α, CSFs, and IL-1 itself.

IL-1 receptors are present on almost all cell types examined and two forms have been identified: the type I receptor (80,000 daltons) and the type II receptor (60,000 daltons). Both forms of the IL-1 receptor consist of an extracellular IL-1 binding domain, a membrane-spanning domain, and a cytoplasmic domain, which is critical for signal transduction. Interestingly, only the type I IL-1 receptor is capable of transducing a signal following ligand binding. The type II IL-1 receptor may serve as a decoy for IL-1 or serve as a precursor for a soluble form of the receptor.

Interferon-Gamma

IFN-γ, a pleiotropic cytokine with antiviral activity, antiproliferative effects, and immunomodulatory effects, is produced predominantly by activated T cells (for review see 76). These immune effects include the ability to enhance the functional activity of macrophages, promotion of T- and B-cell differentiation, and the modulation of both class I and class II MHC expression on a wide variety of cells. IFN-γ is considered the most potent inducer of class II MHC antigen expression on most cell types, however, for B cells, the cytokine IL-4 is the primary inducer of class II MHC (for review see 60). The IFN-γ receptor is composed of two distinct, species-specific polypeptides. A 90,000 dalton α chain is necessary and sufficient for IFN-γ binding, but it is not sufficient for induction of the biological response. The recently cloned IFN-γ receptor 3 chain is essential for signal transduction.

Tumor Necrosis Factors Alpha and Beta

TNF-α is a 17,000 dalton peptide produced primarily by activated macrophages and is the principal mediator of the host response to gram-negative bacteria (for review see 145). Activated macrophages are the major cellular source for TNF-α, although other cell types such as T cells, mast cells, microglia, and astrocytes can be stimulated to secrete TNF-α. TNF-α is an active participant in inflammatory responses, and in particular, can alter vascular endothelial cell function. Specifically, TNF-α enhances the permeability of endothelial cells (23) and enhances local adhesion of neutrophils, lymphocytes, and monocytes to the surface of endothelial cells (129), thereby facilitating transendothelial cell migration of polymorphonuclear leukocytes and immune cells and the formation of leukocyte-rich inflammatory infiltrates. TNF-α can modulate immune responses by affecting the expression of class I and class II MHC molecules on a variety of cell types, and it can stimulate many cell types to produce numerous cytokines, including IL-1, IL-6, CSFs, and TNF-α itself. TNF-α is produced predominantly as a secreted protein, although a membrane-anchored form of TNF-α has been identified on the surface of macrophages that has lytic activity and may play an important role in intercellular communication (84).

There are two distinct TNF-α receptors: the 55,000 dalton (TNF-R1) and the 75,000 dalton (TNF-R2) forms (101,152,165). The cytoplasmic portions of the two TNF receptors have differences, suggesting that the two receptors may activate distinct intracellular signaling pathways. The TNF-R1 is responsible for mediating the effects of TNF-γ on apoptosis, cytokine production, and induction of a number of gene products, while the function of the TNF-R2 is mainly related to T-cell development and the proliferation of cytotoxic T-cells. Almost all cell types express either the 55,000 or 75,000 dalton TNF receptor, and many cells can express both forms of the TNF receptor.

TNF-β is genetically related to TNF-α, but is produced primarily by antigen-activated T cells (for review see 128). TNF-α and TNF-β share approximately 30% amino acid residue homology, bind to the same receptors, and produce similar, but not identical, biological effects. One of the major biological functions of TNF-β is its ability to kill a wide variety of cell types via the process of apoptosis (DNA fragmentation).

Interleukin-6

IL-6, similar to IL-1 and TNF-α, is a pleiotropic cytokine involved in the regulation of inflammatory and immunologic responses (for review see 182). IL-6, a 26,000 dalton molecule, is secreted by a wide range of activated cells, including fibroblasts, monocytes, B cells, endothelial cells, T cells, microglia, and astrocytes. The two best-described functions of IL-6 are on hepatocytes and B cells. IL-6 stimulates hepatocytes to synthesize several plasma proteins, such as fibrinogen and C-reactive protein, which contribute to the acute-phase response. IL-6 serves as the principal cytokine for inducing terminal differentiation of activated B cells into immunoglobulin-secreting plasma cells. IL-6 can also act as a costimulator of T helper–cell activation.

The IL-6 receptor has an external ligand-binding domain and associates with a 130,000 dalton protein (gp130) that does not bind IL-6 itself, but is responsible for initiating signal transduction.

Transforming Growth Factor Beta

TGF-β is a dimeric protein of approximately 28,000 daltons that is synthesized by almost all cell types. It is normally secreted in a latent form that must be activated by proteases (for review see 106). The TGF-β family is comprised of several members showing high structural homology. Three closely related TGF-β genes have been identified in mammals; they are TGF-β1, TGF-β2, and TGF-β3. The actions of TGF-β are highly pleiotropic and include inhibiting the proliferation of many cell types (epithelial, endothelial, lymphoid, and hematopoietic cells), promoting the growth of new blood vessels (angiogenesis), serving as a chemotactic factor for macrophages, and inhibiting immune and inflammatory responses. TGF-β has been demonstrated to inhibit the production of numerous cytokines and is thought to function as a negative regulator of immune responses.

Colony-Stimulating Factors

The group of cytokines that has potent stimulatory effects on the growth and differentiation of bone marrow progenitor cells is collectively called *colony-stimulating factors* (CSFs). By stimulating the growth and differentiation of bone marrow cells, CSFs act to provide inflammatory leukocytes. We will consider four CSFs in this discussion (for review see 61). Interleukin-3 (IL-3), also known as *multi-CSF,* is produced by T helper cells and acts on the most immature bone marrow progenitors to induce the expansion of cells that differentiate into all known mature cell types. Granulocyte-macrophage colony-stimulating factor (GM-CSF) is a 22,000 dalton glycoprotein produced by a number of activated cells, including T cells, macrophages, endothelial cells, fibroblasts, and astrocytes. GM-CSF acts on bone marrow progenitor cells already committed to differentiate to granulocytes and monocytes. GM-CSF can also interact with various mononuclear phagocytes, including microglia, to induce their activation. Macrophage colony-stimulating factor (M-CSF), also called *CSF-1,* is made by macrophages, endothelial cells, and fibroblasts. M-CSF acts primarily on progenitor cells already committed to develop into monocytes; these progenitor cells are more mature than the targets for GM-CSF. Granulocyte colony-stimulating factor (G-CSF) is made by the same cells that produce GM-CSF, activated T cells, macrophages, endothelial cells, and fibroblasts. It acts primarily on bone marrow progenitors already committed to develop into granulocytes.

Having reviewed the salient features of the cytokines of interest, the next sections will describe the known biological effects of these cytokines on glial cells, the ability of glial cells to produce cytokines, and the role of these cytokines in the development and progression of CNS disease.

Interleukin-1 and Glial Cells

Biological Action of IL-1 on Glial Cells

As mentioned above, IL-1 affects a wide range of target cells and is considered an important mediator of inflammatory responses, including those occurring within the CNS. Since one response to brain injury is proliferation of astrocytes, IL-1 was tested for its capacity to induce proliferation of these cells. Purified IL-1 was shown to have a mitogenic effect on astrocyte growth in vitro (58), while IL-1 directly injected into the brain can stimulate astrogliosis (59). These results suggest that IL-1 may contribute to astroglial scarring in damaged mammalian brain. Both activated astrocytes and microglia have been shown to secrete IL-1 in vitro, which will be discussed in more detail below. These cells would provide an endogenous brain source of IL-1, which could promote astrogliosis within the CNS.

A variety of CNS cells have been shown to produce cytokines in response to IL-1. IL-1 stimulation of primary rat astrocytes primes them for the secretion of TNF-α (28) and induces IL-6 (14,48,167) and TGF-β (35); primary human astrocytes produce IL-6, IL-8, TNF-α, and CSFs in response to IL-1 (2,91); and human astroglial cell lines will produce CSFs (49,180), TNF-α (17), IL-6 (196), and IL-8 (79) in response to IL-1. With respect to microglia and oligodendrocytes, IL-1 induces TGF-β expression by these cells (35). These are all cytokines involved in mediating immune reactions and inflammatory responses, thus their production by resident brain cells can contribute to these processes within the CNS.

Little is currently known about the signal transduction pathway(s) elicited by cytokine interaction with glial cells. Recent studies from our laboratory have been directed towards understanding the molecular and intracellular signaling events involved in IL-1-induced TNF-α gene expression in astrocytes. In human astroglioma cells, IL-1 induces transcriptional activation of the TNF-α gene, and the half-life of IL-1-induced TNF-α mRNA is quite short, on the order of 30 min (17). This time frame is in keeping with the half-life of TNF-α mRNA derived from other cell types (26,161) and illustrates the point that TNF-α mRNA expression is quite transient. We have also shown that IL-1-induced TNF-α gene expression in astroglioma cells is dependent upon protein kinase C (PKC) activation in that two PKC inhibitors, H7 and staurosporine, abrogate IL-1-induced TNF-α expression, and depletion of PKC activity by prolonged treatment with a high concentration of phorbol myristate acetate (PMA) renders the astroglioma cells incapable of producing TNF-α in response to IL-1 (18). These data demonstrate that IL-1 induces TNF-α gene expression in astroglioma cells in a PKC dependent manner. In primary rat astrocytes, TNF-α production is induced by a combined treatment of IFN-γ plus IL-1β. Neither IFN-γ or IL-1β alone is an effective stimulus for TNF-α secretion (28). We have recently determined that PKC activity is required for IFN-γ/IL-1β induction of TNF-α gene expression in primary rat astrocytes, and that PKC activity is critical for transcriptional activation of the TNF-α gene (29).

IL-1β-induced IL-6 expression in primary rat astrocytes occurs at the transcriptional level, and the nuclear factor kappa B (NF-κB)-like binding site is required for IL-1β induction of IL-6 promoter activity (167). IL-1β treatment of astrocytes leads to a rapid activation of a nuclear protein that specifically complexes with the NF-κB-like binding region in the IL-6 promoter, suggesting an involvement of an NK-κB-like protein in IL-6 gene expression. Additionally, PKC activity is required for IL-1β induction of IL-6 in astrocytes (121).

Components of the complement cascade have been implicated in the pathology of several neurological autoimmune diseases such as MS, EAE, and Guilain-Barré syndrome (GBS) (for review see 162). For example, the levels of terminal complement components have been shown to fluctuate in MS disease exacerbations and remissions, suggesting C9 consumption. Recent studies have indicated that astrocytes can serve as a local endogenous source of some of the complement components, notably C3, the central component of the complement cascade (96). In particular, IL-1 can enhance C3 expression in both human astroglioma cells and primary rat astrocytes (8,54,147). C3 is an important effector required for bacterial opsonization, activation of macrophages, and anaphylactic reactions, and its expression by astrocytes in response to IL-1 may contribute to inflammatory processes within the CNS (for review see 5).

IL-1 can also modulate the expression of adhesion molecules on both endothelial cells and astrocytes. IL-1 treatment of endothelial cells results in increased adhesion for neutrophils, eosinophils, and lymphocytes (129), and IL-1 increases the expression of intercellular adhesion molecule-1 (ICAM-1) on both human and rat astrocytes (51,163). In CNS diseases such as MS and EAE, initiating events are thought to involve changes at the BBB, resulting in increased vascular permeability. Increased expression of adhesion molecules on endothelial cells and astrocytes may be important for leukocyte homing and adhesion and the establishment of inflammatory infiltrates within the CNS. In this regard, the expression of two molecules associated with cell adhesion, a murine lymph node, high endothelial venule marker, MECA-325, and the murine homologue of ICAM-1, has been correlated with chronic relapsing EAE in the SJL mouse (25). During disease, up-regulated expression of these two molecules occurred in the CNS and was correlated with inflammatory cell infiltration. Expression decreased during remission and increased again with each subsequent relapse. MECA-325 was detected on postcapillary venules, while ICAM-1 was found on endothelial cells, perivascular cells, and astrocytes.

IL-1 Expression by Glial Cells

IL-1 production by glial cells of the CNS was originally suggested by a study in which cultured murine astrocytes, upon stimulation with LPS, secreted an IL-1-like factor (42). This finding was later confirmed using astrocyte cultures of $>95\%$ purity, and LPS-stimulated astrocytes expressed mRNA for both IL-1α and IL-1β (103). Several human astroglioma cell lines can constitutively secrete IL-1, and both PMA and LPS enhance IL-1 production by these cell lines (41,89,184). Additionally, primary cultures of human fetal astrocytes produce IL-1 upon stimulation with LPS (184). Rat, murine, and human microglia produce IL-1 in response to LPS stimulation (27,56,66,91,103), and virally transformed microglia clones produce IL-1 (142). Interestingly, the IL-1 protein is mostly cell associated on human fetal microglia (91). There has been some controversy as to whether primary cultures of astrocytes do in fact produce IL-1, the concern being that contaminating microglia in these cultures may be the source of IL-1. The fact that several astroglioma cell lines produce IL-1 suggests that cells of astrocytic lineage can secrete this particular cytokine. The use of double labeling immunohistochemistry to positively identify cells in vivo expressing IL-1 has demonstrated that both astrocytes and microglia express IL-1, but that astrocytes are the more frequent producer of this cytokine in diseased brain (34). These data indicate that astrocytes are in fact a source of IL-1 in the CNS, although they may not be the exclusive CNS source of this cytokine. Oligodendrocytes also appear to be capable of producing IL-1 based on the observation that human oligodendroglioma cell lines produce IL-1 in vitro (111) and oligodendrocytes in diseased brain stain positively for IL-1 (34). These data indicate that there are three endogenous sources of IL-1 within the CNS: activated astrocytes, microglia, and oligodendrocytes. For a summary of IL-1 effects in the CNS, see Table 11-1.

Table 11-1 Interleukin-1 and Glial Cells

Astrocytes

Induce proliferation of neonatal astrocytes, human astroglioma cells

Induce ICAM-1 expression on primary human and rat astrocytes

Induce IL-6 expression by primary rat and human astrocytes, human astroglioma cell lines

Induce TNF-α expression in conjunction with IFN-γ by neonatal rat astrocytes

Induce TNF-α and IL-8 expression in human astroglioma cell lines

Induce G-CSF and GM-CSF expression in human astroglioma cell lines, primary human astrocytes

Induce M-CSF and IL-8 expression in primary human astrocytes

Induce TGF-β1 protein expression by neonatal rat astrocytes

Enhance expression of C3 complement component in rat astrocytes, human astroglioma cells

Make IL-1α and IL-1β in response to LPS simulation

Human glioblastoma cells constitutively secrete IL-1; stimulation with LPS or PMA enhances expression

Microglia

Induce TFG-β1 protein expression by rat microglia

Make IL-1α and IL-1β in response to LPS stimulation

Oligodendrocytes

Induce TGF-β1 protein expression by rat oligodendrocytes

Human oligodendroglioma cell lines secrete IL-1

Enhance ICAM-1 expression on human adult oligodendrocytes

Involvement of IL-1 in Neurological Disease States

Role of IL-1 in EAE and MS

The best-characterized experimental model for CNS autoimmune disease is EAE. This disease is induced by injection of spinal cord components such as myelin basic protein (MBP) or proteolipid protein (PLP) with adjuvant, or transfer of encephalitogenic MBP or PLP-specific T cells to naive recipients. EAE is characterized by an inflammatory infiltration of the CNS by activated T lymphocytes and macrophages, and acute, chronic, or chronic relapsing paralysis. The mediators of this disease are MBP or PLP reactive CD4+ T helper cells that are class II MHC restricted (for review see 197). It has been proposed that antigen-specific autoimmune T cells are responsible for initiation of disease and that perpetuation of disease may be the result of an influx into the CNS of largely nonantigen-specific inflammatory cells (33).

Because of the known inflammatory effects of IL-1 and the knowledge that glial cells can produce IL-1 within the CNS, there has been interest in the role of IL-1 in EAE. IL-1 has been shown to serve as a cofactor for in vitro activation of encephalitogenic T cells, thereby enhancing the adoptive transfer of EAE (104), and guinea pigs with chronic EAE have elevated levels of IL-1 in their cerebrospinal fluid (171).

More recently, Jacobs et al. (77) demonstrated that in vivo administration of IL-1α enhanced the severity and chronicity of clinical paralysis associated with EAE, whereas treatment of animals with soluble mouse IL-1 receptor (an IL-1 antagonist) significantly delayed the onset of EAE, reduced the severity of paralysis and weight loss, and reduced the duration of disease. These results suggest a role for IL-1 in inflammatory CNS disease states such as EAE. There have been conflicting reports as to whether IL-1 is present in the brains of animals with EAE. In a model of chronic relapsing EAE (CREAE) induced in Biozzi AB/H mice with autologous spinal cord homogenate, IL-1 was detected in the brains of these animals in both the acute and relapsing phases of disease (4), along with the cytokines TNF-α, IL-2, IL-3, and IFN-γ. The cell type(s) expressing the cytokines was not determined. Similarly, a study by Kennedy et al. (81) examining EAE induced in SJL/J mice by adoptive transfer of MBP-sensitized lymph node cells demonstrated that mRNA for IL-1 was detected in the acute phase of disease, and mRNA levels remained elevated during the early chronic state. mRNA for other cytokines such as IL-2, IL-4, IL-6, IL-10, and IFN-γ were also detected in this model of EAE. In contrast, Merrill et al. (109) did not detect IL-1 in the brains of SJL/J and B10.PL mice that were immunized with MBP peptides. This would suggest that the method of immunization by which EAE is induced may influence cytokine expression in the brain, or, alternatively, the different results may be due to the different procedures utilized for detecting cytokine expression.

In MS, peripheral blood macrophages can secrete IL-1 constitutively, which suggests that they have been activated in vivo (112). Also, IL-1+ microglial cells have been identified in chronic active plaques in the brains of patients with MS (70,72). Because IL-1 does have multiple effects on glial cells, such as expression of adhesion molecules, cytokine induction, and proliferation, the inhibition of IL-1 activity may prevent further CNS inflammation and injury. It is speculated that the use of soluble IL-1 receptors or the IL-1 receptor antagonist may be therapeutically beneficial in diseases like MS.

IL-1 in Other Neurological Diseases

IL-1+ cells have been identified in the brains of patients with AIDS dementia complex (181) and Alzheimer's disease (62). In both these diseases, the IL-1 appears to be localized in microglia and macrophages.

In a rabbit model of bacterial meningitis, intracisternal administration of recombinant IL-1 produced a significant inflammatory response within the cerebrospinal fluid (140), and in the rat, IL-1 induced meningeal inflammation and BBB permeability (136). In human studies, IL-1 concentrations in the nanogram range were detected in the cerebrospinal fluid of 95% of children with bacterial meningitis (118). Thus, IL-1 appears to be a potent mediator of meningitis and BBB injury, and production of IL-1 by resident glial cells of the CNS could contribute to this disease process.

Interferon Gamma and Glial Cells

Biological Action of IFN-γ on Glial Cells

The cytokine IFN-γ is the product of activated T cells and has a wide range of immunoregulatory functions. IFN-γ is present in the CNS only in disease states in which the BBB has been disrupted and activated T cells have infiltrated into that site. IFN-γ is a potent modulator of MHC antigen expression in a number of cell types, including astrocytes, oligodendrocytes, and microglia. The preceding chapter provides a comprehensive overview of MHC antigen expression in the CNS, so the effect of IFN-γ on glial cell MHC expression will be briefly discussed here.

Cells in the brain express extremely low levels of class I MHC antigens, which have a critical role in the regulation of immune responses. IFN-γ induces an increase in the expression of class I MHC antigens on astrocytes, oligodendrocytes, and microglia both in vitro and in vivo (68,170,192,193). The implication of enhanced class I MHC expression on these cells is that they can be rendered susceptible to lysis by class I–restricted cytotoxic T lymphocytes (164).

Class II MHC molecules have a key role in regulating the immune response by presenting antigen to T helper cells, resulting in their activation and differentiation (for review see 60,174). Astrocytes and microglia do not constitutively express class II MHC antigens, however, IFN-γ can induce class II molecules on these cells in vitro (38,40,135,168,192,193). Although class II expression on astrocytes has been conclusively demonstrated in vitro, in vivo studies have generated conflicting results, which will be discussed later. In vitro, class II MHC+ astrocytes and microglia can present antigen to T cells in an MHC-restricted manner, resulting in T-cell activation (38,40,50,144). The implication of class II expression on both astrocytes and microglia is that these cells may stimulate the development of aberrant immune responses within the CNS.

Molecules other than class II MHC are involved in antigen presentation; these include adhesion molecules such as ICAM-1 and VCAM-1, as well as co-stimulatory molecules like B7-1 (CD80) and B7-2 (CD86) (for review see 63a,78a,114a,191a). There are differences between astrocytes and microglia with respect to their ability to express B7-1 and B7-2 co-stimulatory molecules (162a), which can also influence their ability to effectively present antigen to T-cells.

Recent studies from our laboratory have focused on understanding the intracellular and molecular events involved in IFN-γ induction of class II MHC expression by primary rat astrocytes. Our results indicate that IFN-γ induced PKC activity, tyrosine kinase activity, and enhanced sodium influx (via the Na^+/H^+ antiporter) are required for class II MHC gene expression in the astrocyte (16,93). Much effort has been directed toward the identification of *cis*-regulatory elements involved in class II MHC gene expression. The cloning and sequencing of MHC class II genes have led to the identification of conserved sequences located between 50 and 160 base pairs upstream of the transcriptional start site of all class II promoters. Four discrete elements have been described: from 5′ to 3′, they are the W, X1, X2, and Y boxes, respectively (for review see 174). Analysis of several murine and human class II promoters has demonstrated that the conserved W, X1, X2, and Y boxes are necessary elements for constitutive and IFN-γ-mediated expression of class II MHC in various cell lines. Few studies, however, have been done with primary cell cultures. We have previously shown that primary astrocytes express class II MHC mRNA and protein in response to IFN-γ in a time- and dose-dependent manner (13, 185). We have extended these studies to examine the molecular mechanism(s) by which IFN-γ regulates class II expression in primary astrocytes. These studies indicate that IFN-γ acts at the transcriptional level to induce class II expression in astrocytes, and that the W, X1, X2, and Y elements are all essential for IFN-γ inducibility of the class II gene. We have found an IFN-γ-enhanced DNA binding protein with specificity for the X2 element that is produced by astrocytes, which we have tentatively named *IFN-γ-enhanced factor X* (IFNEX) (116,125).

Although class II expression on astrocytes has been conclusively demonstrated in vitro, in vivo studies have generated conflicting results. Direct injection of IFN-γ into the brains of mice induced class II antigens on astrocytes, indicating that astrocytes have the potential to express these antigens in vivo (192,193). Many laboratories have examined whether astrocytes express class II antigens in a variety of CNS immune-mediated disease states to better understand the possible role of the astrocyte as a local antigen-presenting cell. In CNS tissue from animals with EAE (67,107), patients with MS (72,92), and patients with ADC (181), class II-positive astrocytes are rare in contrast to the appearance of numerous class II–positive microglia. A recent study (183) demonstrated that upon intrathecal injection of IFN-γ, there was a progressive appearance of class II MHC–positive cells within the CNS, which may determine antigen recognition during different phases of inflammatory disease. The number of class II–positive microglia increased substantially after IFN-γ injection, while astrocytes expressed class II antigens at a later time point, with a low density and patchy distribution. Since both astrocytes and microglia can express class II MHC antigens in vitro after IFN-γ treatment, this suggests that class II expression on astrocytes in vivo may differ from that of microglia. A potential explanation for the paucity of class II–positive astrocytes in disease states compared with class II–positive microglia may be due to differential regulation of class II expression in these two glial cell types. In vitro studies support this speculation in that IFN-γ induction of class II MHC expression on astrocytes can be inhibited by a number of different factors, including IL-1, TGF-β, norepinephrine, glutamate, and cAMP agonists, as well as by direct contact with neurons, whereas microglial class II expression induced by IFN-γ is unaffected by these same mediators (52,90,124,150,166,175). Thus, expression of class II on astrocytes in vivo may be more susceptible to down-regulation by endogenous neurotransmitters like norepinephrine and glutamate, and cytokines such as IL-1 and TGF-β, and expression may be more transient on the astrocyte compared with microglia.

IFN-γ can increase the expression of ICAM-1 on human astrocytes, in a similar fashion to TNF-α and IL-1 enhancement of ICAM-1 (51). Interestingly, in rat astrocytes, IFN-γ is a weaker inducer of ICAM-1 expression than is TNF-α or IL-1 (163). Primary rat astrocytes express high-affinity TNF-α receptors, which are increased in number upon exposure to IFN-γ (13). Because IFN-γ and TNF-α often synergize in mediating biological effects, the ability of IFN-γ to increase TNF-α receptor expression may contribute, in part, to the synergy observed between these two cytokines. IFN-γ does not appear to directly induce cytokine production by astrocytes but provides a "priming signal" that renders the astrocyte responsive to a subsequent exposure to other cytokines. For example, neither IFN-γ nor IL-1β alone induces TNF-α production by primary rat astrocytes, but they act together in a synergistic fashion to induce TNF-α expression (28). More importantly, astrocytes pretreated with IFN-γ and then exposed to IL-1β produce more TNF-α compared with the simultaneous addition of both cytokines, whereas cells pretreated with IL-1β and then exposed to IFN-γ produce negligible levels of TNF-α. This suggests that IFN-γ generates a priming signal for the astrocytes that then increases their sensitivity to a subsequent exposure to IL-1β. These studies also emphasize the complexity of cytokine interactions, demonstrating that different responses are dependent upon the temporal sequence of cytokine encounter. The nature of the IFN-γ-induced priming signal(s) is unknown at this time. IFN-γ can enhance expression of the complement component C3 in both human astroglioma cells and primary rat astrocytes (7,147). This is particularly interesting as IFN-γ either inhibits or has a minimal effect on C3 expression in other cell types such as hepatocytes, monocytes, and endothelial cells. Thus the IFN-γ-mediated increase in C3 gene expression may be unique to the astrocyte.

Adult and neonatal rat microglia express Fc receptors, and treatment with IFN-γ significantly increases Fc receptor expression (194). Fc receptor expression on microglia suggests that these cells may be actively involved in antibody-mediated immune reactions within the CNS. See Table 11-2 for a summary of IFN-γ mediated effects on glial cells.

Involvement of IFN-γ in Neurological Disease States

Role of IFN-γ in EAE and MS

Due to its ability to modulate expression of MHC antigens and adhesion molecules on glial and endothelial cells, and to activate monocyte and macrophages, IFN-γ has been proposed in the pathogenesis of MS. In clinical trials, administration of IFN-γ to relapsing-remitting MS patients caused exacerbation of disease (127). In MS patients, IFN-γ+ cells have been localized to the plaque region (72,178), although the identity of the IFN-γ+ cells is unknown. Studies on the association of IFN-γ with MS demonstrated that peripheral blood lymphocytes from MS patients produced significantly more IFN-γ than normal control cells (8a,114), and that there were increased numbers

Table 11-2 Interferon-γ and Glial Cells

Astrocytes

Increase class I MHC expression on primary astrocytes

Induce class II MHC expression on primary astrocytes, human glioma cells

Induce ICAM-1 expression on primary human and rat astrocytes

Increase TNF-α receptor expression on primary astrocytes, human glioma cells

Prime rat astrocytes for TNF-α production

Prime rat astrocytes for IL-6 production

Enhance expression of the complement component C3 in primary astrocytes, human glioma cells

Microglia

Increase class I MHC expression

Increase class II MHC expression

Induce TNF-α expression

Increase Fc receptor expression

Induce ICAM-1 expression

Oligodendrocytes

Increase class I MHC expression

---

of cells from cerebrospinal fluid secreting IFN-γ in MS patients (122a). Furthermore, peripheral blood cells that expressed IFN-γ mRNA and secreted IFN-γ were significantly higher in MS patients during relapse or in those patients with severe disability (100a,101a). These findings collectively suggest that IFN-γ has a role in promoting MS disease progression.

Interestingly, IFN-γ appears to play a protective role in different models of EAE. Treatment of mice with neutralizing antibody against IFN-γ caused an increase in disease severity and mortality (21,37), while treatment with IFN-γ itself resulted in reduced morbidity and mortality (21). IFN-γ applied locally into the ventricular system of the CNS resulted in complete suppression of EAE in Lewis rats, while administration of anti-IFN-γ antibody prior to the onset of clinical symptoms resulted in a more severe disease course (187). IFN-γ is found in the CNS of mice with EAE (4,81,109), and expression persists into the early chronic/remission stage (81). The reasons for the contradictory actions of IFN-γ in EAE as compared to MS are unknown at this time.

TNF-α and TNF-β in the CNS

Biological Effects of TNF-α and TNF-β on Glial Cells

TNF-α is a pleiotropic cytokine synthesized by a wide variety of cell types and is recognized to be an important mediator of inflammatory and immune responses in a variety of tissues. TNF-α has a diverse range of functions in the CNS because of its direct effects on astrocytes and oligodendrocytes.

Perhaps most relevant to CNS disease is the ability of TNF-α to mediate myelin and oligodendrocyte damage in vitro (158) and its ability to cause cell death of rat oligodendrocytes in vitro (143). This aspect of TNF-α activity may contribute directly to myelin damage and/or the demyelination process observed in diseases such as MS and ADC. TNF-β, the cytokine which is genetically and functionally related to TNF-α, exerts a more potent cytotoxic effect toward oligodendrocytes than does TNF-α, and it mediates its effect via apoptosis (156). Thus, both TNF-α and TNF-β can cause death of the oligodendrocyte, the myelin-producing cell of the CNS.

TNF-α has multiple effects on the astrocyte which are noncytotoxic in nature, and it may function in an autocrine fashion because astrocytes express specific high-affinity receptors for TNF-α (13) and secrete TNF-α upon activation by a variety of stimuli (17,28,91,97,184). TNF-α induces class I MHC expression on cultured human and mouse astrocytes (88,108) making the astrocytes susceptible targets for class I–restricted cytotoxic T cells (164). TNF-α alone has no effect on class II MHC expression by astrocytes, but it acts to enhance class II MHC expression initially induced by either IFN-γ or virus (13,105,185). The mechanism(s) underlying the effect of TNF-α on class II MHC expression is partially understood at this time. TNF-α acts by increasing IFN-γ-induced transcription of the class II gene rather than having an effect on class II mRNA stability (126,185). Elements within the W, X1, X2, and Y sequences of the class II MHC promoter are critical for TNF-α enhancement of IFN-γ-induced class II gene expression. TNF-α alone does not induce any nuclear proteins that bind to the class II promoter; however, combined treatment of astrocytes with both IFN-γ and TNF-α induces a DNA protein complex designated as *TIC-X* (TNF-α-induced complex X), which is distinct from the IFN-γ induced nuclear protein IFNEX (116,125,126). We believe that expression of TIC-X contributes to the ability of TNF-α to enhance IFN-γ-induced class II expression in astrocytes. TNF-α has also been shown to induce proliferation of both primary bovine astrocytes (157) and human astroglioma cell lines (19,87). As mentioned previously, astrocyte proliferation leads to the reactive gliosis associated with various neurological diseases, and TNF-α appears to contribute to this process. As described for IL-1, TNF-α acts in a similar manner to enhance expression of the C3 complement component in both rat astrocytes and human astroglioma cells (8,54,147), and it induces ICAM-1 expression on human and rat astrocytes (51,163).

TNF-α is a potent inducer of cytokine production in astrocytes. Primary astrocytes and human astroglioma cell lines produce three CSFs upon stimulation with TNF-α; GM-CSF, G-CSF, and M-CSF (2,49,103,179). These cytokines can augment inflammatory responses due to their leukocyte chemotactic properties, which would promote migration of granulocytes and macrophages to inflammatory sites within the CNS. Additionally, GM-CSF and M-CSF can induce the proliferation and activation of microglia (50,57). The disease AIDS dementia complex is due to HIV-1 infection of the

CNS, and in particular, infection of macrophages/microglia within this site (191). GM-CSF and M-CSF have been shown to enhance production of HIV-1 in primary human monocytes/macrophages (83); thus, these two cytokines may contribute to HIV replication in the CNS. TNF-α also induces IL-6 expression by both primary rat and human astrocytes (2,14,48). Similar to IL-1β, TNF-α activates IL-6 gene expression in primary rat astrocytes via an NF-κB-like binding protein (167). Finally, TNF-α induces expression of its own gene in primary rat astrocytes, which suggests a positive feedback loop for TNF-α expression (11).

TNF-α Expression by Glial Cells

Resident glial cells are capable of producing TNF-α upon exposure to multiple stimuli. Primary rat astrocytes express TNF-α in response to treatment with LPS (28,97,143), exposure to the cytokines IFN-γ, IL-1β, and TNF-α (11,28), and exposure to the neurotropic virus, Newcastle disease virus (97). Primary rat astrocytes, in addition to producing soluble TNF-α, can express a membrane-bound form of TNF-α upon activation (Chung and Benveniste, unpublished observation). As mentioned previously, we have demonstrated that PKC activity is required for IFN-γ/IL-1β induction of the TNF-α gene in primary rat astrocytes, and that PKC activity is critical for transcriptional activation of the TNF-α gene (129). Lieberman et al. (98) have shown that the induction of TNF-α mRNA in rat astrocytes stimulated with Newcastle disease virus is dependent on PKC activity and that inhibition of PKC accelerated the decay of TNF-α mRNA up to tenfold, while having little effect on TNF-α gene transcription. Thus, PKC activity in this system is needed for TNF-α mRNA stability. The inhibition of PKC activity affected an early step in the mRNA degradation process by increasing the rate at which poly(A) was removed from the TNF-α message (99). The data from these two studies suggest that the mode of action of PKC activity for cytokine-induced vs. virus-induced TNF-α expression differs, which may reflect differences in *trans*-acting factors that act at either the transcriptional or post-transcriptional level.

Primary human astrocytes produce TNF-α in response to LPS (184), and human astroglioma cell lines are capable of expressing TNF-α upon stimulation with LPS (184), IL-1β (17), and PMA plus calcium ionophore (18). Mouse and human microglia secrete TNF-α in response to LPS (27,50,65,91) and IFN-γ (50). Hetier et al. (65) also demonstrated that murine microglia express a membrane-bound form of TNF-α. These data collectively indicate that both activated astrocytes and microglia can produce TNF-α within the CNS.

Controversy exists as to whether astrocytes really express TNF-α in light of the findings by Hetier et al. (65), in which only murine microglia, not astrocytes, were shown to express TNF-α mRNA upon stimulation with LPS by in situ hybridization. A number of possibilities exist for this finding: *(1)* LPS is a very weak inducer of TNF-α expression by astrocytes (91), thus other stimuli should be tested in this system; and *(2)*

Table 11-3 Tumor Necrosis Factor and Glial Cells

Astrocytes

Increase class I MHC expression on primary astrocytes

Enhance class II MHC expression induced by IFN-γ or virus on primary astrocytes

Induce ICAM-1 expression on primary human and rat astrocytes

Induce proliferation of adult astrocytes, human astroglioma cell lines

Induce IL-6 production by primary rat and human astrocytes

Induce G-CSF and GM-CSF production by primary rat and human astrocytes, human astroglioma cell lines

Induce M-CSF and IL-8 production by primary human astrocytes, human astroglioma cells

Enhance expression of C3 complement component in rat astrocytes, human astroglioma cells

Primary rat and human astrocytes make TNF-α in response to LPS, virus, IFN-γ/IL-1, TNF-α

Human astroglioma cells make TNF-α in response to IL-1, PMA, calcium ionophore, TNF-α

Microglia

Microglia make TNF-α in response to LPS or IFN-γ

Oligodendrocytes

Cell death by apoptosis (DNA fragmentation)

Myelin damage

---

murine astrocytes may be poor producers of TNF-α as compared to rat astrocytes. Since astroglioma cell lines and primary human astrocytes produce TNF-α, this indicates that astrocytes have the capacity to secrete this cytokine. Table 11-3 summarizes the effects of TNF-α on glial cells.

Involvement of TNF in Neurological Disease States

Role of TNF-α and TNF-β in EAE and MS

Evidence for an involvement of TNF-α and TNF-β in EAE was obtained from studies demonstrating that the ability of encephalitogenic T-cell clones to transfer disease was positively correlated with the amount of TNF-α and TNF-β cytotoxic activity associated with these cells (133). Two groups have demonstrated that antibody to TNF-α/TNF-β could prevent the transfer of EAE by encephalitogenic T cells in SJL/J mice (146,155). Administration of soluble TNF-receptors (sTNF-R) also has a beneficial effect in EAE. Treatment with bivalent sTNF-R1 and sTNF-R2 inhibited the development of actively induced EAE in Biozzi AB/H mice and adoptive transfer induced EAE in SJL/J mice (4a,157a,158a). Interestingly, intracranial injection of sTNF-R was more effective in inhibiting disease than systemic administration, suggesting that the majority of TNF-α production/activity occurred within the CNS (4a). Kuroda and

Shimamoto (85) demonstrated that intraperitoneal injections of TNF-α resulted in a significant prolongation of clinical EAE in Lewis rats. In contrast, the disease course of EAE in SJL/J mice actively immunized with spinal cord homogenate was not affected by treatment with antibody against TNF (172). These differences may be due to the route of EAE induction. The above findings indicate that under certain conditions, TNF-α and TNF-β play an important role in EAE. Adding to these observations are the findings by Chung et al., (30) that astrocytes from EAE-susceptible and -resistant rat strains differ in their ability to express TNF-α protein. Astrocytes from Lewis rats (susceptible) produce TNF-α in response to IFN-γ/IL-1β while astrocytes from brown Norway rats (resistant) do not. The capacity for TNF-α production by Lewis astrocytes, especially in response to disease-related cytokines such as IFN-γ and IL-1, may contribute to disease susceptibility and to the inflammation and demyelination associated with EAE.

In vivo studies suggest that TNF-α/TNF-β may be implicated in MS. TNF-α+ astrocytes and macrophages have been identified in the brains of MS patients, particularly in the plaque region, an area showing extensive inflammatory cell infiltration (71). Selmaj et al. (154), have determined that both TNF-α and TNF-β are present in MS plaque regions and that TNF-α is localized within astrocytes, whereas TNF-β is associated with microglia and T cells. Increased cerebrospinal fluid levels of TNF-α have been documented in patients with MS (102,159), and a strong correlation exists between cerebrospinal fluid levels of TNF-α and disruption of the BBB in active MS patients (160). Other studies have failed to demonstrate TNF-α in the cerebrospinal fluid of MS patients (53). The failure to detect TNF-α may be due to differences in the patients examined or to the instability of TNF-α in the cerebrospinal fluid if not treated with a protease inhibitor. Additionally, TNF-α may only be present locally in the CNS during different stages of MS and not detectable in cerebrospinal fluid.

TNF in Other Neurological Diseases

Elevated levels of TNF have been demonstrated in the cerebrospinal fluid of AIDS patients, and TNF-α staining in brains from AIDS patients localizes with some endothelial cells and astrocytes, but mostly with macrophages/microglia (181). TNF-α has been shown to activate and enhance HIV-1 replication in macrophages (123,132), and thus may contribute to the pathogenesis of ADC. Astrocytes have a direct role in this process as TNF-α produced by these cells induces the expression of HIV-1 in macrophages (186).

TNF-α is detected in the cerebrospinal fluid of both mice and humans with bacterial meningitis, but not viral meningitis (94). In a rabbit model of bacterial meningitis, intracisternal administration of purified rabbit TNF-α produced significant cerebrospinal fluid inflammation (140). These studies suggest that TNF-α plays an important role in the initial events of meningeal inflammation.

Interleukin-6 and Glial Cells

Biological Action of IL-6 on Glial Cells

IL-6 is a pleiotropic cytokine involved in the regulation of inflammatory and immunologic responses. IL-6 has a mitogenic effect on bovine astrocytes (157), that may contribute to astrogliosis. Astrocytes respond to IL-6 by secreting nerve growth factor, which induces neural differentiation (48). IL-6 directly affects neurons by inducing differentiation and neurite extension and also increases the number of voltage-dependent sodium channels on these cells (151). IL-6 has been demonstrated to inhibit TNF-α production by monocytes (1). Since astrocytes can secrete TNF-α, and TNF-α induces IL-6 production by astrocytes (see below), IL-6 may be involved in the negative regulation of TNF-α expression in the CNS. We have recently demonstrated that IL-6 does in fact inhibit TNF-α expression by astrocytes (15). We have also recently shown that IL-6 inhibits ICAM-1 expression by astrocytes and microglia (163b), indicating that IL-6 has immunosuppressive effects on glial cells.

IL-6 Expression by Glial Cells

IL-6 is produced within the CNS by both astrocytes and microglia. Primary human, murine, and rat astrocytes can secrete IL-6 in response to a number of stimuli, including virus, IL-1, TNF-α, IFN-γ plus IL-1, LPS, calcium ionophore, norepinephrine (NE), and TGF-β (2,11,14,48,97,120), and human astroglioma cell lines express IL-6 mRNA in response to IL-1 (196). Mouse microglia will secrete IL-6 upon infection with virus or stimulation with the cytokine M-CSF (48), rat microglia express IL-6 upon stimulation with LPS (120), and microglial cell clones transformed by the *v-myc* oncogene constitutively secrete IL-6 (142). Similar to IL-1 and TNF-α, there are two endogenous CNS sources for IL-6, astrocytes, and microglia. These two CNS cell types are responsive to different stimuli for IL-6 production as both rat and murine microglia do not produce IL-6 in response to IL-1, TNF-α, or NE, whereas astrocytes do (48,120).

The molecular mechanism(s) by which IL-1β and TNF-α activate IL-6 expression has been examined by transient transfection of the IL-6 promoter linked to a reporter gene in primary rat astrocytes. Both IL-1β and TNF-α act at the transcriptional level to induce IL-6 gene expression, and use of deletion mutants revealed that the NF-κB-like binding site is required for cytokine induction of IL-6 promoter activity (167). Nuclear proteins isolated from IL-1β or TNF-α-treated astrocytes are specific for the NF-κB-like binding site within the IL-6 promoter, and it appears that the action of IL-1β and TNF-α is mediated by post-transcriptional activation of preexisting cytoplasmic NF-κB. Additionally, PKC activity is required for both IL-1β and TNF-α induction of IL-6 expression in astrocytes (121). See Table 11-4 for a summary of IL-6 effects on glial cells.

Table 11-4 Interleukin-6 and Glial Cells

Astrocytes

Induce proliferation of astrocytes

Enhance NGF production by primary astrocytes

Rat astrocytes make IL-6 in response to LPS, IL-1, TNF-α, IFN-γ/IL-1, virus, calcium ionophore, norepinephrine, TGF-β

Human glioma cells make IL-6 in response to IL-1

Primary human astrocytes make IL-6 in response to IL-1β or TNF-α

Inhibit TNF-α production by astrocytes

Inhibit ICAM-1 expression

Microglia

Microglia make IL-6 in response to M-CSF, virus

Inhibit ICAM-1 expression

Involvement of IL-6 in Neurological Disease States

Role of IL-6 in EAE and MS

Increased IL-6 levels have been found in the cerebrospinal fluid of mice suffering acute EAE, and the authors suggest that local production of IL-6 is responsible since serum levels of IL-6 were not elevated (55). IL-6 mRNA levels increase rapidly during acute EAE in SJL/J mice and decline when clinical symptoms resolve (81). In contrast, IL-6 protein is not found in the CNS of SJL/J mice which acquire EAE through MBP peptide immunization (109). Again, the different methods of immunization and analysis may account for the conflicting results.

One of the hallmarks of MS is intrathecal B-cell activation as evidenced by elevation of the cerebrospinal fluid IgG index and the presence of oligoclonal IgG bands in the cerebrospinal fluid (177). Since IL-6 is one of the cytokines involved in the terminal differentiation of activated B cells into immunoglobulin-secreting plasma cells (117), there has been interest in determining whether elevated IL-6 levels could be responsible for local B-cell responses within the CNS. Results from these studies have been rather confusing; two groups report that IL-6 is not detected in MS cerebrospinal fluid (47,73), while two more recent studies suggest that IL-6 is elevated in MS cerebrospinal fluid (102) and MS plasma (46). These latter findings suggest that there is a heightened systemic B-cell response in MS. IL-6 immunoreactivity has been detected at the lesion edge of burnt out plaques in MS brain, rather than in active plaques, suggesting an involvement of IL-6 in resolution of disease (108a).

IL-6 In Other Neurological Diseases

Elevated CNS IL-6 levels have been documented in other neurological diseases, such as bacterial and viral meningitis (47,73,188), CNS neoplasma (95), systemic lupus erythematosus with neurological involvement (69), and ADC (181). IL-6 has been shown to up-regulate production of HIV in infected cells of the monocytic lineage (130); thus, intracerebral production of IL-6 by both astrocytes and microglia may contribute to HIV replication within the CNS.

Transforming Growth Factor Beta and Glial Cells

Biological Action of TGF-β on Glial Cells

TGF-β is produced by a wide variety of both normal and malignant cells and can act as either an inhibitor or stimulator of various cell functions, such as proliferation or cytokine production. TGF-β can modulate the activity of both astrocytes and microglia. TGF-β1 and TGF-β2 can inhibit IFN-γ-induced class II MHC expression on both human astroglioma cells and rat astrocytes (124,153,198), inhibit proliferation of rat astrocytes (100,115,176), inhibit C3 expression by human astroglioma cells and primary astrocytes (6), inhibit or induce cytokine production by astrocytes and microglia (11,169), and can act as a chemotactic agent for both rat astrocytes and microglia (115,195). We have also recently demonstrated that TGF-β inhibits ICAM-1 expression by astrocytes in a stimulus-specific manner; TNF-α and IL-1β induced ICAM-1 expression is inhibited by TGF-β, while IFN-γ induced ICAM-1 expression is unaffected (163a). Primary rat astrocytes have been shown to express multiple subtypes of TGF-β receptors (type I, type II, and type III) (115). Since TGF-β is produced by glial cells (see below), locally produced TGF-β may contribute to the recruitment and activation of glial cells (both astrocytes and microglia) at local inflammatory sites within the CNS.

TGF-β Expression by Glial Cells

TGF-β is not normally found in adult or fetal human brain (22). TGF-β-like activity has been detected from a number of human glial tumors and astroglioma cell lines (22,31,32), which suggests that astrocytes may be a source of TGF-β within the CNS. The human glioblastoma cell lines tested could produce both latent and active forms of TGF-β and exhibited heterogeneity with respect to the isoform of TGF-β expressed (22,32). Primary astrocytes are also capable of expressing TGF-β, although there is some controversy regarding the isotype expressed. Unstimulated rat astrocytes produce undetectable levels of TGF-β, however, treatment with exogenous TGF-β1 causes the astrocyte to secrete nanogram levels of TGF-β into the supernatant (189). In situ hybridization conclusively identified the astrocyte as the cell in primary culture expressing TGF-β. This same group later demonstrated that rat astrocytes constitutively express mRNA for TGF-β1, which is increased upon exposure to exogenous TGF-β1, indicating that TGF-β1 levels can be regulated in an autocrine manner (115). da Cunha and Vitkovic (35) have also shown that primary rat astrocytes constitutively express mRNA for TGF-β1 but do not constitutively secrete TGF-β1 protein. However, upon stimulation with IL-1, the astrocytes secrete a latent form of TGF-β1. Interestingly, TGF-β1 mRNA levels do not increase, suggesting a post-transcriptional level of regulation for TGF-β1 expression. Further work from the Vitkovic laboratory has demonstrated that both primary rat oligodendrocytes and microglia can secrete TGF-β1 upon stimulation with IL-1α (34). Constam et al. (32) report that both astrocytes and microglia can constitutively secrete TGF-β; the astrocytes express mRNA for TGF-β1, β2, and β3, but only secrete TGF-β2 while microglia express mRNA for only TGF-β1. These results differ from the studies of Morganti-Kossmann et al. (115) and da Cunha et al. (34,35), as these two groups found that astrocytes can secrete the TGF-β1 isoform. It is possible that TGF-β1 is secreted only upon stimulation of the astrocytes by such agents as IL-1 or TGF-β1, and not under constitutive conditions. Taken together, the above studies indicate that all three glial cell types—astrocytes, oligodendrocytes, and microglia—are capable of secreting TGF-β, although they may produce different isoforms. Because TGF-β exerts many immunosuppressive effects, TGF-β produced by glial cells may act to restrict and/or down-regulate inflammatory processes within the CNS. See Table 11-5 for a summary of TGF-β influences on glial cells.

Table 11-5 Transforming Growth Factor Beta and Glial Cells

Astrocytes

Express types I, II, and III TGF-β receptors

Chemotactic for astrocytes

Inhibit proliferation of rat astrocytes

Inhibit IFN-γ-induced class II MHC expression on human glioma cells, rat astrocytes

Inhibit TNF-α and IL-1β-induced ICAM-1 expression on human glioma cells, rat astrocytes

Inhibit GM-CSF secretion by IL-1β stimulated human glioma cells

Human astroglioma cells and neonatal rat astrocytes express TGF-β mRNA constitutively

TGF-β mRNA expression enhanced by TGF-β, LPS, EGF, FGF

Astrocytes secrete TGF-β1 protein in response to IL-1α, TGF-β1

Primary astrocytes express TGF-β1, β2, β3 mRNA constitutively, but secrete only the latent form of TGF-β2

TGF-β1 and β2 inhibit TNF-α expression by astrocytes

TGF-β1 and β2 induce IL-6 expression by astrocytes

Microglia

Chemotactic for microglia

Secrete TGF-β1 protein in response to IL-1α

Constitutively express TGF-β1 mRNA and secrete TGF-β1 protein in latent form

TGF-β inhibits cytokine production and class II MHC expression by murine microglia

Oligodendrocytes

Secrete TGF-β1 protein in response to IL-1α

Promote oligodendrocyte differentiation

TGF-β inhibits TNF-α-mediated oligodendrocyte killing

Involvement of TGF-β in Neurological Disease States

Role of TGF-β in EAE and MS

Three studies have demonstrated that TGF-β improves the clinical course of EAE in SJL/J mice (78,86,138). Injection of TGF-β1 could delay, but not suppress, development of EAE; however, TGF-β1 could prevent the incidence of relapse in these mice (86). Racke et al. (138) demonstrated that TGF-β1 inhibited the activation of MBP-specific lymph node cells in vitro, which reduced that capacity of these cells to transfer EAE. Additionally, injection of TGF-β1 resulted in an improved clinical course, even when administered during ongoing disease. This improvement in clinical disease was accompanied by a reduction in CNS damage and in the expression of two accessory molecules, class II MHC and LFA-1. Johns et al. (78) showed that in vivo injection of TGF-β1 reduced the incidence of clinical disease, as well as the severity of inflammation and demyelination within the CNS. In addition, TGF-β1, β2, and β3 were present in inflammatory lesions within the brain. Conversely, injection of anti-TGF-β antibodies resulted in an increase in severity and duration of disease (137). The mechanism(s) by which TGF-β modulates the disease course of EAE is currently unknown; however, possibilities are that the protective effect of TGF-β is exerted at the level of the target organ (CNS), and/or that TGF-β inhibits both the production of TNF-α and its effects within the CNS (11,149). A recent study by Fabry et al. (37a), documented that TGF-β inhibited the migration of lymphocytes into the CNS in animals with EAE.

With respect to MS, one study demonstrated that TGF-β activity could be detected in the blood of MS patients with active disease, and within this group of patients, TGF-β activity was significantly correlated to the period of regression of symptoms (9). In studies to examine TGF-β production by cells from MS patients, a number of investigators have shown that TGF-β expression correlates with disease recovery and/or stable disease (32a,100a,114,141a,b). These data suggest that TGF-β may contribute to regression of exacerbations in MS. A phase I clinical trial to assess the effect of TGF-β2 in MS patients began in April, 1994 (Dr. Joseph Carlino, Celtrix Pharmaceuticals).

TGF-β In Other Neurological Diseases

TGF-β1 has been identified in the brains of patients with AIDS, but not in control brain tissue (189). The TGF-β staining was localized to macrophages, microglia, and astrocytes, especially in areas of diseased brain. Moreover, HIV-1-infected monocytes secreted a factor which induced cultured astrocytes to secrete TGF-β. This factor, in all likelihood, is TGF-β itself (80). TGF-β in turn suppresses HIV replication in primary macrophages (131). Thus, HIV-1-induced TGF-β production by macrophages may act in an autocrine manner to inhibit HIV replication or in a paracrine fashion to induce astrocytes to produce TGF-β. By either pathway, TGF-β may play an important role as a regulator of HIV expression in infected macrophages and/or microglia.

Colony-stimulating Factors

Biological Action of CSFs on Glial Cells

Colony-stimulating factors are cytokines that regulate the survival, proliferation, and differentiation of hematopoietic cells, including mononuclear phagocytes. Because activation of microglia, the macrophage of the brain, is an important early response to brain trauma, there has been interest in how the activation and differentiation of microglia is induced. Numerous studies have examined the ability of CSFs to stimulate biologic activity of microglia. Frei et al. (50) demonstrated that both IL-3 and GM-CSF induced murine microglia to proliferate. Furthermore, in vitro studies by Giulian and Ingeman (57) also showed that rat microglia could proliferate in response to IL-3, GM-CSF, and M-CSF, and that both IL-3 and GM-CSF induced more rapid phagocytosis by microglia. They also performed in vivo experiments in which recombinant forms of GM-CSF, IL-3, M-CSF or G-CSF were infused into the cerebral cortex of rats. Both GM-CSF and IL-3 stimulated the appearance of microglia at the site of injection and the phagocytic capability of these cells. M-CSF has also been show to induce microglia to produce IL-6 (48). The biological effect of M-CSF on microglia is explained by the fact that microglia express the functional receptor for M-CSF, which is the *c-fms* protooncogene (63). These findings indicate that some of the CSFs can enhance inflammatory responses within the CNS by activation of microglia.

CSF Expression by Glial Cells

Astrocytes appear to be the major source of CSFs within the brain. Initial studies by Frei et al. (44,45) indicated that astrocytes were capable of producing IL-3. IL-3 activity in these studies was assessed by the induction of macrophage and microglia proliferation. Further studies by this same group, using more sensitive techniques such as Northern blotting, demonstrated that astrocytes express mRNA for both GM-CSF and G-CSF and secrete these two CSFs (103). mRNA for IL-3 was not detected in astrocytes. Thus the macrophage and microglial proliferation is most likely attributable to GM-CSF and G-CSF, rather than IL-3. Unstimulated astrocytes do not constitutively express these CSFs, but are induced by both TNF-α and LPS (103,122). Human astroglioma cell lines can also express GM-CSF and G-CSF in vitro upon stimulation with IL-1 and TNF-α (49,179,180). Interestingly, GM-CSF cannot be detected in vivo, which may be due to the fact that astroglioma cells also produce TGF-β2, which, in vitro, can inhibit GM-CSF production (49). Thus, the ability to detect GM-CSF in vivo may be dependent upon the time of sampling, or it may not be possible, due to the presence of immunosuppressive cytokines like TGF-β. Normal human astrocytes were recently shown to produce GM-CSF, M-CSF, and G-CSF in response to both IL-1 and TNF-α (2). Unstimulated human astrocytes constitutively expressed mRNA for M-CSF, but they had to be induced by IL-1 or TNF-α to express transcripts for GM-CSF or G-CSF. Similar observations have been made for murine astrocytes (63,173). Microglia can be induced to express mRNA for both M-CSF and G-CSF upon stimulation with LPS (103,173), although measurements for protein expression have not been performed. These findings, taken in concert, indicate that astrocytes are the principal source of CSFs within the CNS, and that these factors can activate numerous biological properties of microglia which are related to inflammatory processes. See Table 11-6 for a summary of CSFs and glial cells.

Cells of the monocyte/macrophage series are important in mediating the disease process of EAE since in vivo depletion of these cells protects against EAE in the rat (24,74). There is only one report on the expression of CSFs in EAE, that being an examination of M-CSF and its receptor, c-fms, in Lewis rats with EAE (75). In this study, a low basal level of M-CSF mRNA was detected in unimmunized animals, and in those immunized with myelin, higher levels of M-CSF mRNA were detected during the preclinical period (days 6 and 8), which peaked immediately before maximal expression of disease. Expression of M-CSF mRNA declined to baseline values when the animals recovered. Expression of the receptor for M-CSF, c-fms, was elevated immediately before disease onset and peaked at the height of clinical symptoms. Interesting, c-fms mRNA expression remained elevated after resolution of the acute phase of EAE. These results indicate that production of a factor that affects monocyte growth, survival, and differentiation (M-CSF) occurs within the CNS of animals with EAE and correlates with disease progression and recovery.

Summary and Conclusion

This chapter has summarized studies showing that cells of the immune system and glial cells of the CNS use many of the same cytokines as communication signals. Activated astrocytes and microglia are the principal sources of these cytokines, although oligodendrocytes are capable of expressing IL-1 and TGF-β. The glial cells respond to these cytokines by changes in gene expression which include *(1)* regulation of proliferation and differentiation, *(2)* induction and enhancement of the expression of cell-surface antigens (class I MHC, class II MHC, ICAM-1), and *(3)* stimulation of the secretion of other cytokines. Some of these changes allow for physical contact between the two systems; i.e., as when class II MHC+ microglia and/or astrocytes present foreign antigens to T helper cells, or when class I MHC+ microglia, astrocytes, and oligodendrocytes serve as target cells for cytotoxic T cells. The secretion of cytokines by glial cells and immune cells allows for bidirectional communication mediated by

Table 11-6 Colony-Stimulating Factors and Glial Cells

Granulocyte-Macrophage Colony-Stimulating Factor

Astrocytes

Murine astrocytes make GM-CSF in response to LPS or TNF-α

Human astroctyes make GM-CSF in response to TNF-α or IL-1β

Glioblastoma/astrocytoma cell lines secrete GM-CSF upon stimulation with IL-1 or TNF-α

Microglia

Proliferate in response to GM-CSF

Increases phagocytic properties of microglia

Stimulates appearance of macrophages within the brain

Inhibit class II MHC expression

Granulocyte Colony-Stimulating Factor

Astrocytes

Murine astrocytes make G-CSF in response to LPS or TNF-α

Human astrocytes make G-CSF in response to TNF-α or IL-1β

Glioblastoma/astrocytoma cell lines secrete G-CSF in response to IL-1 or TNF-α

Microglia

Express G-CSF mRNA upon stimulation with LPS

Macrophage Colony-Stimulating Factor (CSF-1)

Astrocytes

Murine astrocytes and two astrocytic cell lines express M-CSF mRNA constitutively

Primary human astrocytes constitutively express M-CSF, which is enhanced in response to IL-1 and TNF-α

Microglia

Proliferate in response to M-CSF

Undergo morphological changes in response to M-CSF

Express receptors for M-CSF *(c-fms)*

Express M-CSF mRNA upon stimulation with LPS

Induce microglia to produce IL-6

Inhibit class II MHC expression

Interleukin-3 (Multi-CSF)

Microglia

Proliferate in response to IL-3

Increase phagocytic properties of microglia

Stimulate appearance of macrophages within the brain

Induce morphological changes in microglia

445

soluble factors. There is a complex circuitry of interactions mediated by cytokines, especially in the event of BBB damage and lymphoid/mononuclear cell infiltration into the CNS. The secretion of IFN-γ by infiltrating activated T cells may be the initiating signal for glial cell activation by inducing astrocytes and microglia to express class I and II MHC antigens, and priming these cells for subsequent cytokine production. In addition, infiltrating activated macrophages produce cytokines such as IL-1, TNF-α, and IL-6, which, in concert with IFN-γ, would trigger glial cells to produce their own cytokines. The activation of astrocytes and microglia to secrete cytokines may contribute to the propagation of intracerebral immune and inflammatory responses initiated by immune cells. The ongoing cytokine cascades in the CNS could ultimately be down-regulated and suppressed, due to the presence of immunosuppressive cytokines such as TGF-β, or perpetuated, leading to disease progression. Whether immune and inflammatory responses within the CNS are propagated or suppressed depends on a number of factors including *(1)* the activational status of these cells, *(2)* cytokine receptor levels on glial and immune cells, *(3)* the presence of cytokines with both immune-enhancing and immune-suppressing effects (IFN-γ, IL-1, TNF-α, IL-6, TGF-β, CSFs), *(4)* the concentration and location of these cytokines in the CNS, and *(5)* the temporal sequence in which a particular cell is exposed to numerous cytokines. The ultimate outcome of immunologic and inflammatory events in the CNS will be determined in part by an interplay of the above parameters. Members of the chemokine family have recently been suggested to contribute to disease development within the CNS (75,141), while other cytokines with immunosuppressive effects such as IL-10 and IL-4 have been implicated in mediating recovery from EAE (81,82). These cytokines will undoubtedly influence the action of the cytokines that have been reviewed in this chapter and will warrant further investigation.

Many of the studies sited in this chapter reflect the capacity of cultured primary murine, rodent, and human cells or human glial cell lines to function in vitro. These studies provide important information on how these cells can respond to a variety of agents. They also provide useful working models for understanding further the nature of the second messenger signals utilized by glial cells, delineating *cis*-acting DNA regulatory elements and nuclear proteins involved with MHC and cytokine expression by glial cells, and characterizing the types of cytokine receptors found on glial cells. The in vitro studies suffer, however, from the fact that the cells have been taken out of their natural microenvironment. In vivo studies can address the capacity of cells to express cytokines or surface antigens in their normal setting, or in the case of EAE or MS, during ongoing disease. Many of the in vivo studies have demonstrated that particular glial cells can express certain genes, which correlate well with in vitro results. One example in which in vitro and in vivo studies have yielded conflicting data is astrocyte class II MHC expression. In vitro, astrocytes express class II MHC antigens upon stimulation with IFN-γ (40), however, in vivo, class II–positive astrocytes are rare. These in vivo findings may be due to the fact that astrocyte class II expression is subject to down-regulation by endogenous agents such as norepinephrine and glutamate (52,90). Thus, in vitro findings provide information as to the individual agents that can either stimulate or inhibit class II expression on astrocytes, and such studies allow for a more complete understanding of how these agents may act collectively in vivo.

In vivo studies are increasingly oriented towards examining cytokine expression in a number of disease states, and the use of more sensitive techniques such as in situ hybridization and polymerase chain reaction will provide definitive data on this topic. The recent study by Saeki et al. (148), which demonstrated the development of MS-like pathology in SCID mice by intracisternal injection of mononuclear cells from cerebrospinal fluid of MS patients, provides a very nice model system in which to identify cytokines responsible for the inflammatory processes in the CNS.

Thus, the combined use of both in vitro and in vivo systems, and extrapolation between the two, will provide an understanding of the mechanism(s) by which cytokines influence glial cell function and ultimately contribute to disease progression and/or recovery.

Acknowledgments

I thank Ms. Sue Wade for superb secretarial and editorial assistance in preparing this manuscript. This work was supported by National Multiple Sclerosis Society Grants 2205-B-5 and 2269-B-5, and National Institutes of Health Grants NS-29719, NS-31096, MH-50421, and MH-55795.

References

1. Aderka D, Le J, Vilcek J. IL-6 inhibits lipopolysaccharide-induced tumor necrosis factor production in cultured human monocytes, U937 cells, and in mice. J Immunol 143:3517–3523, 1989.
2. Aloisi F, Care A, Borsellino G, Gallo P, Rosa S, Bassani A, Cabibbo A, Testa U, Levi G, Peschle C. Production of hemolymphopoietic cytokines (IL-6, IL-8, colony-stimulating factors) by normal human astrocytes in response to IL-1β and tumor necrosis factor-α. J Immunol 149:2358–2366, 1992.
3. Arai K, Lee F, Miyajima A, Miyatake S, Arai N, Yokota T. Cytokines: coordinators of immune and inflammatory responses. Annu Rev Biochem 59:783–836, 1990.
4. Baker D, O'Neill JK, Turk JL. Cytokines in the central nervous system of mice during chronic relapsing experimental allergic encephalomyelitis. Cell Immunol 134:505–510, 1991.
4a. Baker D, Butler D, Scallon BJ, O'Neill JK, Turk JL, Feldmann M. Control of established experimental allergic encephalomyelitis by inhibition of tumor necrosis factor (TNF) activity within the central nervous system using monoclonal antibodies and TNF receptor-immunoglobulin fusion proteins. Eur J Immunol 24:2040–2048, 1994.
5. Barnum SR. Biosynthesis and regulation of complement by cells of the central nervous

system. In: Complement Profiles, JM Cruse, RE Lewis Jr, ed. Karger, Basel, 1993, p 76–95.

6. Barnum SR, Jones JL. Transforming growth factor-β1 inhibits inflammatory cytokine-induced C3 gene expression in astrocytes. J Immunol 152:765–773, 1994.

7. Barnum SR, Jones JL, Benveniste EN. Interferon-gamma regulation of C3 gene expression in human astroglioma cells. J Neuroimmunol 38:275–282, 1992.

8. Barnum SR, Jones JL, Benveniste EN. Interleukin-1 and tumor necrosis factor mediated regulation of C3 gene expression in human astroglioma cells. Glia 7:225–236, 1993.

8a. Beck J, Rondot P, Catinot L, Falcoff E, Kirchner H, Wietzerbin J. Increased production of interferon gamma and tumor necrosis factor precedes clinical manifestation in multiple sclerosis: Do cytokines trigger off exacerbations? Acta Neurol Scand 78:318–323, 1988.

9. Beck J, Rondot P, Jullien P, Wietzerbin J, Lawrence DA. TGF-β-like activity produced during regression of exacerbations in multiple sclerosis. Acta Neurol Scand 84:452–455, 1991.

10. Benacerraf B. Role of MHC gene products in immune regulation. Science 212:1229–1238, 1981.

11. Benveniste EN, Kwon JB, Chung WJ, Sampson J, Pandya K, Tang L-P. Differential modulation of astrocyte cytokine gene expression by TGF-β. J Immunol 153:5210–5221, 1994.

12. Benveniste EN, Merrill JE, Kaufman SE, Golde DW, Gasson JC. Purification and characterization of human T-lymphocyte derived glial growth promoting factor. Proc Natl Acad Sci USA 82:3930–3934, 1985.

13. Benveniste EN, Sparacio SM, Bethea JR. Tumor necrosis factor-α enhances interferon-γ mediated class II antigen expression on astrocytes. J Neuroimmunol 25:209–219, 1989.

14. Benveniste EN, Sparacio SM, Norris JG, Grenett HE, Fuller GM. Induction and regulation of interleukin-6 gene expression in rat astrocytes. J Neuroimmunol 30:201–212, 1990.

15. Benveniste EN, Tang LP, Law RM. Differential regulation of astrocyte TNF-α expression by the cytokines TGF-β, IL-6 and IL-10. Intl J Dev Neuroscience 13:341–349, 1995.

16. Benveniste EN, Vidovic M, Panek RB, Norris JG, Reddy AT, Benos DJ. Interferon-γ induced astrocyte class II major histocompatibility complex gene expression is associated with both protein kinase C activation and Na+ entry. J Biol Chem 266:18119–18126, 1991.

17. Bethea JR, Chung IY, Sparacio SM, Gillespie GY, Benveniste EN. Interleukin-1β induction of tumor necrosis factor-alpha gene expression in human astroglioma cells. J Neuroimmunol 36:179–191, 1992.

18. Bethea JR, Gillespie GY, Benveniste EN. Interleukin-1β induction of TNF-α gene expression: involvement of protein kinase C. J Cell Physiol 152:264–273, 1992.

19. Bethea JR, Gillespie GY, Chung IY, Benveniste EN. Tumor necrosis factor production and receptor expression by a human astroglioma cell line. J Neuroimmunol 30:1–13, 1990.

20. Bignami A, Eng LF, Dahl D, Uyeda CT. Localization of the glial fibrillary acidic protein in astrocytes by immunofluorescence. Brain Res 43:429–435, 1972.

21. Billiau A, Heremans H, Vandekerckhove F, Dijkmans R, Sobis H, Meulepas E, Carton H. Enhancement of experimental allergic encephalomyelitis in mice by antibodies against IFN-γ. J Immunol 140:1506–1510, 1988.

22. Bodmer S, Strommer K, Frei K, Siepl C, de Tribolet N, Heid I, Fontana A. Immunosuppression and transforming growth factor-β in glioblastoma. J Immunol 143:3222–3229, 1989.

23. Brett J, Gerlach H, Nawroth P, Steinberg S, Godman G, Stern D. Tumor necrosis factor/cachectin increases permeability of endothelial cell monolayers by a mechanism involving regulatory G proteins. J Exp Med 169:1977–1991, 1989.

24. Brosnan CF, Bornstein MB, Bloom BR. The effects of macrophage depletion on the clinical and pathologic expression of experimental allergic encephalomyelitis. J Immunol 126:614–620, 1981.

25. Cannella B, Cross AH, Raine CS. Upregulation and coexpression of adhesion molecules correlate with relapsing autoimmune demyelination in the central nervous system. J Exp Med 172:1521–1524, 1990.

26. Chantry D, Turner M, Abney E, Feldmann M. Modulation of cytokine production by transforming growth factor-β. J Immunol 142:4295–4300, 1989.

27. Chao CC, Hu S, Close K, Choi CS, Molitor TW, Novick WJ, Peterson PK. Cytokine release from microglia: differential inhibition by pentoxifylline and dexamethasone. J Infect Dis 166:847–853, 1992.

28. Chung IY, Benveniste EN. Tumor necrosis factor-α production by astrocytes: induction by lipopolysaccharide, IFN-γ and IL-1β. J Immunol 144:2999–3007, 1990.

29. Chung IY, Kwon J, Benveniste EN. Role of protein kinase C activity in tumor necrosis factor-α gene expression: involvement at the transcriptional level. J Immunol 149:3894–3902, 1992.

30. Chung IY, Norris JG, Benveniste EN. Differential tumor necrosis factor α expression by astrocytes from experimental allergic encephalomyelitis-susceptible and -resistant rat strains. J Exp Med 173:801–811, 1991.

31. Clark WC, Bressler J. Transforming growth factor-β-like activity in tumors of the central nervous system. J Neurosurg 68:920–924, 1988.

32. Constam DB, Philipp J, Malipiero UV, ten Dijke P, Schachner M, Fontana A. Differential expression of transforming growth factor-β1, -β2, and -β3 by glioblastoma cells, astrocytes, and microglia. J Immunol 148:1404–1410, 1992.

32a. Correale J, Gilmore W, McMillan M, Li S, McCarthy K, Le T, Weiner LP. Patterns of cytokine secretion by autoreactive proteolipid protein-specific T cell clones during the course of multiple sclerosis. J Immunol 154:2959–2968, 1995.

33. Cross AH, Cannella B, Brosnan CF, Raine CS. Homing to central nervous system vasculature by antigen-specific lymphocytes. Lab Invest 63:162–170, 1990.

34. da Cunha A, Jefferson JA, Jackson RW, Vitkovic L. Glial cell-specific mechanisms of TGF-β1 induction by IL-1 in cerebral cortex. J Neuroimmunol 42:71–86, 1993.

35. da Cunha A, Vitkovic L. Transforming growth factor-beta (TGF-β1) expression and regulation in rat cortical astrocytes. J Neuroimmunol 36:157–169, 1992.

36. de Giovine FS, Duff GW. Interleukin 1: the first interleukin. Immunol Today 11:13–14, 1990.

37. Duong TT, St. Louis J, Gilbert JJ, Finkelman FD, Strejan GH. Effect of anti-interferon-γ and anti-interleukin-2 monoclonal antibody treatment on the development of actively and passively induced experimental allergic encephalomyelitis in the SJL/J mouse. J Neuroimmunol 36:105–115, 1992.

37a. Fabry Z, Topham DJ, Fee D, Herlein J, Carlino JA, Hart MN, Sriram S. TGF-β2 decreases migration of lymphocytes in vitro and homing of cells into the central nervous system in vivo. J Immunol 155:325–332, 1995.

38. Fierz W, Endler B, Reske K, Wekerle H, Fontana A. Astrocytes as antigen presenting cells. I. Induction of Ia antigen expression on astrocytes by T cells via immune interferon and its effect on antigen presentation. J Immunol 134:3785–3793, 1985.

39. Fontana A, Dubs R, Merchant R, Balsiger S, Grob PJ. Glia cell stimulating factor (GSF): a new lymphokine. part 1: cellular sources and partial purification of murine GSF, role of cytoskeleton and protein synthesis in its production. J Neuroimmunol 2:55–71, 1982.

40. Fontana A, Fierz W, Wekerle H. Astrocytes present myelin basic protein to encephalitogenic T-cell lines. Nature 307:273–276, 1984.

41. Fontana A, Hengartner H, de Tribolet N, Weber E. Glioblastoma cells release interleukin-1 and factors inhibiting interleukin-2-mediated effects. J Immunol 132:1837–1844, 1984.

42. Fontana A, Kristensen F, Dubs R, Gemsa D, Weber E. Production of prostaglandin E and an interleukin-1-like factor by cultured astrocytes and C6 glioma cells. J Immunol 129:2413–2419, 1982.

43. Fontana A, Otz U, DeWeck AL, Grob PJ. Glia cell stimulating factor (GSF): a new lymphokine. Part 2: cellular sources and partial purification of human GSF. J Neuroimmunol 2:73–81, 1982.

44. Frei K, Bodmer S, Schwerdel C, Fontana A. Astrocytes of the brain synthesize Interleukin-3-like factors. J Immunol 135:4044–4047, 1985.

45. Frei K, Bodmer S, Schwerdel C, Fontana A. Astrocyte-derived interleukin 3 as a growth factor for microglial cells and peritoneal macrophages. J Immunol 137:3521–3527, 1986.

46. Frei K, Fredrikson S, Fontana A, Link H. Interleukin-6 is elevated in plasma in multiple sclerosis. J Neuroimmunol 31:147–153, 1991.

47. Frei K, Leist TP, Meager A, Gallo P, Leppert D, Zinkernagel RM, Fontana A. Production of B cell stimulatory factor-2 and interferon-γ in the central nervous system during viral meningitis and encephalitis. Evaluation in a murine model infection and in patients. J Exp Med 168:449–453, 1988.

48. Frei K, Malipiero UV, Leist TP, Zinkernagel RM, Schwab ME, Fontana A. On the cellular source and function of interleukin-6 produced in the central nervous system in viral diseases. Eur J Immunol 19:689–694, 1989.

49. Frei K, Piani D, Malipiero UV, Van Meir E, de Tribolet N, Fontana A. Granulocyte-macrophage colony-stimulating factor (GM-CSF) production by glioblastoma cells. J Immunol 148:3140–3146, 1992.

50. Frei K, Siepl C, Groscurth P, Bodmer S, Schwerdel C, Fontana A. Antigen presentation and tumor cytotoxicity by interferon-γ-treated microglial cells. Eur J Immunol 17:1271–1278, 1987.

51. Frohman EM, Frohman TC, Dustin ML, Vayuvegula B, Choi B, Gupta A, van den Noort S, Gupta, S. The induction of intercellular adhesion molecule 1 (ICAM-1) expression on human fetal astrocytes by interferon-γ, tumor necrosis factor-γ, lymphotoxin, and interleukin-1: relevance to intracerebral antigen presentation. J Neuroimmunol 23:117–124, 1989.

52. Frohman EM, Vayuvegula B, Gupta S, van den Noort S. Norepinephrine inhibits γ interferon-induced major histocompatibility class II (Ia) antigen expression on cultured astrocytes via β₂-adrenergic signal transduction mechanisms. Proc Natl Acad Sci USA 85:1292–1296, 1988.

53. Gallo P, Piccinno MG, Krzalic L, Tavolato B. Tumor necrosis factor alpha (TNFα) and neurological diseases: failure in detecting TNFα in the cerebrospinal fluid from patients with multiple sclerosis, AIDS dementia complex, and brain tumors. J Neuroimmunol 23:41–44, 1989.

54. Gasque P, Julen N, Ischenko AM, Picot C, Mauger C, Ghauzy C, Ripoche J, Fontaine M. Expression of complement components of the alternative pathway by glioma cell lines. J Immunol 149:1381–1387, 1992.

55. Gijbels K, Van Damme J, Proost P, Put W, Carton H, Billiau A. Interleukin 6 production in the central nervous system during experimental autoimmune encephalomyelitis. Eur J Immunol 20:233–235, 1990.

56. Giulian D, Baker TJ, Shih L, Lachman LB. Interleukin-1 of the central nervous system is produced by ameboid microglia. J Exp Med 164:594–604, 1986.

57. Giulian D, Ingeman JE. Colony-stimulating factors as promoters of ameboid microglia. J Neurosci 8:4707–4717, 1988.

58. Giulian D, Lachman LB. Interleukin-1 stimulation of astroglial proliferation after brain injury. Science 228:497–499, 1985.

59. Giulian D, Woodward J, Young DG, Krebs JF, Lachman LB. Interleukin-1 injected into mammalian brain stimulates astrogliosis and neovascularization. J Neurosci 8:2485–2490, 1988.

60. Glimcher LH, Kara CJ. Sequences and factors: a guide to MHC class II transcription. Annu Rev Immunol 10:13–49, 1992.

61. Golde DW, Gasson JC. Hormones that stimulate the growth of blood cells. Sci Am July:62–70, 1988.

62. Griffin WST, Stanley LC, Ling C. Brain interleukin 1 and S-100 immunoreactivity are elevated in Down syndrome and Alzheimer disease. Proc Natl Acad Sci USA 86:7611–7615, 1989.

63. Hao C, Guilbert LJ, Fedoroff S. Production of colony-stimulating factor-1 (CSF-1) by mouse astroglia *in vitro*. J Neurosci Res 27:314–323, 1990.

63a. Harlan DM, Abe R, Lee KP, June CH. Potential roles of the B7 and CD28 receptor families in autoimmunity and immune evasion. Clin Immunol Immunopathol 75:99–111, 1995.

64. Hauser SL, Bhan, AK, Gilles FH, Hoban CJ, Reinherz EL, Schlossman SF, Weiner HL. Immunohistochemical staining of human brain with monoclonal antibodies that identify lymphocytes, monocytes and the Ia antigen. J Neuroimmunol 5:197–205, 1983.

65. Hetier E, Ayala J, Bousseau A, Denefle P, Prochiantz A. Amoeboid microglial cells and not astrocytes synthesize TNF-α in Swiss mouse brain cell cultures. Eur J Neurosci 2:762–768, 1990.

66. Hetier E, Ayala J, Denefle P, Bousseau A, Rouget P, Mallat M, Pronchiantz A. Brain macrophages synthesize interleukin-1 and interleukin-1 mRNAs *in vitro*. J Neurosci Res 21:391–397, 1988.

67. Hickey WF, Osborn JP, Kirby WM. Expression of Ia molecules by astrocytes during acute experimental allergic encephalomyelitis in the Lewis rat. Cell Immunol 91:528–535, 1985.

68. Hirayama M, Yokochi T, Shimokata K, Iida M, Fujuki N. Induction of human leukocyte antigen-A, B, C and -DR on cultured human oligodendrocytes and astrocytes by human γ-interferon. Neurosci Lett 72:369–374, 1986.

69. Hirohata S, Miyamoto T. Elevated levels of interleukin-6 in cerebrospinal fluid from patients with systemic lupus erythematosus and central nervous system involvement. Arthritis Rheum 33:644–649, 1990.

70. Hofman FM, Hinton DR, Baemayr J, Weil M, Merrill JE. Lymphokines and immunoregulatory molecules in subacute sclerosing panencephalitis. Clin Immunol Immunopathol 58:331–342, 1991.

71. Hofman FM, Hinton DR, Johnson K, Merrill JE. Tumor necrosis factor identified in multiple sclerosis brain. J Exp Med 170:607–612, 1989.

72. Hofman FM, VonHanwher R, Dinarello C, Mizel S, Hinton D, Merrill JE. Immunoregulatory molecules and IL-2 receptors identified in multiple sclerosis brain. J Immunol 136:3239–3245, 1986.

73. Houssiau FA, Bukasa K, Sindic CJM, Van Damme J, Van Snick J. Elevated levels of the 26K human hybridoma growth factor (interleukin 6) in cerebrospinal fluid of patients

with acute infection of the central nervous system. Clin Exp Immunol 71:320–323, 1988.

74. Huitinga I, van Rooijen N, de Groot CJA, Uitdehaag BMJ, and Dijkstra CD. Suppression of experimental allergic encephalomyelitis in Lewis rats after elimination of macrophages. J Exp Med 172:1025–1033, 1990.

75. Hulkower K, Brosnan CF, Aquino DA, Cammer W, Kulshrestha S, Guida MP, Rapoport DA, Berman JW. Expression of CSF-1, *c-fms,* and MCP-1 in the central nervous system of rats with experimental allergic encephalomyelitis. J Immunol 150:2525–2533, 1993.

76. Ijzermans JNM, Marquet RL. Interferon-gamma: a review. Immunobiology 179:456–473, 1989.

77. Jacobs CA, Baker PE, Roux ER, Picha KS, Toivola B, Waugh S, Kennedy MK. Experimental autoimmune encephalomyelitis is exacerbated by IL-1α and suppressed by soluble IL-1 receptor. J Immunol 146:2983–2989, 1991.

78. Johns LD, Flanders KC, Ranges GE, Sriam S. Successful treatment of experimental allergic encephalomyelitis with transforming growth factor-β1. J Immunol 147:1793–1796, 1991.

78a. June CH, Bluestone JA, Nadler LM, Thompson CB. The B7 and CD28 receptor families. Immunol Today 15:321–331, 1994.

79. Kasahara T, Mukaida N, Yamashita K, Yagisawa H, Akahoshi T, Matsushima K. IL-1 and TNF-α induction of IL-8 and monocyte chemotactic and activating factor (MCAF) mRNA expression in a human astrocytoma cell line. Immunology 74:60–67, 1991.

80. Kekow J, Wachsman W, McCutchan JA, Cronin M, Carson DA, Lotz M. Transforming growth factor-β and non-cytopathic mechanisms of immunodeficiency in human immunodeficiency virus infection. Proc Natl Acad Sci USA 87:8321–8325, 1990.

81. Kennedy MK, Torrance DS, Picha KS, Mohler KM. Analysis of cytokine mRNA expression in the central nervous system of mice with experimental autoimmune encephalomyelitis reveals that IL-10 mRNA expression correlate with recovery. J Immunol 149:2496–2505, 1992.

82. Khoury SJ, Hancock WW, Weiner HL. Oral tolerance to myelin basic protein and natural recovery from experimental autoimmune encephalomyelitis are associated with downregulation of inflammatory cytokines and differential upregulation of transforming growth factor β, interleukin 4, and prostaglandin E expression in the brain. J Exp Med 176:1355–1364, 1992.

83. Koyanagi Y, O'Brien WA, Zhao JQ, Golde DW, Gasson JC, Chen ISY. Cytokines alter production of HIV-1 from primary mononuclear phagocytes. Science 241:1673–1675, 1988.

84. Kriegler M, Perez C, DeFay K, Albert I, Lu SD. A novel form of TNF/cachectin is a cell surface cytotoxic transmembrane protein: ramifications for the complex physiology of TNF. Cell 53:45–53, 1988.

85. Kuroda Y, Shimamoto Y. Human tumor necrosis factor-α augments experimental allergic encephalomyelitis in rats. J Neuroimmunol 34:159–164, 1991.

86. Kuruvilla AP, Shah R, Hochwald GM, Liggitt HD, Palladino MA, Thorbecke GJ. Protective effect of transforming growth factor β_1 on experimental autoimmune diseases in mice. Proc Natl Acad Sci USA 88:2918–2921, 1991.

87. Lachman LB, Brown, DC, Dinarello CA. Growth promoting effect of recombinant interleukin-1 and tumor necrosis factor for a human astrocytoma cell line. J Immunol 138:2913–2916, 1987.

88. Lavi E, Suzumura A, Murasko DM, Murray EM, Silberg DH, Weiss SR. Tumor necrosis factor induces expression of MHC class I antigens on mouse astrocytes. J Neuroimmunol 18:245–253, 1988.

89. Lee JC, Simon PL, Young PR. Constitutive and PMA-induced interleukin-1 production by the human astrocytoma cell line T24. Cell Immunol 118:298–311, 1989.

90. Lee SC, Collins M, Vanguri P, Shin ML. Glutamate differentially inhibits the expression of class II MHC antigens on astrocytes and microglia. J Immunol 148:3391–3397, 1992.

91. Lee SC, Liu W, Dickson DW, Brosnan CF, Berman JW. Cytokine production by human fetal microglia and astrocytes: differential induction by lipopolysaccharide and IL-1β. J Immunol 150:2659–2667, 1993.

92. Lee SC, Moore GRW, Golenwsky G, Raine CS. Multiple sclerosis: a role for astroglia in active demyelination suggested by class II MHC expression and ultrastructural study. J Neuropathol Exp Neurol 49:122–136, 1990.

93. Lee Y-J, Panek RB, Huston M, Benveniste EN. Role of protein kinase C and tyrosine kinase activity in IFN-γ induced expression of the class II MHC gene. Am J Physiol: Cell Physiol 268:C127–C137, 1995.

94. Leist TP, Frei K, Kam-Hansen S, Zinkernagel RM, Fontana A. Tumor necrosis factor α in cerebrospinal fluid during bacterial, but not viral, meningitis. J Exp Med 167:1743–1748, 1988.

95. Leppert D, Frei K, Gallo P, Yasargil MG, Hess K, Baumgartner G, Fontana A. Brain tumors: detection of B-cell stimulatory factor-2/interleukin-6 in the absence of oligoclonal bands of immunoglobulins. J Neuroimmunol 24:259–264, 1989.

96. Levi-Strauss M, Mallat M. Primary cultures of murine astrocytes produce C3 and factor B, two components of the alternative pathway of complement activation. J Immunol 139:2361–2366, 1987.

97. Lieberman AP, Pitha PM, Shin HS, Shin ML. Production of tumor necrosis factor and other cytokines by astrocytes stimulated with lipopolysaccharide or a neurotropic virus. Proc Natl Acad Sci USA 86:6348–6352, 1989.

98. Lieberman AP, Pitha PM, Shin ML. Protein kinase regulates tumor necrosis factor mRNA stability in virus-stimulated astrocytes. J Exp Med 172:989–992, 1990.

99. Lieberman AP, Pitha PM, Shin ML. Poly(A) removal is the kinase-regulated step in tumor necrosis factor mRNA decay. J Biol Chem 267:2123–2126, 1992.

100. Lindholm D, Castren E, Kiefer R, Zafra F, Thoenen H. Transforming growth factor-β1 in the rat brain: increase after injury and inhibition of astrocyte proliferation. J Cell Biol 117:395–400, 1992.

100a. Link J, Söderström M, Olsson T, Höjeberg B, Ljungdahl A, Link H. Increased transforming growth factor-β, interleukin-4, and interferon-γ in multiple sclerosis. Ann Neurol 36:379–386, 1994.

101. Loetscher H, Pan YE, Lahm HW, Gentz R, Brockhaus M, Tabuchi H, Lesslauer W. Molecular cloning and expression of the human 55 kd tumor necrosis factor receptor. Cell 61:351–359, 1990.

101a. Lu C-Z, Jensen MA, Arnason BGW. Interferon-γ and interleukin-4-secreting cells in multiple sclerosis. J Neuroimmunol 46:123–128, 1993.

102. Maimone D, Gregory S, Arnason BGW, Reder AT. Cytokine levels in the cerebrospinal fluid and serum of patients with multiple sclerosis. J Neuroimmunol 32:67–74, 1991.

103. Malipiero UV, Frei K, Fontana A. Production of hemopoietic colony-stimulating factors by astrocytes. J Immunol 144:3816–3821, 1990.

104. Mannie MD, Dinarello CA, Paterson PY. Interleukin 1 and myelin basic protein synergistically augment adoptive transfer activity of lymphocytes mediating experimental autoimmune encephalomyelitis in Lewis rats. J Immunol 138:4229–4235, 1987.

105. Massa PT, Schmipl A, Wecker E, ter Meulen V. Tumor necrosis factor amplifies virus-mediated Ia induction on astrocytes. Proc Natl Acad Sci USA 84:7242–7245, 1987.

106. Massague J. The transforming growth factor-β family. Annu Rev Cell Biol 6:597–632, 1990.

107. Matsumoto Y, Kawai K, Fujiwara M. *In situ* Ia expression on brain cells in the rat: autoimmune encephalomyelitis-resistant strain (BN) and susceptible strain (Lewis) compared. Immunology 66:621–627, 1989.

108. Mauerhoff T, Pujol-Borrell R, Mirakian R, Bottazzo GF. Differential expression and regulation of major histocompatibility complex (MHC) products in neural and glial cells of the human fetal brain. J Neuroimmunol 18:271–291, 1988.

108a. Merrill JE. Proinflammatory and antiinflammatory cytokines in multiple sclerosis and central nervous system acquired immunodeficiency syndrome. J Immunother 12:167–170, 1992.

109. Merrill JE, Kong DH, Clayton J, Ando DG, Hinton DR, Hofman FM. Inflammatory leukocytes and cytokines in the peptide-induced disease of experimental allergic encephalomyelitis in SJL and B10.PL mice. Proc Natl Acad Sci USA 89:574–578, 1992.

110. Merrill JE, Kutsunai S, Mohlstrom C, Hofman F, Groopman J, Golde DW. Proliferation of astroglia and oligodendroglia in response to human T-cell derived factors. Science 224:1428–1431, 1984.

111. Merrill JE, Matsushima K. Production of and response to interleukin-1 by cloned human oligodendroglioma cell lines. J Biol Regul Homeost Agents 2:77–86, 1988.

112. Merrill JE, Strom SR, Ellison GW, Myers LW. *In vitro* study of mediators of inflammation in multiple sclerosis. J Clin Immunol 9:84–96, 1989.

113. Moench TR, Griffin DE. Immunocytochemical identification and quantitation of the mononuclear cells in the cerebrospinal fluid, meninges, and brain during acute viral meningoencephalitis. J Exp Med 159:77–88, 1984.

114. Mokhtarian F, Shi Y, Shirazian D, Morgante L, Miller A, Grob D. Defective production of anti-inflammatory cytokine, TGF-β by T cell lines of patients with active multiple sclerosis. J Immunol 152:6003–6010, 1994.

114a. Mondino A, Jenkins MK. Surface proteins involved in T cell costimulation. J Leukoc Biol 55:805–815, 1994.

115. Morganti-Kossmann MC, Kossmann T, Brandes ME, Mergenhagen SE, Wahl SM. Autocrine and paracrine regulation of astrocyte function by transforming growth factor-β. J Neuroimmunol 39:163–174, 1992.

116. Moses H, Panek RB, Benveniste EN, Ting JP-Y. Usage of primary cells to delineate IFN-γ responsive DNA elements in the HLA-DRA promoter and to identify a novel IFN-γ enhanced nuclear factor. J Immunol 148:3643–3651, 1992.

117. Muraguchi A, Hirano T, Tang B, Matsuda T, Horii Y, Nakajima K, Kishimoto T. The essential role of B cell stimulatory factor 2 (BSF-2/IL-6) for the terminal differentiation of B cells. J Exp Med 167:332–344, 1988.

118. Mustafa MM, Lebel MH, Ramilo O, Olsen KD, Reisch JS, Beutler B, McCracken GH Jr. Correlation of interleukin-1β and cachectin concentrations in cerebrospinal fluid and outcome from bacterial meningitis. J Pediatr 115:208–213, 1989.

119. Navia BA, Jordan BD, Price RW. The AIDS dementia complex. Ann Neurol 19:517–524, 1986.

120. Norris JG, Benveniste EN. Interleukin-6 production by astrocytes: induction by the neurotransmitter norepinephrine. J Neuroimmunol 45:137–146, 1993.

121. Norris JG, Tang L-P, Sparacio SM, Benveniste EN. Signal transduction pathways mediating astrocyte IL-6 induction by IL-1β and tumor necrosis factor-α. J Immunol 152:841–850, 1994.

122. Ohno K, Suzumura A, Sawada M, Marunouchi T. Production of granulocyte/macrophage

colony-stimulating factor by cultured astrocytes. Biochem Biophys Res Commun 169:719–724, 1990.

122a. Olsson T, Zhi WW, Hojeberg B, Kostulas V, Ping JY, Anderson G, Ekre HP, Link H. Autoreactive T lymphocytes in multiple sclerosis determined by antigen-induced secretion of interferon-γ. J Clin Invest 86:981–985, 1990.

123. Osborn L, Kunkel S, Nabel GJ. Tumor necrosis factor α and interleukin 1 stimulate the human immunodeficiency virus enhancer by activation of the nuclear factor κB. Proc Natl Acad Sci USA 86:2336–2340, 1989.

124. Panek RB, Lee Y-J, Benveniste EN. TGF-β suppression of IFN-γ induced class II MHC gene expression does not involve inhibition of phosphorylation of JAK1, JAK2 or STAT1α or modification of IFNEX expression. J Immunol 154:610–619, 1995.

125. Panek RB, Lee Y-J, Lindstrom-Itoh Y, Ting JP-Y, Benveniste EN. Characterization of astrocyte nuclear proteins involved in IFN-γ and TNF-α mediated class II MHC gene expression. J Immunol 153:4555–4564, 1994.

126. Panek RB, Moses H, Ting JP-Y, Benveniste EN. Tumor necrosis factor α response elements in the HLA-DRA promoter: identification of a tumor necrosis factor α-induced DNA-protein complex in astrocytes. Proc Natl Acad Sci USA 89:11518–11522, 1992.

127. Panitch HS, Hirsch RL, Schindler J, Johnson KP. Treatment of multiple sclerosis with gamma interferon: exacerbations associated with activation of the immune system. Neurology 37:1097–1102, 1987.

128. Paul NL, Ruddle NH. Lymphotoxin. Annu Rev Immunol 6:407–438, 1988.

129. Pohlman TH, Stanness KA, Beatty PG, Ochs HD, Harlan JM. An endothelial cell surface factor(s) induced *in vitro* by lipopolysaccharide, interleukin 1, and tumor necrosis factor-alpha increases neutrophil adherance by a cd18-dependent mechanism. J Immunol 136:4548–4553, 1986.

130. Poli G, Bressler P, Kinter A, Duh E, Timmer WC, Rabson A, Justement JS, Stanley S, Fauci AS. Interleukin 6 induces human immunodeficiency virus expression in infected monocytic cells alone and in synergy with tumor necrosis factor α by transcriptional and post-transcriptional mechanisms. J Exp Med 172:151–158, 1990.

131. Poli G, Kinter AL, Justement JS, Bressler P, Kehrl JH, Fauci AS. Transforming growth factor β suppresses human immunodeficiency virus expression and replication in infected cells of the monocyte/macrophage lineage. J Exp Med 173:589–597, 1991.

132. Poli G, Kinter A, Justement JS, Kehrl JH, Bressler P, Stanley S, Fauci AS. Tumor necrosis factor α functions in autocrine manner in the induction of human immunodeficiency virus expression. Proc Natl Acad Sci USA 87:782–785, 1990.

133. Powell MB, Mitchell D, Lederman J, Buckmeier J, Zamvil SS, Graham M, Ruddle NH, Steinman L. Lymphotoxin and tumor necrosis factor-alpha production by myelin basic protein-specific T cell clones correlates with encephalitogenicity. Int Immunol 2:539–544, 1990.

134. Prineas JW, Wright RG. Macrophages, lymphocytes and plasma cells in the perivascular compartment in chronic multiple sclerosis. Lab Invest 38:409–421, 1978.

135. Pulver M, Carrel S, Mach JP, de Tribolet N. Cultured human fetal astrocytes can be induced by interferon-γ to express HLA-DR. J Neuroimmunol 14:123–133, 1987.

136. Quagliarello VJ, Wispelwey B, Long WJ, Scheld WM. Recombinant human interleukin-1 induces meningitis and blood-brain barrier injury in the rat. J Clin Invest 87:1360–1366, 1991.

137. Racke MK, Cannella B, Albert P, Sporn M, Raine CS, McFarlin DE. Evidence of endogenous regulatory function of transforming growth factor-β1 in experimental allergic encephalomyelitis. Int Immunol 4:615–620, 1992.

138. Racke MK, Jalbut SD, Cannella B, Albert PS, Raine CS, McFarlin DE. Prevention and treatment of chronic relapsing experimental allergic encephalomyelitis by transforming growth factor-β1. J Immunol 146:3012–3017, 1991.

139. Raine CS. Biology of disease: analysis of autoimmune demyelination: its impact upon multiple sclerosis. Lab Invest 50:608–635, 1984.

140. Ramilo OS, Saez-Llorens S, Mertsola J, Jafari H, Olsen KD, Hansen EJ, Yoshinaga M, Ohkawara S, Nariuchi H, McCracken GH. Tumor necrosis factor α/cachetin and interleukin 1β initiate meningeal inflammation. J Exp Med 172:497–507, 1990.

141. Ransohoff RM, Hamilton TA, Tani M, Stoler MH, Shick HE, Major JA, Estes ML, Thomas DM, Tuohy VK. Astrocyte expression of mRNA encoding cytokines IP-10 and JE/MCP-1 in experimental autoimmune encephalomyelitis. FASEB J 7:592–600, 1993.

141a. Rieckmann P, Albrecht M, Kitze B, Weber T, Tumani H, Broocks A, Lüer W, Helwig A, Poser S. Tumor necrosis factor-α messenger RNA expression in patients with relapsing-remitting multiple sclerosis is associated with disease activity. Ann Neurol 37:82–88, 1995.

141b. Rieckmann P, Albrecht M, Kitze B, Weber T, Tumani H, Broocks A, Lüer W, Poser S. Cytokine mRNA levels in mononuclear blood cells from patients with multiple sclerosis. Neurology 44:1523–1526, 1994.

142. Righi M, Mori L, De Libero G, Sironi M, Biondi A, Mantovani A, Donini SD, Ricciardi-Castagnoli P. Monokine production by microglial cell clones. Eur J Immunol 19:1443–1448, 1989.

143. Robbins DS, Shirazi Y, Drysdale BE, Lieberman A, Shin HS, Shin ML. Production of cytotoxic factor for oligodendrocytes by stimulated astrocytes. J Immunol 139:2593–2597, 1987.

144. Rott O, Tontsch U, Fleischer B. Dissociation of antigen-presenting capacity of astrocytes for peptide-antigens versus superantigens. J Immunol 150:87–95, 1993.

145. Ruddle NH. Tumor necrosis factor (TNF-α) and lymphotoxin (TNF-β). Curr Opin Immunol 4:327–332, 1992.

146. Ruddle NH, Bergman CM, McGrath KM, Lingenheld EG, Grunnet ML, Padula SJ, Clark RB. An antibody to lymphotoxin and tumor necrosis factor prevents transfer of experimental allergic encephalomyelitis. J Exp Med 172:1193–1200, 1990.

147. Rus HG, Kim LM, Niculescu FI, Shin ML. Induction of C3 expression in astrocytes is regulated by cytokines and Newcastle disease virus. J Immunol 148:928–933, 1992.

148. Saeki Y, Mima T, Sakoda S, Fujimura H, Arita N, Nomura T, Kishimoto T. Transfer of multiple sclerosis into severe combined immunodeficiency mice by mononuclear cells from cerebrospinal fluid of patients. Proc Natl Acad Sci USA 89:6157–6161, 1992.

149. Santambrogio L, Hochwald GM, Saxena B, Leu C-H, Martz JE, Carlino JA, Ruddle NH, Palladino MA, Gold LI, Thorbecke GJ. Studies on the mechanisms by which transforming growth factor-β (TGF-β) protects against allergic encephalomyelitis: antagonism between TGF-β and tumor necrosis factor. J Immunol 151:1116–1127, 1993.

150. Sasaki A, Levison SW, Ting JPY. Differential suppression of interferon-γ-induced Ia antigen expression on cultured rat astroglia and microglia by second messengers. J Neuroimmunol 29:213–222, 1990.

151. Satoh T, Nakamura S, Taga T, Matsuda T, Hirano T, Kishimoto T, Kaziro Y. Induction of neuronal differentiation in PC12 cells by B-cell stimulatory factor 2/interleukin 6. Mol Cell Biol 8:3546–3549, 1988.

152. Schall TJ, Lewis M, Koller KJ, Lee A, Rice GC, Wong GH, Gatanaga T, Granger GA, Lentz R, Raab H, Kohr WJ, Goeddel DV. Molecular cloning and expression of a receptor for human tumor necrosis factor. Cell 61:361–370, 1990.

153. Schluesener HJ. Transforming growth factors type β1 and β2 suppress rat astrocyte autoantigen presentation and antagonize hyperinduction of class II major histocompatibility complex antigen expression by interferon-γ and tumor necrosis factor-α. J Neuroimmunol 27:41–47, 1990.

154. Selmaj K, Raine CS, Cannella B, Brosnan CF. Identification of lymphotoxin and tumor necrosis factor in multiple sclerosis lesions. J Clin Invest 87:949–954, 1991.

155. Selmaj K, Raine CS, Cross AH. Anti-tumor necrosis factor therapy abrogates autoimmune demyelination. Ann Neurol 30:694–700, 1991.

156. Selmaj K, Raine CS, Farooq M, Norton WT, Brosnan CF. Cytokine cytotoxicity against oligodendrocytes: apoptosis induced by lymphotoxin. J Immunol 147:1522–1529, 1991.

157. Selmaj KW, Farooq M, Norton WT, Raine CS, Brosnan CF. Proliferation of astrocytes *in vitro* in response to cytokines. A primary role for tumor necrosis factor. J Immunol 144:129–135, 1990.

157a. Selmaj K, Papierz W, Glabinski A, Kohno T. Prevention of chronic relapsing experimental autoimmune encephalomyelitis by soluble tumor necrosis factor receptor I. J Neuroimmunol 56:135–141, 1995.

158. Selmaj KW, Raine CS. Tumor necrosis factor mediates myelin and oligodendrocyte damage *in vitro*. Ann Neurol 23:339–346, 1988.

158a. Selmaj KW, Raine CS. Experimental autoimmune encephalomyelitis: immunotherapy with antitumor necrosis factor antibodies and soluble tumor necrosis factor receptors. Neurology 45:S44–S49, 1995.

159. Sharief MK, Phil M, Hentges R. Association between tumor necrosis factor-α and disease progression in patients with multiple sclerosis. N Engl J Med 325:467–472, 1991.

160. Sharief MK, Thompson EJ. *In vivo* relationship of tumor necrosis factor-α to blood-brain barrier damage in patients with active multiple sclerosis. J Neuroimmunol 38:27–34, 1992.

161. Sherman ML, Datta R, Hallahan DE, Weichselbaum RR, Kufe DW. Regulation of tumor necrosis factor gene expression by ionizing radiation in human myeloid leukemia cells and peripheral blood monocytes. J Clin Invest 87:1794–1797, 1991.

162. Shin ML, Koski CL. The complement system in demyelination. In: Myelin: Biology and Chemistry, R Martenson, ed. CRC Press, Boca Raton, pp 801–831, 1992.

162a. Shrikant P, Benveniste EN. The central nervous system as an immunocompetent organ: role of glial cells in antigen presentation. J Immunol 157:1819–1822, 1996.

163. Shrikant P, Chung IY, Ballestas M, Benveniste EN. Regulation of intercellular adhesion molecule-1 gene expression by tumor necrosis factor-α, interleukin-1β, and interferon-γ in astrocytes. J Neuroimmunol 51:209–220, 1994.

163a. Shrikant P, Lee SJ, Kalvakalanu I, Ransohoff RM, Benveniste EN. Stimulus-specific inhibition of ICAM-1 gene expression by TGF-β. J Immunol 157:892–900, 1996.

163b. Shrikant P, Weber E, Jilling T, Benveniste EN. ICAM-1 gene expression by glial cells: differential mechanisms of inhibition by interleukin-10 and interleukin-6. J Immunol 155:1489–1501, 1995.

164. Skias DD, Kim D, Reder AT, Antel JP, Lancki DW, Fitch FW. Susceptibility of astrocytes to class I MHC antigen-specific cytotoxicity. J Immunol 138:3254–3258, 1987.

165. Smith CA, Davis T, Anderson D, Solam L, Beckmann MP, Jerzy R, Dower SK, Cosman D, Goodwin, RG. A receptor for tumor necrosis factor defines an unusual family of cellular and viral proteins. Science 248:1019–1023, 1990.

166. Smith ME, McFarlin DE, Dhib-Jalbut S. Differential effect of interleukin-1β on Ia expression in astrocytes and microglia. J Neuroimmunol 46:97–104, 1993.

167. Sparacio SM,, Zhang Y, Vilcek J, Benveniste EN. Cytokine regulation of interleukin-6 gene

expression in astrocytes involves activation of an NF-κB-like nuclear protein. J Neuroimmunol 39:231–242, 1992.

168. Suzumura A, Mezitis SGE, Gonatas NK, Silberberg DH. MHC antigen expression on bulk isolated macrophage-microglia from newborn mouse brain: Induction of Ia antigen expression by γ-interferon. J Neuroimmunol 15:263–278, 1987.

169. Suzumura A, Sawada M, Yamamoto H, Marunouchi T. Transforming growth factor-β suppresses activation and proliferation of microglia *in vitro*. J Immunol 151:2150–2158, 1993.

170. Suzumura A, Silberberg DH, Lisak RP. The expression of MHC antigens on oligodendrocytes: Induction of polymorphic H-2 expression by lymphokines. J Neuroimmunol 11:179–190, 1986.

171. Symons JA, Bundick RV, Suckling AJ, Rumsby MG. Cerebrospinal fluid interleukin 1-like activity during chronic relapsing experimental allergic encephalomyelitis. Clin Exp Immunol 68:648–654, 1987.

172. Teuschler C, Hickey WF, Korngold R. An analysis of the role of tumor necrosis factor in the phenotypic expression of actively induced experimental allergic orchitis and experimental allergic encephalomyelitis. Clin Immunol Immunopathol 54:442–453, 1990.

173. Thery C, Hetier E, Evrard C, Mallat M. Expression of macrophage colony-stimulating factor gene in the mouse brain during development. J Neurosci Res 26:129–133, 1990.

174. Ting JP-Y, Baldwin AS. Regulation of MHC gene expression. Curr Opin Immunol 5:8–16, 1993.

175. Tontsch U, Rott O. Cortical neurons selectively inhibit MHC class II induction in astrocytes but not in microglial cells. Int Immunol 5:249–254, 1993.

176. Toru-Delbauffe D, Baghdassarian-Chalaye D, Gavaret JM, Courtin F, Pomerance M, Pierce M. Effects of transforming growth factor β1 on astroglial cells in culture. J Neurochem 54:1056–1061, 1990.

177. Tourtellotte WW, Ma IB. Multiple sclerosis: the blood-brain barrier and the measurement of *de novo* central nervous system IgG synthesis. Neurology 28:76–83, 1978.

178. Traugott U, Lebon P. Interferon-γ and Ia antigen are present on astrocytes in active chronic multiple sclerosis lesions. J Neurol Sci 84:257–264, 1988.

179. Tweardy DJ, Glazer EW, Mott PL, Anderson K. Modulation by tumor necrosis factor-α of human astroglial cell production of granulocyte-macrophage colony-stimulating factor (GM-CSF) and granulocyte colony-stimulating factor (G-CSF). J Neuroimmunol 32:269–278, 1991.

180. Tweardy DJ, Mott PL, Glazer EW. Monokine modulation of human astroglial cell production of granulocyte colony-stimulating factor and granulocyte-macrophage colony stimulating factor. I. Effects of IL-1α and IL-1β. J Immunol 144:2333–2241, 1990.

181. Tyor WR, Glass JD, Griffin JW, Becker PS, McArthur JC, Bezman L, Griffin DE. Cytokine expression in the brain during the acquired immunodeficiency syndrome. Ann Neurol 31:349–360, 1992.

182. van Snick JV. Interleukin-6: an overview. Annu Rev Immunol 8:253–278, 1990.

183. Vass K, Lassmann H. Intrathecal application of interferon gamma. Am J Pathol 137:789–800, 1990.

184. Velasco S, Tarlow M, Olsen K, Shay JW, McCracken GH, Nisen PD. Temperature-dependent modulation of lipopolysaccharide-induced interleukin-1β and tumor necrosis factor α expression in cultured human astroglial cells by dexamethasone and indomethacin. J Clin Invest 87:1674–1680, 1991.

185. Vidovic M, Sparacio SM, Elovitz M, Benveniste EN. Induction and regulation of class II

MHC mRNA expression in astrocytes by IFN-γ and TNF-α. J Neuroimmunol 30:189–200, 1990.

186. Vitkovic L, Kalebic T, da Cunha A, Fauci AS. Astrocyte-conditioned medium stimulates HIV-1 expression in a chronically infected promonocyte clone. J Neuroimmunol 30:153–160, 1990.

187. Voorthuis JAC, Uitdehaag BMJ, De Groot CJA, Goede PH, van der Meide PH, Dijkstra CD. Suppression of experimental allergic encephalomyelitis by intraventricular administration of interferon-gamma in Lewis rats. Clin Exp Immunol 81:183–188, 1990.

188. Waage A, Halstensen A, Shalaby R, Brandtzaeg P, Kierulf P, Espevik T. Local production of tumor necrosis factor α, interleukin 1, and interleukin 6 in meningococcal meningitis. J Exp Med 170:1859–1867, 1989.

189. Wahl SM, Allen JB, Francis NM. Macrophage- and astrocyte-derived transforming growth factor β as a mediator of central nervous system dysfunction in acquired immune deficiency syndrome. J Exp Med 173:981–991, 1991.

190. Wang Y, Nesbitt JE, Fuentes NL, Fuller GM. Molecular cloning and characterization of the rat liver IL-6 signal transducing molecule, gp130. Genomics 14:666–672, 1992.

191. Watkins BA, Dorn HH, Kelly WB, Armstrong RC, Potts BJ, Michaels F, Kufta CF, Dubois-Dalcq M. Specific tropism of HIV-1 for microglial cells in primary human brain cultures. Science 249:549–553, 1990.

191a. Wingren AG, Parra E, Varga M, Kalland T, Sjögren H-O, Hedlund G, Dohlsten M. T cell activation pathways: B7, LFA-3, and ICAM-1 shape unique T cell profiles. Crit Rev Immunol 15:235–253, 1995.

192. Wong GHW, Bartlett PF, Clark-Lewis I, Battye F, Schrader JW. Inducible expression of H-2 and Ia antigens on brain cells. Nature 310:688–691, 1984.

193. Wong GHW, Clark-Lewis I, Harris AW, Schrader JW. Effect of cloned interferon-γ on expression of H-2 and Ia antigens on cell lines of hemopoietic, lymphoid, epithelial, fibroblastic and neuronal origin. Eur J Immunol 14:52–56, 1984.

194. Woodroofe MN, Hayes GM, Cuzner ML. Fc receptor density, MHC antigen expression and superoxide production are increased in interferon-gamma-treated microglia isolated from adult rat brain. Immunology 68:421–426, 1989.

195. Yao J, Harvath L, Gilbert DL, Colton CA. Chemotaxis by a CNS macrophage, the microglia. J Neurosci Res 27:36–42, 1990.

196. Yasukawa K, Hirano T, Watanabe Y, Muratani K, Matsuda T, Nakai S, Kishimoto T. Structure and expression of human B cell stimulatory factor-2 (BSF-2/IL-6). EMBO J 6:2939–2945, 1987.

197. Zamvil SS, Steinman L. The T lymphocyte in experimental allergic encephalomyelitis. Annu Rev Immunol 8:579–621, 1990.

198. Zuber P, Kuppner MC, de Tribolet N. Transforming growth factor-β2 down-regulates HLA-DR antigen expression on human malignant glioma cells. Eur J Immunol 18:1623–1626, 1988.

12

CD4 Effector Cells in Autoimmune Diseases of the Central Nervous System

HARTMUT WEKERLE

Historically, the concept of autoimmunity was focused on the interaction of humoral autoantibodies with the body's own tissues. With the availability of appropriate assay systems, many different organ-specific autoantibodies were demonstrated, both in health and in disease. Soon, however, it became evident that few of these autoantibodies were truly pathogenic. Mere binding of an antibody to a tissue determinant was rarely sufficient to cause tissue damage. Hence, in a number of organ-specific autoimmune diseases mechanisms other than autoantibodies must be responsible for generating the pathogenic lesions. But these alternative mechanisms remained elusive for a long time as there was no system to detect them.

The solution came from neuroimmunology, from studies of experimental autoimmune encephalomyelitis (EAE). Autoimmune reactions damaging central nervous system (CNS) tissues were experimentally produced for the first time in the 1930s when Rivers and colleagues inoculated monkeys with brain matter from the same species. The treated primates predictably developed paralytic disease, which correlated with histological infiltration of the brain and spinal cord (176). As will be shown below, further refinement of this disease model led to the discovery of autoimmune, tissue-specific T cells as the pathogenic agents of autoimmune diseases in the CNS and in many other organs.

CD4 + T Cells Are Responsible for the Autoimmune Effects in EAE and EAN

Pioneering studies by Paterson (156), Koprowski et al. (105), and Aström and Waksman (5) indicated that tissue-specific autoimmune disease can be transferred by immune lymphocytes isolated from animals with experimental autoimmune encephalomyelitis (EAE) or neuritis (EAN). Humoral autoantibodies, in contrast, did not produce transferred disease. These studies relied on cell transfer between outbred animals, and thus had to cope with the problem of histoincompatibility between graft and host. This problem was overcome by the use of inbred animals, such as Lewis rats, which provided the basis for a more detailed analysis of the cellular mechanisms of autoimmune disease (157).

Several lines of experimental evidence indicated that the effector lymphocytes required for the development of EAE and EAN are T lymphocytes. First, it was observed that rats (66) or mice (16) depleted of T lymphocytes, were resistant to active induction of EAE using conventional immunization protocols. Reconstitution with T cells restored inducibility of EAE (154,203). Second, cell transfer studies combined with the use of monoclonal antibodies (MAb) specific for T-cell subset markers helped to further identify the encephalitogenic effector T cells. Transfer of unseparated, in vivo primed lymphocytes, which had been reactivated in vitro by confrontation with the encephalitogen, myelin basic protein (MBP), showed that the pathogenic potential was associated with T cells carrying markers of the CD4+ subset (84,165). The ultimate proof of the effector function of CD4+ T cells was provided by Ben-Nun et al., who succeeded in isolating permanent T-cell lines which were exclusively specific for MBP, and which transferred a highly acute EAE to naive histocompatible recipient rats (13). These T-cell lines were derived from Lewis rats that had developed EAE after immunization with MBP in Freund's complete adjuvant (FCA). They recognized their target epitope in the molecular context of MHC class II antigens and expressed the CD4 membrane marker (9).

The key role of CD4+ autoaggressive T cells in the pathogenesis of EAE was ultimately corroborated by therapeutic experiments designed to suppress clinical EAE by transferring (monoclonal) antibodies against CD4 determinants (20,25,226). Autoaggressive CD4+ T-cell lines with analogous properties were shown to mediate a broad spectrum of organ-specific autoimmune diseases, including experimental autoimmune neuritis (119), uveitis (with pinealitis) (33), adjuvant arthritis (87), collagen–type II arthritis (86), thyroiditis (126), and myocarditis (231), to name just a few.

Antigen Recognition by Encephalitogenic Rodent T Cells

Encephalitogenic CNS Antigens

One of the most resistant dogmas in neuroimmunology stated that myelin basic protein is the only encephalitogenic brain autoantigen. This was based mainly on the fact that in many species studied, EAE could be readily induced by simple immunization against homologous or heterologous MBP in strong immune adjuvant (101). Furthermore, attempts to identify additional (myelin) encephalitogens did not yield generally accepted, unequivocal results.

One mundane reason for MBP's privileged situation in neuroimmunology is its convenient molecular properties. All isoforms of MBP are all of relatively small molecular weight (171) and are located at the inner membrane face of myelin lamellae (153). MBP is a bulk component of myelin proteins, is of basic charge, and is readily soluble in water. These latter properties, make it easy to purify amounts, amply sufficient for immunologic study (50).

Purification of other myelin proteins is not that simple, because they are hydrophobic proteins, or only expressed in trace amounts. Fortunately, T-cell technology combined with molecular genetics offered new approaches to identify new encephalitogenic brain structures. Proteolipid protein (PLP), an integral membrane protein of the CNS, but not PNS myelin (31), became the second encephalitogenic myelin protein. Although heralded in an early study by Waksman et al. (225), unequivocal proof for the encephalitogenic potential of PLP was provided by the transfer of EAE to Lewis rats by T-cell lines that responded to PLP while ignoring MBP (242). Such proof was also provided by the induction of EAE in SJL/J mice by immunization with a synthetic PLP peptide analog (216). In the mean time, a number of additional PLP epitopes were found in different mouse strains (68,217,239) and in the Lewis rat (248). The lesion produced by immunization with PLP peptides and by transfer of PLP peptide-reactive T-cell lines closely resembled the inflammation seen in murine MBP-induced EAE (196,197). PLP-specific CD4+ T cell lines transferred chronic relapsing EAE (CREAE) (223). Especially intriguing was the discovery of intermolecular determinant spreading in CREAE. CREAE was induced in SJL/J mice by immunization with MBP or by transferring MBP-specific T cells. Surprisingly, in the relapse phases the animals developed substantial T-cell reactivity against PLP. The PLP-specific T cell must have been newly recruited during the course of the disease, presumably by endogenous myelin (39,162). Such events could take place in human relapsing MS as well.

Using the approach which had established the encephalitogenic potential of PLP, ever-increasing numbers of CNS proteins were identified as encephalitogens recognizable by autoaggressive CD4+ T lymphocytes. A most intriguing example is the myelin-oligodendrocyte glycoprotein (MOG), which was discovered by Linington et al. using a MAb raised against unfractionated myelin (121). MOG is a minor protein component of CNS myelin, and it is not produced in the PNS. It is located on the surface membrane of the myelin sheath and also on the oligodendrocyte soma (26). MOG is a glycosylated member of the immunoglobulin gene family with one transmembrane domain (61); interestingly, both in humans and in mice, its gene is encoded within the MHC (166).

Due to its exposed location on myelin surface, MOG has turned out to be a paramount target structure for demyelinating humoral autoantibodies. Transfer of anti-MOG MAb into rodents undergoing actively induced (187) or passively transferred EAE (118) causes myelin destruction in large perivascular, confluent areas of host white matter. Anti-MOG autoantibodies seem to be also responsible for demyelination noted in chronic relapsing EAE variants (120).

Using synthetic peptide analogs of the rat MOG extracellular domain, Linington et al. isolated encephalitogenic T-cell lines from primed Lewis rats. The T cells were CD4+, and they recognized the peptide in correct context of class II (RT1.B^1). The pattern of cytokines secreted by MOG-specific T cells classified them as Th1-like, including interleukin (IL)-2, interferon (INF)-γ, but not IL-4. The disease mediated was clinically mild, although it was associated with a considerable inflammatory response within the CNS, including opening of the endothelial blood-brain barrier (BBB). The lesions of MOG-specific transfer-EAE were distributed throughout the CNS but completely spared the periperal nervous system (PNS). Interestingly, the CNS infiltrates contained far fewer activated macrophages (stained by MAb ED1) than comparable MBP-induced lesions (117).

Very recently, it became clear that the ability to induce autoimmune encephalitis is by no means restricted to myelin proteins; it may be a much more general property of many, if not all, CNS components. T-cell lines responding against the astroglial calcium-binding protein S100β were raised from primed and in naive Lewis rats. These CD4+ T cells transferred a CNS autoimmune disease spreading throughout the white and gray matter areas of the entire CNS, but interestingly, they also regularly involved the eye through uveitis and retinitis, and somewhat less prominently, they involved peripheral nerves (103). This tissue distribution follows the location of S100β-expressing glia cells, which include, besides CNS astrocytes, Müller cells in the eye and Schwann cells (6). Like in MOG-induced EAE and in S100β-mediated panencephalitis, the mild clinical course is in striking contrast to the large infiltrations noted in the affected tissues. Again, a deficit of activated macrophages may be responsible for this unexpected disparity.

All this new work indicates that MBP is not the only encephalitogenic brain component, but it may be a particular one. In principle, numerous proteins within the myelinated areas but also outside of myelin may be target structures of autoimmune attacks in the CNS. A similar situation seems to emerege in autoimmune diseases of the PNS, where, in addition to the "classic" neuritogen, the peripheral myelin protein P2 (24), additional myelin autoantigens have been identified, including PO protein (32,139) and myelin-associated glycoprotein (MAG) (Linington, personal communication). Responses against a large number of different myelin and nonmyelin antigens could well be involved in human inflammatory brain disease of thus far undetermined origin.

Epitope Dominance

T cells do not recognize antigens as native proteins but rather as molecular complexes formed by antigenic peptide fragments embedded in the central groove of major histocompatibility complex (MHC) class I or class II products. In many responses to foreign antigens, *multiple* peptide sequences, which may be distributed along the entire protein length, are recognized by complementary T-cell clones participating in the response (63).

The MBP-specific, encephalitogenic CD4+ T-cell response in the Lewis rat and in PL/J or B10.PL mice is characterized, however, by unusually strict *epitope dominance*. In the Lewis rat, the overwhelming majority of all encephalitogenic, MBP-specific T-cell clones recognize one or a few epitopes nested within MBP sequence 68-88 (9,71,100,222). This peptide is presented in the context of the RT1.B product of the rat MHC class II gene region (9,54,145). Of interest, most T cells show marked hetero-clisity between rat and guinea pig MBP. The majority of the T cells that have been selected for *rat* MBP (or the MBP peptide p68-88) respond better to the guinea pig homologous sequence than to the rat peptide (Wekerle, unpublished data). Although rare exceptions from this antigen recognition rule have been reported (147,148), there is no doubt about the dominant recognition of MBP sequence 68-88/I-A in the enceph-alitogenic T-cell response of the Lewis rat.

An epitope dominance of similar stringency was seen with encephalitogenic T cells in the PL/J mouse or its congenic strain B10.PL. T cells from these mice recognize N-terminal epitopes of MBP (58) located within sequence 1-10 (244) and presented in the context of I-A^u molecules (41,245). Minor T-cell response components may, in addition, recognize other peptides in context of I-E^u (246).

In the SJL/J mouse, the T-cell response to MBP clearly is more complex. Several epitopes have been specified in the MBP sequence 87-104 (104), and further epitopes are located in additional regions (57,183).

Even in the most extreme cases, epitope dominance is not absolute. When followed over time, the highest proportion of T cells recognizing the dominant epitope is seen in early, active phases of EAE. Later, after resolution of the clinical and histological signs, epitope specificity of the anti-MBP response tends to flatten. T cells recognizing minor MBP epitopes get demonstrable at significant frequency (140,220). Lehmann et al. analyzed this process, which they termed *epitope spreading,* in (SJL/J × PL/J)F1 hybrid mice immunized with guinea pig MBP. While the initial T-cell response was directed against the classic dominant MBP epitope Ac1-11, at least three additional, previously "cryptic" epitopes became demonstrable after another 40 days (113). A number of mechanisms were invoked to explain the changed epitope recognition pat-tern. They include changes in relevant antigen-presenting cells (APCs), such as changed processing machinery, expression of MHC, and cell adhesion molecules that could alter the hierarchy of presented autoantigens. The recent observations of selec-tive T-cell apoptosis within encephalitic CNS target tissue, however, may provide an alternative though not mutually exclusive explanation. Pender et al. reported that in actively induced EAE of Lewis rats, infiltrated lesion areas contained numerous cells in apoptosis, and they identified these elements as T cells (159). This was extended by Schmied et al., who applied a double labeling method allowing identification of cellu-lar apoptosis by in situ nick translation and characterization of the cell involved by immunocytochemistry. Indeed, in T-cell line transferred EAE as well, most of the parenchymal T cells were undergoing *programmed cell death* (189). And it should be stressed that many of the parenchymal infiltrate T cells (as opposed to T cells infiltrating periovascular regions) are encephalitogenic T cells using Vβ8.2+ T-cell receptors (TcR) (110,215). The first wave of encephalitogenic T cells specific for the immunodominant MBP epitope would be deleted by apoptosis in the CNS until exhaustion. T-cell clones specific for minor epitopes would then have their day and dominate the repertoire of late EAE. Support for this hypothesis comes from the lack of epitope spreading in T-cell responses against foreign peptide antigens, such as lysozyme (60).

Epitope dominance in the encephalitogenic T-cell response is now the target of studies designed to examine the use of blocking agents to prevent pathogenic autoimmune recognition steps. Attempts to interfere with autoimmune recognition by MAb binding to relevant MHC class II products (92,145,200) were successful, but the lack of antigen specificity and potential side effects may limit clinical use of this approach. More recently, several groups have explored possibilities to specifically block encephalitogenic T-cell recognition by synthetic peptide. The ideal blocking peptide would be a nonimmunogenic peptide homolog of the dominant encephalitogenic epitope. Due to individual amino acid exchanges, it would firmly bind to the relevant MHC class II molecule required for antigen presentation, but yet it would not be recognized by the TcR (109,194,241). Indeed, peptide analogs have been constructed which successfully force out encephalitogenic peptide in equimolar concentrations (55). Interestingly, EAE inducibility by entire MBP can be blocked by in vivo treatment with one inhibitor peptide (229), and there is the possibility that at least in some cases the peptide inhibitors perform an active regulatory mechanism, rather than merely binding competition (228).

Biased Usage of T-Cell Receptor Variable Genes

Epitope dominance is not the only unusual feature of encephalitogenic T-cell responses in the Lewis rat and the PL/J mouse. Highly restrictive usage of TcR Vβ genes by MBP-specific T cells is the second remarkable feature of this autoimmune reaction.

In general, immune responses against conventional foreign peptide sequences often involve T cells using a more or less variegated spectrum of TcR V genes (93). In contrast, in these strains of rodents, almost all encephalitogenic T cells use the same or very similar genes to construct their antigen receptors. Acha-Orbea et al. (1) and Urban et al. (219) reported that in PL/J and B10.PL mice (both H-2u haplotype), almost all encephalitogenic, MBP-reactive T cells use the TcR Vβ8.2 gene. The selection of Vα genes (Vα2 and Vα4) was also biased, though less absolute.

Astoundingly, exactly the same TcR gene usage was noted in the Lewis rat (27,35). As mentioned above, the epitope recognized by encephalitogenic Lewis rat T cells (sequence 68-88) differs completely from the epitope of the PL/J and B10.PL mouse

(Ac1-11), and naturally, the restricting class II products differ between the two species. T cells from the Louvain strain of rat (RT1ʷ) recognize a C-terminal sequence of human MBP and use TcR V genes similar to, but distinct from those used in the Lewis rat (Vβ8.5/Vα2.3) (75).

Biased selection of Vβ8.2 for encephalitogenic T cells could have occurred on several levels. First, for unknown reasons, Vβ8.2 using T cells could have overgrown other clones during the establishment of T-cell lines in vitro. Second, expansion of such T cells might follow active immunization of donor animals in vivo. Third, and most interesting, preferential usage of Vβ8.2 could be a genetically controlled feature of the natural T-cell repertoire developing in the animals concerned.

To distinguish between these alternatives, Lannes-Vieira et al. used a primary cloning technique (163) to isolate MBP-specific T cells from the thymuses of naive, unprimed Lewis rats (110a). The existence of encephalitogenic T-cell clones in naive rats had been proven before in bulk cultures (188).

With this approach, a panel of MBP-reactive T-cell lines could be cloned. These cells recognized the dominant epitope p68-88 presented in the correct class II context. Furthermore, the T cells were able to transfer EAE to Lewis rats after activation in vitro. Most important, however, in the present context, the majority of these T-cell lines utilized a TcR undistinguishable from receptors used by conventional T-cell lines isolated from primed lymph nodes. Vβ8.2 was the predominant Vβ gene used, and some of the CDR3 (complementarity determining region 3) sequences, which determine peptide specificity of a TcR, were seen before in other conventional T-cell collections (64,247). Preferential utilization of Vβ8.2 by encephalitogenic T cells is therefore a hallmark of the normal repertoire of the naturally developing Lewis rat immune system.

Recent work in a different system suggests that positive selection mechanisms in intrathymic T-cell differentiation are involved in Vβ8.2 usage. Kääb et al. (95a) followed V gene usage in MBP-specific Lewis rat T cells developing in a xenogeneic environment, that of immunodeficient SCID mice. SCID mice are immunologically handicapped by a mutation that interferes with proper rearrangement of immunoglobulin and T-cell receptor variable regions. Hence they are devoid of any mature T and B cell and are unable to reject pathogenic agents or foreign tissues (18). Hemopoietic stem cells from normal rat embryos transferred to a SCID mouse host will differentiate to mature T and B lymphocytes (210), including encephalitogenic, PLP-specific T cells (91).

Kääb et al. (95a) analysed the MBP-specific T-cell repertoire in SCID chimeras reconstituted with stem cells from fetal Lewis rat livers. They found that, as expected, all the CD4+ T cells recovered were of rat origin. All of these were restricted by rat, but in no case by mouse MHC class II products. These MBP-specific, chimera-derived rat T cells recognized the dominant MBP peptide p68-88, but there was no preferential usage of Vβ8.2. TcR analysis using a panel of rat Vβ-specific MAbs indicated random utilization of the Vβ genes tested. A different situation was seen in a second type of rat/SCID mouse chimeras. These chimeras were reconstituted not only by fetal Lewis rat liver but in addition by fetal Lewis thymus lobes grafted under the mouse's kidney capsule. In these double-reconstituted chimeras, the CD4+ MBP-specific T-cell repertoire again recognized the dominant epitope, but used preferentially Vβ8.2-like T cells derived from the intact rat immune system.

These recent results suggest that acquisition of dominant usage of Vβ genes by MBP-specific Lewis rat T cells is, as pointed out above, a property of the natural repertoire and that it requires an intact thymus microenvironment to properly develop. One might speculate that expression of suitable MHC class II determinants on a thymic stroma cell is the key prerequisite in a positive selection step to generate this biased TcR utilization.

Biased usage of individual Vβ elements by pathogenic, autoimmune T cells opens novel approaches to immunospecific therapies of autoimmune disease. Indeed, in rodent EAE models that show Vβ8.2 preponderance in MBP-induced EAE, TcR-targeted therapies have been extremely successful. In B10.PL (H-2^u) mice, for example, which preferentially use Vβ8.2 (and Vβ13) in their encephalitogenic response, pretreatment with anti-Vβ MAbs prevented EAE induction by immunization. MAb therapy of established EAE reduced the severity and duration of the disease (243).

A second kind of TcR-directed immunotherapy was inaugurated in 1989 by the groups of Brostoff and Vandenbark. This strategy relies on the active immunization of Lewis rats with peptides representing epitopes typical for encephalitogenic TcR. These were either homologs of the CDR3 (VDJ) region (88) or of the CDR2 region of MBP-specific T-cell clones (221).

In both systems, vaccination prevented subsequent inducibility of EAE by active immunization. Later reports described therapeutic effects on *established* disease (149). TcR peptide vaccination is clearly an intriguing approach to specifically treat T-cell mediated autoimmune disease, but it seems to be somewhat capricious. Some groups reported undesirable exacerbations following vaccination (45), others had to change the immunization protocol to see an effect (132,202), while a third group of laboratories was disappointed by a lack of effect (95,205). The mechanism of TcR peptide vaccination has not been definitely established so far. TcR-binding antibodies (74) as well as activation of regulatory T cells have been invoked, but direct evidence for cellular interactions has come only recently from a vaccination model using CDR1 peptides of Vβ8.2 in the Lewis rat (22).

The therapeutic potential of TcR vaccination strategies for human disease is enormous. Unquestionably, however, application of this strategy is absolutely limited to disorders that involve T-cell responses with known Vβ gene preference. How generally, then, is Vβ preference observed in tissue-specific autoimmune disease?

In the SJL/J mouse, MBP-specific T cells definitely use a broader repertoire of Vβ elements than T cells from PL/J mice. In SJL/J mice, MBP-specific T cells show a certain preference to Vβ17, but this is by no means absolute. As shown by Sakai et al., most Vβ17+ encephalitogenic T cells recognize an epitope located in sequence

89-101, while their Vβ17− counterparts may additionally respond to a nested peptide from 89-100 (181). The Vβ17− SJL T cells, which represent about 50% of the entire MBP-specific repertoire, may use Vβ4 or Vβ6 (204). It is thus not surprising that treatment of SJL/J mice with anti-Vβ17 MAbs did not suppress EAE induction (181). The SJL response against another major encephalitogenic protein, PLP, is probably even more diverse than the anti-MBP response, with at least 4 different Vβ elements used by T cells specific for one epitope (106).

In the Lewis rat, Vβ selectivity differs fundamentally between epitopes on the same MBP molecule, and it varies over the course of the encephalitogenic response. Comparable to the decay of the immunodominance of epitope 68-88 (vide supra), selective usage of Vβ8.2 decreases over time (146). Similar mechanisms could account for both changes. There are, however, profound differences between T-cell responses against diverse MBP epitopes. In contrast to the Vβ8.2-biased response against the dominant epitope p68-88, T cells recognizing a minor epitope p87-99 use a broader repertoire of Vβ elements (65,207).

Studies of other models of organ-specific autoimmunity gave contradictory results. In experimental autoimmune uveoretinitis (EAU), for example, there are reports confirming dominance of Vβ8 family elements in uveitogenic T lines recognizing two distinct retinal autoantigens (48,69); others saw a broader repertoire (53). Incidentally, attempts to prevent EAU induction by TcR Vβ8.2 peptide vaccination were not very successful (99). In experimental autoimmune neuritis mediated by T cells reacting against the peripheral myelin protein P2, preferential Vβ8.2 usage observed by one group (36) could not be confirmed by others (94).

These few examples suggest that biased utilization of individual Vβ elements by tissue-specific, autoimmune T cells is not exclusively limited to the MBP response in Lewis rats and PL/J mice. On the other hand, a number of other autoimmune models do not show this feature. Applicability of TcR-directed therapies therefore must be determined in each individual case by an analysis of the autoimmune T-cell repertoire.

Activation of Potentially Pathogenic T Cells Is a Prerequisite for Induction of Autoimmune Disease.

Encephalitogenic T-cell lines can be readily derived from MBP-primed (13), EAE-resistant (10,11), and even unprimed rats (140,188). This is a very important observation with a profound impact on our understanding of the immune system. Since in mature T cells, the V region genes of the TcR are stable and fail to undergo somatic mutation (42), progenitors of this T-cell line having identical recognition properties must have been preformed in the donor's immune repertoire. In other words, *potentially autoaggressive* T-cell clones are regular members of the *healthy* immune system. Why else would the self tissue-specific CD4+ T cell clones cause "spontaneous" autoimmune disease? How are these immunological "time bombs" kept in check so safely?

One answer is that in order to attack the myelinated parts of the CNS, encephalitogenic T cells must be activated. It has been known for a long time that direct transfer of EAE by in vivo primed lymphocyte populations required enormous cell doses, and that the number of pathogenic effector T lymphocytes can be drastically reduced by in vitro prestimulation with MBP before transfer (46,85,174). The requirement of effector cell activation is dramatically evident in T-cell line mediated EAE. MBP-specific T-cell lines, which have been freshly activated either by properly presented MBP peptides or by the mitogen concanavalin A, transfer clinical EAE at doeses as low as 1×10^4/adult recipient. Resting cells from the same lines are ineffective even in transfers of 5×10^7 (142). The state of activation must be maximal, since the encephalitogenic capacity is lost within 2–3 days after antigen stimulation (234).

The crucial role of effector T-cells activation is underscored by the favorable therapeutic effect of MAb recognizing T-cell activation markers. A MAb against an (undefined) activation marker of Lewis rat, MBP-specific T-line cells reliably prevents development of and mitigates established T-cell mediated EAE (186). Similarly, ligation of the receptor for IL-2, again, a marker of *activated* rodent T cells, with MAbs (47,49) or immunotoxins (15,177) is a highly efficient remedy for T-line mediated EAE, but less for actively induced EAE. Corresponding results were reached in EAN (72).

More recently, transgenic mice were constructed whose T cells expressed receptors predominantly specific for organ-specific autoantigens. Induction of local immunopathological tissue damage by activation of potentially self-destructive T cells was achieved in two similar transgenic mouse models. Transgenic mice expressing a protein of lymphocytic choriomeningitis virus (LCMV) targeted to their pancreatic β-cells do not show any endocrine or histological abnormalities. When the transgenic mice are infected with LCMV, LCMV-specific CD8+ T cells are activated in the peripheral immune system. These cells then attack truly infected tissues, as well as the virus glycoprotein transgenic pancreas islet cells, an inflammatory destruction that ultimately results in diabetes mellitus (152). Even more striking were the activation effects in double transgenic mice expressing LCMV antigen in the islet β-cells, along with TcR genes for this antigen on all T cells. Again, only activation of resting autoreactive T cells, in these cases by LCMV infection, triggers autoaggressive islet destruction in a previously tolerant animal (150).

The transgenic mouse models described above represent autoreactivity on a CD8 T-cell level. CD4 T-cell transgenic mice were produced more recently by inserting into the germ line the α- and β-chains of TcRs recognizing MBP. Among transgenic mice with a wild-type genetic background, a minor proportion developed spontaneous CNS inflammation (presumably EAE) when kept under conventional dirty conditions (67). The incidence of spontaneous EAE reached 100% in truly "monoclonal" TcR transgenic mice, which had been produced by back-crossing transgenic mice with MBP-specific TcR into a mouse strain incapable of forming their own mature T- and B-cell receptors (like SCID mice). These animals possess solely mature T cells with the transgenic, MBP-specific TcR; consequently there is no regulatory lymphocyte interaction to suppress their activation by infectious agents, etc. (108).

Thus, the mere presence of autoimmune CD4+ T-cell clones is not sufficient to cause autoimmune disease. To be able to attack self target tissues, the autoimmune T cells must be driven into a state of high activation. Several potential mechanisms of activation can be envisaged. *Molecular mimicry* and activation by *superantigens* are currently popular concepts. In the course of an infection, T-cell clones specific for a given self peptide–MHC complex could be erroneously triggered by peptides whose key structural features resemble those of the encephalitogen but which are components of the infectious agents (151). As a classic example, Fujinami and Oldstone described the induction of EAE in some rabbits using a synthetic peptide representing a sequence shared by MBP and the polymerase of hepatitis B virus (59). In the case of EAU, mimicry response have been reported between the uveitogenic S antigen and yeast (193) and hepatitis B virus products (234).

The profound effect of bacterial superantigens on T-cell mediated organ-specific autoimmunity has been noted by numerous investigators. In most cases, however, the superantigens protected against autoimmune disease rather than precipitating it. Pretreatment with staphylococcal enterotoxins, an activator of several TcR Vβ isotypes, profoundly decreases susceptibility to EAE in Lewis rats (7,179) and in PL/J mice (62,97,173,199).

But more recently, activation of encephalitogenic T cells by superantigens was noted in a number of situations. Endogenous, viral superantigens (Mls antigens) activate appropriate encephalitogenic T cells in mouse systems, but this activation may not suffice to transfer over clinical disease (121,182). Also, rat MBP-specific T-cell lines were readily activated by bacterial superantigen (179). Induction of autoimmune disease by superantigens has been reported only recently. Depending on the dosage and the timing of superantigen treatment, EAE relapses were elicited in mice with actively induced or passively transfereed EAE (21,185).

A third possibility to accidentally activate potential autoimmune T-cell clones could be provided by local microenvironments favoring general T-cell activation. Such processes have been described during infectious disease. The animal model studied most thoroughly is subacute encephalomyelitis induced in the Lewis rat after infection with coronavirus. Watanabe et al. isolated MBP-specific T-lymphocyte lines from Lewis rats with ongoing subacute coronavirus encephalomyelitis (227). The lymphocyte lines established were not distinguishable from MBP-specific T-cell lines isolated from MBP-primed, autoimmune rats. The lines were CD4+ and recognized MBP but no viral products in the context of the correct MHC class II. Most importantly, these MBP T cells, which probably were virally infected themselves, were able to transfer "classical" EAE to naive recipients. In striking contrast, CD4+ T cells reactive against coronavirus antigens mediated protection against viral encephalitis rather than exacerbating it (230). In addition, the same group obtained similar results in a measles-dependent rat encephalomyelitis model (116).

It appears that in both models, the virus infection triggered an MBP-directed T-cell response, which in turn was responsible for an EAE component of the disease. It is of interest that the coronavirus activates astrocytes to express class II antigens independent of interferon production (128), and that a similar effect is seen in measles-infected glia cell cultures (129). Autoimmunization of T cells in an especially proinflammatory milieu may also underlay activation of T cells against "new" myelin autoantigens, as described in CREAE (vide supra).

Regulatory Mechanisms Safeguarding Self-tolerance Against CNS Autoantigens

As stressed above, the identification of autoreactive, potentially autoimmune T-lymphocyte clones in the normal immune repertoire was one of the most surprising findings in autoimmune research. The presence of autoimmune T-cell clones in the healthy organism as first described in naive Lewis rats (188,232) is by no means a feature restricted to inbred rodents. The normal human immune system contains numerous T-cell clones specific for different autoantigens, including MBP (29,127,155,164), the PNS myelin protein P2 (28), and the nicotinic acetylcholine receptor of the neuromuscular end plate (134,184,198). Neonatal peripheral blood seems to contain particularly high levels of autoreactive T cells (56).

Although cell activation is critically required to unleash the autoaggressive potential of autoreactive T lymphocytes, one would not expect that self-tolerance is maintained by mere exclusion of activating factors. Intuitively, participation of active, self-tolerogenic regulatory mechanisms seems to be a more satisfactory explanation. Indeed, over the past few years, several lines of indirect evidence have provided fresh support to cellular regulation in self tolerance. There is evidence for regulatory cells recognizing the *autoantigen*, and for regulatory cells recognizing determinants on the autoimmune *effector cells.*

Evidence for cellular down-regulation of CD4+ self-reactive T lymphocytes is old and diverse. Studies from Swanborg's group indicated that pretreatment with either soluble MBP (211) or MBP in Freund's incomplete adjuvant (237) protected Lewis rats against subsequent active induction of EAE, and that protection could be transferred to naive recipient rats by T cells from primed lymph nodes. This group also found suppressor cells in immune organs of rats recovering from an actively induced EAE episode (236). Others found suppressor T cells in thymuses and spleens of rats with acute EAE (2). However, control of autoimmune T cells by suppressor cells turned out to be a capricious phenomenon, which was not demonstrated in all experimental situations and by all groups (240), and thus the number of reports describing suppression in autoimmunity decreased for some time.

More recently, autoantigen-specific down-regulatory T cells have reemerged, mainly in the context of oral therapy strategies designed to protect against induction of EAE or other organ-specific autoimmune diseases. Oral instillation of soluble MBP in rats leads to a remarkably firm state of resistance against active induction of EAE (17,83).

Several mechanisms seem to account for orally induced protection. One group of investigators used limiting dilution technology to enumerate MBP-reactive T cells in orally treated rats. In these studies, the number of T cells reacting against MBP was decreased, which, according the authors' interpretation, was due to specific, but partly reversible, anergy of MBP-specific T cells (238). Anergy, however, is not the only mechanism of oral immunotherapy. Using a similar system, Weiner and associates obtained evidence for active cellular suppression. T-cell fractions were isolated from the spleens and mesenteric lymph nodes of orally treated rats, which transferred protection against EAE. Depletion of CD4+ T cells from these populations decreased their therapeutic effect, which was interpreted as evidence for CD8+ suppressor T cells (115). Later work showed that the orally induced suppressor T cells require antigen-dependent activation to act optimally and that they produce soluble suppressive factors (138), including transforming growth factor (TGF)-β (137).

Most recently, Weiner and colleagues isolated MBP-specific T-cell clones from the intestines of orally tolerized SJL/J mice. These T cells protected recipient mice against EAE induction, but on the other hand, had TcR and membrane properties which could not be distinguished from encephalitogenic effector cells. However, instead of secreting the Th1-like cytokine pattern (IL-2, IFN-γ, and TNF), these gut-derived T suppressor cells produced a TH2-like spectrum of cytokines (IL-4, IL-10, and TGF-β) (34).

A second category of down-regulatory T lymphocytes which may participate in the control of autoreactive T lymphocytes recognizes determinants on the membrane of encephalitogenic effector T cells rather than autoantigen epitopes.

The first evidence in favor of an anti-T-cell regulatory network was provided by Ben-Nun's classic vaccination studies. This work showed that transfer of irradiated samples of encephalitogenic T lymphocytes into a compatible naive rat did not result in EAE, but on the contrary, rendered the recipient resistant against later active induction of EAE (8,14). When T-cell vaccination was first observed, Ben-Nun et al. postulated activation of counterregulatory lymphocyte circuits as the underlying principle. Indeed, suppressive T cells were isolated and characterized in two distinct situations.

Lohse et al. found that activated CD4+ T lymphocytes have the capacity to recruit another set of lymphocytes which then exerts an inhibitory effect on the primary T lymphocytes. This interaction, which was not antigen specific but depended on the activated state of the recruiting cells, was termed *ergotypic*. In the original experiments, the anti-ergotypic T cells were activated in vitro and, when transferred to naive hosts, mediated protection against actively induced EAE as well as against T-cell transferred EAE (122). The target structure recognized by anti-ergotypic T cells is uncertain, but it is a membrane component which can be isolated by detergent solubilization but is not secreted by the living cell (123).

Target cell-specific counterreactive T lymphocytes were isolated from Lewis rats recovering from T-line mediated EAE. Such T cells were CD8+ and responded by proliferation only when confronted in vitro with the original CD4+ T-cell line that primed the donor rat (114,208). An analysis of counterregulatory CD8+ T-cell lines revealed their highly specific and efficient suppressive potential. CD8+ T cells primed by an individual CD4+ encephalitogenic T-cell line, S1, were exclusively cytotoxic against S1 T cells. Furthermore, when transferred into naive rats, they strongly protected against EAE transferred by S1 T cells, but not against unrelated T lymphocytes (208). Anti-T cell responses are induced readily in adult rats. In neonatal recipients, however, which will not undergo EAE because of their lack of myelin (218), encephalitogenic T cells cause a profound, life-long tolerance against the transferred T line (172).

It was tempting to correlate the high degree of target specificity of the T line-specific CD8+ T-cell response with "anti-idiotypic" (i.e., TcR-specific) immune regulation. Unfortunately, several findings argue against this attractive possibility. Clearly, the cytotoxic T cells cannot be directed against Vβ sequences of their target T cells, because the anti-S1 T-cell response discriminated between distinct Vβ8.2+ CD4+ T-cell lines. Furthermore, it should be noted that not all T cells are able to elicit a cytotoxic reaction (206).

Recently evidence was found of TcR-specific regulatory T cells in myelin-specific T-cell responses. Kumar and Sercarz isolated anti-idiotypic T cells from a PL/J mouse recovering from MBP-induced EAE. These T cells were CD4+, and they recognized epitopes of the TcR Vβ8.2 sequence (used preferentially by encephalitogenic, MBP-specific T cells in the PL/J mouse, vide supra) in the context of MHC class II. Transfers of these T cells resulted in a reduced incidence of EAE and decreased T-cell reactivity against the dominant MBP epitope Ac1-11 (107).

Although the evidence of regulatory T-cell circuits controlling organ-specific autoimmunity is complex and often confusing, there are additional findings that keep the search attractive and promising. Partial immunosuppression of Lewis rats with cyclosporin A leads to the generation of spontaneous relapses after a first bout of actively induced EAE. Spontaneous relapses in normal Lewis rats are extremely rare, which suggests that drug treatment interfered with some (cellular) regulatory mechanisms (52,161,169).

This point has become more distinct in two mouse systems. Depletion of CD8 T cells in PL/J mice by large doses of MAbs, for example, interfered with the development of resistance after one bout of actively induced EAE. According to one interpretation, this treatment eliminated counterregulatory CD8+ T cells which under normal conditions would prevent elicitation of a second EAE episode (90). This was corroborated by a study of transgenic knock-out mice with a disrupted CD8 gene. In CD8−/− PL/J mice EAE can be readily induced by conventional immunization. The actual clinical bout may be somewhat milder than in wild-type animals, but the occurrence of spontaneous relapses is drastically increased. Again, this was interpreted as evidence of CD8 T cells having a role in down-regulating autoimmune activation (102).

Generation of Autoimmune Lesions in the CNS

Encephalitogenic CD4+ T Cells in CNS Infiltrates

As described in detail elsewhere (Chapter 19), the CNS lesion of EAE is characterized by three main features: (1) predominantly mononuclear cell infiltrates, which are concentrated around postcapillary microvessels and within the meninges, but which also enter the CNS parenchyma; (2) disruption of the endothelial blood-brain barrier with vasogenic edema, fibrin deposits, and in some cases, hemorrhage; and (3) activation of local glia cells, which are predominantly astrocytes and microglial elements.

The blood-derived infiltrates definitely contain the encephalitogenic CD4+ effector cells, but it is equally well established that these effectors form only a minority among all infiltrating cells. This was made evident first by transfer experiments. Encephalitogenic T-line cells were activated in vitro, labeled with isotopes (the isotope of choice is ^{14}C-TdR, which does not leak from the cells, and in contrast to ^{3}H−TdR, does not lead to cellular suicide), and transferred to proper recipient animals. Autoradiography of the subsequently induced EAE lesions documents that only few infiltrate cells are labeled, i.e., derived from the pathogenic T-cell line (38,135,136). It is noteworthy that the immigration of the effector T cells occurs within a few hours after intravenous transfer, thus preceding onset of clinical EAE by more than 48 hours. (79,135,136).

These observations were confirmed by polymerase chain reaction (PCR) studies. In early, preclinical phases of T-line transferred EAE, PCR amplification of CNS material yielded almost exclusively Vβ elements used by the transferred T-line lymphocytes. With the onset of clinical disease (which commonly coincides with heavy round-cell infiltration [78]) the demonstrable Vβ repertoire dramatically broadened (98).

More detailed investigations of the migration pathways of encephalitogenic T cells in vivo became possible with the availability of a new panel of rat Vβ-specific MAbs (213). Immunocytochemical studies revealed that in Lewis rat EAE mediated by Vβ8.2 T cells, the encephalitogenic T cells had a propensity to infiltrate the CNS parenchyma, but not the perivascular cuffs or the meninges. In Lewis rats immunized with MBP, the T cells contained within the infiltrates of the spinal cord were up to 80% Vβ8.2+, while the proportion of these T cells in the perivascular cuffs corresponded roughly to their proportion in the normal T-cell repertoire (5–10%) (215). Very similar cell frequencies was observed in T-cell line-transferred Lewis rat EAE (110).

There is evidence that the CD4+ encephalitogenic T-line cells are autonomous in producing clinical EAE and that they do not require substantial contributions by the infiltrate T cells derived from the host. Building upon the studies by Paterson and Harvey, who used unselected primed T-cell populations (158), the T-line transfer studies by Sedgwick et al. (190) and Wekerle et al. (233) showed that immune depletion of recipient Lewis rats by (sub)lethal irradiation by no means abrogates the encephalitogenic effect of transferred activated MBP specific T line cells, but may even enhance it further. As expected, instead of perivascular infiltrates, the CNS infiltrates are limited to few activated lymphocytes scattered through the myelinated parenchyme.

These studies strongly argue against the participation of unspecific lymphoid cells in generation of the EAE lesion, which is in contrast to the formation of delayed type hypersensitivity reaction (190). The participation of radioresistant host populations, is however, not ruled out in any of the model systems described. Especially macrophages are strong candidates to act as amplifiers in the generation of the EAE lesions. Depletion of macrophages from rats by toxic silica dust (23,37,73) or liposome encapsulated toxic material (89) profoundly interferes with inducibility of EAE or EAN.

6.2 Effector Mechanisms

If the encephalitogenic T cells are indeed largely autonomous in producing clinical EAE, by which mechanisms do they cause the destructive effects? Direct cytotoxic attack against CNS antigen presenting glia cells is as possible mechanism, but an indirect effect via recruitment and activation of ancillary inflammatory cells could have a major role as well.

Cytotoxic T lymphocytes destroy their target cells by more than one mechanism. Besides the cytotoxic granule protein perforin (167), the fas antigen dependent apoptosis pathways, along with TNFα/β secretion may account of cytotoxic target cell killing (99,124). Both mechanisms may have a role in EAE. On the one hand, especially CD4+ CTL seem to kill their target with strong participation of the Fas apoptosis pathway (201). On the other hand, in the EAE lesion both perforin and TNF are significantly expressed (76).

In the rat (209), and in the mouse as well (51), encephalitogenic, MBP specific T cells are strongly cytotoxic against any APC capable of presenting the relevant MBP epitope in a recognizable fashion. At least in the rat, T lines with specificity for other neural antigens, as the neuritogenic P2 protein of peripheral nerve myelin are also killers (235), whereas T cells specific for foreign antigens lack cytotoxic potential (209). The cytotoxic capacity of the MBP specific T lines was unexpected, since, as pointed out before, they are all members of the CD4+ T cell subset, which contains mainly T helper cells, along with T cell effectors of delayed type hypersensitivity (DTH).

The cytotoxic potential of MBP specific rat T lines was found to be inseparably associated with the capacity of mediating clinical EAE in vivo. So far no myelin-specific encephalitogenic, or neuritogenic T cell line was seen, which lacked cytotoxic activity in vitro (209). Interestingly, however, S100β specific T cells, which mediate a severe histological autoimmune panencephalitis with paradoxically mild clinical effects were non-cytotoxic (103). The speculation may not be too bold that the cytotoxic interactions seen so readily in culture may have a role in producing pathogenic defects in the CNS in vivo, as well. Cytotoxic cell-to-cell interactions in vivo are hard to demonstrate by conventional morphology (4). Even in the case of organ rejection, which certainly involves large scale cytotoxic target cell destruction elaborate technology is required for visualization (70). In EAE lesions of Lewis rats, apoptotic cell death has been demonstrated in the CNS (160), but more detailed investigations revealed that a large proportion of the degenerating cells were in fact infiltrate cells, mainly T cells (159,189), wity some participation of macrophages (144).

As an alternative to contact dependent cytotoxicity, encephalitogenic changes could be effected via cytotoxic cytokines secreted either directly by effector T cells, or by recruited macrophages. Indeed, tumor necrosis factors-α and -β (TNF-α, -β) are produced by encephalitogenic T cells (43,77,212), which produce cytokine patterns qualifying them as Th1 cells (3,141). In fact, antibodies against TNF-β were reported to efficiently reduce clinical EAE (180). The same holds true for TNF-α by MAbs (192), pentoxifylline (143,178), or by recombinant TNF-receptor protein (W.E.F. Klinkert, manuscript submitted), which all significantly reduce initiation and development of EAE in vivo.

Still the critical target cell of encephalitogenic T lymphocytes remains to be identified. As pointed out, in vitro experiments have established that astrocytes (209) and endothelial cells (133,175,191) can be induced to express (auto-)antigens and to serve as targets to cytotoxic encephalitogenic T cells. Due to their central role in CNS physiology, astrocytes are especially attractive candidates for EAE target cells. Indeed, local astrocytes are profoundly affected by encephalitogenic mechanisms, both very early in the development of the lesion (40), and in later stages (30,125,195). In situ expression of MHC class II antigens on astrocytes, a prerequisite for antigen presentation to T lymphocytes, has, however, been a matter of dispute. Class II–expressing astrocytes have been described by some authors (81,112,214,224), but not by others (19,131,170). It is possible that astrocytic MHC expression is very low and that technical problems are responsible for their discrepant demonstrability. In any event, it should be kept in mind that only very few membrane-bound MHC class II peptide complexes may be sufficient for antigen presentation to T cells (44).

Intriguing results concerning the EAE glial target cells have been obtained in EAE of bone marrow chimeric rats. Several groups showed that attack of the CNS by encephalitogenic T cells depends on compatibility with the grafted bone marrow rather than with the recipient (80,82,130). These results emphasize the importance of a newly identified bone marrow–derived perivascular monocyte (111) which may have a role in initiating antigen-dependent inflammatory processes within the CNS. If indeed the lesions of bone marrow chimeras are identical with the one seen in intact T-cell recipients, the mechanisms affecting endothelium and astrocytes would have to be redefined.

As discussed above, there is good evidence that infiltrating macrophages have a key role in the development of EAE lesions. An amplifying role of inflammatory macrophages has been strongly supported by functional and immunocytochemical analyses of new encephalitis models compared with the classic MBP–EAE paradigm. Autoimmune encephalitides mediated by T cells specific for MOG or S100β typically show mild clinical courses with very intensive CNS infiltration. Immunocytochemical examination of these lesions has revealed in both cases a deficit of activated macrophages stained by MAb marker ED1 (103,117). In striking contrast, the infiltrate of MBP-mediated EAE is characterized by large proportions of ED1+ macrophages, which usually outnumber infiltrating T cells (117,168).

What remains is for researchers to directly investigate the mechanisms (probably involving cytokines) by which the initial encephalitogenic T effector cells recruit macrophages to the lesion site and activate them to help attack the local tissue.

Summary and Conclusions

There is no doubt that in experimental autoimmune diseases of the CNS, CD4+ T lymphocytes are the initiators and main effector cells responsible for the pathogenic lesions. These cells arise in the thymus, presumably as the result of positive selection through self peptides, but without subsequent deletion in a negative selection stage.

The number of potentially encephalitogenic brain autoantigens is continually increasing. Encephalitogenic myelin proteins include internal membrane components (MBP), integral membrane proteins (PLP), and members of the immunoglobulin gene superfamily (MOG, MAG). In addition, nonmyelin antigens such as the astroglial S100β protein have been identified as an encephalitogen.

Encephalitogenic T cells produce their effect within the CNS probably through a combination of distinct mechanisms. Direct cytotoxic attack against brain structures may contribute to pathogenesis, as do recruitment and activation of ancillary macrophages.

Recognition of unusually dominant encephalitogenic peptide epitopes and a strongly biased usage of TcR genes by encephalitogenic T cells in several model systems have raised hopes that novel immunospecific strategies might be designed. Unfortunately, so far, these features have not been found in human CNS-specific T-cell responses. Direct adaptation of these strategies toward the cure of MS does not appear to be realistic at present. But new evidence of regulatory lymphocyte circuits involved in safeguarding immunological self-tolerance in the CNS may provide alternative approaches to immunotherapies of autoimmune demyelination.

References

1. Acha-Orbea H, Mitchell DJ, Timmermann L, Wraith DC, Tausch GS, Walsor MK, Zamvil SS, McDevitt HO, Steinman L. Limited heterogeneity of T cell receptors from lymphocytes mediating autoimmune encephalomyelitis allows specific immune intervention. Cell 54:263–273, 1988.

2. Adda DH, Béraud E, Depieds R. Evidence for suppressor cells in Lewis rats' experimental allergic encephalomyelitis. Eur J Immunol 7:620–623, 1977.

3. Ando DG, Clayton J, Kono D, Urban JL, Sercarz EE. Encephalitogenic T cells in the B10.PL model of experimental allergic encephalomyelitis (EAE) are of the Th1 lymphokine subtype. Cell Immunol 124:132–143, 1989.

4. Ando K, Guidotti LG, Wirth S, Ishikawa T, Missale G, Moriyama T, Schreiber RD, Schlicht H-J, Huang S-N, Chisari FV. Class I-restricted cytotoxic T lymphocytes are directly cytopathic for their target cells in vivo. J Immunol 152:3245–3253, 1994.

5. Aström K-E, Waksman BH. The passive transfer of experimental allergic encephalomyelitis and neuritis with living lymphoid cells. J Pathol Bacteriol 83:89–107, 1962.

6. Baimbridge KG, Celio MR, Rogers JH. Calcium-binding proteins in the nervous system. Trends Neurosci 15:303–308, 1992.

7. Ben-Nun A. Staphylococcal enterotoxin B as a potent suppressant of T cell proliferative responses in rats. Eur J Immunol 21:815–818, 1991.

8. Ben-Nun A, Cohen IR. Vaccination against autoimmune encephalomyelitis (EAE): attenuated autoimmune T lymphocytes confer resistance to induction of active EAE but not to EAE mediated by the intact T lymphocyte line. Eur J Immunol 11:949–952, 1981.

9. Ben-Nun A, Cohen IR. Experimental autoimmune encephalomyelitis (EAE) mediated by T cell lines: process of selection of lines and characterization of the cells. J Immunol 129:303–308, 1982.

10. Ben-Nun A, Cohen IR. Spontaneous remission and acquired resistance to autoimmune encephalomyelitis (EAE) are associated with suppression of T cell reactivity: Suppressed EAE effector cells recovered as T cell lines. J Immunol 128:1450–1457, 1982.

11. Ben-Nun A, Eisenstein S, Cohen IR. Experimental autoimmune encephalomyelitis (EAE) in genetically resistant rats: PVG rats resist active induction of EAE but are susceptible to and can generate EAE effector T cell lines. J Immunol 129:918–919, 1982.

12. Ben-Nun A, Lando Z, Dorf ME, Burakoff SJ. Analysis of cross-reactive antigen-specific T cell clones. Specific recognition of two major histocompatibility complex (MHC) and two non-MHC antigens by a single clone. J Exp Med 157:2147–2153, 1983.

13. Ben-Nun A, Wekerle H, Cohen IR. The rapid isolation of clonable antigen-specific T lymphocyte lines capable of mediating autoimmune encephalomyelitis. Eur J Immunol 11:195–199, 1981.

14. Ben-Nun A, Wekerle H, Cohen IR. Vaccination against autoimmune encephalomyelitis using attenuated cells of a T lymphocyte line reactive against myelin basic protein. Nature 292:60–61, 1981.

15. Béraud E, Lorberboum-Galski H, Chan C-C, Fitzgerald D, Pastan I, Nussenblatt RB. Immunospecific suppression of encephalitogenic activated T lymphocytes by chimeric cytotoxin IL-2-PE40. Cell Immunol 133:379–389, 1991.

16. Bernard CCA, Leydon J, Mackay IR. T cell necessity in the pathogenesis of experimental autoimmune encephalomyelitis in mice. Eur J Immunol 6:655–660, 1976.

17. Bitar D, Whitacre CC. Suppression of experimental autoimmune encepholomyelitis by the oral administration of myelin basic protein. Cell Immunol 112:364–370, 1988.

18. Bosma MJ, Carroll AM. The SCID mouse mutant: definition, characterization, and potential uses. Annu Rev Immunol 9:323–350, 1991.

19. Boyle EA, McGeer PL. Cellular immune response in multiple sclerosis plaques. Am J Pathol 137:575–584, 1990.

20. Brinkman CJJ, Ter Laak HJ, Hommes OR. Modulation of experimental allergic encephalomyelitis in Lewis rats by monoclonal anti-T cell antibodies. J Neuroimmunol 7:207–214, 1985.

21. Brocke S, Gaur A, Piercy C, Gautam AM, Gijbels K, Fathman CG, Steinman L. Induction of relapsing paralysis in experimental autoimmune encephalomyelitis by bacterial super-antigen. Nature 365:642–644, 1993.

22. Broeren CPM, Lucassen MA, Van Stipdonk MJB, Van der Zee R, Boog CJP, Kusters JG, Van Eden W. CDR1 T-cell receptor β-chain peptide induces major histocompatibility complex class II-restricted T-T cell interactions. Proc Natl Acad Sci USA 91:5997–6001, 1994.

23. Brosnan CF, Bornstein MB, Bloom BR. The effects of macrophage depletion on the clinical and pathologic expression of experimental allergic encephalomyelitis. J Immunol 126:614–620, 1981.

24. Brostoff SW, Burnett P, Lampert PW, Eylar EH. Isolation and characterization of the protein from sciatic nerve myelin responsible for allergic neuritis. Nature 235:210–212, 1972.

25. Brostoff SW, Mason DW. Experimental allergic encephalomyelitis: successful treatment in vivo with a monoclonal antibody that recognizes T helper cells. J Immunol 133:1938–1942, 1984.

26. Brunner C, Lassmann H, Waehneldt TV, Matthieu J-M, Linington C. Differential ultrastructural localization of myelin basic protein, myelin/oligodendrocyte glycoprotein, and 2′, 3′-cyclic nucleotide 3′-phosphodiesterase in the CNS of adult rats. J Neurochem 52:296–304, 1989.

27. Burns FR, Li X, Shen N, Offner H, Chou YK, Vandenbark AA, Heber-Katz E. Both rat and mouse T cell receptors specific for the encephalitogenic determinant of myelin basic protein use similar Vα and Vβ chain genes even though the major histocompatibility complex and encephalitogenic determinants being recognized are different. J Exp Med 169:27–39, 1989.

28. Burns J, Krasner J, Rostami A, Pleasure D. Isolation of P2 protein-reactive T-cell lines from human blood. Ann Neurol 19:391–393, 1986.

29. Burns J, Rosenzweig A, Zweiman B, Lisak RP. Isolation of myelin basic protein-reactive T cell lines from normal human blood. Cell Immunol 81:435–440, 1983.

30. Cammer W, Tansey TA, Brosnan CF. Reactive gliosis in the brains of Lewis rats with experimental allergic encephalomyelitis. J Neuroimmunol 27:111–120, 1990.

31. Campagnoni AT, Macklin WB. Cellular and molecular aspects of myelin protein gene expression. Mol Neurobiol 2:41–89, 1988.

32. Carlo DJ, Karkhanis YD, Bailey PJ, Wisniewski HM, Brostoff SW. Experimental allergic neuritis: evidence for involvement of the P0 and P2 proteins. Brain Res 88:580–584, 1975.

33. Caspi RR, Roberge FG, McAllister CG, El-Sayed M, Kuwabara T, Gery I, Hanna E, Nussenblatt RB. T cell lines mediating experimental autoimmune uveoritinitis (EAU) in rats. J Immunol 136:928–933, 1986.

34. Chen Y, Kuchroo VK, Inobe J-i, Hafler DA, Weiner HL. Regulatory T cell clones induced by oral tolerance: suppression of autoimmune encephalomyelitis. Science 265:1237–1240, 1994.

35. Chluba J, Steeg C, Becker A, Wekerle H, Epplen JT. T cell receptor β chain usage in myelin basic protein-specific rat T lymphocytes. Eur J Immunol 19:279–284, 1989.

36. Clark L, Heber-Katz E, Rostami A. Shared T-cell receptor gene usage in experimental allergic neuritis and encephalomyelitis. Ann Neurol 31:587–592, 1992.

37. Craggs RI, King RHM, Thomas PK. The effect of suppression of macrophage activity on the development of experimental allergic neuritis. Acta Neuropathol 62:316–323, 1984.

38. Cross AH, Cannella B, Brosnan CF, Raine CS. Homing to central nervous system vascula-

ture by antigen-specific lymphocytes. I. Localization of ^{14}C-labelled cells during acute, chronic, and relapsing experimental allergic encephalomyelitis. Lab Invest 63:162–170, 1990.

39. Cross AH, Tuohy VK, Raine CS. Development of reactivity to new myelin antigens during chronic relapsing autoimmune demyelination. Cell Immunol 146:261–269, 1993.

40. D'Amelio FE, Smith ME, Eng LF. Sequence of tissue responses in the early stages of experimental allergic encephalomyelitis (EAE): immunohistochemical, light microscopic, and ultrastructural observations in the spinal cord. Glia 3:229–240, 1990.

41. Davis CB, Mitchell DJ, Wraith DC, Todd JA, Zamvil SS, McDevitt HO, Steinman L, Jones PP. Polymorphic residues on the I-Aβ chain modulate the stimulation of T cell clones specific for the N-terminal peptide of the autoantigen myelin basic protein. J Immunol 143:2083–2093, 1989.

42. Davis MM, Bjorkman PJ. T-cell antigen receptor genes and T-cell recognition. Nature 334:395–402, 1988.

43. Day MJ, Mason DW. Loss of encephalitogenicity of a myelin basic protein-specific T cell line is associated with a phenotypic change but not with alteration in production of interleukin-2, γ-interferon or tumour necrosis factor. J Neuroimmunol 30:53–59, 1990.

44. Demotz S, Grey HM, Sette A. The minimal number of class II MHC-antigen complexes needed for T cell activation. Science 249:1028–1030, 1990.

45. Desquenne-Clark L, Esch TR, Otvos L, Heber-Katz E. T-cell receptor peptide immunization leads to enhanced and chronic experimental allergic encephalomyelitis. Proc Natl Acad Sci USA 88:7219–7223, 1991.

46. Driscoll BF, Kies MW, Alvord EC. Enhanced transfer of experimental allergic encephalomyelitis with strain 13 guinea pig lyumph node cells: requirement for culture with specific antigen and allogeneic peritoneal exudate cells. J Immunol 125:1817–1822, 1980.

47. Duong TT, St. Louis J, Gilbert JJ, Finkelman FD, Strejan GH. Effect of anti-interferon-y and anti-interleukin-2 monoclonal antibody treatment on the development of actively and passively induced experimental allergic encephalomyelitis. J Neuroimmunol 36:105–115, 1992.

48. Egwuagu CE, Mahdi RM, Nussenblatt RB, Gery I, Caspi RR. Evidence for selective accumulation of Vβ8$^+$ T lymphocytes in experimental autoimmune uveoretinitis induced with two different retinal antigens. J Immunol 151:1627–1636, 1993.

49. Engelhardt B, Diamantstein T, Wekerle H. Immunotherapy of experimental autoimmune encephalomyelitis (EAE). Differential effect of anti-IL-2 receptor antibody therapy on actively induced and T-line mediated EAE of the Lewis rat. J Autoimmun 2:61–74, 1989.

50. Eylar EH, Kniskern PJ, Jackson JJ. Myelin basic protein. Methods Enzymol 32B:323–341, 1974.

51. Fallis RJ, McFarlin DE. Chronic relapsing experimental allergic encephalomyelitis: cytotoxicity effected by a class II-restricted T cell line specific for an encephalitogenic epitope. J Immunol 143:2160–2165, 1989.

52. Feurer C, Chow LH, Borel J-F. Preventive and therapeutic effects of cyclosporin and valine-dihydro-cyclosporin in chronic relapsing experimental allergic encephalomyelitis in the Lewis rat. Immunology 63:219–223, 1988.

53. Fling SP, Gold DP, Gregerson DS. Multiple, autoreactive TCR Vβ genes utilized in response to a small pathogenic peptide of an autoantigen in EAU. Cell Immunol 142:275–286, 1992.

54. Fontana A, Fierz W, Wekerle H. Astrocytes present myelin basic protein to encephalitogenic T cell lines. Nature 307:273–276, 1984.

55. Franco A, Southwood S, Arrhenius T, Kuchroo VK, Grey HM, Sette A, Ishioka GY. T cell receptor antagonist peptides are highly effective inhibitors of experimental allergic encephalomyelitis. Eur J Immunol 24:940–946, 1994.

56. Fredrikson S, Sun J-B, Huang W-X, Olsson T, Link H. Cord blood contains high numbers of autoimmune T cells recognizing multiple myelin proteins and acetylcholine receptor. J Immunol 151:2217–2224, 1993.

57. Fritz RB, Skeen MJ, Chou C-HJ, Zamvil SS. Localization of the encephalitogenic epitope for the SJL mouse in the N-terminal region of myelin basic protein. J Neuroimmunol 26:239–243, 1990.

58. Fritz RB, Skeen MJ, Ziegler HK. Influence of the H-2^u haplotype on immune function in F1 hybrid mice. I. Antigen presentation. J Immunol 134:3574–3579, 1985.

59. Fujinami RS, Oldstone MBA. Amino acid homology between the encephalitogenic site of myelin basic protein (MBP) and virus: mechanism for autoimmunity. Science 230:1043–1046, 1985.

60. Gammon G, Geysen HM, Apple RJ, Pickett E, Palmer M, Ametani A, Sercarz EE. T cell determinant structure: cores and determinant envelopes in three mouse major histocompatibility complex haplotypes. J Exp Med 173:609–617, 1991.

61. Gardinier MV, Amiguet P, Linington C, Matthieu J-M. Myelin/oligodendrocyte glycoprotein is a unique member of the immunoglobulin superfamily. J Neurosci Res 33:177–187, 1992.

62. Gaur A, Fathman CG, Steinman L, Brocke S. SEB induced anergy: modulation of immune response to T cell determinants of myoglobin and myelin basic protein. J Immunol 150:3062–3069, 1993.

63. Germain RN. MHC-dependent antigen processing and peptide presentation: Providing ligands for T lymphocyte activation. Cell 76:287–299, 1994.

64. Gold DP, Offner H, Sun D, Wiley S, Vandenbark AA, Wilson DB. Analysis of T cell receptor β chains in Lewis rats with experimental allergic encephalomyelitis: conserved complementary determining region 3. J Exp Med 174:1467–1476, 1991.

65. Gold DP, Vainiene M, Celnik B, Wiley S, Gibbs C, Hashim GA, Vandenbark AA, Offner H. Characterization of the immune response to a secondary encephalitogenic epitope of basic protein in Lewis rats. II. Biased T cell receptor Vβ expression predominates in spinal cord infiltrating T cells. J Immunol 148:1712–1717, 1992.

66. Gonatas NK, Howard JC. Inhibition of experimental allergic encephalomyelitis in rats severely depleted of T cells. Science 186:839–841, 1974.

67. Goverman J, Woods A, Larson L, Weiner LP, Hood L, Zaller DM. Transgenic mice that express a myelin basic protein-specific T cell receptor develop spontaneous autoimmunity. Cell 72:551–560, 1993.

68. Greer JM, Kuchroo VK, Sobel RA, Lees MB. Identification and characterization of a second encephalitogenic determinant of myelin proteolipid protein (residues 178–191) for SJL mice. J Immunol 149:783–788, 1992.

69. Gregerson DS, Fling SP, Merryman CF, Zhang X, Li X, Heber-Katz E. Conserved T cell receptor V gene usage by uveitogenic T cells. Clin Immunol Immunopathol 58:154–161, 1991.

70. Hameed A, Truong LD, Price V, Kruhenbuhl O, Tschopp J. Immunohistochemical localization of granzyme B antigen in cytotoxic cells in human tissues. Am J Pathol 138:1069–1075, 1991.

71. Happ MP, Heber-Katz E. Differences in the repertoire of the Lewis rat T cell response to self and non-self myelin basic proteins. J Exp Med 167:502–513, 1988.

72. Hartung H-P, Schäfer B, Diamantstein T, Fierz W, Heininger K, Toyka KV. Suppression of

P2-T cell line mediated experimental autoimmune neuritis by interleukin-2 receptor targeted monoclonal antibody ART-18. Brain Res 489:120–128, 1989.

73. Hartung H-P, Schäfer B, Heininger K, Stoll G, Toyka KV. The role of macrophages and eicosanoids in the pathogenesis of experimental allergic neuritis. Brain 111:1039–1059, 1988.

74. Hashim G, Vandenbark AA, Galang AB, Diamanduros T, Carvalho E, Srinivasan J, Jones R, Vainiene M, Morrison WJ, Offner H. Antibodies specific for Vβ8 receptor peptide suppress experimental autoimmune encephalomyelitis. J Immunol 144:4621–4627, 1990.

75. Hashim G, Vandenbark AA, Gold DP, Diamanduros T, Offner H. T cell lines specific for an immunodominant epitope of human basic protein define an encephalitogenic determinant for experimental autoimmune encephalomyelitis-resistant Lou/M rats. J Immunol 146:515–520, 1991.

76. Held W, Meyermann R, Qin Y, Mueller C. Perforin and tumor necrosis factor α in the pathogenesis of experimental allergic encephalomyelitis: comparison of autoantigen induced and transferred disease in Lewis rats. J Autoimmun 6:311–322, 1993.

77. Hershkoviz R, Mor F, Gilat D, Cohen IR, Lider O. T cells in the spinal cord in experimental autyoimmune encephalomyelitis are matrix adherent and secrete tumor necrosis factor alpha. J Neuroimmunol 37:161–166, 1992.

78. Hickey WF, Gonatas NK, Kimura H, Wilson DB. Identification and quantitation of T lymphocyte subsets found in the spinal cord of the Lewis rat during acute experimental allergic encephalomyelitis. J Immunol 131:2805–2809, 1983.

79. Hickey WF, Hsu BL, Kimura H. T lymphocyte entry into the central nervous system. J Neurosci Res 28:254–260, 1991.

80. Hickey WF, Kimura H. Perivascular microglial cells of the CNS are bone-marrow derived and present antigen in vivo. Science 239:290–293, 1988.

81. Hickey WF, Osborn JP, Kirby WM. Expression of Ia molecules by astrocytes during acute experimental allergic encephalomyelitis in the Lewis rat. Cell Immunol 91:528–535, 1985.

82. Hinrichs DJ, Wegmann KW, Dietsch GN. Transfer of experimental allergic encephalomyelitis to bone marrow chimeras: endothelial cells are not the restricting element. J Exp Med 166:1906–1911, 1987.

83. Higgins PJ, Weiner HL. Suppression of experimental autoimmune encephalomyelitis by oral administration of myelin basic protein and its fragments. J Immunol 140:440–445, 1988.

84. Holda JH, Swanborg RH. Autoimmune effector cells. II. Transfer of experimental allergic encephalomyelitis with a subset of T lymphocytes. Eur J Immunol 12:453–455, 1982.

85. Holda JH, Welch AM, Swanborg RH. Autoimmune effector cells. I. Transfer of experimental allergic encephalomyelitis with lymphoid cells cultured with antigen. Eur J Immunol 10:657–659, 1980.

86. Holmdahl R, Klareskog L, Rubin K, Larsson E, Wigzell H. T lymphocytes in collagen II-induced arthritis in mice. Characterization of arthritogenic collagen II-specific T cell line and clones. Scand J Immunol 22:295–306, 1985.

87. Holoshitz J, Naparstek Y, Ben-Nun A, Cohen IR. Lines of T lymphocytes mediate or vaccinate against autoimmune arthritis. Science 219:56–58, 1983.

88. Howell MD, Winters ST, Olee T, Powell HC, Carlo DJ, Brostoff SW. Vaccination against experimental allergic encephalomyelitis with T cell receptor peptides. Science 246:668–670, 1989.

89. Huitinga I, Van Rooijen N, De Groot, CJA, Uitdehaag BMJ, Dijkstra CD. Suppression of

experimental allergic encephalomyelitis in Lewis rats after elimination of macrophages. J Exp Med 172:1025–1033, 1990.

90. Jiang H, Zhang S-L, Pernis B. Role of CD8+ T cells in murine experimental allergic encephalomyelitis. Science 256:1213–1215, 1992.

91. Jones RE, Bourdette DN, Whitham RH, Offner H, Vandenbark AA. Induction of experimental autoimmune encephalomyelitis in severe combined immunodeficient mice reconstituted with allogeneic and xenogeneic hematopoietic cells. J Immunol 150:4620–4629, 1993.

92. Jonker M, Van Lambalgen R, Mitchell DJ, Durham SK, Steinman L. Successful treatment of EAE in rhesus monkeys with MHC class II specific monoclonal antibodies. J Autoimmun 1:399–414, 1988.

93. Jorgensen JL, Reay PA, Ehrich EW, Davis MM. Molecular components of T-cell recognition. Annu Rev Immunol 10:835–873, 1992.

94. Jung S, Hartung H-P, Toyka KV. Shared T-cell receptor gene usage in experimental allergic neuritis and encephalomyelitis. Ann Neurol 34:113, 1993.

95. Jung S, Schluesener HJ, Toyka KV, Hartung H-P. Modulation of EAE by vaccination with T cell receptor peptides: Vβ8 T cell receptor peptide-specific CD4+ lymphocytes lack direct immunoregulatory activity. J Neuroimmunol 45:15–22, 1993.

95a. Kääb G, Brandl G, Marx A, Wekerle H, Bradl M. The myelin basic protein specific T cell repertoire in (transgenic) Lewis rat/SCID mouse chimeras: Preferential Vβ8.2 T cell receptor usage depends on an intact Lewis thymic microenvironment. Eur J Immunol 26:981–988, 1996.

96. Kägi D, Vignaux F, Ledermann B, Bürki K, Depraetere V, Nagata S, Hengartner H, Golstein P. Fas and perforin pathways as major mechanisms of T cell mediated cytotoxicity. Science 265:528–530, 1994.

97. Kalman B, Lublin FD, Lattime E, Joseph J, Knobler RL. Effects of staphylococcal enterotoxin B on T cell receptor Vβ utilization and clinical manifestations of experimental allergic encephalomyelitis. J Neuroimmunol 45:83–88, 1993.

98. Karin N, Szafer F, Mitchell D, Gold DP, Steinman L. Selective and nonselective stages in homing of T lymphocytes to the central nervous system during experimental allergic encephalomyelitis. J Immunol 150:4116–4124, 1993.

99. Kawano Y, Sasamoto Y, Kotake S, Thurau SR, Wiggert B, Gery I. Trials of vaccination against experimental autoimmune uveoretinitis with a T cell receptor peptide. Curr Eye Res 10:173–177, 1991.

100. Kibler RF, Fritz RB, Chou FC-H, Chou C-HJ, Peacocke NY, Brown NM, McFarlin DE. Immune response of Lewis rats to peptide C1 (residues 68-88) of guinea pig and rat myelin basic proteins. J Exp Med 146:1323–1331, 1977.

101. Kies MW. Species-specificity and localization of encephalitogenic sites in myelin basic protein (MBP). Springer Semin Immunopathol 8:295–303, 1985.

102. Koh D-R, Fung-Leung W-P, Ho A, Gray D, Acha-Orbea H, Mak TW. Less mortality but more relapses in experimental allergic encephalomyelitis in CD8−/− mice. Science 256:1210–1213, 1992.

103. Kojima K, Berger T, Lassmann H, Hinze-Selch D, Zhang Y, Gehrmann J, Wekerle H, Linington C. Experimental autoimmune panencephalitis and uveoretinitis in the Lewis rat transferred by T lymphocytes specific for the S100β molecule, a calcium binding protein of astroglia. J Exp Med 180:817–829, 1994.

104. Kono DH, Urban JL, Horvath SJ, Ando DG, Saavedra R, Hood L. Two minor determinants of myelin protein induce experimental allergic encephalomyelitis in SJL/J. J Exp Med 168:213–228, 1988.

105. Koprowski H, Paraf A, Billingham R, Jervis G. Etudes sur le mécanisme de l'encéphalite allergique chez le rat. C R Acad Sci III 250:2956, 1960.

106. Kuchroo VK, Sobel RA, Laning JC, Martin CA, Greenfield E, Dorf ME, Lees MB. Experimental allergic encephalomyelitis mediated by cloned T cells specific for a synthetic peptide of myelin proteolipid protein. Fine specificity and T cell receptor Vβ usage. J Immunol 148:3776–3782, 1992.

107. Kumar V, Sercarz EE. The involvement of T cell receptor peptide-specific regulatory CD4$^+$ T cells in recovery from antigen-induced autoimmune disease. J Exp Med 178:909–916, 1993.

108. Lafaille J, Nagashima K, Katsuki M, Tonegawa S. High incidence of spontaneous autoimmune encephalomyelitis in immunodeficient anti-myelin basic protein T cell receptor mice. Cell 78:399–408, 1994.

109. Lamont AG, Sette A, Fujinami RS, Colon SM, Miles C, Grey HM. Inhibition of experimental autoimmune encephalomyelitis induction in SJL/J mice by using a peptide with high affinity for IA^s molecules. J Immunol 145:1687–1683, 1990.

110. Lannes-Vieira J, Gehrmann J, Kreutzberg GW, Wekerle H. The inflammatory lesion of T cell line transferred experimental autoimmune encephalomyelitis of the Lewis rat: distinct nature of parenchymal and perivascular infiltrates. Acta Neuropathol 87:435–442, 1994.

110a. Lannes-Vieira J, Goudable B, Drexler K, Gehrmann J, Torres-Nagel NE, Hünig T, Wekerle H. Encephalitogenic, myelin basic protein specific T cells from naive rat thymus: preferential use of the T cell receptor gene Vβ8.2 and expression of the CD4$^-$CD8$^-$ phenotype. Eur J Immunol 25:611–616, 1995.

111. Lassmann H, Zimprich F, Vass K, Hickey WF. Microglial cells are a component of the perivascular glia limitans. J Neurosci Res 28:236–243, 1991.

112. Lee S, Moore GRW, Golenowsky G, Raine CS. Multiple sclerosis: a role for astroglia in active demyelination suggested by class II MHC expression and ultrastructural study. J Neuropathol Exp Neurol 49:122–136, 1990.

113. Lehmann PV, Forsthuber T, Miller A, Sercarz EE. Spreading of T-cell autoimmunity to cryptic determinants of an autoantigen. Nature 358:155–157, 1992.

114. Lider O, Reshef T, Béraud E, Ben-Nun, A, Cohen IR. Anti-idiotypic network induced by T-cell vaccination against experimental autoimmune encephalomyelitis. Science 239: 181–183, 1988.

115. Lider O, Santos LMB, Lee CSY, Higgins PJ, Weiner HL. Suppression of experimental autoimmune encephalomyelitis by oral administration of myelin basic protein. II. Suppression of disease and in vitro immune responses is mediated by antigen specific CD8$^+$ T lymphocytes. J Immunol 142:748–752, 1989.

116. Liebert UG, Hashim GA, ter Meulen V. Characterization of measles virus-induced cellular autoimmune reactions against myelin basic protein in Lewis rats. J Neuroimmunol 29:139–147, 1990.

117. Linington C, Berger T, Perry L, Weerth S, Hinze-Selch D, Zhang Y, Lu H-C, Lassmann H, Wekerle H. T cell specific for the myelin oligodendrocyte glycoprotein (MOG) mediate an unusual autoimmune inflammatory response in the central nervous system. Eur J Immunol 23:1364–1372, 1993.

118. Linington C, Bradl M, Lasssmann H, Brunner C, Vass K. Augmentation of demyelination in rat acute allergic encephalomyelitis by circulating mouse monoclonal antibodies directed against a myelin/oligodendrocyte glycoprotein. Am J Pathol 130:443–454, 1988.

119. Linington C, Izumo S, Suzuki M, Uyemura K, Meyermann R, Wekerle H. A permanent rat

T cell line that mediates experimental allergic neuritis in the Lewis rat in vivo. J Immunol 133:1946–1950, 1984.

120. Linington C, Lassmann H. Antibody responses in chronic relapsing experimental allergic encephalomyelitis: correlation of serum demyelinating activity with antibody titer to myelin/oligodencrocyte glycoprotein (MOG). J Neuroimmunol 17:61–70, 1987.

121. Linington C, Webb M, Woodhams PL. A novel myelin-associated glycoprotein defined by a mouse monoclonal antibody. J Neuroimmunol 6:387–396, 1984.

122. Lohse AW, Mor F, Karin N, Cohen IR. Control of experimental autoimmune encephalomyelitis by T cells responding to activated T cells. Science 244:820–822, 1989.

123. Lohse AW, Spahn TW, Wölfel T, Herkel J, Cohen IR, Meyer zum Büschenfelde K-H. Induction of the anti-ergotypic response. Int Immunol 5:533–539, 1993.

124. Lowin B, Hahne M, Mattmann C, Tschopp J. Cytolytic T-cell cytotoxicity is mediated through perforin and Fas lytic pathways. Nature 370:650–652, 1994.

125. Ludowyk PA, Hughes W, Hugh A, Willenborg DO, Rockett KA, Parish CR. Astrocyte hypertrophy: an important pathological feature of chronic experimental autoimmune encephalitis in aged rats. J Neuroimmunol 48:121–134, 1993.

126. Maron R, Zerubavel R, Friedman A, Cohen IR. T lymphocyte line specific for thyroglobulin produces or vaccinates against autoimmune thyroiditis in mice. J Immunol 131:2316–2322, 1983.

127. Martin R, Jaraquemada D, Flerlage M, Richert JR, Whitaker J, Long EO, McFarlin DE, McFarland HF. Fine specificity and HLA restriction of myelin basic protein-specific cytotoxic T cell lines from multiple sclerosis patients and healthy individuals. J Immunol 145:540–548, 1990.

128. Massa PT, Dörries R, ter Meulen V. Viral particles induce Ia antigen expression on astrocytes. Nature 320:543–546, 1986.

129. Massa PT, Schimpl A, Wecker E, ter Meulen V. Tumor necrosis factor amplifies measles virus-mediated Ia induction on astrocytes. Proc Natl Acad Sci USA 84:7242–7245, 1987.

130. Matsumoto Y, Fujiwara M. Adoptively transferred experimental allergic encephalomyelitis in chimeric rats: identification of transferred cells in the lesions of the central nervous system. Immunology 65:23–29, 1988.

131. Matsumoto Y, Hara N, Tanaka R, Fujiwara M. Immunohistochemical analysis of the rat central nervous system during experimental allergic encephalomyelitis, with special reference to Ia-positive cells with dendritic morphology. J Immunol 136:3668–3676, 1986.

132. Matsumoto Y, Tsuchida M, Hanawa H, Abo T. T cell receptor peptide therapy for autoimmune encephalomyelitis: stronger immunization is necessary for effective vaccination. Cell Immunol 153:468–478, 1994.

133. McCarron RM, Racke M, Spatz M, McFarlin DE. Cerebral vascular endothelial cells are effective targets for in vitro lysis by encephalitogenic T lymphocytes. J Immunol 147:503–508, 1991.

134. Melms A, Malcherek G, Hern U, Wiethölter H, Müller CA, Schoepfer R, Lindstrom J. T cells from normal and myasthenic individuals recognize the human acetylcholine receptor: heterogeneity of antigenic sites on the α-subunit. Ann Neurol 31:311–318, 1992.

135. Meyermann R, Lampert PW, Korr H, Wekerle H. T line mediated EAE. A morphological study of the developing lesions [Abstract]. J Neuropathol Exp Neurol 44:320, 1985.

136. Meyermann R, Lampert PW, Korr H, Wekerle H. The blood-brain-barrier: a strict border to lymphoid cells? In: Stroke and Microcirculation, 1st ed, J Cervos-Navarro, JR Ferszt, eds. Raven Press, New York, 1987, pp 289–296.

137. Miller A, Lider O, Roberts AB, Sporn MB, Weiner HL. Suppressor T cell generated by oral tolerization to myelin basic protein suppress both the *in vitro* and *in vivo* immune re-

sponses by the release of transforming growth factor β after antigen-specific triggering. Proc Natl Acad Sci USA 89:421–425, 1992.

138. Miller A, Lider O, Weiner HL. Antigen-driven suppression after oral administration of antigens. J Exp Med 174:791–798, 1991.

139. Milner P, Lovelidge CA, Taylor WA, Hughes RAC. P0 myelin protein produces experimental allergic neuritis in Lewis rats. J Neurol Sci 79:275, 1987.

140. Mor F, Cohen IR. Shifts in the epitopes of myelin basic protein recognized by Lewis rat T cells before, during and after the induction of experimental autoimmune encephalomyelitis. J Clin Invest 92:2199–2206, 1993.

141. Mustafa M, Vingsbo C, Olsson T, Höjeberg B, Holmdahl R. The major histocompatibility complex influences myelin basic protein 63-88-induced T cell cytokine profile and experimental autoimmune encephalomyelitis. Eur J Immunol 23:3089–3095, 1993.

142. Naparstek Y, Ben-Nun A, Holoshitz J, Reshef T, Frenkel A, Rosenberg M, Cohen IR. T lymphocyte line producing or vaccinating against autoimmune encephalomyelitis (EAE). Functional activation induces peanut agglutinin receptors and accumulation in the brain and thymus of line cells. Eur J Immunol 13:418–423, 1983.

143. Nataf S, Louboutin JP, Chabannes D, Fève JR, Muller JY. Pentoxifylline inhibits experimental allergic encephalomyelitis. Acta Neurol Scand 88:97–99, 1993.

144. Nguyen KB, McCombe PA, Pender MP. Macrophage apoptosis in the central nervous system in experimental autoimmune encephalomyelitis. J Autoimmun 7:145–152, 1994.

145. Offner H, Brostoff SW, Vandenbark AA. Antibodies against I-A and I-E determinants inhibit the activation and function of encephalitogenic T-lymphocyte lines. Cell Immunol 100:364–373, 1986.

146. Offner H, Buenafe AC, Vainiene M, Celnik B, Weinberg AD, Gold DP, Hashim G, Vandenbark AA. Where, when, and how to detect biased expression of disease-relevant Bβ genes in rats with experimental autoimmune encephalomyelitis. J Immunol 151:506–517, 1993.

147. Offner H, Hashim G, Celnik B, Galang A, Li X, Burns FR, Sheng N, Heber-Katz, E. T cell determinants of myelin basic protein include a unique encephalitogenic I-E restricted epitope for Lewis rats. J Exp Med 170:355–368, 1989.

148. Offner H, Hashim G, Chou YK, Celnik B, Jones R, Vandenbark AA. Encephalitogenic T cell clones with variant receptor specificity. J Immunol 141:3828–3832, 1988.

149. Offner H, Hashim GA, Vandenbark AA. T cell receptor peptide therapy triggers autoregulation of experimental encephalomyelitis. Science 251:430–432, 1991.

150. Ohashi PS, Oehen S, Buerki K, Pircher H, Ohashi CT, Odermatt B, Malissen B, Zinkernagel RM, Hengartner H. Ablation of "tolerance" and induction of diabetes by virus infection in viral antigen transgenic mice. Cell 65:305–317, 1991.

151. Oldstone MBA. Molecular mimicry and autoimmune disease. Cell 50:819–820, 1987.

152. Oldstone MBA, Nerenberg M, Southern P, Price J, Lewicki H. Virus infection triggers insulin-dependent diabetes mellitus in a transgenic model: Role of anti-self (virus) immune response. Cell 65:319–331, 1991.

153. Omlin FX, Webster HdeF, Palkovits CG, Cohen SR. Immunocytochemical localization of basic protein (MBP) in the major dense line regions of central and peripheral myelin. J Cell Biol 95:242–248, 1982.

154. Ortiz-Ortiz L, Nakamura RM, Weigle WO. T cell requirement for experimental allergic encephalomyelitis in the rat. J Immunol 117:576–579, 1976.

155. Ota K, Matsui M, Milford EL, Mackin GA, Weiner HL, Hafler DA. T-cell recognition of an immunodominant myelin basic protein epitope in multiple sclerosis. Nature 346:183–187, 1990.

156. Paterson PY. Transfer of allergic encephalomyelitis in rats by means of lymph node cells. J Exp Med 111:119–135, 1960.

157. Paterson PY, Bell J. Studies. J Immunol 89:72–79, 1962.

158. Paterson PY, Harvey JM. Irradiation potentiation of cellular transfer of EAE: time course and locus of effect in irradiated recipient Lewis rats. Cell Immunol 41:256–263, 1978.

159. Pender MP, McCombe PA, Yoong G, Nguyen KB. Apoptosis of αβ T lymphocytes in the nervous system in experimental autoimmune encephalomyelitis: its possible implications for recovery and acquired tolerance. j Autoimmun 5:401–410, 1992.

160. Pender MP, Nguyen KB, McCombe PA, Kerr JFR. Apoptosis in the nervous system in experimental allergic encephalomyelitis. J Neurol Sci 104:81–87, 1991.

161. Pender MP, Stanley GP, Yoong G, Nguyen KB. The neuropathology of chronic relapsing experimental allergic encephalomyelitis induced in the Lewis rat by inoculation with whole spinal cord and treatment with cyclosporin A. Acta Neuropathol 80:172–183, 1990.

162. Perry LL, Barzaga-Gilbert E, Trotter JL. T cell sensitization to proteolipid protein in myelin basic protein-induced relapsing experimental allergic encephalomyelitis. J Neuroimmunol 33:7–15, 1991.

163. Pette M, Fujita K, Kitze B, Whitaker JN, Albert E, Kappos L, Wekerle H. Myelin basic protein-specific T lymphocyte lines from MS patients and healthy individuals. Neurology 40:1770–1776, 1990.

164. Pette M, Fujita K, Wilkinson D, Altmann DM, Trowsdale J, Giegerich G, Hinkkanen A, Epplen JT, Kappos L, Wekerle H. Myelin autoreactivity in multiple sclerosis: recognition of myelin basic protein in the context of HLA-DR2 products by T lymphocytes of multiple sclerosis patients and healthy donors. Proc Natl Acad Sci USA 87:7968–7972, 1990.

165. Pettinelli CB, McFarlin DE. Adoptive transfer of experimental allergic encephalomyelitis in SJL/J mice after in vitro activation of lymph node cells with myelin basic protein: requirement for Lyt-1+2- T lymphocytes. J Immunol 127:1420–1423, 1981.

166. Pham-Dinh D, Mattei M-G, Nussbaum J-L, Roussel G, Pontarotti P, Roeckel N, Mather IH, Artzt K, Fischer Lindahl K, Dautigny A. Myelin/oligodendrocyte glycoprotein is a member of a subset of the immunoglobulin superfamily encoded within the major histocompatibility complex. Proc Natl Acad Sci USA 90:7990–7994, 1993.

167. Podack ER, Hengartner H, Lichtenheld MG. A central role of perforin in cytolysis? Annu Rev Immunol 9:129–148, 1991.

168. Polman CH, Dijkstra CD, Sminia T, Koetsier JC. Immunohistological analysis of macrophages in the central nervous system of Lewis rats with experimental allergic encephalomyelitis. J Neuroimmunol 11:215–222, 1986.

169. Polman CH, Matthaei I, De Groot CJA, Koetsier JC, Sminia T, Dijkstra CD. Low-dose cyclosporin A induces relapsing remitting experimental allergic encephalomyelitis in the Lewis rat. J Neuroimmunol 17:209–216, 1988.

170. Poltorak M, Freed WJ. Immunological reactions induced by intracerebral transplantation: evidence that host microglia, but not astroglia are the antigen presenting cells. Exp Neurol 103:222–233, 1989.

171. Pribyl TM, Campagnoni CW, Kampf K, Kashima T, Handley VW, McMahon J, Campagnoni AT. The human myelin basic protein gene is included within a 179-kilobase transcription unit: expression in the immune and central nervous system. Proc Natl Acad Sci USA 90:10695–10699, 1993.

172. Qin Y, Sun D, Wekerle H. Immune regulation in self tolerance: Functional elimination of

self-reactive, counterregulatory CD8$^+$ T lymphocyte circuit by neonatal transfer of encephalitogenic CD4$^+$ T cell lines. Eur J Immunol 22:1193–1198, 1992.

173. Racke MK, Quigley L, Cannella B, Raine CS, McFarlin DE, Scott DE. Superantigen modulation of experimental allergic encephalomyelitis: activation or anergy determines outcome. J Immunol 152:2051–2059, 1994.

174. Richert JR, Driscoll BF, Kies MW, Alvord EC. Adoptive transfer of experimental allergic encephalomyelitis: incubation of rat spleen cells with specific antigen. J Immunol 122:494–496, 1979.

175. Risau W, Engelhardt B, Wekerle H. Immune function of the blood brain barrier: incomplete presentation of protein (auto-) antigens by rat brain microvascular endothelium in vitro. J Cell Biol 110:1757–1766, 1990.

176. Rivers TM, Sprunt DH, Berry GP. Observations on attempts to produce acute disseminated encephalomyelitis in monkeys. J Exp Med 58:39–53, 1933.

177. Rose JW, Lorberboum-Galski H, Fitzgerald D, McCarron R, Hill KE, Townsend JJ, Pastan I. Chimeric cytotoxin IL2-PE40 inhibits relapsing experimental allergic encephalomyelitis. J Neuroimmunol 32:209–217, 1991.

178. Rott O, Cash E, Fleischer B. Phosphodiesterase inhibitor pentoxifylline, a selective suppressor of T helper type-1, but not type-2 associated lymphokine production, prevents induction of experimental autoimmune encephalomyelitis in Lewis rats. Eur J Immunol 23:1745–1751, 1993.

179. Rott O, Wekerle H, Fleischer B. Protection from experimental allergic encephalomyelitis by application of a bacterial superantigen. Int Immunol 4:347–354, 1992.

180. Ruddle NH, Bergman CM, McGrath KM, Lingenheld EG, Grunnet ML, Padula SJ, Clark RB. An antibody to lymphotyoxin and tumor necrosis factor prevents transfer of experimental allergic encephalomyelitis. J Exp Med 172:1193–11200, 1990.

181. Sakai K, Sinha AA, Mitchell DJ, Zamvil SS, Rothbard JB, McDevitt HO. Involvement of distinct murine T-cell receptors in the autoimmune encephalitogenic response to nested epitopes of myelin basic protein. Proc Natl Acad Sci USA 85:8608–8612, 1988.

182. Sakai K, Tabira T, Kunishita T. Recognition of alloantigens and induction of experimental allergic encephalomyelitis by a murine encephalitogenic T cell clone. Eur J Immunol 17:955–960, 1987.

183. Sakai K, Zamvil SS, Mitchell DJ, Lim M, Rothbard J, Steinman L. Characterization of a major T cell epitope in SJL/J mice with synthetic oligopeptides of myelin basic protein. J Neuroimmunol 19:21–32, 1988.

184. Salvetti M, Jung S, Chang S-F, Will H, Schalke BCG, Wekerle H. Acetylcholine receptor-specific T lymphocyte clones in the normal human immune repertoire: target epitopes, HLA restriction, and membrane phenotypes. Ann Neurol 29:508–516, 1991.

185. Schiffenbauer J, Johnson HM, Butfilowski EJ, Wegrzyn L, Soos, JM. Staphylococcal enterotoxins can reactivate experimental allergic encephalomyelitis. Proc Natl Acad Sci USA 90:8543–8546, 1993.

186. Schluesener H, Brunner C, Vass K, Lassmann H. Therapy of rat autoimmune disease by a monoclonal antibody specific for T lymphoblasts. J Immunol 137:3814–3920, 1986.

187. Schluesener HJ, Sobel RA, Linington C, Weiner HL. A monoclonal antibodfy against a myelin oligodendrocyte glycoprotein induces relapses and demyelination in central nervous system autoimmune disease. J Immunol 139:4016–4021, 1987.

188. Schluesener HJ, Wekerle H. Autoaggressive T lymphocyte lines recognizing the encephalitogenic region of myelin basic protein: in vitro selection from unprimed rat T lymphocyte populations. J Immunol 135:3128–3133, 1985.

189. Schmied M, Breitschopf H, Gold R, Zischler H, Rothe G, Wekerle H, Lassmann H.

Apoptosis of T lymphocytes—a mechanism to control inflammation in the brain. Am J Pathol 143:446–452, 1993.

190. Sedgwick J, Brostoff SW, Mason DW. Experimental allergic encephalomyelitis in the absence of a classical delayed-type hypersensitivity reaction. Severe paralytic disease correlates with the presence of interleukin-2 receptor-positive cells infiltrating the central nervous system. J Exp Med 165:1058–1075, 1987.

191. Sedgwick JD, Hughes CC, Male DK, MacPhee IAM, ter Meulen V. Antigen-specific damage to brain vascular endothelial cells mediated by encephalitogenic and non-encephalitogenic CD4$^+$ T cell lines in vitro. J Immunol 145:2474–2481, 1990.

192. Selmaj K, REaine CS, Cross AH. Anti-tumor necrosis factor therapy abrogates auto-immune demyelination. Ann Neurol 30:694–700, 1991.

193. Singh VK, Yamaki K, Donoso LA, Shinohara T. Molecular mimicry. Yeast histone H3-induced experimental autoimmune uveitis. J Immunol 142:1512–1516, 1989.

194. Smilek DE, Wraith DC, Hodgkinson S, Dwivedy S, Steinman L, McDevitt HO. A single amino acid change in a myelin basic protein peptide confers the capacity to prevent rather than induce experimental autoimmune encephalomyelitis. Proc Natl Acad Sci USA 88:9633–9637, 1991.

195. Smith ME, Somera FP, Eng LF. Immunocytochemical staining for glial fibrillary acidic protein and the metabolism of cytoskeletal proteins in experimental allergic encepha-lomyelitis. Brain Res 264:241–253, 1983.

196. Sobel RA, Kuchroo VK. The immunopathology of acute experimental allergic encepha-lomyelitis induced with myelin proteolipid protein. J Immunol 149:1444–1451, 1992.

197. Sobel RA, Tuohy VK, Lu Z, Laursen RA, Lees MB. Acute experimental allergic encepha-lomyelitis in SJL/J mice induced by a synthetic peptide of myelin proteolipid protein. J Neuropathol Exp Neurol 49:468–479, 1990.

198. Sommer N, Harcourt GC, Willcox N, Beeson D, Newsom-Davis J. Acetylcholine receptor-reactive T lymphocytes from healthy subjects and myasthenia gravis patients. Neurology 41:1270–1276, 1991.

199. Soos JM, Schiffenbauer J, Johnson HM. Treatment of PL/J mice with the superantigen, staphylococcal enterotoxin B, prevents development of experimental allergic encepha-lomyelitis. J Neuroimmunol 43:39–44, 1993.

200. Sriram S, Steinman L. Anti-I-A antibody suppresses active encephalomyelitis: Treatment model for diseases linked to Ir genes. J Exp Med 158:1362–1367, 1983.

201. Stalder T, Hahn S, Erb P. Fas antigen is the major target molecule for CD4$^+$ T cell-mediated cytotoxicity. J Immunol 152:1127–1133, 1994.

202. Stevens DB, Karpus WJ, Gould KE, Swanborg RH. Studies of Vβ8 T cell receptor peptide treatment in experimental autoimmune encephalomyelitis. J Neuroimmunol 37:123–129, 1992.

203. Stohl W, Gonatas NK. Detection of the precursor and effector cells of experimental allergic encephalomyelitis in the thoracic duct of the rat. Cell Immunol 43:471–477, 1980.

204. Su X-M, Sriram S. Analysis of TCR Vβ gene usage and encephalitogenicity of myelin basic protein peptide p91-103 reactive T cell clones in SJL mice: lack of evidence for V gene hypothesis. Cell Immunol 141:485–495, 1992.

205. Sun D. Synthetic peptides representing sequence 39 to 59 of rat Vβ8 TCR fail to elicit regulatory T cells reactive with Vβ8 TCR on rat encephalitogenic T cells. Cell Immunol 141:200–210, 1992.

206. Sun D, Ben-Nun A, Wekerle H. Regulatory circuits in autoimmunity: Recruitment of counterregulatory CD8$^+$ T cells by encephalitogenic CD4$^+$ T line cells. Eur J Immunol 18:1993–2000, 1988.

207. Sun D, Gold DP, Smith L, Brostoff S, Coleclough C. Characterization of rat encephalitogenic T cells bearing non-Vβ8 T cell receptors. Eur J Immunol 22:591–594, 1992.

208. Sun D, Qin Y, Chluba J, Epplen JT, Wekerle H. Suppression of experimentally induced autoimmune encephalomyelitis by cytolytic T–T-cell interactions. Nature 332:843–845, 1988.

209. Sun D, Wekerle H. Ia-restricted encephalitogenic T lymphocytes mediating EAE lyse autoantigen-presenting astrocytes. Nature 320:70–72, 1986.

210. Surh CD, Sprent J. Long-term xenogeneic chimeras. Full differentiation of rat T and B cells in SCID mice. J Immunol 147:2148–2154, 1991.

211. Swierkosz JE, Swanborg RH. Suppressor cell control of the unresponsiveness to experimental allergic encephalomyelitis. J Immunol 115:631–633, 1975.

212. Tokuchi F, Nishizawa M, Nihei J, Motoyama K, Nagashima K, Tabira T. Lymphokine production by encephalitogenic and non-encephalitogenic T cell clones reactive to the same antigenic determinant. J Neuroimmunol 30:71–79, 1990.

213. Torres-Nagel NE, Gold DP, Hünig T. Identification of rat Tcrb-V 8.2, 8.5, and 10 gene products by monoclonal antibodies. Immunogenetics 37:305–308, 1993.

214. Traugott U, Scheinberg LC, Raine CS. On the presence of Ia-positive endothelial cells and astrocytes in multiple sclerosis lesions and its relevance to antigen presentation. J Neuroimmunol 8:1–14, 1985.

215. Tsuchida M, Matsumoto Y, Hirahara H, Hanawa H, Tomiyama K, Abo T. Preferential distribution of Vβ8.2-positive T cells in the central nervous system of rats with myelin-basic protein induced autoimmune encephalomyelitis. Eur J Immunol 23:2399–2406, 1993.

216. Tuohy VK, Lu Z, Sobel RA, Laurson RA, Lees MB. A synthetic peptide from myelin proteolipid protein induces experimental allergic encephalomyelitis. J Immunol 141:1126–1130, 1988.

217. Tuohy VK, Sobel RA, Lu Z, Laursen RA, Lees MB. Myelin proteolipid protein: minimum sequence requirements for active induction of autoimmune encephalomyelitis in SWR/J and SJL/J mice. J Neuroimmunol 39:67–74, 1992.

218. Umehara F, Goto M, Qin Y, Wekerle H, Meyermann R. Experimental autoimmune encephalomyelitis (EAE) in the maturing central nervous system: transfer of myelin basic protein-specific T line lymphocytes to neonatal Lewis rats. Lab Invest 62:147–155, 1990.

219. Urban JL, Kumar V, Kono DH, Gomez C, Horvath SJ, Clayton J, Ando DG, Sercarz EE, Hood L. Restricted use of T cell receptor V genes in murine autoimmune encephalomyelitis raises possibilities for antibody therapy. Cell 54:577–592, 1988.

220. Vainiene M, Offner H, Morrison WJ, Wilkinson M, Vandenbark AA. Clonal diversity of basic protein specific T cells in Lewis rats recovered from experimental autoimmune encephalomyelitis. J Neuroimmunol 33:207–216, 1991.

221. Vandenbark AA, Hashim G, Offner H. Immunization with a synthetic T-cell receptor V-region peptide protects against experimental autoimmune encephalomyelitis. Nature 341:541–544, 1989.

222. Vandenbark AA, Offner H, Reshef T, Fritz RB, Chou C-HJ, Cohen IR. Specificity of T lymphocyte lines for peptides of myelin basic protein. J Immunol 139:229–233, 1985.

223. Van der Veen RC, Trotter JL, Clark HB, Kapp JA. The adoptive transfer of chronic relapsing experimental allergic encephalomyelitis with lymph node cells sensitized to myelin proteolipid protein. J Neuroimmunol 21:183–191, 1989.

224. Vass K, Lassmann H. Intrathecal application of interferon gamma: Progressive appearance of MHC antigens within the rat nervous system. Am J Pathol 137:789–800, 1990.

225. Waksman BH, Porter H, Lees MB, Adams RD, Folch J. A study of the chemical nature of

components of bovine white matter effective in producing allergic encephalomyelitis in the rabbit. J Exp Med 100:4451–471, 1954.

226. Waldor MK, Sriram S, Hardy R, Herzenberg LA, Lanier L, Lim M, Steinman L. Reversal of experimental allergic encephalomyelitis with a monoclonal antibody to a T cell subset marker (L3T4). Science 227:415–417, 1985.

227. Watanabe R, Wege H, ter Meulen V. Adoptive transfer of EAE-like lesions from rats with coronavirus-induced demyelinating encephalomyelitis. Nature 305:150–151, 1983.

228. Wauben, MHM, Boog CJP, Van der Zee R, Joosten I, Schlief A, Van Eden W. Disease inhibition by major histocompatibility complex peptide analogues of disease-associated epitopes: more than blocking alone. J Exp Med 176:667–677, 1992.

229. Wauben MHM, Kozhich A, Joosten I, Schlief A, Boog CJP, Van Eden W. Inhibition of entire myelin basic protein-induced experimental autoimmune encephalomyelitis in Lewis rats by major histocompatibility complex class II-binding competitor peptides. Eur J Immunol 24:1053–1060, 1994.

230. Wege H, Schliephake A, Körner H, Flory E, Wege HA. An immunodominant CD4+ T cell site on the nucleocapsid protein of murine coronavirus contributes to protection against encephalomyelitis. J Gen Virol 74:1287–1294, 1993.

231. Wegmann KW, Zhao W, Griffin AC, Hickey WF. Identification of myocarditogenic peptides derived from cardiac myosin capable of inducing experimental allergic myocarditis in the Lewis rat. The utility of a class II binding motif in selecting self-reactive peptides. J Immunol 153:892–900, 1994.

232. Wekerle H. In vitro induction of immunological memory against testicular autoantigen. Nature 267:357–358, 1977.

233. Wekerle H, Engelhardt B, Risau W, Meyermann R. Passage of lymphocytes across the blood-brain barrier in health and disease. In: Pathophysiology of the Blood-Brain Barrier, 1st ed, BB Johansson, C Owman, H Widner, eds. Elsevier, Amsterdam, 1990, pp 439–445.

234. Wekerle H, Fierz W. T lymphocyte autoimmunity in experimental autoimmune encephalomyelitis. Concepts Immunopathol 2:102–127, 1985.

235. Wekerle H, Pette M, Fujita K, Nomura K, Meyermann R. Autoimmunity in the nervous system: functional properties of an encephalitogenic protein. Prog Immunol 7:813–820, 1989.

236. Welch AM, Holda JH, Swanborg RH. Regulation of experimental allergic encephalomyelitis. II. Appearance of suppressor cells during remission phase of the disease. J Immunol 125:186–189, 1980.

237. Welch AM, Swanborg RH. Characterization of suppressor cells involved in regulation of experimental allergic encephalomyelitis. Eur J Immunol 6:910–912, 1976.

238. Whitacre CC, Gienapp IE, Orosz CG, Bitar DM. Oral tolerance in experimental autoimmune encephalomyelitis. III. Evidence for clonal anergy. J Immunol 147:2155–2163, 1991.

239. Whitham RH, Jones RE, Hashim GA, Hoy CM, Wang R-Y, Vandenbark AA, Offner H. Location of a new encephalitogenic epitope (residues 43 to 64) in proteolipid protein that induces relapsing experimental autoimmune encephalomyelitis in PL/J and (SJL × PL) F1 mice. J Immunol 147:3803–3808, 1991.

240. Willenborg DO, Sjollema P, Danta G. Immunoregulation of passively induced allergic encephalomyelitis. J Immunol 136:1676–1681, 1986.

241. Wraith DC, Smilek DE, Mitchell DJ, Steinman L, McDevitt HO. Antigen recognition in autoimmune encephalomyelitis and the potential for peptide-mediated immunotherapy. Cell 59:247–255, 1989.

242. Yamamura T, Namikawa T, Endoh M, Kunishita T, Tabira T. Passive transfer of experimental allergic encephalomyelitis induced by proteolipid apoprotein. J Neurol Sci 76:269–275, 1986.

243. Zaller DM, Osman G, Kanagawa O, Hood L. Prevention and treatment of murine experimental allergic encephalomyelitis with T cell receptor Vβ-specific antibodies. J Exp Med 171:1943–1955, 1990.

244. Zamvil SS, Mitchell DJ, Moore AC, Kitamura K, Steinman L, Rothbard JB. T-cell epitope of the autoantigen myelin basic protein that induces encephalomyelitis. Nature 324:258–260, 1986.

245. Zamvil SS, Mitchell DJ, Moore AC, Schwarz AJ, Stiefel W, Nelson PA, Rothbard JB, Steinman L. T cell reactivity for class II (I-A) and the encephalitogenic N-terminal epitope of the autoantigen myelin basic protein. J Immunol 139:1075–1079, 1987.

246. Zamvil SS, Mitchell DJ, Powell MB, Sakai K, Rothbard JB, Steinman L. Multiple discrete encephalitogenic epitopes of the autoantigen myelin basic protein include a determinant for I-E class II restricted T cells. J Exp Med 168:1181–1186, 1988.

247. Zhang X-M, Heber-Katz E. T cell receptor sequences from encephalitogenic T cells in adult Lewis rats suggest an early ontogenic origin. J Immunol 148:746–752, 1992.

248. Zhao W, Wegmann KW, Trotter JL, Ueno K, Hickey WF. Identification of an N-terminally acetylated encephalitogenic epitope in myelin proteolipid apoprotein for the Lewis rat. J Immunol 153:901–909, 1994.

13

Direct Cell-Mediated Responses in the Nervous System: CTL vs. NK Activity, and Their Dependence Upon MHC Expression and Modulation

WENDY S. ARMSTRONG
LOIS A. LAMPSON

The immune and inflammatory systems include a wealth of effector cells and mechanisms. Their normal roles in the nervous system, and the extent to which they can be exploited clinically, are still being defined. This chapter compares two forms of direct cell-mediated attack against infected or neoplastic cells: the antigen-specific attack mediated by cytotoxic T lymphocytes (CTL), and the broader recognition mediated by natural killer (NK) cells.

In the following sections, the CTL and NK responses are discussed separately and then compared. The role that products of the major histocompatibility complex (MHC) may play in each response, with emphasis on implications for neural tissue, is explored.

Turning from theoretical concerns to observations of function in vivo, we review evidence that each mechanism can act in the nervous system. A model system for probing the cell-mediated response to microscopic disease, such as disseminated tumor, is described. Finally, the question of whether cell-mediated effector mechanisms must be detrimental to postmitotic cells is addressed.

Placing the CTL and NK Responses Within the Immune/Inflammatory Network

The CTL and NK responses normally function as part of a complex interactive network. Pathological changes in the body (such as injury or infection) are recognized by two interlocking systems. The inflammatory response includes cell types, such as monocytes and neutrophils, with broad recognition for different classes of pathogens, such as bacteria or parasites. More specific recognition, for example, of a particular pathogen, is mediated by the immune response.

Classically, the immune response has been divided into antibody-mediated and cell-mediated arms. Antibody production and cell-mediated immunity are mediated by B and T lymphocytes, respectively. The CTL response is one of the major forms of T cell-mediated immunity. The NK response is the most recently identified component of the immune/inflammatory network (57,172). It combines properties of both cell-mediated immunity and more general inflammatory functions, as will be brought out in this chapter.

Normally, the immune and inflammatory responses are inseparable. The cells influence each others' migration patterns and effector mechanisms through direct contact and through secreted cytokines. Although lymphocytes can move through tissue independently of other inflammatory cells, they also enter as part of a normal inflammatory cascade. Although lymphocytes can recognize their targets specifically, the final effect on the target may be mediated by a nonspecific inflammatory cell. It is within this richly interactive network that the CTL and NK responses function in vivo, as described below.

The CTL Response

Relationship to Other Immune Effector Mechanisms

The immune response is characterized by its exquisite antigen specificity and memory. Antibody molecules, the humoral arm of the response, can bind to free antigen or cell-associated antigen. T lymphocytes, which mediate the cellular arm of the immune response, must recognize cell-associated antigen. Not only must the antigen be cell-associated, but it must be complexed to a protein coded in the major histocompatibility complex (MHC). This is what is meant by defining the antigen-specific T-cell response as *MHC-restricted.*

T cells, T cell-mediated effector functions, and MHC proteins may each be grouped into two broad classes (179). T cells have long been divided, on empirical grounds, according to their expression of the surface proteins CD4 or CD8. The classic division of the T-cell effector functions has been into direct cytotoxicity and helper functions. The division of the MHC proteins into the class I and class II families is based on their structure.

Two predominant groupings of the subdivisions of T cells, effector mechanisms and MHC proteins are well established, based on empirical findings. Direct cytotoxicity is most commonly mediated by CD8+, MHC class I–restricted cytotoxic T lymphocytes (Tc or CTL). Regulatory T-cell functions are most commonly mediated by CD4+ MHC class II–restricted helper-inducer T cells (Th), which secrete immunoactive cytokines.

Recent work provides fresh support for these traditional groupings (179). It is now appreciated that CD8 and MHC class I proteins bind to each other. Interactions between CD8 on the T cell and class I molecules on the target cell help to stabilize CTL–target binding. Similarly, CD4 and MHC class II proteins bind to each other and can help to stabilize the interaction between Th and the corresponding antigen-expressing cell.

It is now appreciated that antigen that is synthesized within a cell, such as virus or tumor antigen, is most likely to be presented complexed to a class I MHC protein. According to the classical scheme, recognition of the antigen by class I–restricted lytic CTL would result in elimination of the infected or neoplastic cell.

Cells that ingest antigen, such as phagocytes, are most likely to present the ingested antigen complexed to a class II MHC protein. Recognition of the antigen by class II–restricted cytokine-secreting Th leads to modulation of the immune response, rather than lysis of the antigen-presenting cell.

There are many exceptions to this general scheme. For example, CD8+ class I–restricted cells also secrete regulatory cytokines (as discussed below), and direct lysis can be mediated by CD4+ class II–restricted cells (155). Yet the scheme is still valuable as a statement of the best understood pathways and as a guide through the literature. The CTL response, including aspects of the Th response that help to initiate and regulate it, is described in more detail in the following sections; Th are discussed from other viewpoints elsewhere in this volume.

Specificity and Memory of CTL

The T-cell response, for both CTL and Th, is clonal. Each T cell displays a characteristic receptor (TcR), which is also displayed by subsequent daughter cells. A given antigen may be recognized by a number of different T cells, each bearing a different TcR.

While the TcR defines the specificity of a T-cell clone, other cell surface molecules contribute to the T cell–target interaction. T-cell membrane proteins known by the collective term *CD3* are required for signal transduction leading to T-cell activation. Together with the TcR, these form the *TcR–CD3 complex* (1). Still other cell surface molecules act to stabilize T cell–target adhesion. The T-cell membrane proteins CD8 and CD4, discussed above, are examples.

Following stimulation by antigen, the clones of responding T cells are expanded, contributing to a more efficient response at the next exposure (Fig. 13-1A). Both activated effector cells and memory cells are produced; the lineage relationships are still being defined. Qualitative differences between naive and activated or memory T-cell populations also contribute to the greater efficiency of a subsequent response (59,86). For example, activated T cells are more likely to leave the blood circulation and enter the tissues (86), including neural tissue (64,84).

A. CTL RESPONSE   B. NK RESPONSE

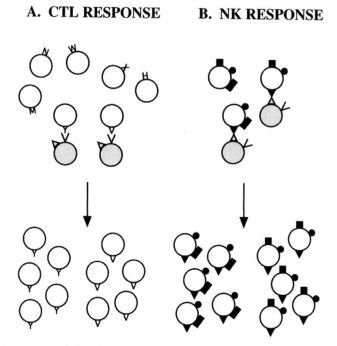

Fig. 13-1. Comparison of clonal expansion in the CTL and NK responses. A: CTL response. Above the arrow: each CTL (white circles) has a narrow specificity. In the illustration, two CTL have reacted to the antigenic determinant depicted as a *V* on the gray target cell. Below the arrow: the clonal expansion of the two responding CTL is depicted. As shown, each daughter cell displays the same narrow specificity as the original responding cell. B: NK response. Above the arrow: each NK effector (white circles) has a broad specificity. It is thought that a given cell may use more than one recognition structure, and different cells may express different combinations of structures. Three recognition structures are depicted as dark shapes on each NK effector, with different combinations shown on the different cells. In the illustration, two of the NK effectors recognize the gray target cell. Note that they do not recognize the antigenic determinant seen by the CTL (panel A), but a different structure. Below the arrow: following clonal expansion, the daughter cells still display broad reactivity patterns.

MHC Restriction of the CTL Response

T cells do not recognize foreign antigen alone. Rather, the foreign antigen must appear on a cell surface in the context of an appropriate product of the major histocompatibility complex. This requirement is referred to as *MHC restriction.* Formation of the peptide–MHC complex normally requires degradation of the foreign molecule, producing a fragment of the appropriate size to fit within the peptide-binding groove of the MHC protein.

Two major classes of MHC proteins can serve as restricting elements in the T-cell response. These are the class I MHC proteins, called *HLA-A, B, C* in humans and *H-2* in the mouse; and the class II MHC proteins, called *HLA-D* or *Ia* in humans and *Ia* in the mouse. Class I molecules, composed of a polymorphic heavy chain and an invariant light chain (b2-microglobulin), are of particular importance in presentation of internal antigen. Class II molecules, composed of two polymorphic chains, α and β, that are of similar size, are used most commonly in presentation of ingested antigen.

The MHC proteins are highly polymorphic. In humans, three different genes code for the variable heavy chain of the HLA-A, B, and C molecules, respectively. Within the population as a whole, there are multiple alleles at each locus. All three gene products are codominantly expressed. An individual may therefore express as many as six different class I alleles (if heterozygous at HLA-A, B, and C). Similar polymorphism is found among the class II molecules (HLA-DP, DQ, and DR in human), with the added complexity that both of the component chains are polymorphic.

The class I and class II families each have a characteristic structure for the peptide-binding groove. A particular MHC protein can accommodate many different peptides, although only one can fit in the groove at a time. A single peptide may fit the binding groove of more than one MHC protein, including both class I and class II proteins (179).

The chance that an individual will respond to a foreign antigen is enhanced by the possibility of forming multiple peptides from a single protein, by the expression of multiple MHC alleles within the individual, and by the likelihood of several possible MHC–peptide interactions for a given peptide (179). The chance that a foreign antigen will be recognized within the population as a whole is further enhanced by the extensive polymorphism of the MHC proteins (97).

Formation of the Antigen–MHC Complex

The antigen–MHC complex is formed intracellularly. The processing pathways have been analyzed most extensively for the production of MHC–peptide complexes. It is not clear to what extent other kinds of molecules might be able to be presented in the peptide-binding groove.

Peptide–MHC complexes may be formed by two pathways (Fig. 13-2). The *cytosolic pathway* is the predominant one for molecules that are synthesized within the cell. It usually involves complexing to class I MHC molecules. Nascent proteins within the cytosol (for example, following synthesis on free ribosomes) are degraded into fragments of the appropriate size, approximately nine amino acids (30,40), which are then transported into the endoplasmic reticulum (ER). Complexing to MHC proteins, usually class I, occurs in the ER. The binding of the antigen fragment is thought to stabilize the two-chain class I molecule (29) (Fig. 13-2A). Although it is not the dominant pathway, MHC class II molecules can also complex with antigen through the cytosolic pathway (109).

The *endosomal pathway* is the predominant one for ingested protein. Antigen may be ingested by cells with phagocytic capabilities either nonspecifically or specifically. Specific uptake, which is more efficient, occurs when an antigen has been coated (opsonized) by specific antibodies or by complement fragment C3b. A phagocyte may

ANTIGEN PRESENTATION TO T CELLS

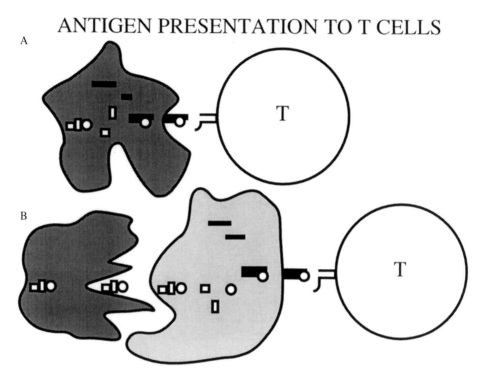

Fig. 13-2. Pathways for MHC-restricted expression of internal antigen. The figure illustrates two mechanisms by which internal proteins can serve as T-cell target antigens. A: In the *direct* or *cytosolic* pathway, a fragment of an intracellular protein is complexed to the MHC protein within the target cell itself. The protein and its fragments are shown as white shapes within the dark antigen-synthesizing cell. The antigen–MHC complex is then displayed at the cell surface, where it can be recognized by a responding T cell. A class I MHC protein is the usual restricting element. The two chains of the class I molecule are shown as black rectangles. B: In the *indirect* or *endosomal* pathway, the target cell, or its products, are ingested by a phagocyte. The antigenic fragments are complexed to MHC proteins within the phagocyte, which then presents the antigen to a responding T cell. A class II MHC protein is the usual restricting element. In the figure, antigen is released by the dark antigen-synthesizing cell, then picked up and degraded by the light gray phagocyte. An antigenic fragment is complexed to the two-chain class II MHC protein, depicted by black rectangles. The antigen–MHC complex is then displayed at the surface of the phagocyte.

then recognize the opsonized antigen by its own receptors for complement or immunoglobulin (1). Regardless of the method of uptake, the antigen enters the cell in endocytotic vesicles. It is processed by cellular proteases in intracellular vesicles which then merge with vesicles containing nascent MHC proteins. The resultant antigen–MHC complex is then transported to and displayed at the cell surface (117,179). MHC class II proteins are the usual restriction element for external antigen (Fig. 13-2B). Yet, class I molecules can also serve as restricting elements (130).

Discrimination between self and foreign peptide. Peptides derived from native and foreign molecules alike can be complexed to MHC proteins (6,17). Although self-proteins are presumably far more abundant in a normal cell, this balance may change in pathological conditions, such as following transformation or viral infection, where the cell actively synthesizes foreign antigen. Other factors, besides relative abundance, that may favor formation of complexes between MHC proteins and foreign peptides rather than self-peptides are still being defined.

When self peptides are complexed to MHC proteins, this need not lead to autoimmune reactivity. The specificity of the response is controlled by the specificity of the TcR on the responding T-cell clones (Fig. 13-1A). Autoreactive clones may be eliminated or inactivated by more than one mechanism, during development or later, either in the thymus or in the peripheral tissues (15,37). Autoimmunity represents a failure or reversal of these mechanisms.

Examples: T-cell recognition of viral or tumor antigen. Viral or tumor antigen can potentially be recognized by MHC-restricted T cells in two ways. The antigen may be presented as an antigen–MHC complex on the surface of the cell in which the antigen was synthesized. This would be the normal mechanism for recognition of the infected or neoplastic *target cell* by activated CTL, usually employing a class I MHC molecule as the restriction element (Fig. 13-2A).

Viral or tumor antigen may also be presented as an antigen–MHC complex on the surface of a secondary cell. For example, this may occur following phagocytosis of the cell in which the antigen was first synthesized or of its released or secreted products (Fig. 13-2B). A class II MHC protein is the usual restricting element in this case. This pathway is particularly important when the secondary cell can serve as an *antigen-presenting cell (APC),* presenting its antigen to MHC-restricted helper/inducer T cells.

Th are important in initiating or amplifying a CTL response, as discussed below. Th also have effector functions in their own right. Th recognition of antigen–MHC on the secondary cell may lead to damage of adjacent cells, once an immune–inflammatory cascade has been initiated. Damage to cells that are adjacent to an antigen-bearing cell, referred to as a *bystander* effect, is the underlying mechanism of the delayed-type hypersensitivity (DTH) response. Defining the relative contributions, or therapeutic potential, of direct CTL and indirect Th attack against infected, neoplastic, or transplanted neural cells is an area of current interest (61,63, discussed below).

Summary. The cytosolic pathway is the primary pathway for presentation of endogenous peptides, such as viral gene products or tumor antigens, usually in the context of class I MHC proteins. This is the main pathway by which target cells present their antigen to CTL.

The endosomal pathway is the major pathway for presentation of ingested antigen, usually in the context of class II MHC proteins. Viral or tumor antigen may be presented through this pathway if the infected or neoplastic cell, or its products, have been ingested by other cells. This is the main pathway for stimulation of Th, which play a key role in initiation of the CTL response (Fig. 13-3).

CELLS THAT MAY PARTICIPATE IN INITIATING THE CTL RESPONSE

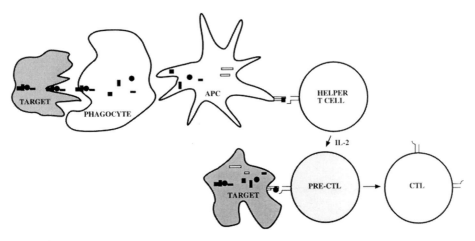

Fig. 13-3. Complexity of cell interactions in the initiation of the CTL response. The figure illustrates the number of different cell types that may participate in initiating a CTL response. Top line: a phagocyte has ingested and broken down the target cell antigen (shown as black shapes). Antigenic fragments, released by the phagocyte, are taken up by a dendritic cell, which is a more efficient antigen-presenting cell (APC) than the phagocyte. The antigen is complexed with an MHC protein, usually class II MHC, within the APC. The two chains of the class II molecule are shown as open rectangles. The antigen–MHC complex is then presented on the surface of the APC to a helper T cell (Th). This activates the helper T cell, causing it to secrete CTL-activating cytokines such as IL-2. Although not depicted here, phagocytes can also present antigen directly, as shown in Fig. 13-2. Bottom line: A pre-CTL has recognized an antigen–MHC complex, usually involving class I MHC, on the surface of the target cell. The two chains of the class I molecule are shown as open rectangles within the target. The combined signals provided by antigen recognition and helper-secreted cytokine cause the pre-CTL to differentiate into a fully mature CTL. The mature CTL then circulates through the tissues, where it can attack other target cells bearing the appropriate antigen–MHC complex.

Implications: CTL Target Antigens Need Not Be Cell Surface Proteins

In the past, it was assumed that only cell surface molecules could be recognized by CTL. This assumption was first challenged by experimental evidence that internal viral antigens can be targets of CTL attack (157). The emerging picture of antigen–MHC complexing, stimulated by the early studies of viral antigens, now provides a conceptual basis for the original findings. Once it is appreciated that the complex between antigen and MHC protein forms inside the cell, it is easier to understand how any protein that is synthesized or ingested by the cell may have the potential to serve as a T-cell target antigen (Fig. 13-2). Internal components of tumor cells, infected cells, or transplanted cells are all potential targets of CTL attack (70,71,157).

T-cell Recognition in Graft Rejection: A Special Case

MHC-incompatible grafts provide a special case where the MHC molecule itself is foreign. The structural basis for the recognition of MHC differences in an *allograft* (a graft between two individuals of the same species) or a *xenograft* (a graft between two different species) is now being reevaluated in light of new understanding of the role and formation of the MHC–antigen complex (15,39,92,102,162). For both allografts and xenografts, the MHC proteins are just one potential target for graft rejection. Any foreign molecule present in the graft or produced by the grafted cell is a potential antigen (71,162).

There are many possible sources of restricting molecules in the complex setting of a tissue graft. In grafts within the same species, the graft and donor may share one or more MHC haplotypes. In that case, a grafted cell may present its own antigen to a host T cell, and so be susceptible to direct CTL attack.

Even where graft and donor do not share MHC haplotypes, or come from different species, restricting MHC molecules may still be provided by host cells which have ingested the antigen. In this case, donor cells could be damaged through a Th-mediated or bystander response (63).

There has been increasing interest in grafting genetically modified cells into the nervous system. It is important to appreciate that any product of the modified cells that is foreign to the host, even an internal molecule, is a potential target of graft rejection (70,71,157).

Other Aspects of the CTL Response

Factors Determining Target Susceptibility to CTL Attack

The ability to express MHC molecules at the surface is a necessary requirement for a cell to be a CTL target, but it is not the only requirement. The capacity to form antigen–MHC complexes, the expression of appropriate accessory and adhesion molecules, and susceptibility to the CTL lytic mechanism also determine a cell's susceptibility to CTL attack. A cell that lacked any of these elements would be protected from CTL-mediated cytotoxicity, even if it expressed a viral, tumor-associated, or other foreign antigen (60).

Experimental examples of CTL-resistant cells have been described. These include cultured CNS neurons and neuroblastoma and glioma cell lines (50,51,54,88,89,171). The different experimental systems illustrate the different potential sites of regulation. Down-regulation of MHC class I synthesis, defects in peptide processing or antigen–MHC complex formation, lack of accessory adhesion molecules, and resistance to a major T-cell lytic mechanism are among the factors that may contribute to a cells' resistance to CTL attack (28,33,50,51,54,88,89,171,179). The extent to which normal, infected, or neoplastic neural cells might be resistant to CTL attack in vivo is a question of current interest. A more subtle expression of this resistance is suggested by evidence that CTL may be able to affect their targets without lysing them (112), as discussed below.

Cell–Cell Interactions in Initiation of the CTL Response

Although the final effector of the CTL response is the cytotoxic T lymphocyte, other cells participate in the initiation of the response (Fig. 13-3). In the course of differentiating into a fully functional CTL, the CTL precursor *(pre-CTL* or *naive CTL)* normally makes its first contact with antigen in the presence of an activated helper-inducer T cell, Th. The activated Th secretes cytokines that contribute to the activation of the CTL (1) (Fig. 13-3, bottom line).

The Th is itself activated by recognition of an antigen–MHC complex on the surface of an antigen-presenting cell (APC) (Fig. 13-3, top line). Two properties define the APC. Like the target cells described above, an APC presents antigen to T cells in an MHC-restricted fashion. Usually, class II MHC proteins are the restricting element. The second defining property is the ability of the APC to deliver a stimulating signal to the bound Th. Delivery of the Th activating signal is referred to as *costimulation* or *signal two,* presentation of the antigen to the Th being *signal one.* It is thought that if a Th receives only signal one, it is made tolerant or anergic to the antigen, instead of undergoing activation (169).

Activated Th in turn secrete cytokines that activate adjacent pre-CTL which have recognized antigen–MHC on an antigen-bearing cell (Fig. 13-3, bottom line). Direct recognition between the Th and pre-CTL is not required. Rather, it is the physical proximity of the cells that allows the Th-secreted cytokines to stimulate the pre-CTL (Fig. 13-3).

Some APC have a relatively limited potential to process antigen but can ingest antigen that has been previously digested by other cells. The reciprocal properties of macrophages and dendritic cells provide an example of the interplay that is possible. Of the two cell types, macrophages process antigen efficiently but are relatively inefficient as antigen-presenting cells. Dendritic cells, while relatively inefficient in antigen processing, are particularly efficient antigen-presenting cells (38) (Fig. 13-3).

Site of initial CTL stimulation in vivo. The greatest probability for juxtaposition of the different cell types that may participate in initiating a CTL response is in organized lymphoid tissue. It has often been suggested that lack of a conventional lymphatic drainage in the brain prevents CNS antigen from gaining access to organized lymphoid tissue. Yet potential routes of antigen egress from the brain are increasingly appreciated (20; see Chapter 4). One route involves antigen movement from the interstitial fluid to the CSF, and ultimate egress from the brain with the bulk flow of the CSF (20). Antigen may also be carried from the brain following ingestion by phagocytes. This potential route of egress is suggested by the accumulation of antigen-laden phagocytes in the perivascular spaces of degenerating white matter (69).

Thus, antigen is able to leave the brain by more than one route, enabling initiation of a CTL response in organized lymphoid tissue. Once stimulated, the circulating CTL are able to respond to MHC–antigen expressed by targets within the CNS, without participation of other cell types (59).

Summary: potential complexity of the CTL response. Initiating a CTL response may involve the participation of five different cell types (Fig. 13-3):

1. The antigen-processing cell (for example, a macrophage).
2. The antigen+/MHC+ antigen-presenting cell (APC), which may or may not be the same as the antigen-processing cell (for example, a macrophage or a dendritic cell).
3. The antigen-specific, MHC-restricted, cytokine-secreting helper-inducer T cell (Th).
4. The antigen-specific, MHC-restricted, naive cytotoxic T cell (naive or pre-CTL).
5. The antigen+/MHC+ target cell.

More complex schemes are also possible. The important point here is that, once appropriately stimulated, the effector CTL can respond directly to antigen–MHC on the target cell (59).

Each of the participating cells may play other regulatory and effector roles in the immune/inflammatory cascade, over and above the function in the MHC-restricted CTL response stressed here (61,63a). The special property of the activated CTL is that it is able to move through the body and mediate a direct, specific attack against antigen+/MHC+ target cells at distant sites (63a,64).

CTL Migration into the Brain and Other Tissues

An important consequence of T-cell activation, for both CTL and Th, is the establishment of long-lived, recirculating populations that move between the lymphoid and peripheral tissues. The brain, like other tissues, is surveyed as part of the normal recirculation pathways (64,84,86).

The blood-brain barrier does not prevent CTL from entering the CNS. It was originally thought that the blood-brain barrier prevented T-cell migration into the CNS. It is now appreciated that T-cell migration is active, not passive, and so is not impeded by the endothelial tight junctions that constitute the blood-brain barrier as classically defined (60,62,126). Rather, T cells leave CNS vessels, like other vessels, if appropriate molecular signals are presented at the site.

Activated and naive T cells have different migratory characteristics, and the activated cells are more likely to enter the nonlymphoid tissues, including the brain (64,84,86). T-cell movement can also be influenced by activating endothelial cells, for example, by injection of proinflammatory cytokines (64,139).

Thus, T-cell entry into the brain, just as in the rest of the body, is under regulatory control and can be influenced by the same cytokines that are active elsewhere. The extent to which selective signals may influence the entry of particular leukocyte sub-populations into the brain, or entry into the brain as opposed to other tissues, are areas of current interest (62,64).

The CTL Response: Summary

In the CTL response, the effectors directly attack antigen-bearing target cells. The response is antigen-specific, MHC restricted, and clonal. It displays immune memory. Although the final effector is the CTL, other cell types participate in initiating the response. Once stimulated, CTL recirculate and can enter nonlymphoid organs, including the brain. NK activity, described below, differs from the CTL response in many of these aspects.

NK Activity

Natural killer (NK) activity is characterized by its broad specificity and the speed with which it is initiated. Like CTL, NK cells are able to kill infected and neoplastic cells. Yet they display neither the fine antigen specificity nor the memory of the CTL response.

The defining properties of the NK response are that the effector cells are able to kill their targets without prior exposure to the target, MHC restriction, or participation of other cell types. The fact that prior exposure to the target is not needed is reflected in the designation *natural* killer activity. It is this property that permits the rapid response that is the hallmark of NK activity.

NK activity is assumed to be of particular importance during the first exposure to a cell-associated foreign antigen, before T cells specific for that antigen have been activated. Peak NK activity in vivo may be reached several days earlier than the peak of the primary CTL response (158). NK activity is also of potential importance where MHC-restricted CTL may not function efficiently. This is of interest in the nervous system and other tissues where MHC molecules are not detected on many of the parenchymal cells or their derivative tumors (60,61,63a,139,170). NK activity is of special interest in AIDS, where it may be affected later than Th-dependent CTL initiation, or other Th-dependent responses.

Heterogeneity of NK Activity

"NK activity" encompasses several effector mechanisms (158). NK cells may kill their targets directly. This may involve insertion of pore-forming proteins (perforins) into the target membrane. Cytokines, either secreted by NK cells or by adjacent cells, may alter the anti-target activity of the NK cells or affect the NK susceptibility of the target. The most active cytokines include γ-interferon (IFN-γ), which is produced by both activated NK cells and activated T cells; IFN-α, often produced by adjacent cells rather than the NK effector itself; and interleukin (IL)-2, secreted by activated T cells (158).

NK effectors can also mediate antibody-dependent cell-mediated cytotoxicity (ADCC) (57,158,172). Antibody molecules can bind through their constant *(Fc)* domains to Fc receptors on an NK effector. After an antibody has bound to a target cell surface antigen, recognition by an NK Fc receptor can focus NK attack against the target cell. Preexisting "natural antibodies" can serve to focus an NK attack. Where new antibody must be produced, this effector mechanism would not be as rapid as the others described.

None of these effector mechanisms is unique to NK cells. For example, CTL can affect their targets via perforin-mediated lysis or cytokine action, and monocytes can mediate ADCC. It is the MHC-unrestricted broad recognition and the sensitization-independent, accessory cell–independent rapidity of the response that characterize NK activity, rather than a specific effector mechanism.

The Changing Definition of "NK Cell"

Until recently, *NK activity* defined a function rather than a cell type (128). Large granular lymphocytes (LGLs), monocytes, natural cytotoxic (NC) cells, and even T cells can all display MHC-independent, sensitization-independent cytotoxic activity against infected or neoplastic cells. More recently, the term *NK cell* has been restricted to a defined population of LGL (158). Even among these, subpopulations with different characteristic profiles of cell surface antigens can mediate NK activity (158). As the terminology changes, it is important to stress that many different cells are capable of "natural" cytotoxic activity that is not MHC restricted.

In the experiments discussed below, *NK activity* refers to the MHC-unrestricted cytotoxicity displayed by the populations used in the individual studies, often peripheral blood lymphocytes (PBL). The LGL population denoted by the more restricted use of the term *NK cell* is a major population, but not the only population, contributing to the NK activity of normal PBL (158).

Specificity and Memory of the NK Response

NK–target recognition is thought to be qualitatively different from the recognition between a TcR and its corresponding peptide–MHC complex. The current model is that a small number of structures can serve as targets for NK recognition (Fig. 13-1B). A particular target cell may display one or more of these. A source of complexity is that there are many NK effector subpopulations, and each may recognize a different set of target structures. Ljunggren and Kärre (80) refer to this as a "multiple choice" model of NK activity, stressing the heterogeneity of NK effector populations and the potential heterogeneity of mechanisms used by a single effector population. Many examples of this heterogeneity, at multiple levels of the NK/target interaction, are found in the comprehensive review by Trinchieri (158). Even taking this complexity into account, the number of NK recognition structures is thought to be smaller, by several orders of magnitude, than the number of different TcR that can identify different conventional antigens (158) (Fig. 13-1).

Like CTL, NK cells may proliferate after recognizing their targets. Yet the effects on the specificity repertoires of the resulting daughter cells are thought to be very different in the two responses. Each expanded CTL clone retains the same fine specificity as the original responding cell (Fig. 13-1A). In contrast, the NK daughter cells are thought to retain the broad reaction potential that defines NK activity (Fig. 13-1B) (158).

Increased production of NK cells from bone marrow precursors also contributes to the expanded NK population following NK activation in vivo (158). This population would presumably include NK cells with a range of receptor combinations (Fig. 13-1B, top). The lack of clonal expansion (in the sense it is displayed by T cells), coupled with the short life of NK cells (158), explains why the NK response does not display the memory of the CTL response.

Like CTL, NK cells may change their phenotype and become more efficient effectors following interaction with their target cells (56,173). Yet the nature of their recognition and the cells' short life-span still mean that there will be a lack of memory upon second exposure to the same antigen.

How the NK Response May Be Targeted to Specific Cells

It is important to appreciate how much target specificity can be achieved by broadly reactive effector mechanisms. Several mechanisms may help to focus an NK response.

Concentration of NK activity at a particular site occurs once the immune–inflammatory cascade has been initiated. This may occur as part of a specific immune response or in response to a more nonspecific event, such as trauma. Accumulation of NK effectors, including monocytes and other potential effectors, is part of the normal inflammatory sequence.

A more specific focusing can also occur. For example, although NK effectors may not discriminate between cells infected with related viruses, they can discriminate between infected and uninfected cells (158). This level of discrimination would contribute to selective target damage, once NK effectors have accumulated at a given site. NK effectors may also be directed to specific individual targets by means of the ADCC (antibody-dependent) effector mechanism.

The focusing of broadly reactive effector mechanisms is of special interest as one attempts to understand how immune or inflammatory mechanisms could contribute to or exacerbate what was initially a nonimmunologic insult. Cases where immune exacerbation is thought to contribute to the clinical course include trauma-induced paralysis, stroke, and perhaps Alzheimer's or Parkinson's disease.

An example of the possible interplay between specific and nonspecific factors is suggested by studies of the neurodegenerative disease, amyotrophic lateral sclerosis (ALS). ALS is characterized by selective loss of motor neurons in the brain and spinal cord. The etiology is not understood. Analysis of immune parameters in affected spinal cord suggests one scenario by which, following an initial nonimmunologic insult, the immune–inflammatory cascade might contribute to the characteristic pattern of selective damage (69). A similar argument has been made for the focusing of NK activity against selected peripheral neurons (41).

Molecular Bases of NK Recognition

It is thought that NK cells recognize broad classes of targets. For example, whereas CTL can discriminate between cells infected with closely related viruses, NK cells are though to discriminate between infected and noninfected cells in a more general way.

The molecular bases of NK recognition are still being defined, and several candidate structures are being investigated (52,132). It appears that a variety of recognition pathways are possible, with different NK subpopulations expressing different receptor subsets (52) (Fig. 13-1B, top). Not only cell surface interactions between the NK cell and its target but also target susceptibility to the various NK effector mechanisms are important in determining the specificity patterns (158).

Many aspects of NK/target recognition and signal transduction are shared with CTL or other cells, just as the ultimate effector mechanisms are shared. For example, CD2, an adhesion molecule that can mediate polyclonal T-cell activation, and CD16, the low-affinity Fc receptor for immunoglobulin, can both mediate NK activation (4,52, 158,167). Although NK cells do not express the complete TcR–CD3 receptor complex, they can express the zeta chain subunit, which has been implicated in signal transduction via CD2 or CD16 (4,52,167).

The Paradoxical Role of the MHC in NK Recognition

NK activity is not MHC restricted, and cells without detectable MHC expression can be targets of NK attack. For some target cells, MHC expression on the target is not only unnecessary, it appears to inhibit the NK response. It is hypothesized that, for certain NK–target combinations, NK activity is triggered when the NK cells recognizes "lack of self-MHC" on the target. This idea, of special interest because of the low baseline MHC expression in neural tissue, is discussed more fully below, after other aspects of NK biology are considered.

Other Aspects of the NK Response

The migratory characteristics of the different NK effectors and precursors, and their potential control by immunoactive cytokines, are just now being defined. It has been suggested that NK activity against tumor may be most active against blood-borne metastatic cells, rather than tumor growing within the tissues (158,160).

Although NK activity does not require the participation of additional cell types, both the effectors and their targets are susceptible to regulation by cytokines. Within the brain, potential sources of regulatory cytokines include endogenous cells, inflammatory cells, and, in pathological tissue, damaged, infected, neoplastic, or transplanted cells (67,161).

When NK cells are cultured in vitro with IL-2 or other activating regimens, the resultant populations may display more efficient cytotoxic activity. These populations include lymphokine-activated killer (LAK) cells, adherent LAK (A-LAK) cells, and other related cells (172,173). The different LAK variants have displayed anti-tumor activity outside the brain when injected in large doses. Their efficacy against CNS tumors has been controversial. The entry and movement of the cells in the brain, as well as their efficacy against tumor within the brain parenchyma, are points of current interest (48,61,98,139,170,173).

NK Activity in Graft Rejection

Many different interactions are possible between NK cells and cells of a different MHC phenotype. NK cells are not MHC restricted. They can attack infected or neoplastic targets with nonidentical MHC phenotypes, or with no detectable MHC expression.

Although NK activity is not MHC restricted, NK cells do respond to MHC differences. NK cells can reject allografts of lymphoid or hematopoietic cells. Indeed, the need to explain NK-mediated rejection of bone marrow grafts ("hybrid resistance") underlies the initial proposal that NK cells recognize lack of self MHC, as discussed below.

Recent work raises questions about the relationship between NK recognition of bone marrow allografts and other forms of NK–target interaction. A set of polymorphic cell surface molecules (the hematopoietic histocompatibility [Hh] molecules), different from the MHC proteins, has been defined that can serve as targets for NK recognition of bone marrow allografts in the mouse (13,105,138). The interplay between this recognition system and those mediating NK recognition of tumor or infected cells, and the ways that NK cells might recognize grafts of other cell types, are still being defined. The question is tied to questions about the significance and mechanism of lack of self-MHC as a recognition signal. It remains possible that allo-MHC is simply seen as lack of self-MHC for some NK–target combinations (111).

Questions about the relationship between NK recognition of bone marrow allografts and other kinds of targets have a practical implication. Many studies of human NK activity involve effectors and target cells from different individuals. Interpretation of these studies is complicated by incomplete understanding of the basis for NK-mediated allorecognition, particularly for lymphoid or hematopoietic targets.

Synthesis: Comparison Between the CTL and NK Responses

The NK response is marked by its relative simplicity compared to the CTL response. It is not MHC restricted and does not require prior exposure to the target cell. Although NK cells are regulated by cytokines, cytokine secretion by other cells is not required to initiate the response.

The simplicity of the NK response permits rapid response to a new viral infection or tumor during the days before a full CTL response can develop. In addition, the lack of MHC restriction provides a potential mechanism for surveillance of cells that do not express MHC proteins, do not efficiently form antigen–MHC complexes, or for some other reason are not susceptible to MHC-restricted CTL attack.

Some of the same properties that underlie the efficiency of the NK response also underlie its differences from the CTL response in terms of target specificity and memory. NK cells are thought to recognize broad classes of targets, as opposed to the exquisite specificity of the CTL response. Short-lived, broadly reactive NK cells do not display the immunologic memory of CTL.

Although the requirements for initiation are different, the effector mechanisms used by NK and CTL overlap. NK and CTL effectors can both lyse their targets directly and can both influence their targets, directly or indirectly, by secreting immunoactive cytokines. This means that the complementarity of the two mechanisms is not complete. For example, tumor resistance to perforin-mediated lysis (25,54) would affect both NK and CTL susceptibility.

Similarities between stimulated CTL and NK effectors are of interest in AIDS. Although Th are important in the initiation of the CTL response, activated CTL are able to attack their targets without further participation of Th (see above). Where Th function is preferentially lost, NK and memory CTL activity, and their possible clinical enhancement, are of special interest.

The complementary properties of the CTL and NK responses do provide a fuller range of surveillance than either alone. For example, where reduced MHC expression protects infected or transformed cells from CTL attack, NK activity may spontaneously eliminate the target, or may be manipulated to do so.

Where NK cells recognize lack of self-MHC, CTL and NK activity may be not only complementary but mutually exclusive. This possibility, and its relevance to neural tissue, are discussed below.

The Paradoxical Role of the MHC in NK Recognition

An aspect of NK recognition that has received great attention is the possibility that target MHC expression may be inversely related to NK susceptibility. The experimental evidence for this idea, its possible structural basis, and its applicability to neural targets, are reviewed here.

Background

In the late 1950s investigators began describing the puzzling observation that F1 hybrids reject parental bone marrow grafts, an effect that became known as *hybrid resistance* (13). One theory that arose from this observation was the *missing self* hypothesis. This suggests that F1 rejection of parental targets may result from the parental cells' lack of a "self" determinant, namely the other parent's MHC haplotype. A variety of experiments revealed that the rejection in hybrid resistance could be mediated by NK cells (13,80).

As described above, recognition of an alternative set of polymorphic proteins (the Hh molecules), different from the classic MHC molecules, may underlie the phenomenon of hybrid resistance (13,105,138). Yet recognition of lack of self-MHC has retained its interest as an explanation for NK recognition in other contexts. The question has almost always been posed in terms of class I molecules.

The molecular mechanisms by which lack of self-MHC could trigger NK recognition are not yet understood. Recognition of lack of self-MHC is not implicated for all target cell types. Even among lymphoid and hematopoietic targets, the most consistent evidence for MHC–NK reciprocity is found with B-cell lines (Table 13-1). The relationship between the roles of Hh-1 and of recognition of lack of self-MHC in lymphoid targets must still be defined. Current knowledge about lack of self-MHC recognition, with emphasis on points of relevance to neural tissue, is reviewed below.

How Might NK Effectors Recognize "Lack of Self-MHC"?

Ljunggren and Kärre (80) have reviewed two general mechanisms through which MHC molecules could affect NK susceptibility. In the *target interference* model, the MHC molecule physically hinders an interaction between the NK cell and its receptor on the target cell. In the *effector inhibition* model, recognition of the MHC molecule causes an inhibitory signal to be delivered to the NK effector. Effector inhibition is most consistent with cases where regulation of NK susceptibility occurs after, or is independent of, NK binding (53,81). Where regulation occurs at the NK–target binding step (110,151), either effector inhibition or target interference can be envisioned. The underlying assumption of both models is that NK cells will attack potential targets, unless the attack is inhibited by self-MHC expression on the target cell.

Recent work implicates the peptide-binding groove of the MHC molecule in the interaction between a class I+ target and an NK cell (33,53,152). For example, Storkus and colleagues have proposed a physical association between MHC molecules and NK target structures (NKTS), one that involves residues in the peptide-binding groove (152). According to the model, NKTS that are bound to MHC proteins are no longer free to bind to NK cells. Reducing the number of free MHC molecules or filling their binding grooves with peptide would increase the number of free NKTS. This in turn would increase NK–target binding.

Experimental work implicating the peptide binding groove in NK–target recognition is illustrated by the studies by Storkus et al. of a human B-cell line, into which they is illustrated by the studies by Storkus et al. of a human B-cell line, into which they introduced different human class I MHC haplotypes by transfection (152). Several different haplotypes reduced the cells' susceptibility to NK lysis. The protective effect was mapped to the a1/a2 domains of the HLA heavy chain, which form the peptide-binding groove. One haplotype, HLA-A2, failed to confer protection. HLA-A2 could be made protective by altering one amino acid to a residue that was common to many of the protective haplotypes, opening a previously blocked side-pocket of the antigen-binding cleft (152).

The potential importance of peptide is also stressed by Chadwick and Miller, who suggest NK susceptibility may be changed by changing the repertoire of peptides in the MHC binding groove (16). The importance of peptide is again suggested by Franksson et al., who have studied targets with a defect in the peptide transporter gene, resulting in defective ability to form peptide–MHC complexes (33).

These models are still under active investigation. The important point here is that they do offer examples at the structural level of possible relationships between NK cells and target class I molecules. With reference to the two general mechanisms discussed above, most of the structural work could be compatible with either target interference or target inhibition.

Implications of Lack of Self-MHC as a Potential Basis for NK Recognition

Reduced MHC expression is seen in certain viral infections and in some tumors, and non-self MHC may be expressed by transplants. Where lack of self-MHC can be a basis for NK recognition, this could contribute to NK susceptibility of the infected, neoplastic, or transplanted cells.

The role of lack of self-MHC as a basis for NK recognition in vivo must still be defined. One model is based on the traditional assumption that MHC class I expression is "ubiquitous." According to this model, all normal nucleated cells express MHC class I proteins, and so are protected from NK attack. Viral infection or neoplastic changes that reduce or alter class I expression would concomitantly increase NK susceptibility.

Appreciation of the heterogeneity of MHC distribution in vivo (37,63) suggests that a more complex model is needed, that relative MHC levels cannot be the only factor. In

Table 13-1 Evidence For and Against Inverse Correlation Between MHC Class I Expression and Susceptibility to NK-Mediated Lysis[a]

Reference	Cell Type[b]	Method of MHC Modulation[c]	Effector Cell Type	Inverse Correlation Seen?
Targets of hematopoietic origin				
Sugawara et al. (154)	B-cell lymphoma (EBV)	Acid treatment (d)	NK[d]	Yes
Quillet et al. (123)	**Burkitt's lymphoma** (DAUDI)	**Gene transfection**	NK[d] / LAK[i]	**Yes** / **Yes**
Öhlén et al. (110)	B-lymphoblastoid line (EBV)	Deletion mutants (d)	NK[d] / LAK[i]	Yes / Yes
Storkus et al. (151)	**B-lymphoblastoid line** (EBV)	**Gene transfection**	NK[d] / LAK[i]	**Yes** / No
Migita et al. (100)	Erythroleukemia (K562); T-cell leukemia (MOLT-3, -4)	Phorbol esters +/− cytokine	NK[d]; LAK[i] / NK[d]; LAK[i]	Yes / Yes
Reiter et al. (127)	Erythroleukemia (K563)	Cytokine / Vesicle fusion	NK[h] / NK[h]	Yes / No
Leiden et al. (75)	Erytholeukemia (K562); T-cell leukemia (MOLT-4)	Cytokine (K562 only) / **Gene transfection**	NK[d] and NK cell line / NK[d] and NK cell line	Yes / **No**
Maziarz et al. (96)	Erythroleukemia	Cytokine / **Gene transfection** / Transfection + cytokine	NK[d]	Yes / **No** / Yes[k]
Sugawara et al. (154)	T-cell leukemia (MOLT-4); myeloid cell line (U937)	Acid treatment (d)	NK[d]	Yes
Tsai et al. (159)	Murine T-cell lymphoma (viral) (YAC-1)	Cytokine	LAK[j]	Yes
Ljunggren et al. (81)	Murine T-cell lymphoma (viral) (YAC-1)	**Gene transfection** / Transfection + cytokine	NK[f]	**No** / Yes
Targets of non-lymphoid origin				
Algarra et al. (2)	Murine fibrosarcoma (chemical)	Subclones / Cytokine	NK[f] / NK[f]	Yes / Yes

512

Study	Tumor	Treatment[a]	Effector cells	Modulation
Dennert et al. (23)	Murine lung carcinoma	**Gene transfection**	NK[g]	**No**
		DMSO	NK[g]	No
		Gene transfection + DMSO	NK[g]	No
Blottière et al. (14)	Rat colon carcinoma (chemical)	Variants selected for NK or LAK resistance	NK[d]	No
			LAK[j]	No
		Cytokine	NK[d]	No
Targets of neuroectodermal origin				
Maio et al. (90)	**Melanoma**	**Gene transfection**	NK[d]	**Yes**
			LAK[i]	No
Versteeg et al. (166)	Melanoma	Introduced *c-myc* (d)	NK[d]	Yes
		c-myc + cytokine	NK[d]	Yes
Tsai et al. (159)	Murine melanoma (B16)	Cytokine	LAK[j]	Yes
Stam et al. (147)	Small cell lung carcinoma (SCLC)	Cytokine	NK[d]	Yes
		Gene transfection	NK[d]	**No**
Main et al. (89)	Peripheral primitive neuroectodermal tumor (PNET) (CHP-100)	Cytokine	NK[d]	No

[a] Representative experiments were chosen that meet these criteria: the experiment was internally controlled, comparing variants, subclones, or modification of a single cell line; it was shown that the treatment used did modulate class I MHC levels; class I levels were measured using monomorphic reagents able to detect the multiple classical class I genes (HLA-A, B, C in humans); if subclones were compared, multiple examples, with varying class I levels, were evaluated.

[b] Unless otherwise specified, cells listed are human tumor-derived cell lines. Murine lines are from spontaneously arising tumors, unless otherwise specified.

[c] MHC modulation produced an up-regulation except where denoted by (d). This indicates down-regulation.

[d] NK cells derived from peripheral blood lymphocytes (PBL).

[e] NK cells derived from splenocytes.

[f] NK cells derived from splenocytes boosted with tilerone to activate Nk cells.

[g] NK cells derived from hosts boostd with poly I:C to activate NK cells.

[h] NK cells derived from PBL +/− incubation with IFN-α.

[i] LAK cells obtained by incubating PBL with IL-2.

[j] LAK cells obtained by incubating splenocytes with IL-2.

[k] Correlation only seen at highest levels of class I expression.

analysis of tissue sections, different cell types in situ display varying levels of MHC class I expression, including lack of detectable expression in normal neural cells (neurons, astrocytes, oligodendrocytes) and skeletal muscle fibers (36,45,69; see below) (Fig. 13-4). This implies a more limited role for lack of self-MHC as the sole basis for NK attack. Experimental work exploring the relationship between MHC expression and NK susceptibility, stressing neural targets, is reviewed below.

Defining the Relationship Between MHC Expression and NK Susceptibility in Neural Tissue

Clinical Significance

Defining the relationship between MHC expression and NK susceptibility is important for planning strategies of immunoregulation in neural tissue, particularly when a greater response is desirable. Here, two aspects of the question are stressed. One concerns the effects of NK cells in normal brain. Most cells in the normal brain do not show detectable MHC expression. If this alone can render a cell an NK target, then introducing NK cells into the brain would lead to widespread destruction of neural cells.

A second aspect of the question concerns the number of effector mechanisms that can be active against a single abnormal target at the same time. As discussed above, target MHC expression is essential for the CTL response. If lack of self-MHC is a dominant basis for NK recognition, this implies a reciprocal relationship between a target cell's CTL and NK susceptibility. The goals and methods of immunoregulation could be very different depending on whether CTL and NK susceptibility are mutually exclusive or can both be up-regulated simultaneously.

Experimental Models Used to Define the MHC–NK Relationship

Most published studies examining the relationship between NK susceptibility and MHC expression involve in vitro systems, with tumor-derived cell lines serving as the targets. The cell lines offer the advantages of homogeneous target populations whose MHC expression can be readily manipulated. Separate studies are required to determine whether individual findings reflect properties of the cell or tumor of origin in situ.

Representative findings with tumor and lymphoblastoid cell lines are summarized in Table 13-1. Several points stand out from the table. One is the difference between direct introduction of MHC proteins by gene transfection and more indirect methods of class I modulation, such as cytokine treatment. In several cases, the more indirect modulation is consistent with an inverse correlation between MHC expression and NK susceptibility, whereas the direct introduction of the MHC gene does not show it.

A second point revealed by Table 13-1 is the variation in reactivity that is displayed

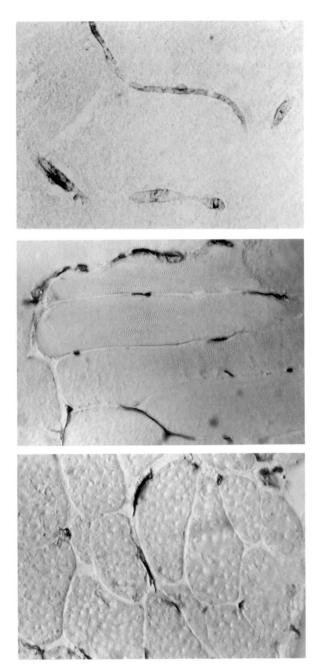

Fig. 13-4. Immune quiescence is not unique to brain. The immune quiescence of normal brain and muscle are illustrated. Top panel: human brain. Lower panels: human skeletal muscle, shown predominantly in longitudinal section (middle panel) or in cross-section (bottom panel). In each case, MHC expression is limited to the endothelial cells (stained dark with anti-MHC monoclonal antibody) and is not seen on parenchymal cells. No inflammatory cells are seen. (Top panel adapted from Lampson and Hickey, J Immunol 136:4054–4062, 1986 (68); lower panels adapted from Lampson et al., Ann Neurol 28:365–372, 1990 (69), both by permission.)

by different cell types. For cell lines of B-cell or melanoma origin, most treatments, including gene transfection, do show an inverse correlation between MHC expression and NK susceptibility. Gene transfection does not confirm the inverse correlation for the other cell types tested.

A third point suggested by Table 13-1 is the difference between NK and LAK activity. Even for B-cell lymphoma and melanoma, the inverse correlation between MHC expression and NK activity may not be retained when LAK rather than NK cells are used as the effector population. In this context, it should be noted that many studies of "NK" activity have used cells from donors whose NK activity had first been stimulated in vivo, as indicated in the footnotes to Table 13-1.

A final point concerns the MHC–NK relationship for tumors of neural origin or for those commonly found in the brain. B-cell lymphoma is increasingly common within the CNS, particularly in AIDS patients, other immunosuppressed patients, and the elderly. Melanoma is one of the most common sources of brain metastases. As shown in Table 13-1, cell lines derived from both tumor types do show a reciprocal relationship between MHC expression and NK (but not LAK) susceptibility. Among the cell lines of neuroectodermal origin in Table 13-1 (bottom of Table 13-1), only melanoma consistently shows the inverse relationship.

Cell lines from other common primary CNS tumors or metastases have not been evaluated for MHC–NK reciprocity in the same internally controlled way. Surveys of cell lines derived from neuroectodermal tumors, including primary CNS tumors, have not revealed a striking reciprocal relationship between MHC expression and NK susceptibility (116,88,89). As previous authors have pointed out, other variables, including the differentiation state of the tumor, may obscure potential effects of MHC levels. More generally, the authors of almost every study cited in Table 13-1 acknowledge the multiplicity of factors, including both receptor and effector heterogeneity, that must contribute to determining NK susceptibility. Some specific aspects of this complexity are discussed in greater detail below.

Reasons for Divergent Experimental Findings

Limitations of protocols for achieving MHC modulation. One source of divergent findings lies in the mechanisms used to modulate MHC expression on the target cell. In many cases, the altered MHC expression is not the only variable. Multiple changes would be expected from most of the methods of MHC modulation listed in Table 13-1, with the exception of gene transfection. A common example is found in the many studies, including our own, in which IFN-γ has been used to up-regulate MHC expression on the target cells, and then the IFN-treated and control cells are compared for their NK susceptibility (Table 13-1). MHC up-regulation is only one of myriad changes seen following exposure to IFN-γ. In some cases, IFN-γ treatment has been explicitly shown to alter NK susceptibility independently of MHC upregulation (75,90,96,127).

Studies where MHC expression has been increased by gene transfection are better controlled, but still do not lead to uniform results (Table 13-1). Results have again varied with the effector–target combination. In some cases, the results have varied with the particular MHC haplotype introduced (152). In other cases, combining increased MHC expression with IFN-γ treatment revealed a reciprocal relationship that was not otherwise seen (81,96).

Heterogeneity among targets and effectors. A major source of discordant data is likely to be heterogeneity among and within different NK effector populations. As discussed above, NK effectors are heterogeneous and are subject to regulation by other cells. The NK target structures are not yet defined. It is likely that more than one set of recognition molecules and more than one regulatory mechanism are involved, with different combinations important for different effectors and different effector–target combinations.

A special problem arises when PBL are used as the source of NK cells in examining a target from a different individual, as is often the case in human studies. Typically, the basic plan of the in vitro studies is to increase MHC expression on the target and ask if that reduces susceptibility to NK lysis. As discussed above, the molecular basis for NK rejection of allotargets is not known. When the NK cells and targets are from different individuals, the presence of allo-MHC, and its possible alteration by the experimental protocol, complicate interpretation of the results.

Specific Examples From Within a Single Experimental System

Dose-dependent effects. In their studies of B-cell targets, Storkus et al. established a dose–response curve for the level of NK protection as a function of the amount of class I target expression (150). At the low end of the curve, MHC expression below a threshold level did not protect against NK-mediated lysis. As the authors discuss, this could be one reason that reciprocity between MHC levels and NK susceptibility may be difficult to demonstrate when the target cell has a low baseline MHC expression. The point is relevant here because of the low baseline MHC levels of many neural cell lines and of neural cells in vitro and in situ (51,54,60,63,65,68,69,116,139,170,171).

At the high end of the dose–response curve, a plateau was reached where complete inhibition of NK activity was still not achieved, yet additional MHC expression did not lead to additional protection from NK attack (150). This adds to the body of evidence implying multiple NK–target recognition systems, which may have different relative importance for different target cell types. Predominance of MHC-independent recognition systems is indicated in studies where neural cell lines show NK susceptibility regardless of their MHC levels (88,89).

Haplotype-specific effects. The finding that a particular haplotype, HLA-A2, did not protect against NK susceptibility has an implication over and above its importance in helping to define the structural basis for the protection seen with other haplotypes (152). HLA-A2 is one of the most common class I haplotypes in the population. If

HLA-A2, and perhaps other common haplotypes, do not protect against NK attack, this would be relevant for the NK response to both neural and non-neural targets.

Effector heterogeneity. In one study where increased MHC expression protected against NK activity, the result was only seen with NK effectors and not with LAK effectors (151). This again points to the heterogeneity of the NK response and to the importance of different NK–target recognition mechanisms in different circumstances.

Summary: MHC/NK Reciprocity

Elucidation of the relationship between MHC expression and NK activity has been hampered by the complexities of the different experimental systems used. Recent work suggests possible structural bases for MHC influence on NK susceptibility. At the same time, the recent work also suggests ways of understanding why the level of MHC expression need not determine NK susceptibility in all cases. This background lays the foundation for interpreting studies of MHC expression, NK susceptibility, and CTL susceptibility in the response to neural antigen, as reviewed below.

Relationship Among MHC Expression, NK and CTL Susceptibility in the Response to Neural Targets

Cell Lines Studied in vitro

NK and CTL susceptibility of neural cell lines with varying levels of MHC expression. Our laboratory has examined neural cell lines, including lines derived from neuroblastoma, a tumor of the sympathetic neuroblast, and from different glial sources. The panel included cells with varying levels of class I MHC expression (88,89). Regardless of the MHC levels, all of the cell lines were sensitive to NK-mediated lysis. The cells remained sensitive following IFN-γ-induced increases in class I expression. Many of the same cell lines were resistant to allo-killing by CTL directed against their class I antigens. The target cells remained CTL resistant, even after IFN-γ treatment had increased their class I levels (88,89).

In follow-up studies, the resistance to CTL activity was shown to be at the target recognition stage. When CTL–target conjugates were formed artificially, all targets were lysed by the CTL (89). Lack of accessory adhesion molecules or inability to form adequate numbers of appropriate peptide–MHC complexes are two possible explanations for the ineffective target recognition (33,50,89,171). A third possibility comes from the fact that the CTL were raised against B cells of appropriate MHC phenotype rather than the neuroblastoma cells. Recent studies suggest that tissue-specific peptide in the MHC groove can be part of the recognition complex for allo-specific CTL (92,102).

The next step will be to determine which additional manipulations are required to achieve CTL-mediated lysis of the MHC+ neural targets. It will be of special interest to determine whether these manipulations concomitantly alter the cells' susceptibility to NK-mediated lysis.

Conclusions from the studies of neural cell lines. The studies described above do show a reciprocity between CTL and NK susceptibility, but it was not correlated with the levels of MHC expression on the target cells. Cells with various levels of class I MHC expression were NK targets and were resistant to CTL-mediated allo-killing.

Few other studies have evaluated both CTL and NK susceptibility after MHC manipulation of neural targets. Studies of MHC effects on NK susceptibility alone are consistent with what was found for neuroblastoma and other neural cell lines, as reviewed below.

Relationship between MHC expression and NK susceptibility in SCLC lines. Cell lines derived from small-cell lung cancer (SCLC), a tumor of neuroendocrine origin, are similar to neuroblastoma lines in their weak expression of MHC class I molecules and their potential for IFN-γ-induced class I up-regulation (27). Stam et al. (147) increased class I expression on SCLC cell lines by exposure to IFN-γ, or by transfection with class I genes. They found reduced NK susceptibility in the cells treated with IFN-γ, but unchanged or enhanced NK susceptibility in the transfected cells.

This work again demonstrates that the levels of MHC molecules alone do not determine a cell's NK susceptibility. It also illustrates that the effects of IFN-γ on NK susceptibility may be independent of the IFN's effects on MHC expression (147).

Other tumor-derived lines. Pena et al. (116) examined cell lines derived from primary human brain tumors and from brain metastases. Among four meningiosarcoma lines, the highest NK susceptibility was seen in a line with no detectable class I expression. Yet two other lines with no detectable class I expression showed low NK susceptibility. Five lines derived from brain metastases (from melanoma or sarcomas) showed various levels of class I expression and NK susceptibility, with no correlation between the two variables.

Each of four lines derived from high-grade astrocytoma showed no detectable class I expression and relatively high NK susceptibility. Two lines derived from lower grade astrocytoma, including one with no detectable class I expression, showed lower NK susceptibility (116).

The authors also examined the effect of IFN-γ on lines from each tumor category. They report that exposure to IFN-γ reduced NK susceptibility without changing class I levels (116).

These data again illustrate that MHC levels alone do not determine NK susceptibility, and that IFN-γ may affect MHC expression and NK susceptibility independently (116). As the authors point out, the data suggest the importance of cell type as a variable. Of particular interest here, low class I expression did not predict high NK susceptibility.

In vitro studies of MHC/NK reciprocity: summary and implications. Studies of cell lines derived from neural tumors or from brain metastases do not show a simple predictive relationship between MHC class I expression and NK susceptibility. Cells with either high or low MHC expression can be NK targets. Exposure to IFN-γ can both increase a target cell's MHC expression and reduce its NK susceptibility, but these effects can be independent.

Where NK and CTL susceptibility were compared directly, reciprocity was seen in that all of the cells were NK targets and all were resistant to CTL-mediated allo-killing. Yet, the susceptibility patterns were independent of the targets' levels of MHC expression (88,89).

MHC/NK Reciprocity Analyzed in vivo

Positive examples of reciprocity between MHC expression and NK susceptibility in non-neural targets. These two examples, which do not involve neural tissue, illustrate that an inverse relationship between target MHC expression and NK susceptibility can be detected in vivo in some experimental systems. They also illustrate the techniques that have been used to reveal it.

Algarra et al. (2) examined two murine fibrosarcoma subclones with different levels of MHC class I expression. In vitro, the subclones showed an inverse correlation between their sensitivity to NK lysis and their levels of class I expression. The inverse correlation was reflected in the patterns of growth following subcutaneous tumor implantation in syngeneic mice, where the cells with greater class I expression showed the most aggressive growth. The differences in growth were abolished in NK-depleted mice, implicating NK activity in the anti-tumor response.

In a second example, Glas et al. (35) studied a murine lymphoma mutant that no longer expressed b2-m, the invariant light chain of all MHC class I molecules. The mutant had reduced tumorigenicity compared to the parent tumor. Tumorigenicity was restored after restoration of the b2-m gene by transfection. The results were unchanged in T cell–deficient mice, implying that T cells did not mediate the anti-tumor activity. Both the b2-m loss mutant and the b2-m reconstituted lines formed tumors in NK-depleted mice, implying that NK activity contributed to control of tumor growth.

There have been few comparable studies of the relationship between MHC expression and NK susceptibility for neural tumors or tumors growing in the brain. The work that is available suggests that the tumor site may be as important as properties of the tumor cell itself in determining NK susceptibility, as reviewed below.

Neural tumor growing in the periphery. A number of human neural cell lines have been found to be sensitive to NK killing in vitro, regardless of their levels of MHC expression (88,89). In follow-up studies, well-characterized immunodeficient mice were used to determine whether the same behavior would be displayed in vivo. One of the previously-studied lines, the MHC+, NK-sensitive line CHP-100, was injected by different routes into NK-deficient beige mice, T cell–deficient nude mice, or doubly deficient beige/nudes (160).

In this case, the primary tumors did not grow in the way suggested by the in vitro findings. In vitro, NK activity, but not T cell–mediated allo-killing, lysed the tumor cells. Despite the in vitro findings, tumor only grew in T cell–deficient mice. That is, T cells did contribute to the control of tumor growth. When T cell–deficient and doubly deficient mice were compared, the level of host NK activity still did not affect the growth of primary tumor at the site of subcutaneous injection (160).

The evidence for T-cell activity in vivo was not surprising, given the potential contribution of T cell–mediated effector mechanisms that had not been measured in the in vitro studies. Of greater interest was the finding that NK activity did not appear to contribute to control of tumor growth at the primary site. Rather, the only suggestion of an NK-related effect was in the tumor distribution following intravenous injection. Metastases were more widespread and more frequent in the doubly deficient hosts than in the nude hosts (160).

Taken together, the findings in the immunodeficient mice are consistent with work in other contexts, implying that NK surveillance is particularly important for blood-borne targets (158,160). Complementary studies, of tumor growing in the brain itself as compared to other sites, also point to the target site as a critical factor in determining NK efficacy, as discussed below.

Non-neural tumor growing in the brain. Ljunggren et al. (82) implanted MHC class I+ and class I− variants of a T-cell lymphoma line into the mouse brain or into peripheral sites. Previous studies had demonstrated that rejection in peripheral tissues was mediated by NK cells. After subcutaneous or intraperitoneal injection into syngeneic mice, the class I+ line grew preferentially. This result was consistent with the model that NK activity controlled tumor growth and that the class I− variant was the better NK target. Following intracranial injection, however, no difference in growth between the two cell lines was seen. When the protocol was changed to favor T cell–dependent anti-tumor activity, the two lines did show differences in intracranial growth. The class I− line grew more efficiently, which is consistent with the model that lack of class I would protect the cells from MHC-restricted T-cell attack.

In interpreting their results, Ljunggren and colleagues suggest that NK activity may be suppressed in the brain, or NK migration into the brain may be reduced, as compared with the other tissues studied (82). It will be of interest to see how manipulation of NK migration into the brain will affect the growth of tumors that are known to be NK susceptible in other contexts (66).

Summary. The studies in this section suggest that the target site may be at least as important as properties of the target cell itself in determining NK susceptibility. A reciprocity between NK and CTL activity was seen in that CTL activity could be demonstrated at sites where NK activity could not. These include the site of primary tumor growth in the studies of Turner et al. (160), and the brain itself in the studies of Ljunggren et al. (82). The work raises the possibility that therapeutic manipulation of NK migration or function may be necessary to achieve NK activity against infected or neoplastic cells within the brain (66,139).

The Relationships Between MHC Expression and NK Susceptibility in Neural Tissue: Synthesis and Clinical Implications

Lack of self-MHC does not appear to be the dominant basis for NK recognition of neural targets. Studies of neural cell lines in vitro do not show a consistent reciprocal relationship between target MHC levels and NK susceptibility. In vivo, the target cell type and site appear to be at least as important as target MHC levels in determining NK susceptibility.

Independence of MHC expression and NK susceptibility has two positive clinical implications. It implies that normal neural cells need not necessarily be vulnerable to NK attack, even though they do not show detectable MHC expression. It implies that MHC-restricted CTL activity and NK activity need not be mutually exclusive for abnormal neural targets. Rather, it might be possible to enhance both CTL and NK responses against the same infected or neoplastic neural cells. Further insight into these clinical predictions comes from studies where CTL and NK activity were examined independently, as discussed below.

Examples of CTL and NK Responses, and Their Control, Within the CNS

In the sections above, CTL and NK activity were discussed with special reference to the role of the MHC. In the following sections, CTL and NK responses in the brain are reviewed from a broader perspective. The baseline level of each activity; pathological or experimental situations where the levels may change; and specific examples, stressing beneficial responses to viral infection or tumor, are reviewed.

Baseline Potential for CTL and NK Activity Within the Brain

The normal brain and spinal cord are immunologically quiescent, with minimal expression of properties that would favor either CTL or NK responses (Figure 13-4, top). Few leukocytes of any kind are seen. Those that are found are usually associated with the walls of the larger vessels (64,69).

MHC expression is also down-regulated. Strong MHC expression, particularly MHC class I, would imply susceptibility to CTL attack. Strong class II expression is usually taken to imply potential to act as an APC. In standard microscopic assays, few cells in the normal brain show MHC expression of either type, and those that do are usually not neural cells (neurons, astrocytes, or oligodendrocytes). In most cases, the only detectable MHC expression is the class I expression of endothelial cells (Fig. 13-4, top), and the class II expression of phagocytes in the choroid plexus (epiplexus cells) and meninges, individual cells in the perivascular space, and variable numbers of parenchymal microglia (36,63,68,95,139).

Immune Quiescence Is Not Unique to the Brain

The immunohistologic picture of normal brain is not unique to that organ. Rather, undetectable MHC expression and few infiltrating leukocytes are characteristic of many parenchymal cells outside of connective tissue, lymphoid tissue, or sites of hematopoiesis. Skeletal muscle provides a well-characterized example. In normal tissue, MHC proteins are not detected in skeletal muscle fibers and few infiltrating leukocytes are seen (Fig. 13-4, lower panels). Yet both MHC up-regulation and inflammation may be seen in pathological situations, just as in the brain (45,69). For studies of immunoregulation, skeletal muscle, as a large volume of immunologically quiescent tissue, can be a useful standard of comparison to CNS (5).

Summary: Baseline Potential for CTL and NK Activity

The normal brain is quiescent with respect to both CTL and NK activity, a quiescence that is seen in other tissues as well. Changes that are observed in pathologic or experimental situations, and the extent to which they could facilitate CTL or NK activity in the CNS, are reviewed below.

Changes Affecting the Potential for a CTL Response Within the Brain

The minimal requirements for a CTL response in the brain are activated CTL and susceptible target cells bearing the corresponding antigen–MHC complex. Situations in which these elements are found are reviewed below.

T-cell Entry and MHC+ Potential Target Cells

Inflammatory cells can enter the brain from the cerebral vessels. The efficiency of T-cell entry can be increased by activating the cells themselves or by activating vascular endothelium. Activation of cerebral endothelial cells can be achieved by exposure to immunoactive cytokines, for example, following intracerebral injection of IFN-γ or TNF-α (64,139). Trauma alone, such as a needle wound, can increase entry of activated T cells in the region of insult (64,58,78,143).

Although MHC expression is not detected in most cells of the normal brain, increased expression is seen in pathological or experimental circumstances. As described above, either class I or class II MHC molecules may be the restricting element for CTL. Although the role of class I is usually stressed, class II expression is often more prominent in the CNS (63,67).

The range of cell types showing increased MHC expression is limited. In appropriate circumstances, MHC class I or class II expression may be seen in endothelial cells, individual perivascular cells, microglia, neoplastic cells, transplanted cells, and inflammatory cells. Under the same conditions, MHC class I or II expression is usually still not detected in neurons, astrocytes, or oligodendrocytes in situ (reviewed in 63).

The quantitative difference between the strong MHC expression seen non-neural cells and the lack of detectable expression by most neural cells is provocative. Yet, lack of MHC staining in situ does not necessarily imply that neural cells cannot be CTL targets. The number of MHC molecules needed to present antigen to CTL may be below the detection limit of the assays currently used for MHC analysis in situ (18,54,114,142). Functional studies that imply CTL activity against neural cells in situ are reviewed in subsequent sections.

Changes Affecting the Potential for an NK Response

The minimal requirements for NK activity are NK cells themselves and NK-susceptible targets, such as infected or neoplastic cells. Neither accessory cells nor target MHC expression is required.

Few studies have aimed at evaluating or enhancing NK migration into the brain. Studies in other contexts suggest that, as for T cells, entry of NK cells into tissue can be enhanced by activating the NK cell or by activating the vascular endothelium (158). The studies of Ljunggren et al. (82) suggest that, without manipulation, NK cells may not enter the brain, or may not function there, as efficiently as in other tissues. Preliminary work suggests that intracerebral injection of proinflammatory cytokines may increase NK entry into the CNS (66,139). Functional studies are now required to more fully characterize these cells and their efficacy against CNS targets.

Examples of CTL and NK Activity Within the Brain: CTL

Criteria for Evidence of an MHC-restricted CTL Response in vivo

As discussed above, T cells are able to mediate MHC-unrestricted "natural" killer activity, as well as MHC-restricted responses. In reviewing the recent literature, examples were sought where the response has been shown to be both antigen-specific and MHC restricted in vivo. More often, the antigen specificity and MHC restriction have been studied only in vitro, either before injecting the cells into adoptive hosts or after isolating them from the brain or CSF. Stressed here are reports where the specificity and restriction were confirmed in vivo.

The studies that most fully meet the criteria for in vivo analysis come from the body of work on lymphocytic choriomeningitis virus (LCMV). The criteria are also partially fulfilled by studies of several other viruses, as listed in Table 13-2. Selected aspects of the CTL response that have been revealed by study of the response to neural viruses are discussed below.

Table 13-2 CTL and NK Activity in CNS Viral Infection[a]

Virus (host) (references)	Neural Target Cell[b]	Effector	Affects Clinical Course	Virus Cleared in Vivo	Target Cell Death in Vivo	Specificity Shown in Vivo	MHC-Restriction Shown in Vivo	MHC Class I Up-Regulation in Vivo
LCMV (mouse) (3, 9, 103, 112, 146)	Neurons	CTL[c] NK cells	Yes[e,f] No[e,g,h]	Yes[e,i]	No	Yes	Yes	No[l]
Measles (rat) (87, 113)	Neurons	CTL[d]	No[g]	Yes[g]				Yes[m]
Sindbis (mouse) (42, 43, 76)	Neurons	T cells NK cells	No[h] No[h]	No[h] No[h]				
MHV/JHM strain (mouse) (156, 175, 178)	Neurons, astrocytes, oligodendrocytes	CTL[c]	Yes[e]	Yes[g]	Yes[j]	[k]	Yes	
MuLV (mouse) (44, 129)	Astrocytes	CTL[c]	Yes[e]	No[e]	No[e]	Yes	Yes	

[a] Abbreviations: LCMV, lymphocytic choreomeningitis virus; MHV, murine hepatitis virus; MuLV, murine leukemia virus. Blank = not reported.

[b] Only response to neural target cells is included in table.

[c] CTL activity of transferred cells confirmed in vitro.

[d] OX8+ cells depleted, which could include NK effectors as well as CTL.

[e] Shown by adoptive transfer.

[f] CTL exacerbate or ameliorate disease, depending on experimental conditions.

[g] Shown by depletion studies.

[h] Shown in immunodeficient mice.

[i] Clearance from specific cell type shown by microscopic analysis.

[j] Individual dead or damaged cells not identified; contribution of dead or damaged inflammatory cells not evaluated.

[k] Specificity shown in vitro but not evaluated in vivo.

[l] When virus infected neural targets, parenchymal MHC up-regulation was not seen. Class I up-regulation was seen in areas of infection when leptomeninges, choroid plexus, and ependyma were infected, although MHC expression was not localized to individual cells, and contribution of MHC+ inflammatory cells was not evaluated (103).

[m] Diffuse stain, not localized to individual cells.

The CTL Response to Virus Within the Brain: the LCMV Response

Several features of the well-characterized LCMV response have helped refine understanding of CTL activity in the brain. The reported studies take advantage of two different patterns of LCMV infection. In immunologically normal, previously unexposed adult mice, intracerebral injection of LCMV causes an acute fatal choriomeningitis, *acute LCMV disease*. Viral antigen is seen in the meninges, choroid plexus, and ependymal lining of the ventricles (103,134). Inflammatory cells are seen at the same sites. The inflammatory response, rather than the viral infection per se, leads to the fatal outcome, although the exact mechanism is not clear. CTL contribute to the fatal inflammatory response (24,103,134).

Immunosuppressed mice show a different pattern, one of *persistent infection*. Following intracerebral injection of LCMV, they contract a mild acute disease and then become persistently infected, with viral antigen found predominantly in neurons (112). The inflammatory response is minimal during persistent infection, and the presence of virus does not cause neuronal cell death or other gross pathology. CTL can contribute to clearance of virus from infected neurons (112).

The two LCMV models focus attention on the range of possible outcomes, from beneficial to deleterious, of cell-mediated immune activity directed against virus or other antigen within the CNS. Insights into other aspects of the response are reviewed below.

Lessons from the LCMV Response

Differential MHC upregulation in different cell types. During acute LCMV disease, MHC class I expression is up-regulated in the same areas where viral antigen and inflammation are seen—within the meninges and choroid plexus and in the ependymal lining of the ventricles. The MHC up-regulation is dependent upon the inflammatory response. If inflammation is prevented, viral infection alone does not lead to class I upregulation (103). In persistent LCMV disease, when the virus is predominantly localized to neurons, neither parenchymal class I up-regulation nor intraparenchymal inflammatory cells are seen (103,112).

Limitation of MHC up-regulation to non-neural cells is seen in other contexts as well (reviewed in 63). For example, differential MHC expression is also seen in studies of cytokine-mediated MHC regulation. Following intracerebral injection of IFN-γ, MHC up-regulation is seen in endothelial cells, ependymal cells, and microglia, but not neurons, astrocytes, or oligodendrocytes (139). In contrast, evidence for MHC up-regulation by neural cells themselves has been seen in measles virus infection (113) and following transplantation (below). However, in most cases, including that of measles infection (113), definitive localization of the MHC molecules to the neural cells has not yet been reported.

Desirable and undesirable consequences of CTL activity. An important aspect of CNS immunobiology brought out by the LCMV model is the range of possible consequences of CTL action in the brain. Depending upon the experimental conditions, CTL can mediate viral clearance or can initiate an inflammatory response which itself is the cause of fatal CNS pathology (9,24,112). More broadly still, CTL may affect viral clearance and the clinical course independently, and need not have an effect upon either one (Table 13-2). Additional examples of CNS antiviral responses that may be beneficial or harmful are found in the different possible outcomes of infection with Theiler's virus (79). Consequences of T-cell activity against human CNS viral infection have been reviewed by Johnson (49).

A more subtle point concerns the range of possible CTL effects on the target cell per se, particularly whether target lysis is an inevitable consequence of CTL attack. An intriguing aspect of persistent LCMV disease is that virus is cleared from infected neurons by a CTL-dependent mechanism without obvious neuronal drop-out or other gross evidence of target cell damage (112).

Questions about the mechanism of viral clearance. In most of the examples given in Table 13-2, the precise way in which the implicated effector mechanism leads to virus clearance is not yet known. Many of the outstanding questions are illustrated by LCMV disease. Although transfer of CTL can lead to viral clearance from neurons in LCMV disease, several aspects of the mechanism are not yet well understood. CTL-mediated viral clearance may be seen in the absence of obvious inflammation, detectable MHC up-regulation, or target cell death (112).

These observations may have a quantitative explanation. Many of the cells at a site of inflammation are nonspecific. A much smaller number of cells may be sufficient to mediate T-cell activity (135). A level of inflammation that is readily detected by conventional histological stains may not be required. This may be particularly relevant for viral clearance from the CNS, which follows an indolent course as compared to most other tissues (112). Similarly, the minimal number of MHC proteins required to render a cell susceptible to CTL-mediated attack may well be below the threshold detectable by conventional staining techniques (18,54,114,142).

Non-lytic CTL activity. While quantitative arguments may help to explain the limited MHC expression and inflammation associated with LCMV clearance from neurons, another kind of explanation has been sought for the finding of viral clearance without obvious target cell death. One mechanism that has been proposed is viral clearance mediated by cytokine release (74,112). Although cytokine-mediated clearance is not established in the LCMV model, it is consistent with studies in other contexts showing that cytokines such as interferon can influence viral infection without killing the infected cell (22). It is also consistent with work in other contexts showing that the outcome of a potentially lytic event can be influenced by properties of the target cell (77,136).

Although viral clearance without target cell death appears to contradict the definition of a "CTL" response, this reflects the historical development of the terminology, rather than current understanding of CTL biology. Traditionally, CTL activity in vitro has been defined by target cell damage or lysis, most commonly measured by release of ingested [51]Cr. This measure of CTL function has fit the traditional demarcation of CTL as lytic cells and Th as cytokine producers. More recent work draws attention to the potential diversity of all cell-mediated responses. It is now appreciated that CTL, Th, and NK cells can each mediate both direct lysis and cytokine release and can secrete many of the same cytokines, including IFN-γ and TNF.

A possible alternative to nonlytic CTL activity is that CTL clear virus from non-neural cells, and complementary, CTL-independent mechanisms clear virus from infected neurons. Yet it is still necessary to explain how virus is cleared from the neurons without their death. The recent work of D. Griffin and colleagues implying antibody-mediated viral clearance without concomitant target lysis (76) is one example of the more general question. Regardless of the mechanism, it is important to stress the possibility of viral clearance or other immune activity without target cell death (104,124).

Work by Keane and colleagues suggests that CNS neurons may be resistant to at least one of the lytic mechanisms used by CTL (54). This fits well with the idea of a limited CTL attack on infected neurons, one that stops short of target cell death. Although this kind of mechanism is particularly attractive in the case of postmitotic neurons, a nonlytic mechanism has also been implicated in the CTL response to other kinds of cells (74). A more general view would be that cell lysis is just one of the possible ways in which CTL can affect their targets or influence viral replication within the target cell (77,112,136). An intriguing possibility is that the effects of the CTL–target interaction are controlled, in part, by the strength of the interaction, with low target MHC levels favoring a nonlytic outcome.

The CTL Response to Virus in the CNS: Summary

Taken together, the published studies do provide direct evidence that antigen-specific, MHC-restricted CTL can affect the course of viral infection in the brain (Table 13-2). MHC up-regulation can be detected in the brain after viral infection or in other circumstances. The level and role of MHC expression in neural cells themselves (neurons, astrocytes, and oligodendrocytes) are still controversial (63). Directly or indirectly, CTL are able to mediate the clearance of virus from infected neurons under delicately controlled conditions, without conventionally detected intraparenchymal inflammation or target MHC expression, and without massive target cell death (103,112).

The CTL Response to Tumor in the CNS

Macroscopic tumor. A wealth of descriptive studies have defined T-cell subpopulations in human brain tumors. In most studies of primary tumors, "CTL" outnumber Th (131,133,168). In one study of brain metastases, the opposite trend was reported, with Th outnumbering "CTL" (149). The basic procedure in these studies has been to use antibody staining of tissue sections or of cells from dissociated tumor to define the surface characteristics of the component cells. The strength of this approach is that, when applied to tissue sections, it gives the most direct information about the distribution of the T-cell populations in relation to tumor. The weakness is that the functional potential of the cells may be ambiguous.

Typically, CTL and Th in humans are identified by their characteristic accessory molecules, CD8 and CD4, respectively. An example of the factors that complicate interpretation is that CD8+ T cells may have either CTL or suppressor activity. This ambiguity is acknowledged by the cells' usual designation as "cytotoxic/suppressor" cells, when identified by CD8 expression (131,133,149,168).

Direct evidence of effector function is much sparser. The evidence that is available, from in vitro analysis of cells isolated from the tumor mass, often suggests immunosuppression rather than anti-tumor activity. T-cell clones isolated from gliomas may be anergic (99). This may reflect immunosuppressive factors secreted by the tumor cells. One current line of research is to try to overcome this suppressive environment. Approaches include isolating and restimulating tumor-infiltrating lymphocytes (TILs), introducing fresh effector populations, or using injected cytokines or cytokine-producing cells to change the regulatory environment in situ (reviewed in 61,63a).

Microscopic tumor. Cell-mediated immunotherapy is likely to have the greatest chance of success at sites of microscopic tumor (63a,64). Not only should the concentration of secreted immunosuppressive factors be reduced, as compared to within a large tumor mass, but a more favorable ratio of effector cells to target cells may be achievable.

The potential for motile immune or inflammatory cells to attack microscopic tumor becomes of increasing interest as conventional therapies permit greater success at removing or inactivating a discrete tumor mass (63a,64,83). Cell-mediated attack of microscopic tumor is of particular interest in astrocytoma and in CNS lymphoma (the predominant CNS tumor of AIDS). Both tumors have a characteristic infiltrative mode of spread, with individual tumor cells moving amid functional brain tissue.

Of necessity, most studies of both human and animal tumors have focused on analysis of a visualizable tumor mass. Insights that have come from an animal model where individual tumor cells and responding cells could be identified in tissue sections (Fig. 13-5) are reviewed below.

An internal protein can be a tumor antigen. Traditionally, it has been assumed that a tumor antigen must be a cell surface molecule. Yet, the mechanism of antigen–MHC complexing implies that any protein synthesized by a tumor cell, including internal protein, can serve as a tumor target antigen. The *lacZ* reporter system has been used to illustrate this directly in a brain tumor model.

Tumor cell lines were made to express the *lacZ* reporter gene, coding for *E. coli*–derived β-galactosidase (b-gal). The b-gal is expressed as a cell-filling cytoplasmic protein, which serves to identify tumor cells in other contexts (73) (Fig. 13-5). Here, b-gal was used as a well-defined tumor antigen. Immunization with b-gal protein was found to be at least as efficient as immunization with tumor homogenate in preventing

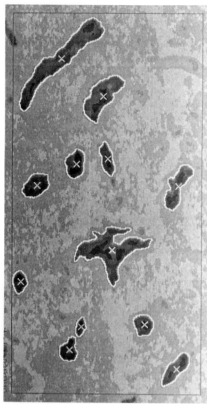

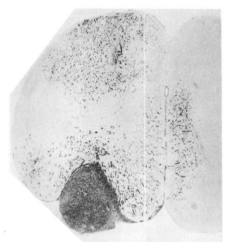

Fig. 13-5. An experimental model that facilitates visualization and quantitative analysis of leukocyte–target interactions in the brain. Left panel: the 9L/lacZ cell line, expressing the *lacZ* reporter gene, was injected stereotactically into the rat brain. Histochemical stain reveals (dark) lacZ+ cells growing as a tumor in the brain. Right panel: a digitized image of microscopic tumor such as that shown (at lower magnification) in the left panel. The image is used as the basis for quantitative image analysis, for example, to determine tumor areas. Figure adapted from Lampson et al., Cancer Res 53:176–182, 1993 (70), by permission.)

tumor growth. Specificity was shown in two ways: immunization with unrelated antigens did not confer protection, and immunization with b-gal did not protect against the b-gal-negative parent line (70).

This work confirms that immunization can influence tumor growth in the brain. Protection occurs despite the brain's normal immunologically quiescent status and despite the immunosuppressive environment that brain tumors may create (32,99). The work draws attention to the full range of molecules, including aberrant growth factors, oncogene products, or suppressor gene products, regardless of their location in the tumor cell, that may be exploited as targets for cell-mediated immune attack (70).

Increasing the frequency of leukocyte/target interactions. Studies of identifiable tumor cells bearing the b-gal marker (Fig. 13-5), have facilitated analysis of tumor-leukocyte interactions. Double-labeling techniques reveal inflammatory cells adjacent to individual tumor cells, even on the opposite side of the brain from the site of tumor implantation (73). This implies that, in aiming to facilitate leukocyte-target interactions for therapy of disseminated tumor, one would be enhancing a process that does occur physiologically.

In parallel studies, it was found that intracerebral injection of proinflammatory cytokines can increase the numbers of inflammatory or responding cells that come into contact with CNS tumor, and that entry and migration of different subpopulations can be controlled selectively (64,66,139). This work lays a foundation for functional studies of CTL and other effectors against disseminated or microscopic tumor in the brain.

Immune modulation need not be inhibited by tumor growth. In studies of tumor-free rats, it was shown that injected cytokines could affect immune parameters (139,141,148,165). The next step was to ask whether the same effects could occur in the presence of growing tumor. In practice, it was found that IFN-γ-mediated changes in MHC expression and leukocyte entry can occur in the presence of growing tumor, even if the IFN has been injected into the midst of an established tumor mass (61,72,170). Thus, although brain tumors may well create an immunosuppressive environment (32,61,99), it need not prevent cytokine-mediated changes in immune parameters (63a). The effects of IFN-γ or other cytokines on the cell-mediated response to microscopic disease must now be evaluated.

Conclusions: potential of the CTL response against CNS tumor. Cell-mediated activity should be of particular value against microscopic or disseminated CNS tumor that cannot be imaged or selectively attacked by other means. Studies of CNS viral infection demonstrate that CTL can be active in the brain (Table 13-2). Studies in humans and laboratory animals show that CTL do have access to CNS tumor. Techniques for enhancing CTL–tumor interactions and CTL activity in the brain are now being developed, paving the way for efforts to enhance anti-tumor function (64,99). As new techniques provide ways of amplifying or modifying the intrinsic activities of migratory cells, the cells become of increasing interest as vehicles, as well as effectors in their own right (63a,64).

Undesirable Responses: Graft Rejection

While the therapeutic potential of neural grafts is widely appreciated, perception of the importance of graft rejection has been changing. For many years it was widely assumed that the brain was "immunologically privileged," and that grafts in the brain would not be rejected. This assumption was made despite the fact that, even in the classic paper in which they described the brain's "immune privilege," Barker and Billingham also described its limitations. Indeed, they foresaw many of the issues and questions that are still being addressed in this field (11). In recent years, there has been a growing appreciation that allografts and xenografts to the CNS can indeed be rejected, even in the "doubly privileged" (106) case where a neural graft is placed within the CNS (8,21,34,47,55,85,106,125,145,153,174).

Points of general agreement, and outstanding questions, regarding the role of the MHC and cell-mediated immunity in rejection of grafts to the CNS are reviewed below. As in the work reviewed, the emphasis is on the immune response to grafts of neural tissue, including pieces of tissue from fetal or adult donors, tissue homogenates that have been enriched for particular cell types (12,119), and neural cell lines (5,122).

It is now accepted that, once stimulated, immune mechanisms can lead to rejection of grafts in the brain, just as at other sites. When the only immune challenge is the placement of the graft in the brain, initiation of an immune response may be relatively slow, as compared to grafts placed at other sites, such as skin. Peripheral sensitization leads to accelerated rejection of the CNS graft. Most often, the peripheral sensitization has been achieved by placing a graft of donor tissue in the host skin. Regardless of whether the skin graft is placed before, at the same time as, or after the CNS graft, rejection of the CNS graft is accelerated. Even established CNS grafts will be rejected if the host receives a skin graft from the same donor (11,34,47,85,106,145).

There is general agreement that MHC disparity between donor and host can lead to graft rejection, but that this is not the only relevant variable (21,47,125,174). Other antigens can be targets of graft rejection (47,125), even where there is no MHC disparity (5,71,145). Although graft rejection is expected to be most efficient when products of the major histocompatibility complex are targeted, any foreign protein, including internal proteins, has the potential to be recognized as a transplantation antigen (71).

MHC modulation in CNS grafts: evidence and functional consequences. It is frequently observed that MHC expression is up-regulated in the vicinity of a graft to the CNS (119,120,121,144,176). Increased MHC expression may be seen within grafted neural tissue and also within adjacent tissue. Graft-associated MHC up-regulation is not a unique property of neural grafts or grafts to neural tissue; rather, it is seen in other contexts as well (101).

In the case of neural tissue, localization of enhanced MHC expression has been difficult to establish. Host and donor MHC+ inflammatory cells, MHC+ microglia of host and donor origin, and MHC+ endothelial cells of host and donor origin can all to contribute to the observed strong MHC expression (5,120). In the presence of increased MHC expression by so many non-neural cell types, it has been difficult to assess the MHC expression of neural cells themselves. Several investigators report that they do not find MHC up-regulation in large numbers of host or donor neurons, astrocytes or oligodendrocytes following transplantation (reviewed in 63,119).

MHC localization is simplified in xenografts of purified cells or cell lines. In grafts of human neural cell lines into the adult rat brain, no alteration of MHC expression was detected in the donor human cells. With time, MHC+ host inflammatory cells and MHC+ host microglia were abundant within the graft and in its vicinity. This work illustrates the extent to which MHC expression can be increased in the region of a graft even without increased expression by the grafted neural cells themselves (5). Of course, it does not rule out the possibility of neural MHC modulation in grafted neural cells in other cases.

Although it is often assumed that enhanced MHC expression facilitates graft rejection, this has not been thoroughly investigated. The effect and importance of increased MHC expression is likely to vary for different MHC+ cell types; it may not necessarily be an important factor in each case. For example, two human cell lines with different levels of MHC expression were rejected at the same rate from the brains of adult rat hosts (5).

Current questions about the effector cell types and mechanisms mediating CNS graft rejection. Questions regarding the effect of enhanced MHC expression are tied to more general questions about the nature of the effector mechanisms that contribute to CNS graft rejection. This is a topic of ongoing research for transplantation in general (7,19,93,94). The relative importance of different mechanisms must vary with the composition of the graft, the host site (121,153), and the nature of the antigenic disparity between host and donor. The way in which host T cells recognize MHC-disparate donor cells is another topic of current research for transplantation in general. In the case of CNS grafts, uncertainty about the localization of enhanced MHC expression adds an additional layer of complexity.

Even where T cells have been shown to mediate CNS graft rejection, the actual effector mechanisms must still be defined. Nicholas, Arnason, and colleagues have shown that both CD4+ T cells and CD8+ T cells can contribute to rejection of neural grafts placed within the CNS (106–108). As discussed in the initial sections of this chapter, each kind of T-cell can attack targets directly or indirectly and by MHC-unrestricted as well as MHC-restricted mechanisms. The effector mechanisms of greatest importance in vivo must still be defined.

The implications of the limited MHC expression that is usually observed in neural cells per se must also be defined. Interpretation has been complicated by differences in sensitivity when MHC expression is defined by binding studies as opposed to functional analysis. For example, studies in vitro demonstrate that astrocytes are susceptible to T cell–mediated allo-killing, even when the astrocytes' levels of MHC expression are below the limits of detection by immunocytochemistry or FACS analysis (142).

The dominant effector mechanisms mediating CNS graft rejection need not be the same for every cell type, nor for every part of a cell. Histologic observations in vivo suggest that grafted neurons may be spared from cell-mediated lysis (10). This is consistent with reports previously discussed of viral clearance without neuronal death (76,112), and it raises similar questions about the possible consequences of cell-mediated attack. The potential importance of the cellular point of attack is suggested by studies of Manning and colleagues, who used cultured sympathetic neurons as the target (91). Target lysis was observed when allo-specific CTL were applied to the cell bodies but not when the CTL were applied to the processes (91).

Undesirable responses: summary and conclusions. CNS grafts provide additional examples of some of the outstanding questions about the cell-mediated response to neural antigen in general: Which cells express the MHC molecules? What is the balance between direct and indirect attack? What is the balance between MHC-restricted and MHC-unrestricted attack? As for desirable responses to viral or tumor antigen, discussed above, the answers in the context of graft rejection are just now being defined.

The effector cascade in CNS autoimmune reactions is equally complex. Perhaps the important lesson to draw here is that an effective desirable response, such as an anti-tumor response, may have to include a complex mix of effector cells and mechanisms as well.

Overview: CTL Activity Within the CNS

There is good evidence that classical antigen-specific, MHC-restricted CTL can act within the CNS (Table 13-2). Because the antigen–MHC complex forms internally, internal proteins can be targets of the CTL response. The mechanisms by which CTL affect their targets in situ, including possible nonlytic mechanisms, and the way beneficial CTL activity can be enhanced against infected or neoplastic cells, are areas of active research. There is much less firm knowledge about the role or potential of NK activity in the CNS, as discussed below.

Evaluation of NK Activity Within the Nervous System

Few studies have directly evaluated NK function within the brain. Available information about NK activity in viral infection, anti-tumor responses, deleterious responses, and normal neural tissue are reviewed below.

Changing the host's NK activity was found to alter the course of the acute CNS inflammatory response that follows intracerebral inoculation of Theiler's murine encephalitis virus (TMEV). Virus titers in the brain were not affected (115). This suggests an indirect effect on the course of infection, rather than a direct effect of NK activity on infected targets per se. Alteration of NK activity was not found to have a major influence on the course of LCMV disease (3).

NK cells have been detected as a minor inflammatory population in some human CNS tumors, and their functional activity has been confirmed in vitro (131,149,163, 164). The cells' potential for tumor control in situ is not yet known. In a mouse model, Ljunggren et al. (82) were unable to demonstrate NK-mediated attack of intracerebral tumor, although the same cells were susceptible to NK attack in other tissues. When LAK cells and IL-2 are injected together into an intracerebral tumor bed, necrosis is seen at the injection site, but not beyond it (98). Taken together, these studies point to the need for more knowledge about NK migration and activation in situ as essential aspects of evaluating NK efficacy against tumor in the CNS (66,82,98,139,173). The procedures used to date have suggested a greater potential for control of local (98) or leptomeningeal disease (140) than of disseminated tumor within the CNS parenchyma.

For grafts outside the CNS, NK cells can contribute to graft rejection, for example, by attacking donor endothelial cells (31,46). The possible role of NK cells has not yet been a major focus of study for CNS grafts. As other, more dominant anti-graft effector mechanisms are brought under control, it will be of interest to learn if NK activity alone can mediate intracerebral graft rejection.

In most studies of cell-mediated autoimmune disorders or of potential immune–inflammatory exacerbation of nonimmune insults, attention has also focused on T cell-mediated responses, rather than NK activity. There has been recent interest in ways that MHC-unrestricted T cells may contribute to myelin destruction in multiple sclerosis (MS) (137,177), and evidence of NK-mediated destruction of peripheral nerve in a rat model was recently described (41).

Although few studies have demonstrated significant NK activity in the brain, in many cases there was no evidence that the cells were present or functional. This leaves open the question of whether NK cells might be harmful to normal neural cells. The question follows from the hypothesis that lack of self-MHC may trigger NK activity and the observation that most neural cells do not show detectable MHC expression.

The view that normal neurons are in fact safe from NK attack is consistent with the evidence, reviewed above, that levels of MHC expression alone do not determine NK susceptibility for neural cells (Table 13-1). It is also consistent with the evidence reviewed above that cell-mediated effectors may influence their targets without necessarily causing target cell death, and that even infected neurons may be resistant to lytic attack.

Conclusions: NK Activity Within the CNS

The available data suggests that NK activity need not be deleterious to normal neural cells, despite their undetectable MHC expression. The work draws attention to the possibility that increasing NK migration or activation therapeutically may be necessary for achieving NK activity against infected or neoplastic cells within the brain.

The extent to which NK or CTL use nonlytic mechanisms to affect their targets is a question of current interest. A model system that facilitates quantitative in situ analysis of this and other questions about the cell-mediated response to neural targets is described below.

Visualization and Quantitative Analysis of Individual Leukocyte/Target Interactions Within the Brain

A model system that facilitates quantitative analysis of leukocyte/target interactions in situ is illustrated in Fig. 13-5. To allow identification of target cells, cell lines were made to constitutively express the *lacZ* reporter gene. The reporter gene product, *E.*

coli-derived β-galactosidase (b-gal), is detected histochemically on tissue sections. The intense cell-filling blue-green stain permits single target cells to be unambiguously identified (Fig. 13-5). Leukocyte subpopulations, MHC expression, and other features of interest can be identified by monoclonal antibody double-labeling on the same slides (73). To gain insight into immunoregulation in different anatomic regions (64), stereotactic injection is used to deliver target cells, effector cells, and activating cytokines to selected sites.

The reporter gene product can be exploited in several additional ways, complementing its use as a marker for individual cells. The contrast between b-gal$^+$ cells and background facilitates computer-assisted image analysis of the location and number of target cells, changes in immune parameters, and leukocyte–target interactions. The marker protein itself can serve as a well-defined tumor antigen. When the marker protein is the antigen, its loss can be a convenient indicator of antigenic modulation, a concern for all forms of therapy against metabolically active targets (61,63a,64,70).

Variations of this system have been used to study the cell-mediated response to both microscopic tumor and transplanted tissue within the CNS. Examples from studies of internal antigen, cytokine-mediated changes in MHC expression and leukocyte migration, and leukocyte–target interactions have been included in the preceding sections (64,70,71,73).

Are CTL and NK Responses Deleterious in the Brain?

There is a widespread perception that cell-mediated immune responses in the brain must be detrimental, that "if the brain isn't immunologically privileged, it should be." Observations that have had led to this opinion, and arguments against it, are reviewed below.

Many of the most widely studied neural immune reactions are indeed detrimental. These include the autoimmune responses seen in experimental allergic encephalomyelitis (EAE) and thought to be the etiology of MS; the unwanted rejection of neural transplants; and instances where it is the T-cell response to virus, rather than viral infection per se, that leads to the observed CNS pathology.

Positive aspects of the immune response to antigen in the brain have received less attention. Beneficial aspects of the response are suggested by the number of different opportunistic infections seen in AIDS patients (118) or others with suppressed cell-mediated immunity. Although all of the contributing factors are still being defined, it is likely that reduced immune surveillance within the brain itself contributes to the CNS pathology.

One approach to CNS immunobiology stems from the traditional view that class I MHC expression is "ubiquitous." The argument made is that neural cells are unique in their lack of detectable class I expression and that this is necessary to protect them from CTL attack. Protection is necessary, according to this argument, because neurons are postmitotic and so it is better to retain infected neurons than to lose them. The potentially fatal damage that can result from an uncontrolled inflammatory response within the confines of the skull is seen as yet another reason for thinking that a CTL response must be detrimental within the brain.

Current understanding suggests alternative interpretations of the brain's characteristic pattern of MHC expression. As discussed above, parenchymal cells of many normal tissues fail to show detectable MHC class I expression; it is not solely a property of irreplaceable or postmitotic cells (Fig. 13-4). An alternative interpretation is that MHC expression is under regulatory control in all tissues, with neural tissue at the low end of the spectrum of normal baseline activity.

Recent work also suggests more positive ways of viewing the consequences of cell-mediated activity within the brain. Although new neurons are not formed in the human adult, new connections can be formed, a plasticity that could help to compensate for destruction of small numbers of infected neurons. While an uncontrolled inflammatory response is indeed dangerous within the skull, that level of inflammation may not necessarily be required (135).

Finally, although plasticity may compensate for some neuronal loss, recent evidence suggests that neuronal loss need not necessarily occur. Accumulating evidence that cell-mediated responses can affect their targets without lysing them provides a compelling argument in favor of the potential benefits of physiologic or therapeutic CTL and NK responses within the brain.

Summary and Conclusions

The CTL and NK responses are complementary in many ways. The NK response to the first appearance of an infected or transformed cell is rapid, occurring before the CTL response or other antigen-specific mechanisms can be initiated. It is MHC unrestricted and may even be inhibited by target MHC expression for particular NK–target combinations.

The CTL response, in contrast, is MHC restricted, and its initiation requires participation of accessory cells and their stimulatory cytokines. Although slower to reach its peak, the CTL response displays much finer antigenic specificity than the NK response. Upon second exposure to the same antigen, the CTL response, but not the NK response, displays immune memory.

Both CTL and NK effector cells can interact directly with their targets. Both CTL and NK cells can also affect their targets indirectly by secreting cytokines. Whether direct CTL or NK activity must lead to the lysis of the target is a question of current interest (25,104,125).

CTL can contribute to control of viral infections in the nervous system, although many questions about the mechanism remain. In different circumstances, CTL may control infection or may themselves be the cause of the observed pathology. The role of

CTL in graft rejection and their potential role in tumor immunity are less well understood.

The extent to which NK activity occurs or can be exploited in the CNS is still being defined. NK cells are only a minor population in tumor infiltrates, and NK activity has not been found to play a major role in control of viral infections. Although MHC expression may inhibit NK susceptibility for some NK–target combinations, there is at present no evidence for this relationship against neural targets. It may well be possible to exploit CTL and NK activity simultaneously against infected or neoplastic cells within the brain. Interest in enhanced NK and memory CTL activity is further increased by the possibility that each may be preferentially retained in AIDS.

Acknowledgements

The secretarial assistance of Ms. Nicole Walcott and Ms. Len Martyr is greatly appreciated. Work from the authors' laboratory was supported by awards to L.A.L. from NINDS, the National Multiple Sclerosis Society, the National Muscular Dystrophy Association, the American Cancer Society, the John Alden Trust, the Alex Coffin Fund for Brain Tumor Research, the Fuller Foundation, Inc., and the Marcus Foundation. W.S.A. is the recipient of a Carl Walter Fellowship from Harvard Medical School.

References

1. Abbas AK, Lichtman AH, Pober JS. Cellular and Molecular Immunology. WB Saunders, Philadelphia, 1991.
2. Algarra I, Ohlen C, Perez M, Ljunggren H-G, Klein G, Garrido F, Kärre K. NK sensitivity and lung clearance of MHC-class-I-deficient cells within a heterogeneous fibrosarcoma. Int J Cancer 44:675–680, 1989.
3. Allan JE, Doherty PC. Natural killer cells contribute to inflammation but do not appear to be essential for the induction of clinical lymphocytic choriomeningitis. Scand J Immunol 24:153–162, 1986.
4. Anderson P, Caligiuri M, Ritz J, Schlossman SF. CD3-negative natural killer cells express ζ TCR as a part of a novel molecular complex. Nature 341:159–162, 1989.
5. Armstrong WS. Evaluation of MHC expression in xenografts of human neural cell lines. M.D. dissertation, Harvard Medical School, Boston MA 1994.
6. Babbitt BP, Matsueda G, Haber E, Unanue ER, Allen PM. Antigenic competition at the level of peptide-Ia binding. Proc Natl Acad Sci USA 83:4509–4513, 1986.
7. Bach FH. Reconsideration of the mechanism of first-set vascularized allograft rejection: some concluding remarks. Hum Immunol 28:263–269, 1990.
8. Backes MG, Lund RD, Langenaur CF, Kunz HW, Gill TJ III. Cellular events associated with peripherally induced rejection of mature neural xenografts placed into neonatal rat brains. J Comp Neurol 295:428–437, 1990.
9. Baenziger J, Hengartner H, Zinkernagel RM, Cole GA. Induction or prevention of immunopathological disease by cloned cytotoxic T cell lines specific for lymphocytic choriomeningitis virus. Eur J Immunol 16:387–393, 1986.

10. Banerjee R, Lund RD, Radel JD. Anatomical and functional consequences of induced rejection of intracranial retinal transplants. Neuroscience 56:939–953, 1993.

11. Barker CF, Billingham RE. Immunologically privileged sites. Adv Immunol 25:1–54, 1977.

12. Bartlett PF. Allograft rejection overcome by immunoselection of neuronal precursor cells. Prog Brain Res 82:153–160, 1990.

13. Bennett M. Biology and genetics of hybrid resistance. Adv Immunol 41:333–445, 1987.

14. Blottière HM, Zennadi R, Burg C, Douuillard J-Y, Meflah K, Le Pendu J. Relationship between sensitivity to natural killer cells and MHC class-I antigen expression in colon carcinoma cell lines. Int J Cancer 50:659–664, 1992.

15. Carbone FR, Bevan MJ. Major histocompatibility complex control of T cell recognition. In: Fundamental Immunology, 2nd ed, WE Paul, ed. Raven Press, New York, 1989, pp 541–567.

16. Chadwick BS, Miller RG. Hybrid resistance in vitro: possible role of both class I MHC and self peptides in determining the level of target cell sensitivity. J Immunol 148:2307–2313, 1992.

17. Chicz RM, Urban RG, Lane WS, Gorga JC, Stern LJ, Vignali DAA, Strominger JL. Predominant naturally processed peptides bound to HLA-DR1 are derived from MHC-related molecules and are heterogeneous in size. Nature 358:764–768, 1992.

18. Christinck ER, Luscher MA, Barber BH, Williams DB. Peptide binding to class I MHC on living cells and quantitation of complexes required for CTL lysis. Nature 352:67–70, 1991.

19. Colvin RB. Cellular and molecular mechanisms of allograft rejection. Annu Rev Med 41:361–375, 1990.

20. Cserr HF, Knopf PM. Cervical lymphatics, the blood-brain barrier and the immunoreactivity of the brain: a new view. Immunol Today 13:507–512, 1992.

21. Date I, Kawamura K, Nakashima H. Histological signs of immune reactions against allogeneic solid fetal neural grafts in the mouse cerebellum depend on the MHC locus. Exp Brain Res 73:15–22, 1988.

22. De Maeyer E. The antiviral activity of interferons. In: Interferons and Other Regulatory Cytokines. E. De Maeyer, J De Maeyer-Guignard, eds. John Wiley and Sons, New York, 1988, pp 114–133.

23. Dennert G, Landon C, Lord EM, Bahler DW, Frelinger JG. Lysis of a lung carcinoma by poly I:C-induced natural killer cells is independent of the expression of class I histocompatibility antigens. J Immunol 140:2472–2475, 1988.

24. Doherty PC. Cell-mediated immunity in virus infections of the central nervous system. Ann NY Acad Sci 540:228–239, 1988.

25. Doherty PC. Cell-mediated cytotoxicity. Cell 75:607–612, 1993.

26. Doherty PC, Allan JE, Lynch F, Ceredig R. Dissection of an inflammatory process induced by CD8[+] T cells. Immunol Today 11:55–59, 1990.

27. Doyle A, Martin WJ, Funa K, Gazdar A, Carney D, Martin SE, Linnoila I, Cuttitta F, Mulshine J, Bunn P, Minna J. Markedly decreased expression of class I histocompatibility antigens, protein, and mRNA in human small-cell lung cancer. J Exp Med 161:1135–1151, 1985.

28. Drew PD, Lonergan M, Goldstein ME, Lampson LA, Ozato K, McFarlin DE. Regulation of MHC class I and b2-microglobulin gene expression in human neuronal cells. Factor binding activity to conserved *cis*-acting regulatory sequences correlates with expression of the genes. J Immunol 150:3300–3310, 1993.

29. Elliott T, Cerundolo V, Elvin J, Townsend A. Peptide-induced conformational change of the class I heavy chain. Nature 351:402–406, 1991.

30. Elliott T, Townsend A, Cerundolo V. Naturally processed peptides. Nature 348:195–197, 1990.

31. Elsen M, Soares M, Latinne D, Cornet A, Bazin H. Role of activated natural killer and CD4+, CD8+ cells in the cellular rejection of a discordant xenograft. Transplant Proc 25:447–449, 1993.

32. Fontana A, Frei K, Bodmer S, Hofer E. Immune-mediated encephalitis: on the role of antigen-presenting cells in brain tissue. Immunol Rev 100:185–201, 1987.

33. Franksson L, George E, Powis S, Butcher G, Howard J, Kärre K. Tumorigenicity conferred to lymphoma mutant by major histocompatibility complex-encoded transporter gene. J Exp Med 177:201–205, 1993.

34. Freed WJ. Substantia nigra grafts and Parkinson's disease: from animal experiments to human therapeutic trials. Restorative Neurol Neurosci 3:109–134, 1991.

35. Glas R, Sturmhöfel K, Hämmerling GJ, Kärre K, Ljunggren H-G. Restoration of a tumorigenic phenotype by β_2-microglobulin transfection to EL-4 mutant cells. J Exp Med 175:843–846, 1992.

36. Grabowska A, Lampson LA. Expression of class I and II major histocompatibility complex (MHC) antigens in the developing CNS. J Neural Transplant Plast 3:204–205, 1992.

37. Grabowska A, Lampson LA. MHC expression in nonlymphoid tissues of the developing embryo: strongest class I or class II expression in separate populations of potential antigen-presenting cells in the skin, lung, gut, and inter-organ connective tissue. Dev Comp Immunol 19:425–450, 1995.

38. Hamilos DL. Antigen presenting cells. Immunol Res 8:98–117, 1989.

39. Heath WR, Hurd ME, Carbone FR, Sherman LA. Peptide-dependent recognition of H-2K^b by alloreactive cytotoxic T lymphocytes. Nature 341:749–752, 1989.

40. Henderson RA, Michel H, Sakaguchi K, Shabanowitz J, Appella E, Hunt DF, Engelhard VH. HLA-A2.1-associated peptides from a mutant cell line: a second pathway of antigen presentation. Science 255:1264–1266, 1992.

41. Hickey WF, Ueno K, Hiserodt JC, Schmidt RE. Exogenously induced, natural killer cell-mediated neuronal killing: a novel pathogenetic mechanism. J Exp Med 176:811–817, 1992.

42. Hirsch RL. Natural killer cells appear to play no role in the recovery of mice from Sindbis virus infection. Immunology 43:81–89, 1981.

43. Hirsch RL, Griffin DE. The pathogenesis of Sindbis virus infection in athymic nude mice. J Immunol 123:1215–1218, 1979.

44. Hoffman PM, Cimino EF, Robbins DS. Effects of viral specific cytotoxic lymphocytes on the expression of murine leukemia virus induced neurologic disease. J Neuroimmunol 33:157–165, 1991.

45. Hohlfeld R, Engel AG. Immune responses in muscle. Semin Neurosci 4:249–255, 1992.

46. Inverardi L, Samaja M, Marelli F, Bender JR, Pardi R. Cellular early immune recognition of xenogeneic vascular endothelium. Transplant Proc 4:459–461, 1992.

47. Isono M, Poltorak M, Kulaga H, Adams AJ, Freed WJ. Certain host-donor rat strain combinations do not reject brain allografts after systemic sensitization. Exp Neurol 122:48–56, 1993.

48. Jaaskelainen J, Kalliomaki P, Paetau A, Timonen T. Effect of LAK cells against three-dimensional tumor tissue: in vitro study using multi-cellular human glioma spheroids as targets. J Immunol 142:1036–1045, 1989.

49. Johnson RT. Viral Infections of the Nervous System. Raven Press, New York, 1982.

50. Joly E, Mucke L, Oldstone MBA. Viral persistence in neurons explained by lack of major histocompatibility class I expression. Science 253:1283–1285, 1991.

51. Joly E, Oldstone MBA. Neuronal cells are deficient in loading peptides onto MHC class I molecules. Neuron 8:1185–1190, 1992.
52. Kärre K, Hansson M, Kiessling R. Multiple interactions at the natural killer workshop. Immunol Today 12:343–345, 1991.
53. Kaufman DS, Schoon RA, Leibson PJ. MHC class I expression on tumor targets inhibits natural killer cell-mediated cytotoxicity without interfering with target recognition. J Immunol 150:1429–1436, 1993.
54. Keane RW, Tallent MW, Podack ER. Resistance and susceptibility of neural cells to lysis by cytotoxic lymphocytes and by cytolytic granules. Transplantation 54:520–526, 1992.
55. Kerr RSC, Bartlett PF. The immune response to intraparenchymal fetal CNS transplants. Transplant Proc 21:3166–3168, 1989.
56. Kiessling R, Eriksson E, Hallenbeck LA, Welsh RM. A comparative analysis of the cell surface properties of activated *vs* endogenous mouse natural killer cells. J Immunol 125:1551–1556, 1980.
57. Kiessling R, Wigzell H. Surveillance of primitive cells by natural killer cells. Curr Top Microbiol Immunol 92:107–123, 1981.
58. Konno H, Yamamoto T, Suzuki H, Yamamoto H, Iwasaki Y, Ohara Y, Terunuma H, Harata N. Targeting of adoptively transferred experimental allergic encephalitis lesion at the sites of Wallerian degeneration. Acta Neuropathol 80:521–526, 1990.
59. Kos FJ, Mullbacher A. Specific epitope-induced conversion of CD8+ memory cells into effector cytotoxic T lymphocytes in vitro: presentation of peptide antigen by CD8+ T cells. Eur J Immunol 22:1595–1601, 1992.
60. Lampson LA. Molecular bases of the immune response to neural antigens. TINS 10:211–216, 1987.
61. Lampson LA. Cell-mediated immunotherapy directed against disseminated tumor in the brain. In: Astrocytomas: Diagnosis, Treatment and Biology, P McL Black, WC Schoene, LA Lampson, eds. 1993, Boston, Blackwell Scientific, 261–289.
62. Lampson LA. Mechanisms and control of cell migration in the adult CNS. Brain Pathol 4:123–124, 1994.
63. Lampson LA. Interpreting MHC class I expression and class I/class II reciprocity in the CNS: reconciling divergent findings. Microsc Res Tech 32:267–285, 1995.
63a. Lampson LA. Immunobiology of brain tumors: Antigens, effectors, and delivery to sites of microscopic tumor in the brain. P McL Black, JS Loeffler, eds., 1997, Cancer of the Nervous System, Boston, Blackwell, pp 874–906.
64. Lampson LA, Chen A, Vortmeyer AO, Sloan AE, Ghogawala Z, Kim L. Enhanced T cell migration to sites of microscopic CNS disease: Complementary treatments evaluated by 2- and 3-D image analysis. Brain Pathol 4:125–134, 1994.
65. Lampson LA, Fisher CA, Whelan JP. Striking paucity of HLA-A, B, C, and β_2-microglobulin on human neuroblastoma cell lines. J Immunol 130:2471–2478, 1983.
66. Lampson L, Ghogawala Z, Chen A, Kim L, Jenkins J. Enhancing interaction between CNS lymphoma and therapeutic cells. Cancer Res 35:516, 1994.
67. Lampson LA, Grabowska A, Whelan JP. Class I and II MHC expression and its implications for regeneration in the nervous system. Prog Brain Res 103:307–317, 1994.
68. Lampson LA, Hickey WF. Monoclonal antibody analysis of MHC expression in human brain biopsies: Tissue ranging from "histologically normal" to that showing different levels of glial tumor involvement. J Immunol 136:4054–4062, 1986.
69. Lampson LA, Kushner PD, Sobel RA. Major histocompatibility complex antigen expression in the affected tissues in amyotrophic lateral sclerosis. Ann Neurol 28:365–372, 1990.

70. Lampson LA, Lampson MA, Dunne AD. Exploiting the *lacZ* reporter gene for quantitative analysis of disseminated tumor growth within the brain: Use of the *lacZ* gene product as a tumor antigen, for evaluation of antigenic modulation, and to facilitate image analysis of tumor growth in situ. Cancer Res 53:176–182, 1993.

71. Lampson LA, Lampson MA, Dunne AD. Defining the range of cellular components, including internal antigens, that can serve as targets of graft rejection. J Neural Transplant Plast 3:240–241, 1992.

72. Lampson LA, Lampson MA, Dunne AD, Sethna MP. Tumor/cytokine interactions within the brain: Interactions between gamma interferon and visualizable brain tumor cells. Neurology 41 (Suppl 1):302, 1991.

73. Lampson LA, Wen P, Roman VA, Morris JH, Sarid JA. Disseminating tumor cells and their interactions with leukocytes visualized in the brain. Cancer Res 52:1018–1025, 1992.

74. Lehmann-Grube F, Moskophidis D, Lohler J. Recovery from acute virus infection. Role of cytotoxic T lymphocytes in the elimination of lymphocytic choriomeningitis virus from spleens of mice. Ann NY Acad Sci 532:238–256, 1988.

75. Leiden JM, Karpinski BA, Gottschalk L, Kornbluth J. Susceptibility to natural killer cell-mediated cytolysis is independent of the level of target cell class I HLA expression. J Immunol 142:2140–2147, 1989.

76. Levine B, Hardwick JM, Trapp BD, Crawford TO, Bollinger RC, Griffin DE. Antibody-mediated clearance of alphavirus infection from neurons. Science 254:856–860, 1991.

77. Levine B, Huang Q, Isaacs JT, Reed JC, Griffin DE, Hardwick JM. Conversion of lytic to persistent alphavirus infection by the *bcl*-2 cellular oncogene. Nature 361:739–742, 1993.

78. Levine S. Hyperacute, neutrophilic, and localized forms of experimental allergic encephalomyelitis: a review. Acta Neuropathol (Berl) 28:179–189, 1974.

79. Lindsley MD, Thiemann R, Rodriguez M. Cytotoxic T cells isolated from the central nervous systems of mice infected with Theiler's virus. J Virol 65:6612–6620, 1991.

80. Ljunggren H-G, Kärre K. In search of the 'missing self': MHC molecules and NK cell recognition. Immunol Today 11:237–244, 1990.

81. Ljunggren H-G, Sturmhöfel K, Wolpert E, Hämmerling GJ, Kärre K. Transfection of b$_2$-microglobulin restores IFN-mediated protection from natural killer cell lysis in YAC-1 lymphoma variants. J Immunol 145:380–386, 1990.

82. Ljunggren H-G, Yamasaki T, Collins P, Klein G, Kärre K. Selective acceptance of MHC class I-deficient tumor grafts in the brain. J Exp Med 167:730–735, 1988.

83. Loeffler JS, Alexander E III, Hochberg FH, Wen PY, Morris JH, Schoene WC, Siddon RL, Morse RH, Black PM. Clinical patterns of failure following stereotactic interstitial irradiation for malignant gliomas. Int J Radiat Oncol Biol Phys 19:1445–1462, 1990.

84. Ludowyk PA, Willenborg DO, Parish CR. Selective localisation of neuro-specific T lymphocytes in the central nervous system. J Neuroimmunol 37:237–250, 1992.

85. Lund RD, Rao K, Kunz HW, Gill TJ III. Immunological considerations in neural transplantion. Transplant Proc 21:3159–3162, 1989.

86. Mackay CR. T-cell memory: the connection between function, phenotype and migration pathways. Immunol Today 12:189–192, 1991.

87. Maehlen J, Olsson T, Löve A, Klareskog L, Norrby E, Kristensson K. Persistence of measles virus in rat brain neurons is promoted by depletion of CD8$^+$ T cells. J Neuroimmunol 21:149–155, 1989.

88. Main EK, Lampson LA, Hart MK, Kornbluth J, Wilson DB. Human neuroblastoma cell lines are susceptible to lysis by natural killer cells but not by cytotoxic T lymphocytes. J Immunol 135:242–246, 1985.

89. Main EK, Monos DS, Lampson LA. IFN-treated neuroblastoma cell lines remain resistant

to T cell-mediated allo-killing, and susceptible to non-MHC-restricted cytotoxicity. J Immunol 141:2943–2950, 1988.

90. Maio M, Altomonte M, Tatake R, Zeff RA, Ferrone S. Reduction in susceptibility to natural killer cell-mediated lysis of human FO-1 melanoma cells after induction of HLA class I antigen expression by transfection with β_2m gene. J Clin Invest 88:282–289, 1991.

91. Manning PT, Johnson EM Jr, Wilcox CL, Palmatier MA, Russell JH. MHC-specific cytotoxic T lymphocyte killing of dissociated sympathetic neuronal cultures. Am J Path 128:395–409, 1987.

92. Marrack P, Kappler J. T cells can distinguish between allogeneic major histocompatibility complex products on different cell types. Nature 332:840–843, 1988.

93. Mason D. The roles of T cell subpopulations in allograft rejection. Transplant Proc 20:239–242, 1988.

94. Mason DW, Morris PJ. Effector mechanisms in allograft rejection. Annu Rev Immunol 4:119–145, 1986.

95. Mattiace LA, Davies P, Dickson DW. Detection of HLA-DR on microglia in the human brain is a function of both clinical and technical factors. Am J Pathol 136:1101–1114, 1990.

96. Maziarz RT, Mentzer SJ, Burakoff SJ, Faller DV. Distinct effects of interferon-γ and MHC class I surface antigen levels on resistance of the K562 tumor cell line to natural killer-mediated lysis. Cell Immunol 130:329–338, 1990.

97. McMichael A. Natural selection at work on the surface of virus infected cells. Science 260:1771–1772, 1993.

98. Merchant RE, Ellison MD, Young HF. Immunotherapy for malignant glioma using human recombinant interleukin-2 and activated autologous lymphocytes: a review of pre-clinical and clinical investigations. J Neurooncol 8:173–188, 1990.

99. Miescher S, Whiteside TL, de Tribolet N, Von Fliedner V. *In situ* characterization, clonogenic potential, and antitumor cytolytic activity of T lymphocytes infiltrating human brain cancers. J Neurosurg 68:438–448, 1988.

100. Migita K, Eguchi K, Akiguchi I, Ida H, Kawakami A, Ueki Y, Kurata A, Fukuda T, Nagataki S. Synergistic effects of phorbol ester and interferon-α: target cell class I HLA antigen expression and resistance to natural killer and lymphokine-activated killer cell-mediated cytolysis. Cell Immunol 134:325–335, 1991.

101. Milton AD, Fabre JW. Massive induction of donor-type class I and class II major histocompatibility complex antigens in rejecting cardiac allografts in the rat. J Exp Med 161:98–112, 1985.

102. Molina IJ, Huber BT. The expression of a tissue-specific self-peptide is required for allorecognition. J Immunol 144:2082–2088, 1990.

103. Mucke L, Oldstone MBA. The expression of major histocompatibility complex (MHC) class I antigens in the brain differs markedly in acute and persistent infections with lymphocytic choriomeningitis virus (LCMV). J Neuroimmunol 36:193–198, 1992.

104. Mullbacher A, Ada GL. How do cytotoxic T lymphocytes work *in vivo*? Microb Pathog 3:315–318, 1987.

105. Murphy WJ, Kumar V, Bennett M. Natural killer cells activated with interleukin 2 *in vitro* can be adoptively transferred and mediate hematopoietic histocompatibility-1 antigen-specific bone marrow rejection *in vivo*. Eur J Immunol 20:1729–1734, 1990.

106. Nicholas MK, Arnason BGW. Immunologic considerations in transplantation to the central nervous system. In: Frontiers in Clinical Neuroscience, FJ Seil, ed. Alan R. Liss, New York, 1989.

107. Nicholas MK, Arnason BGW. A role for CD8+ T lymphocytes late in the rejection of

intraventricular fetal neocortical fragment allografts in the mouse. In: Pathophysiology of the Blood-brain Barrier, BB Johansson, Ch Owman, H Widner, eds. Elsevier, Amsterdam, 1990, pp 573–586.

108. Nicholas MK, Chenelle AG, Brown MM, Stefansson K, Arnason BGW. Prevention of neural allograft rejection in the mouse following in vivo depletion of L3T4+ but not LYT-2+ T-lymphocytes. Prog Brain Res 82:161–167, 1990.

109. Nuchtern JG, Biddison WE, Klausner RD. Class II MHC molecules can use the endogenous pathway of antigen presentation. Nature 343:74–76, 1990.

110. Öhlén C, Bejarano MT, Gronberg A, Torsteinsdottir S, Franksson L, Ljunggren HG, Klein E, Klein G, Karre K. Studies of sublines selected for loss of HLA expression from an EBV-transformed lymphoblastoid cell line: changes in sensitivity to cytotoxic T cells activated by allostimulation and natural killer cells activated by IFN or IL-2. J Immunol 142:3336–3341, 1989.

111. Öhlén C, Kling G, Hoglund P, Hansson M, Scangos G, Bieberich C, Jay G, Karre K. Prevention of allogeneic bone marrow graft rejection by H-2 transgene in donor mice. Science 246:666–668, 1989.

112. Oldstone MBA, Blount P, Southern PJ, Lampert PW. Cytoimmunotherapy for persistent virus infection reveals a unique clearance pattern from the central nervous system. Nature 321:239–243, 1986.

113. Olsson T, Maehlen J, Löve A, Klareskog L, Norrby E, Kristensson K. Induction of class I and class II transplantation antigens in rat brain during fatal and non-fatal measles virus infection. J Neuroimmunol 16:215–224, 1987.

114. O'Malley MB, MacLeish PR. Induction of class I major histocompatibility complex antigens on adult primate retinal neurons. J Neuroimmunol 43:45–58, 1993.

115. Paya CV, Patick AK, Leibson PJ, Rodriguez M. Role of natural killer cells as immune effectors in encephalitis and demyelination induced by Theiler's virus. J Immunol 143:95–102, 1989.

116. Peña J, Alonso C, Solana R, Serrano R, Carracedo J, Ramirez R. Natural killer susceptibility is independent of HLA class I antigen expression on cell lines obtained from human solid tumors. Eur J Immunol 20:2445–2449, 1990.

117. Peters PJ, Neefjes JJ, Oorschot V, Ploegh HL, Geuze HJ. Segregation of MHC class II molecules from MHC class I molecules in the Golgi complex for transport to lysosomal compartments. Nature 349:669–676, 1991.

118. Petito CK, Cho E-S, Lemann W, Navia BA, Price RW. Neuropathology of acquired immunodeficiency syndrome (AIDS): an autopsy review. J Neuropathol Exp Neurol 45:635–646, 1986.

119. Pollack IF, Lee LH-C, Zhou HF, Lund RD. Long-term survival of mouse corpus callosum grafts in neonatal rat recipients, and the effect of host sensitization. J Neurosci Res 31:33–45, 1992.

120. Poltorak M, Freed WJ. Immunological reactions induced by intracerebral transplantation: evidence that host microglia but not astroglia are the antigen-presenting cells. Exp Neurol 103:222–233, 1989.

121. Poltorak M, Freed WJ. BN rats do not reject F344 brain allografts even after systemic sensitization. Ann Neurol 29:377–388, 1991.

122. Poltorak M, Isono M, Freed WJ, Ronnet GV, Snyder SH. Human cortical neuronal cell line (HCN-1): further in vitro characterization and suitability for brain transplantation. Cell Transplant 1:3–15, 1992.

123. Quillet A, Presse F, Marchiol-Fournigault C, Harel-Bellan A, Benbunan M, Ploegh H, Fradelizi D. Increased resistance to non-MHC-restricted cytotoxicity related to HLA A, B expression. J Immunol 141:17–20, 1988.

124. Ramsay AJ, Ruby J, Ramshaw IA. A case for cytokines as effector molecules in the resolution of virus infection. Immunol Today 14:155–157, 1993.
125. Rao K, Lund RD, Kunz HW, Gill TJ III. The role of MHC and non-MHC antigens in the rejection of intracerebral allogeneic neural grafts. Transplantation 48:1018–1021, 1989.
126. Rapoport SI. Blood-brain Barrier in Physiology and Medicine. Raven Press, New York, 1976.
127. Reiter Z, Fischer DG, Rubinstein M. The protective effect of interferon against natural killing activity is not mediated via the expression of class I MHC antigens. Immunol Lett 17:323–328, 1988.
128. Reynolds CW, Ortaldo JR. Natural killer activity: the definition of a function rather than a cell type. Immunol Today 8:172–174, 1987.
129. Robbins DS, Hoffman PM. Virus-specific cytotoxic lymphocyte response in a neurotropic murine leukemia virus infection. J Neuroimmunol 31:9–17, 1991.
130. Rock KL, Gamble S, Rothstein L. Presentation of exogenous antigen with class I major histocompatibility complex molecules. Science 249:918–926, 1990.
131. Rossi ML, Hughes JT, Esiri MM, Coakham HB, Brownell DB. Immunohistological study of mononuclear cell infiltrate in malignant gliomas. Acta Neuropathol 74:269–277, 1987.
132. Ryan JC, Niemi EC, Goldfien RD, Hiserodt JC, Seaman WE. NKR-P1, an activating molecule on rat natural killer cells, stimulates phosphoinositide turnover and a rise in intracellular calcium. J Immunol 147:3244–3250, 1991.
133. Sawamura Y, Abe H, Aida T, Hosokawa M, Kobayashi H. Isolation and *in vitro* growth of glioma-infiltrating lymphocytes, and an analysis of their surface phenotypes. J Neurosurg 69:745–750, 1988.
134. Schwendemann G, Lohler J, Lehmann-Grube F. Evidence for cytotoxic T-lymphocyte–target cell interaction in brains of mice infected intracerebrally with lymphocytic choriomeningitis virus. Acta Neuropathol 61:183–195, 1983.
135. Sedgwick J, Brostoff S, Mason D. Experimental allergic encephalomyelitis in the absence of a classical delayed-type hypersensitivity reaction. J Exp Med 165:1058–1075, 1987.
136. Sellins KS, Cohen JJ. Cytotoxic T lymphocytes induce different types of DNA damage in target cells of different origins. J Immunol 147:795–803, 1991.
137. Selmaj K, Brosnan CF, Raine CS. Expression of heat shock protein-65 by oligodendrocytes in vivo and in vitro: implications for multiple sclerosis. Neurology 42:795–800, 1992.
138. Sentman CL, Kumar V, Koo G, Bennett M. Effector cell expression of NK1.1, a murine natural killer cell-specific molecule, and ability of mice to reject bone marrow allografts. J Immunol 142:1847–1853, 1989.
139. Sethna MP, Lampson LA. Immune modulation within the brain: recruitment of inflammatory cells and increased major histocompatibility antigen expression following intracerebral injection of interferon-γ. J Neuroimmunol 34:121–132, 1991.
140. Shimizu K, Okamoto Y, Miyao Y, Yamada M, Ushio Y, Hayakawa T, Ikeda H, Mogami H. Adoptive immunotherapy of human meningeal gliomatosis and carcinomatosis with LAK cells and recombinant interleukin-2. J Neurosurg 66:519–521, 1987.
141. Simmons RD, Willenborg DO. Direct injection of cytokines into the spinal cord causes autoimmune encephalomyelitis-like inflammation. J Neurol Sci 100:37–42, 1990.
142. Skias DD, Kim D-K, Reder AT, Antel JP, Lancki DW, Fitch FW. Susceptibility of astrocytes to class I MHC antigen-specific cytotoxicity. J Immunol 138:3254–3258, 1987.
143. Sloan AE, Lampson LA. Localization of inflammation to the cerebral hemispheres with minimal tissue damage in EAE, in both susceptible (LEW) and relatively resistant (CDF) rat strains. Neurology 42 (Suppl 3):347, 1992.
144. Sloan DJ, Baker BJ, Puklavec M, Charlton HM. The effect of site of transplantation and

histocompatibility differences on the survival of neural tissue transplanted to the CNS of defined inbred rat strains. Prog Brain Res 82:141–152, 1990.

145. Sloan DJ, Wood MJ, Charlton HM. The immune response to intracerebral neural grafts. TINS 14:341–346, 1991.

146. Speiser DE, Kyburz D, Stübi U, Hengartner H, Zinkernagel RM. Discrepancy between in vitro measurable and in vivo virus neutralizing cytotoxic T cell reactivities. J Immunol 149:972–980, 1992.

147. Stam NJ, Kast WM, Voordouw AC, Pastoors LB, Van Der Hoeven FA, Melief CJM, Ploegh HL. Lack of correlation between levels of MHC class I antigen and susceptibility to lysis of small cellular lung carcinoma (SCLC) by natural killer cells. J Immunol 142:4113–4117, 1989.

148. Steiniger B, van der Meide PH. Rat ependyma and microglia cells express class II MHC antigens after intravenous infusion of recombinant gamma interferon. J Neuroimmunol 19:111–118, 1988.

149. Stevens A, Klöter I, Roggendorf W. Inflammatory infiltrates and natural killer cell presence in human brain tumors. Cancer 61:738–743, 1988.

150. Storkus WJ, Alexander J, Payne JA, Cresswell P, Dawson JR. The a1/a2 domains of class I HLA molecules confer resistance to natural killing. J Immunol 143:3853–3857, 1989.

151. Storkus WJ, Alexander J, Payne JA, Dawson JR, Cresswell P. Reversal of natural killing susceptibility in target cells expressing transfected class I HLA genes. Proc Natl Acad Sci USA 86:2361–2364, 1989.

152. Storkus WJ, Salter RD, Alexander J, Ward FE, Ruiz RE, Cresswell P, Dawson JR. Class I-induced resistance to natural killing: identification of nonpermissive residues in HLA-A2. Proc Natl Acad Sci USA 88:5989–5992, 1991.

153. Streilein JW. Transplantation immunobiology in relation to neural grafting: lessons learned from immunologic privilege in the eye. Int J Devl Neurosci 6:497–511, 1988.

154. Sugawara S, Abo T, Itoh H, Kumagai K. Analysis of mechanisms by which NK cells acquire increased cytotoxicity against class I MHC-eliminated targets. Cell Immunol 119:304–316, 1989.

155. Sun D, Wekerle H. Ia-restricted encephalitogenic T lymphocytes mediating EAE lyse autoantigen-presenting astrocytes. Nature 320:70–72, 1986.

156. Sussman MA, Shubin RA, Kyuwa S, Stohlman SA. T-cell-mediated clearance of mouse hepatitis virus strain JHM from the central nervous system. J Virol 63:3051–3056, 1989.

157. Townsend A, Bodmer H. Antigen recognition by class I-restricted T lymphocytes. Annu Rev Immunol 7:601–624, 1989.

158. Trinchieri G. Biology of natural killer cells. Adv Immunol 47:187–376, 1989.

159. Tsai L, Öhlen C, Ljunggren H-G, Kärre K, Hansson M, Kiessling R. Effect of IFN-γ treatment and in vivo passage of murine tumor cell lines on their sensitivity to lymphokine-activated killer (LAK) cell lysis in vitro; association with H-2 expression on the target cells. Int J Cancer 44:669–674, 1989.

160. Turner WJD, Chatten J, Lampson LA. Human neuroblastoma cell growth in xenogeneic hosts: comparison of T cell-deficient and NK-deficient hosts, and subcutaneous or intravenous injection routes. J Neurooncol 8:121–132, 1990.

161. Unsicker K, Grothe C, Westermann R, Wewetzer K. Cytokines in neural regeneration. Curr Opin Neurobiol 2:671–678, 1992.

162. Van Twuyver E, Mooijaart RJ, Kast WM, Melief CJ, de Waal LP. Different requirements for the regulation of transplantation tolerance induction for allogeneic versus xenogeneic major histocompatibility complex antigens. Hum Immunol 29:220–228, 1990.

163. Vaquero J, Coca S, Escandon J, Magallon R, Martinez R. Immunohistochemical study of IOT-10 natural killer cells in brain metastases. Acta Neurochir 104:17–20, 1990.

164. Vaquero J, Coca S, Oya S, Martinez R, Ramiro J, Salazar FG. Presence and significance of NK cells in glioblastomas. J Neurosurg 70:728–731, 1989.

165. Vass K, Lassmann H. Intrathecal application of interferon gamma: progressive appearance of MHC antigens within the rat nervous system. Am J Pathol 137:789–800, 1990.

166. Versteeg R, Peltenburg LTC, Plomp AC, Schrier PI. High expression of the *c-myc* oncogene renders melanoma cells prone to lysis by natural killer cells. J Immunol 143:4331–4337, 1989.

167. Vivier E, Rochet N, Ackerly M, Petrini J, Levine H, Daley J, Anderson P. Signaling function of reconstituted CD16: zeta: gamma receptor complex isoforms. Int Immunol 4:1313–1323, 1992.

168. Von Hanwehr RI, Hofman FM, Taylor CR, Apuzzo MLJ. Mononuclear lymphoid populations infiltrating the microenvironment of primary CNS tumors. J Neurosurg 60:1138–1147, 1984.

169. Weaver CT, Unanue ER. The costimulatory function of antigen-presenting cells. Immunol Today 11:49–55, 1990.

170. Wen PY, Lampson MA, Lampson LA. Effects of γ-interferon on major histocompatibility complex antigen expression and lymphocytic infiltration in the 9L gliosarcoma brain tumor model: implications for strategies of immunotherapy. J Neuroimmunol 36:57–68, 1992.

171. White LA, Keane RW, Whittemore SR. Differentiation of an immortalized CNS neuronal cell line decreases their susceptibility to cytotoxic T cell lysis *in vitro*. J Neuroimmunol 49:135–43, 1994.

172. Whiteside TL, Herberman RB. The biology of human natural killer cells. Ann Ist Super Sanita 26:335–348, 1990.

173. Whiteside TL, Herberman RB. Extravasation of antitumor effector cells. Invasion Metastasis 12:128–146, 1992.

174. Widner H, Brundin P. Immunological aspects of grafting in the mammalian central nervous system. A review and speculative synthesis. Brain Res Revs 13:287–324, 1988.

175. Williamson JSP, Stohlman SA. Effective clearance of mouse hepatitis virus from the central nervous system requires both CD4$^+$ and CD8$^+$ T cells. J Virol 64:4589–4592, 1990.

176. Wood MJA, Sloan DJ, Dallman MJ, Charlton HM. A monoclonal antibody to the interleukin-2 receptor enhances the survival of neural allografts: a time-course study. Neuroscience 49:409–418, 1992.

177. Wucherpfennig KW, Newcombe J, Li H, Keddy C, Cuzner ML, Hafler DA. γδ T-cell receptor repertoire in acute multiple sclerosis lesions. Proc Natl Acad Sci USA 89:4588–4592, 1992.

178. Yamaguchi K, Goto N, Kyuwa S, Hayami M, Toyoda Y. Protection of mice from a lethal coronavirus infection in the central nervous system by adoptive transfer of virus-specific T cell clones. J Neuroimmunol 32:1–9, 1991.

179. Yewdell JW, Bennink JR. The binary logic of antigen processing and presentation to T cells. Cell 62:203–206, 1990.

14

Neuroendocrine–Immune Interactions

DOUGLAS A. WEIGENT
J. EDWIN BLALOCK

Historical Survey

That the mind might influence the well-being of an individual is an almost timeless concept with obvious implications for infection and immunity. Perhaps the first evidence that this could occur in part through an action of the central nervous system (CNS) on the immune system came with the observation of Metal'nikov and Chorine (90), later confirmed and extended by Ader and Cohen (for review, see 1), that Pavlovian conditioning methods could be used to modulate the immune system. The first mechanism by which the CNS might affect the immune system came from Selye's classic observations of thymic involution during "stress" (110). With a better understanding of the mechanism of stress arose the still somewhat dominant idea that adrenal glucocorticoids are solely responsible for neuroendocrine control of immunity (33). This was supported by the immunosuppressive activity of glucocorticoids (29). More recent studies have clearly shown that glucocorticoids are not the sole players in immune neuroendocrine communication since stressed adrenalectomized animals are functionally immunosuppressed (80). An important role for the pituitary gland in the development and regulation of the immune system was next observed in the impaired lymphoid cell numbers and function in hypopituitary mice (6,7). This observation was confirmed and extended by the finding of similar immunologic dysfunction in hypophysectomized mice and rats which are corrected by pituitary grafts (for review, see 105).

Direct evidence for CNS regulation of immune function came with the demonstration that electrolytic lesions of various brain areas could either facilitate or inhibit

548

immune reactivity (31). Interestingly, the effects of the brain lesions were ablated by removal of the pituitary gland (for review, see 105). Thus, it appeared as if CNS recognition of an immunologic stress was transduced into neural-immune stimuli through an action involving the pituitary and adrenal glands.

While these discoveries constituted in part the foundation for the pathways of communication from the CNS to the immune system, an equally exciting series of experiments pointed to this information flow as being bidirectional rather than unidirectional (13). Largely due to the work of Besedovsky, Sorkin, and colleagues, hormonal and neuronal changes were observed coincident with the generation of an immune response (for review, see 13). For instance, an increase in circulating glucocorticoids and the firing rate of hypothalamic neurons was observed after antigenic challenge. Collectively, this work led to the idea that the immune system could exert a regulatory influence on the neuroendocrine system and that this might be a feedback mechanism by which the immune system regulates itself. Although these studies clearly demonstrated that there was crosstalk between the immune and neuroendocrine systems, an integrated hormonal–molecular mechanism by which this could occur was lacking. Insights into this mechanism began with our discovery that certain brain and pituitary peptides, such as corticotropin (ACTH) and endorphins, were actually synthesized by lymphocytes (for review, see 17). Furthermore, these neuropeptides acted upon lymphocytes which were demonstrated to express receptors for them (70). Conversely, pituitary cells were first found to be acted upon by interleukins (IL) 1 and 6 (131), and we predicted that cytokines would be produced by cells of the neuroendocrine system (15). These observations were formulated into the very simple biochemical mechanism of shared receptors and ligands as the means of communication between the immune and neuroendocrine system (14). These findings ultimately led to our conclusion that the immune system is a sensory organ for stimuli not recognized by the nervous system (14). Thus immune rather than neural recognition of viruses, bacteria, tumor cells, or antigens could lead to physiologic changes as a result of leukocyte release of shared peptides acting on receptors common to the immune and neuroendocrine systems.

At this time, concepts based upon the above historical foundations are under intense investigation. As will be described in more detail below, more additional information has been accumulated in a relatively short period of time. This data in turn has led to a clearer understanding of how the immune system interfaces with other physiologic systems.

Basic Scientific Discoveries

Actions of Neuroendocrine Hormones and Neuropeptides on the Immune System

A great deal of data has been published to support the idea that neuroendocrine polypeptide hormones and neuropeptides can regulate the immune response (69). The effects can be positive or negative and all the major immune cell types appear to be influenced (Table 14-1). It is very likely that the neuroendocrine hormones and neuro-peptides produced by lymphocytes perform most functions in an autocrine or paracrine fashion within the immune system as opposed to the endocrine effects of molecules released from the pituitary. The in vitro studies describing the effects of neuroendocrine hormones on lymphoid cells are briefly described below for ACTH and endorphins, thyroid stimulating hormone (TSH), prolactin (PRL), and growth hormone (GH).

The evidence that ACTH and endorphin-like activities were made by lymphocytes prompted a study of the effect of ACTH on antibody production (70). It was discovered that ACTH profoundly inhibited antibody production. ACTH's ability to suppress the antibody response to T-dependent antigens (Ag) was more effective than T-independent Ag, suggesting that ACTH may interfere with the production or action of helper T-cell signals. ACTH 1-24, like ACTH 1-39, has full steroidogenic activity, yet had no effect on antibody production, suggesting that the immunoregulatory effects of ACTH may

Table 14-1 Major Effects of Neuroendocrine Hormones and Neuropeptides on Cells of the Immune System

Hormone	Immunologic Function
ACTH	Suppression of antibody synthesis
	Suppression of IFN-γ synthesis and IFN-γ-mediated macrophage activation
	Suppress MHC class II expression by macrophages
	Stimulates B-cell proliferation
	Stimulate NK-cell activity
Endorphin	Enhance the generation of cytotoxic T cells and NK-cell activity
	Modulate T-cell proliferation
	Modulate antibody synthesis
	Chemotactic for monocytes and neutrophils
TSH	Enhances antibody synthesis
GH	Enhances the generation of cytotoxic T cells
	Stimulates the production of superoxide anion by macrophages
	Stimulates erythroid colony formation
PRL	Comitogenic with ConA and induces IL-2 receptors
	Activates PKC
AVP	Replacement of IL-2 requirement for IFN-γ synthesis
SOM	Suppression of T-cell proliferation
	Inhibits the secretion of IFN-γ and colony-stimulating factor
GHRH	Stimulate lymphocyte proliferation
	Inhibit NK activity
	Inhibit chemotactic response

be associated with different structural parts of ACTH than those involved in steroidogenesis. ACTH has also been shown to stimulate the growth and differentiation of enriched cultures of human tonsillar B cells (2). More recently, ACTH has been shown to suppress MHC class II expression by murine peritoneal macrophages (136); stimulate natural killer (NK) cell activity (88); modulate the rise in intracellular-free calcium concentration after T-cell activation (77); suppress the production of interferon (IFN)-γ (71); and function as a late-acting B-cell growth factor that can synergize with IL-5 (21). Thus ACTH appears to influence the immune response at several key stages (Table 14-1).

The endogenous opiates β-, γ- and α-endorphin are also contained in the polyprotein proopiomelanocortin (POMC) and have been shown to modulate the activity of cells in the immune system (25,70). α-endorphin is a potent inhibitor of the anti-sheep red blood cell (SRBC) plaque-forming cell (PFC) response while β- and γ-endorphin are mild inhibitors (70). Many other aspects of immunity are modulated by the opiate peptides, including *(a)* enhancement of the natural cytotoxicity of lymphocytes and macrophages toward tumor cells; *(b)* enhancement or inhibition T-cell mitogenesis; *(c)* enhancement of T-cell rosetting; *(d)* stimulation of human peripheral blood mononuclear cells; and *(e)* inhibition of major histocompatibility (MHC) class II antigen expression (for review, see 25).

The early observation that hypothyroidism was observed in athymic mice suggested a relationship between the thyroid gland and the immune system (100). Later it was shown that TSH could augment both T-dependent and T-independent antibody production (69). TSH had to be present in the medium during the first 24–48 hours of culture for enhancement of the antibody response to occur. In additional studies, it was shown that thyrotropin releasing hormone (TRH) also enhanced the antibody plaque-forming cell response and induced splenocyte production of TSH (84). This enhancement by TRH was specifically blocked by antibodies to the TSH β-subunit, which demonstrated that the action of TRH was through its ability to induce TSH production by lymphocytes. This was the first demonstration that a pituitary hormone could function as an autocrine or paracrine regulator of the immune system (84). Subsequently, studies have suggested that TSH may elevate cAMP levels in B-cell lines and may also influence differentiation (59).

In addition to TSH, evidence has accumulated that suggest PRL has important immunoregulatory activities (for review, see 49). Animal studies have shown that lymphoid hyperplasia results from the injection of PRL, and that a reduction in PRL levels by bromocryptive diminishes T-cell responsiveness and function (12). In vitro studies show that PRL is comitogenic with concanavalin A and induces IL-2 receptors on the surface of lymphocytes (92). PRL stimulates ornithine decarboxylase and activates protein kinase C, which are important enzymes in the differentiation, proliferation, and function of lymphocytes.

A number of observations indicate that GH has an important influence on the maintenance of humoral and cell-mediated immunity (for review, see 81). Treatment of hypophysectomized animals with GH stimulated the expression of the *c-myc* oncogene and DNA synthesis and reversed the involution of the spleen and thymus (93). These growth-promoting effects may influence all the lymphoid cell types and may be the principal mechanism by which GH enhances the function of the immune system. Moreover, GH promotes engraftment of human T cells in severe combined immunodeficient (SCID) mice (94). Overall, GH also appears to modulate the cytolytic activity of T cells, antibody synthesis, granulocyte differentiation, tumor necrosis factor (TNF)-α production by macrophages (Table 14-1). Our own studies show that leukocyte-derived GH plays an important role in lymphocyte proliferation as well as in the inducing synthesis of leukocyte-derived insulin-like growth factors (8,130).

Substances from the anterior pituitary are not unique in possessing the ability to affect the immune system. The posterior pituitary releases arginine vasopressin (AVP), which is produced in the hypothalamus and subsequently transported to the pituitary where it stimulates the release of ACTH and enhances the corticotropin-releasing hormone (CRH)-mediated ACTH release (115). This hormone, in addition to its antidiuretic and vasopressor activities, also influences the immune response. AVP plays an important role in enhancing IFN-γ production by providing a costimulatory signal to lymphocytes that is able to replace IL-2. Overall, the effects of AVP appear to be positive and opposite to those of ACTH on T-cell function.

The influence of hypothalamic hormones on immunity is being extensively investigated and includes studies of CRH, growth hormone–releasing hormone and somatostatin (SOM). SOM has potent inhibitory effects on immune responses (116). SOM has been shown to significantly inhibit Molt-4 lymphoblast proliferation and phytohemagglutinin antigen (PHA) stimulation of human T lymphocytes (99). In addition, nanomolar concentrations of SOM inhibit the proliferation of both spleen- and Peyer's patch–derived lymphocytes. Other immune responses, such as staphylococcus enterotoxin A (SEA)–stimulated IFN-γ secretion, endotoxin-induced leukocytosis, and colony-stimulating activity release are also inhibited by SOM (for review, see 69).

Evidence has been obtained indicating that GHRH may be involved in immunomodulation (127). GHRH has been shown to stimulate lymphocyte proliferation, inhibit NK activity, and inhibit the chemotactic response (134). Our own studies have identified a specific GHRH receptor on immune cells, and we have measured an increase in Ca^{2+} uptake, thymidine incorporation, and the levels of GH RNA in such cells after treatment with GHRH. Since leukocytes can function as a source of immunoreactive (ir)GH, this suggests the possibility that irGHRH synthesis by leukocytes may function in an autocrine manner as a signal for the synthesis of leukocyte-derived irGH. It has also been reported that CRH is able to influence immune function (for review, see 62). The most important function of CRH may be to stimulate production of immunoreactive POMC peptides after stimulation with CRH. Thus the effects of ACTH and endorphins discussed above may be initiated in the immune system via hypothalamic releasing hormones. Along another line, some studies suggest that CRH modulates the immune response to stress in the rat by inhibiting lymphocyte proliferation and natural killer cell activity (67). Overall, it appears that hypothalamic and pituitary hormones have significant enhancing and inhibitory effects on the immune system.

Receptors for Neuroendocrine Peptide Hormones and Neuropeptides in the Immune System

The interaction between the immune and neuroendocrine system is mediated by signal molecules that interact with specific cell-surface receptors. A growing body of evidence supports the presence of neuroendocrine hormone and neuropeptide receptors on lymphocytes. These receptors appear to be similar to their neuroendocrine counterparts (Table 14-2). Some of the evidence is briefly discussed below.

The presence of ACTH receptors have been described on the surface of both T and B lymphocytes (27). They possess both high- and low-affinity binding sites. Interestingly, nonstimulated thymocytes possess few receptors (27). It appears that B lymphocytes possess three times the number of high-affinity binding sites as compared to T lymphocytes (27). Treatment of lymphocytes with the mitogen ConA increases the number of high-affinity ACTH receptors on these cells by two- to three-fold (27). ConA stimulation of thymocytes results in a 100-fold increase in the high-affinity ACTH receptor binding site. ACTH binding to its receptor initiates a signal transduction pathway that involves cyclic AMP and mobilization of Ca^{2+}. Activation of the high-affinity site increases calcium flux, while ACTH binding to the low-affinity receptor is thought to affect regulatory elements in the adenylate system (68). This mechanism in cells of the immune system is similar to the one advanced for the actions of ACTH in the stimulation of steroidogenesis in adrenal cells.

Table 14-2 Neuroendocrine Peptide Receptors on Cells of the Immune System[a]

Receptor	Immunocyte Source	Kd (nM)	Number of Sites
ACTH	Rat spleen T and B cells	90	(low) 1,000–4,000
		4	(high) 30,000–40,000
β-endorphin	Mouse spleen	4	0.1–0.3 fmol/10^6 cells
GH	Human PBL	1–10	6,000–8,000
PRL	Human PBL	1.7	360
TSH	Mouse cell line	1–3	25–50 fmol/mg
SOM	Human PBL (activated)	11	7×10^5 cells
CRH	Human PBL	0.26	8.74 fmol/mg
GHRH	Rat spleen	2.5	35 fmol/10^6 cells
TRH	Mouse Molt 4 T-cell line	20 (low)	—
LHRH	Rat thymocytes	84	14 fmol/mg

[a]For a more detailed review and description of how the values were obtained, see Azad et al. (4).

Opioid receptors were first identified in neuronal tissue and are designated into four distinct classes termed μ, δ, ε, and κ, based on ligand-binding characteristics. The characterization of immunocyte opioid receptors is still in progress, but the same four classes defined by neuronal tissue binding have been identified on cells of the immune system (25). The lymphocyte receptors for the opioid peptides appear to share many of the unique features with those described for neuronal tissue. These characteristics include molecular size, immunogenicity, and the use of specific intracellular signaling pathways (25). The opioid receptors in the immune system are apparently linked to the production of IL-2, since β-endorphin has been shown to up-regulate this cytokine (50).

Thyrotropin (TSH) receptors have been identified on lymphoid cell lines and murine splenocytes. The murine spleen TSH receptor is specific to B lymphocytes and B-cell lines, including a pre-B cell and immunoglobulin (IgM- and IgG-secreting cell lines (53,59). The expression of the TSH receptor is elevated with activation of the cell. Murine splenocytes enriched for T and B cells display no measurable TSH receptors; however, liposaccharide (LPS)-stimulated B cells express high-affinity receptors, while SEA-stimulated T cells do not (56). This work has been confirmed in human immune cells (30). In one report, TSH stimulated Ig production and increased intracellular cAMP levels in mouse lymphocytes, while in another study done on human immune cells, no change was seen in adenylate cyclase activity after TSH treatment (30,59).

The results of previous studies showed that PRL and GH stimulated lymphocyte proliferation, suggesting that cells of the immune system have receptors for PRL and GH (for review, see 49). More detailed analysis has shown that saturable, high-affinity PRL receptors are found on T, B, and large granular lymphoid (LGL) cells (106). High concentrations of cyclosporin decrease PRL receptor expression while low concentrations increase the number of cell surface PRL receptors (107). Specific oligonucleotide primers based on the rat liver PRL receptor sequence have been used in the polymerase chain reaction (PCR) to detect mRNA for the PRL receptor in the Nb2 T-cell line, thymocytes, and splenocytes (132). GH receptors have been identified on both thymocytes and lymphocytes with high-affinity binding constants at a concentration of 6,000–8,000 binding sites per cell. Human IM-9 lymphocytes have been used for the radioreceptor assay of GH and biochemical studies of the hormone receptor. In this system, lymphocyte-derived GH has been shown to bind to the GH receptor on lymphocytes, which suggests that this molecule may serve an autocrine or paracrine role in immunity (26). Additional studies show that phorbol esters reduce human GH (hGH)-stimulated growth of IM-9 lymphocytes by down-regulation of GH receptors (121). It appears that phosphorylation of a receptor-associated protein by protein kinase C may be involved in this receptor's regulation. Recent findings in rat tissues suggest that two or more GH receptor RNA molecules are present in tissues from normal and hypophysectomized rats. The levels of these RNAs are under differential hormonal regulation in liver, muscle, and fat, but specific cells of the immune system have not yet been examined. Interestingly, the molecular structure of the GH receptor and the PRL receptor identifies them as members of a new receptor superfamily that includes several cytokine receptors (10). No signal transducing domain has yet been identified, and it is possible these receptors may interact with other membrane proteins that function as mediators of signal transduction.

Other neuroendocrine receptors have been identified on cells of the immune system, although they are less well characterized. These include receptors for AVP and hypothalamic releasing factors. AVP receptors have been categorized into V1 receptors causing calcium mobilization or V2 receptors which stimulate cAMP production (41). Cells of the immune system appear to have novel V1-like receptors as determined by the blocking ability of different V1 and V2 antagonists (69). CRH mediates a variety of effects on cells of the immune system that take place through specific cell receptors. Cell-surface high-affinity CRH receptors coupled to the adenylate cyclase system are found on macrophage-enriched populations and on B lymphocytes (123,124). GHRH receptors have also been identified on cells of the immune system. These latter receptor binding sites are saturable and are found on both thymocytes and splenic lymphocytes. The results of chemical cross-linking studies using $[^{125}I]$GHRH show that thymocytes possess two such binding sites with molecular weights of 42 and 27 kDa. Following GHRH binding to its receptor, there is a rapid increase in intracellular Ca^{2+} which is associated with the stimulation of lymphocyte proliferation (52). Additionally, luteinizing hormone-releasing hormone (LHRH) receptors have been functionally identified on thymocytes (18).

Several studies have demonstrated that cells of the immune system express receptors for SOM (64,108). Recently, one group has described the existence of distinct subsets of SOM receptors on the Jurkat line of human leukemic T cells and U266 IgG-producing human myeloma cells (42). They showed that these cells have both high- and low-affinity receptors with K_d values in the pM and nM range, respectively. The authors speculate that two subsets of receptors may account for the biphasic concentration-dependent nature of the effects of SOM in some systems. Finally, leukocytes have been shown to respond to TRH treatment as well as producing TSH mRNA and protein. More recent work has shown the presence of two receptor types for TRH present on T cells (56). One of these sites satisfies the criteria for a classical TRH receptor and is involved in the release of IFN-γ from T cells (54).

Overall, it appears that numerous types of neuroendocrine receptors exist on cells of the immune system. Many of these receptors have characteristics which are nearly identical to those receptors found on neuroendocrine tissue. It appears from recent data obtained from patients with neuroendocrine disorders that receptors for ACTH, CRH, TRH, and GHRH that are rendered less responsive to stimulation in the neuroendocrine system are also blunted in the immune system. This result is consistent with their structural similarity and their expression and function being subject to similar influences.

Production of Neuroendocrine Peptide Hormones by the Immune System

The first neuroendocrine hormone identified as being produced in the immune system was corticotropin (ACTH) (for review, see 17). Lymphoid cells were observed to produce ACTH following viral infection or interaction with LPS (112) and, more recently, after exposure to CRH (115). Leukocyte-derived endorphins were shown to be coordinately produced along with ACTH probably from the common precursor, proopiomelanocortin (POMC) (57). The shared characteristics between immune system and pituitary-derived ACTH and endorphins include shared antigenicity as determined with monospecific antibodies against synthetic peptide hormones; identical retention times on reverse-phase, high-pressure liquid chromatographic (HPLC) columns; identical molecular weights; and shared biological activities and the presence of POMC-related mRNA in lymphocytes and macrophages. The identity between pituitary and leukocyte ACTH has been established by showing that the amino acid and nucleotide sequences in mice are identical (113). Cells of the immune system also synthesize enkephalins, since abundant levels of preproenkephalin mRNA has been found in activated but not resting T helper cells (135). ACTH secretion from lymphocytes has also been shown to occur after thymopentin treatment in vitro (23). Along similar lines, POMC mRNA increased in the spleen during development of adjuvant-induced arthritis in which ACTH and circulating levels of corticosteroid are elevated but hypothalamic expression of CRH is reduced (120). In this latter model, IL-1 is increased and is thought to play an important role in mediating the increase in the systemic levels of ACTH synthesized by the pituitary and spleen. It has been shown that CRH acts by stimulating monocytes to produce the cytokine IL-1 (131). IL-1 then activates B lymphocytes to secrete the POMC-derived β-endorphin. β-endorphin synthesis in turn was sensitive to inhibition by dexamethasone through its ability to inhibit IL-1 rather than β-endorphin itself (78). Supporting this model, lymphocyte production of β-endorphin has been demonstrated in vivo after subcutaneous administration of CRH to rats (79). Thus it appears that CRH and IL-1 play pivotal roles in the production of POMC products and in the interaction between the neuroendocrine and immune systems.

In addition to responding to TSH, certain cells of the immune system also produce immunoreactive TSH (for review, see 16 and 17). This response was initially observed in human peripheral blood cells after exposure to a T-cell mitogen. TSH is also produced by human T-cell leukemia cell lines (55). One of these cell lines expressed mRNA, but not protein, for the TSH β-subunit, whereas the other cell line expressed intact TSH that could be induced by TRH and inhibited by triiodothyronine (T_3). TSH-β mRNA has been observed in mouse lymphocytes as well.

The expression of prolactin (PRL) was originally thought to be restricted only to the pituitary; however, several reports now suggest that murine splenic lymphocytes may also synthesize or contain PRL (for review, see 46). Initially, it was reported that lymphocytes transcribe a PRL-like mRNA transcript of about 10 kb in spleen cells after stimulation with ConA (63). In support of these results, PRL-like molecules were detected in the supernatant of stimulated cells using the NB2 cell growth assay. Western blot analysis of lymphocyte lysates using antisera to PRL showed a protein with a molecular weight of 48 kDa, compared to pituitary PRL of 23 kDa (82). In contrast to these data, another report suggested that PRL in lymphocytes resulted from internalization of the hormone from fetal bovine serum in culture medium (28). In a series of molecular studies, PRL gene expression has been evaluated in detail in IM-9 cells, a human B-lymphoblastoid cell line. These studies have detected PRL mRNA in cells and detected the protein in the medium by bioassay and immunoassay. The hPRL secreted by these cells is indistinguishable from pituitary hPRL by immunological, biological, and electrophoretic criteria. Analysis of the PRL mRNA transcript from IM-9 lymphocytes revealed that it was 150 nucleotides longer than pituitary PRL mRNA in the 5′ untranslated region. Primer extension analysis has shown that a new transcription initiation site exists 5–7 Kb upstream of exon 1 of the pituitary PRL gene (35). The proximal and distal pituitary-1 binding sites which are important in regulating gene expression are part of a new intron spliced out of the primary mRNA transcript. The release of PRL in this cell line is inhibited by dexamethasone but unaffected by other factors that regulate pituitary PRL secretion, including TRH, vasoactive intestinal peptide (VIP), T_3, and dopamine. The IM-9 cell line, although unresponsive to many PRL secretogogues, does respond to short-term treatment with phorbol ester in the same manner as the pituitary lactotroph. These differences in the pattern of regulation could be due to tissue-specific parameters manifested by the nonendocrine nature of synthesis of PRL by the immune system. New insights on the regulation of PRL gene expression in IM-9 cells will help determine the role of PRL in regulating immune function.

Recent work by ourselves and others has established that cells of the immune system also produce GH (for review, 127). The difference between other neuroendocrine hormones and GH is that once animals are sacrificed and tissues removed from animals, the leukocytes spontaneously produce and secrete an immunoreactive GH that is similar to pituitary GH by both immunologic and biologic techniques (126). GH mRNA can be detected after 4 hours of in vitro culture in cells from spleen, thymus, bone marrow, and peripheral blood. The mRNA has the same molecular weight as pituitary GH mRNA and is translated into a 22-kDa biologically active irGH. Additional studies utilizing reverse transcription and polymerase chain reaction to generate cDNA molecules resulted in a single major DNA band corresponding in length to the distance between the 5′ ends of the two GH primers and identical to the product obtained when pituitary RNA was used as the template. The DNA band specifically hybridized to a GH-specific probe after Southern transfer. The similarity of the samples amplified by PCR from leukocytes and the pituitary was confirmed by restriction enzyme analysis. The cloning and sequencing of leukocyte GH cDNA showed that there were only four nucleotide differences throughout the molecule. These differences may be sequencing errors or they may encode two different amino acids from pituitary GH—one near the amino terminal and the other near the carboxy terminal end of the protein. Overall, the studies suggest that an almost identical GH molecule is produced by leukocytes. The significance of the amino acid differences and whether they are allelic differences or sequencing errors is unclear. The production of GH by leukocytes has been confirmed by two independent groups using normal and transformed cell lines (61,74).

The secretion of GH by immune cells appears to have similarities (induction by GHRH) and differences (no effect with GH or somatostatin) when compared to that described for the pituitary (127). Since it had been shown that cells of the immune system manufacture neuroendocrine hormones and that hypothalamic releasing hormones have direct effects upon the immune system, we and others hypothesized that immune cells might produce releasing factors. In general, it appears that cells of the immune system have the ability to produce hypothalamic releasing factors similar in structure and function to those originally identified in the neuroendocrine system (for review, see 129). The first report on this topic described the presence of corticotropin releasing factor mRNA and irCRH in nonstimulated human peripheral blood lymphocytes and neutrophils (118). In situ hybridization demonstrated CRH mRNA in both T and B lymphocytes. Northern blot analysis detected a CRH-like mRNA of around 1.7 Kb in comparison with a 1.5 Kb mRNA species associated with human hypothalamic CRH. Although the lymphocyte-derived material reacts with anti-CRH antiserum, the irCRH is not identical with CRH-41, since dilution curves in a radioimmunoassay (RIA) are not parallel and the leukocyte irCRH is more labile. In this initial report, no biological function studies were reported (118). However, the demonstration that lymphocytes can produce POMC peptides after stimulation with CRH, in conjunction with other studies showing potent direct immunosuppressive effects of CRH on lymphocytes, suggests that the lymphocyte product could exert direct immunomodulatory effects in an autocrine manner or indirectly influence immune function through the induction of POMC intermediates. The second hypothalamic releasing factor identified as being produced by cells of the immune system was GHRH (130). Our studies in the rat showed that lymphocyte GHRH-related RNA was polyadenylated and of the same molecular mass as hypothalamic GHRH RNA. Antibody affinity chromatography followed by size separation columns demonstrated two peaks of irGHRH. The smaller peak (5 kDa) was de novo synthesized, could bind to the GHRH receptor, and increased GH mRNA synthesis in lymphocytes and pituitary cells. This finding was the first demonstration that lymphocyte-derived GHRH was active on pituitary cells. In subsequent studies, we have shown that hypothalamic GHRH has an effect on leukocytes and that cells of the immune system have receptors for GHRH similar to those described on pituitary cells. Our work in the rat has been confirmed in human PBL with one important difference: our results suggest that irGHRH has a molecular weight similar to that of hypothalamic GHRH in the rat, whereas in the human the data suggest a molecular weight of approximately 50 kD (119).

In another series of studies, rat splenic lymphocytes were shown to contain an immunoreactive, bioactive luteinizing hormone-releasing hormone (LHRH) (39). Increasing amounts of lymphocyte irLHRH displaced ^{125}I-LHRH from LHRH antibodies in an RIA with kinetics parallel to that obtained with synthetic hypothalamic LHRH. The lymphocyte product stimulated the release of LH in a dose-dependent fashion and could be significantly inhibited by an LHRH antagonist (4). These same authors, using reverse transcription and the polymerase chain reaction, synthesized a 375 base pair cDNA both from lymphocytes and from the hypothalamus that hybridized to a specific LHRH cDNA probe (for review, see 17). A more recent report has confirmed this finding and has also shown that the cDNA sequence of hypothalamic and lymphocyte LHRH are identical (86).

In addition to GHRH and CRH, the hypothalamus-derived inhibiting hormone, somatostatin, has been identified in platelets, mononuclear leukocytes, mast cells, and polymorphonuclear leukocytes (17). Although the amino acid sequences have not been fully defined, the SOM from these hematologic sources appears to be larger than the CNS-produced neuropeptide and has a similar, but not identical, amino acid composition (51). In conclusion, cells of the immune system can serve as a source of neuroendocrine hormones and neuropeptides. Although the molecules appear to be predominantly the same or very similar to their CNS counterparts, they are in some respects regulated differently than what has been reported for the corresponding neuroendocrine substances.

Actions of Cytokines on the Neuroendocrine System

The effects of cytokines on neuroendocrine function have not been completely elucidated, but accumulating evidence suggests important roles for cytokines in linking the immune and neuroendocrine systems (Table 14-3). In this respect, the actions of IL-1, IL-2, IL-6, TNF, and IFN-γ have been the most thoroughly studies (66). The cytokine IL-1 has a number of biologic activities, including pronounced effects on the nervous and neuroendocrine systems. It is now clear that IL-1 can activate the hypothalamic-pituitary-adrenal (HPA) axis (111). This cytokine appears to act directly on the central nervous system, on the pituitary, and on the adrenal gland itself. Intravenous injection of IL-1, β induces a rapid rise in plasma ACTH; moreover, an intracerebroventricular injection elicits an even greater plasma ACTH increase, suggesting a site of action of IL-1 in the CNS (108). The effect of IL-1 can be abolished by pretreatment with anti-CRH-antisera, indicating that CRH mediates the action of IL-1 (108). An increase in

Table 14-3 Major Effects of Cytokines on the Neuroendocrine System

Axis	Cytokine	Effect
Hypothalamic-pituitary-adrenal	IL-1, IL-6, TNF-α	Enhances the release of CRH
	IL-1, IL-2	Enhances the release of ACTH
Hypothalamic-pituitary-thyroid	IL-1	Enhances TSH release inhibiting factor (SOM)
	TNF-α	Decreased TRH content
Hypothalamic-pituitary-gonadal	IL-1	Inhibits GnRH release

CRH has been reported in the pituitary portal vessels after intravenous injection of IL-1 in rats. Such injections also result in an increase in hypothalamic CRH content and CRH mRNA. Thus it seems clear that IL-1 stimulates an increase in the synthesis and release of CRH. The exact nature of the effects of IL-1 on the pituitary is controversial; however, by using in vitro methods several investigators have shown IL-1 has stimulatory effects on ACTH release from murine pituitary cells and the pituitary adenoma cell line AtT-20 (48). Since IL-1 receptor antibody was reported to block the release of ACTH induced by lipopolysaccharide, it is surmised that CRH may mediate the IL-1-induced ACTH release by enhancing expression of IL-1 receptors on pituitary cells (103). Also, endotoxin may induce production of cytokines in the neuroendocrine system which contribute in turn to its overall activation and secretion of ACTH. Among the other cytokines studied, IL-2, IL-6, and TNF-α have similar effects on ACTH release (66). The ACTH-stimulating effect of IL-6 and TNF-α could be blocked by an anti-CRH antiserum, whereas the effect of IL-2 on plasma ACTH was not abolished by such antisera (66). These results suggest that ACTH release is mediated by a different mechanism for IL-2 than that for IL-1, IL-6, and TNF-α.

IL-1, IL-6, and TNF have also been studied for their effect on GH and PRL release by pituitary cells in vitro (66). The results have been varied and may be due to different experimental conditions. In one study, the intracerebroventricular injection of low doses of IL-1 or TNF caused significant increases in GH and PRL (101). Since low doses were used, it is likely that the hypothalamus is the site of action. In another recent report, IL-1 β was observed to stimulate the release of GHRH and somatostatin from rat hypothalamus in vitro, whereas TNF and IL-6 had no effect (65). Intravenous injection of IL-1 β into intact animals also caused an increase in plasma oxytocin and vasopressin, but IL-6 had no effect (95). The site of action of IL-1 producing these changes is thought to be the neurohypophysis. Prostaglandins may be involved since pretreatment of animals with aspirin blocked IL-1-induced elevation of serum vasopressin levels (95).

The effects of cytokines on the neuroendocrine system have been investigated in hopes of elucidating the clinically observed decrease in thyroid hormones during illness. Subcutaneous injection of IL-1 β decreased plasma T_4, T_3, and TSH levels (36). Since depression of T_4 and T_3 occurred more rapidly than TSH-lowering, it suggested a direct action of IL-1 on the thyroid. In a separate study, it was observed that T_4 and T_3 responses to TSH were impaired in IL-1-treated rats (47). These results lend further support to the belief that IL-1 has inhibitory effects on the thyroid. IL-1 has been shown to enhance the synthesis of somatostatin, a TSH-release-inhibiting factor, by hypothalamic neurons, which also raises the possibility that the hypothalamus is one of the sites of IL-1 action (109). Interestingly, TNF-α has actions similar to those of IL-1 in depressing T_3, T_4, and TSH levels in plasma (97). Since TNF-α decreased the hypothalamic content of thyrotropin-releasing hormone, it appears that this cytokine, too, may act on the hypothalamus. In contrast to some of the above observations, in vitro studies tended to show an increase in TSH following IL-1 or TNF treatment (98), although this effect appears to be minimal. Direct inhibitory actions of cytokines on thyroid cells has also been reported. In these instances, it seems clear that IL-1, TNF, and IFN-γ directly inhibit thyroid hormone biosynthesis and secretion, and cell growth induced by TSH (133).

The thyroid is not alone among endocrine organs in its responsiveness to the effects produced by cytokines. It has been observed that infection and inflammation are sometimes accompanied by an inhibition of reproductive function (66). Intra-cerebroventricular injection of IL-1 α caused an inhibition of plasma LH (104). Moreover, several studies suggest that intracerebroventricularly injected IL-1 inhibits gonadotropin-releasing hormone release via a mechanism involving endogenous opioids since naloxone reversed the inhibitory effect (72). Cytokines also act directly on the gonad. IL-1, TNF-α, and IFNs exert gonadal inhibitory effects and are thought to act as paracrine or autocrine regulators in gonadal function (76).

Receptors for Cytokines in the Neuroendocrine System

The exact mechanisms by which cytokines stimulate the synthesis and secretion of neuroendocrine hormones are still largely unknown, but reports have been published that identify cytokine receptors in neuroendocrine tissue (5,89). The primary site of action of IL-1 appears to be the hypothalamus, but the data supporting the presence of IL-1 receptors in the hypothalamus is controversial. Using autoradiographic techniques, the binding of radioactive IL-1 was found to be high in neuron-rich brain areas (43). The signal demonstrated moderately high binding in the ventromedial hypothalamus but only low density of IL-1 binding in the median eminence and anterior hypothalamus. Although the molecular weight of the brain-associated IL-1 receptor is similar to the receptor described in the immune system, the Kd values are different (43). IL-1 receptors on mouse AtT-20 mouse pituitary tumor cells are up-regulated following treatment with CRH (125). Early studies in rat brain reported a diffuse distribution of CNS IL-1 receptors, yet studies in the mouse described a relatively restricted receptor localization in the anterior pituitary (43). Such discrepancies may result from differences in the species of IL-1 used, the animals studied, and the type of IL-1 receptor examined. More recently, an in situ histochemical analysis using ^{35}S-labeled antisense cRNA probe for the IL-1 receptor revealed distinct regions for the presence of the IL-1 receptor in the dentate gypus, choroid plexus, and the anterior pituitary gland (32). The absence of signal in the hypothalamus may be because of another IL-1 receptor subtype or because IL-1 receptors are synthesized outside the hypothalamus and transported to axon terminals in this region. Another study has reported that the hypothalamus contains a high density of IL-1 receptors (89), but these findings are not universally obtained. Thus it appears that if present in the hypothalamus, this cytokine receptor is of low density or its integrity is modified during tissue preparation.

Production of Cytokines by the Neuroendocrine System

The production of cytokines by the neuroendocrine system is an area for extensive future study. It is now well known that IL-1 is produced by astrocytes and brain macrophages in response to endotoxins (11). TNF-α and IL-6 are produced in the brain in response to lipopolysaccharide or IL-1 (85). Furthermore, nerve fibers containing an IL-1β-like material have been detected in the human hypothalamus, which suggests that IL-1 is produced in neurons and that it may act as a neuromodulator (20). Further studies should clarify the production of cytokines by neuroendocrine tissues, what role they play locally, or how they react in concert with circulating levels of cytokines.

Controversies

Authenticity of Neuroendocrine Hormones and Neuropeptides Produced by Cells of the Immune System

Since the early observation that cells of the immune system could produce an ACTH-like molecule after viral infection, the controversy over the relationship of this newly identified molecule to its neuroendocrine counterpart has continued unabated. Overall, the reagents that have been used have allowed investigators to make direct comparisons to the neuroendocrine hormone. Thus efforts to detect ACTH-producing cells using immunofluorescent staining techniques or purification of immunoreactive molecules on antibody affinity columns have employed highly specific antibodies against purified neuroendocrine hormones. In addition, RNA and cDNA analysis and bioactivity studies for the presence of ACTH have usually studied the lymphocyte immunoreactive material and made comparisons to neuroendocrine hormones by the standard bioassay procedures or published sequence information. At this time, a convincing case can be made to support the presence of ACTH in cells of the immune system. The ACTH protein from lymphocytes has been sequenced and a cDNA synthesized from the RNA and sequenced (113). In both cases, the lymphocyte product was shown to be identical to that produced in the neuroendocrine system (113). Likewise, the cDNA for hypothalamic and thymic LHRH have been shown to be identical (86).

At the present time, although most of the evidence supports the idea that other neuroendocrine hormones and neuropeptides produced by lymphocytes are similar and probably identical to the corresponding neuroendocrine products, the evidence is not yet as thorough as the case for ACTH. We attempted to sequence the GH molecule made by lymphocytes but were unsuccessful due to the molecule being blocked at the N-terminus. Nevertheless, other data discussed elsewhere in this chapter strongly suggest that the molecules are the same. We have preliminary cDNA sequence data to show that the GH molecule produced by lymphocytes is the same as that produced by somatotrophs in the pituitary. To our knowledge, no publications exist that include sequence data for the protein or cDNA molecules for lymphocyte-derived TSH, LH, follicle-stimulating hormone (FSH), or GHRH. In one report on CRH, the available evidence suggests that the molecule may be different since nonparallel curves were obtained by RIA (118). Further studies are needed, and this information should be available in the near future.

Amount of Hormones Produced by Cells of the Immune System

In light of reports that lymphocytes produced neuroendocrine hormones, several investigators have attempted to quantitate the actual amount made and secreted (Table 14-4). Overall, it appears that cells of the neuroendocrine system have the capacity to produce and secrete much larger amounts of hormones than lymphocytes on a per-cell basis. However, one needs to bear in mind that in intact animals, the number of lymphocytes greatly exceeds the quantity of neuroendocrine cells. Thus, the immune system has the potential to produce and secrete a sizable amount of hormone. Some data are available for ACTH, GH, CRH, and GHRH, which are briefly discussed below.

The levels of ACTH produced by lymphocytes has been studied in both primary lymphoid cell cultures and cell lines. In humans, lymphocytes were observed to produce approximately 10 pg/10^7 cells; another report found slightly higher values of 29 pg/10^7 cells (22,45). Several cell lines from patients with lymphoid or myeloid malignancies produced 135–208 pg/10^7 cells after overnight culture (22). The levels of TSH and TRH produced by immune cells have not yet been defined. The levels of GH secreted by lymphocytes have been reported by several groups and may vary between 10 and 100 pg/10^7 cells for normal and transformed cell lines (61,73). The levels of PRL have been studied mostly in a cell line (IM-9-P-3) where 4 ng/10^7 cells were reported (34). It appears that although lymphocytes produce neuroendocrine hormones at much lower levels, sufficient amounts appear to be secreted to stimulate biological processes.

Table 14-4 Quantification of Neuroendocrine Hormone Immunoreactivity in Cells of the Immune System

Hormone	Amount Produced Lymphocyte (pg/10^7)	Bioactive[a]
ACTH	29	+
PRL (IM9-P3)	4,000	+
GH	10–100	+
CRH	1.0	ND
GHRH	130–350	+
LHRH	202	ND

[a]+, The lymphocyte derived hormone is biologically similar to its neuroendocrine counterpart in a bioassay; ND, not determined.

The amount of releasing hormones produced by immune cells is quite comparable to that found in the hypothalamus. In our studies, rat lymphocytes released 200 pg/mg protein of irGHRH, compared to 1,000 pg/mg protein for the hypothalamus (128). In the human, 130 pg/10^7 cells were detected in resting lymphocytes; after activation in mixed lymphocyte culture, the value rose to 350 pg/10^7 cells (119). Activated human lymphocytes also released GHRH at a concentration of 51 pg/10^7 cells into the medium after a 24-hour culture incubation period (119). Similar levels of irLHRH have been detected. Interestingly, the levels of CRH are approximately 100 times less than those found for GHRH or LHRH in immune cells (118). This may be a result of rapid secretion of this hormone since only intracellular levels have been measured. Alternatively, the actual lymphocyte inducer of CRH may not have been identified yet, so maximum levels have not been measured, or immune cells may merely synthesize less CRH.

Paracrine and Autocrine vs. "Endocrine" Role for Immune System-derived Peptides

The idea that neuroendocrine hormones produced by lymphocytes function in paracrine and/or autocrine roles (rather than endocrine) is supported by the low levels of hormone produced by immune cells. It remains uncertain whether the hormone products of leukocytes are secreted or sequestered within the cells of origin. In the case of GH, it appears that approximately 10% of spleen cells are positive by immunofluorescence for GH, whereas only 0.1% of the spleen cells are secreting GH as determined by the reverse hemolytic plaque assay (73). Thus, by all measures, more of the hormone appears to remain intracellular and may be released to function in an autocrine manner. Interestingly, PRL molecules produced by a human B-lymphoblastoid cell line are secreted at a much higher level (50 ng/10^6 cells) than GH (35). Lymphocyte proliferation can be blocked by the exogenous addition of antibodies to PRL (60). We and others have shown that antibodies to GH do not block the proliferation of lymphocytes in vitro, however, antisense oligodeoxynucleotides that would bind to GH mRNA can block proliferation and the production of lymphocyte-derived GH (130). These data suggest an autocrine role for lymphocyte-derived GH. Whether such lymphocyte hormones are secreted or sequestered has important implications for the role of leukocyte-derived peptides in regulating the function of other cells. Several groups have had problems measuring extracellular levels of such hormones because low levels are produced in vitro and/or the degree of secretion is not maximized in vitro. In this regard, it has been proposed, and experimentally supported, that lymphocytes release sufficient ACTH to stimulate steroidogenesis in vivo (114). In this important study, three- to four-fold increases in serum corticosterone levels were observed 8 hours after infection with Newcastle disease virus (NDV). The increase in serum corticosterone could be blocked by dexamethasone treatment of hypophysectomized mice (114). Subsequent studies in mice and rats suggested that the production of ACTH by lymphocytes was not sufficient to stimulate the adrenal gland in the absence of the pituitary (see below). The ability of lymphocyte-derived neuroendocrine hormones to mediate an endocrine response should continue to be studied in the future with regard to lymphocyte ACTH as well as GH, PRL, and TSH to determine whether they also may serve as endocrine sources of neuroendocrine hormones.

Taken together, the data suggest that some immunocompetent cells can synthesize neuroendocrine-derived peptides, may release very small amounts of these peptides, and may respond to these peptides in either an autocrine or paracrine fashion by altering immune function. The evidence that they are regulated by the same mechanisms that control pituitary POMC peptide secretion is convincing. Thus, neuroendocrine-immune interactions may have important functions in response to stress or infection. Lymphocyte-derived neuroendocrine peptides appear to exert direct effects on the immune system itself, while the interaction with their neuroendocrine system may be mediated largely by cytokines.

Hypothalamic vs. Pituitary Site of IL-1 Action

One of the most heated debates has followed our initial discovery that IL-1 caused ACTH release from pituitary cells in vitro (131). Although some were initially unable to reproduce this finding, the basic observation has now been reproduced by several laboratories (for review, see 111). This led to tests of the in vivo site of action of IL-1 on the hypothalamic pituitary axis. Virtually all studies suggested that the hypothalamus was the site of IL-1 action and that increased pituitary ACTH and adrenal glucocorticoid levels resulted from IL-1-induced CRH release (111). The evidence supporting this conclusion was the ability of antibody to CRH or a CRH antagonist to block IL-1 mediated release of ACTH and glucocorticoids. These findings, however, do not explain the protracted ACTH response on account of IL-1, as compared to the brief response due to CRH. We suspect that IL-1 acts at both the hypothalamus and the pituitary, with the initial ACTH response being due to CRH release and the protracted ACTH response due to an action of IL-1 on the pituitary. A recent observation may explain how this could occur. De Sousa and others have shown that CRH can up-regulate the expression of IL-1 receptors on pituitary cells (83,125). Thus the controversy could be resolved if the direct pituitary action of IL-1 is dependent on CRH-mediated IL-1 receptor expression on the pituitary. If this is true, it would explain why CRH antagonists completely block ACTH and glucocorticoid release as if the pituitary gland were not involved.

Animal Models and Human Disease Relevance

Certain experimental models and clinical observations would seem to support the view that leukocyte-derived hormones can act on typical neuroendocrine targets. The finding that cells of the immune system are a source of secreted ACTH suggested that stimuli which elicit the leukocyte-derived hormone should not require a pituitary gland for an ACTH-mediated increase in corticosteroids (114). This seemed to be the case when virus infection (in vitro inducer of leukocyte ACTH) of hypophysectomized mice caused a time-dependent increase in corticosterone production which was inhibitable by dexamethasone (114). Unless such mice were pretreated with dexamethasone, their spleens were positive for ACTH by immunofluorescence (114). A more recent study has strongly suggested that B lymphocytes can be responsible for extrapituitary ACTH and glucocorticoid production (9). In this report, hypophysectomized chickens were shown to produce ACTH and corticosterone in response to *Brucella abortus*. This ACTH and corticosterone response was ablated if B lymphocytes were deleted by bursectomy prior to hypophysectomy (9). Two laboratories have been unable to reproduce a pituitary-independent ACTH response in mice and rats, respectively (37,96). They speculate that the positive results were due to incomplete hypophysectomies, yet it is difficult to understand why these animals would segregate to the experimental and not the control groups. This potentially important question of pituitary-independent ACTH responses obviously needs further study to reconcile the conflicting results. In certain instances, similar positive results have, however, been observed in humans. For example, when children who were pituitary ACTH-deficient were pyrogen tested (typhoid vaccine, another in vitro inducer of leukocyte ACTH), they showed an increase in the percentage of ACTH-positive mononuclear leukocytes (91). Both the response in hypophysectomized mice and hypopituitary children peaked at approximately 6–8 hours after administration of virus and typhoid vaccine, respectively. These findings might explain the earlier observation of bacterial polysaccharide (Piromen)-induced cortisol responses in 7 out of 8 patients who underwent pituitary stalk sectioning (122). Such studies have been furthered by the report of Fehm et al. (44) that corticotropin-releasing factor (CRF) administration to pituitary ACTH-deficient individuals results in both an ACTH and a cortisol response.

Gram-negative bacterial infections and endotoxin shock may represent yet another situation in which leukocyte hormones act on the neuroendocrine system. For instance, endorphins have been implicated in the pathophysiology associated with these maladies since the opiate antagonist, naloxone, improved survival rates and blocked a number of cardiopulmonary changes associated with these conditions (102). Furthermore, two separate pools of endorphins have been observed following endotoxin, bacterial LPS, administration, and it was suggested that one pool might originate in the immune system (24). Considering the potent immunological effects of endotoxin, as well as its ability to induce in vitro leukocyte production of endorphins, cells of the immune system seem the most likely source of endogenous opiates that are observed during gram-negative sepsis and endotoxin shock. Consistent with this idea is the observation that lymphocyte depletion, like naloxone treatment, blocked a number of endotoxin-induced cardiopulmonary changes (19). Our interpretation of these results is that lymphocyte depletion removes the source of the endorphins while naloxone blocks their effector function. In a different approach, LPS-resistant inbred mice, which have essentially no pathophysiologic response to LPS, were shown to have a defect in leukocyte processing of POMC to endorphins. If leukocyte-derived endorphins were administered to such LPS-resistant mice, they then showed much of the pathophysiology associated with LPS administration to sensitive mice (58). A final and exciting new development in the opioid field has come with the demonstration that activation of endogenous opioids in rats by a cold water swim results in a local antinociception in the inflamed tissue apparently results from production by immune cells of endogenous opioids which interact with opioid receptors on peripheral sensory nerves (117).

Hormone replacement therapy in hypophysectomized rodents and dwarf animals has provided evidence for PRL and GH involvement in immunity (for review, see 49). Antibody formation and the development of contact sensitivity were restored in hypophysectomized rats by the injection of rat PRL or GH. The anemia observed for hypophysectomized rats could be corrected by either bovine PRL or GH. The decrease in NK cells in hypophysectomized mice was partially prevented by ovine GH. Macrophages isolated from the peritoneal cavity of hypophysectomized rats showed a decrease in TNF-α production, which could be restored by the exogenous administration of GH. Most interesting in this study was the observation that simultaneous administration of antiserum to TNF-α and GH blocked macrophage cytotoxicity (38). These results suggest that the enhanced macrophage cytotoxicity observed after GH treatment was due to production of TNF-α. Studies in dwarf animals treated with GH or PRL show that these hormones were effective in restoring thymus and spleen weights and antibody production to those of normal animals. Other studies in thymectomized mice and in the nude rat suggest that the thymus may be an important site of action for these hormones (40,100). In humans, although improved growth responses have been observed after treatment with GH, consistent results have not been observed, and often a decrease in the proliferative response to PHA has been observed. The exception to this appears to be the increase in NK cell activity of GH-impaired individuals (87).

It is clear from all the studies to date that PRL and GH have important and sometimes similar effects on the immune system. Both animal studies and the available clinical data in humans suggest that absence of either PRL or GH can lead to deficiencies in both cell-mediated and humoral immunological functions. The deficiencies can be corrected by replacement therapy with PRL or GH. Several studies point toward the presence of functional receptors for PRL and GH on cells of the immune system, the physiological significance of which will continue to be explored. The production of these same or similar hormones by immune cells further reflects the complexity behind the study of the exact role of these hormones and the control of their receptors in the immune system.

Conclusions

For far too long, the immune system has been viewed in isolation from the rest of the body's organ systems. It seems evident from the above discussion that the immune and neuroendocrine systems share many ligands and receptors that result in constant and important bidirectional communication. Indeed, we have postulated that a new and important function for the immune system is to serve as a sensory organ for noncognitive stimuli such as infectious agents. What we now seem to be witnessing is the reintegration of an important organ system into the physiologic context of the whole animal. This undoubtedly is going to lead to a more basic understanding of physiology and to profound changes in the practice of medicine. To completely understand the process of immune neuroendocrine cross talk will require the continued pursuit of ligands and receptors that are shared by the two systems, as well as an understanding of similarities and differences in their regulation. New immunologic functions will likely be assigned to neuropeptides and hormones and novel neuroendocrine properties of cytokines will be discovered. Ultimately, it will be a challenge for physiologists to assimilate this information into functions of the animal as a whole. This in turn should lead to novel techniques for the treatment and diagnosis of human disease of immune and neuroendocrine origin. Two recent findings vividly point to future possibilities. One is the observation that CRH is a proinflammatory agent in the periphery (75), and the second is the dramatic prolongation of renal allografts in rats treated with the opiate antagonist, naltrindole (3). A few years ago it would have seemed unthinkable that in the near future we may treat peripheral inflammation with an antagonist of a hypothalamic releasing hormone and use an opiate antagonist in tissue transplantation.

References

1. Ader R, Cohen N. Conditioned immuno-pharmacological responses. In: Psychoneuro-immunology, R Ader, ed. Academic Press, Orlando, 1981, pp 281–320.
2. Alvarez-Mon A, Kehrl JH, Fauci AS. A potential role for adrenocorticotropin in regulating human B lymphocyte functions. J Immunol 135:3823–3826, 1985.
3. Arakawa K, Akami T, Okamoto M, Oka T, Nagase H, Matsumoto S. The immunosuppressive effect of δ-opioid receptor antagonist on rat renal allograft survival. Transplantation 53:951–953, 1992.
4. Azad, N, Jurgens, J, Young MR, Reda D, Duffner, L, Kirsteins L, Emanuele NV, Lawrence AM. Presence of luteinizing hormone-releasing hormone in rat thymus. Prog Neuro Endocrin Immunol 4:113–120, 1991.
5. Ban E, Milon G, Prudhomme N, Fillion G, Haour F. Receptors for interleukin-1 (α and β) in mouse brain: mapping and neuronal localization in hippocampus. Neuroscience 43:21–30, 1991.
6. Baroni C. Thymus, peripheral lymphoid tissue and immunological responsiveness of the pituitary dwarf mice. Experientia 23:282–283, 1967.
7. Baroni C, Fabris N, Bertoli G. Age dependence of the primary immune response in the hereditary pituitary dwarf and normal Snell-Bagg mouse. Experientia 23:1059–1060, 1967.
8. Baxter JB, Blalock JE, Weigent DA. Characterization of immunoreactive insulin-like growth factor-I from leukocytes and its regulation by growth hormone. Endocrinology 129:1727–1734, 1991.

9. Bayle JE, Guellati M, Ibos F, Roux J. Brucella abortus antigen stimulates the pituitary-adrenal axis through the extrapituitary B lymphoid system. Prog Neuro Endocrin Immunol 4:99–105, 1991.

10. Bazan JF. A novel family of growth factor receptors: a common binding domain in the growth hormone, prolactin, erythropoietin and IL-6 receptors, and the p75 IL-2 receptor β-chain. Biochem Biophys Res Commun 164:788–795, 1989.

11. Benveniste EN. Cytokines: influence on glial cell gene expression and function. In: Neuroimmunoendocrinology, 2nd rev ed, JE Blalock, ed. Chem Immunol 52:106–153, 1992, Karger, Basel.

12. Bernton EW, Meltzer MS, Holaday JW. Suppression of macrophage activation and T-lymphocyte function in hyoprolactinemic mice. Science 239:401–404, 1988.

13. Besedovsky HO, Sorkin E. Immunologic-neuroendocrine circuits: physiological approaches. In: Psychoneuroimmunology, R Ader, ed. Academic Press, Orlando, 1981 pp 545–571.

14. Blalock JE. The immune system as a sensory organ. J Immunol 132:1067–1070, 1984.

15. Blalock JE. Relationships between neuroendocrine hormones and lymphokines. In: Lymphokines, E Pick ed. Academic Press, Orlando, 1984, pp 1–13.

16. Blalock JE. A molecular basis for bidirectional communication between the immune and neuroendocrine systems. Physiol Rev 69:1–32, 1989.

17. Blalock JE. Production of peptide hormones and neurotransmitters by the immune system. In: Neuroimmunoendocrinology, 2nd rev ed, JE Blalock, ed. Chem Immunol 52:1–19, 1992, Karger, Basel.

18. Blalock JE, Costa O. Immune neuroendocrine interactions: implications for reproductive physiology. Ann NY Acad Sci 564:261–266, 1989.

19. Bohs CT, Fish JC, Miller TH, Traber DL. Pulmonary vascularresponse to endotoxin in normal and lymphocyte depleted sheep. Circ Shock 6:13–21, 1979.

20. Breder CD, Dinarello CA, Sapler CB. Interleukin-1 immunoreactive innervation of the human hypothalamus. Science 240:321–324, 1988.

21. Brooks WH, Walmann M. Adrenocorticotropin functions as a late-acting B cell growth factor and synergizes with IL-5. FASEB J Vol 3 A1471, 1989.

22. Buzzetti R, McLoughlin L, Lavender PM, Clark AJL, Rees LH. Expression of pro-opiomelanocortin gene and quantification of adrenocorticotropic hormone-like immunoreactivity in human normal peripheral mononuclear cells and lymphoid and myeloid malignancies. J Clin Invest 83:733–737, 1989.

23. Buzzetti R, Valente L, Barletta C, Scavo D, Pozzilli P. Thymopentin induces release of ACTH-like immunoreactivity by human lymphocytes. J Clin Lab Immunol 29:157–159, 1989.

24. Carr DB, Bergland R, Hamilton A, Blume H, Kasting N, Arnold M, Martin MB, Rosenblatt M. Endotoxin stimulated opioid peptide secretion: two secretory pools and feedback control in vivo. Science 217:845–848, 1982.

25. Carr DJJ. The role of endogenous opioids and their receptors in the immune system. Soc Exp Biol Med 198:710–720, 1991.

26. Carr DJJ, Weigent DA, Blalock JE. Hormones common to the neuroendocrine and immune systems. Drug Des Del 4:187–195, 1989.

27. Clarke BL, Bost KL. Differential expression of functional adrenocorticotropic hormone receptors by subpopulations of lymphocytes. J Immunol 143:464–469, 1989.

28. Clevenger CV, Russell DH, Appasamy PM, Prystowsky MB. Regulation of interleukin-2 driven T-lymphocytes. Proc Natl Acad Sci USA 87:6460–6464, 1990.

29. Cohen JJ, Crnic LS. Glucocorticoids, stress and the immune response. In: Immunophar-

macology and the Regulation of Leukocyte Function, ed. DR Webb, Dekker, New York, 1982, pp 61–91.

30. Coutelier J-P, Kehrl JH, Bellur SS, Kohn LD, Notkins AL, Prabhakar BS. Binding and functional effects of thyroid stimulating hormone on human immune cells. J Clin Immunol 10:204–210, 1990.

31. Cross RJ, Markesbery WR, Brooks WH, Roszman TL. Hypothalamic-immune interactions. Neuromodulation of natural killer activity by elsioning of the anterior hypothalamus. Immunology 51:399–405, 1984.

32. Cunningham ET Jr, Wada E, Carter DB, Tracey DE, Battey JF, DeSouza EB. In situ histochemical localization of type 1 interleukin-1 receptor messenger RNA in the central nervous system, pituitary, and adrenal gland of the mouse. J Neurosci 12:1101–1114, 1992.

33. Cupps TR, Fauci AS. Corticosteroid-mediated immunoregulation in man. Immunol Rev 65:133–155, 1982.

34. DiMattia GE, Gellersen B, Bohnet HG, Freisen HG. A human B-lymphoblastoid cell line produces prolactin. Endocrinology 122:2508–2517, 1988.

35. DiMattia GE, Gellersen B, Duckworth ML, Friesen HG. Human prolactin gene expression: the use of an alternative noncoding exon in decidua and the IM-9-P3 lymphoblast cell line. J Biol Chem 2165:16412–16421, 1990.

36. Dubuis JM, Dayer, JM, Siegris-Kaiser CA, Burger AG. Human recombinant interleukin-1β decreases plasma thyroid hormone and thyroid stimulating hormone levels in rats. Endocrinology 123:2175–2181, 1988.

37. Dunn AJ, Powell ML, Gaskin JM. Virus-induced increases in plasma corticosterone. Science 238:1423–1425, 1987.

38. Edwards CK III, Lorence RM, Dunham DM, Arkins S, Yunger LM, Greager JA, Walter RJ, Dantzer R, Kelley KW. Hypophysectomy inhibits the synthesis of tumor necrosis factor α by rat macrophages: partial restoration by exogenous growth hormone or interferon beta. Endocrinology 128:989–996, 1991.

39. Emanuele NV, Emanuele MA, Tentler J, Kirsteins L, Azad N, Lawrence AM. Rat spleen lymphocytes contain an immunoreactive and bioactive luteinizing hormone-releasing hormone. Endocrinology 126:2482–2486, 1990.

40. Fabris N, Pierpaoli W, Sorkin E. Hormones and the immunological capacity. IV: Restorative effects of developmental hormones of lymphocytes on the immunodeficiency syndrome of the dwarf mouse. Clin Exp Immunol 9:227–240, 1971.

41. Fahrenholz F., Kajro E, Muller M, Boer R, Lohr R, Grzonka Z. Iodinated photoreactive vasopressin antagonist: labelling of hepatic vasopressin receptor subunits. Eur J Biochem 161:321–328, 1986.

42. Pais S, Annibale B, Boirivant M, Santoro A, Pallone F, Delle Fave G. Effects of somatostatin on human intestinal lamina propria lymphocytes. Modulation of lymphocyte activation. J Neuroimmunol 31:211–219, 1991.

43. Farrar WL, Kilian PL, Ruff, MR, Hill JM, Pert CB. Visualization and characterization of interleukin-1 receptors in brain. J Immunol 139:459–463, 1987.

44. Fehm HL, Holl R, Spath-Schwalbe E, Voigt KH, Born J. Ability of human corticotropin releasing factor (hCRF) to stimulate cortisol secretion independent from pituitary ACTH. Life Sci 42:679–686, 1988.

45. Ferreira JA, Carstens ME, Taljaard JJF. Quantitative determination of lymphocyte ACTH 1–39. Neuropeptides 15:11–15, 1990.

46. Friesen HG, DiMattia GE, Too CKL. Lymphoid tumor cells as models for studies of prolactin gene regulation and action. Prog Neuro Endocrin Immunol 4:1–9, 1991.

47. Fujii T, Sato K, Ozawa M, Kasono K, Imamura H, Kanaji Y, Tsushima T, Shizume K. Effect of interleukin-1 (IL-1) on thyroid hormone metabolism in mice: stimulation by IL-1 of iodothyronine 5-deiodinating activity (type 1) in the liver. Endocrinology 124:167–174, 1989.

48. Fukata J, Usui T, Naitoh Y, Nakai Y, Imura H. Effects of recombinant human interleukin-1α, -1β, 2 and 6 on ACTH synthesis and release in the mouse pituitary tumor cell line AtT-20. J Endocrinol 122:33–39, 1989.

49. Gala RR. Prolactin and growth hormone in the regulation of the immune system. Proc Soc Exp Biol Med 198:513–527, 1991.

50. Gilmore W, Weiner LP. Beta-endorphin enhances interleukin-2 (IL-2) production in murine lymphocytes. J Neuroimmunol 18:125–138, 1988.

51. Goetzl EJ, Sreedharan SP, Turck CW. Structurally distinctive vasoactive intestinal peptides from rat basophilic leukemia cells. J Biol Chem 263:9083–9086, 1988.

52. Guarcello V, Weigent DA, Blalock JE. Growth hormone releasing hormone receptors on thymocytes and splenocytes from rats. Cell Immunol 136:291–302, 1991.

53. Habaud O, Lissitzky S. Thyrotropin-specific binding to human peripheral blood monocytes and polymorphonuclear leukocytes. Mol Cell Endocrinol 7:79–87, 1977.

54. Harbour DV, Hughes TK. Thyrotropin releasing hormone (TRH) induces gamma interferon release. FASEB J5:A5884, 1991.

55. Harbour DV, Kruger TE, Coppenhaver D, Smith EM, Meyer WJ. Differential expression and regulation of thyrotropin (TSH) in T cell lines. Mol Cell Endocrinol 64:229–241, 1989.

56. Harbour DV, Leon S, Keating C, Hughes TK. Thyrotropin modulates B-cell function through specific bioactive receptors. Prog Neuro Endocrin Immunology 3:266–276, 1990.

57. Harbour DV, Smith EM, Blalock JE. A novel processing pathway for proopiomelanocortin in lymphocytes: endotoxin induction of a new pro-hormone cleaving enzyme. J Neurosci Res 18:95–101, 1987.

58. Harbour DV, Smith EM, Blalock JE. Splenic lymphocyte production of an endorphin during endotoxic shock. Brain Behav Immun 1:123–133, 1987.

59. Harbour DV, Wilhite JE. Expression of bioactive TSH receptors on B cells. FASEB J5:A480, 1989.

60. Hartmann DP, Holaday JW, Bernton EW. Inhibition of lymphocyte proliferation by antibodies to prolactin. FASEB J 3:2194–2202, 1989.

61. Hattori N, Shimatsu A, Sugita M, Kumagai S, Imura H. Immunoreactive growth hormone (GH) secretion by human lymphocytes: augmented release by exogenous GH. Biochem Biophys Res Commun 168:396–401, 1990.

62. Heijnen CJ, Kavelaars A, Ballieux RE. Corticotropin-releasing hormone and proopiomelanocortin-derived peptides in the modulation of the immune function. In: Psychoneuroimmunology, 2nd ed, R Ader, DL Felten, N Cohen, eds. Academic Press, Orlando, 1991, pp 429–446.

63. Hiestand PC, Mekler P, Nordmann R, Grieder A, Permmongkol C. Prolactin as a modulator of lymphocyte responsiveness provides a possible mechanism of action for cyclosporin. Proc Natl Acad Sci USA 83:2599–2603, 1986.

64. Hiruma K, Nakamura KH, Sumida T, Maeda T, Tomioka H, Yoshida S, Fujita T. Somatostatin receptors on human lymphocytes and leukaemia cells. Immunol 71:480–485, 1990.

65. Honegger J, Spagnoli A, D'urso R, Navarra P, Tsagarakis S, Besser GM, Grossman AB. Interleukin-1β modulates the acute release of growth hormone-releasing hormone and

somatostatin from rat hypothalamus in vitro, whereas tumor necrosis factor and inter-leukin-6 have no effect. Endocrinology 129:1275–1282, 1991.

66. Imura N, Fukata J-I, Mori T. Cytokines and endocrine function: an interaction between the immune and neuroendocrine systems. Clin Endocrinol 35:107–115, 1991.

67. Jain R, Zwickler D, Hollander CS, Brand H, Saperstein A, Hutchinson B, Brown C, Audhya T. Corticotropin-releasing factor modulates the immune response to stress in the rat. Endocrinology 128:1329–1336, 1991.

68. Johnson EW, Blalock JE, Smith EM. ACTH receptor-mediated induction of leukocyte cyclic AMP. Biochem Biophys Res Commun 157:1205–1211, 1988.

69. Johnson HM, Downs MO, Pontzer CH. Neuroendocrine peptide hormone regulation of immunity. In: Neuroimmunoendocrinology, 2nd rev ed, JE Blalock, ed. Chem Immunol 52:49–83, 1992, Karger, Basel.

70. Johnson HM, Smith EM, Torres BA, Blalock JE. Neuroendocrine hormone regulation of in vitro antibody production. Proc Natl Acad Sci USA 79:4171–4174, 1982.

71. Johnson HM, Torres BA, Smith EM, Lion LD, Blalock JE. Regulation of lymphokine (γ-interferon) production by corticotropin. J Immunol 1332:246–250, 1984.

72. Kalra PS, Fuentes M, Sahu A, Kalra SP. Endogenous opioid peptides mediate the interleukin-1-induced inhibition of luteinizing hormone (LH)-releasing hormone and LH. Endocrinology 127:2381–2386, 1990.

73. Kao T-L, Harbour DV, Meyer WJ III. Immunoreactive growth hormone production by cultured lymphocytes. Ann NY Acad Sci 650:179–181, 1992.

74. Kao T-L, Harbour DV, Smith EM, Meyer WJ III. Immunoreactive growth hormone produc-tion by cultured lymphocytes. Endocrine Society, 71st Annual Meeting, Seattle WA, 1989, Abstract 343.

75. Karalis K, Sano H, Redwin J, Listwak S, Wilder RL, Chrousos GP. Autocrine or paracrine in-flammatory actions of corticotropin-releasing hormone in vivo. Science 254:421–423, 1991.

76. Kauppila A, Cantell K, Janne O, Kokko E, Vihko R. Serum sex steroid and peptide hormone concentrations, and endometrial estrogen and progestin receptor levels during administration of human leukocyte interferon. Int J Cancer 29:291–294, 1982.

77. Kavelaars A, Ballieux RE, Heijnen C. Modulation of the immune response by pro-opiomelanocortin derived peptides. Brain Behav Immun 2:57–66, 1988.

78. Kavelaars A, Ballieux RE, Heijnen CJ. The role of IL-1 in the corticotropin-releasing factor and arginine-vasopressin-induced secretion of immunoreactive beta-endorphin by human peripheral blood mononuclear cells. J Immunol 142:2338–2342, 1989.

79. Kavelaars A, Berkenbosch F, Croiset G, Ballieux RE, Heijnen CJ. Induction of beta-endorphin secretion by lymphocytes after subcutaneous administration of corticotropin-releasing factor. Endocrinology 126:759–764, 1990.

80. Keller SE, Weiss JM, Schleifer SJ, Miller NE, Stein M. Stress-induced suppression of immunity in adrenalectomized rats. Science 221:1301–1304, 1983.

81. Kelley KW. Growth hormone, lymphocytes, and macrophages. Biochem Pharmacol 35:705–713, 1989.

82. Kenner JR, Holaday JW, Bernton EW, Smith PF. Prolactin-like protein in murine lympho-cytes: morphological and biochemical evidence. Prog Neuro Endocrin Immunol 3:188–195, 1990.

83. Kobayashi H, Fukata J, Tominaga T, Murakami N, Fukushuima M, Ebisui O, Segaua H, Nakai Y, Imura H. Regulation of interleukin-1 receptors on AtT-20 mouse pituitary tumour cells. FEBS Lett 298:100–104, 1992.

84. Kruger TE, Smith LR, Harbour DV, Blalock JE. Thyrotropin: an endogenous regulator of the immune response. J Immunol 142:744–747, 1989.

85. Lieberman AP, Pitha PM, Shin HS, Shin ML. Production of tumor necrosis factor and other cytokines by astrocytes stimulated with lipopolysaccharide or a neurotropic virus. Proc Natl Acad Sci USA 86:6348–6352, 1989.

86. Maier CC, Marchetti B, LeBoeuf RD, Blalock JE. Thymocytes express a mRNA that is identical to hypothalamic luteinizing hormone-releasing hormone mRNA. Cell Mol Neurobiol 12:447–454, 1992.

87. Matsuura M, Kikkawa Y, Kitagawa T, Tanaka S. Modulation of immunological abnormalities of growth hormone-deficient children by growth hormone treatment. Acta Paediatr Jpn 31:53–57, 1989.

88. McGlone JJ, Lumpkin EA, Norman RL. Adrenocorticotropin stimulates natural killer cell activity. Endocrinology 129:1653–1658, 1991.

89. Merrill JE. Bellini, Carpaccio, and receptors in the central nervous system. J Cell Biochem 46:191–198, 1991.

90. Metal'nikov S, Chorine V. Role des reflexes conditionnels dans l'immunite. Ann Inst Pasteur (Paris) 40:893–900, 1926.

91. Meyer WJ III, Smith EM, Richards GE, Cavallo A, Morrill AC, Blalock JE. In vivo immunoreactive ACTH production by human leukocytes from normal and ACTH-deficient individuals. J Clin Endocrinol Metabol 64:98–105, 1988.

92. Mukherjee P, Mastro AM, Hymer WC. Prolactin induction of interleukin-2 receptors on rat splenic lymphocytes. Endocrinology 126:88–94, 1990.

93. Murphy LJ, Bell GI, Friesen HG. Growth hormone stimulates sequential induction of c-myc and insulin-like growth factor I expression in vivo. Endocrinology 120:1806–1812, 1987.

94. Murphy WJ, Durum SK, Longo DL. Human growth hormone promotes engraftment of murine or human T cells in severe combined immunodeficient mice. Proc Natl Acad Sci USA 89:4481–4485, 1992.

95. Naito Y, Fukata J, Shindo K, Ebisui O, Murakami N, Tominaga T, Nakai Y, Mori K, Kasting NW, Imura H. Effects of interleukins on plasma arginine vasopressin and oxytocin levels in conscious, freely moving rats. Biochem Biophys Res Commun 174:1185–1195, 1991.

96. Olsen NJ, Nicholson WE, DeBold CR, Orth DN. Lymphocyte-derived adrenocorticotropin is insufficient to stimulate adrenal steroidogenesis in hypophysectomized rats. Endocrinology 130:2113–2119, 1992.

97. Ozawa M, Sato K, Han DC, Kawakami M, Tsushima T, Shizume K. Effects of tumour necrosis factor-α/cachetin on thyroid hormone metabolism in mice. Endocrinology 123:1461–1467, 1988.

98. Pang XP, Hershman JM, Mirell CJ, Pekary AE. Impairment of hypothalamic-pituitary-thyroid function in rats treated with human recombinant tumor necrosis factor-α (cachectin). Endocrinology 125:76–84, 1989.

99. Payan DG, Hess CA, Goetzl EJ. Inhibition by somatostatin of the proliferation of T-lymphocytes and Molt-4 lymphoblasts. Cell Immunol 84:433–438, 1984.

100. Pierpaoli W, Baroni C, Fabris N, Sorkin E. Hormones and immunological capacity. II: Reconstitution of antibody production in hormonally deficient mice by somatotropic hormone, thyrotropic hormone and thyroxine. Immunology 16:217–230, 1969.

101. Rettori V, Milenkovic L, Beutler BA, McCann SM. Hypothalamic action of cachectin to alter pituitary hormone release. Brain Res Bull 23:471–475, 1989.

102. Reynolds DG, Guill NV, Vargish T, Hechner RB, Fader AI, Holaday JW. Blockage of opiate receptors for naloxone improves survival and cardiac performance in canine endotoxic shock. Circ Shock 7:39–48, 1980.

103. Rivier C, Chizzonite R, Vale W. In the mouse, the activation of the hypothalamic-pituitary-

adrenal axis by a lipopolysaccharide (endotoxin) is mediated through interleukin-1. Endocrinology 125:2800–2805, 1989.

104. Rivier C, Vale W. In the rat, interleukin-1α acts at the level of the brain and the gonads to interfere with gonadotropin and sex steroid secretion. Endocrinology 124:2105–2109, 1989.

105. Roszman TL, Brooks WH. Signaling pathways of the neuroendocrine-immune network. In: Neuroimmunoendocrinology, 2nd rev ed, JE Blalock, ed. Chem Immunol 52:170–190, 1992, Karger, Basel.

106. Russell DH, Kibler R, Matrisian L, Larson DF, Poulos B, Magun BE. Prolactin receptors on human T and B lymphocytes: antagonism of prolactin binding by cyclosporin. J Immunol 134:3027–3030, 1985.

107. Russell DH, Matrisian L, Kibler R, Larson DF, Poulos B, Magun BE. Prolactin receptors on human lymphocytes and their modulation by cyclosporin. Biochem Biophys Res Commun 121:899–906, 1984.

108. Sapolsky R, Rivier C, Yamamoto G, Plotsky P, Vale W. Interleukin-1 stimulates the secretion of hypothalamic corticotropin-releasing factor. Science 238:522–524, 1987.

109. Scarborough DE, Lee SL, Dinarello CA, Reichlin S. Interleukin-1β stimulates somatostatin biosynthesis in primary culture of fetal rat brain. Endocrinology 124:549–551, 1989.

110. Selye H. Thymus and adrenals in the response of the organism to injuries and intoxications. Br J Exp Pathol 17:234–238, 1936.

111. Smith, EM. Hormonal activities of cytokines. In: Neuroimmunoendocrinology, 2nd rev ed, JE Blalock, ed. 52:154–169, 1992, Karger, Basel.

112. Smith EM, Blalock JE. Human lymphocyte production of ACTH and endorphin-like substances: Association with leukocyte interferon. Proc Natl Acad Sci USA 78:7530–7534, 1981.

113. Smith EM, Galin FS, LeBoeuf RD, Coppenhaver DH, Harbour DV, Blalock JE. Nucleotide and amino acid sequence of lymphocyte-derived corticotropin: endotoxin induction of a truncated peptide. Proc Natl Acad Sci USA 87:1057–1060, 1990.

114. Smith EM, Meyer WJ, Blalock, JE. Virus-induced increases in corticosterone in hypophysectomized mice: a possible lymphoid adrenal axis. Science 218:1311–1313, 1982.

115. Smith EM, Morrill AC, Meyer WJ, Blalock JE. Corticotropin releasing factor induction of leukocyte-derived immunoreactive ACTH and endorphins. Nature 322:881–882, 1986.

116. Stanisz AM, Befus D, Bienenstock J. Differential effects of vasoactive intestinal peptide, substance P, and somatostatin on immunoglobulin synthesis and proliferation by lymphocytes from Peyer's patches, mesenteric lymph nodes, and spleen. J Immunol 136:152–156, 1986.

117. Stein C, Hassan AHS, Przewlocki R, Gramsch C, Peter K, Herz A. Opioids from immunocytes interact with receptors on sensory nerves to inhibit nociception in inflammation. Proc Natl Acad Sci USA 87:5935–5939, 1990.

118. Stephanou A, Jessop DS, Knight RA, Lightman SL. Corticotrophin-releasing factor-like immunoreactivity and mRNA in human leukocytes. Brain Behav Immun 4:67–73, 1990.

119. Stephanou A, Knight RA, Lightman SL. Production of a growth hormone-releasing hormone-like peptide and its mRNA by human lymphocytes. Neuroendocrinology 53:628–633, 1991.

120. Stephanou A, Sarlis NJ, Knight RA, Chowdrey HS, Lightman SL. Response of pituitary and spleen pro-opiomelanocortin mRNA, and spleen and thymus interleukin-1β mRNA to adjuvant arthritis in the rat. J Neuroimmunol 37:59–63, 1992.

121. Suzuki K, Suzuki S, Saito Y, Ikebuchi H, Terao T. Human growth hormone-stimulated growth of human cultured lymphocytes (IM-9) and its inhibition by phorbol diesters

through down-regulation of the hormone receptors. J Biol Chem 265:11320–11327, 1990.

122. Van Wyk JJ, Dugger GS, Newsome JF, Thomas PZ. The effect of pituitary stalk section in the adrenal function of women with cancer of the breast. J Clin Endocrinol Metab 20:157–172, 1960.

123. Webster EL, Battaglia G, DeSouza EB. Functional corticotropin releasing factor (CRF) receptors in mouse spleen: evidence for adenylate cyclase studies. Peptides 10:395–402, 1989.

124. Webster EL, DeSouza EB. Corticotropin-releasing factor receptors in mouse spleen: identification, autoradiographic localization, and regulation by divalent cations and guanine nucleotides. Endocrinology 122:609–617, 1988.

125. Webster EL, Tracey DE, DeSouza EB. Upregulation of interleukin-1 receptors in mouse AtT-20 pituitary tumor cells following treatment with corticotropin-releasing factor. Endocrinology 129:2796–2798, 1991.

126. Weigent DA, Baxter JB, Wear WE, Smith LR, Bost KL, Blalock JE. Production of immunoreactive growth hormone by mononuclear leukocytes. FASEB J 2:2812–2818, 1988.

127. Weigent DA, Blalock JE. Growth hormone and the immune system. Prog Neuro Endocrin Immunol 3:231–241, 1990.

128. Weigent DA, Blalock JE. Immunoreactive growth hormone releasing hormone in rat leukocytes. J Neuroimmunol 29:1–13, 1990.

129. Weigent DA, Blalock JE. Endogenous "neural and endocrine factors" made by immune cells. In: The Molecular Basis of Neuro-Immune Interactions, S Hauser, D Payan, eds. Pergamon Press, Oxford, 1996.

130. Weigent DA, LeBoeuf RD, Blalock, JE. An antisense oligonucleotide to growth hormone mRNA inhibits lymphocyte proliferation. Endocrinology 128:2053–2057, 1991.

131. Woloski BMRNJ, Smith EM, Meyer WJ III, Fuller GM, Blalock JE. Corticotropin-releasing activity of monokines. Science 230:1035–1037, 1985.

132. Yu-Lee L-Y, Stevens AM, Hrachovy JA, Schwarz LA. Prolactin-mediated regulation of gene transcription in lymphocytes. Ann NY Acad Sci 594:146–155, 1990.

133. Zakarija M, McKenzie JM. Influence of cytokines on growth and differentiated function of FRTL5 cells. Endocrinology 125:1260–1265, 1989.

134. Zelazowski P, Dohler KD, Stepien H, Pawlikowski M. Effect of growth hormone releasing hormone on human peripheral blood leukocyte chemotaxis and migration in normal subjects. Neuroendocrinology 50:236–239, 1989.

135. Zurawski G, Benedik M, Kamp BJ, Abrams JS, Zurawski SM, Lee FD. Activation of mouse T-helper cells induces abundant pre-proenkephalin mRNA synthesis. Science 232:772–775, 1986.

136. Zwilling BS, Lafuse WP, Brown D, Pearl D. Characterization of ACTH mediated suppression of MHC class II expression by murine peritoneal macrophages. J Neuroimmunol 39:133–138, 1992.

15

Establishment and Control of Viral Infections of the Central Nervous System

JÜRGEN SCHNEIDER-SCHAULIES
UWE G. LIEBERT
RÜDIGER DÖRRIES
VOLKER TER MEULEN

Viral CNS infections can be viewed as a competitive process in which several factors interact simultaneously. Not only the properties encoded by the viral agent but also the ability of host cell or tissue to react against the infection in addition to nonspecific and specific immune responses are important aspects that determine the outcome of the ensuing disease and the consequences for the entire host organism. On the one hand, for acute lytic virus infections of the CNS, a rapid and efficient elimination of the pathogenic agent is necessary because nerve cells lack the capacity for regeneration. On the other hand, the structure of the CNS, the restricted expression of major histocompatibility complex (MHC) antigens on glial cells and neurons, and the lack of lymphatic drainage facilitate the chances for viruses to persist or at least temporarily escape immune surveillance.

Viral infections of the CNS are rare but nevertheless medically important complications of systemic viral infections. They do not result per se from a pathogen's specific tropism for neural tissue since viruses associated with CNS disorders usually infect humans without involvement of this organ. Some viruses, e.g., certain enteroviruses, only lead to diseases when the brain or spinal cord is invaded. Other viruses, such as herpes simplex or mumps viruses, usually cause rather mild illnesses that may become severe when the CNS is also infected. Many neurotropic viruses more readily invade the CNS of the young, for the following obvious reasons: immaturity of the immune response, reduced capacity to produce interferon, dependence of susceptibility to viral infection on the stage of cell differentiation, and the age-specific nature and distribution of receptor protein. The efficiency with which a virus can multiply infection in the CNS and the effectiveness of the host immune response determine the extent of injury suffered by the host. This chapter discusses those aspects of viral pathogenesis in which CNS infections differ from systemic viral infections, rather than attempting to provide a complete overview of all the different virus infections of the CNS (see Table 15-1).

Entry Mechanisms of Viruses into the CNS

The CNS is usually not the primary site of viral replication. After infection and multiplication in the periphery are followed by viremia, viral particles or infected mononuclear cells invade the CNS by various pathways. The major route is hematogenous via the bloodstream (62). The blood-brain barrier (BBB) formed by endothelial cells of the cerebral microvasculature, astrocyte foot processes, and the basal lamina usually prevents viral particles from entering the CNS directly. The brain is, however, relatively easily accessible to activated lymphocytes and macrophages, which, if infected, may serve also as vehicles transporting viruses across the barrier (compare Induction of Cytokine Expression in the Brain). This transport mechanism for viruses, also referred to as the *Trojan horse* mechanism, is responsible for CNS

Table 15-1 Selected Viruses Causing CNS Diseases

Virus	Family (Genome)	Host (Model)	Pathological Changes in the CNS	References
Herpes simplex	Herpesviridae (dsDNA)	Human (mouse)	Acute cytolytic infection or latent infection of neurons	29,31,32,44,170,102,111, 116,138,145,159,174
LCM	Arenaviridae (ssRNA)	Mouse	Lymphocytic choriomeningitis	3,12,109,110,112,121,190
MHV-JHM	Coronaviridae (+ssRNA)	Mouse	Encephalomyelitis	23,38,42,59,72,125, 126,157,184,188,192
Measles	Paramyxoviridae (−ssRNA)	Human (mouse, rat)	Acute encephalitis or subacute sclerosing panencephalitis (SSPE)	9,17,22,41,49,54,34,88, 95,119,150,151,153, 156,157,173,181
Polio	Picornaviridae (+ssRNA)	Human (mouse)	Poliomyelitis or aseptic meningitis	4,55,58,66,70,71,76,103, 105,134,143,165
Rabies	Rabdoviridae (−ssRNA)	Human (mouse, rat)	Infection of neurons	10,28,33,75,118,176
Sindbis	Togaviridae (+ssRNA)	Human (mouse)	Human: no CNS disease Mouse: encephalitis	79,80,81,179
Theiler's	Picornaviridae (−ssRNA)	Mouse	Acute or chronic encephalomyelitis	8,20,24,90,101,104,117, 123,127,130,139,140, 141,186,187,194

infections with several viruses, among them paramyxoviruses, such as canine distemper, measles, and mumps (43,189), and lentiviruses, including human immunodeficiency virus (HIV)-1, simian immunodeficiency virus (SIV), and visna virus (50,115). Other viruses invade the CNS by direct infection of endothelial cells, a mechanism proposed for poliovirus (18), Sindbis virus (61), Semliki Forest virus (124) and murine retroviruses (171). Viruses can also invade the CNS via the stroma of the choroid plexus by infection of endothelial cells or by passive transport into the cerebrospinal fluid (CSF), where ependymal cells of the ventricle walls provide the basis for further spread in the CNS. This entry mechanism has been suggested for mumps virus (52), and eastern and western equine encephalitis virus (91).

The second major pathway of CNS infection is provided by direct infection of neurons at nerve endings in the periphery and subsequent retrograde axonal transport into the CNS. Herpes viruses (48,96), poliovirus (142), and rabies virus (60,113) have been shown to use the neural route of CNS invasion. In the case of herpes simplex virus (HSV) infection of humans, the primary sites of replication are the epithelial cells of the skin or mucosa before the virus enters peripheral ganglia. It has been demonstrated that axonal transport of herpes and rabies viruses occurs also in tissue culture of primary neurons and can be specifically inhibited in vitro and in vivo (74,78,93,94). This neural pathway of entry using direct cellular connections into the CNS keeps viruses hidden from the immune system until the CNS infection is established. Once in the CNS, the cellular tropism and the replication cycle of viruses determine the efficiency of the developing immune response (Fig. 15-1).

Virus–Cell Interactions in the CNS

The interaction of infectious viruses with susceptible cells lead in general to cell destruction, persistent infection, or cell transformation. This is largely determined by the genetic constitution of the host cell and by the type of viral agent. After infectious virus has reached the CNS, a disease develops only if viral spread within the CNS is accomplished and sufficient numbers of susceptible cells are infected, leading to brain dysfunction. In this respect, a number of unique features of the CNS are noteworthy. First, the nervous system contains a highly differentiated cell population with complex, functionally integrated cell-to-cell connections and highly specialized cytoplasmic membranes. This probably results in the great variability in virus receptor sites on cells and in their capacity to replicate viruses. Second, CNS tissue is unique in its high metabolic rate and relative lack of capacity to regenerate. While persistent infection by a noncytopathogenic virus in cells of an organ with a low energy requirement and high rate of regeneration may be tolerated, in CNS tissue such infections may interfere with normal function, especially when neurons are affected. Third, the privileged site of the brain, its relative isolation from the immune system, is another feature that plays an important role in the establishment and pathogenesis of CNS infections (62).

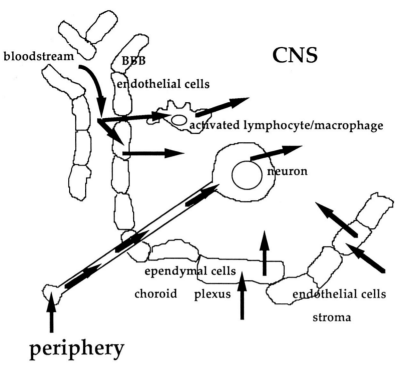

Fig. 15-1. Routes of viral entry into the CNS. Viruses gain access to the CNS via transport in lymphocytes and macrophages, infection of endothelial and ependymal cells, and axonal retrograde transport.

Acute Cytolytic Infections

Acute cytolytic infections inevitably lead to cell death and to the release of progeny virus. Cell destruction is induced by the products of the viral genome or their effect on the regulatory mechanism of the cell. For some viruses, such as herpes and polio-myelitis virus, the molecular events taking place during a lytic infection have been well described for tissue culture systems and it would be logical to assume that similar processes occur in CNS infections (103,170).

One of the most severe acute viral infections of the CNS is caused by herpes simplex virus, which results either from a primary infection or reactivation of a latent virus infection. Productive replication in brain tissue leads to cell destruction, the extent and pathology of which depend on the effectiveness of the host defense mechanism. Central phenomena for CNS infection with HSV include the neuroinvasiveness and neuro-virulence of the virus. Extensive molecular biological studies have defined several regions on the viral genome as specific contributors to these processes (170). HSV consists of a 152 kb linear double-stranded DNA in four isomeric arrangements that codes for 77 genes, 74 of which are present in one copy per genome. Of the 74 different HSV genes, 37 have been deleted without losing the capacity of the virus to replicate in cell cultures. These genes are referred to as *supplemental essential genes,* which are associated with the function of virus entry, sorting, augmenting precursor pool or repair of DNA, and shut-off of host macromolecular metabolism. Although the role of these 37 genes for the biological properties of HSV has not been fully defined, there is evidence that some of these dispensable genes are linked directly to the neuroinvasiveness and neurovirulence of this virus (29,31,174). Obviously, for the survival of HSV in a human population the virus only requires a certain set of genes, since infection of the CNS is a dead end for the pathogen. However, the capacity of this agent to cause CNS disease is related to additional genes that allow the virus to invade the CNS, to replicate in a variety of different brain cells, and to spread efficiently from cell to cell. It has been observed that the genes dispensable for HSV replication in dividing cells, such as the thymidine kinase gene, are required for infection of nondividing or polarized cells. Marker rescue experiments also suggest a relationship between the viral DNA-polymerase, and neuroinvasiveness and neurovirulence (31). The majority of viral deletion mutants have shown to have a reduced capacity to invade the CNS and to replicate in brain cells. Furthermore, changes in the genes coding for structural glycoproteins D, C, and B, as well as immediate early genes and the long-terminal repeat region are involved (29,174). Once infection of neurons has occurred, one of two mutually exclusive events will take place. Only if immediate early genes, which regulate the viral lytic cascade, are repressed, will the neuronal destruction and killing be prevented. The price the infected cell must pay is the establishment of viral latency with potential reactivation of viral multiplication.

Another destructive infection of CNS tissue is observed during poliomyelitis (103). The portal of entry for poliovirus is the alimentary tract, as experimental studies in monkeys have shown. The virus replicates first in the tonsils, lymph nodes of the neck, Peyer's patches, and the small intestine. Viremia subsequently develops, which can lead to an infection of the target organ, the spinal cord, or brain. Alternatively, poliovirus may spread along the axons of peripheral nerves to the CNS, as has been demonstrated in experimental infection (76,103). This latter route of virus infection may occur in children who have had an infection at the time of tonsillectomy or in patients who receive an injection of an irritating material during a period of high poliovirus prevalence. Once poliovirus has entered the CNS, neuronal tissue is damaged or completely destroyed as a consequence of intracellular replication. The anterior horn cells of the spinal cord are most prominently involved, resulting in a flaccid paralysis. However, in severe cases posterior horn lesions can be found and the virus may also spread to the brain.

Poliovirus, of which three serotypes exist, is a member of the enterovirus genus, which contains an RNA genome of a single-strand, positive-sense molecule. This genome closely resembles a cellular messenger RNA in structure and function (70,143,175). The fine structure of poliovirus has been determined by X-ray crystallography (55).

The replication of poliovirus begins with its binding to a specific cellular receptor, which is a typical transmembrane protein belonging to a previously unrecognized member of the immunoglobulin (Ig) superfamily (105). It is of interest to note that receptor mRNA can be detected in many tissues that do not bind the poliovirus or support its replication. Since it has been shown in tissue culture that several alternatively spliced mRNAs of the receptor exist, it is conceivable that not all expressed forms of the receptor protein can function as a receptor for poliovirus (71,105). In addition, another surface molecule of human cells, CD44, has recently been found to be functionally associated with the infection of cells with poliovirus and might determine the cellular tropism of the virus, although poliovirus does not bind directly to CD44 (165).

To understand the neurovirulence of poliovirus, nucleotide sequencing and gene cloning were carried out to identify the genetic differences between wild-type virulent strains of poliovirus and the live-attenuated strains used as vaccines (4). The most significant changes were observed in the 5' nontranslated region (NTR) at positions 480, 481, and 472 in poliovirus types 1, 2, and 3, respectively. These mutations could be linked to the ability of the different virus strains to replicate in mouse brain or in neuroblastoma cells in culture (76). Detailed investigation of the structure and function of the mutated NTR region revealed that attenuating mutations in the vaccine strains act through the disruption of a stem structure in the region of positions 470–540. Computer-generated analysis suggested that the greater the disruption of the stem, the greater the temperature sensitivity and the extent of attenuation. The intracellular functions of these mutations have not yet been identified completely, but the data available suggest that the 5' NTR interacts with cellular factors influencing the tropism of the virus. Understanding of the intracellular events may eventually provide an explanation as to why motor neurons are the specific target cells for these particular enteroviruses. The tissue tropism, neurovirulence, and species specificity of the poliovirus infection are currently being studied in a transgenic mouse model (58,134).

The control of poliovirus infection in an organism depends on the immune system. The humoral immune response is most important in this process, since persistent poliovirus infections are not known and viral membrane changes, as seen, for example, in budding viruses, are not observed. Although the virus–cell interaction in this disease is to some extent well understood, the host factors, which in most cases prevent poliovirus from entering the CNS and infecting the neural tissue, are still unknown.

Persistent Infections

Within the group of persistent virus infections, a variety of virus–cell and virus–host interactions exists which forms the basis for different disease processes. First, latent viral infections are characterized by intermittent episodes of viral replication and formation of infectious virus (recurrence). This may remain clinically silent or result in overt clinical disease (recrudescence). In between such episodes, the virus remains within the host in a quiescent form. Second, in chronic viral infections, virus can be reproducibly and continuously recovered from the host. Overt clinical disease may or may not develop. In some cases, disease is caused not by the replication of virus, but by the action of the immune system, or immunopathologically. Third, in slow virus infections prior to clinical manifestation, a long incubation period of months to years is followed by a slowly progressive disease course that is usually fatal. During the incubation period, the concentration of virus in the infected organism increases until disease becomes manifest.

As an example to illustrate that closely related viruses may induce acute as well as persistent CNS infections, Theiler's murine encephalomyelitis virus (TMEV) infection in mice will be discussed in some detail. This infection has been used to serve as a model for such diverse human diseases as poliomyelitis and multiple sclerosis (MS). TMEV is a member of the cardiovirus genus of the Picornaviridae and the structure of its RNA genome is very similar to the human polioviruses. There are two groups of known isolates that cause either acute, rapidly fatal encephalitis (virulent strains GDVII and FA), or biphasic chronic persistent diseases with demyelination (so-called avirulent strains To, BeAn, DA). Despite their different biological properties, both strains are highly homologous with 95% identity at the genome and 90% at the protein level (127,128). Through generation of chimeric viruses containing genomic mixtures of the two virus groups, as well as through generation or isolation of mutant strains that have reverted to an avirulent phenotype, regions of the genome associated with neurovirulence and persistence have been mapped, to the 5' NTR and to the L/P1/2A region coding for the capsid protein VP1 (24,101). These regions are similar to those of poliovirus. Isolation of monoclonal antibody (MAb) escape mutants with a single amino acid change in the VP1 underline the importance of this protein for the viral phenotype (194).

Acute, fatal infection with the virulent strains of TMEV predominantly affects neurons in the cerebral cortex and the ventral horns of the spinal cord (as in poliovirus infections). The principal portal of entry into the CNS is by axonal transport, although endothelial cell infection has also been shown (193). In contrast, a persistent infection primarily of oligodendrocytes develops in most mice surviving the infection with avirulent strains of TMEV in which infectious virus is associated with demyelinating lesions (186). Here the entry of virus into the CNS might involve macrophages as "Trojan horse" since TMEV has been shown to persist in macrophages in vitro and macrophage-like cells constitute about 10% of infected cells in the brain (8). The mechanism of persistence may involve interferon-induced blockage of viral RNA replication at the level of negative-strand RNA synthesis (141) and the generation of antigenic variants by antibody escape.

The susceptibility to TMEV infection is associated with the MHC class I locus H-2D and two non-MHC genes encoded on chromosomes 3 and 6 (104,139). It has been shown that CD8+ T cells are involved in antiviral immunity during acute infection.

These cells may play a role in immune surveillance of persistently infected CNS cells, but they are not vital for recovery from acute infection (20). Essential for the control of TMEV infection are CD4+ T cells, as has been shown by depleting this cell type, or by inhibiting its function in vivo using anti-CD4 or anti-Ia blocking MAbs, respectively (187). On the other hand, TMEV-specific CD4+ T cells apparently lead to immunopathology, i.e., demyelination in this model. Essentially three possibilities exist to explain this pathological response. First, the CD4 cells directly damage MHC class II expressing glial cells. Second, they induce mononuclear cell infiltraiton and activate macrophages, which can lead to damage of myelinated nerves in the so-called by-stander effect. Third, during the infection, T cells with autoimmune properties against nerve cell antigens could be induced, which might exacerbate ongoing pathology or induce new lesions.

In the human nervous system only the latent and the slow virus type of infection is found. The classical latent infection is caused by herpes simplex virus types 1 and 2. HSV is transmitted from human to human by skin or mucous membrane contact and has the ability to remain latent in the nervous system for the lifetime of the host. Its occurrence is not restricted to sensory neurons and it has also been detected in neurons of peripheral nerve ganglia, the adrenal medulla, retina, and the CNS (170). Although known for 20 years, latency in sensory neurons has only recently been studied successfully and partially characterized with the detection of a unique transcription unit. The establishment of the latent phase is a function controlled and executed by the neuron rather than by the virus itself. This is conceivable, because viruses selected for their ability to replicate still establish latent infection, and mutants with deletion of the immediate-early transcript regulator gene ICP4 persist in neurons (159). Although no infectious virus can be isolated during latency, viral genomes can be detected as multiple extrachromosomal DNA copies characteristically represented as covalently closed circles associated with nucleosomes (32,102,111,138). The only viral RNA transcripts detected in latently infected neurons are the so-called latency-associated transcripts (LATs) (44). Analyses of viruses encoding for mutant LAT genes showed that replication competence in tissue culture cells and the establishment of latent infections in vivo is not affected. A functional role for the LAT genes during reactivation has recently been suggested by showing that LAT minus mutants were reactivated normally from sacral ganglia, but only slowly from trigeminal ganglia (145). Although open reading frames are present within LAT sequences, it is not known whether proteins are expressed. While the underlying molecular events that trigger viral reactivation are still unknown, clinical observations have shown that recurrence is associated with physical or emotional stress, immune suppression, UV light, or nerve damage. For the immune system, HSV in latently infected neurons is refractory and cannot be cleared from those cells. The role of the immune system in controlling HSV infection is not entirely clear, because recurrences can be observed even in the presence of an apparently normal cell-mediated and humoral immune response. While there seems to be no impact on nerve function during silent periods of latency, reactivation of HSV leads to the destruction of infected neurons. Since only a low number of neurons within one nerve are infected and in only a very small proportion of those neurons is HSV reactivation successful, there is usually no functional defect observed.

The best-studied slow virus disease of humans associated with a conventional virus is subacute sclerosing panencephalitis (SSPE) (173). The disease develops on the basis of a persistent measles virus (MV) infection in brain cells months to years after acute measles. How and when the virus reaches the CNS as well as the mechanisms that trigger the disease remain unknown. The broad tropism of MV for human tissue seems to be determined by its receptor usage. Recently, the complement receptor CD46 has been identified as receptor for MV (34,114). In addition, a second molecule is involved in the susceptibility of cells for MV forming a complex with CD46 (37,149). Both molecules are widely expressed in the human body and may well mediate the infection of various brain cells with MV. The persistent infection is characterized by a restricted measles virus gene expression at several stages (17,155). Electron microscopical studies revealed the presence of viral nucleocapsids in neurons and other cells of the CNS in the absence of viral budding from these cells. It was found that the viral envelope proteins are markedly underexpressed or absent in infected brain cells. Transcriptional efficiencies of the corresponding mRNAs are reduced, leading to a steep expression gradient for the virus-specific monocistronic transcripts and, in some cases, an increased number of bicistronic transcripts has been observed. Mutations and hypermutations in various genes of cloned SSPE viruses have been found to prevent a complete replicative cycle of measles virus and might contribute to the establishment of persistence (8,27,53,135). In addition, at least three further mechanisms may contribute to the restriction of MV gene expression, thus supporting the establishment of persistence. First, high levels of intrathecal antibodies causing antibody-induced antigenic modulation; second, a brain cell–specific restriction of MV mRNA expression; and third, the presence of (interferon) IFN-α/β and interferon-inducible gene products in SSPE brains. In spite of the massive immune response during SSPE, clearance of virus from the CNS is not observed. In tissue culture experiments and in the rat model, antibody-induced antigenic modulation with MAbs to MV hemagglutinin caused the down-regulation of viral RNA and protein expression. Complete clearance of virus is not achieved, since removal of antibodies led to reactivation of the viral infection from low copy numbers of persisting viral genomes (15,87,153). Similar experiments have recently been described with Sindbis virus in immunodeficient SCID-mice, where infectious viral particles are cleared from the CNS by antiviral antibodies, but viral RNA can persist for months in mouse brains (79,80,81). Intrinsic brain cell–specific mechanisms leading to a restriction of MV expression were found in the rat model, in primary rodent astrocytes, and human glioblastoma cell lines (151,152,154). The induction of cytokines by MV infection of brain cells, especially of type-I interferon, leads to further antiviral activity (46,54) and might cause the selection of interferon-resistant MV strains persisting in the brain (26). Recently, evidence has been provided that the interferon-inducible Mx protein inhibits the expression of MV in human monocytes and neural cells (156,157). Although the inhibition was determined in a cell type-specific manner to occur at the transcriptional or post-translational level, the mechanism of Mx action is still unknown.

Impact on Specific Neural Cell Functions

Before discussing the immune response against viral infections in the CNS, we should briefly mention a few direct consequences of the virus–cell interaction on the function of the infected cell itself. Such consequences may be severe, even if only restricted areas of the CNS are involved and particularly when brain cells are affected, the function of which is vital for the host. In rat astrocytoma cells persistently infected with MV it has been demonstrated that this infection strongly reduces the cAMP response following the addition of catecholamines, and that not only the density of β-adrenergic receptors is decreased by 50% but also coupling of the receptor to G-proteins is affected (51,73). The endothelin-1-induced Ca^{2+} signal was absent in cells persistently infected with MV and 95% of the binding sites for endothelin-1 were lost (172). Furthermore, anti-MV antibodies, which are present in high concentrations in SSPE brain, influenced the inositol-phosphate signal transduction pathway in these cells (185).

A further example for direct disturbance of brain cell functions is the infection with rabies virus (RV). This virus may cause a nonlytic infection of brain cells that rapidly leads to the death of the infected individual. The cytopathic effects in the CNS may vary considerably depending on the strain of RV; little is known about the immune response during human rabies infections (10,118). In contrast to the limited cytopathology, the death of the infected individual seems to be caused by interference of the virus with neuronal cell functions in vital centers of the brain regulating sleep, body temperature, and respiration (176). In experimental rabies infections it was observed that the uptake and release of gamma-amino-n-butyric acid (GABA) was reduced by 45% in rabies-infected embryonic rat cortical neurons (75) and that binding of 5-hydroxytryptamine to serotonin receptor subtypes is reduced by 50% in infected rat brains (28). It is conceivable that disturbances of specialized receptor systems for neurotransmitter and neurohormone turnover, as well as for the generation of chemical signals and electrical potentials, might be the major cause of death in the viral infection rather than cytopathic effects or immunopathogenesis.

Induction of Cytokine Expression in the Brain

In response to a viral infection, cytokines are secreted within the CNS either from infected brain cells or from lymphomononuclear cell infiltrates. Cytokines serve as important factors for the induction of MHC molecules and the stimulation of the humoral and cell-mediated immune response by acting on cells of the immune system as well as surrounding brain cells, thereby inducing antiviral proteins like Mx or the expression of surface recognition molecules like MHC antigens (25,129). There is an increasing number of studies measuring cytokine levels in human diseased brains. For example, in brains of SSPE patients, elevated levels of IFN-α/β, and IFN-γ and tumor necrosis factor (TNF)-α positive cells have been detected (30,54,63). In the brains of HIV-1-infected patients, where essentially CD4-positive microglial cells take up and propagate the virus, these cells have been found to be the source of intrathecal synthesis of IL-1, IL-6, granulocyte-macrophage colony-stimulating factor (GM-CSF), and TNF-α (65,107). Especially TNF-α and IL-1 have pleiotropic, or even toxic effects in the CNS, including regulation of body temperature and sleep, stimulation of surface molecules, chronic inflammatory effects, and the stimulation of proliferation and differentiation of glial cells (47,97,106,129). Since these two cytokines and MHC class II antigens were increased in gliotic areas of HIV brains, a potential role for the immune system in the pathogenesis of HIV encephalopathy has been suggested (179). Furthermore, TNF-α, IFN-γ, and IFN-β can contribute to selective virus elimination by interacting directly with infected brain cells (67,92,147).

The data obtained so far from human brains reflect late or final stages of disease processes and little is known about the expression of cytokines and their cellular sources during early phases of an infection, when virus is spreading in the brain. To study the role of cytokines in the development of viral CNS infections, animal models, particularly with RNA viruses, have been investigated with respect to cytokine expression. Induction of IL-1α, IL-2, IL-6, TNF-α, and IFN-γ mRNA synthesis has been found in Borna disease virus (BDV)-infected rat brains within 2 weeks after intranasal infection. IL-2 and IFN-γ mRNA expression correlated well with the appearance of CD4+ and CD8+ lymphocytes during the early stages of BDV infection (164). Interesting differences in the cytokine expression of acute and persistent infections in the CNS have also been found. In the CSF of mice persistently infected with lymphocytic choriomeningitis virus (LCMV), significant levels of IL-6 could be detected in high-responder (NMRI) but not in low-responder (CBA/J) mouse strains. In contrast, after acute intracerebral infection, both strains contained high levels of IL-6 in the CSF and serum (110). The source of IL-6 in mouse brains has been identified to be astrocytes and microglial cells infected with LCMV or vesicular stomatitis virus (45). In tissue cultures of rat astrocytes, Newcastle disease virus has been shown to induce TNF-α and -β, IL-6, and IFN-α and -β shortly after primary infections (82). Infection of human astrocytoma cells with measles virus also resulted in a transient expression of a similar set of cytokines, namely IL-1, IFN-β, IL-6, and TNF-α (150). In contrast to the acute cytolytic infection, astrocytoma cells persistently infected with measles virus continuously produced IL-6 and IFN-β, whereas TNF-α and IL-1β were hardly detectable. However, the pathways for induction of TNF-α and IL-1β expression in these cells were found not to be suppressed by the persistent infection, and additional stimuli like diacylglycerol and calcium ionophore could induce overexpression of these cytokines (150). These findings suggest that the induction of certain cytokines may play an important role for activation of the humoral and cell-mediated antiviral immune response, as well as for the pathogenesis observed during a particular viral CNS infection.

MHC Expression in the Brain and Its Relation to Viral Infection

Since astrocytes and microglial cells are important antigen presenting cells in the CNS, it is interesting that virus infections can lead to, or increase the level of MHC class II expression on the surface of these cells. This process can be observed in the absence of IFN-γ as a direct effect of the infection, as shown for murine coronavirus J. Howard Mueller virus (JHMV)- or MV-infected astrocytes (98,99). Interestingly, in the TMEV model it was shown that MHC induction was IFN-γ dependent and did not result from mere TMEV infection. It was found that the susceptibility to immunopathology depends on the mouse strains. MHC class II was readily inducible in the susceptible SJL and CBA strains but not in the resistant Balb/c mice (117). In contrast, in BN rats, which live well with experimental JHMV or MV infections, a constitutive high MHC class II expression in the brain was detected, while in Lewis rats, in which MHC class II expression occurred as a consequence of the viral infection, immunopathological (autoimmune) processes are observed in a significant proportion of the animals. This illustrates that early presence of immunoregulatory molecules in the brain may serve a protective purpose, while the same process could lead to pathology and disease when MHC molecules are expressed several days or weeks later (161).

Generally, induction of MHC molecules on neural cells, where they are usually absent or expressed at low levels, is one of the prerequisites for efficient cell-mediated defense against intracellular pathogens in the brain. That this is not sufficient, however, to result in viral elimination, is well illustrated by observations of brain tissue from patients with progressive multifocal leukoencephalopathy, a slow papovavirus infection predominantly of oligodendrocytes with extensive demyelination and bizarre glial cell changes. Here, both MHC class I and II are expressed in the lesions, yet viral clearance does not occur, probably because there are no reactive T cells generated and the patients generally are immunosuppressed. This may allow for the establishment of persistent and ultimately chronic viral infection with progressive disease (1).

The Humoral Immune Response in the CNS

It has been shown that the control of virus infection depends on the generation of both humoral and cell-mediated immune responses. Antibodies, which attack predominantly extracellular virus particles released from infected cells, are essential to limit the spread of virus in the host. However, the failure to clear varicella zoster, cytomegalovirus, or measles virus infections in cell-mediated immunodeficiency states suggests that T-cell responses may be more important than antibody in overcoming several virus infections. In this context it is important to remember that the immune response to viral infections of the CNS is probably initiated in peripheral lymphoid tissue followed by entry of activated (end-differentiated) T cells into the cerebrospinal fluid, meninges, and brain parenchyma (162). To study these aspects of viral CNS infections, the use of animal model systems is a necessity.

Inhibition of Virus Entry into the Brain and Blockade of Intracerebral Viral Spread

Virus-specific antibodies are the main tool of the infected host to prevent extracellular hematogenous viral spread from primary sites of infection to other organs during viremia (166). Since virtually all viral CNS infections are preceded by primary peripheral infection, it is clear that virus neutralization and opsonization during viremia is one of the most efficient defense reactions to prevent viral entry into the CNS. This was shown, first, for agammaglobulinemic patients who suffer more frequently from persistent CNS infections as compared to fully immunocompetent hosts (167), and second, by the preventive effect of peripheral virus-specific antibodies for neuroinvasion in perinatal viral hosts whose immune system is not yet fully developed. Experimentally, the lethal encephalomyelitis induced by the murine coronavirus JHM (JHMV) in newborn or suckling rats was prevented by nursing the babies with milk from JHMV immunized mothers (126,184). Identical findings were recently published in a mouse model of murine retrovirus-induced neurological diseases (144). Baldridge and co-workers (12) demonstrated protection from LCMV-induced teratogenic effects in neonatals nursed by immunized mothers or injected with LCMV-specific neutralizing MAbs. Moreover, experimental virus infections of the CNS in immunocompetent hosts remain regularly subclinical if a strong virus-neutralizing antibody response is mounted (66,136,158,177).

Nevertheless, viruses manage to circumvent extracerebral neutralization and succeed in entering the CNS. In cases where viruses use retrograde transport along the axonal routes of peripheral nerves, the virus is inaccessible to the immune system as it disappears in the nerve cell, and the immune system is no longer aware of the invading agent. Neither virus-specific antibodies nor cytotoxic T lymphocytes (CTL) can prevent the axonal transport of the virus to the CNS, especially because nerve cells most likely are unable to up-regulate MHC class I molecules (108). In addition, by using leukocytes as "Trojan horses," viruses can escape neutralization by antibodies. Although there is so far no direct experimental evidence for this hypothesis, it is a likely way of bypassing the BBB unrecognized by peripheral virus-specific antibodies. With the infection of peripheral recirculating monocytes, these viruses enhance the probability to reach the perivascular space in the CNS, because in contrast to ramified microglia, the perivascular type of this cell is frequently exchanged by peripheral monocytes (160,163).

After infection of resident target cells, the virus has the chance to replicate and spread in the CNS, as long as the infected host does not succeed in recruiting immune effector cells into the brain parenchyma. Among these effector cells, plasma cells of B-lymphocyte lineage home toward virus-infected sites of the tissue (36), where they secrete virus-specific antibodies (158). Cytotoxic T lymphocytes provide an early virus-specific defense mechanism in the brain parenchyma. Nevertheless, although they can eliminate virus-infected cells by lysis very efficiently, they are unable to prevent formation of secondary virus-infected foci in the tissue through extracellular spread of the virus. This needs intracerebral secretion of virus-specific antibodies in close spatial arrangement to infected sites of the tissue. As has been shown in several animal models of virus induced encephalitis, these antibodies will significantly restrict extracellular viral spread in the CNS (7,38,123,125,158,191). Most interestingly, not only is extracellular spread limited by virus-specific antibodies, but dissemination from cell to cell, e.g., fusion, can be interrupted by antibodies, as shown for mice infected with rabies virus (33). The underlying molecular mechanism is not fully understood, but it is suggested that upon uptake of antibody-complexed virus into the infected nerve cell, viral RNA transcription is severely disturbed. In line with this concept are the data obtained in vitro and in vivo with antibody-induced antigenic modulation (15,87,153; compare 3.2), which demonstrate abrogation of measles virus transcription by antiviral antibodies. These findings were further extended by data from immunodeficient SCID mice infected with Sindbis virus (81). In this model system, intracerebral replication of the virus was prevented by passive immunization of the animals with virus-specific antibodies in the absence of T lymphocytes. Morphological studies by immune electron microscopy supported the view that viral replication is disturbed on the transcriptional or translational level, because the typical arrangement of virus-specific proteins in perinuclear cytopathic vacuoles and the amount of rough endoplasmatic reticulum was drastically reduced in antibody-treated neurons after virus infection.

Although it is generally assumed that the protective effect of a virus neutralizing antibody in the CNS is mainly due to binding of its F_{ab}-part to viral epitopes necessary for infection of the target cell, recent data strongly suggest an important contribution of the F_c-part of the antibody molecule to its protective capacity. Schlesinger and co-workers (148) have shown that a MAb specific for the yellow fever virus (YFV) nonstructural protein NS1 protects mice only from encephalitis when given as an intact molecule but not as F(ab)$_2$-fragment, although this fragment can neutralize YFV infectivity in vitro. Moreover, protection was limited to a MAb of the IgG$_{2a}$ subclass; neither IgG$_1$ or IgG$_{2b}$ MAbs that were able to neutralize YFV in vitro were able to protect the animals from acute encephalitis. Since NS1 is expressed on the surface of YFV infected cells and since the protective property of the MAb is independent of the complement system, it seems likely that only binding of a distinct IgG subclass to NS1 allows recognition by Fc receptor (FcR) expressing cells. In this context, it is of note that in Semliki Forest virus (SFV) infection of mice, IgG2a is the dominant subclass in the CSF for a long time after infection (122) and that most virus-specific antibody-secreting cells (AbSC) from the CNS of Sindbis virus–infected animals secrete the IgG2a subclass (178). Similarly, effective protection from LCMV induced encephalitis depends on IgG2a (11). Although these findings suggest an important role for IgG2a in protection from virally induced CNS disease in the mouse, it is clearly not a general principle, since in rabies virus–infected mice protection from lethal disease is achieved by IgG1 and IgG2a subclasses (33).

Successful action of the afferent arm of the humoral immune response requires very rapid recruitment of virus-specific AbSC into the brain parenchyma. This is usually achieved if viral CNS infection occurs concomitantly with the acute peripheral infection because in this case, preexisting AbSC can immediately enter the brain tissue, allowing early restriction of viral distribution. In contrast, when viral CNS infection occurs late after primary infection or remains unrecognized by the immune system, the immune response has to be initiated in local secondary lymphatics, such as the cervical lymph nodes (CLNs). This gives the virus considerably more time to travel through the tissue, until humoral effector systems reach the brain parenchyma. Speed of AbSC recruitment is also determined by the genetic background of the host, as is clearly evident from studies of coronavirus JHM-induced encephalomyelitis in rats. While clinically resistant brown Norway (BN) rats rapidly recruit virus-specific AbSC into infected areas of the brain, clinically highly susceptible Lewis (LEW) rats exhibit a significant delay in this process (158). The differences are explained by a more rapid differentiation of virus-specific CD4+ T helper cells in CLNs of BN rats as compared to LEW animals (59).

Of equal importance are the specificity and effectiveness of the recruited humoral response. As seen in severe acute Sindbis virus encephalitis in mice, the vast majority of AbSC extracted from the brains of these animals within the first few days postinfection is not of viral specificity (179). In the JHMV rat model, an individual plasma cell from the brain of infected but clinically healthy BN rats synthesizes approximately 5 times more virus-specific antibodies as compared to a plasma cell from the CNS of infected and severely diseased LEW rats (158). As a consequence, effective virus-neutralizing antibody titers appear late in the CSF of the latter animal strain.

The effect of a late or a rather unspecific recruitment of humoral immunity to the CNS is often disastrous. Viral spread within the CNS can result in destruction of important neural cells and/or disturbances of vital functions of the CNS. Moreover, large infected areas will cause a more vigorous infiltration of virus-specific T cells as is usually seen in cases of limited viral spread. This may end in severe enhancement of neurological disease and even cause rapid death. This intimate relationship between virus-specific antibody response and T cell–mediated immunopathology was observed in acute LCMV-induced encephalitis of mice. In this model, passive administration of MAbs between 1 day before and 2 days after viral infection resulted in protection of mice from lethal encephalitis. This was accompanied by a diminished CTL response and clearance of the virus from the brain with less tissue damage than is usually seen in unprotected mice (190).

Similar results were obtained in the measles encephalitis model in rats and mice (41,88). Here the induction of MV-neutralizing antibodies may completely suppress the development of disease in weanling animals (22,95), and maternal antibodies transferred during gestation are protective in newborn animals. These findings are consistent with the resistance to encephalitis observed in BN rats that mount an early and high-level, MV-specific humoral immune response (88). The inevitably fatal acute disease can also be prevented by passive immunization of newborn animals with neutralizing monoclonal antibodies, albeit at the price of converting the infection into one of a persistent nature (87,131). Thus, the presence of mere antibody, even if neutralizing the infectivity of virus, may be generally insufficient to eliminate measles virus from the infected brain as long as no MV-reactive T cells are available. On the contrary, even without available virus-neutralizing antibodies, animals can be protected. This was demonstrated by immunization with recombinant vaccinia viruses expressing either the internal nucleocapsid (N) protein, or hemagglutinin (H) or fusion (F) glycoprotein, which prevented the disease that results from subsequent challenge with MV in nonimmunized rats, as well as in mMT mice (69) that have an inherent defect for antibody production (13,22,41; Liebert and Geißendörfer, unpublished results).

Enhancement of Viral Pathogenesis by Humoral Effector Systems

In general, humoral immunity does not contribute to the pathology of viral CNS infection. Nevertheless, there are theoretical considerations and experimental data obtained in vitro that do not strictly rule out disease-enhancing properties of humoral immune responses. Intrathecal antibody synthesis may help to augment viral pathogenesis by antibody-dependent enhancement (ADE). This phenomenon refers to the uptake of antibody-complexed viral particles by cells that do not necessarily express a virus-specific receptor. Adhesion to the target cell is achieved either by binding to the FcR, or in the case of activation of the complement cascade, by antibody-complexed particles through attachment via the C3 receptor. In vitro, the latter seems to occur more readily than FcR binding. Nevertheless, in both cases cells of the monocyte–macrophage lineage are prime targets for ADE (57). Therefore, in the CNS, microglial cells should be preferentially prone to ADE.

Theoretically, presence of virus-specific antibodies in the CNS could allow a complement-dependent immunological effector mechanism to operate, namely, antibody-activated cytolytic action of complement. So far, there are very little in vivo data supporting this hypothesis. On the one hand, in the rat model of JHMV-induced demyelination, enrichment of complement components and immunoglobulin was found in infected areas of the brain (192), and activation of the complement cascade in CSF has been demonstrated in patients suffering from HIV-1 infection (132). On the other hand, investigations in Theiler's virus–induced demyelinating encephalitis of mice have shown enhancement of tissue lesions in complement-depleted mice as compared to untreated animals (140). This argues strongly against antibody- and complement-mediated pathology. In line with these findings is the observation that there is no evidence for antibody-mediated tissue destruction in the CNS of AIDS patients (77). Thus, the question of antibody- and complement-mediated cytotoxicity as a relevant in vivo mechanism of tissue-destructive virus elimination is still open and a matter of conflicting debate.

However, indirect tissue destruction might occur during viral encephalitis. Activation of macrophages or microglia may be triggered by engagement of the FcR, which is expressed at high densities on these cells. Binding of immune complexes to the FcR of macrophages can stimulate these cells to release toxic substances that will cause severe bystander destruction of "innocent," healthy cells in the surroundings of virus-infected areas. This assumption is supported by the observation in vitro of macrophage-dependent oligodendroglia cell degeneration in mixed glial cell cultures that were treated with immune complexes formed by canine distemper virus (CDV) and CDV-specific antibodies (21).

Viral Persistence and Virus-specific Antibodies

Incomplete elimination of virus from the CNS will result in persistent infection. Usually, a long-lasting intrathecal antibody synthesis with specificity for viral proteins accompanies viral persistence (168,179) and efficiently prevents reactivation of the infection (79). Over time, there is selection of the best-fitting antibody clones to the virus. Thus high-avidity antibodies eventually prevail, and the respective clones are preferentially recruited to the CNS. In this case, isoelectric focusing of cerebrospinal fluid specimens will show a restricted "oligoclonal pattern" of antibody clones as compared to the polyclonal distribution detectable in paired serum specimens. Presence of these oligoclonal bands can continue over decades after primary infection of the CNS; therefore, it is used as diagnostic marker in viral CNS infections (39).

Beside the fact that intrathecal virus-specific antibody synthesis is a relevant indicator of viral CNS infection, long-lasting presence of these antibodies in high titers is thought to interfere with viral replication, thereby probably contributing to selection of virus variants. Direct evidence for selection of neurotropic variants by antibodies has been provided by the demonstration of changes in the cell tropism of neurotropic JHMV when grown in the presence of virus-neutralizing MAbs (23). Furthermore, in the CNS of mice inoculated with both the neurotropic virus and the MAb, viral target cells were primarily oligodendrocytes. This was in striking contrast to animals inoculated exclusively with virus alone, where neurons were the major target. Recently this observation was further extended by work in a rat model of MV-induced encephalitis

(88).When given intraperitoneally (i.p.), MV-neutralizing MAbs modified the disease process in these animals (see Inhibition of Virus Entry into the Brain and Blockade of Intracerebral Viral Spread) and occasionally prevention of the usually necrotizing encephalitis was seen in unprotected rats. However, MV variants emerged that were no longer neutralized by the i.p. administered MAb, but they were with other MAbs (83). From these data it has to be concluded that only rapid and effective elimination of virus-infected CNS cells will prevent long-lasting antibody-controlled persistence of the virus and thereby the potentially dangerous development of viral variants with altered neurotropism.

The Cell-mediated Immune Response

In contrast to the effect of antibody-mediated antiviral mechanisms, which at least in vivo act predominantly either against the virus itself or interact with cell surface molecules without damaging the cell integrity, the T cell–mediated immune protection is generally mediated by cell destruction, i.e., pathology. In experimental infection of mice with the lymphocytic choriomeningitis virus, the number of infected brain cells has been shown to constitute an important factor directing beneficial or harmful effects mediated by effector lymphocyte activity (3). Since a timely T-cell immune response encounters a limited number of infected cells, the pathology inflicted should be little in most instances of acute viral encephalitis, and the beneficial effects will usually outweigh the harmful effects of the cell-mediated immune response. Paradoxically, the elaborate system of the host immune response to viral infection that may be protective outside the CNS can be destructive when operating within this isolated, regeneration-deficient compartment where cell lysis, complement activation, and cytokines may injure the host while helping to clear virus, particularly in a persistent infection. This also illustrates the importance of the balance between the kinetics of immune responses and the virus host interaction. The outcome of a viral infection is also determined in part by the type of neural cell infected. This is an important factor in the pathogenesis of disease, not only for the potential injury caused by viral infection per se but also for the potential interactions of the infected cells with effector cells of the immune system.

The Role of CD4+ and CD8+ T Cells

Although both CD4+ as well as CD8+ T cells can be relatively easily isolated and grown in culture from the CSF of patients with viral encephalitis and meningoencephalitis, their relative importance in, and contribution to, combating an infection is uncertain. From observations made in several animal models it appears that the presence and function of CD4+ rather than CD8+ T cells is required to overcome viral CNS infections. This is in contrast to the situation in other organs where, during acute and chronic viral hepatitis, cytotoxic MHC class I–restricted CD8+ T cells attack virus-infected hepatocytes and thus mediate protection as well as immunopathology, or cell destruction (5).

Results obtained in the Theiler's virus model in mice argue against the hypothesis that the ability to generate CD8+ T cells mediates resistance. In C57B1/10 mice, which develop an acute encephalitis followed by subsequent clearance of virus from CNS, as well as in SJL mice, which experience a persistent viral infection with demyelination, there are CD8+ CTL in the CNS (90). Furthermore, β2-microglobulin-deficient transgenic mice that lack both MHC class I and functional CD8+ cells develop persistent encephalitis with extensive demyelination, but neither antibody titer nor viral persistence was significantly affected (130). Therefore, CD8+ T cells do not directly contribute to demyelination and obviously also do not eliminate virus or prevent establishment of persistence.

To analyze the role of T cells in overcoming measles virus infection in the rodent MV encephalitis model, lymphocyte subpopulations were depleted by in vivo application of MAbs directed against the CD4 or CD8 surface molecules of lymphocytes (13,41), or MV-primed T cells were intravenously transferred into MV-infected rats (133). Both approaches rendered comparable results and demonstrated that CD4+ cells are apparently indispensable in achieving viral clearance from the CNS, while CD8+ cells were not vital for recovery from the acute infection. When CD8+ T cells are depleted, rats are still completely protected by adoptive transfer of immune (primed by viral antigen) CD4+ T cells recognizing MV-N, H, or F proteins even in rats without local production of neutralizing antibody (86). From these results it was concluded that both CD8+ T cells and antibodies are not necessary for efficient elimination of MV and protection from disease in the encephalitis model. The results were surprising, because the susceptibility of mice to MV encephalitis correlates with their ability to generate a MHC class I (L^d)–restricted, CD8+ T cell–mediated cytotoxic immune response (119). Furthermore, a mouse strain, Balb/c^{dm2}, which carries a genomic deletion encompassing the H-2L^d gene locus, thus failing to express L^d (169) but is otherwise genetically identical to MV-resistant Balb/c mice, also eliminates MV efficiently from the CNS, although no MV-reactive CD8+ T cells are primed in these mice. The apparent explanation for the observation that CD8+ cells are dispensable in combating MV CNS infection is that these cells are unable to interact with neurons that do not express MHC class I even after MV infection.

At this point it has to be remembered that in different species, different virus-specific immune effector cells are generated to control viral infections in the periphery, and even within a single species there is no unique T-cell subset used in antiviral defense. In many different murine virus infections, including HSV, influenza A virus, LCMV, and mouse pox virus, the importance of CD8+ CTL to combat infection has been consistently shown (2,6,16,109,116,121). However, the clearance of murine hepatitis virus from the brain by CD8+ T cells was found to require CD4 help (42,72,183,188), and in the protective immunity to retroviruses both CD8+ and CD4+ T cells were partially effective, but only the combination of both led to full protection (56). Recovery from acute murine cytomegalovirus infection can proceed in the absence of the CD8+ subset and is mediated by CD4+ T cells which develop a compensatory protective activity that is absent in normal mice (64). CD4+ T cells appear to be required for maintenance of the spontaneous recovery from Friend virus–induced leukaemia (137). These examples illustrate that there is no general assignment of a determinative role in vivo to either T-lymphocyte subset in the recovery from viral infections. Instead, a detailed examination is required for every virus infection in relation to its susceptible host, and hardly any prediction can be made even for related viruses. It appears, however, that in the CNS, antiviral cell-mediated activity is largely dependent on CD4+ T cells.

Mechanisms of T Cell–Mediated Antiviral Activity

The mechanism of the antiviral activity of CD4+ T cells in vivo has not been completely elucidated. A detailed characterization in vitro revealed that all protective T-cell lines produce high amounts of IL-2, IFN-γ, and TNF-α but not IL-4 or IL-6, defining them as TH1 cells (40, observations 133). In this context it is interesting that the predominant generation of TH2 cells, which is seen both after natural MV infection and vaccination against measles in humans, has led to the hypothesis that the lack of virus-specific TH1 cells may contribute to the immunosuppression seen after infection or vaccination (49,181). Data obtained in the mouse model are consistent with this concept, as they are for the highly susceptible C3H mouse strain in which TH2 CD4+ T-cell lines can be isolated, but not TH1 cells. If cytokines secreted by TH1 cells are important, two requirements must be fulfilled. First, virus-primed T cells have to invade the CNS and home toward sites of infection, and second, blocking cytokine function should abolish protection. By exploiting a genetic marker, it was shown in adoptive transfer experiments in MV-infected rats, as well as in mice, that MV-specific CD4+ T cells from a donor animal enter the brain of the host. These cells accumulated in infected areas, whereas in an immunocompetent animal they never comprised more than 5% of all infiltrating T cells (Liebert et al., unpublished results). It is unlikely that MHC class II–restricted cytolysis plays a major role in eliminating MV from the brain, because the major cell population in the infected rodent brain are neurons that do not express MHC class II molecules. In this context it is interesting that in the LCMV-infection model, virus-specific MHC class II–restricted cytolytic lymphocytes induced immunopathological foci in the brain (112). The observed paucity of virus-specific donor T cells in the brains of MV-infected mice and rats leads to the conclusion that recruitment of further cells is essential for combat of virus in an infected brain. Along these lines it was shown experimentally that the neutralization of IFN-γ by administration of anti-IFN antibody rendered all mice susceptible to MV-induced acute encephalitis. Irrespective of the mouse strain, anti-IFN-treated animals died from infection, which suggests that cytokines may play an important role in the immune surveillance of the CNS. The mechanism of cytokine action is conceivably to assist in the recruitment of effector cells into the CNS. For example, IFN-γ and TNF-α enhance the expression of VCAM-1 on brain endothelial cells to which stimulated T cells bind before they enter the brain and encounter viral antigen, which leads to further events of activation and the secretion of cytokines (14). The prime source of IFN-γ and TNF-α in MV infection of the murine CNS is apparently CD4+ T cells, at least under protective conditions. The potential contribution of other cytokines and the role of mononuclear phagocytes, which are consistently present in infected foci, are not yet characterized.

In the Theiler's encephalitis model in mice it was shown that the susceptibility to infection is MHC associated and maps to the class I locus H-2D (117). In susceptible strains of mice, CD8+ T cells apparently fail to recognize viral antigens in the context of MHC class I, and so the virus persists and eventually causes disease. In in vivo depletion experiments using anti CD8-antibody it was shown that virus clearance is delayed and demyelinating disease develops. These data show that CD8+ T cells are not involved in immunopathology (i.e., demyelination) and are also not vital for recovery from acute infection. They may contribute, however, to antiviral immunity in acute infection and immune surveillance of persistently infected cells. Observations made in β2-microglobulin-deficient transgenic mice suggest that CD8+ T cells may play a role in clearing viral persistence from glial cells (130). Similar to the measles model, CD4+ cells are essential for controlling the early stages of infection. Depletion studies of CD4+ cells in the Theiler's virus model suggest that the major role of CD4+ T cells in Picornavirus infections is probably to provide help for B lymphocytes and thus enable the production of neutralizing antibody (180,187). Little is known about the possible antiviral activity of CD4+ T cells in Theiler's virus infection. However, experiments in which the MHC II–restricted CD4+ T-cell function was suppressed have resulted in a reduction in the incidence of demyelinating disease. Following TMEV infection and initial T-cell infiltration into the CNS, MHC class II induction on astrocytes is a key step allowing local antigen presentation and amplification of immunopathological responses within the CNS and hence development of demyelinating disease (19). A bystander effect caused by the induction of mononuclear cell infiltration and activation of macrophages, which in turn can lead to damage on myelin sheaths, is probably responsible for the observed immunopathology.

Another possibility involves T cells reactive against brain cell antigens, which could be induced during the course of infection and may serve to exacerbate ongoing pathology or to initiate new lesions. An argument against a role for autoimmune T cells in the induction of demyelination in Theiler's virus infection is the observation that tolerance induced to myelin antigens blocked the induction of experimental allergic encephalitis (EAE) but did not affect the development of demyelinating disease in Theiler's virus–infected mice (68). In rats infected with JHMV or MV, however, myelin basic protein (MBP)-reactive CD4+ T cells have been detected that could transfer EAE to naive uninfected animals (85,182). In rats rendered tolerant to MBP, not only EAE but also the precipitation of subacute measles encephalitis (SAME) was suppressed (89). In the following section, MV infection in a rat model in relation to EAE will be briefly presented and the mechanisms by which measles virus may alter host reactivity against self-antigens discussed.

Virus-induced Cell-mediated Autoimmune Reactions Against Brain Antigens

A cofactor role for MV in the development of EAE was suggested by early observations that showed that the course of EAE and its severity were potentiated in MV-infected hamsters (100). Interestingly, the molecular pathology of one form of SAME (type 2) in Lewis rats is characterized by a persisting inflammatory process in the CNS in the absence of MV antigen or viral nucleic acid. The lesions are very similar to those of rats receiving MBP-specific CD4+ T lymphocytes, and the infiltrates reveal a similar composition of lymphocyte subpopulations in SAME type 2 and EAE, with a dominance of CD4+ T cells over CD8+ cells and a high proportion of macrophages (84,85). Oligoclonal immunoglobulins with restricted heterogeneity were detected in the cerebrospinal fluid of these animals, which probably react with brain antigens (35). Splenic lymphocytes and superficial cervical lymph node cells isolated from these animals were found to proliferate in vitro in the presence of MBP or PLP (85). The intravenous transfer of MBP-reactive, MHC class II–restricted CD4+ T-cell lines isolated from bulk cell populations induced a disease in naive syngeneic recipients with clinical and histopathological signs identical to T cell–mediated EAE. The analysis of the antigenic fine specificity revealed that MBP-specific T cells from MV-infected as well as from MBP-challenged rats displayed an identical pattern of reactivity to a panel of synthetic peptides (84). The high degree of antigenic specificity was further supported by the failure of the T-cell lines to proliferate in the presence of disrupted measles virions, isolated MV proteins, or other control antigens or peptide sequences. Vice versa, MV-specific T-cell lines did not proliferate when MBP or synthetic MBP peptides were added to the cultures. The disease induced was clearly not due to activation of MV in the brain of immunized Lewis rats, because virus could not be isolated from brain material and measles antigen was not detectable (89). The interaction between MBP peptide and MV infection was not observed when rats were infected intraperitoneally or when inactivated MV was used. Obviously, at least initially, some viral replication in the brain is required to enhance the vulnerability of the brain to autoimmune aggression. If autoimmune mechanisms participate in the pathogenesis of virus-induced encephalomyelitis, susceptibility to measles encephalitis and EAE should parallel different rat strains, depending on the genetic background. This is indeed the case, as BN rats, which are resistant to EAE, did not develop a subacute clinical disease, although they are generally able to replicate MV (88). The susceptibility of rats to the development of MV-induced CNS changes and disease is multifactorial, with the development of a MBP-specific cell-mediated immunity (CMI) response representing a major factor.

There are several possibilities of how a virus can induce a strong CMI response to brain antigen. First, while viruses multiply in living cells, during replication they incorporate host antigens in the envelope. In the context of viral proteins, modified or newly exposed cellular antigens could be recognized as foreign by the host and might elicit an immune reaction in the same manner as any other previously unencountered protein (146). Furthermore, viruses with tropism towards lymphocytes and macrophages might interact with the immune regulatory system in such a way that lymphocyte subpopulations are destroyed or autoreactive lymphocyte clones generated and/or expanded. The prime example is Epstein-Barr virus, which infects and transforms B lymphocytes. Under certain conditions these immortalized cells secrete autoantibodies that react with cellular constituents (146). Immune responses raised against certain viral antigens may cross-react with normal host-cell antigens and lead to autoimmunity by molecular mimicry (120). Although definite experimental evidence for either of these mechanisms leading to disease has not been obtained, one cannot single out any one factor leading to such diverse immune reactions. It is more conceivable that diseases result from the sequelae of a number of different virus-induced changes, each one a relatively common event.

Consequences of Antiviral Mechanisms in the CNS

In summary, immune responses generated in the periphery meet extraordinary difficulties when it comes to combating CNS virus infections. In most cases where neurons are infected, direct interaction of T cells with the infected host cell is not possible due to the lack of MHC expression. In any case, this would not be desirable, because any immune response, while being beneficial and effective in the periphery, inflicts enormous pathology when attacking cells that lack the capacity to regenerate. Hence, a rapid elimination of virus (infected cells) is necessary, whereas a delayed immune response may allow the virus to spread in the CNS and, even if ultimately effective against the virus, may be destructive to the host. Thus, precautions are built into the system to prevent potentially damaging and disease-inducing immune responses during persistent infections in which the virus at least temporarily does not destroy its host cell. The fine regulation of the intracerebral immune surveillance has yet to be elucidated. However, it is clear that to the advantage of the host, a delicate balance is normally maintained between the requirements for the morphological and functional integrity of the CNS and the pretension of the immune system to combat virus and eliminate virus-infected cells.

Currently the data obtained regarding viral infection of the CNS indicate the following conclusions: (1) The immune response to viral infections of the CNS is initiated in peripheral lymphoid tissues, followed by entry of activated end-differentiated T and B cells into the cerebrospinal fluid, meninges, and brain parenchyma. *(2)* During viral infections, cytokines are induced in a differential way in different strains of mice and in different cell types of the same mouse strain or of human. *(3)* Together with interferon-induced proteins such as Mx, these factors contribute to the establishment of persistent infections, which may depend on down-regulation of replication of certain viruses by lack of factors and/or restriction of viral gene expression. *(4)* During viral infections, MHC class I or II antigens are expressed on astrocytes and oligodendrocytes and extensively on microglial cells that present viral antigen produced by infected cells. *(5)* Full development of the inflammatory response requires virus-specific T cells, but natural killer (NK) cells, γ/δ T cells, mononuclear phagocytes, B cells, and plasma cells participate in a bystander response. *(6)* In many viral systems including the experimental coronavirus JHMV and MV models, T cells are required for viral elimination, but clearance of virus may also depend on the timely presence of virus-specific antibodies, such as shown in the Sindbis model where passive transfer of antibody to a surface viral glycoprotein eliminated virus by a noncomplement-mediated, noncytolytic mechanism. *(7)* In a situation where a virus infection encounters a virgin (unprimed) immune system, a synergistic interaction of all major cell types of the adaptive immune system is required for both limitation of virus spread within the CNS and ultimate elimination of virus from brain cells. *(8)* However, immunopathology and/or autoimmunity may result from inopportune or inefficient T-cell responses generated after the viral agent has succeeded in establishing a persistent infection in brain cells as a result of immune-mediated damage during attempted viral clearance.

Acknowledgements

The preparation of this manuscript was supported by the Deutsche Forschungsgemeinschaft and Bundesministerium für Forschung und Technologie.

References

1. Achim CL, Wiley CA. Expression of major histocompatibility complex antigens in the brains of patients with progressive multifocal leukoencephalopathy. J Neuropathol Exp Neurol 51:257–263, 1992.
2. Ahmed R, Butler LD, Bhatti L. T4+ T helper cell function in vivo: differential requirement for induction of antiviral cytotoxic T-cell and antibody response. J Virol 62:2102–2106, 1988.
3. Allan JE, Dixon JE, Doherty PL. Nature of the inflammatory process in the central nervous system of mice infected with LCM. Curr Top Microbiol Immunol 134:131–143, 1987.
4. Almond JW. Poliovirus neurovirulence. Semin Neurosci 3:101–108, 1991.
5. Almond PS, Bumgardner GL, Chen S, Platt J, Payne WD, Matas AJ. Immunogenicity of class I+, class II− hepatocytes. Transplant Proc 23:108–109, 1991.

6. Askonas BA, Taylor PM, Esquivel F. Cytotoxic T cells in influenza infection. Ann NY Acad Sci 532:230, 1988.

7. Atherton SS. Protection from retinal necrosis by passive transfer of monoclonal antibody specific for herpes simplex virus glycoprotein D. Curr Eye Res 11:45–52, 1992.

8. Aubert C, Chamorro M, Brahic M. Identification of Theiler's virus infected cells in the central nervous system of the mouse during demyelinating disease. Microb. Pathog 3:319–326, 1987.

9. Baczko K, Liebert UG, Billeter MA, Cattaneo R, Budka H, ter Meulen V. Expression of defective measles virus genes in brain tissue of patients with subacute sclerosing panencephalitis. J Virol 59:472–478, 1986.

10. Baer GM, Bellini WJ, Fishbein DB. Rhabdoviruses. In: Virology, 2nd ed, BN Fields, DM Knipe, eds. Raven Press, New York, 1990, pp 883–930.

11. Baldridge JR, Buchmeier MJ. Mechanisms of antibody-mediated protection against lymphocytic choriomeningitis virus infection: mother-to-baby transfer of humoral protection. J Virol 66:4252–4257, 1992.

12. Baldridge JR, Pearce BD, Parekh BS, Buchmeier MJ. Teratogenic effects of neonatal Arenavirus infection on the developing rat cerebellum are abrogated by passive immunotherapy. Virology 197:669–677, 1993.

13. Bankamp B, Brinckmann UG, Reich A, Niewiesk S, ter Meulen V, Liebert UG. Measles virus nucleocapsid protein protects rats from encephalitis. J Virol 65:1695, 1991.

14. Baron JL, Madri JA, Ruddli NH, Hashim G, Janeway CA. Surface expression of $\alpha4$ integrin by CD4 T cells is required for their entry into brain parenchyma. J Exp Med 177:57–68, 1993.

15. Barrett PN, Koschel K, Carter M, ter Meulen V. Effect of measles virus antibodies on a measles SSPE virus persistently infected C6 rat glioma call line. J Gen Virol 66:1411–1421, 1985.

16. Bender B, Croghant T, Zhang L, Small P. Transgenic mice lacking class I major histocompatibility complex-restricted T cells have delayed viral clearance and increased mortality after influenza virus challenge. J Exp Med 175:1143, 1992.

17. Billeter MA, Cattaneo R. Molecular biology of defective measles viruses persisting in the human central nervous system. In: The Paramyxoviruses, D Kingsbury, ed. Plenum Press, New York, 1991, pp 323–345.

18. Blinzinger K, Simon J, Magrath D, Boulger L. Poliovirus crystals within the endoplasmic reticulum of endothelial and mononuclear cells in the monkey spinal cord. Science 163:1336–1337, 1969.

19. Borrow P, Nash AA. Susceptibility to Theiler's virus-induced demyelinating disease correlates with astrocyte class II induction and antigen presentation. Immunology 76:133–139, 1992.

20. Borrow P, Tonks P, Welsh CJ, Nash AA. The role of CD8+ T cells in the acute and chronic phases of Theiler's murine encephalomyelitis virus-induced disease in mice. J Gen Virol 73:1861–1865, 1992.

21. Botteron C, Zurbriggen A, Griot C, Vandevelde M. Canine distemper virus-immune complexes induce bystander degeneration of oligodendrocytes. Acta Neuropathol (Berl) 83:402–407, 1992.

22. Brinckmann UG, Bankamp B, Reich A, ter Meulen V, Liebert UG. Efficacy of individual measles virus structural proteins in the protection of rats from measles virus encephalitis. J Gen Virol 72:2491–2500, 1991.

23. Buchmeier M, Lewicki H, Talbot P, Knobler R. Murine hepatitis virus-4 (strain JHM) induced neurologic disease is modulated in vivo by monoclonal antibody. Virology 132:261–270, 1984.

24. Calenoff MA, Faaberg KS, Lipton HL. Genomic regions of neurovirulence and attenuation in Theiler's murine encephalomyelitis virus. Proc Natl Acad Sci USA 87:978–982, 1990.
25. Campbell IL. Cytokines in viral diseases. Curr Opin Immunol 3:486–491, 1991.
26. Carrigan D, Knox KK. Identification of interferon-resistant subpopulations in several strains of measles virus: positive selection by growth of the virus in brain tissue. J Virol 64:1606–1615, 1990.
27. Cattaneo R, Rebmann G, Schmid A, Baczko K, ter Meulen V, Billeter M. Altered transcription of a defective measles virus genome derived from a diseased human brain. EMBO J 6:681–687, 1987.
28. Ceccaldi PE, Fillion MP, Ermine A, Tsiang H, Fillion G. Rabies virus selectively alters 5-HT1 receptor subtypes in rat brain. Eur J Pharmacol 245:129–138, 1993.
29. Chou J, Kern ER, Whitley RJ, Roizman B. Mapping of herpes simplex virus-1 neurovirulence to gamma 134.5, a gene nonessential for growth in culture. Science 250:1262–1266, 1990.
30. Cosby SL, Macquaid S, Taylor MJ, Bailey M, Rima BK, Martin SJ, Allen IV. Examination of eight cases of multiple sclerosis and 56 neurological and non-neurological controls for genomic sequences of measles virus. J Gen Virol 70:2027–2036, 1989.
31. Day SP, Lausch RN, Oakes JE. Evidence that the gene for herpes simplex virus type 1 DNA polymerase accounts for the capacity of an intertypic recombinant to spread from eye to central nervous system. Virology 163:166–173, 1988.
32. Deshmane SJ, Fraser JW. During latency, herpes simplex virus type I DNA is associated with nucleosomes in a chromatin structure. J Virol 63:943–947, 1989.
33. Dietzschold B, Kao M, Zheng YM, Chen ZY, Maul G, Fu ZF, Rupprecht CE, Koprowski H. Delineation of putative mechanisms involved in antibody-mediated clearance of rabies virus from the central nervous system. Proc Natl Acad Sci USA 89:7252–7256, 1992.
34. Dörig RE, Marcil A, Chopra A, Richardson CD. The human CD46 molecule is a receptor for measles virus (Edmonston strain). Cell 75:295–305, 1993.
35. Dörries R, Liebert UG, ter Meulen V. Comparative analysis of virus-specific antibodies and immunglobulins in serum and cerebrospinal fluid of subacute measles virus-induced encephalomyelitis (SAME) in rats and subacute sclerosing panencephalitis (SSPE). J Neuroimmunol 19:339–352, 1988.
36. Dörries R, Schwender S, Imrich H, Harms H. Population dynamics of lymphocyte subsets in the central nervous system of rats with different susceptibility to coronavirus-induced demyelinating encephalitis. Immunology 74:539–545, 1991.
37. Dunster LM, Schneider-Schaulies J, Löffler S, Lankes W, Schwartz-Albiez R, Lottspeich F, ter Meulen V. Moesin: a cell membrane protein linked with susceptibility to measles virus infection. Virology 198:265–274, 1994.
38. Fazakerley JK, Parker SE, Bloom F, Buchmeier MJ. The V5A13.1 envelope glycoprotein deletion mutant of mouse hepatitis virus type-4 is neuroattenuated by its reduced rate of spread in the central nervous system. Virology 187:178–188, 1992.
39. Felgenhauer K, Reiber H. The diagnostic significance of antibody specificity indices in multiple sclerosis and herpes virus induced diseases of the nervous system. Clin Investig 70:28–37, 1992.
40. Finke D, Brinckmann UG, ter Meulen V, Liebert UG. Gamma interferon is a mediator of antiviral defense in experimental measles virus-induced encephalitis. J Virol 69:5469–5474, 1995.
41. Finke D, Liebert UG. CD4+ T cells are essential in overcoming experimental murine measles encephalitis. Immunology 83:184–189, 1994.
42. Flory E, Pfleiderer M, Stuhler A, Wege H. Induction of protective immunity against

coronavirus-induced encephalomyelitis: evidence for an important role of CD8$^+$ T cells in vivo. Eur J Immunol 23:1757–1761, 1993.

43. Fournier JG, Tardieu M, Lebon P, Robain O, Ponsot G, Rozenblatt S, Bouteille M. Detection of measles virus RNA in lymphocytes from peripheral blood and brain perivascular infiltrates of patients with subacute sclerosing panencephalitis. N Engl J Med 313:910–915, 1985.

44. Fraser NW, Block TM, Spivack JG. The latency-associated transcripts of herpes simplex virus: RNA in search of function. Virology 191:1–8, 1992.

45. Frei K, Malipiero UV, Leist TP, Zinkernagel RM, Schwab ME, Fontana A. On the cellular source and function of interleukin-6 produced in the central nervous system in viral diseases. Eur J Immunol 19:689–694, 1989.

46. Fujii N, Oguma K, Kimura K, Yamashita T, Ishida S, Fujinaga K, Yashiki T. Oligo-2′,5′-adenylate synthetase activity in K562 cell lines persistently infected with measles or mumps virus. J Gen Virol 69:2085–2091, 1988.

47. Giulian D, Lachman LB. Interleukin-1 stimulation of astroglial proliferation after brain injury. Science 228:497–499, 1985.

48. Goodpasture E. The axis cylinders of peripheral nerves as portals of entry to the central nervous system for the virus of herpes simplex in experimentally infected rabbits. Am J Pathol 1:11–28, 1925.

49. Griffin DE, Ward BJ. Differential CD4 T cell activation in measles. J Infect Dis 168:275–281, 1993.

50. Haase AT. Pathogenesis of lentivirus infections. Nature 322:130–136, 1986.

51. Halbach M, Koschel K. Impairment of hormone dependent signal transfer by chronic SSPE virus infection. J Gen Virol 42:615–619, 1979.

52. Herndon RM, Johnson RT, Davis LE, Descalzi LR. Ependymitis in mumps virus meningitis: electron microscopic studies of cerebrospinal fluid. Arch Neurol 30:475–479, 1974.

53. Hirano A. Subacute sclerosing panencephalitis virus dominantly interferes with replication of wild-type measles virus in a mixed infection: implication for viral persistence. J Virol 66:1891–1898, 1992.

54. Hofman FM, Hinton DR, Baemayr J, Weil M, Merrill JE. Lymphokines and immunoregulatory molecules in subacute sclerosing panencephalitis. Clin Immunol Immunopathol 58:331–342, 1991.

55. Hogle JM, Chow M, Filman DJ. Three-dimensional structure of Poliovirus at 2.9 Å resolution. Science 229:1358–1367, 1985.

56. Hom RC, Finberg RW, Mullaney S, Rupprecht RM. Protective cellular retroviral immunity requires both CD4$^+$ and CD8$^+$ T cells. J Virol 65:220–224, 1991.

57. Homsy J, Meyer M, Tateno M, Clarkson S, Levy JA. The Fc and not CD4 receptor mediates antibody enhancement of HIV infection in human cells. Science 244:1357–1360, 1989.

58. Horie H, Koike S, Kurata T, Sato-Yoshida Y, Ise I, Ota Y, Abe S, Hioki K, Kato H, Taya C, Nomura T, Hashizume S, Yonekawa H, Nomoto A. Transgenic mice carrying the human poliovirus receptor: new animal model for study of poliovirus neurovirulence. J Virol 68:681–688, 1994.

59. Imrich H, Schwender S, Hein A, Dörries R. Cervical lymphoid tissue but not the central nervous system supports proliferation of virus-specific T lymphocytes during coronavirus-induced encephalitis in rats. J Neuroimmunol 53:73–81, 1994.

60. Iwasaki Y, Liu D, Yamamoto T, Konno H. On the replication and spread of rabies virus in the human central nervous system. J Neuropathol Exp Neurol 44:185–195, 1985.

61. Johnson RT. Virus invasion of the central nervous system. A study of Sindbis virus infection of the mouse using fluorescent antibody. Am J Pathol 46:929–943, 1965.

62. Johnson RT. Viral Infections of the Nervous System. Raven Press, New York, 1982.

63. Joncas JH, Robillard LR, Boudreault A, Leyritz M, McLaughlin BJM. Interferon in serum and cerebrospinal fluid in subacute sclerosing panencephalitis. Can Med Assoc J 115:309–315, 1976.

64. Jonjic S, Pavic I, Lucin P, Rukavina D, Koszinowski U. Efficacious control of cyto-megalovirus infection after long-term depletion of CD8+ T lymphocytes. J Virol 64: 5457–5464, 1990.

65. Jordan CA, Watkins BA, Kufta C, Dubois-Dalque M. Infection of brain microglial cells by human immunodeficiency virus type 1 is CD4 dependent. J Virol 65:736–742, 1991.

66. Jubelt B, Ropka SL, Goldfarb S, Waltenbaugh C, Oates RP. Susceptibility and resistance to poliovirus-induced paralysis of inbred mouse strains. J Virol 65:1035–1040, 1991.

67. Karupiah R, Woodhams GCE, Blanden RV, Ramshaw IA. Immunobiology of infection with recombinant vaccinia virus encoding murine IL-2. Mechanisms of rapid viral clearance in immunocompetent mice. J Immunol 147:4327–4332, 1991.

68. Kennedy MK, Tan LJ, dal Canto MC, Tuohy VK, Lu ZJ, Trotter JL, Miller SD. Inhibition of murine relapsing experimental autoimmune encephalomyelitis by immune tolerance to proteolipid protein and its encephalitogenic peptides. J Immunol 144:909–915, 1990.

69. Kitamura D, Roes J, Kuhn R, Rajewski K. A B cell-deficient mouse by targeted disruption of the membrane exon of the immunoglobulin mu chain gene. Nature 350:423–426, 1991.

70. Kitamura N, Semler BL, Rothberg PG, Larsen GR, Adler CJ, Dorner AJ, Emini EA, Hanecak R, Lee JJ, van der Werf S, Anderson CW, Wimmer E. Primary structure, gene organization and polypeptide expression of poliovirus RNA. Nature 291:547–553, 1981.

71. Koike S, Horie H, Ise I, Okitsu A, Yoshida N, Iizuka N, Takeuchi K, Tagegami T, Nomoto A. The poliovirus receptor protein is produced both as membrane-bound and secreted forms. EMBO J 9:3217–3224, 1990.

72. Körner H, Schliephake A, Winter J, Zimprich F, Lassmann H, Sedgwick J, Siddell S, Wege H. Nucleocapsid or spike protein-specific CD4+ T lymphocytes protect against coronavirus-induced encephalomyelitis in the absence of CD8+ T cells. J Immunol 147:2317–2323, 1991.

73. Koschel K, Münzel P. Persistent paramyxovirus infections and behaviour of β-adrenergic receptors in C6 rat glioma cells. J Gen Virol 47:513–517, 1980.

74. Kristensson K, Lycke E, Ryotta M, Svennerholm B, Vahlne A. Neuritic transport of herpes simplex virus in rat sensory neurons in vitro. Effects of substances interacting with micro-tubular function and axonal flow (nocodazde, taxol and erythro-9-3(2-hydroxynonyl) adenine). J Gen Virol 67:2023–2028, 1986.

75. Ladogana A, Bouzamondo E, Pochiari M, Tsiang H. Modification of tritiated γ-amino-n-butyric acid transport in rabies virus-infected primary cortical cultures. J Gen Virol 75:623–627, 1994.

76. La Monica N, Almond JW, Rancaniello VR. A mouse model for poliovirus neurovirulence identifies mutations that attenuate the virus for humans. J Virol 61:2917–2920, 1987.

77. Lenhardt TM, Wiley CA. Absence of humorally mediated damage within the central nervous system of AIDS patients. Neurology 39:278–280, 1989.

78. Lentz TL, Burrage TL, Smith AL, Crick J, Tignor GH. Is the acetylcholine receptor a rabies virus receptor? Science 215:182–184, 1982.

79. Levine B, Griffin DE. Persistence of viral RNA in mouse brains after recovery from acute Alphavirus encephalitis. J Virol 66:6429–6435, 1992.

80. Levine B, Griffin DE. Molecular analysis of neurovirulent strains of Sindbis virus that evolve during persistent infection of scid mice. J Virol 67:6872–6875, 1993.

81. Levine B, Hardwick JM, Trapp BD, Crawford TO, Bollinger RC, Griffin DE. Antibody-mediated clearance of alphavirus infection from neurons. Science 254:856–860, 1991.

82. Lieberman AP, Pitha PM, Shin HS, Shin ML. Production of tumor necrosis factor and other cytokines by astrocytes stimulated with lipopolysaccharide or a neurotropic virus. Proc Natl Acad Sci USA 86:6348–6352, 1989.

83. Liebert UG, Flanagan SG, Löffler S, Baczko K, ter Meulen V, Rima BK. Antigenic determinants of measles virus hemagglutinin associated with neurovirulence. J Virol 68:1486–1493, 1994.

84. Liebert UG, Hashim GA, ter Meulen V. Characterization of measles virus-induced cellular autoimmune reactions against myelin basic protein in Lewis rats. J Neuroimmunol 29:139–147, 1990.

85. Liebert UG, Linington C, ter Meulen V. Induction of autoimmune reactions to myelin basic protein in measles virus encephalitis in Lewis rats. J Neuroimmunol 17:103–118, 1988.

86. Liebert UG, Reich A, Bankamp B, Brinckmann UG, ter Meulen V. Control of measles virus infections by virus-specific CD4⁺ T cells. In: Viruses and Cellular Immuneresponses, DB Thomas, ed. Marcel Dekker, New York, Basel, Hong Kong, 1993, pp 279–291.

87. Liebert UG, Schneider-Schaulies S, Baczko K, ter Meulen V. Antibody-induced restriction of viral gene expression in measles encephalitis in rats. J Virol 64:706–713, 1990.

88. Liebert UG, ter Meulen V. Virological aspects of measles virus induced encephalomyelitis in Lewis and BN rats. J Gen Virol 68:1715–1722, 1987.

89. Liebert UG, ter Meulen V. Synergistic interaction between measles virus infection and MBP peptide-specific T cells in the induction of EAE in Lewis rats. J Neuroimmunol 46:217–224, 1993.

90. Lindsley MD, Thiemann R, Rodriguez M. Cytotoxic T cells isolated from the central nervous systems of mice infected with Theiler's virus. J Virol 65:6612–6620, 1991.

91. Liu C, Voth D, Rodina P, Shauf L, Gonzalez G. A comparative study of the pathogenesis of western equine and eastern equine encephalomyelitis virus infections in mice by intracerebral and subcutaneous inoculations. J Infect Dis 122:53–63, 1970.

92. Lucchiari MA, Modolell M, Eichmann K, Pereira CA. In vivo depletion of interferon-γ leads to susceptibility of A/J mice to mouse hepatitis virus 3 infection. Immunobiology 185:475–482, 1993.

93. Lycke E, Kristensson K, Svenerholm B, Vahlne A, Ziegler R. Uptake and transport of herpes simplex virus in neurites of rat dorsal root ganglia cells in culture. J Gen Virol 65:55–64, 1984.

94. Lycke E, Tsiang H. Rabies virus infection of cultured rat sensory neurons. J Virol 61:2733–2741, 1987.

95. Malvoisin E, Wild F. Contribution of measles virus fusion protein in protective immunity: anti-F monoclonal antibody neutralize virus infectivity and protect mice against challenge. J Virol 64:5160–5162, 1990.

96. Martin X, Dolivo M. Neuronal and transneuronal tracing in the trigeminal system of the rat using the herpes virus suis. Brain Res 273:253–276, 1983.

97. Martiney JA, Berman JW, Brosnan CF. Chronic inflammatory effects of interleukin-1 on the blood-retina barrier. J Neuroimmunol 41:167–176, 1992.

98. Massa PT, Dörries R, ter Meulen V. Viral antigens induce Ia antigen expression on astrocytes. Nature 320:543–546, 1986.

99. Massa PT, Schimpl A, Wecker E, ter Meulen V. Tumor necrosis factor amplifies measles virus-mediated Ia induction on astrocytes. Proc Natl Acad Sci USA 84:7242–7245, 1987.

100. Massanari RM, Paterson PY, Lipton HL. Petentiation of experimental allergic encepha-

lomyelitis in hamsters with persistent encephalitis due to measles virus. J Infect Dis 139:297–303, 1979.

101. McAllister A, Tangy F, Aubert C, Brahic M. Genetic mapping of the ability of Theiler's virus to persist and demyelinate. J Virol 64:4252–4257, 1990.

102. Mellerick DM, Fraser NW. Physical state of the latent herpes simplex genome in a mouse model system: evidence suggesting an episomal state. Virology 158:265–275, 1987.

103. Melnick JL. Enteroviruses: polioviruses, Coxsackieviruses, ecchoviruses and newer enteroviruses. In: Virology, 2nd ed, BN Fields, DM Knipe, et al., eds. Raven Press, New York, 1990, pp 549–604.

104. Melvold RW, Jokinen DM, Miller SD, dal Canto MC, Lipton HL. Identification of a locus on mouse chromosome 3 involved in differential susceptibility to Theiler's murine encephalomyelitis virus-induced demyelinating disease. J Virol 64:686–690, 1990.

105. Mendelsohn C, Wimmer E, Rancianello V. Cellular receptor for poliovirus: molecular cloning, nucleotide sequence, and expression of a new member of the immunoglobulin superfamily. Cell 56:855–865, 1989.

106. Merrill JE. Effects of interleukin-1 and tumor necrosis factor-α on astrocytes, microglia, oligodendrocytes, and glial precursor in vitro. Dev Neurosci 13:130–137, 1991.

107. Merrill JE, Chen ISY. HIV-1, macrophages, glial cells, and cytokines in AIDS nervous system disease. FASEB J 5:2391–2397, 1991.

108. Momburg F, Koch N, Möller P, Moldenhauer G, Hämmerling GJ. In vivo induction of H-2K/D antigens by recombinant interferon-γ. Eur J Immunol 16:551–557, 1986.

109. Moskophidis D, Cobbold P, Waldmann H, Lehmann-Grube F. Mechanism of recovery from acute virus infection: treatment of lymphocytic choriomeningitis virus-infected mice with monoclonal antibodies reveals that Lyt-2$^+$ T lymphocytes mediate clearance of virus and regulate the antiviral antibody response. J Virol 61:1867–1874, 1987.

110. Moskophidis D, Frei K, Löhler J, Fontana A, Zinkernagel RM. Production of random classes of immunoglobulins in brain tissue during persistent viral infection paralleled by secretion of interleukin-6 (IL-6) but not IL-4, IL-5, and gamma interferon. J Virol 65:1364–1369, 1991.

111. Moss H. The herpes simplex virus type 2 alkaline DNase activity is essential for replication and growth. J Gen Virol 67:1173–1178, 1986.

112. Muller D, Koller BH, Whitton JL, Lapan KE, Brigman KK, Frelinger JA. LCMV-specific, class II-restricted cytotoxic T cells in b$_2$-microglobulin-deficient mice. Science 255: 1576–1578, 1992.

113. Murphy FA, Bauer SP. Early street rabies virus infection in striated muscle and later progression to the central nervous system. Intervirology 3:256–268, 1974.

114. Naniche D, Varior-Krishnan G, Cervoni F, Wild F, Rossi B, Rabourdin-Combe C, Gerlier D. Human membrane cofactor protein (CD46) acts as a cellular receptor for measles virus. J Virol 67:6025–6032, 1993.

115. Narayan O, Clements JE. Biology and pathogenesis of lentiviruses. J Gen Virol 70:1617–1639, 1989.

116. Nash AA, Jayasuriya A, Phelan J, Cobbold SP, Waldmann H, Prospero T. Different roles for L3T4$^+$ and Lyt 2$^+$ T cells subsets in the control of an acute herpes simplex virus infection of the skin and nervous system. J Gen Virol 68:825–833, 1987.

117. Nash AA, Leung KN, Wildy P. The T cell-mediated immune response of mice to herpes simplex virus. In: The Herpesviruses, vol. 4, B Roizman, C Lopez, eds. Plenum Press, New York, 1985, pp 87–102.

118. Nathanson N, Gonzales-Scarano F. The Natural History of Rabies Virus, 2nd ed, GM Baer, ed. CRC Press, Boston, 1991, pp 145–161.

119. Niewiesk S, Bankamp B, Brinckmann UG, Sirak S, ter Meulen V, Liebert UG. Susceptibility to measles-induced encephalitis in mice correlates with impaired antigen presentation to CTL. J Virol 67:75–81, 1993.

120. Oldstone MBA. Molecular mimicry as a mechanism for the cause and a probe uncovering etiologic agent(s) of autoimmune disease. Curr Top Microbiol Immunol 145:127–135, 1989.

121. Oldstone MBA, Blount P, Souther PJ, Lampert PW. Cytoimmunotherapy for persistent virus infection reveales an unique clearance pattern from the central nervous system. Nature 321:239, 1986.

122. Parsons LM, Webb HE. IgG subclass responses in brain and serum in Semliki Forest virus demyelinating encephalitis. Neuropathol Appl Neurobiol 18:351–359, 1992.

123. Patick AK, Lindsley MD, Rodriguez M. Differential pathogenesis between mouse strains resistant and susceptible to Theiler's virus-induced demyelination. Semin Virol 1:281–288, 1990.

124. Pathak S, Webb HE. Possible mechanism for the transport of Semliki Forest virus into andwithin the mouse brain: an electron microscopic study. J Neurol Sci 23:175–184, 1974.

125. Perlman S, Jacobsen G, Afifi A. Spread of a neurotropic murine coronavirus into the CNS via the trigeminal and olfactory nerves. Virology 170:556–560, 1989.

126. Perlman S, Schelper R, Bolger E, Ries D. Late onset, symptomatic, demyelinating encephalomyelitis in mice infected with MHV-JHM in the presence of maternal antibody. Microb Pathogen 2:185–194, 1987.

127. Pevear DC, Borkowski J, Calenoff M, Oh CK, Ostrowski B, Lipton HL. Insights into Theiler's virus neurovirulence based on a genomic comparison of the neurovirulent GDVII and less virulent BeAn strains. Virology 165:1–12, 1988.

128. Pevear DC, Calenoff M, Rozhon E, Lipton HL. Analysis of the complete nucleotide sequence of the picornavirus Theiler's murine encephalomyelitis virus indicates that it is closely related to cardioviruses. J Virol 61:1507–1516, 1987.

129. Plata-Salaman CR. Immunoregulators in the central nervous system. Neurosci Biobehav Rev 15:185–215, 1991.

130. Pullen LC, Miller SD, dal Canto MC, Kim BS. Class I-deficient resistant mice intracerebrally inoculated with Theiler's virus show an increased T cell response to viral antigens and susceptibility to demyelination. Eur J Immunol 23:2287–2293, 1993.

131. Rammohan KW, Dubois-Dalcq M, Rentier B, Paul J. Experimental models to study measles virus persistence in the nervous system. Prog Neuropathol 5:343–372, 1983.

132. Reboul J, Schuller E, Pialoux G, Rey MA, Lebon P, Allinquant B, Brun-Vezinet F. Immunoglobulins and complement components in 37 patients infected by HIV-1 virus: comparison of general (systemic) and intrathecal immunity. J Neurol Sci 89:243–252, 1989.

133. Reich A, Erlwein O, Niewiesk S, ter Meulen V, Liebert UG. CD4+ T cells control measles virus infection of the central nervous system. Immunology 76:185–191, 1992.

134. Ren R, Costantini F, Gorgacz EJ, Lee JJ, Rancaniello VR. Transgenic mice expressing a human poliovirus receptor: a new model for poliomyelitis. Cell 63:353–362, 1990.

135. Rima BK, Davidson WB, Martin SJ. The role of defective interfering particles in persistent infection of Vero cells by measles virus. J Gen Virol 35:89–97, 1977.

136. Rima BK, Duffy N, Mitchell WJ, Summers BA, Appel MJ. Correlation between humoral immune responses and presence of virus in the CNS in dogs experimentally infected with canine distemper virus. Arch Virol 121:1–8, 1991.

137. Robertson MN, Spangrude GJ, Hasenkrug K, Perry L, Nishio J, Wehrly K, Chesebro B.

Role and specificity of T-cell subsets in spontaneous recovery from Friend virus-induced leukemia in mice. J Virol 66:3271–3277, 1992.

138. Rock DL, Fraser NW. Latent herpes simplex virus type 1 DNA contains two copies of the virion DNA joint region. J Virol 55:849–852, 1985.

139. Rodriguez M, Leibowitz J, David CS. Susceptibility to Theiler's virus-induced demyelination. Mapping of the gene within the H-2D region. J Exp Med 163:620–631, 1986.

140. Rodriguez M, Lucchinetti CF, Clark RJ, Yakash TL, Markowitz H, Lennon VA. Immunoglobulins and complement in demyelination induced by Theiler's virus. J Immunol 140:800–806, 1988.

141. Roos RP, Firestone S, Wollman R, Variakojis D, Arnason BGW. The effect of short-term and chronic immunosuppression on Theiler's virus demyelination. J Neuroimmunol 2:223–234, 1982.

142. Sabin AB. Pthogenesis of poliomyelitis. Reappraisal in the light of new data. Science 123:1151–1157, 1956.

143. Sabin AB, Boulger LR. History of Sabin attenuated poliovirus oral live vaccine strains. J Biol Stand 1:115–118, 1973.

144. Saha K, Hollowell D, Wong PK. Mother-to-baby transfer of humoral immunity against retrovirus-induced neurologic disorders and immunodeficiency. Virology 198:129–137, 1994.

145. Sawtell NM, Thompson RL. Herpes simplex virus type 1 latency-associated transcription unit promotes anatomical site-dependent establishment and reactivation from latency. J Virol 66:2157–2169, 1992.

146. Schattner A, Rager-Zisman B. Virus induced autoimmunity. Rev Infect Dis 12:204–222, 1990.

147. Schijns VE, Van der Neut R, Haagmans BL, Bar DR, Schellekens H, Horzinek MC. Tumour necrosis factor-alpha, interferon-gamma and interferon-beta exert antiviral activity in nervous tissue cells. J Gen Virol 72:809–815, 1991.

148. Schlesinger JJ, Foltzer M, Chapman S. The Fc portion of antibody to yellow fever virus NS1 is a determinant of protection against YF encephalitis in mice. Virology 192:132–141, 1993.

149. Schneider-Schaulies J, Dunster LM, Schwartz-Albiez R, Krohne G, ter Meulen V. Physical association of moesin and CD46 as a receptor complex for measles virus. J Virol 69:2248–2256, 1995.

150. Schneider-Schaulies J, Schneider-Schaulies S, ter Meulen V. Differential induction of cytokines by primary and persistant MV-infection in human glial cells. Virology 195:219–228, 1993.

151. Schneider-Schaulies S, Liebert UG, Baczko K, Cattaneo R, Billeter M, ter Meulen V. Restriction of measles virus gene expression in acute and subacute encephalitis of Lewis rats. Virology 171:525–534, 1989.

152. Schneider-Schaulies S, Liebert UG, Baczko K, ter Meulen V. Restricted expression of measles virus in primary rat astroglial cells. Virology 177:802–806, 1990.

153. Schneider-Schaulies S, Liebert UG, Segev Y, Rager-Zisman B, Wolfson M, ter Meulen V. Antibody-dependent transcriptional regulation of measles virus in persistently infected neural cells. J Virol 66:5534–5541, 1992.

154. Schneider-Schaulies S, Schneider-Schaulies J, Bayer M, Löffler S, ter Meulen V. Spontaneous and differentiation-dependent regulation of measles virus expression in human glial cells. J Virol 67:3375–3383, 1993.

155. Schneider-Schaulies S, Schneider-Schaulies J, Dunster LM, ter Meulen V. Measles virus gene expression in neural cells. Current Topics in Microbiology and Immunology, 191:101–116. Eds: V ter Meulen and MA Billeter, Springer-Verlag, New York, 1995.

156. Schneider-Schaulies S, Schneider-Schaulies J, Schuster A, Bayer M, Pavlovic J, ter Meulen V. Cell type specific MxA-mediated inhibition of measles virus transcription in human brain cells. J Virol 68:6910–6917, 1994.

157. Schnorr JJ, Schneider-Schaulies S, Simon-Jödicke A, Pavlovic J, Horisberger MA, ter Meulen V. MxA-dependent inhibition of measles virus glycoprotein synthesis in a stably transfected human monocytic cell line. J Virol 67:4760–4768, 1993.

158. Schwender S, Imrich H, Dörries R. The pathogenic role of virus-specific antibody-secreting cells in the central nervous system of rats with different susceptibility to coronavirus-induced demyelinating encephalitis. Immunology 74:533–538, 1991.

159. Sedarati F, Margolis TP, Stevens JG. Latent infection can be established with drastically restricted transcription and replication of the HSV-1 genome. Virology 192:687–691, 1993.

160. Sedgwick J. Schwender S, Imrich H, Dörries R, ter Meulen V, Butcher GW. Isolation and direct characterization of resident microglia cells from the normal and inflamed central nervous system. Proc Natl Acad Sci USA 88:7438–7442, 1991.

161. Sedgwick JD, Dörries R. The immune system response to viral infection of the CNS. Semin Neurosci 3:93–100, 1991.

162. Sedgwick JD, Mößner R, Schwender S, ter Meulen V. MHC-expressing non-hematopoietic astroglial cells prime only CD8+ T lymphocytes: astroglial cells as perpetuators but not initiators of CD4+ T cell responses in the central nervous system. J Exp Med 173:1235–1246, 1991.

163. Sedgwick JD, Schwender S, Gregersen R, ter Meulen V. Resident macrophages (ramified microglia) of the adult brown Norway rat central nervous system are constitutively major histocompatibility complex class II positive. J Exp Med 177:1145–1152, 1993.

164. Shankar V, Kao M, Hamir AN, Sheng H, Koprowski H, Dietzschold B. Kinetics of virus spread and changes in levels of several cytokine mRNAs in the brain after intranasal infection of rats with Borna disease virus. J Virol 66:992–998, 1992.

165. Shepley MP, Rancaniello VR. A mouse antibody that blocks polivirus attachment recognizes the lymphocyte homing receptor CD44. J Virol 68:1301–1308, 1994.

166. Sissons JGP, Oldstone MBA. Host response to viral infections. In Virology, BN Fields et al., eds. Raven Press, New York, 1985, pp 265–279.

167. Smith TW, De Girolami U, Hickey WF. Neuropathology of immunosuppression. Brain Pathol 2:183–194, 1992.

168. Sonnerborg AB, von Sydow MA, Forsgren M, Strannegard OO. Association between intrathecal anti-HIV-1 immunoglobulin G synthesis and occurrence of HIV-1 in cerebrospinal fluid. AIDS 3:701–705, 1989.

169. Stephan D, Sun H, Fischer-Lindahl K, Meyer E, Hämmerling G, Hood L, Steinmetz M. Organisation and evolution of D region class I genes in the mouse major histocompatibility complex. J Exp Med 163:1227–1244, 1986.

170. Stevens JG. HSV-1 neuroinvasiveness. Intervirology 35:152–163, 1993.

171. Swarz JR, Brooks BR, Johnson RT. Spongiform polioencephalomyelopathy caused by a murine retrovirus. II. Ultrastructural localization of virus replication and spongiform changes in the central nervous system. Neuropathol Appl Neurobiol 7:365–380, 1981.

172. Tas PW, Koschel K. Loss of the endothelin signal pathway in C6 rat glioma cells persistently infected with measles virus. Proc Natl Acad Sci USA 88:6736–6739, 1991.

173. ter Meulen V, Stephenson JR, Kreth HW. Subacute sclerosing panencephalitis. In: Comprehensive Virology, vol 18, H Fraenkel-Conrat, RR Wagner, eds. 1983, pp 105–159.

174. Thompson RL, Rogers SK, Zerhusen MA. Herplex simplex virus neurovirulence and

productive infection of neural cells is associated with a function which maps between 0.82 and 0.832 map units ion the HSV genome. Virology 172:435–450, 1989.

175. Toyoda H, Kohara M, Kataoka Y, Suganuma T, Omata T, Imura N, Nomoto A. Complete nucleotide sequences of all three poliovirus serotype genomes. Implication for genetic relationship, gene function and antigenic determinants. J Mol Biol 174:561–585, 1984.

176. Tsiang H. Pathopysiology of rabies virus infection of the nervous system. Adv Virus Res 42:375–411, 1993.

177. Tyler KL, Virgin HW 4th, Bassel Duby R, Fields BN. Antibody inhibits defined stages in the pathogenesis of Reovirus serotype 3 infection of the central nervous system. J Exp Med 170:887–900, 1989.

178. Tyor WR, Griffin DE. Virus specificity and isotype expression of intraparenchymal antibody-secreting cells during Sindbis virus encephalitis in mice. J Neuroimmunol 48:37–44, 1993.

179. Tyor WR, Wesselingh S, Levine B, Griffin DE. Long term intraparenchymal Ig secretion after acute viral encephalitis in mice. J Immunol 149:4016–4020, 1992.

180. Virelizier JL. Cellular activation and human immunodeficiency virus infection. Curr Opin Immunol 2:409–413, 1989.

181. Ward BJ, Griffin DE. Changes in cytokine production after measles virus vaccination: predominant production of IL-4 suggests induction of a Th2 response. Clin Immunol Immunopathol 67:171–177, 1993.

182. Watanabe R, Wege H, ter Meulen V. Adoptive transfer of EAE-like lesions from rats with corona virus induced demyelinating encephalomyelitis. Nature 305:150–153, 1983.

183. Wege H, Schliephake A, Korner H, Flory E, Wege H. An immunodominant CD4⁺ T cell site on the nucleocapsid protein of murine coronavirus contributes to protection against encephalomyelitis. J Gen Virol 74:1287–1294, 1993.

184. Wege H. Watanabe R, Koga M, ter Meulen V. Coronavirus JHM-induced demyelinating encephalomyelitis in rats: influence of immunity on the course of disease. Prog Brain Res 59:221–231, 1983.

185. Weinmann-Dorsch C, Koschel K. Coupling of viral membrane proteins to phosphat-idylinositide signalling system. FEBS L 247:185–188, 1990.

186. Welsh CJ, Tonks P, Borrow P, Nash AA. Theiler's virus: an experimental model of virus-induced demyelination. Autoimmunity 6:105–112, 1990.

187. Welsh CJ, Tonks P, Nash AA, Blakemore WF. The effect of L3T4 T cell-depletion on the pathogenesis of Theiler's murine encephalomyelitis virus infection in CBA mice. J Gen Virol 68:1659–1667, 1987.

188. Williamson J, Stohlmann S. Effective clearance of mouse hepatitis virus from the central nervous system both requires CD4⁺ and CD8⁺ T cells. J Virol 64:4589–4592, 1990.

189. Wolinsky JS, Klassen T, Baringer JR. Persistence of neuroadapted mumps virus in brains of newborn hamsters after intraperitoneal inoculation. J Infect Dis 133:260–267, 1976.

190. Wright KE, Buchmeier MJ. Antiviral antibodies attenuate T-cell-mediated immunopathology following acute lymphocytic choriomeningitis virus infection. J Virol 65:3001–3006, 1991.

191. Yokomori K, Baker SC, Stohlman SA, Lai MM. Hemagglutinin-esterase-specific monoclonal antibodies alter the neuropathogenicity of mouse hepatitis virus. J Virol 66:2865–2874, 1992.

192. Zimprich F, Winter J, Wege H, Lassmann H. Coronavirus induced primary demyelination: indications for the involvement of a humoral immune response. Neuropathol Appl Neurobiol 17:469–484, 1991.

193. Zurbriggen A, Fujinami RS. Theiler's virus infection in nude mice: viral RNA in vascular endothelial cells. J Virol 62:3589–3596, 1988.

194. Zurbriggen A, Hogle JM, Fujinami RS. Alteration of amino acid 101 within capsid protein VP-1 changes the pathogenicity of Theiler's murine encephalomyelitis virus. J Exp Med 170:2037–2049, 1989.

16

Transplantation into the Central Nervous System

MACIEJ POLTORAK
WILLIAM J. FREED

What Is Neural Transplantation?

Neural transplantation may be defined as implantation of living neuronal or non-neuronal tissue into a host nervous system. The implanted tissue may be grafted in the form of fragments of dissected tissue or as a cell suspension. There are many possible placement sites for such grafts within the nervous system. From a practical point of view, the most important distinction is between grafts that are implanted into the brain parechyma (intraparenchymal) or into the ventricular system (intraventricular). Neural tissue is often employed as a graft, although non-neural tissue, e.g., adrenal medulla, is also widely utilized. Embryonic neuronal tissues, and especially embryonic neurons, survive transplantation much better than neonatal tissues and are most widely used for neural transplantation. There are no convincing data showing survival of transplanted adult neurons.

The first trials of grafting procedures within the central nervous system (CNS) started at the beginning of this century. It was not until the end of the 1970s, however, that realization of the potential of neural grafting fueled massive research in this area (for historical review, see 8,26). Experiments showing that embryonic brain tissue grafts could produce a functional alleviation of behavioral deficits in an animal model of Parkinson's disease eventually led to numerous trials of both embryonic ventral mesencephalon and adrenal medulla transplantations for the treatment of Parkinson's disease in humans. There are several other potential applications of transplantation for the treatment of neurological disorders. The neuroendocrinological diseases are obvious choices, since often in these diseases there are known defects of distinct, small numbers of cells. Substitution of these cells by transplanted normal cells may alleviate the disease. Moreover, transplants might also be applied in a variety of other neurological disorders, including epilepsy, intractable pain, progressive supranuclear palsy, and others (for review, see 22). The ultimate goal of neural transplantation would be to repair or replace defective tissue in neurological disease and traumatic injury, including stroke and spinal cord injury.

The specific purpose of experimental or clinical neural transplantation requires the use of many different types of tissue. The advantage of fetal neurons, the most commonly used tissue, as compared to other types of cells, is that fetal neuronal cells have the potential ability to produce appropriate neurotransmitters or trophic substances. They can extend processes, make synapses and, to some degree, functionally integrate with the host tissue. Fetal neurons as transplants in humans, however, have many limitations, in particular, the restricted source of tissue with its complex legal and ethical problems, as well as limitations related to the immunological barrier (for review, see 21).

Non-neuronal tissue can also be used for transplants in some circumstances. In humans, adrenal medulla intracerebral autografts have been used for the treatment for Parkinson's disease. The adrenal medulla is considered as non-neuronal tissue even though this tissue is derived from the neural crest. Although the functional effects of adrenal medulla grafts may be less than those of ventral mesencephalon grafts, the limited tissue source and problems of rejection can be avoided by the use of autografts (for review, see 24). Adrenal medulla grafts have also been used for chronic pain.

Tumor cell lines are often transplantated to the CNS. Because the proliferation of cell lines is an unwanted feature, the transplanted cell lines must be rendered amitotic or cell division controlled in some manner. Cells may be genetically modified or cell growth controlled by encapsulation. The obstacles to development of genetically modified cells suitable for human transplantation are considerable. Besides safety mechanisms to prevent cell division, genetically modified cells must possess other desirable characteristics including the capability to produce useful neurotransmitters, trophic factors, or enzymes. This requirement can be achieved by incorporation of a gene of interest. At the present time, the main cell sources for genetic alteration are fibroblasts and glial cells. A human neuronal nontumor cell line has only recently been established (82). This cell line may be suitable for human neuronal transplantation (73). If cell lines can be genetically altered to contain specific genes, such cells could potentially be useful as neuronal substitutes for transplantation in certain neurodegenerative and neurotraumatic disorders.

Survival of the Graft and the Rejection Response

The term *graft survival,* although often used, is almost never defined. In terms of embryonic neural grafting, one can define graft survival as appropriate development of the implanted tissue without evidence of structural damage.

In contrast, rejection can be described as an immunological response that produces damage or death of the implanted tissue. It is obvious that such a definition is very vague. We know that within the CNS, immunological reactions against grafted tissue generally occur more slowly than in the periphery, and therefore the assessment of rejection vs. survival is often difficult.

When embryonic neuronal tissue is grafted, this tissue is taken from an intact brain. Obviously, this procedure itself damages the grafted tissue. Moreover, any grafting technique that is used to implant tissue induces further damage. Neuronal tissue is fragile, and whether implanted to a homotopic or heterotopic site within the CNS, it always shows some signs of degeneration unrelated to immune rejection responses. Further damage may take place due to factors such as failure of vascularization or neurotoxicity. Consequently, significant damage of the implanted tissue and even complete graft failure is often associated with the grafting technique and not with a rejection response.

The differentiation between graft damage arising through these nonimmunological factors and that due to immunological reactions can be illustrated by comparing syngrafts (nonimmunological damage) with allografts or xenografts. By using this comparison, immunological rejection can be measured by comparing any immunological reactions or damage in allografts or xenografts in excess of those observed in the syngraft paradigm.

The Concept of Immunological Privilege of the Brain

Experimental neural transplantation has been performed since the beginning of our century. It has become apparent that some grafted tissues can survive in the host brain but are readily rejected when transplanted elsewhere. Enhanced graft survival is observed not only in the brain but also within several other sites which include the anterior chamber of the eye, cornea, hamster cheek pouch, testicle, prostate, uterus, and others (3). The concept of the CNS as an *immunologically privileged site* emerged from the pioneering studies of Medawar (56), who demonstrated that the rejection of brain allografts is an immunological phenomenon. He showed that skin allografts survived in the brains of host rabbits, but not if the hosts had previously received orthotopic skin grafts from the same donors. In other words, in the brain, the allografts did not themselves induce rejection, but were nonetheless susceptible to rejection induced by other means. Medawar (56) thought that since lymphatic drainage is required to create immunological reactions, a lack of lymphatics within the brain was the basis for the unresponsiveness of the host to transplanted tissue.

Soon, however, it was realized that intracerebral grafted tissue does sensitize the host and that brain grafts are therefore able to induce an immunological response (77,86,103). Some of these studies noted, however, that despite host sensitization, brain grafts may survive within the host brain for a prolonged period of time. In another experiment, Geyer and Gill (27) used inbred rat strains to supplement these observations and demonstrated that such sensitization is related to the antigenic disparity between donor and host.

Since it had been shown that both efferent and afferent arcs of immunological reactions may be present after intracerebral transplantation, the reason the host brain permits enhanced graft survival was still not clear. Initially, the quite obvious separation of the CNS from the immunological system was considered to be a major contributor to CNS graft survival. It was reasoned that since the blood-brain-barrier (BBB) largely excludes intravascular proteins and lymphocytes (as it was also once believed) from the brain parenchyma, therefore, the BBB may protect the graft from immune attack.

It is now recognized that the brain should not be regarded as a categorically immunologically privileged site for transplantation. Allogenic, and particularly xenogenic tissue, can induce in the host immune system reactions against grafted tissue. In view of possible graft applications in human disorders, and the obvious difficulties in finding suitable sources of donor tissue, an understanding of the immunological processes within the host brain after allo- or xenotransplanations is essential.

This chapter does not cover all known available literature on the topic. Instead, we have attempted to present a short overview and synthesis of the data on immunological reactions after intracerebral transplantation in view of recent advances in immunology, with an emphasis on well-established facts. Other very good general reviews on this subject include papers by Widner and Brundin (98); Nicholas and Arnason (60); Lund et al. (51); and Sloan et al. (89).

Review of Basic Scientific Findings

Immunological Status of the Adult (Host) and Embryonic (Donor) Brain

The relevant immunological status of the brain tissue that is involved in allograft rejection may be considered from two points of view. The first concerns properties of the donor tissue itself, i.e., what factors within the donor tissue may induce the general immune (rejection) response? The second point of view deals with the host brain tissue and its complex accessibility and potential to express an immune (rejection) response. Both depictions, naturally, are to some degree interrelated.

From an immunological point of view, the most important issue for the survival of grafts in the host is their histocompatibility. The most pertinent antigen systems, where compatibility between the donor and host is required, are the major histocompatibility complex (MHC) and ABO (blood group antigens) systems.

In the ABO system, vascularized grafted tissue containing red blood cells incompatible with the host promptly induces a hyperacute rejection response because of the presence of preexisting antibodies. The role of blood-group compatibility in brain transplantation has not yet been fully addressed.

CNS Tissue Expresses Unusually Low Levels of MHC Class I Antigens

Compatibility between the donor and host of MHC class I and class II antigens is the single-most important characteristic determining the outcome of grafting procedures in the periphery. Under normal conditions, neither neurons, astrocytes, oligodendrocytes, nor resting microglia synthesize MHC class I antigens in detectable quantities. Within the brain parenchyma, only endothelial cells of blood vessel walls consistently express MHC class I antigens. It is obvious that since there are no substantial MHC antigens on grafted neuronal tissue, allogenic grafts would not be recognized by host effector cells as non-self target tissue. Generally, however, the synthesis of MHC by any cell is under the regulatory control of the immunological system. Expression of MHC class I antigens can be increased by stimulation of cells with lymphokines, primarily interferon gamma (INF-γ). Even though CNS cells do not normally express MHC class I antigens, it has been shown that the majority of cell types from the CNS are able to synthesize detectable amounts of MHC class I antigens in culture after appropriate stimulation (38,102). It is still controversial whether neurons can become MHC class I antigen positive (see Fig. 16-1).

The CNS Lacks MHC Class II Positive Cells

Similarly, although some data indicate the presence of rare MHC class II+ cells (45), parenchymal brain tissue in the normal state does not express MHC class II antigen immunoreactivity (32), and therefore does not contain the appropriate fixed antigen-presenting cells (APCs). These scarce APCs are only present within the meninges and choroid plexus (34). The relative lack of APCs within the CNS would imply that foreign-grafted antigens could not be presented to effector cells and consequently that there would not be a reaction against the allogenic grafts.

However, as with MHC class I antigen expression, it has been shown that induction of MHC class II antigens in cultured CNS cells occurs after lymphokine stimulation. In culture, MHC class II molecules have been reported on many CNS cells, with the notable exception of neurons. There are no convincing data showing MHC class II antigens on neurons following stimulation with lymphokines.

The CNS Possesses a Blood-Brain Barrier

The brain parenchyma is unique as compared to peripheral tissue since it is divided from the blood environment by the BBB, which acts to prevent a free exchange of chemicals and macromolecules between the vascular interior and the brain parenchyma. Thus, the BBB may contribute to the protection of grafted tissue from the rejection response.

The Brain Possesses Limited Lymphatic Drainage

Obviously, brain tissue does not contain typical lymphatics, but this does not mean that the proteins from the CNS area do not penetrate to the peripheral lymph nodes (10,100;

Brain Parenchyma, Normal Tissue

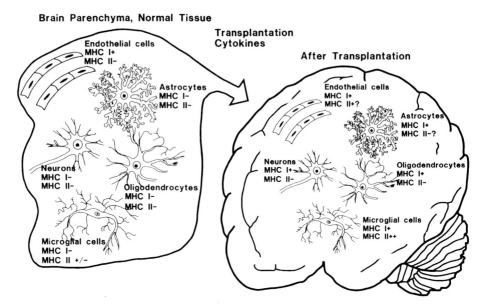

Fig. 16-1. Expression of MHC molecules by major cell types present in the brain. Under normal conditions, brain cells, with some exceptions, do not express MHC class I and MHC class II antigens. After implantation to the host CNS, cells within the grafted brain tissue, and particularly allogenic and xenogenic tissue, start to express both MHC class I and MHC class II antigens on their surface. Expression of MHC molecules may also be induced by other forms of immune response not related to graft rejection, including nonspecific brain injury. Such events may also result in expression of MHC molecules by host cells as well. The degree of MHC antigen expression varies widely, depending on the donor cell type as well as on other factors related to the induction of immune responses. Expression of MHC molecules is likely to be induced by cytokines. Microglial cells and endothelial cells are likely to express MHC molecules and may play important roles in CNS graft rejection.

see Chapter 4). The flow of brain parenchymal interstitial fluid has some preferential channels. It is thought that molecular transport is achieved by means of the cerebrospinal fluid (CSF). The bulk of the CSF gets into the blood circulation via the arachnoid villi in the dural sinus, but some molecules, especially larger ones, flow into the peripheral lymph. By this route, the passage of fluid is primarily from the subarachnoid space surrounding the olfactory bulb and nerves, down to the interstitial spaces of the nasal submucosa, and from there to the lymphatic system. The nasal submucosa is the final common route for fluid flow from both the direct subpial and subarachnoid spaces.

When radioactive albumin is injected into the animal brain, the amount of albumin collected in the cervical lymph nodes is greater after intraparenchymal injection than after intraventricular injection (10). These data may suggest that antigens present in the ventricular system, which communicates directly with the subarachnoid space, are mainly removed through arachnoid villi to the circulating blood. Antigens present in the brain parenchyma are cleared through subpial space to the nasal submucosa and finally to the lymph nodes.

Some authors suggest that the brain possesses so-called prelymphatics in close proximity to blood vessels (15). In fact, thin-walled canals in the perivascular space have been reported in brains of patients diagnosed with various neurological disorders including multiple sclerosis (MS) (75). It seems, however, that even if these canals are physiologically functional, they do not convey fluid to the lymphatic system.

In general, therefore, it appears that there is an afferent lymphatic drainage for the CNS, but it is clear that it is less efficient than the peripheral lymphatic system. An impaired afferent lymphatic drainage would suggest that the graft antigens and activated host APCs may not migrate to the host peripheral lymph nodes, and it is possible, therefore, that the immune rejection response is not initiated or amplified by this means (see Chapter 4).

Passenger Leucocytes

Another issue involves the contribution of so-called passenger leukocytes to allograft rejection. These donor bone marrow–derived cells are present in most peripheral tissues and are capable of activating host lymphocytes. In many circumstances these cells appear to be an important factor promoting graft rejection. It is commonly believed that the predepletion of these passenger cells from grafted tissue greatly enhances the survival of allografts. In the case of cerebral embryonic allografts, it is possible that the implanted tissue is nearly devoid of passenger cells, since at this point of embryogenesis the animals do not contain fully reactive lymphocytes.

Specifics of Transplantation Models

Neural transplants have a greater range of anatomical variation and specific properties as compared to transplants of other tissue in the periphery (see Fig. 16-2). Grafts usually consist of embryonic CNS tissue. There are many exceptions, however, such as adult adrenal medulla, sympathetic ganglia, tumor cells, and immortalized cell lines, some of which may have proposed clinical applications. Other exceptions, such as adult skin grafts, pancreas, or thyroid tissue are mainly placed to the CNS for experimental purposes. Neural transplants are generally placed in the CNS of adult hosts, although often grafts are implanted into neonatal hosts as well. The specificity of neural transplantation in the CNS is a factor which can play an important role in the immunological rejection response.

The survival of grafted neuronal tissue is correlated with its age (87). Generally, young embryonic tissue survives better than older embryonic or neonatal donor tissue. Neurons survive transplantation best when they are still dividing or shortly after cell division is complete and they have not yet entered the postmitotic phase of differentiation. In many

SPECIAL PROPERTIES OF CNS TRANSPLANTATION SITES

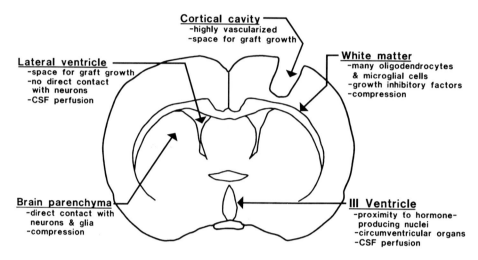

Fig. 16-2. The CNS is not a homogeneous organ. There are several specific sites that can be used for CNS transplantation, each of which has unique special properties. Each transplantation site has distinct advantages and disadvantages for grafting purposes, some of which influence the probability that grafts will induce or succumb to immune responses.

circumstances, the survival of younger tissue depends more on its ability to overcome physiological constraints after implantation (e.g., requirements for trophic factors and contacts with other cells) and its ability to integrate with the host, rather than true immunological antigenicity. In contrast to younger tissue, differentiated mature neurons do not generally survive transplantation to the adult CNS. Dissecting tissue from the donor CNS damages neuronal processes and removes the tissue from the action of trophic factors. Glial cells are more likely than neurons to survive transplantation when tissue from donors of later gestational stages is used. There are no data which specifically show that the lack of survival of mature neurons is due to immunologically mediated events, but it is possible that there are immunological factors in older tissue which contribute to the decline in survival.

The age of the host at the time of graft implantation is important. In some experiments, neonatal host animals are employed. In these circumstances, the survival rate of allogenic as well as xenogenic grafts is higher than for comparable adult hosts (50). The lack of an evident immune rejection response in rodent hosts is limited to the first postnatal week (50). There is no direct evidence for the mechanisms involved in the prolonged survival of grafts placed in a neonatal host CNS. It is possible that, in a manner similar to the induction of neonatal tolerance, survival is due to deletion of the immature host T cells that recognize donor MHC. Another possibility is that the healing of the disrupted BBB subsequent to implantation, and its return to normal function after grafting procedures, occurs while the neonatal hosts are still immunologically immature (67). Disruption of the BBB in nonimmunosuppressed neonatal hosts with previously established neuronal xenografts provokes rapid graft rejection (68,69).

Astrogliosis and Microgliosis

It is expected that when grafts are implanted, they will always damage the host parenchyma to some degree. When transplanted to the host hippocampal region, embryonic tissue induces detectable astrocytic reactions as soon as 6 hours after implantation (97). By 1 week after transplantation, host astrocytes start to differentiate to reactive astrocytes and concentrate around the transplant region. Furthermore, host astrocytes from surrounding regions migrate towards the grafted tissue to form a thick and often continuous border around the transplant. This type of "scar" can be observed for a very long period of time after transplantation (97). Moreover, it has been established not only that host astrocytes migrate to the graft but also that donor astrocytes migrate out from the graft to surrounding host tissue, forming a halo around the transplant (48,76,104). It is possible that certain immunological factors may be involved in this glial migration. When autonomic ganglia grafts, which do not contain classical astrocytes, are implanted into the ventricle, the migration of host astrocytes to the grafts is much stronger for allogenic grafts as compared to autografts (84). The presence of reactive astrocytosis around the grafts seems to depend on implantation technique. Embryonic spinal cord transplants do not induce astrocytosis when placed into the ventricles or into an intracephalic cavity (78). Intraparenchymal cerebellar grafts induce much stronger astrocytic reactions than similar grafts in the lateral ventricles (72).

After brain damage, usually both astrogliosis and microgliosis are present. Although astrocytes are easily distinguishable by immunostaining with glial fibrillary acidic protein (GFAP), immunological markers for microglial are not well defined. In fact, there are no immunological markers that are uniquely specific for microglia since all cross-react with macrophages and monocytes. Microglial cells are of bone-marrow origin (36), and during early development populate the CNS, forming the so-called resting microglial cells. These cells are specialized brain macrophages and share some markers with the macrophage–monocyte cell lineage (65). In adult brain, after parenchymal damage, recruitment of new macrophages from the blood circulation takes place (through the damaged BBB) and resident microglial cells differentiate towards so-called reactive microglia. Additionally, an influx of reactive astrocytes occurs after the tissue insult (30). The activated astrocytes produce certain growth factors, including interleukin (IL)-3, which can, in turn, potentiate the mitogenic activity of microglial cells (25). On the other hand, it is possible that macrophages invading the damaged tissue influence astrocyte proliferation by releasing IL-1 (29).

The host brain damage due to grafting procedures and the graft itself seem to induce a specific sequence of events. The initial reactions that are found a few hours after transplantation involve macrophages. Probably, a leaking BBB is responsible for large infiltrations of macrophages, which differentiate toward ameboid macrophages, around small vessels. These macrophages phagocytose necrotic host and donor tissue (47). Next, microglial cells residing in the host respond by surrounding the graft and lesion. They begin to retract processes to form reactive microglia (70). Whether there is proliferation of resident microglial cells is still disputed. However, in neonatal and adult T-cell deficient host animals, it has been shown that retinal xenografts are populated by microglia almost exclusively derived from the host (66). In the case of syngenic grafts, these microglial and blood-derived macrophage reactions disappear slowly.

Astrocytes also undergo temporally restricted changes associated with brain grafting (1). First, there is a period of so-called reactive gliosis, when the host astrocytes surrounding the grafted tissue increase in size and expression of GFAP. It has been suggested that, in the case of graft rejection, these events are followed by destruction of astrocytes of donor origin, and next accompanied by damage of donor neuronal as well as astroglial cells (1). Earlier data suggested that in culture, under certain circumstances astrocytes can act as APCs (19). It is doubtful that these APC astrocytes play a significant role in graft rejection. It seems that the phenomena involving astrocytes are secondary to the function of microglia and macrophages. However, activated astrocytes express MHC class I antigens (see below), so that astrocytes may become a target for host immunocompetent cells. Although neurons are not necessarily a primary target for the host immune response, they may nonetheless be damaged by bystander phenomena.

Thus, implantation of tissue into the brain will always induce astrocytic and resident microglial reactions, with an invasion of newly recruited blood-derived macrophages as well.

Breakdown of the Host Blood-Brain Barrier

There is no doubt that the implantation of any tissue into the brain causes damage to host tissue and disruption of blood vessels. This is observed particularly after intraparenchymal transplantation. Not only is the integrity of the BBB disturbed around the grafts but in fact, host blood vessels have direct access to the implants. These factors invariably produce edema surrounding the grafts. Under normal conditions, in the case of grafts that are not rejected, this breakdown of the host BBB is transient, and after a few days a normal functional host BBB is restored (13).

To understand the role of the donor BBB, we need to comprehend that the BBB consists primarily of endothelial cells connected by tight junctions. During embryogenesis, brain vessels (nonleaky) develop from leaky peripheral vessels which sprout into the brain parenchyma. Brain tissue, particularly astrocytes surrounding sprouting vessels, are implicated in the generation of the functional BBB (40). Angiogenesis, and sprouting of leaky vessels into the brain parenchyma, strongly suggest that at least a short period of time exists during which the sprouting vessels are permeable. These events take place early in embryogenesis, in rats, around gestational day 15. Thus, when fragments of embryonic neuronal tissue taken before days 13–14 of gestation in rodents are implanted, this tissue probably contains sprouting leaky vessels, whereas grafted tissue taken after 15–16 gestational days may contain vessels which have become nonleaky.

It has been suggested that the BBB is leaky in the area within the brain parenchyma surrounding embryonic cortex implants (83). However, recent data indicate that this dysfunction of the BBB at the neuronal graft site is transient. Healthy neuronal tissue grafts, implanted either as blocks or as cell suspensions, do not show BBB disturbances (12,13). Implantation of non-neuroglial tissue to the host brain parenchyma does, however, result in a permeable BBB (83). The leaky vessels of these peripheral tissue grafts do not acquire a functional BBB.

The role of the intact BBB as a factor in restricting access of immune system functions to transplanted tissue is a complex issue. There are two sets of rather contradictory data. In one group of studies, the importance of breakdown of the BBB for the induction and occurrence of immune rejection responses against CNS grafts has been demonstrated (58,68,69). These data are difficult to understand in view of new evidence showing that even the intact BBB is permeable to activated lymphocytes, which circulate and maintain surveillance in the CNS (37,96). On the other hand, it has been known for a long time that transplanted non-neural tissues, often highly immunogenic, and without a BBB, are not rejected readily in the brain (34). It is possible that integrity of the BBB is required for the survival of certain types of CNS grafts (e.g., xenografts), but that for other types of grafts permeability of the BBB is induced during graft rejection.

Up-regulation of MHC Class I Antigen Expression in Donor and Host Tissue

Normal neuronal tissue expresses very low levels of MHC immunoreactivity (35,85). The level of MHC induction after a brain lesion or syngenic transplantation exhibits a temporally related pattern of expression. It appears quickly, within days after the lesion, has a peak of expression with a duration of several days to 2 or 3 weeks, has a variable plateau, and the expression of MHC antigens disappears relatively late. This picture reflects direct damage of host tissue, that is, reactions that occur due to damage itself, and does not include the additional immunogenic factors that arise when a foreign target is found within the host tissue.

What type of cells express MHC antigens? MHC class I antigens are induced on astrocytes and microglial cells. As discussed above, both astrogliosis and microgliosis are present within the host and donor tissue after grafting. Whether neurons are able to express MHC class I is still controversial. Neurons in culture do not appear to be able to express MHC class I antigens even after very strong stimulation with lymphokines (4,5). There are, however, data suggesting that axotomy induces MHC class I expression on neurons (52), although this result is disputed by others (93). Using light microscopy, it is extremely difficult or impossible to clearly demonstrate in situ what kinds of cells express MHC class I after grafting. Ultrastructually, however, Lawrence et al. (47) were able to show direct contact between T lymphocytes and neurons, indirectly implying that neurons can bear MHC class I antigens. More precise studies using immunolabeling on the electron-microscopic level could resolve this question. It is possible that an immunological disparity between donor and host additionally stimulates neuronal tissue to express MHC class I antigens, whereas following tissue damage alone, the increase in expression of MHC antigens may be weak. Furthermore, in culture many neuroblastoma and neuronal cell lines express MHC class I antigens and their MHC immunoreactivity is enhanced after stimulation with Interferon (INF)-γ (44,73).

After CNS transplantation of syngenic, allogenic, or xenogenic tissue, MHC class I antigens appear within CNS grafts and the surrounding host tissue. Usually, however, syngenic grafts induce only transient and rather weak enhancement of MHC class I antigens (54). In the case of allografts and xenografts, the up-regulation of MHC class I antigens is stable and pronounced (54). It seems probable that in all types of grafts, expression of MHC class I antigens is initially induced by tissue damage and ischemia during implantation procedures. In the case of syngenic grafts, the up-regulation of MHC expression follows a natural course similar to that seen after a brain lesion and gradually disappears. In the case of allografts and xenografts, however, the original MHC class I antigen induction may be sustained through release of lymphokines by effector cells which are in turn activated by foreign allogenic and xenogenic MHC class I antigens. The released lymphokines in turn stimulate host and donor tissue to additional up-regulation of MHC class I antigens. This positive feedback could be a major element leading to persistent enhancement of MHC class I antigens within the allogenic and xenogenic grafted neuronal tissue.

Up-regulation of MHC Class II Antigen Expression in Donor and Host Tissue

Graft implantation always induces an influx of blood-derived macrophages. These cells constitutively express MHC class II antigens. In the case of nonrejected grafts there is no large accumulation of cells, and the MHC class II positive macrophages usually extend out only to the damaged brain tissue. However, in the case of rejected grafts, the MHC class II antigen-positive macrophages infiltrate the grafts in large numbers, usually accompanied by perivascular cuffing of small vessels (47,54,68,70). It appears that the number of these cells within the graft correlates inversely with graft survival (69,70).

MHC class II antigen–positive macrophages which migrate into the host brain originate from bone marrow. Aside from the presence of these cells, recent data have demonstrated other parenchymal cell populations that induce MHC class II molecules following brain damage resulting from transplantation procedures (47,70). In fact, simple insult to the brain tissue, without a transplantation procedure, produces enhancement of MHC class II antigen expression within the injured tissue (93). There is still some controversy surrounding the type of cells that show MHC class II up-regulation. Earlier light microscopy studies of human multiple sclerosis brains suggested that GFAP-positive astrocytes express MHC class II molecules (94). Other data suggest that microglia can also express MHC class II antigens in brains of patients with multiple sclerosis (33) or in brains that have sustained neuronal injury (93). In intracerebral transplantation it is not possible to completely exclude other possibilities, but it clearly seems that GFAP+ astrocytes are not the main source of MHC class II+ cells (70).

Microglial cells are widely distributed in normal brain and in fact, are most dense in the cortex. After brain damage, reactive microglial cells associated with longitudinal myelinated neuronal tracts tend to express MHC class II antigens. This effect appears to involve activation of the local microglia due to damage of host neuronal fibers during implantation of the tissue (70,93). Furthermore, populations of nonmicroglia-derived macrophages with phagocytic abilities are found within the ventricular system, i.e., in the supraependymal and epiplexus cells. MHC class II expression is also enhanced on these cells, possibly as a result of the introduction of tissue debris into the ventricular system after transplantation (70).

It should be emphasized that induction of MHC class II antigens is not entirely an immunologically specific event. It is likely that expression of MHC class II antigens by these two cell populations is induced by injury-related mechanisms and not by rejection-related events, although the influx of MHC class II+ cells may facilitate graft rejection. It should also be kept in mind that the presence of MHC class II+ cells indicates that these cells may be capable of presenting antigens; however, MHC antigen expression is only one of the attributes an APC must possess to perform its function. It does not mean that these cells are actually functioning as APCs. After intracerebral allotransplantation and xenotransplantation, therefore, both injury-induced and foreign-graft induced MHC class II+ cells are found (47,70).

In one important study, Lawrence et al. (47) transplanted syngenic hippocampal formation tissue to one side of the brain and allogenic tissue to the other side. Comparing one side to the other, he suggested that MHC class II+ microglia form characteristic satellite clusters surrounding individual neurons in allogenic tissue, whereas this phenomenon was not found within the grafted syngenic tissue.

There are many studies suggesting that endothelial cells may be involved in antigen presentation, since they can up-regulate MHC class II synthesis in vitro (53,55,95). However, recent data demonstrate that in pure cultures, endothelial cells express MHC class II antigens in response to INF-γ but are unable to induce antigen-specific proliferation of syngeneic T lymphocytes (79). These data indirectly suggest that antigen presentation of foreign or transplanted tissue by donor endothelial cells may not have functional significance.

Vascularization of Grafted Tissue: Vessels from Host or from Implants?

To better understand vascularization within the grafted tissue, normal development of mammalian brain vessels should be examined. Brain vessels do not develop from preexisting capillaries. Brain tissue is invaded by sprouting capillaries from outside the brain. Migratory angioblasts radially invade brain tissue, penetrating deep into the brain parenchyma from the mesenchymal leptomenigeal plexus and subsequently branching. In rodents, these events occur at approximately days 13–14 of gestation (2). The endothelial proliferation is continuous in rats, with the greatest growth occurring at around 1 week postnatally, followed by markedly decreased growth after this period of life (81).

These data suggest that the implanted tissue from rodent embryos after gestational days 13–14 already possesses vessels of donor origin. It is possible that grafted tissue from earlier gestational stages does not contain donor blood vessels (assuming that the implanted tissue was stripped of leptomeningeal membranes). This situation is only rarely considered, and it should be acknowledged that the majority of grafted tissues will already contain some donor vessels.

Moreover, the origin of the blood vessels within the grafted tissue is influenced by other important factors, such as the site of the implanted tissue. Whether the grafts are placed within the ventricular system or within the brain parenchyma could affect the origin of vessels. We know that generally, grafts within the ventricular system (particularly in the lateral ventricles) can grow to quite large dimensions, but they are more poorly integrated with the host tissue than are intraparenchymal grafts (72). Grafts may even be free-floating within the ventricular system. The relative lack of graft–host integration might suggest that a graft within the ventricular system would tend to contain primarily vessels of donor origin. Indeed, recent data suggest that this is true (12). On the other hand, in the case of well-integrated intraparenchymal grafts, it would be expected that vessels of both host and donor origin would be found within the graft. Moreover, it has been shown that endothelial cells from intraparenchymal hippocampal grafts migrate to the host and therefore both the graft itself and the host tissue surrounding the graft contain mosaic vessels consisting of host and donor endothelial cells (46). The budding of host vessels into the implants is profuse. Even when neonatal brain tissue is implanted, in only about half of it can donor vessels be detected. Host vessels are always found, suggesting that the process of donor vessel budding is slow and that the tissue probably requires additional blood vessels supplied by the host.

Angiogenesis and anastomosis are affected by many factors that can appear within the graft or its surrounding host brain tissue after implantation. Such factors as fibroblast growth factor (FGF) (80), transforming growth factor-β (TGF-β), and others enhance angiogenesis (91). Moreover, the presence of direct or indirect damage to brain areas where the grafted tissue is placed may influence angiogenesis. Other factors, e.g., type of graft, or whether the graft consists of solid fragments of tissue or dissociated cells, probably have minor influences. Because the dissociation of brain fragments would disrupt vessels, it is expected that angiogenesis from dissociated endothelial cells would be less robust than that from intact vessels. In fact, both donor and host vessels may contribute to the vascularization of grafted cell suspensions.

Lymphocyte Homing and Passage

Under normal conditions, the brain parenchyma is almost entirely devoid of resting lymphocytes, and only a small number of lymphocytes are present within the CSF. Recent data suggest that normally activated lymphocytes cross the "intact" BBB, as opposed to mature lymphocytes (37,96). This passage is independent of whether the immunocompetent cells are specifically or nonspecifically activated.

Adhesion of lymphocytes and macrophages to the surfaces of endothelial cells is the first event in their passage into the brain parenchyma. This leucocyte passage is mediated by many families of extracellular and cell surface proteins, including integrins. Lymphocyte passage and interactions with endothelial cells is discussed in more detail in Chapter 7.

The role of allogenic MHC antigens on endothelial cells in lymphocyte CNS homing is undetermined. Clearly, however, the presence or absence of donor vessels within transplanted tissue could have consequences for immunological reactions against the grafts. Host effector cells should recognize non-self MHC alloantigens on donor vessels, but would not respond to self MHC class I antigens on host vessels. Recognition of "non-self" antigens could induce the release of lymphokines, which stimulate the integrin–endothelium interaction. This in turn might very well accelerate both lymphocyte passage to the grafted tissue and host allograft recognition of implanted vascularized tissue. The MHC–antigen interaction itself is not sufficient to stabilize the binding of T lymphocytes, and the previously mentioned nonantigen-specific adhesion pathways are essential to complete the response.

Because passage of activated lymphocytes is not blocked by brain endothelial cells there is a continuous surveillance of the CNS by activated lymphocytes (37). In the case of CNS transplantation, activated lymphocytes constantly pass the BBB and reach the host brain parenchyma and grafted tissue. It is possible that this phenomenon has a pivotal role in the generation of an immune response against CNS tissue grafts. The role of lymphocyte homing and passage after intracerebral grafting, however, is not yet fully understood.

Allografting with Additional Systemic Sensitization of the Host with Donor Tissue

Evidence that the efferent arc of the immune response in the CNS is functionally intact initially came from studies of allografting combined with supplemental systemic sensitization of the host with donor tissue. This model was first described by Medawar (56). Generally, this model consists of the establishment of a neuronal allograft in the host brain, combined with challenge of the host with donor antigens administered in the periphery. This systemic immunization of the host animal can be performed either prior or subsequent to transplantation. This paradigm has some special properties. Generally, brain neuronal allograft rejection, if it occurs, is relatively slow as compared to the rejection of peripheral grafts. In this model, the immune responses against brain allografts are amplified in the host peripheral lymphoid organs by systemic immunization with donor tissue. We know that activated immunocompetent cells constantly survey the CNS; thus, following systemic sensitization, immunocompetent cells sensitized to donor antigens enter the host brain to produce reactions within the graft. By using a variety of species, strains, and transplantation models, many studies have since confirmed that accelerated rejection of brain allografts within the CNS indeed occurs using both prior and subsequent systemic sensitization (20,34,41,51). It is reasoned that host systemic stimulation with donor antigens produces sensitized immunocompetent cells and that the grafted tissue thus becomes a target of these cells. After the discovery that embryonic brain tissue indeed acquires the MHC class I antigens after intracerebral transplantation (54), it became obvious that the grafted tissue can become a direct target for host immunocompetent cells. In fact, numerous studies have confirmed that intracerebral allotransplantation across MHC antigen differences induces MHC class I antigen expression in grafted tissue in situ (1,16,18,54,59,64,67). The up-regulation of MHC class I antigens within the grafted tissue is a necessary condition for graft rejection.

It is well known that intracerebral grafts may be more slowly rejected than peripheral grafts. It has been shown that in large allografts, areas of neuronal tissue with normal appearance are often intermixed with areas demonstrating varying phases of immunological response (46). It has been reasoned that these patches of cell infiltration are evidence of a host rejection response. However, whether these supposed rejection responses against the grafted tissue are perpetuated, invariably resulting in destruction of the graft, is unclear. Moreover, it appears there are at least two different forms of immune response against intracerebral allografted tissue with differing outcomes (see Mechanisms of Graft Rejection).

Using this immune response–amplifying transplantation paradigm, we (23,39,71) studied several combinations of host and donor rat strains. Interestingly, rejection responses vary considerably, depending on which host–donor combinations are used. Systemic sensitization with BN-RT1^n tissue results in the rejection of established BN-RT1^n neuronal allografts in the lateral ventricle of host F344-RT1^l rats (23); however, if the host and donor strains are reversed, a similar sensitization-induced brain graft rejection does not occur (71). A similar asymmetry was observed in another experiment, when BN-RT1^n donor grafts were efficiently rejected in LEW-RT1^l hosts, while LEW-RT1^l grafts in BN-RT1^n hosts were not (39). These differences in terms of intensity of immune rejection response cannot be explained entirely in terms of genetic disparity between the donor and host strains. Despite complete genetic disparity in both MHC and minor histocompatibility antigens, for some rat strain combinations, brain allografts can survive for prolonged periods of time even after sensitization with donor tissue.

From these results, it appears that immunogenicity of the donor tissue is an important factor in neural graft rejection. There are several factors, however, that may contribute to differences in graft rejection between rat strains. There is a very low degree of graft versus host disease (GvHD) induction between some of the rat strains (7). Also, there is a relative lack of suppressor cells in the host rats, particularly in the BN-RT1^n strain which in turn is responsible for a low mixed lymphocyte response (MLR) (7). Additional factors, including host MHC allele and host susceptibility to autoimmune disease, may also be influential.

Interestingly, when astrocyte aggregates are implanted to the anterior chamber of the eye of experimental allergic encephalitis (EAE)-susceptible mice, these transplants show a strong response similar to the EAE inflammatory response after sensitization with myelin basic proteins (49). Although myelination does not occur in embryonic brain tissue, adult brain tissue which is sometimes used for sensitization does express myelin basic protein. It is conceivable that sensitization with such adult brain tissue would result in an autoimmune reaction that could contribute to rejection of CNS grafts in susceptible strains of animals (and humans). It should be strongly emphasized, however, that the majority of available data are obtained from experiments performed in rodents. In general, rodents may be relatively resistant to CNS immune phenomena, including graft rejection as well as autoimmune responses. Thus, whether these results can be fully applied to human intracerebral transplantation is unclear, and more data on immune responses to CNS grafts in primates should be acquired.

Evidence of Host Sensitization with Grafted Brain Tissue

Older studies used the survival rate of skin allografts or other relatively insensitive immunological methods as measures of systemic sensitization (for review, see 20). The first evidence that brain tissue is able to induce systemic sensitization came from studies in which donor brain tissue was systemically injected. Often, sensitization was not detected with grafting to the brain alone. With the use of more sophisticated techniques, it has been demonstrated that sensitization to donor brain tissue in secondary lymphoid organs of the host can occur after allotransplantation (99). The question remains, how is this sensitization achieved? It appears that implantation of tissue within the brain produces immunologic activation within the cervical lymphatic nodes (101). These lymph nodes provide a local amplification of the immune response to allografted tissue and are the final terminus of the relatively limited, CNS lymphatic drainage. When neuronal grafts are rejected, specific, systemic sensitization can subsequently be detected in the spleen and peripheral blood (99). Therefore, there is no doubt that, at least when the grafts are rejected, intracerebrally grafted allogenic neuronal tissue is able to induce a systemic immunological response after transplantation in some circumstances.

Mechanisms of Graft Rejection

Our current hypothesis for graft rejection involves the possibility that grafted neuronal tissue can elicit two different kinds of immune responses. One would involve primarily microglial cells and blood-derived macrophages. The second type of rejection is characterized by additional involvement of cytotoxic and helper T cells and includes T-cell infiltrations within the grafted tissue. The latter type of response results in rejection and graft destruction, whereas the first type of response may produce some tissue damage but is not sufficient to produce complete graft destruction.

It is known that peripheral allograft rejection is mediated by host T-cell populations and that both T helper (CD4) cells and cytotoxic (CD8) lymphocytes are required for rejection to occur. Although the kinetics of the immune response to intracerebral grafts are generally much slower than against allografts transplanted into the periphery, both T helper cells and cytotoxic lymphocytes are found in rejected brain allografts (54). During rejection of brain allografts, there appears to be an initial infiltration of T helper cells, followed by an increase in cytotoxic lymphocytes (59,63,64). Interestingly, when T helper cells are inactivated by antibodies, neuronal grafts survive well and do not show any signs of rejection; however, when the cytotoxic lymphocytes are removed, the brain allografts undergo rejection similar to that seen in control grafts (62). These data suggest that T helper cells are of primary importance for rejection of brain allografts.

Phenotypic analysis of rejected grafts indicates that the relative number of cytotoxic lymphocytes in the grafts increases with the progression of rejection. Moreover, when mononuclear cells are isolated from brain allograft infiltrations, the cytotoxic lymphocytes are found to be sensitized to host MHC antigens and are able to lyse appropriate target cells in vitro (61). Therefore, it seems that T helper cells are essential for initiation of the immune rejection response to brain allografts. Later in the rejection response, cytotoxic lymphocytes may contribute to the process of graft destruction. Rejected allografts always show strongly enhanced MHC class I and II immunoreactivities. Within rejected CNS grafts, there is always a large influx of T cells consisting of cytotoxic and helper lymphocytes. Activated microglial cells and macrophages are also present. Host animals with rejected CNS allografts demonstrate blood lymphocyte activation. The cellular events involved in this type of immunological reaction, including T-cell infiltration, are similar for most cases of strongly rejected grafts.

It has been mentioned that grafted allogenic neuronal tissue demonstrates increased expression of MHC class I antigen, and that damage of the host brain during implantation procedures and injury of the grafted tissue itself also induces increased MHC class I antigen expression. Moreover, up-regulation of MHC class II antigen expression on microglial cells, which can potentially function as antigen-presenting cells, can be induced by nonspecific damage of the host or donor brain tissue. Increased expression of both MHC class I and II antigens within the grafted tissue, however, does not necessarily predict allograft rejection. Using CNS allotransplantation combined with systemic donor tissue-induced host sensitization, in certain rat strain combinations, allografts express increased MHC class I and II immunoreactivity without apparent immunological rejection responses and without lymphocytic infiltration (39,71). Therefore, it seems that in these rat strain combinations, simple up-regulation of MHC antigen expression within the grafted tissue is not sufficient to induce a brain allograft rejection response.

After host sensitization with donor tissue, in some rat strain combinations, allografts show increased cellular density, as compared to sham-sensitized allografts. Nevertheless, T-cell infiltration is not detected within the allografted tissue. In these cases, the infiltrating cells consisted primarily of activated microglial cells and blood-derived macrophages (39). These data support the hypothesis that even with systemic sensitization some CNS allografts do not induce T cell-mediated immune rejection responses. This form of reaction is mediated primarily by microglial cells and macrophages. Such immune responses are generally not sufficient, however, to produce complete graft destruction. This category of response correlates with a relative absence of host lymphocyte activation.

Thus, it seems that there are two types of immune response to CNS tissue allografts. In one, the lymphocyte-mediated response, the presence of an infiltration of cytotoxic lymphocytes is obvious. Graft rejection is very efficient. For CNS allografts this type of immune response is not usually seen under normal conditions, that is, without additional systemic sensitization. The second, more frequently seen type, can be called the *macrophage/microglia-mediated response*. This response is characterized by the presence of microglia and blood-derived macrophages, with a relative lack of lymphocytes. This latter type of immune response is generally not sufficient to actually destroy the graft.

MHC Disparity Between Donor and Host and Influence of the Implantation Site

Obviously, the most important factor predicting the rejection of peripheral grafts is MHC disparity between the donor and host. The circumstances are more complicated in the case of brain allografts, and there are many conflicting data. While not universally acknowledged, it appears that when there is a difference between the donor and host in only MHC class I or only MCH class II antigens, the rejection response is weak, whereas the combination of both a MHC class I and class II disparity produces a strong rejection response (16,27,28,54,60). A disparity between minor histocompatibility factors induces only a minimal rejection response (60). Nevertheless, the classical measures of genetic disparity between the donor and host are not always complete predictors of brain graft rejection, since for certain donor–host rat strain combinations, even with complete MHC and minor histocompatibility mismatches, rejection is not observed. On the other hand, the intensity of MLR and GvHD responses may be a better prognosis of the graft rejection response. Immunogenicity of the donor tissue and the host predisposition to immune rejection also have a major influence on the rejection response.

There is some evidence that estrogens are involved in the mechanism of the immune response. Many years ago, it was been found that female rats reject skin grafts more readily than do males of the same strain. Moreover, females may reject skin grafts from males within the same inbred strain of animals (11,31,42). The available studies on brain grafting do not yet address this issue.

It is likely that the specific location of implanted neuronal tissue influences the immunological response. One of the first studies (57) suggested that grafts placed within the brain parenchyma survived better than those placed within the ventricular system. After this initial report there were no further attempts to study the issue in more detail. Recently, Sloan et al. (88) directly compared the survival of neonatal cortex grafts transplanted to the brain parenchyma, lateral ventricle, and third ventricle of adult rats. These authors suggested that the ventricular placement of allografts induced more MHC class I and leukocyte common–antigen positive cell infiltrations, than when allografts were implanted within the brain parenchyma. It has also been shown that MHC class I expression on grafts placed in the third ventricle is much greater than similar grafts in the lateral ventricle, even for comparisons within a single animal (71). On the other hand, many studies in animals have successfully used an intraventricular approach and have demonstrated excellent survival of neuronal as well as non-neuronal allografts. Theoretically, the immune response could be influenced by MHC class II+ macrophages present within the choroid plexus and pial membranes and on ependymal cells (9,34). Up-regulation of MHC class II expression has been shown on the supraependymal cells after neuronal transplantation (70). The very low numbers of these macrophages normally present in the ventricular system casts some doubt over whether their presence conveys any functional immunological impact. There are numerous factors related to the specifics of various CNS transplantation sites (see Fig. 16-3), and other possibilities should also be taken into account.

Active Immunosuppression

The favorable rate of graft survival within the brain, the basis for which is unclear, has provoked many explanatory hypotheses. One of these is the concept of the presence within the brain of local immunosuppression. Generally, the phenomenon of active immunosuppression is connected with immunological tolerance. Some time ago, it was suggested that the brain environment contains or produces immunosuppressive factors. Recent trends hint at locally released cytokines such as TGF-β. This hypothesis has still not been elaborated in detail.

Another explanation for the properties of the brain as a favorable site for transplantation is the suggestion that the introduction of antigens via the intravascular route favors the development of tolerance rather than sensitization (92). It has been suggested that this is due to aberrant presentation of graft antigens to the host immune system. It has been advocated that CNS grafts, through sensitization restricted to vascular routes, induce

Forms of CNS Grafts

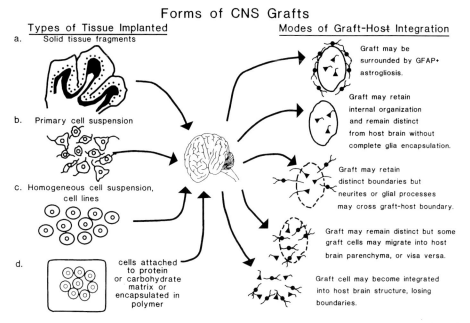

Types of Tissue Implanted

a. Solid tissue fragments

b. Primary cell suspension

c. Homogeneous cell suspension, cell lines

d. cells attached to protein or carbohydrate matrix or encapsulated in polymer

Modes of Graft-Host Integration

Graft may be surrounded by GFAP+ astrogliosis.

Graft may retain internal organization and remain distinct from host brain without complete glia encapsulation.

Graft may retain distinct boundaries but neurites or glial processes may cross graft-host boundary.

Graft may remain distinct but some graft cells may migrate into host brain parenchyma, or visa versa.

Graft cell may become integrated into host brain structure, losing boundaries.

Fig. 16-3. There are several forms of CNS grafts, each differing in the form in which the tissue is transplanted and in the mode of the graft–host interrelationship. In practical terms, there are four forms in which tissue may be implanted. For example, in studies of transplanted fetal tissue, attention is largely focused on the neuronal population, although several cell types are present in these grafts.

After transplantation there are several distinct forms of graft–host integration that may be observed. The mode of host–graft intergration may vary, depending on the graft type as well as other factors, including the development of an immune response, age of donor, and location within the host brain. In some cases, grafts may be almost entirely isolated from the host brain parenchyma by a barrier of glial processes, while in other cases, it may not be possible to precisely define graft–host boundaries because of migration of cells from graft to host and vice versa, and because of the crossing of the graft–host boundary by cellular processes. Both the type of graft and the form of graft–host integration are factors that influence the form and development of immune responses.

proliferation of suppressor T cells in the spleen, and that these suppressor cells produce an active immune response that is protective rather than destructive. Most of these data were obtained after transplantation of cell lines into the anterior chamber of eye and so far have not yet been extended to intracerebral neural tissue transplantation (also Chapter 17).

Xenotransplantation

Intracerebral grafting is no longer entirely an experimental procedure. At least several hundred transplantations have been performed on humans. The difficulties in obtaining

Different Forms of Cellular Infiltration into CNS Grafts

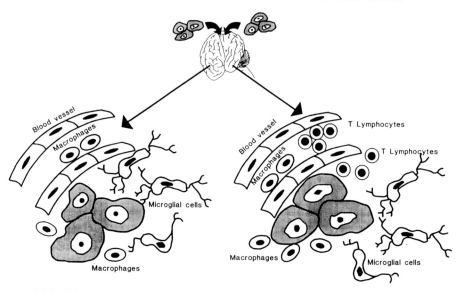

Fig. 16-4. After allogenic neural transplantation, two major forms of cellular infiltration into the graft may be observed. One consists of microglial cells and blood-derived macrophage infiltrations. These reactions are presumably mediated primarily by cytokines. In the second form of infiltration, in addition to the influx of blood-derived macrophages and microglial cells, large numbers of blood-derived T lymphocytes, including both T-helper and cytotoxic cells, are present. This type of infiltration, a classic rejection response, ultimately results in complete graft destruction in virtually all cases.

human embryonic tissue, ethical problems, and other limitations have attracted attention to other tissue possibilities, including cross-species grafting or the use of various types of substitute cells. Generally, the mechanisms of immunological rejection response after allotransplantation appear to be different than those involved in xenotransplantation. For most species combinations, the major barrier for successful peripheral xenotransplantation seems to be the existence of naturally occurring preformed antibodies. Both IgM and IgG classes of immunoglobulin are represented, and there is no agreement whether IgM or IgG is prevalent. Although the antigen targets for these antibodies have not yet been completely identified, they are primarily membranes of endothelial cells. These antibodies induce hyperacute rejection of vascularized organs by induction of platelet aggregation and an increase in thromboxanes with all its consequences. Moreover, complement activation occurs, which potentiates destruction of transplanted xenogenic cells. Plasmapheresis and ex vivo xenoantibody absorption can increase survival time.

As compared to vascularised peripheral xenografts, survival of intracerebral xenografts is sometimes observed. Depending on the model of transplantation used the results vary, from complete xenograft destruction to survival rates of close to 90%. It is well established that the survival rate for intracerebral xenografts is lower than for allografts, and that the survival rate can be increased by immunosuppression. Nevertheless, many researchers have reported quite good xenograft survival without immunosuppressive treatment. A relative resistance of xenografts to rejection seems to occur primarily with small intraparenchymal neural xenografts. In contrast, relatively strong rejection reactions may be observed against intraventricular xenografts. This phenomenon may be due in part to the presence of predominantly host-derived vasculature in intraparenchymal neuronal grafts as compared to mainly donor-derived endothelial cells in the intraventricular xenografts, as discussed above. Recently, it has been shown that systemic removal of host CD4+ lymphocytes increase the survival of xenografts. Neural xenograft survival can also be increased by treatment with MHC class I antibodies (64b). Nevertheless, it appears that even with immunosuppressive treatment, the survival rate of neuronal xenografts is low and unpredictable. In view of the shortage of human embryonic neural tissue, xenotransplantation would seem to be an obvious and desirable choice. Given the current level of knowledge about the issue, however, clinical CNS xenotransplantation procedures should be approached with great caution.

Immunosuppression for Brain Grafting

It can be concluded that intracerebral allografts, and especially xenografts under certain conditions, can induce a rejection response. The factors that predict rejection, as compared to survival, are not entirely understood. Immunosuppressive treatment decreases the immune rejection response. Many studies have employed cyclosporin A to improve both intracerebral xenograft and allograft survival (14,17,18). The effectiveness of treatment varies depending on the transplantation model. In peripheral transplantation, cyclosporin A must usually be administered continuously, throughout the entire life of the host. Cyclosporin A, although highly lipophylic, does not penetrate easily into the brain tissue unless the BBB is compromised (6). In practical terms, this means that cyclosporin A must produce its immunosuppressive effect mainly in the periphery. In the case of neural tissue allografts, the BBB is compromised primarily during the first few weeks, and it becomes intact thereafter. It is thus possible, especially in view of relatively good survival of CNS allografts, that immunosuppression can be reduced after an initial short period of treatment. Moreover, it is tempting to speculate that the reduction of immunosuppression might allow the induction of specific host immunosuppression phenomena to occur. Cyclosporin A could be initiated again in the event of a recurrent rejection phase and additional breakdown of the BBB. This type of immunosuppression regime has already been applied for human patients following transplantation of embryonic human substantia nigra for the treatment of Parkinson's disease (90).

Another approach to immunosuppression is the application of blocking antibodies against various immunocompetent cells. The interaction of different antibodies with MHC antigens and lymphocyte populations could influence the outcome of transplantation. The issue is complex. In peripheral systems, it has been postulated that, by using monoclonal antibodies, the depletion of antigen-presenting cells expressing MHC class II molecules may prevent rejection of grafts, although the results of such studies have been variable (74). Systemic depletion of cytotoxic lymphocytes does not enhance brain allograft survival. In contrast, removal of T helper cells with monoclonal antibodies alone or antibodies conjugated with toxins can increase the survival of neural tissue allografts (62). Antibodies against the IL-2 receptors are used to prevent allograft rejection in the periphery (43). Recent trials have been completed with antibodies against the IL-2 receptors after intracerebral transplantation (89).

Neuronal allografts can induce an immune rejection response. It is not yet possible, however, to predict whether rejection will occur for any specific donor-host combination or graft type. Although certain immunological laws apply—for instance, increased MHC disparity between donor and host increases the probability that a reaction will occur—these "laws" are not absolute, since several other factors significantly influence intracerebral neural allografting. The use of some form of immunosuppression in human allotransplantation, at least for a limited period of time, would seem to be an essential precautionary measure.

Summary and Conclusions

The brain is a relatively, but not entirely, immunologically privileged site for neuronal transplantation. It is probable that several properties of brain tissue are implicated in enhanced CNS graft survival. The CNS possesses a BBB and limited lymphatic drainage, and brain tissue expresses low levels of MHC class I antigens and lacks APCs. Nevertheless, allogenic neuronal tissue implanted to the host brain can induce a specific immune rejection response. The BBB is not an impenetrable obstacle for immunocompetent cells, since activated lymphocytes readily cross the barrier. Protection from a rejection response by an intact BBB is also not absolute. Tissue implantation always induces BBB damage, at least for a short period of time. Although the brain has a relative absence of afferent lymphatics, foreign antigens can and do migrate to the peripheral cervical lymphoid nodes initiating or amplifying immune rejection responses. Moreover, after transplantation, allogenic neural tissue may start to up-regulate the expression of donor MHC class I antigens.

Under these circumstances, all of the conditions required for graft rejection may be functional. Thus, grafted tissue can then be recognized as foreign by effector cells and it becomes a direct target for host cytotoxic lymphocytes. Neuronal allografts are invaded by blood-derived MHC class II+ cells. Microglia of the host brain tissue surround the implants and the allografts themselves demonstrate up-regulation of MHC class II antigen synthesis. These cells act as facultative APCs. Foreign antigens, therefore, can be presented by both blood-derived macrophages and activated microglia to T helper cells. As a consequence, an immune reaction against allografted tissue takes place. The question, therefore, is, why these immune reactions do not invariably culminate in CNS graft destruction?

It is possible that there are multiple mechanisms of immune responses to CNS grafts. One form features limited T-cell infiltration into the grafted tissue and a predominance of blood-derived macrophages and activated microglial cells. This type of response is probably mediated primarily by microglial and macrophage cytokines. However, this immune response is usually not efficient and does not produce complete graft destruction. Immune responses that result in vigorous allograft rejection are mediated by T-cell populations. In addition to microglial and macrophage infiltrations, in these cases, a massive influx of T cells consisting of both helper and cytotoxic lymphocytes is present and allograft destruction is virtually complete.

It might be suggested that the immune rejection response against intracerebrally allografted tissue differs from that observed against peripheral transplants only by the speed of appearance and the rate of progress of the immune response. On the other hand, there is much well-documented data suggesting prolonged survival of allogenic neural tissue without a detectable rejection response. The reasons for enhanced graft survival within the host brain are still unclear. Some attractive hypotheses explaining this phenomenon by local or systemic immunosuppression are not yet confirmed. It is possible that, if events required to stimulate CNS graft rejection do not take place during the early post-transplantation period while nonspecific activation of MHC expression and BBB leakiness are seen, then CNS allografts will survive indefinitely.

In conclusion, the immune response to grafted neuronal tissue within the CNS depends on many known and unknown factors. The well-established major contributors include: immunogenic disparity between host and donor; donor tissue origin and its immunogenecity; host susceptibility to immune reactions; host brain tissue damage during the transplantation procedure; degree of impairment of the BBB; and, at least in some circumstances, active systemic suppressor responses. At the current level of knowledge, the occurrence of an immune rejection response against implanted neural allogenic tissue seems to be unpredictable, but sometimes it does occur. Therefore, some form of immunosuppressive treatment after intracerebral allotransplantation in human patients is advised.

Acknowledgments

We are grateful to Eleanor H. Cannon-Spoor for editing the manuscript.

Opinions expressed herein are the views of the authors and do not necessarily reflect the offical position of the National Institute of Mental Health or any other part of the United States Department of Mental Health and Human Services.

References

1. Backes MG, Lund RD, Lagenaur CF, Kunz HW, Gill TJ III. Cellular events associated with peripherally induced rejection of mature neural xenografts placed into neonatal rat brains. J Comp Neurol 295:428–437, 1990.
2. Bar T. The vascular system of the cerebral cortex. Adv Anat Embryol Cell Biol 59:1–62, 1980.
3. Barker CF, Billingham RE. Immunologically privileged sites. Adv Immunol 25:1–54, 1977.
4. Bartlett PF, Kerr RSC, Bailey KA. Expression of MHC antigens in the central nervous system. Transplant Proc 21:3163–3165, 1989.
5. Bartlett PF, Rosenfeld J, Bailey KA, Cheesman H, Harvey AR, Kerr RSC. Allograft rejection overcome by immunoselection of neuronal precursor cells. In: Neural Transplantation: from Molecular Basis to Clinical Applications, SB Dunnett, SJ Richards, eds. Elsevier, Amsterdam. Prog Brain Res 82:153–160, 1990.
6. Begley DJ, Squires LK, Zlokovic BV, Mitrovic DM, Hughes CCW, Revest PA, Greenwood J. Permeability of the blood-brain barrier to the immunosuppressive cyclic peptide cyclosporin A. J Neurochem 55:1222–1230, 1990.
7. Bellgrau D, Smilek D, Wilson DB. Induced tolerance in F1 rats to anti-major histocompatibility complex receptors on parietal T cells. J Exp Med 153:1660–1665, 1981.
8. Bjorklund A, Stenevi U. Intracerebral neural grafting: a historical perspective. In: Neural grafting in the Mammalian CNS, A Bjorklund, U Stenevi, eds. Elsevier, Amsterdam, 1985, pp 3–14.
9. Bleir R, Albrecht R. Supraependymal macrophages of third ventricle of hamster: morphological, functional and histochemical characterization in situ and in culture. J Comp Neurol 192:489–504, 1980.
10. Bradbury MWB, Cserr HF, Westrop RJ. Drainage of cerebral interstitial fluid into deep cervical lymph of the rabbit. Am J Physiol 240:F329–F336, 1981.
11. Brent L, Medawar P. Quantitative studies on tissue transplantation immunity: VII. The effect of irradiation. Proc R Soc Lond (Biol) 165:413–424, 1966.
12. Broadwell RD, Charlton HM, Ebert PS, Hickey WF, Shirazi Y, Villegas J, Wolf AL. Allografts of CNS tissue possess a blood-brain barrier. II. Angiogenesis in solid tissue and cell suspension grafts. Exp Neurol 112:1–28, 1991.
13. Broadwell RD, Charlton HM, Ganong WF, Salcman M, Sofroniew M. Allografts of CNS tissue possess a blood-brain barrier. I. Grafts of medial preoptic area in hypogonadal mice. Exp Neurol 105:131–151, 1989.
14. Brundin P, Nilsson OG, Gage FH, Bjorklund A. Cyclosporin A increases survival of cross-species intrastriatal grafts of embryonic dopamine-containing neurons. Exp Brain Res 60:204–208, 1985.
15. Casey-Smith JR, Foldi-Borcsok E, Foldi M. The prelymphatic pathways of the brain as revealed by cervical lymphatic obstruction and the passage of particles. Br J Exp Pathol 57:179–188, 1976.
16. Date I, Kawamura K, Nakashima H. Histological signs of immune reactions against allogeneic solid fetal neural grafts in the mouse cerebellum depend on the MHC locus. Exp Brain Res 73:15–22, 1988.
17. Finsen B, Poulsen PH, Zimmer J. Xenografting of fetal mouse hippocampal tissue to the brain of adult rats: effects of cyclosporin A treatment. Exp Brain Res 70:117–133, 1988.
18. Finsen BR, Pedersen EB, Sorensen T, Hokland M, Zimmer J. Immune reactions against intracerebral murine xenografts of fetal hippocampal tissue and cultured cortical astrocytes

in the adult rat. In: Neural Transplantation: from Molecular Basis to Clinical Applications, SB Dunnett, SJ Richards, eds. Elsevier, Amsterdam, Prog Brain Res 82:111–128, 1990.

19. Fontana A, Fierz W, Wekerle H. Astrocytes present myelin basic protein to encephalitogenic T-cell lines. Nature 307:273–276, 1984.

20. Freed WJ. Functional brain tissue transplantation: reversal of lesion-induced rotation by intraventricular substantia nigra and adrenal medulla grafts, with a note on intracranial retinal grafts. Biol Psychiatry 18:1205–1267, 1983.

21. Freed WJ. Substantia nigra grafts and Parkinson's disease: from animal experiments to human therapeutic trials. Rest Neurol Neurosci 3:109–134, 1991.

22. Freed WJ. Neural transplantation: prospects for clinical use. Cell Transplant 2:13–31, 1993.

23. Freed WJ, Dymecki J, Poltorak M, Rodgers CR. Intraventricular brain allografts and xenografts: studies of survival and rejection with and without systemic sensitization. In: Transplantation in the Mammalian CNS, DM Gash, JR Sladek Jr, eds. Elsevier, Amsterdam. Prog Brain Res 78:233–241, 1988.

24. Freed WJ, Poltorak M, Becker J. Intracerebral adrenal medulla grafts: a review. Exp Neurol 110:139–166, 1990.

25. Frei K, Bodmer S, Schwerdel C, Fontana A. Astrocyte-derived interleukin-3 as a growth factor for microglial cells and peritoneal macrophages. J Immunol 137:3521–3527, 1986.

26. Gash DM. Neural transplants in mammals: a historical overview. In: Neural Transplants: Development and Function, JR Sladek Jr, DM Gash, eds. Plenum Press, New York, 1984, pp 1–12.

27. Geyer SJ, Gill TJ. Immunogenetic aspect of intracerebral skin transplantation in inbred rats. Am J Pathol 3:569–584, 1979.

28. Geyer SJ, Gill TJ, Kunz HW, Moody E. Immunogenetic aspect of transplantation in the rat brain. Transplantation 39:244–247, 1985.

29. Giulian D, Lachman LB. Interleukin-1 stimulates astroglial proliferation after brain injury. Science 228:497–499, 1985.

30. Graeber MB, Kreutzberg GW. Astrocytes increase in glial fibrillary acidic protein during retrograde changes of facial motor neurons. J Neurocytol 15:363–373, 1986.

31. Graff RJ, Lappe MA, Snell GD. The influence of the gonads and adrenal glands on the immune response to skin grafts. Transplantation 7:105–111, 1969.

32. Hart DNJ, Fabre JW. Demonstration and characterization of Ia positive dendritic cells in the interstitial connective tissues of rat heart and others tissues, but not brain. J Exp Med 153:347–361, 1981.

33. Haynes GM, Woodroofe MN, Cuzner ML. Microglia are the major cell type expressing MHC class II in human white matter. J Neurol Sci 80:25–37, 1987.

34. Head JR, Griffin WS. Functional capacity of solid tissue transplants in the brain: evidence for immunological privilege. Proc R Soc Lond (Biol) 224:375–387, 1985.

35. Hickey W, Kimura H. Graft-vs.-host disease elicits expression of class I and II histocompatibility antigens and the presence of scattered T lymphocytes in rat central nervous system. Proc Natl Acad Sci USA 84:2082–2086, 1987.

36. Hickey W, Kimura H. Perivascular microglial cells of the CNS are bone marrow-derived and present antigen in vivo. Science 239:290–292, 1988.

37. Hickey W, Hsu BL, Kimura H. T-lymphocyte entry into the central nervous system. J Neurosci Res 28:254–260, 1991.

38. Hirsch MR, Wietzerbin J, Pierres M, Goridis C. Expression of Ia antigens by cultured astrocytes treated with γ-interferon. Neurosci Lett 41:199–204, 1983.

39. Isono M, Poltorak M, Kulaga H, Adams A, Freed WJ. Certain host-donor rat strain

combinations do not reject brain allografts after systemic sensitization. Exp Neurol 122:48–56, 1993.

40. Janzer RC, Raff MC. Astrocytes induce blood-brain barrier properties in endothelial cells Nature 325:253–257, 1987.

41. Kaplan HJ, Stevens TR. A reconsideration of immunologic privilege within the anterior chamber of the eye. Transplantation 19:302–309, 1975.

42. Kongshavn PAL, Bliss JQ. Sex differences in survival of H-2 incompatible skin grafts in mice treated with antithymocyte serum. Nature 226:451, 1969.

43. Kupiec-Weglinski JW, Diamantstein T, Tilney NL, Strom TB. Therapy with monoclonal antibody to interleukin 2 receptor spares suppressor T cells and prevents or reverse acute allograft rejection in rats. Proc Natl Acad Sci USA, 83:2624–2627, 1986.

44. Lampson LA, Fisher CA. Weak HLA and β2-microglobulin expression of neuronal cell lines can be modulated by interferon. PNAS. 81:6476–6480, 1984.

45. Lampson LA, Hickey WF. Monoclonal antibody analysis of MHC expression in human brain biopsies: tissue ranging from "histologically normal" to that showing different levels of glial tumor involvement. J Immunol 136:4054–4062, 1986.

46. Lawrence JM, Huang SK, Raisman G. Vascular and astrocytic reactions during establishment of hippocampal transplants in adult brain. Neuroscience 3:745–760, 1984.

47. Lawrence JM, Morris RJ, Wilson DJ, Raisman G. Mechanisms of allograft rejection in the rat brain. Neuroscience 37:431–462, 1990.

48. Lindsay RM, Raisman G. An autoradiographic study of neural development, vascularization and glial cell migration from hippocampal transplants labelled in intermediate explant culture. Neuroscience 12:513–530, 1984.

49. Lublin FD, Marini JC, Perreault M, Olender C, D'Impero C, Joseph J, Korngold R, Knobler RL. Autoimmune inflammation of astrocyte transplants. Ann Neurol 31:519–524, 1992.

50. Lund RD, Rao K, Hankin MH, Kunz HW, Gill TJ III. Transplantation of retina and visual cortex to the rat brains of different ages: maturation, connection patterns, and immunological consequences. Ann NY Acad Sci 495:227–241, 1987.

51. Lund RD, Rao K, Kunz HW, Gill TJ III. Neural transplantation and the immune response. In: Neuroimmune Networks: Physiology and Diseases, EJ Goetzl, NH Spector, eds. Alan R. Liss, New York, 1989, pp 269–279.

52. Maehlen J, Schroder HD, Klareskog L, Olsson T, Kristensson K. Axotomy induces MHC class I antigen expression on rat nerve cells. Neurosci Lett 92:8–13, 1988.

53. Male DK, Pryce G, Hughes CCW. Antigen presentation in brain: MHC induction on brain endothelium and astrocytes compared. 60:453–459, 1987.

54. Mason DW, Charlton HM, Jones AJ, Lavy CB, Puklavec M, Simmonds SJ. The fate of allogenic and xenogenic neuronal tissue transplanted into third ventricle of rodents. Neuroscience 19:685–694, 1986.

55. McCarron R, Kempski O, Spatz M, McFarlin DE. Presentation of myelin basic protein by murine cerebral vascular endothelial cells. J Immunol 134:3100–3103, 1985.

56. Medawar PB. Immunity to homologous grafted skin. III. The fate of skin homografts transplanted to the brain, to subcutaneous tissue, and to anterior chamber of the eye. Br J Exp Pathol 29:58–69, 1948.

57. Murphy JB, Sturm E. Conditions determining the transplantability of tissue in the brain. J Exp Med 38:183–197, 1923.

58. Nakashima H, Kawamura K, Date I. Immunological reaction and blood-brain barrier in mouse-to-rat cross-species neural graft. Brain Res 475:232–243, 1988.

59. Nicholas MK, Antel JP, Stefansson K, Arnason BGW. An in vivo and in vitro analysis of

systemic immune function in mice with histologic evidence of neural transplant rejection. J Neurosci Res 18:245–257, 1987.

60. Nicholas MK, Arnason BGW. Immunologic considerations in transplantation to the central nervous system. In: Neural Regeneration and Transplantation, FJ Seil ed. Alan R. Liss, 1989, pp 239–284.

61. Nicholas MK, Arnason BGW. A role for CD8+ T lymphocytes late in the rejection of intraventricular fetal neocortical fragment allografts in the mouse. In: Pathophysiology of the blood-brain barrier, BB Johansson, CH Owman, H Widner, eds. Elsevier, Amsterdam, 1990, pp 573–586.

62. Nicholas MK, Chenelle AG, Brown MM, Stefansson K, Arnason BGW. Prevention of neural allograft rejection in the mouse following in vivo depletion of L3T4+ but not LYT-2+ T lymphocytes. In: Neural Transplantation: from Molecular Basis to Clinical Applications, SB Dunnett, SJ Richards, eds. Elsevier, Amsterdam. Prog Brain Res 82:161–167, 1990.

63. Nicholas MK, Sagher O, Hartley JP, Stefansson K, Arnason BGW. 1988. A phenotypic analysis of T lymphocytes isolated from the brains of mice with allogeneic neural transplants. In: Transplantation in the Mammalian CNS, DM Gash, JR Sladek Jr, eds. Elsevier, Amsterdam. Progr Brain Res 78:249–259, 1988.

64. Nicholas MK, Stefansson K, Antel JP, Arnason BGW. Rejection of fetal neocortical neural transplants by H-2 incompatible mice. J Immunol 139:2275–2283, 1987.

64b. Pakzaban P, Deacon TW, Burns LH, Dinsmore J, Isacson O. A novel mode of immunoprotection of neural xenotransplants: masking of donor major histocompatibility complex class I enhances transplant survival in the central nervous system. Neuroscience 65:983–996, 1995.

65. Perry VH, Gordon S. Macrophages and microglia in the nervous system. TINS 11:273–277, 1988.

66. Perry VH, Lund RD. Microglia in retinae transplanted to the central nervous system. Neuroscience 31:453–462, 1989.

67. Pollack I, Lee LHC, Zhou HF, Lund RD. Long-term survival of mouse corpus callosum grafts in neonatal rat recipients, and effect of host sensitization. J Neurosci Res 31:33–45, 1992.

68. Pollack I, Lund RD. The blood-brain-barrier protects foreign antigens in the brain from immune attack. Exp Neurol 198:114–121, 1990.

69. Pollack I, Lund RD. The MHC antigen expression in spontaneous and induced rejection of neural xenografts. In: Neural Transplantation: from Molecular Basis to Clinical Applications, SB Dunnett, SJ Richards, eds. Elsevier, Amsterdam. Prog Brain Res 82:129–140, 1990.

70. Poltorak M, Freed WJ. Immunological reactions induced by intracerebral transplantation: evidence that host microglia but not astroglia are the antigen-presenting cells. Exp Neurol 103:222–233, 1989.

71. Poltorak M, Freed WJ. BN rats do not reject F344 brain allografts even after systemic sensitization. Ann Neurol 29:377–388, 1991.

72. Poltorak M, Freed WJ, Sternberger LA, Sternberger NH. A comparison of intraventricular and intraparenchymal cerebellar allografts in rat brain: evidence for normal phosphorylation of neurofilaments. J Neuroimmunol 20:63–72, 1988.

73. Poltorak M, Isono M, Freed WJ, Ronnett GV, Snyder SH. Human cortical neuronal cell line (HCN-1): further in vitro characterization and suitability for brain transplantations. Cell Transplant 1:3–15, 1992.

74. Poltorak M, Logan S, Freed WJ. Intraventricular xenografts: chronic injection of antibodies into the CSF provokes granulomatosis reactions but Ia antibodies do not enhance graft survival. Reg Immunol 2:197–202, 1989.

75. Prineas JW. Multiple sclerosis: presence of lymphatic capillares and lympoid tissue in the brain and spinal cord. Science 203:1123–1125, 1979.

76. Raisman G, Lawrence JM, Zhou CF, Lindsay RM. Some neuronal, glial and vascular interactions which occur when developing hippocampal primordia are incorporated into adult host hippocampi. In: Neural grafting in the Mammalian CNS, A Bjorklund, U Stenevi, eds. Elsevier, Amsterdam, 1985, pp 125–150.

77. Raju S, Grogan JB. Immunologic study of the brain as a privileged site. Transplant Proc 9:1187–1191, 1977.

78. Reier PJ, Perlow MJ, Guth L. Development of embryonic spinal cord transplants in the rat. Dev Brain Res 10:2012–219, 1983.

79. Risau W, Engelhardt B, Wekerle H. Immune function of the blood-brain-barrier: incomplete presentation of protein (auto-) antigens by rat brain microvascular endothelium in vitro. J Cell Biol 110:1727–1766, 1990.

80. Risau W, Gautschi-Sova P, Bohlen P. Endothelial cell growth factors in embryonic and adult chick brain are related to human acidic fibroblast growth factors. EMBO J 7:959–962, 1988.

81. Robertson, PL, Du Bois M, Bowman PD, Goldstein GW. Angiogenesis in developing rat brain: an in vivo and in vitro study. Dev Brain Res 23:219–223, 1985.

82. Ronnett GV, Hester LD, Nye JS, Connors K, Snyder SH. Human cortical neuronal cell line: establishment from a patient with uniteral megalencephaly. Science 248:603–605, 1990.

83. Rosenstein JM. Neocortical transplants in the mammalian brain lack blood-brain barrier to macromolecules. Science 235:772–774, 1987.

84. Rosenstein JM, Krum JM, Trapp BD. The astroglial response to autonomic tissue grafts. Brain Res 476:110–119, 1989.

85. Schachner M, Sidman RL. Distribution of H-2 allogen in adult and developing mouse brain. Brain Res 60:191–198, 1973.

86. Scheinberg LC, Kotsilimbas DG, Karpf R, Mayer N. Is the brain an "immunologically privileged site"?. Arch Neurol 15:62–67, 1966.

87. Seiger A, Olson L. Quantification of fiber outgrowth in transplanted central monoamine neurons. Cell Tissue Res 179:285–316, 1977.

88. Sloan DJ, Baker BJ, Puklavec M, Charlton HM. The effect of site of transplantation and histocompatibility differences on the survival of neural tissue transplanted to the CNS of defined inbred rat strains. In: Neural Transplantation: from Molecular Basis to Clinical Applications, SB Dunnett, SJ Richards eds. Prog Brain Res 82:141–152, 1990.

89. Sloan DJ, Wood MJ, Charlton HM. The immune response to intracerebral neural grafts. TINS 14:341–346, 1991.

90. Spencer DD, Robbins RJ, Naftolin F, Marek KL, Vollmer T, Leranth C, Roth RH, Price LH, Gjedde A, Bunney BS, Sass KJ, Elsworth JD, Kier EL, Makuch R, Hoffer PB, Redmond DE. Unilateral transplantation of human fetal mesencephlic tissue into the caudate nucleus of patients with Parkinson's disease. N Eng J Med 327:1541–1548, 1992.

91. Sporn, MB, Roberts AB, Wakefield LD, de Crombrugghe B. Some recent advances in the chemistry and biology of transforming growth factor-β. J Cell Biol 105:1039–1045, 1987.

92. Streilein JW, Niederkorn JY, Shadduck JA. Systemic immune unresponsiveness induced in adult mice by anterior chamber presentation of minor histocompatibility antigens. J Exp Med 152:1121–1125, 1987.

93. Streit WJ, Graeber MB, Kreutzberg GW. Expression of Ia antigen on perivascular and microglial cells after sublethal and lethal motor neuron injury. Exp Neurol 105:115–126, 1989.

94. Traugott U. Multiple sclerosis: relevance of class I and class II MHC-expressing cells to lesion development. J Neuroimmunol 16:283–302, 1987.
95. Traugott U, Raine CS, McFarlin DE. Acute experimental allergic encephalomyelitis in the mouse: immunopathology of the developing lesion. Cell Immunol 91:240–254, 1985.
96. Wekerle H, Linington C, Lassmann H, Meyermann R. Cellular immune reactivity within the CNS. TINS 9:271–277, 1986.
97. Whitaker-Azmitia PM, Ramirez A, Noreika L, Gannon PJ, Azmitia EC. Onset and duration of astrocytic response to cells transplanted into adult mammalian brain, Ann NY Acad Sci 495:10–23, 1987.
98. Widner H, Brundin P. Immunological aspects of grafting in the mammalian central nervous system. A review and speculative synthesis. Brain Res Rev 13:287–324, 1988.
99. Widner H, Brundin P, Bjorklund A, Moller G. Survival and immunogenecity of dissociated allogenic fetal neral dopamine-rich grafts when implanted into the brains of adult mice. Exp Brain Res 76:187–197, 1989.
100. Widner H, Johansson BB, Moller G. Quantitative demonstration of a link between brain parenchyma and the lymphatic system after intracerebral antigen deposition. J Cereb Blood Flow Metab 5:88–89, 1985.
101. Widner H, Moller G, Johansson BB. Immune response in deep cervical lymphnodes and spleen in the mouse after antigen deposition in different intracerebral sites. Scand J Immunol 28:563–571, 1988.
102. Wong GH, Bartlett PF, Clark-Lewis I, Battye F, Schrader JW. Inducible expression of H-2 and Ia antigens on brain cells. Nature 310:688–691, 1984.
103. Zalewski AA, Goshgarian HG, Silvers WK. The fate of neurons and neurilemmal cells in allografts of ganglia in the spinal cord of normal and immunologically tolerant rats. Exp Neurol 59:322–330, 1978.
104. Zhou CF, Lawrence JM, Morris RJ, Raisman G. Migration of host astrocytes into superior cervical sympathetic ganglia autografted into the septal nuclei or choroid fissure of adult rats. Neuroscience 17:815–827, 1986.

17

Immunosuppression: CNS Effects

ROBERT W. KEANE

Substantial evidence has accumulated that immune protection against pathogens in immune-privileged sites is accomplished with a minimum of inflammation. For many years immune privilege was considered a passive process by which foreign antigens were sequestered in sites beyond the capacity of the immune system to recognize them. As extensively outlined in Chapter 3, experimental analysis of this process, particularly in the eye, has not supported the "sequestration" hypothesis, but instead offers a contemporary view that immune privilege is a physiological process in which the immune system is adapted so that active, specific, and selective regulation permits the privileged tissue to survive, even if immune effectors are present (131,132). While certain types of immune effector cells can function within the central nervous system (CNS), other types appear to be profoundly suppressed. Moreover, immunity generated in response to antigens placed in the brain is unusual, and shows enhanced serum antibody response and suppression of delayed type hypersensitivity (DTH) that do not characteristically occur in response to antigens introduced at conventional body sites (36,63,71). These alterations in immune effector modalities by antigenic challenge in the CNS undoubtedly make an important contribution to the phenomenon of immune privilege, and may account, at least in part, for the survival of grafted material. The multifactorial strategies employed by the CNS to suppress immune responses appropriate to its physiological functions and the mechanisms gone awry in CNS diseases will be discussed in this chapter.

Suppression of the Afferent Limb of the Immune Response: Immunization via the CNS

Most analyses of immune responses following administration of antigenic materials into the CNS failed to preserve the blood-brain barrier integrity through the acute insertion into brain tissues of needles or cannulas used to deliver the antigen. The systemic immune responses elicited by antigenic materials introduced into the CNS by these techniques produced variable conclusions and interpretations. Cserr and co-workers (36,63,71) have designed experimental conditions by which cannulae are inserted into the lateral ventricles of the brain 7 days prior to antigen administration to provide time for recovery of the blood-brain barrier, and resolution of edema associated with brain surgery. Studies employing these methods have shown that antigens gain access to the systemic circulation and extracerebral immune organs and that the afferent connection from the CNS to the immune system is intact (36,63,71). Antigen may drain with cerebrospinal fluid (CSF) to regional lymph nodes via passage along certain cranial nerves and spinal roots. Alternatively, antigen may travel to the spleen following drainage across the arachnoid villi to blood (13). These studies show that the connection from the brain to the draining nodes is substantial, and they suggest that the route that an antigen travels along CSF outflow pathways may dramatically influence the systemic immune response. For a more complete discussion of this topic, the reader is referred to Chapter 4.

Specific systemic immune responses elicited by microinjection of soluble antigens into the brain or CSF in animals with normal blood-brain barrier function are antigen-specific suppression of DTH reactions and enhanced serum antibodies (36,63,71). These characteristic immunological responses to antigens injected into brain are similar to those described for anterior chamber–associated immune deviation (ACAID), a well-characterized systemic immunological response elicited by antigens placed in the anterior chamber of the eye (131). However, the two systems differ in that the ACAID response also includes suppression of production of complement-fixing antibodies (132). Collectively, these studies demonstrate a mechanism in the brain and eye that is capable of suppressing the cell-mediated immune response (DTH), but the mechanisms employed by the two compartments may not be identical.

Local Immunosuppression Within the CNS and the Efferent Limb of the Immune Response

Biological Fluids of Immune-Privileged Sites

One strategy employed in immune-privileged sites to suppress immune reactivity is the creation of a local immunosuppressive microenvironment. This inhibitory milieu appears to be contributed in part by immunosuppressive cytokines and substances present in biological fluids that bathe these sites. Immunosuppressive actions have been reported for CSF (brain), aqueous humor (eye) and amniotic fluid (fetal placental unit)—three fluids from immune privileged sites (147). Transforming growth factor-β (TGF-β) (34,132,147), neuropeptides (α-melanocyte-stimulating hormone [134]), vasoactive intestinal peptide (135), calcitonin gene-related peptide (132), and substances of different molecular size (66) have been found in these fluids, and all of these substances have been reported to have immunosuppressive activity. CSF, aqueous humor, and amniotic fluid were analyzed for the capacity to influence the functional properties of T lymphocytes and antigen-presenting cells (154). F 4/80+ peritoneal macrophages were treated overnight with these fluid samples. When peritoneal macrophages were isolated from these cultures and injected intravenously into syngeneic, naive recipients, animals were less effective in displaying antigen-specific DTH than animals injected with peritoneal macrophages that were treated with normal mouse serum or rat thoracic duct lymph (154). Therefore, it has been suggested that these fluids share a similar capacity to alter the functional programs of antigen-presenting cells that leads to suppression of cell-mediated immunity (132,154).

TGF-β can mimic some of the immunosuppressive properties of CSF and aqueous humor, such as the inhibition of antigen- and mitogen-driven T-cell activation, but it spares other important functional properties of T cells (34,132). Peritoneal macrophages treated with antigen and TGF-β are unable to carry out antigen-specific DTH, but this inhibition is removed by neutralizing antibodies against TGF-β. Thus, microenvironments of the brain and eye appear to suppress the efferent limb of the immune response. This suppression may be regulated in part by TGF-β.

Production of Transforming Growth Factor-β within the CNS

The family of TGF-β at present comprises five distinct, yet highly homologous isoforms (8,116). TGF-β1, -β2, and -β3 are found in mammals, whereas TGF-β4 is present in avian species and TGF-β5 is present in amphibians. TGF-β isoforms seems to differ in selective expression, regulation, and biological functions (8,116). The most common reported cellular and humoral effects of TGF-β is inhibitory (8,116).

Until recently, it was not clear whether TGF-β was present in neural tissues, since immunocytochemical studies had demonstrated that TGF-β1 was absent from the CNS and confined to meninges (73,144). With the development of more selective, diagnostic tools, a more refined level of expression and distribution of TGF-β has been reported for the adult rat CNS (141) and glial cells in culture (31,38,39,104,123,158). In the rat brain, TGF-β2 and -β3 was found in large multipolar neurons present in spinal cord, brain stem motor nuclei, hypothalamus, amygdaloid complex, hippocampus, and cerebral cortical layers II, III, and V (141). TGF-β2 and -β3 immunoreactivity entirely overlapped. Most thalamic nuclei, superior colliculi, periaqueductal gray matter and striatum were almost devoid of TGF-β2 and -β3. TGF-β1-like immunoreactivity was confined to the meninges and choroid plexus (141). TGF-β has been reported in fibrous astrocytes and neurons in vivo by electron microscopic examination of immunostained material (141), but this cellular localization has not been verified by the use of cell-type-specific markers for CNS cells. TGF-β receptor type I is expressed in the sensory retina and in the marginal zone of the brain (81a).

As outlined in Chapter 11, there is controversy as to the TGF-β isoform expressed by glial cells in culture. Fontana and co-workers report that astrocytes secrete TGF-β2, while microglia secrete TGF-β1 (31). At the mRNA level, astrocytes express TGF-β1, -β2, and -β3, while microglia harbor only detectable levels of TGF-β1 mRNA (31). Other laboratories (38,39,104,144) report that unstimulated rat astrocytes produce undetectable levels of TGF-β, but can be induced to produce TGF-β1 by treatment with exogenous TGF-β1 (144) or stimulation by IL-1 (39). When appropriately stimulated by IL-1α, both primary rat oligodendrocytes and microglia can secrete TGF-β1 (39). TGF-β1 is chemotactic for astrocytes in a dose-dependent fashion (104) and inhibits astrocyte proliferation (104). Both TGF-β1 and -β2 suppress IFN-γ-induced class II major histocompatibility complex (MHC) expression on both human astroglioma cells and rat astrocytes (123,158). Astrocytes appear to express three distinct subtypes of TGF-β receptors with nearly 10,000 receptors per cell (104), suggesting a signal transduction pathway for TGF-β1. In summary, astrocytes, microglia, and oligodendrocytes are capable of producing TGF-β, but they differ in the isoforms that they express. Furthermore, the cellular source(s) of TGF-β in fluids from immune-privileged sites has not been identified.

As discussed in Chapters 3 and 18, the parenchymal cells of the iris and ciliary body produce TGF-β that suppresses proliferation of T cells (34,132). Moreover, Müller cells (retinal glial cells) have been shown to inhibit lymphoproliferative responses, but this differs from the suppression induced by iris or ciliary cells in that Müller cell inhibition is cell-contact dependent (25,115), and involves reduction of IL-2R expression and IL-2 production by T helper (Th) cells (25). The Müller cell inhibitory substance is a membrane-bound protein and is not related to products of the arachidonic acid metabolic pathway or TGF-β (25).

TGF-β in Immunosuppression of Neurological Disease

Treatment and management of autoimmune demyelinating CNS disease is still a clinical challenge. Immunosuppressive and anti-inflammatory substances are only of limited value and have serious side effects. An alternative approach has been the use of cytokines that suppress inflammation. Since a number of autoimmune disease show periodic exacerbations and remissions, it is possible that abnormal cyclical patterns of immune regulatory cytokines provide the basis for the initiation and subsequent relapsing nature of the disease (9,75,138,145,146,155).

In vivo administration of TGF-β into experimental autoimmune encephalomyelitis (EAE) mice has been shown to be successful in reducing the incidence of clinical disease and the histologic severity of inflammation and demyelination in the brain and spinal cord (84,95,111). However, Weinberg and co-workers (153) have shown that TGF-β administration in EAE may have a biphasic response, with lower dosages enhancing disease and higher dosages inhibiting disease potential. In these studies, it is suggested that TGF-β may promote the development of the helper memory lymphocyte phenotype in vitro and enhance T-cell effector function upon adoptive transfer in vivo in EAE disease (153).

TGF-β has been observed in neuritic plaques of Alzheimer's disease (141a), and identified in brain tissues of AIDS patients (144). In AIDS patients TGF-β was localized to astrocytes and not limited to HIV-positive cells; primary macrophages infected by HIV in vitro were also shown to increase their expression of TGF-β, which triggered the release of TGF-β from cultured astrocytes that were not infected with HIV. TGF-β may recruit HIV-infected cells into the CNS, enabling viral spread and augmenting cytokine production from astrocytes, which can cause neuronal damage. In support of this idea is the report that neuronotoxicity associated with HIV–CNS disease is mediated in part through cytokines and arachidonic acid metabolites produced during cell-to-cell interactions between HIV-infected brain macrophages and uninfected astrocytes (60). For a more detailed discussion of cytokines in HIV neurological disease, see Chapter 20.

The aberrant expression of TGF-β associated with neuropathological conditions of the CNS suggests a vital role of TGF-β in the response to trauma in the CNS. Supporting this idea is the observation that TGF-β_1 mRNA is upregulated in activated astrocytes at the site of injury and in reactive microglia in the zones of neural degeneration (99a,103a). TGF-β has been reported to have beneficial effects on neuronal growth and survival (81b,93a). TGF-β has been reported to have beneficial effects on neuronal growth and survival (81b,93a), while also promoting destructive processes such as neuronal apoptosis (41a). Thus, the multifunctional functions provided by TGF-β indicate an essential role of this cytokine in development and maintenance of neurons and glia in the CNS and in the disease process.

Fas-FasL Pathway

Recent observations have determined that potentially injurious immune reactions in immunologically privileged sites may be prevented by functionally inactivating the responding lymphocytes or by inducing apoptotic cell death (9a,68a). The primary cytolytic mechanism governing lymphocyte apoptosis is triggered by an interaction of Fas (CD95) with its ligand (FasL). Fas antigen is constitutively expressed on a wide variety of cell types or is induced after activation. Conversely, FasL has limited tissue distribution, but is rapidly induced on T-lymphocytes following their activation by antigen. In a recent report, Fas and FasL gene expression was analyzed during mouse development and in adult tissues (56a). Fas mRNA was detected in distinct cell types of the developing sinus, thymus, lung and liver, whereas FasL expression was restricted to submaxillary gland epithelial cells and the developing nervous system. In the adult mouse, RNase protection analysis showed expression of both Fas and FasL on several tissues including the thymus, lung, spleen, small intestine, large intestine, seminal vesicle, prostate, and uterus. Most of the tissues coexpressing Fas and FasL in the adult are characterized by apoptotic cell turnover, some of those tissues expressing FasL are known to be immune privileged.

With respect to the eye and testes, two immunologically privileged sites, it appears that immune privilege is maintained by elimination of its own potentially harmful cells by killing them via the Fas-FasL pathway (9a,68a). Griffith et al. (9a) report that Fas$^+$ lymphoma cells are triggered to undergo apoptosis when exposed to FasL$^+$ cells of the eye, but not from eyes of *gld* mice that do not express FasL. Thus FasL expression on cells of the eye equips the immunologically privileged site to remove by apoptosis Fas$^+$ T-cells that enter the eye. Moreover, lack of FasL expression at this site may interfere with immune privilege. Sertoli cells of the testis may serve a similar function in the testis to destroy Fas$^+$ T-cells that infiltrate this site (68a). It is intriguing that in addition to the eye and testis, other tissues, including the CNS, constitutively express FasL (56a). Whether immune privilege within these compartments is regulated by the Fas-FasL pathway will require further study to confirm this hypothesis.

Gliomas and Glioblastomas

Patients with primary intracranial tumors (gliomas) provide a naturally occurring suppression of host immunocompetence and offer an opportunity to examine neural–immune interactions in relation to tumor immunology (see 52,117 for reviews). Patients with gliomas demonstrate a broad suppression of humoral and cell-mediated immunity (3,16,18,100). Studies investigating impaired T-cell responsiveness to a variety of specific and nonspecific stimuli suggest that the cellular and biochemical dysfunction appears to be related to the production of immunosuppressive mediators by the glioma (19,20,33,52,117,127,156). Serum obtained from patients with these tumors is immunosuppressive when added to mitogen- or antigen-stimulated human lymphocytes (157), while surgical removal of the tumor partially ameliorates suppression (17). It is not clear whether this suppressive factor is directly or indirectly responsible for the immunosuppressed status observed in these patients.

Culture supernatants from cloned human glioblastoma cell lines inhibit IL-2-dependent T-cell proliferation (19,20,47,52,127), the formation of lymphokine-activated killer cells (LAK) and cytotoxic T cells (52), the generation of tumor-infiltrating activated lymphocytes (94), and mitogen- and antigen-dependent T-cell proliferation (19,20,54). Initial studies to isolate and characterize the suppressor factor(s) from culture supernatants of human glioblastoma cell lines have shown that the suppressor factor is a heat- and acid-stable 97-kDA protein, termed *glioblastoma-derived T-cell suppressor factor* (G-TSF) (19,156). G-TSF now appears to be identical to TGF-β2 (20,127).

Human glioblastoma cell lines show heterogeneity in regard to the isoform of TGF-β expressed, but share with astrocytes the inability to release TGF-β3 (31). Both latent and active forms of TGF-β have been identified in the supernatants of glioblastomas (31), and some cell lines can also secrete TGF-α (120). Other reports fail to detect immunosuppressive cytokines in supernatants of glioblastoma cell lines (41), suggesting that cell culture conditions may influence the number and mode of immunosuppressive (or stimulatory) cytokines secreted by glioblastomas. Therefore, a better understanding to the regulation of immunosuppressive cytokines produced by glioblastomas could lead to development of immunobiological response modifiers to improve the immune status of patients (see Chapter 21).

Prostaglandins

Prostaglandins (PGs) are derived from arachidonic acid, a component of cell membrane phospholipids that is released by the action of phospholipase A_2. The release of arachidonic acid may be triggered by hormones, inflammatory or immunological stimuli, or perturbations in the cell membrane in general. PGs are ubiquitously distributed in virtually all mammalian tissues. $PGF_{2\alpha}$ was the first PG to be reported in the ox brain (122), and subsequently the formation of PGs has been demonstrated in brain tissues in vivo and in vitro (126). In the rodent brain, PGD_2 is the major cyclooxygenase metabolite formed, followed by lower concentrations of $PGF_{2\alpha}$, PGE_2, thrombane A_2, and PGI_2 (82,126).

Cultured astrocytes treated with lipopolysaccharide (54) and microglia (55) release significant amounts of PGE_2, which can inhibit the proliferative response of thymocytes and T-cell lines (55). Astrocytes demonstrate heterogeneity in the PG receptors expressed (82). Type-1 astrocytes preferentially express $PGF_{2\alpha}$ receptors, the activation of which leads to phosphoinositide metabolism and $[Ca^{2+}]_i$ elevation. Type-2 astrocytes possess PGE receptors that are linked to cyclic AMP formation (82). Thus, type-1 and type-2 astrocytes are distinct targets for various PGs. Although PGs have been implicated in physiological and pathological responses of the CNS (52), the PGs responsible for these responses remain unclear.

PGs have been shown to be potent inhibitors of class II MHC antigens on macrophages and IFN-γ-induced expression of Ia antigens on brain cells (52,55). It does not appear that the low-level expression of MHC antigens in the brain are due to the continuous release of PGs, but in pathological conditions like multiple sclerosis (MS), an increase in prostaglandins could interfere with intracerebral activation of class II antigen–dependent T-cell mechanisms (52). Further PG release could interfere with immune stimulatory factors such as the interleukins (ILs) synthesized by CNS cells, thus leading to down-regulation of immune responses within the CNS. Numerous effects of IL-1 on the CNS require the activation of the arachidonic acid cascade (15,32,79,140). Adrenocorticotropin (ACTH) secretion induced by IL-1 could be partially or totally blocked by acute PG synthesis inhibition (89,90,103,105,114,151), suggesting that PGs could be mediators of IL-1 action on pituitary–adrenal activity.

Lipocortins

Lipocortins are a family of calcium- and phospholipid-binding proteins that are potential mediators of the anti-inflammatory effects of glucocorticoid hormones. At present, six lipocortins have been identified (109), and they are now recognized to be members of a larger family of structurally homologous, calcium- and phospholipid-binding proteins termed the *annexins* (43). Many studies have demonstrated induction of lipocortin 1 following in vitro and in vivo treatment with glucocorticoids (4,64,128). Lipocortins have been suggested to be anti-inflammatory substances (51,139) that inhibit the release of arachidonic acid from phospholipids and inhibit the formation of prostaglandin, leuko-triene, and platelet-activating factor (37,119). Lipocortins inhibit the activity of the enzyme phospholipase A_2 in vitro, and this inhibition was presumed to be the primary biological anti-inflammatory action. The nature of the interaction and the physiological relevance of the inhibitory effect of lipocortin 1 on phospholipase A_2 activity has been questioned, and the topic remains controversial (65). Putative receptors for lipocortins have been reported on phagocytes that may influence the inflammatory action of these cells by mechanisms independent of inhibition of phospholipase A_2 (65).

Lipocortin 1 suppresses Con A–stimulated T-cell proliferation (77), NK cell activity (72), and IL-1 production by Th cells (76,77). Moreover, lipocortin 1 also induces T suppressor (Ts) cells (77). Macrophage-secreted lipocortin 1 has been associated with cancer in mice (121) and implicated in the teratogenicity of glucocorticoids (69).

High levels of lipocortins concentrations have been found in immunologically privileged sites. In the CNS, lipocortin 1 appears to have powerful effects on the prevention of ischemic (113) and chemically induced neuronal damage (11) and the inhibition of fever (23,40). Lipocortins 1, 2, 4, and 5 are distributed in normal gray and white matter, and are increased in tissue samples from MS patients, especially in plaques (46). If lipocortins do act as endogenous regulators of inflammation, the increased amount of lipocortin in the CNS of MS patients may represent an unsuccessful attempt to overcome the chronic inflammation present in this disease. Lipocortin 1 has been detected in reactive astrocytes (104a), microglia (101a) and in inflammatory infiltrates in EAE (45a). Whether there are specific receptors on phagocytic CNS cells, and whether excess production of this protein and/or its receptor thwarts the ability of the immune system to eliminate pathogens and tumors remains to be determined. Future studies in this field will be fascinating in providing a better understanding played by lipocortins in immune privilege and inflammation of the CNS.

Interleukins

Within the CNS, interleukins (ILs) have been reported in astrocytes (54), microglia (55,61), and neurons (14,49). In cultured astrocytes from rat cerebral cortex, interleukin-1β stimulates proenkephalin gene expression at the mRNA and promoter levels (106), suggesting a cytokine-induced enkephalin peptide release from astrocytes that may interlink the immune system with the pituitary–hypothalamic axis (12).

IL-4 and IL-10 are two immunosuppressive cytokines that may play a role in diminishing DTH reactions and in other Th1 cell-mediated processes (59,80). IL-10 synergizes with IL-4 and TGF-β to inhibit macrophage cytotoxic activity (107). Cytokine mRNA expression has been analyzed by the very sensitive reverse transcription polymerase chain reaction (RT-PCR) technique in spinal cord tissues of mice with EAE (92). Distinct patterns of cytokine gene expression occurred during the acute, recovery, and chronic phases of the disease. The acute phase was characterized by dramatically elevated levels of mRNA for five cytokines (IL-1α, IL-2, IL-4, IL-6, and IFN-γ). With the exception if IL-1α, peak expression of these cytokines occurred before the peak in clinical severity. The recovery phase was characterized by decreased expression of IL-2, IL-4, IL-6, and IFN-γ cytokine mRNA concomitant with a dramatic rise in IL-10 mRNA expression. The chronic phase was characterized by the persistent expression of IL-1α, IFN-γ, and IL-10 mRNA, whereas all the other cytokine mRNA examined returned to baseline level. The differences in the time course of expression of the various cytokine mRNA may be a reflection of the complexity of the immune response within the spinal cord. However, the RT-PCR technique does not allow for identification of the cellular source of the various cytokine mRNA species, and it is possible that the spinal cord tissue analysis performed in this study could represent cytokine gene expression by infiltrating cells as well as by resident cells responding to the inflammation within the CNS (92). Nevertheless, this study raises the possibility that some cytokines (IL-10) could act as down-regulators of the immune response in the CNS and may serve to decrease the levels of inflammatory cytokines in the CNS.

Suppressin

A novel inhibitor of cell proliferation, termed *suppressin* (SPN), has been isolated and purified from bovine pituitaries (24,96,97). SPN is a monomeric polypeptide with an apparent molecular weight of 63 kDa and an isoelectric point of 8.1. SPN is constitutively synthesized by the rat pituitary cell line, GH$_3$ (96), and human peripheral blood lymphocytes (97). Not only do neuroendocrine and lymphoid tissues act as a source of SPN but they also appear to be the predominant target for the effects of this cytokine (24). The structural characteristics of SPN and its target cell specificity indicate that SPN is different from other endogenous inhibitors of cell proliferation like TGF-β, and it may function as an autocrine regulator of cell growth in neuroendocrine and lymphoid tissues (96).

T and B leukemias and lymphomas, neuroblastomas and gliomas, and pituitary tumor cells are highly sensitive to the antiproliferative effects of SPN, whereas the proliferation of fibroblasts and amnionic cells are not (24). SPN inhibits murine lymphocyte proliferation; T cells may be more sensitive to the effects of SPN as compared to B cells. Con-A stimulation of immunoglobulin (Ig) secretion of B lymphocytes is inhibited by SPN. Although all isotypes are suppressed, both IgG- and IgM-secreting B cells are more sensitive to its effects than IgA-secreting B cells (24).

Cell cycle analysis of SPN-treated splenocytes demonstrates that cells are arrested in the G_0–G_1 phase. Moreover, SPN down-regulates RNA, DNA, and protein synthesis, and these effects are reversible when SPN is removed (97). SPN interacts with other cytokines to regulate biological activity. Preincubation of splenic leukocytes with SPN enhances NK activity and potentiates the ability of other lymphokines such as IFN-γ or IL-2 to augment NK activity. This increase in NK activity by SPN may be in part attributed to the induction of IFN-α/β (24). Whether SPN potentially contributes to CNS tumor growth, immune privilege, or disease, remains to be determined.

Interferons

Interferons (IFNs) comprise a group of proteins primarily defined by their antiviral activity, but which also exhibit a wide range of biological and biochemical effects on cells and whole animals. IFNs modulate expression of cell surface antigens of the major histocompatibility complex, which is one of the essential functions by which all three IFN species influence the immune system (50,53,56). Chapters 10, 11, and 13 provide a comprehensive review of IFN-γ regulation of MHC antigen expression on CNS cells, therefore, the production of IFN-α/β by glial cells will be briefly discussed here.

Studies from our laboratory have demonstrated that astrocytes in vitro can be induced to produce IFN-α/β when appropriately stimulated with an IFN super-inducing regimen of cycloheximide, poly rI-rC, and actinomycin D (21,91,136). The response of astrocytes to IFN superinduction increases with the length of time in culture. Astrocytes maintained for 3 weeks in culture produce 35 times more IFN-α/β than astrocytes cultured for shorter periods (91). Although the role of IFN-α/β in the CNS is unclear, IFN-α/β can induce class I MHC antigen expression on a subpopulation of astrocytes (136). Since there is normally low expression on the astrocytes cell surface, this enhanced MHC antigen expression favors interaction with CD8 lymphocytes and renders astrocytes susceptible to T cell-mediated killing (91). This finding may have implications in viral and other diseases of the nervous system in which T cells infiltrate the CNS.

IFN-α/β can antagonize the effects of IFN-γ-induced class II expression and may be a naturally occurring suppressor substance in the brain (150). Studies employing human astrocytes and astrocytoma cells from surgical specimens and nuclear run-on experiments have demonstrated that the inhibitory effect of IFN-β on IFN-γ induction of the class II MHC gene is exerted at the transcriptional level (112). IFN-β does not antagonize IFN-γ induction of class II on human monocytes, which suggests that the inhibition in astrocytes is relatively tissue-specific. However, responses to IFN by macrophages and monocyte lineage cells vary markedly as a function of differentiation (22).

Natural suppressor systems have been extensively studied in tissues such as normal bone marrow (44) and neonatal spleen (6). Natural suppression has been documented during recovery from severe insults to the immune system of normal animals, as demonstrated in total lymphoid or whole body irradiation (152), cyclophosphamide treatment (124), or during graft-versus-host disease (28). Spontaneous production of IFN-β by splenic macrophages has been associated with natural suppressive activity (27), but whether CNS cells elaborate IFN that contributes to immune suppression in the brain has not been adequately addressed.

IFN-γ and IFN-α/β have significant effects on microglial superoxide anion production, IL-1 production, and chemotaxis (30). Microglia treated with IFN-γ and IFN-α/β produce a marked increase in superoxide level and decreased chemotaxic responses. IFN-α/β increased IL-1 activity in microglia, but these changes were only observed in experiments using serum-free medium. Microglial responses to IFN differ from those determined for other monocytic-derived macrophages, and they suggest that IFN in the CNS may inhibit movement and migration of microglia at sites of injury and wound repair (30).

IFNs in Neurological Diseases

During the course of several neurological diseases—some of no apparent viral origin—IFNs have been reported in the circulation, the CNS, and CSF (42,137). It is difficult to discern between the presence of IFNs as a symptom of disease or as active contributors to pathogenesis. This problem is further complicated by the difficulty to define a standard of "normal" production, since even in disease-free individuals there can be differences in production that reach several orders of magnitude (42). Nevertheless, defective or impaired IFN-γ and IFN-α production has been reported in peripheral blood leukocytes from MS patients. Defective IFN-γ production after mitogenic stimulation is not specific to MS patients, since it is also prevalent in peripheral blood leukocytes of patients with a variety of nonimmunological neurological diseases including Alzheimer's and Huntington's chorea (42). Moreover, an impaired IFN-γ response also occurs in patients recovering from surgical removal of brain tumors and cerebrovascular accidents (142,143).

Systemic or intraventricular administration of rat IFN-α/β decreases the severity and symptoms of EAE in rats (1,2,74). This observation may be explained by the fact that IFNs can suppress the expression of DTH. In clinical trials, intrathecal administration of IFN-β to MS patients palliated the severity of symptoms (83,93), whereas administration of IFN-γ caused exacerbation of the disease (108). Two forms of IFN-β, β-seron and avonex, are currently used in therapeutic treatment of MS. Interestingly, contradictory actions of IFN-γ in EAE in mice as compared to those in rats and MS patients have been reported in which IFN-γ exerts an inhibitory effect on the development of EAE (10,45). The reasons for the discrepancies are not known. Many questions about suppressed IFN responses in neurological diseases in general, and their connection to deviant immunity generated by the introduction of antigen into the CNS in particular, are waiting to be answered.

Neurotransmitters and Neuroendocrine Peptide Hormones

Considerable evidence has accumulated that the nervous and immune systems communicate in a bidirectional manner with interactions that are both facilitatory and inhibitory. Cross talk exists between neurally derived substances and lymphokines that result in immune alterations that are generally small in magnitude and duration (118) and contain many feedback loops. As reviewed in Chapters 8 and 14, lymphocytes respond to neural modulation by interacting with specific receptors for neurotransmitters, neurohormones, or neuropeptides (12,62,118). Since the neuroimmune interactions can result in either inhibition or facilitation of lymphocyte function, these modulations in function have been suggested to be initiated by second messengers evoked by neurally derived substances that bind to their receptors on lymphocytes (12,62,118).

With respect to suppression of immune reactivity within the CNS, Frohman and colleagues have demonstrated that the neurotransmitter, norepinephrine, inhibits IFN-γ-induced class II expression on cultured astrocytes (57,58). This inhibition can be attenuated by the β-adrenergic antagonist, propranolol, but not by a β_1-selective antagonist, atenolol, or by the α-adrenergic antagonist, phentolamine (57). Moreover, the β-adrenergic agonist, isoproterenol, suppresses EAE in Lewis rats (26). These results suggest that β_2-adrenergic receptor signal transduction pathways may be responsible for the norepinephrine-mediated inhibition on induced class II expression. β_2-adrenergic signal transduction mechanisms are known to involve the activation of adenylate cyclase and elevations of intracellular cAMP. Treatment of astrocytes with a combination of dibutyrl-cAMP and dipyridimole, a phosphodiesterase inhibitor, attenuated induced class II expression (57,58). Incubation of cells with forskolin, an inducer of cAMP, resulted in a dose-dependent inhibition of class II antigens on astrocytes. In addition, complete inhibition of class II can be achieved with H-7, an inhibitor of protein kinase C, whereas an H-7 analog HA-1004, which is a more selective inhibitor of cGMP and cAMP-dependent kinases, had no effect on class II expression. These data collectively suggest that class II induction in astrocytes by IFN-γ appear to be protein kinase C dependent, and that cAMP, which also down-regulates class II on astrocytes, may not act in a kinase-dependent manner.

Glutamate, an excitatory neutotransmitter, has been shown to profoundly inhibit IFN-γ-induced class II expression on astrocytes (98). Both glutamate and norepinephrine appear to eliminate accumulation of class II MHC mRNA at doses that inhibit the expression of the cell surface protein on astrocytes. The kinetics of class II mRNA induction by IFN-γ in the presence of glutamate suggest that glutamate may act as a transcriptional inhibitor (98).

The inhibitory effects of glutamate and norepinephrine on IFN-γ-induced class II expression astrocytes do not regulate expression of these antigens on microglia, which demonstrate a higher incidence of class II expression in the brain (98). Systemic infusion of IFN-γ selectively induces class II on microglia and not astrocytes, although its in vitro induction is similar for both cell types (130). Thus, neurotransmitters, such as glutamate and norepinephrine, may selectively act as inhibitors of astrocyte class II MHC antigen expression in vivo, but not in microglia.

Ly-6 Products

The Ly-6 locus encodes a group of murine phosphotidylinositol-anchor proteins that share several structural and functional characteristics with Thy-1. Ly-6 products have been implicated in regulation of T-cell activation based on the observation that monoclonal antibodies (MAbs) specific for cell-surface antigen induce T cells to secrete lymphokines and proliferate (29). Recently, it has been shown that Ly-6A/E may also inhibit IL-2 production of T-cell lines and down-regulate T-cell proliferation (29). Ly-6A/E is expressed in brain tissues primarily in the hippocampus and thalamus, while low levels are present in white matter of the folium in the cerebellum (35). Although cultured glial and neuronal cells express marginally detectable levels of Ly-6A/E, astrocytes can be induced to express high levels of Ly-6A/E following incubation with cytokines such as IFN-γ and TNF-α (35). Since Ly-6A/E has been shown to be a sensitive indicator of the onset of graft-versus-host reaction (99) in which mononuclear cells infiltrate the brain and release cytokines that induce Ly-6 expression on astrocytes (35), then it is possible that Ly-6 expression may inhibit IL-2 production in T cells that have infiltrated the CNS, such as those in autoimmune demyelinating, virally induced, and other CNS diseases.

Physiological Adaptations of CNS Cells to Immune Attack

The barely detectable levels of MHC molecules on CNS cells mitigates their ability to initiate and participate in immune reactions. Many studies have demonstrated that cytokines like IFN-γ and TNF-α increase MHC antigen expression on glial cells, but CNS neurons and neuronal cell lines are functionally devoid of MHC molecules and do not up-regulate expression after induction with cytokines (21,50,53,56,91,134). The lack of class I MHC antigens on CNS neurons enables them to escape recognition and destruction by cytotoxic lymphocytes (21,87,88,91). One strategy employed by CNS neurons is that they express low levels of MHC class I-αC, the peptide transporters HAM1 and HAM2, and possibly other genes of the peptide-loading machinery (88). Essentially, neuronal cells are unable to load peptides into the groove of MHC class I molecules for antigen presentation.

Another strategy evolved by CNS neurons is that they are strikingly resistant to perforin, the monomeric pore-forming proteins that are the major cytotoxic constituents of cytotoxic granules (91). Thus, since the immune system is actively suppressed within the nervous system in a multifactorial fashion, CNS neurons have evolved multiple strategies to suppress and prevent destruction by immune-mediated injury. Understanding the mechanisms involved in regulating the immune response against neurons, especially in viral infections of the nervous system, is likely to be of great importance in pathologies of the nervous system.

Immunosuppression in CNS Diseases

Three human neurological diseases, measles (85), AIDS dementia (48,110), and multiple sclerosis (MS) (70), are complicated by frequent opportunistic infections and are of particular importance in this chapter in that they cause alterations in immunosuppression. While the causative agent for measles and AIDS is known (MS is a disease of unknown etiology), the neuropathogenesis of all three diseases remains entirely enigmatic.

Measles

Measles was the first infectious agent shown to cause profound immunosuppression complicated by opportunistic infections, and severe disabling or fatal neurological diseases. Complications still result in over a million deaths per year worldwide (7). Abnormalities in the immune response associated with measles virus infection include suppression of DTH skin responses (133), depression of in vitro lymphoproliferative responses to mitogens (78), decreased natural killer cell activity, and altered cytokine production in vitro (67,68,147,149). Immune activation during this period of immune suppression is suggested by spontaneous proliferation of peripheral blood mononuclear cells and increased plasma levels of sIL-2R, soluble CD8, IFN-γ, neopterin, and β2-microglobulin (147). Recent studies have demonstrated increased production of IL-4 and concomitant suppression of IL-1 and PGE_2 production after measles vaccine, suggesting that preferential stimulation of a Th2 response may be responsible for some of the immunologic abnormalities seen after infection or vaccination (147).

Karp and coworkers (88a) have reported that the profound suppression of cell-mediated immunity accompanying measles involves the down-regulation of IL-12. IL-12 is a cytokine derived principally from monocytes and macrophages and is critical for the generation of cell-mediated immunity. In this study, human monocytes were isolated from normal volunteers, infected with measles virus, and stimulated with bacterial inducers of IL-12 production. Infection of primary monocytes with measles virus down-regulated the stimulated production of IL-12, both at the level of p40 and p70 subunits. Cross-linking of CD46, the complement regulatory protein that is the cellular receptor for measles virus, with antibody or with the complement activation C3b similarly inhibited monocyte IL-12 production, providing a possible mechanism for measles virus-induced immunosuppression. CD46 provides the link between the complement system and the cellular immune responses, and shows that complement activation products can directly regulate the production of IL-12.

Neither measles-derived antigen or RNA has been localized in the brains of patients with fatal encephalomyelitis or the brains of patients dying acutely when virus is readily identifiable in other organs (102). The pathogenesis of measles encephalitis has been assumed to be autoimmune, but how this immune response is generated is not understood, since virus is not found in the nervous system.

A variety of other neurological diseases that differ clinically, pathologically, and virologically are associated with measles. These include postinfectious encephalomyelitis, subacute sclerosing panencephalitis, and inclusion body encephalitis (85). Only postinfectious encephalomyelitis is associated with immune suppression induced by the measles virus.

AIDS Dementia

Pathological abnormalities are reported upon postmortem examination of the CNS in greater than 80% of patients with AIDS, while 40% of these patients manifest signs and symptoms of neurological dysfunction (48,110). As outlined in Chapter 20, the marked CNS dysfunction observed in AIDS patients manifests despite subtle or minimal lesions; it has been suggested that cytokines released from HIV-infected macrophages or brain microglia might be involved in this aspect of AIDS pathology and in the profound systemic immunodeficiency associated with the disease. As discussed previously, TGF-β has been found to be aberrantly expressed in brains of AIDS patients (142), but the role of this cytokine in the immunosuppression and nervous system diseases is yet to be defined (106a).

Multiple Sclerosis

A consistent finding in the peripheral blood of patients with chronic progressive MS has been the loss of functional suppression (50) and low autologous mixed lymphocyte reaction (70). This decrease in suppression in the blood of MS patients may be reflected in the brain. It has been reported that suppressor T cells are absent in MS brains (5) whereas these cells are present in subjects with viral encephalitis (129). Not all MS patients demonstrate low functional suppression, and even some healthy controls have lower levels of suppression. Significance to "normal values" of suppression is complicated because these values vary during the course of sampling. Patients with reduced functional suppression have also been found with systemic lupus erythematosus, myaesthenia gravis, and viral encephalitis (measles) (85). Therefore, a loss of functional suppression may herald the disease and make it highly unlikely that a loss of functional suppression is the only condition necessary for the disease to occur.

Cytokines produced in the CNS by infiltrating macrophages or by CNS microglia or astrocytes may be involved with the pathogenesis of MS (81,101,125). TGF-β has been reported at the lesion edge in MS brains (155), but the significance of this finding in the pathogenesis of the disease and the immune response remains to be determined.

Summary and Conclusions

Immune privilege maintained by the CNS appears to result from the creation of a potent immunosuppressive microenvironment by cells within the brain. This environment has profound effects on the induction of immunity to antigens placed in the CNS and in the expression of systemic immunity. The immunosuppressive properties of the brain microenvironment are mediated by cytokines, especially TGF-β, prostaglandins, and immunosuppressive substances produced by CNS cells during the inflammatory process. The microenvironment alters the functional programs of blood-borne, antigen-presenting cells; whereas alterations of the efferent limb of the immune response results in inhibition of DTH reactions and increased systemic antibody production. Inflammatory responses associated with DTH reactions are accompanied by bystander tissue destruction. Such a strategy within the CNS would be devastating and would distort the delicate microanatomy and architecture of the brain, leading to profound neurological deficits. In order to minimize this potentially life threatening situation, the CNS may possess multiple mechanisms to suppress T cell–mediated inflammation, functionally inactivate the responding lymphocytes or kill the cells by apoptosis. These mechanisms are manifest as immune privilege and ensure that an electrophysiologically active system of neurons in the brain is maintained. Moreover, CNS neurons appear to have evolved physiological adaptations that may contribute to immune privilege. CNS neurons do not express class I or II MHC antigens and are strikingly resistant to alloantigen-specific cytotoxic lymphocytes and to cytolytic granule-mediated lysis, whereas PNS neurons and astrocytes are susceptible to both types of immune attack. Therefore, immune privilege of the CNS may involve adaptations in both the nervous and immune systems to provide immune protection. An understanding of the strategies employed by the CNS and immune systems to generate immunity will add knowledge to our understanding of CNS diseases and make possible manipulations of CNS immune responses for therapeutic paradigms.

References

1. Abreu SL. Suppression of experimental allergic encephalomyelitis by interferon. Immunol Comm 11:1–7, 1982.
2. Abreu SL, Tondreau J, Levine S, Sowinski R. Inhibition of passive localized experimental allergic encephalomyelitis by interferon. Int Arch Allergy Appl Immunol 2:30–33, 1983.

3. Albright L, Seab JA, Ommaya AK. Intracerebral delayed hypersensitivity reactions in glioblastoma multiforme patients. Cancer 39:1331–1336, 1977.

4. Ambrose MP, Hunninghake GW. Corticosteroids increase lipocortin 1 in BAL fluid from normal individuals and patients with lung disease. J Appl Physiol 68:1668–1671, 1990.

5. Antel JP, Arnason BGW, Medoff MW. Suppressor cell function in multiple sclerosis: correlation with clinical disease activity. Ann Neurol 5:338–342, 1978.

6. Argyris BF. Suppressor activity in the spleen of neonatal mice. Cell Immunol 366:354–358, 1978.

7. Assaad F. Measles: summary of worldwide impact. Rev Infect Disease 5:452–459, 1983.

8. Barnard JA, Lyons RM, Moses HL. The cell biology of transforming growth factor β. Biochim Biophys Acta 1032:79–87, 1990.

9. Beck JP, Rondot P, Catinot E, Falcoff H, Kirchner H, Wietzerbin J. Increased production of interferon gamma and tumor necrosis factor precedes clinical manifestation in multiple sclerosis: do cytokines trigger off exacerbations? Acta Neurol Scand 78:318–323, 1988.

9a. Bellgrau D, Gold D, Selawry H, Moore J, Franzusoff A, Duke RC. A role for CD95 ligand in preventing graft rejection. Nature 377:630–632, 1995.

10. Billiau A, Heremans H, Vandekerckhove R, Dijkmans R, Sobis H, Meulepas E, Carton H. Enhancement of experimental allergic encephalomyelitis in mice by antibodies against IFN-γ. J Immunol 140:1506–1510, 1988.

11. Black MD, Reltion JK, Carey F, Crossman AR, Rothwell NJ. Lipocortin-1 inhibits NMDA-induced neuronal damage. Br J Pharmacol 104 (suppl) C34, 1991.

12. Blalock JE. A molecular basis for bidirectional communication between the immune system and neuroendocrine systems. Physiol Rev 69:1–32, 1989.

13. Bradbury MWB, Cserr HF. Drainage of cerebral interstial fluid and of cerebrospinal fluid into lymphatics. In: Experimental Biology of the Lymphatic Circulation, MG Johnston ed. Elsevier, New York, 1985, pp 355–394.

14. Breder CD, Dinarello CA, Saper CB. Interleukin-1 immunoreactive innervation of the human hypothalamus. Science 240:321–324, 1988.

15. Brendan FB, Yates AJP, Mundy GR. Bolus injections of recombinant human interleukin-1 cause transient hypocalcemia in normal mice. Endocrinology 125:2780–2783, 1989.

16. Brooks WH, Caldwell HD, Mortara RH. Immune responses in patients with gliomas. Surg Neurol 2:419–423, 1974.

17. Brooks WH, Latta RB, Mahaley MS, Roszman TL, Dudka L, Skaggs C. Immunobiology of primary intracranial tumors. Part 5. Correlation of a lymphocyte index and clinical status. J Neurosurg 54:331–337, 1981.

18. Brooks WH, Netzley MC, Normansell DE, Horwitz DA. Depressed cell mediated immunity in patients with primary intracranial tumors: characterization of a humoral immunosuppressive factor. J Exp Med 136:1631–1647, 1972.

19. Bodmer S, Siepl C, Fontana A. Immunoregulatory factors secreted by glioblastoma cells: glioblastoma-derived T-cell suppressor factor/transforming growth factor-β2. In: Neuroimmune Networks: Physiology and Diseases, EJ Goetzl, NH Spector, eds. Alan R. Liss, New York, 1989, pp 73–82.

20. Bodmer S, Strommer K, Frei K, Siepl C, De Tribolet N, Heid I, Fontana A. Immunosuppression and transforming growth factor-β in glioblastoma. Preferential production of transforming growth factor-β2. J Immunol 143:3222–3229, 1989.

21. Borgeson M, Tallent MW, Keane RW. Astrocyte modulation of central nervous system immune responses. In: Neuroimmune Networks: Physiology and Diseases, EJ Goetzl, NH Spector, eds. Alan R. Liss, New York, 1989, pp 51–55.

22. Calder VL, Wolswijk G, Noble M. The differentiation of O-2A progenitor cells into

oligodendrocytes is associated with a loss of inducibility of Ia antigens. Eur J Immunol 18:1195–1201, 1988.

23. Carey F, Forder R, Edge MD, Greene AR, Horan MA, Strijbos PJLM, Rothwell NJ. Lipocortin 1 fragment modifies pyrogenic actions of cytokines in rats. Am J Physiol 259:R266–R269, 1990.

24. Carr DJJ, Blalock JE, Green MM, LeBoeuf RD. Immunomodulatory characteristics of a novel antiproliferative protein, suppressin. J Neuroimmunol 30:170–187, 1990.

25. Caspi RR, Roberge FG, Nussenblatt RB. Organ-resident, nonlymphoid cells suppress proliferation of autoimmune T-helper lymphocytes. Science 237:1029–1032, 1987.

26. Chelmicka-Schorr E, Kwasniewski MN, Thomas BE, Arnason BGW. The β-adrenergic agonist isoproterenol suppresses experimental allergic encephalomyelitis in Lewis rat. J Neuroimmunol 25:203–207, 1989.

27. Cleveland MG, Lane RG, Klimpel GR. Spontaneous IFN-β production. A common feature of natural suppressor systems. J Immunol 141:2043–2049, 1988.

28. Cleveland MG, Ramirez RB, Klimpel GR. IFN-β production by macrophages obtained from mice undergoing graft vs host disease. J Immunol 141:3823–3827, 1988.

29. Codias EK, Fleming TJ, Zacharchuk CM, Ashwell JD, Malek TR. Role of Ly-6A/E and T cell receptor-ζ for IL-2 production. Phosphotidylinositol-anchored Ly-6A/E antagonizes T cell receptor-mediated IL-2 production by a ζ-independent pathway. J Immunol 149:1825–1832, 1992.

30. Colton CA, Yao J, Keri JE, Gilbert D. Regulation of microglial function by interferons. J Neuroimmunol 30:89–98, 1992.

31. Constam DN, Philipp J, Malipiero UV, ten Dijke P, Schachner M, Fontana A. Differential expression of transforming growth factor-β1, -β2, and -β3 by glioblastoma cells, astrocytes, and microglia. J Immunol 148:1404–1410, 1992.

32. Cooper KE. The neurobiology of fever: thoughts on recent developments. Annu Rev Neurosci 10:297–324, 1987.

33. Couldwell WT, Dore-Duffy P, Apuzzo MLJ, Antel JP. Malignant glioma modulation of immune function: relative contribution of different soluble factors. J Neuroimmunol 33:89–96, 1991.

34. Cousins SW, McCabe MM, Danielpour D, Streilein JW. Identification of transforming growth factor-beta as an immunosuppressive factor in aqueous humor. Invest Ophthalmol Vis Sci 32:2201–2211, 1991.

35. Cray C, Keane RW, Malek TR, Levy RB. Regulation and selective expression of Ly-6A/E, a lymphocyte activation molecule, in the central nervous system. Mol Brain Res 8:9–15, 1990.

36. Cserr HF, DePasquale M, Harling-Berg CJ, Park JT, Knopf PM. Afferent and efferent arms of the humoral immune response of CSF-administered albumins in a rat model with normal blood-brain barrier permeability. J Neuroimmunol 41:195–202, 1992.

37. Curino G, Flower RJ, Browing JL, Sinclair LK, Pepinsky RB. Recombinant human lipocortin I inhibits thromboxane release from guinea-pig isolated perfused lung. Nature 328:270–272, 1987.

38. daCunha A, Vitkovic L. Transforming growth factor-beta (TGF-β1) expression and regulation in rat cortical astrocytes. J Neuroimmunol 36:157–169, 1992.

39. daCunha AD, Jefferson JA, Jackson RW, Vitkovic L. Glial cell-specific mechanisms of TGF-β1 induction by IL-1 in cerebral cortex. J Neuroimmunol 42:71–86, 1993.

40. Davidson J, Flower RJ, Milton AS, Peers SH, Rotondo D. Antipyretic actions of human recombinant lipocortin-1. Br J Pharmacol 102:7–9, 1991.

41. Daubener W, Zennati SS, Wernet P, Bilzer T, Fischer HG, Hadding U. Human glioblastoma

cell line 86HG39 activates T cells in an antigen specific major histocompatibility complex class II-dependent manner. J Neuroimmunol 41:21–28, 1992.

41a. deLuca A, Weller M, Fontana A. TGF-β-induced apoptosis of cerebellar granule neurons is prevented by depolarization. J Neurosci 16:4174–4185, 1996.

42. DeMaeyer E, DeMaeyer-Guignard J. The presence and possible pathogenic role of interferons in disease. In: Interferons and Other Regulatory Cytokines. John Wiley & Sons, New York, 1988, pp 380–424.

43. Di Rosa M, Flower RJ, Hirata F, Parente L, Russo-Marie F. Nomenclature announcement. Anti-phospholipase proteins. Prostaglandins 28:441–442, 1984.

44. Dorschkind K, Rose C. Physical, biologic, and phenotypic properties of natural regulatory cells in murine bone marrow. Am J Anat 164:1–15, 1982.

45. Duong TT, St. Louis J, Gilbert JJ, Finkelman FD, Strejan GH. Effect of anti-interferon-γ and anti-interleukin-2 monoclonal antibody treatment on the development of actively and passively induced experimental allergic encephalomyelitis in the SJL/J mouse. J Neuroimmunol 36:105–115, 1992.

45a. Elderfield AJ, Bolton C, Flower RJ. Lipocortin 1 (annexin 1) immunoreactivity in the cervical spinal cord of Lewis rats with experimental allergic encephalomyelitis. J Neurol Sci 119:146–153, 1993.

46. Elderfield AJ, Newcombe J, Bolton C, Flower RJ. Lipocortins (annexins) 1, 2, 4 and 5 are increased in the central nervous system in multiple sclerosis. J Neuroimmunol 39:91–100, 1992.

47. Elliot LH, Brooks WH, Roszman TL. Activation of immunoregulatory lymphocytes obtained from patients with malignant gliomas. J Neurosurg 67:231–236, 1987.

48. Fauci AS. The human immunodeficiency virus: infectivity mechanisms of pathogenesis. Science 239:617–622, 1988.

49. Farrar WL, Vinocour M, Hill JM. In situ hybridization histochemistry localization of interleukin-3 mRNA in mouse brain. Blood 73:137–140, 1989.

50. Fierz W, Endler B, Reske K, Wekerle H, Fontana A. Astrocytes as antigen-presenting cells I. Induction of Ia antigen expression on astrocytes by T cells via immune interferon and its effect on antigen presentation. J Immunol 134:3785–3793, 1985.

51. Flower RJ. Lipocortin and mechanism of action of glucocorticoids. Br J Pharmacol 94:987–992, 1988.

52. Fontana A, Bodmer S, Frei K. Immunoregulatory factors secreted by astrocytes and glioblastoma cells. Lymphokines 14:91–121, 1987.

53. Fontana A, Fierz W, Wekerle H. Astrocytes present myelin basic protein to encephalitogenic T-cell lines. Nature 307:273–276, 1984.

54. Fontana A, Kristensen F, Dubs R, Gemsa D, Weber E. Production of prostaglandin E and interleukin-1 like factor by cultured astrocytes and C_6 glioma cells. J Immunol 129:2413–2419, 1982.

55. Frei K, Fontana A. Immune regulatory functions of astrocytes and microglial cell within the central nervous system. In: Neuroimmune Networks: Physiology and Diseases, EJ Goetzl, NH Spector, eds. Alan R. Liss, New York, pp 127–136.

56. Frei K, Siepl C, Groscurth P, Bodmer S, Schwerdel C, Fontana A. Antigen presentation and tumor cytotoxicity by interferon-γ-treated microglial cells. Eur J Immunol 17:1271–1278, 1987.

56a. French LE, Hahne M, Viard I, Radlgruber G, Zanone R, Becker K, Müller C, Tschopp J. Fas and fas ligand in embryos and adult mice: ligand expression in several immune-privileged tissues and coexpression in adult tissues characterized by apoptotic cell turnover. J Cell Biol 133:335–343, 1996.

57. Frohman EM, Vayuvegula B, Gupta S, van den Noort S. Norepinephrine inhibits γ interferon-induced major histocompatibility class II (Ia) antigen expression on cultured astrocytes via β_2-adrenergic signal transduction mechanisms. Proc Natl Acad Sci USA 85:1292–1296, 1988.

58. Frohman EM, Vayuvegula B, van den Noort S, Gupta S. Norepinephrine inhibits gamma-interferon-induced MHC class II (Ia) antigen expression on cultured brain astrocytes. J Neuroimmunol 17:89–101, 1988.

59. Gautam SC, Chikkala NF, Hamilton TA. Anti-inflammatory action of Il-4: negative regulation of contact sensitivity to trinitrochlorobenzene. J Immunol 148:1411–1415, 1992.

60. Genis P, Jett M, Bernton EW, Boyle T, Gelbard HA, Dzenko K, Keane RW, Resnick L, Mizrachi Y, Volsky DJ, Epstein LG, Gendelman HW. Cytokines and arachidonic metabolites produced during HIV-infected macrophage-astroglia interactions: implications for neuro-pathogenesis of HIV disease. J Exp Med 176:1703–1718, 1992.

61. Giulian D, Baker TJ, Shih LN, Lachman LB. Interleukin-1 of the central nervous system is produced by ameboid microglia. J Exp Med 164:594–604, 1986.

62. Goetzl EJ, Adelman DC, Sreedharan SP. Neuroimmunology. Adv Immunol 48:161–190, 1990.

63. Gordon LB, Knopf PM, Cserr HF. Ovalbumin is more immunogenic when introduced into brain or cerebrospinal fluid than into extracerebral sites. J Neuroimmunol 40:81–87, 1992.

64. Goulding NJ, Godolphin JL, Sharland PR, Peers SH, Sampson M, Maddison PJ, Flower RJ. Anti-inflammatory lipocortin-1 production by peripheral blood leucocytes in response to hydrocortisone. Lancet 335:1416–1418, 1990.

65. Goulding NJ, Guyre PM. Regulation of inflammation by lipocortin 1. Immunol Today 13:295–297, 1992.

66. Granstein RD, Staszewski R, Knisely TL, Zeira E, Nazareno R, Latina M, Albert DM. Aqueous humor contains transforming growth factor-β and a small (<3500 daltons) inhibitor of thymocyte proliferation. J Immunol 144:3021–3027, 1990.

67. Griffin DE, Johnson RT, Tamashiro VG, Moench TR, Jauregui E, Lindo de Soriano I, Vaisberg A. In vitro studies of the role of monocytes in the immunosuppression associated with natural measles virus infection. Clin Immunol Immunopathol 45:375–383, 1987.

68. Griffin DE, Moench TR, Johnson RT, Lindo de Soriano I, Vaisberg A. Peripheral blood mononuclear cells during natural measles infection. Cell surface phenotypes and evidence of activation. Clin Immunol Immunopathol 40:305–312, 1986.

68a. Griffith TS, Brunner T, Fletcher SM, Green DR, Ferguson TA. Fas ligand-induced apoptosis as a mechanism of immune privilege. Science 270:1189–1192, 1995.

69. Gupta C, Katsumata M, Goldman AS, Herold R, Piddington R. Glucocorticoid-induced phospholipase A_2-inhibitory proteins mediate glucocorticoid teratogenicity in vitro. Proc Natl Acad Sci USA 81:1140–1143, 1984.

70. Hafler DA, Weiner HL. MS: a CNS and systemic autoimmune disease. Immunol Today 10:104–111, 1989.

71. Harling-Berg CJ, Knopf PM, Cserr HF. Myelin basic protein infused into cerebrospinal fluid suppresses experimental autoimmune encephalomyelitis. J Neuroimmunol 35:45–51, 1991.

72. Hattori T, Hirata F, Hoffman A, Hizuta A, Herberman RB. Inhibition of human natural killer (NK) activity and antibody dependent cellular cytotoxicity (ADCC) by lipo-modulin, a phospholipase inhibitory protein. J Immunol 131:662–665, 1984.

73. Heine UI, Munoz EF, Flanders KC, Ellingsworth LR, Lam HYP, Thompson NL, Roberts AB, Sporn MB. Role of transforming growth factor-β in the development of the mouse embryo. J Cell Biol 105:2861–2876, 1987.

74. Hertz F, Deghenghi R. Effect of rat and β-human interferons on hyperacute experimental allergic encephalomyelitis. Agents Actions 16:397–403, 1985.

75. Hintzen RQ, Polman CH, Lucas CJ, vanLier RAW. Multiple sclerosis: immunological and possible implications for therapy. J Neuroimmunol 39:1–10, 1992.

76. Hirata F. Roles of lipomodulin: a phospholipase inhibitory protein in immunoregulation. Adv Inflammation Res 7:71–77, 1984.

77. Hirata F, Iwata M. Role of lipomodulin, a phospholipase inhibitory protein, in immunoregulation by thymocytes. J Immunol 130:1930–1936, 1983.

78. Hirsch RL, Griffin DE, Johnson RT, Cobb SJ, Lindo de Soriano I, Roedenbeck S, Vaisberg A. Cellular immune responses during complicated and uncomplicated measles virus infection in man. Clin Immunol Immunopathol 31:1–12, 1984.

79. Hori T, Shibata M, Nakashima T, Yamasaki M, Asami A, Asami T, Koga H. Effects of interleukin-1 and arachidonate on the preoptic and anterior hyphothalmic neurons. Brain Res Bull 20:75–82, 1988.

80. Howard M, O'Garra A. Biological properties of interleukin 10. Immunol Today 13:198–200, 1992.

81. Huddlestone JR, Oldstone MBA. T suppressor (Tg) lymphocytes fluctuate in parallel with changes in the clinical course of patients with multiple sclerosis. J Immunol 123:1615–1622, 1979.

81a. Iseki S, Osumi-Yamashita N, Miyazono K, Franzen P, Ichijo H, Ohtani H, Hayashi Y. Eto K Localization of transforming growth factor-β type I and type II receptors in mouse development Exp Cell Res 219:339–347, 1995.

81b. Ishihara A, Saito H, Abe K. Transforming growth factor-β_1 and -β_2 promote neurite sprouting and elongation of cultured rat hippocampal neurons. Brain Res 639:21–25, 1994.

82. Ito S, Sugama K, Inagaki N, Fukui H, Giles H, Wada H, Hayaishi O. Type-1 and type-2 astrocytes are distinct targets for prostaglandins $D_{2\alpha}$, $E_{2\alpha}$, and $F_{2\alpha}$. Glia 6:67–74, 1992.

83. Jacobs L, O'Malley JA, Freeman A, Ekes R, Reese PS. Intrathecal interferon in the treatment of multiple sclerosis. Arch Neurol 42:841–847, 1985.

84. Johns LD, Flanders KC, Ranges GE, Sriram S. Successful treatment of experimental allergic encephalomyelitis with transforming growth factor-β1. J Immunol 147:1792–1796, 1991.

85. Johnson RT. Viruses with dual specificity for the immune and nervous systems. In: Neuroimmune Networks: Physiology and Diseases, EJ Goetzl, NH Spector, eds. Alan R. Liss, New York, 1989, pp 173–178.

86. Johnson RT, Griffin DE, Hirsch RL, Wolinsky JS, Lindo de Soriano I, Roedenbeck S, Vaisberg A. Measles encephalomyelitis: clinical and immunological studies. New Engl J Med 310:137–141, 1984.

87. Joly E, Oldstone MBA. Viral persistence in neurons explained by lack of MHC class I expression. Science 253:1283–1285, 1991.

88. Joly E, Oldstone MBA. Neuronal cells are deficient in loading peptides onto MHC class I molecules. Neuron 8:1185–1190, 1992.

88a. Karp CL, Wysocka M, Wahl LM, Ahearn JM, Cuomo PJ, Sherry B, Trinchieri G, Griffin DE. Mechanism of suppression of cell-mediated immunity in measles virus. Science 273:228–231, 1996.

89. Katsuura G, Arimura A, Koves K, Gottschall PE. Involvement of organum vasculosum of lamina terminalis and preoptic area in interleukin 1 β-induced ACTH release. Am J Physiol 258:E163–E171, 1990.

90. Katsuura G, Gottschall PE, Dahl RR, Arimura A. Adrenocorticotropin release by intracerebroventricular injection of recombinant human interleukin-1 in rats: possible involvement of prostaglandins. Endocrinology 122:1773–1779, 1988.

91. Keane RW, Tallent MT, Podack ER. Resistance and susceptibility of neural cells to lysis by cytotoxic lymphocytes and by cytolytic granules. Transplantation 54:520–526, 1992.

92. Kennedy MK, Torrance DS, Picha KS, Mohler KM. Analysis of cytokine mRNA expression in the central nervous system of mice with experimental autoimmune encephalomyelitis reveals that IL-10 mRNA expression correlates with recovery. J Immunol 149:2496–2505, 1992.

93. Knobler RL. Systemic interferon therapy of multiple sclerosis. The pros. Neurology 38 (suppl 2):58–61, 1988.

93a. Krieglstein K, Suter-Crazzolara C, Fisher WH, Unsicker K. TGF-β superfamily promotes survival of midbrain dopaminergic neurons and protects them against MPP$^+$ toxicity EMBO J. 14:736–742, 1995.

94. Kuppner MC, Hamou MF, Sawamura Y, Bodmer S, de Tribolet N. Inhibition of lymphocyte function by glioblastoma derived transforming growth factor β$_2$. J Neurosurg 71:211–217, 1989.

95. Kuruvilla AP, Shah R, Hochwald GM, Liggit HD, Palladino MA, Thorbecke GJ. Protective effect of transforming growth factor β1 on experimental autoimmune diseases in mice. Proc Natl Acad Sci 88:2918–2921, 1991.

96. LeBoeuf RD, Burns JN, Bost KL, Blalock JE. Isolation, purification, and partial characterization of suppressin, a novel inhibitor of cell proliferation. J Biol Chem 265:158–165, 1990.

97. LeBoeuf RD, Carr DJJ, Green MM, Blalock JE. Cellular effects of suppressin, a biological response modifier of the neuroendocrine and immune system. Prog Neuroendocrinol Immunol 3:176–186, 1990.

98. Lee SC, Collins M, Vanguri P, Shin ML. Glutamate differentially inhibits the expression of class II MHC antigens on astrocytes and microglia. J Immunol 148:3391–3397, 1992.

99. Levy RB, Cotterell AH, Jones M, Malek TR. Graft-versus-host reaction-induced autoimmune modulation. I. Donor-recipient genetic disparity and the differential expression of Lyt-2, L3T4, and Ly-6 during acute reactions in the host thymus. J Immunol 140:1717–1725, 1988.

99a. Logan A, Frautschy SA, Gonzalez A-M, Sporn MB, Baird A. Enhanced expression of transforming growth factor β$_1$ in the rat brain after a localized cerebral injury. Brain Res 587:216–225, 1992.

100. Mahaley MS, Brooks WH, Roszman TL, Bigner D, Dudka L, Richardson S. Immunobiology of primary intracranial tumors. Part 1: studies of the cellular and humoral general immune competence of brain-tumor patients. J Neurosurg 46:467–476, 1977.

101. Maimaone D, Gregory S, Arnason BGW, Reder A. Cytokine levels in the cerebrospinal fluid and serum of patients with multiple sclerosis. J Neuroimmunol 32:67–74, 1991.

101a. McKanna JA. Lipocortin 1 immunoreactivity identifies microglia in adult rat brain. J Neurosci Res 36:491–500, 1993.

102. Moench TR, Griffin DE, Obriecht CR, Vaisberg A, Johnson RT. Distribution of measles virus antigen and RNA in acute measles with and without neurologic involvement. J Infect Dis 158:433–442, 1988.

103. Morimoto A, Murakami N, Nakamori T, Sakata Y, Watanabe T. Possible involvement of prostaglandin E in development of ACTH response in rats induced by human recombinant interleukin-1. J Physiol 411:245–256, 1989.

103a. Morgan TE, Nichols NR, Pasinetti GM, Finch CE. TGF-β$_1$ mRNA increases in macrophage microglial cells of the hippocampus in response to deafferentation and kainic acid-induced neurodegeneration. Exp Neurol 120:291–301, 1993.

104. Morganti-Kossman MC, Kossman T, Brandes ME, Mergenhagen SE, Wahl SM. Autocrine and paracrine regulation of astrocyte function by transforming growth factor-β. J Neuroimmunol 39:163–174, 1992.

104a. Mullens L, Marriott DR, Young KA, Tannahill L, Lightman SL, Wilkins GP. Up-regulation of lipocortin-1 and its mRNA in reactive astrocytes in kainate-lesioned rat cerebellum. J Neuroimmunol 50:25–33, 1994.

105. Murakami N, Watanabe T. Activation of ACTH release is mediated by the same molecule as the final mediator, PGE_2 of the febrile response in rats. Brain Res 478:171–174, 1989.

106. Negro A, Tavella A, Facci L, Callegaro L, Skaper SD. Interleukin-1β regulates proenkephalin gene expression in astrocytes cultured from rat cortex. Glia 6:206–212, 1992.

106a. Nottet SLM, Jett M, Flanagan CR, Zhai Q-H, Persidsky Y, Rizzino A, Bernton EW, Genis P, Baldwin T, Schwartz J, LaBenz CJ, Gendelman HE. A regulatory role for astrocytes in HIV-1 encephalitis. J Immunol 154:3567–3581, 1995.

107. Oswald IP, Gazzinelli RT, Sher A, James SL. Il-10 synergizes with Il-4 and transforming growth factor-β to inhibit macrophage cytotoxic activity. J Immunol 148:3578–3582, 1992.

108. Panitch HS, Hirsch RL, Schindler I, Johnson KP. Treatment of multiple sclerosis with gamma interferon: exacerbations associated activation of the immune system. Neurology 37:1097–1102, 1987.

109. Pepinsky RB, Tizard R, Mattaliano RJ, Sinclair LK, Miller GT, Browning JL, Chow EP, Burne C, Huang K-S, Pratt D, Wachter L, Hession C, Frey AZ, Wallner BP. Five distinct calcium- and phospho-lipid binding proteins share homology with lipocortin 1. J Biol Chem 263:10799–10811, 1988.

110. Price RW, Brew B, Sidtis J, Rosenblum M, Scheck AC, Cleary P. The brain of AIDS: central nervous system HIV-1 infection and AIDS dementia complex. Science 239:586–592, 1988.

111. Racke MK, Dhib-Jalbut S, Cannella B, Albert PS, Raine CS, McFarlin DE. Prevention and treatment of chronic relapsing experimental allergic encephalomyelitis by transforming growth factor-β1. J Immunol 146:3012–3017, 1991.

112. Ransohoff RM, Devajyothi C, Estes ML, Babcock G, Rudick RA, Frohman EM, Barna BP. Inteferon-β specifically inhibits interferon-γ-induced class II major histocompatibility complex gene transcription in a human astrocytoma cell line. J Neuroimmunol 33:103–112, 1991.

113. Relton JK, Strijbos PJLM, O'Shaughnessy CT, Carey F, Forder RA, Tilders FJH, Rothwell N. Lipocortin-1 as an endogenous inhibitor of ischemic damage in the rat brain. J Exp Med 174:305–310, 1991.

114. Rivier C, Vale W. Stimulatory effects of interleukin-1 on adrenocorticotropin secretion in the rat: is it modulated by prostagandins? Endocrinology 129:384–388, 1991.

115. Roberge FG, Caspi RR, Nussenblatt RB. Glial retinal Muller cells produce Il-1 activity and have a dual effect on autoimmune T helper lymphocytes. J Immunol 140:2193–2196, 1988.

116. Roberts AB, Sporn MB. Transforming growth factor-β. In: Handbook of Experimental Pharmcology, Vol 95, Peptides, Growth Factors and Their Receptors, MB Sporn, AB Roberts, eds. Springer-Verlag, New York, 1990, pp 419–472.

117. Roszman T, Elliot L, Brooks W. Modulation of T-cell function by gliomas. Immunol Today 12:370–374, 1991.

118. Roszman TL, Carlson SL. Neural-immune interactions: circuits and networks. Prog NeuroEndocrinImmunol 4:69–78, 1991.

119. Russo-Marie F, Duval D. Dexamethasone-induced inhibition of prostagandin production does not result from direct action on phospholipase activities but is mediated through a steroid-inducible factor. Biochem Biophys Acta 712:177–185, 1982.

120. Rutka JT, Rosenblum ML, Stern R, Ralston HJ, Dougherty D, Giblin J, DeArmond S. Isolation and partial purification of growth factors with TGF-like activity from human malignant gliomas. J Neurosurg 71:875–883, 1989.

121. Sakata T, Owagami S, Tsuruta Y, Teraoka H, Hojo K, Suzuki S, Sato K, Suzuki R. The role of

lipocortin I in macrophage-mediated immunosuppression in tumor-bearing mice. J Immunol 145:387–396, 1990.

122. Samuelsson B. Identification of a smooth muscle-stimulating factor in bovine brain. Biochim Biophys Acta 84:218–219, 1964.

123. Schluesener HJ. Transforming growth factor type β_1 and β_2 suppress rat astrocyte autoantigen presentation and antagonize hyperinduction of class II major histocompatibility complex antigen expression by interferon-γ and tumor necrosis factor-α. J Neuroimmunol 27:41–47, 1990.

124. Segre M, Tomei E, Segre D. Cyclophosphamide-induced suppressor cells in mice: suppression of the antibody response in vitro and characterization of the effector cells. Cell Immunol 91:443–448, 1985.

125. Selmaj K, Nowak Z, Tchorzewski H. Interleukin-1 and interleukin-2 production by peripheral blood mononuclear cells in multiple sclerosis patients. Clin Exp Immunol 72:428–433, 1988.

126. Shimizu T, Wolfe LS. Arachidonic acid cascade and signal transduction. J Neurochem 55:1–15, 1990.

127. Siepl C, Bodmer S, Frei K, MacDonald HR, de Martin R, Hofer E, Fontana A. The glioblastoma-derived T cell suppressor factor/transforming growth factor beta-2 inhibits T cell growth without affecting the interaction of interleukin-2 with its receptor. Eur J Immunol 18:593–600, 1988.

128. Smillie F, Peers SH, Elderfield AJ, Bolton C, Flower RJ. Differential regulation by glucocorticoids of intracellular lipocortin I, II and V in rat mixed peritoneal leukocytes. Br J Pharmacol 97:425P, 1989.

129. Sobel RA, Blanchette BW, Bhan AK, Cohen RB. The immunopathology of acute experimental allergic encephalomyelitis. II. Endothelial cell Ia expression increases prior to inflammatory cell infiltration. J Immunol 132:2402–2408, 1984.

130. Steiniger B, van der Meide PH. Rat ependyma and microglial cells express class II MHC antigens after intravenous infusion of recombinant gamma interferon. J Neuroimmunol 19:111–118, 1988.

131. Streilein JW. Immune regulation and the eye: a dangerous compromise. FASEB J 1:199–208, 1987.

132. Streilein JW, Wilbanks GA, Cousins SW. Immunoregulatory mechanisms of the eye. J Neuroimmunol 39:185–200, 1992.

133. Tamashiro VG, Perez HH, Griffin DE. Prospective study of the magnitude and duration of changes in tuberculin reactivity during complicated and uncomplicated measles. Pediatr Infect Dis J 6:451–454, 1987.

134. Taylor AW, Strelein JW, Cousins SW. Identification of alpha-melanocyte stimulating hormone as a potential immunosuppressive factor in aqueous humor. Curr Eye Res 11:1199–1206, 1992.

135. Taylor AW, Streilein JW, Cousins SW. Immunoreactive vasoactive intestinal peptide contributes to the immunosuppressive activity of normal aqueous humor. J Immunol 154:1080–1086, 1994.

136. Tedeschi B, Barrett JN, Keane RW. Astrocytes produce interferon that enhances expression of H-2 antigens on a subpopulation of brain cells. J Cell Biol 102:2244–2253, 1986.

137. Traugott U, Lebond P. Interferon-gamma and Ia antigen are present on astrocytes in active chronic multiple sclerosis. J Neurol Sci 84:257–262, 1988.

138. Tsukada N, Miyagi K, Masuda M, Yanagisawa N, Yone K. Tumor necrosis factor and interleukin-1 in the CSF and sera of patients with multiple sclerosis. J Neurol Sci 102:230–234, 1992.

139. Ueda R, Hirata F, Harashima M, Ishizaka J. Modulation of the biological activities of IgE-binding factors. I. Identification of glycosylation-inhibiting factor as a fragment of lipomodulin. J Immunol 130:878–884, 1983.

140. Uehara A, Sekiya C, Takasugi Y, Namiki M, Arimura A. Indomethacin blocks the anorexic action of interleukin-1. Eur J Pharmacol 170:257–260, 1989.

141. Unsicker K, Flanders KC, Cissel DS, Lafyatis R, Sporn MB. Transforming growth factor beta isoforms in the adult rat central and peripheral nervous system. Neuroscience 44:613–625, 1996.

141a. vander Wal EA, Gómez-Pinilla F, Constam CW. Transforming growth factor-β_1 is in plaques in Alzheimer and Down pathologies. Neuro Report 4:69–72, 1993.

142. Vervliet G, Carton H, Billiau A. Interferon-γ production by peripheral blood leucocytes from patients with multiple sclerosis and other neurological disease. Clin Exp Immunol 59:391–397, 1985.

143. Vervliet G, Carton H, Meulepas E, Billiau A. Interferon production by cultured peripheral blood leucocytes of MS patients. Clin Exp Immunol 58:116–126, 1984.

144. Wahl SM, Allen JB, McCartney-Francis N, Morganti-Kossman MC, Kossmann T, Ellingsworth L, Mai UEH, Mergenhagen SE, Orenstein JM. Macrophage- and astrocyte derived transforming growth factor β as a mediator of central nervous system dysfunction in acquired immune deficiency syndrome. J Exp Med 173:981–991, 1991.

145. Waksman B. Mechanisms in multiple sclerosis. Nature 318:104–105, 1985.

146. Waksman B, Reynolds WE. Multiple sclerosis as a disease of immune regulation. Proc Soc Biol Med USA 175:282–294, 1984.

147. Ward BJ, Griffin DE. Changes in cytokine production after measles virus vaccination: predominant production of Il-4 suggests induction of a Th-2 response. Clin Immunol Immunopathol 67:171–177, 1993.

148. Ward BJ, Johnson RT, Vaisberg A, Jauregui E, Griffin DE. Spontaneous proliferation of peripheral mononuclear cells in natural measles virus infection: identification of dividing cells and correlation with mitogen responsiveness. Clin Immunol Immunopathol 55:315–326, 1990.

149. Ward BJ, Johnson RT, Vaisberg A, Jauregui E, Griffin DE. Cytokine production in vitro and the lymphoproliferative defect of natural measles virus infection. Clin Immunol Immunopathol 61:236–248, 1991.

150. Watanabe Y, Kawade Y. Suppressive effect of mouse interferon-β on gene expression occurring in concanavalin A-stimulated mouse spleen cells. Immunology 64:739–741, 1988.

151. Watanabe T, Morimoto A, Sakata Y, Murakami N. ACTH response induced by interleukin-1 is mediated by CRF secretion stimulated by hypothalamic PGE. Experientia 46:481–484, 1990.

152. Weigensberg M, Morecki S, Weiss L, Fuks Z, Slavin S. Suppression of cell-mediated immune responses after total lymphoid irradiation (TLI). I. Characterization of suppressor cells of the mixed lymphocyte reaction. J Immunol 132:971–975, 1984.

153. Weinberg AD, Whithman R, Swain SL, Morrison WJ, Wyrick G, Hoy C, Vandenbark AA, Offner H. Transforming growth factor-β enhances the in vivo effector function and memory phenotype of antigen-specific T helper cells in experimental autoimmune encephalomyelitis. J Immunol 148:2109–2117, 1992.

154. Wilbanks GA, Streilein JW. Fluids from immune privileged sites endow macrophages with the capacity to induce antigen-specific immune deviation via a mechanism involving transforming growth factor-β. Eur J Immunol 22:1031–1036, 1992.

155. Wiley CA, Johnston RT, Reingold SC. Neurological consequences of immune dysfunction: lessons from HIV infection and multiple sclerosis. J Neuroimmunol 40:115–120, 1992.

156. Wrann M, Bodmer S, de Martin R, Siepl C, Hofer-Warbinek R, Frei K, Hofer E, Fontana A. T-cell suppressor factor from human glioblastoma is a 12.5-kd protein closely related to transforming growth factor-beta. EMBO J 6:1633–1636, 1987.
157. Young HF, Sakalas R, Kaplan AM. Inhibition of cell-mediated immunity in patients with brain tumors. Surg Neurol 5:19–23, 1986.
158. Zuber P, Kuppner MC, de Tribolet N. Transforming growth factor-β2 down-regulates HLA-DR antigen expression on human glioma cells. Eur J Immunol 18:1623–1626, 1988.

18

Immunology of the Eye

SCOTT W. COUSINS
RICHARD D. DIX

The immunologic responses of the eye are nearly as complex and diverse as those of the central nervous system (CNS). Concepts such as immune privilege, blood-tissue barriers, unique anatomy, and regional specialization are especially relevant to ocular immunology. A comprehensive discussion of all the factors that are important to the understanding of ocular immunology is not possible in this chapter. We will therefore focus on a comparison of the major similarities and differences between the immunologic responses of the eye and those of the CNS. In particular, we will discuss the intraocular immune responses, especially those that are particularly relevant to the CNS. For discussions of the immunologic responses that occur within the cornea, orbit, and other extraocular tissues, the reader is directed to other textbooks (71,140a).

The eye was one of the first organs in which the immunologic basis of disease was suspected. Perhaps one of the first accounts of autoimmunity was given in 1583 by Bartisch, who observed blindness in the second eye after severe injury to the first (111). By the mid-nineteenth century, the syndrome of sympathetic ophthalmia (bilateral ocular inflammation following injury to one eye) was well established (58). Subsequent studies in the early twentieth century demonstrated that immunization with homogenates of whole eyes, or a variety of biochemical extracts, produced ocular autoimmune inflammation. By 1977, the first retinal autoantigen, S antigen, was purified (54,174), leading to the identification and characterization of other relevant autoantigens.

Although these observations suggested that the eye is susceptible to immunologic attack, other lines of investigation indicated that the immunology of the eye is different when compared with other body sites. In the late 1800s, observations that certain mucous membrane xenografts could survive within the anterior chamber anticipated the concept of the eye as an immune-privileged site (171). Experiments by Medawar, Billingham, and others demonstrated that the eye is indeed immunologically different; allografts and histoincompatible tumors were found to grow within the anterior chamber of the eye when similar transplants were rejected at other body sites (15). Unfortunately, several of these early investigations incorrectly attributed immune privilege to blockade of the afferent limb of the immune response, mistakenly believing that communication between the eye and the lymphoid system is lacking (15). During the last two decades, however, immune privilege of the anterior chamber of the eye has been carefully reevaluated in the laboratories of Streilein, Niederkorn, Kaplan, Ferguson, and others, and it is now known that privilege is an *active* immunoregulatory process involving unique interactions between the eye and both afferent and efferent limbs of the immune response (36,132,160). Current investigations are oriented towards a better understanding of the precise cellular and biochemical events that take place within the eye to produce a unique immunologic microenvironment.

Basic Science Discoveries

Normal Ocular Immunologic Microenvironment

Anatomic Considerations

Compartments of the eye. Although a detailed review of the anatomy of the eye is beyond the scope of this review, mention of some basic principles is appropriate (41,161). The external structural integrity of the ocular globe is provided by a tough, collagenous tissue, the sclera. The internal structures of the eye are often grouped into two physiologic and functional sections, the anterior segment and posterior segment (Fig. 18-1).

The anterior segment contains the optical components of the eye (lens and cornea) as well as the iris, ciliary body, and outflow channels. In some respects, analogies can be drawn between functions of the anterior segment of the eye and the production and clearance of cerebrospinal fluid (CSF) within the CNS. The anterior segment contains a fluid-filled space, the anterior chamber (AC). Aqueous humor, which is secreted by the nonpigmented epithelium of the cilary body, is a complex biologic fluid that contains numerous growth factors that come into contact with most of the tissues of the anterior segment. The physiologic basis of the regulation of aqueous humor formation has been an important area of study in recent years, and the roles of neural, hormonal, and intracellular regulation have been extensively explored (23). The aqueous humor circulates from behind the lens, around the iris, and exits through the major outflow channel, the trabecular meshwork. The trabecular meshwork empties into the canals of Schlemn and the aqueous veins, all of which ultimately drain into the extraocular venous circulation. Another outflow channel, accounting for 10 to 20% of aqueous humor

Anterior Segment   Posterior Segment

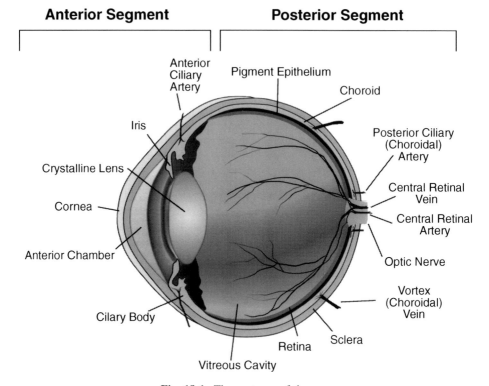

Fig. 18-1. The anatomy of the eye.

clearance, requires the movement of fluid through the ciliary body and through the sclera, ultimately emptying into the orbital extracellular spaces.

The posterior segment contains the vitreous cavity, neurosensory retina, retinal pigment epithelium, and choroid. A large chamber, the vitreous cavity, dominates the innermost aspect of the posterior segment, and this chamber is filled with the vitreous gel. This gel is composed of hyaluronic acid, collagen, and water, and contains small but significant amounts of protein, including immunoregulatory cytokines (35a,85a). The neurosensory retina, which is often considered to be an extension of the CNS, is a three-layered tissue comprised of photoreceptors (rods and cones), an interconnecting (bipolar) layer, and a ganglion cell layer (Fig. 18-2). In addition, several glial cells, including Müller cells and astrocytes, populate the neurosensory retina. The photo-receptors each have a cell body and an outer segment that contains the photodetecting and signal-transducing apparatus of the eye. The outer segments project externally, inserting into a monolayer of supporting epithelium, the retinal pigment epithelium (RPE). Adhesion between these two tissues is based upon physiologic interactions rather than anatomic tight junctions, such that detachment of the neurosensory retina from the RPE can occur, revealing a potential space in which immune responses can take place. It is noteworthy that since the RPE overlies the highly permeable choroidal circulation of the eye to form a blood-ocular barrier, it is analogous to the epithelium of the choroid plexus of the CNS that forms the blood-CSF barrier (79).

The iris, ciliary body, and choroid together comprise the uvea. Conceptually, the anterior and posterior segments are linked together by the uvea, especially by its vasculature, connective tissue, and neuroectodermal derivatives (melanocytes and se-cretory epithelium). The uvea is normally invested with certain populations of leuko-cytes, especially macrophages and dendritic cells, and this tissue is often the site of leukocyte infiltration during inflammation.

Blood supply of the eye. The eye is served by a dual blood supply (41,147) (Fig. 18.1). The retinal circulation is derived from the central retinal artery that enters the eye through the optic nerve; branches of its circulation penetrate into the inner two-thirds of the neurosensory retina, ultimately producing a complex, layered, capillary network with important regional variations. The blood-ocular barrier formed by this vascular system is characterized by nonfenestrated endothelial cells with tight junctions, closely associated with astrocytes and pericytes (Fig. 18-2A) (147). Unfortunately, the ultra-structural and physiologic interactions between these cell types have not received as much attention as in the CNS. Venous drainage is accomplished through the central retinal vein that travels adjacent to the artery.

The second vascular system supplies the uveal tract, the RPE, the outer one-third of the retina, and the anterior segment. This system derives from an orbital arterial system that perforates sclera and sends vessels into the choroid and ciliary body. While the choroid is a complex vascular bed with both high-flow and low-flow vessels, the ultimate microvascular bed is the choriocapillaris. These capillaries form "lobules" that serve localized regions of overlying RPE and retina (Fig. 18-2B). The anterior segment circulation is formed from anterior-extending arterioles of the same vascular bed. The venous circulation exits the eye through the vortex veins, two to five of which perforate the sclera and drain into orbital veins. Although avascular, the lens and cornea are exposed to aqueous humor and tears which supply important nutrients.

Functional Aspects

Blood-ocular barrier to movement of macromolecules. The compartments of the eye (anterior chamber and vitreous cavity), as well as the neurosensory retina, possess a blood-ocular barrier. As with the blood-brain barrier, regional variations in anatomy and physiology are extremely important to its function (79,147). Both physiologically and functionally, the blood-ocular barrier to movement of plasma-derived macro-molecules is quite different when compared with the movement of leukocytes. For example, plasma-derived proteins and intravascularly administered diagnostic dyes are excluded from some of the ocular compartments by the presence of tight junctions between capillary endothelium and the absence of fenestrations (Fig. 18-2).

The blood-ocular barrier to macromolecules is fundamentally different in the neuro-sensory retina as compared to that in the uveal tract. In the retinal circulation, the

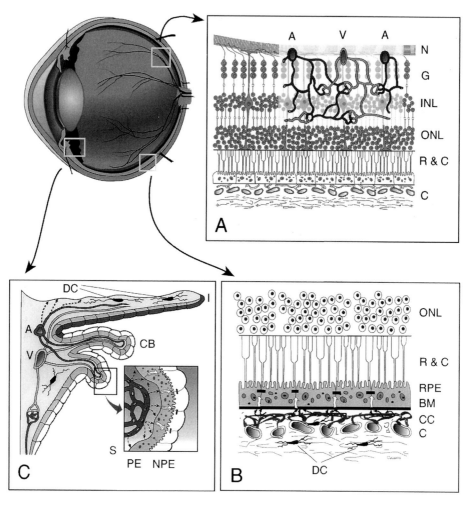

Fig. 18-2. The blood-ocular barriers. A: Barrier of the inner retina. The inner two-thirds of the retina is served by a vascular system similar to the brain, with nonfenestrated capillaries and tight junctions that prevent leakage of macromolecules. Resident antigen-presenting cells or other lymphoid elements have not been observed in this region. However, transmigration of inflammatory cells with perivascular cuffing of the venules (V) can occur during inflammation. The resident glial cells, especially the Müller cell, might be capable of antigen presentation during inflammation. N = nerve fiber layer, G = ganglion cell layer, INL = inner nuclear layer, ONL = outer nuclear layer, R & C = rods and cones, C = choroid. B: Barrier of the outer retina. The rods and cones (R & C) and retinal pigment epithelium (RPE) are served by the choroidal circulation (C). The choriocapillaris (CC), a layer formed by loops of capillaries originating from the choroidal vessels, consists of leaky, fenestrated capillaries. Macromolecules permeate through Bruch's membrane (BM) and between the RPE. Tight junctions at the apex of these cells provide the physiologic barrier. The choroid is richly invested with dendritic cells (DC) and mast cells, and it can become densely infiltrated with lymphocytes during inflammation. The RPE can express cell adhesion molecules during inflammation, perhaps aiding in the transmigration of leukocytes into the retina. ONL = outer nuclear layer. C: Barrier of the anterior uvea. The

blood-ocular barrier exists at the level of tight junctions between adjacent endothelial cells. Retinal pericytes are closely associated with the vascular endothelium. Whether the retinal pericytes are physiologically analogous to the pericytes of the CNS is unknown. In contrast, the vessels of the uveal tract are highly permeable to macromolecules. In the ciliary body, fenestrated capillaries allow relatively high permeability to plasma macromolecules into the interstitial tissue, but a size-dependent concentration gradient is observed; i.e., smaller plasma-derived molecules are present in a higher concentration than are larger molecules (Fig. 18-2C) (189).

The tight junctions between the ciliary pigmented epithelium and nonpigmented epithelium provide a second and more exclusive blood-ocular barrier, preventing interstitial macromolecules from permeating directly through the cilary body into the aqueous humor (Fig. 18-2C). Nevertheless, plasma macromolecules can bypass the nonpigmented epithelium barrier, and via diffusion, they may permeate anteriorly through the uvea to enter the anterior chamber through the anterior iris surface. The vessels of the choriocapillaris are also highly permeable, allowing transudation of most plasma macromolecules into the extravascular spaces. The tight junctions between the RPE probably provide the true physiologic barrier between the choroid and the retina (79,189).

Blood-ocular barrier to migration of leukocytes. One misconception of the blood-ocular barrier is that it presents an absolute barrier to the emigration of leukocytes into the eye. Actually, the normal blood-ocular barrier is relative to and selective of the transmigration of blood-borne leukocytes, implying complicated and regulated physiologic control. Normal ocular tissues, predominantly those of the uveal tract, are richly invested with certain leukocyte subsets, especially macrophages, dendritic cells, and mast cells (108,124). T lymphocytes and B lymphocytes are probably not present within the normal eye, but this issue has not been carefully addressed. Animal studies have shown that macrophages recirculate (158), and a dynamic flux presumably exists, with entry and egress determined by physiologic signals. Since cell transmigration is an

---

leukocytes into the retina. ONL = outer nuclear layer. C: Barrier of the anterior uvea. The anterior uvea (iris and ciliary body) has a complex vascular system. The major arteriole of the iris (A) in the ciliary body stroma gives rise to capillary loops that serve each ciliary body process (CB) and the iris (I), eventually draining into venules (V) that ultimately form sinus-like beds before collecting into the choroidal vortex veins. The stroma is richly invested with macrophages and dendritic cells (DC), many of which are MHC class II positive. Many DC are situated near uveal nerve endings. During inflammation, the stroma can become densely infiltrated with lymphocytes and other inflammatory leukocytes. Inset: Macromolecules freely permeate from leaky, fenestrated capillaries in the stroma (S) of the ciliary body process (although capillaries in the *iris* are nonfenestrated). Macromolecules diffuse between the pigmented epithelial layer (PE) which is anatomically continuous with the RPE. The blood-aqueous barrier is actually formed by tight junctions between the nonpigmented epithelial layer (NPE). During inflammation and after various stimuli, these junctions can uncouple, thereby allowing ready access of blood-derived macromolecules into the aqueous humor. In the normal eye, small amounts of blood proteins can enter into the aqueous humor via diffusion through the iris stroma and anterior iris surface.

active, directive process, the vascular endothelium of the uvea must constitutively express cell adhesion molecules for certain leukocyte subsets (85a), but this expression has not been well characterized (see Chapter 7). The ability of leukocytes to enter the retina through the normal retinal vasculature is also unknown, although transmigration of leukocytes through the retinal vessels, especially the veins, can be observed as an early sign in many experimental models of inflammation (124).

Antigen and leukocyte clearance from the eye. The inner eye does not contain well-developed lymphatics. Rather, the inner eye depends upon the aqueous humor outflow channels for clearance of soluble substances, and endocytosis by trabecular meshwork endothelial cells or macrophages for clearance of particulates. Nevertheless, inoculation of antigen by the AC route results in efficient communication with the systemic immune response (66,181). Intact soluble antigens gain entrance to the venous circulation where they communicate with the spleen. More importantly, antigen-processing by resident macrophages and dendritic cells can occur within the eye, and these cells can recirculate (presumably exiting via the trabecular meshwork) and home to peripheral lymphoid organs (123).

Production of immunosuppressive molecules by ocular tissues. The aqueous humor that fills the AC is actively secreted by the nonpigmented epithelium of the ciliary body, which is analogous to the secretion of CSF by the choroid plexus. Although aqueous humor is relatively protein depleted as compared to serum (about 0.1 to 1% of serum total protein) (41,189), aqueous humor nevertheless contains a complex mixture of biologic factors that are capable of influencing cellular events within the eye. A partial list of these factors is shown in Table 18-1. In particular, transforming growth factor-beta 2 (TGF-β2), a potent cytokine capable of numerous immunoregulatory actions upon local intraocular immune responses, is a constitutive component of aqueous humor and within the anterior uvea (35,77,95). Studies utilizing uveal explants or cultured ciliary body epithelium indicate that the secretory epithelium is probably the source of this TGF-β2 (84). Neuropeptides, presumably released by ocular nerves, have also been detected in aqueous humor (Table 18-1), and they may participate in paracrine interactions with non-neural cells within the AC (168–170). Although less well characterized, the vitreous gel contains molecules similar to those found within the aqueous humor (186).

Immune Privilege of the Eye

Concept of immune privilege. The current concept of immune privilege refers to the phenomenologic observation that tumor implants or allografts survive unexpectedly within an immune-privileged region, while a similar implant or graft is rejected rapidly by immune mechanisms at nonprivileged sites, such as the skin. Like the brain (see Chapters 3 and 19), the eye has also been recognized as an immune-privileged site. For example, when an immunogenic tumor is implanted into a conventional site of a mouse, especially subcutaneously, the tumor will grow for about a week, but it will

Table 18-1 Potential Immunoregulatory Molecules in the Normal Eye

Factor	Location in Eye	Possible Ocular Immunoregulatory Effect
Cytokines		
Transforming growth factor-β	Stroma of ciliary body; vitreous; retina AqH[a] (40–120 pM)	Immunosuppressive Inhibits T-cell proliferation and cytokine production Inhibits macrophage activation and alters macrophage antigen presentation
Neuropeptides		
Substance P	Nerves of anterior segment; retina Aqh (10 pM)	Proinflammatory Chemotactic for macrophage and PMN Enhances neutrophil activation Enhances T-helper/inhibits T-suppressor activation Induces mast cell degranulation
Enkephalins	Retina	Immunosuppressive—inhibits T-cell proliferation
Vasoactive intestinal peptide	Retina; nerves in anterior choroid and ciliary body AqH (10 nM)	Immunosuppressive Modulated lymphocyte homing Inhibits T-cell proliferation and IFN-γ production
Calcitonin gene-related peptide	Nerves of anterior uvea AqH (15–20 pM, increase to 40–45 pM after neural stimulation)	Anti-inflammatory Inhibits oxygen-free radical production Inhibits IFN-γ by T cells
α-melanocyte stimulating hormone	AqH (10–30 pM)	Immunosuppressive Inhibits effects of IL-1 and TNF Inhibits contact hypersensitivity of skin Inhibits PMN migration Inhibits IFN-γ by T cells
Others		
Glucocorticoids	AqH (30 nM)	Immunosuppressive and anti-inflammatory

[a] AqH = Aqueous humor

then be eliminated rapidly by an intense inflammatory response. In contrast, when implanted in the eye, the same tumor will continue to grow without immune rejection (132,160). Ultimately, depending upon the type of tumor, it may grow large enough to extend into the brain or metastasize to other organs, eventually killing the host.

Immune privilege of the anterior chamber. Immune privilege of the eye has been best characterized in the AC, although the vitreious gel appears to function similarly (97). Preliminary results have suggested that the subretinal space may also exhibit immune privilege (96). A wide variety of antigens have been used in studies of immune privilege of the eye, including alloantigens (especially retinal allografts), tumor antigens, haptens, soluble proteins, autoantigens, bacteria, and viruses (160). Collectively, these studies have shown that immune privilege of the eye is an active immunoregulatory process that operates on both the *afferent* (or immunization) and *efferent* (or elicitation) limbs of the ocular immune response. While recent data suggest that immune privilege contributes to a partial blockade of efferent limb elicitation (18,36,38), most studies have focused on the effects of ocular immunization on the afferent limb, which produces a deviant systemic immune response following immunization by the AC route.

Immunization of rats (101), mice (133), and nonhuman primates (adult cynomologus monkeys) (61) via AC injection has been shown to produce an altered form of systemic immunity to that antigen when compared to the immune response following conventional cutaneous immunization. This unique immune response, termed *anterior chamber-associated immune deviation* or *ACAID* (132a), is characterized by a selective reduction of antigen-specific delayed hypersensitivity (DH) responses (160) and a selective diminished production of immunoglobulin (Ig)G2 (182), the complement-fixing IgG isotype in the mouse. In sharp contrast, the production of antigen-specific cytotoxic T-cell precursors and other IgG isotypes continues at levels similar to those found following conventional immunization (160). Hallmark to ACAID is the production of effector suppressor T cells that down-regulate DH responses to the immunizing antigen at *all* body sites (160). Overall, this pattern of immunity results in the production of a noninflammatory response to the antigen, thereby imparting onto the eye a powerful defensive mechanism that protects the delicate visual structures of the organ from destructive immune-mediated inflammation. ACAID may also contribute to organ-specific immunologic tolerance, since immunization by the AC route has been shown to influence the immune response to ocular autoantigens (81). It must be emphasized, however, that one distinct disadvantage to ACAID would be a diminished immune effector response to pathogens or tumors that might invade the eye.

ACAID induction requires participation of both the antigen-containing eye and the spleen for at least 4 to 5 days after ocular immunization (164). An explanation for the requirement of a "splenic-cameral axis" has been suggested by Wilbanks, Mammolenti, and Streilein (180). These investigators demonstrated that the ACAID-inducing signal (at least for soluble protein antigens) originates in the eye, exits the eye, enters the circulation, and ultimately homes to the spleen where the activation of antigen-specific suppressor T cells takes place. The courier for this signal appears to be a macrophage-like cell that must be exposed to the antigen while within the specialized immunosuppressive microenvironment of the eye. Thus, the ACAID-inducing signal is the direct result of immunosuppressive factors found within the aqueous humor, especially TGF-β (183), that act upon the local antigen-presenting cells (mostly macrophages) that are resident in the iris and ciliary body. These aqueous humor/TGF-β-exposed macrophages exit the eye after antigen challenge and travel to the spleen to induce the activation of antigen-specific suppressor T cells. The significance of the selective regulation of IgG2 during ACAID is less certain, but it might be related to the activation of suppressor T cells that are directed toward B-cell activities.

Diminished expression of ocular immune effectors in the anterior chamber. In addition to ACAID, the immunologic microenvironment of the AC appears to inhibit locally the elicitation and function of T cell–mediated effector responses, providing yet another layer of protection against immune-mediated inflammation. For example, the adoptive transfer of primed lymphocytes plus antigen-presenting cells into the AC fails to produce a clinically significant inflammatory response (36,38). To explain these observations, several laboratories have analyzed the immunoregulatory capacity of fluids and cells obtained from the AC for their ability to inhibit lymphocyte functions in vitro or effector functions in vivo. Results have shown that normal aqueous humor is a potent inhibitor of certain in vitro assays of lymphocyte function, including antigen-, mitogen-, and cytokine-induced lymphocyte proliferation (100), and inhibits the production of various T cell–derived cytokines (35,77), especially interferon-gamma (IFN-γ) (168), an important mediator of T cell–mediated inflammation. Aqueous humor also prevents the maturation of effector cytotoxic T cells from the precursor T cells (112). Finally, in addition to its in vitro activities, aqueous humor–derived factors can block the function of T-cell effectors in vivo at extraocular sites. Lymphocytes that have been preincubated in aqueous humor are rendered incapable of eliciting cutaneous DH responses when injected into receptive sites (37). Analysis of the cytokines present in aqueous humor has revealed that TGF-β accounts for a major portion of this functional immunosuppressive activity (37). Furthermore, preliminary data indicate that several immunosuppressive neuropeptides, especially vasoactive intestinal peptide and alpha-melanocyte-stimulating hormone, may also contribute to the immunosuppressive properties of aqueous humor (169).

Ocular Immunologic Microenvironment during Inflammation

Loss of Immune Privilege: Physiologic Changes Associated with Inflammation

Immune privilege of the eye and the ocular immunosuppressive microenvironment are powerful protectors of the eye from inflammatory attack. Nevertheless, they can be modified and overcome by a number of environmental, clinical, and regulatory stimuli, thereby predisposing the eye to inflammation. Traditionally, trauma to the eye has been associated with initiation of ocular inflammation, but the underlying mechanism has yet to be determined. Disruption of the blood-ocular barrier is suspected to be one specific mechanism whereby the immunosuppressive microenvironment of the eye is abrogated. For example, the extremely large, blood-borne protease inhibitor, α_2-macroglobulin, is effectively excluded from aqueous humor by the normal blood-ocular barrier. However, high concentrations of α_2-macroglobulin can be found in the aqueous humor of the eye with breakdown of the blood-ocular barrier (189). α_2-macroglobulin not only transports bioactive interleukin 1 (IL-1) into the eye (thereby promoting inflammation), but α_2-macroglobulin also binds to and neutralizes

TGF-β produced within the eye (thereby preventing local immunosuppression) (94). The presence of persistently altered permeability may therefore indicate that the ocular microenvironment has oriented itself towards a proinflammatory mode, perhaps causing the eye to be at greater risk for recurrent inflammation (167). The influence of other immunoregulatory stimuli in the abrogation of the immunosuppressive microenvironment, such as ocular surgery (4), bacterial toxins (69), exposure to different wavelengths of light (65), and local production of proinflammatory cytokines (162), have also received attention. It appears, however, that the immunologic features that mediate ACAID might be regulated differently from those that regulate effector blockade.

Immunopathogenic Mechanisms in Ocular Inflammation

Role of antibody and B lymphocytes. Traditionally, antibody–antigen interactions have been considered important triggers for ocular inflammation, although antibody-induced phagocytosis or complement-mediated lysis of microorganisms and/or virus-infected cells can occur in the absence of overt inflammation. The ocular deposition of circulating immune complexes (IC) of serum origin probably does not serve as an important stimulus for ocular inflammation (135). Even though some animal models producing intravascular soluble IC overload (e.g., serum sickness) can induce ocular inflammatory manifestations (185), this process is not believed to participate routinely in human ocular inflammation. In contrast, the local formation of IC *within* the eye is thought to be an important stimulus for inflammation. IC formation and concomitant complement activation can induce severe inflammatory reactions (e.g., Arthus reaction) (93) within the ocular compartment under a variety of experimental conditions, including those using autoantigens, protein antigens, and bacterial antigens (3,39,75, 119,120).

Immunoglobulins can be detected within ocular fluids, especially within aqueous humor and vitreous fluid during the course of uveitis or retinitis caused by infectious microorganisms (12,60,104,106,175). The immunoglobulins may originate from one of two sources. They may be of systemic (serum) origin due to compromise of the blood-ocular barrier. Alternatively, in a fashion analogous to intrathecal synthesis within the CNS, immunoglobulins may be synthesized locally within the eye by infiltrating B cells (see Chapter 7). The most common method used to differentiate between local versus systemic origination of intraocular immunoglobulin involves calculation of the Goldmann-Witmer coefficient (12,75a,184), which is generated by comparison of the intraocular fluid to serum ratio of the immunoglobulin in question to the intraocular fluid to serum ratio of total immunoglobulin. Theoretically, a coefficient above 1.0 indicates a local production of immunoglobulins within the eye. This method for demonstrating local intraocular IgG production has been used to assist in the clinical diagnosis of ocular infections with *Toxoplasma gondii,* herpes simplex virus type 1 (HSV-1), varicella-zoster virus, cytomegalovirus (CMV), and Epstein-Barr virus (12,105,106,118,139,166). A method used to quantitate intra-blood-brain barrier synthesis of human immunodeficiency virus type 1 (HIV-1) IgG in AIDS patients with neurologic disease (148) has also been used successfully to demonstrate intraocular HIV-1-specific IgG synthesis during AIDS-related retinitis (53).

More direct measures of intraocular immunoglobulin synthesis have also been described. For example, B-cell and plasma cell infiltrates predominate in certain forms of uveitis, especially in a form of uveitis known as *Fuchs heterochromic iridocyclitis* (130,116a). Oligoclonal bands, similar to those found within the CSF, have been identified in aqueous humor obtained from these eyes. In addition, antigen-specific B cells have been identified and enumerated from ocular tissues in animal models for immunogenic inflammation (130).

Role of cellular immunity: T lymphocytes. As has been demonstrated in the CNS, a role for T lymphocytes in the initiation and/or maintenance of inflammation has been suspected for both infectious diseases and autoimmune diseases of the eye (35a,85a). A detailed discussion of this topic is beyond the scope of this chapter, but certain general principles have emerged. T lymphocytes have been detected in ocular tissues of experimental models for infectious and immunogenic inflammation (135,145), as well as in infiltrates recovered from human eyes with uveitis and various infections (32,102). In addition, intraocular T-cell activation, as detected by DNA synthesis or IL-2 receptor expression by ocular infiltrating T cells, has been shown to occur in some cases (32,102). Recent studies have begun to explore the spectrum of cytokines produced by T cells within the eye during inflammation, and preliminary results suggest that IL-2 and IFN-γ can be detected in some animal models (31) or in some clinical situations (90,126). T cells have also been shown to play a significant role in the evolution of autoimmune diseases of the eye. Experimental autoimmune uveitis (EAU), the classic animal model for ocular T cell–mediated autoimmune disease, is discussed in detail in a later section. Immunosuppressive therapy with cyclosporine A has been shown to be effective in some T-cell dependent animal models as well as in selected cases of human uveitis (134,135).

During ocular infections, especially those caused by viruses, T cells are critically important in providing protection against spread of infection, in regulating the severity of the inflammatory response to infection, and in assisting with the eventual clearance of the infectious agent. Experimental animal models have provided much of our knowledge regarding the role of T cells during retinitis of virus origin in both immunocompetent and immunosuppressed hosts. The role of T cells in the pathogenesis of ocular virus infections has been demonstrated in two animal models for retinal infections, experimental HSV-1 retinitis and experimental murine CMV retinitis, both of which are discussed in later sections.

Other leukocytes. Granulocytes, especially polymorphonuclear leukocytes (PMN), are actively involved in animal models for immune-associated inflammation and ocular infection (35a). For example, PMN infiltrates often predominate in the early phases of acute T cell–mediated immune lesions, especially during T cell–mediated DH reactions in the eye and during T cell–mediated autoimmune inflammation. PMN predominate during virus infections of the eye as well. Thus, at least in animal models of ocular disease, the histologic presence of PMN appears to be a general characteristic of inflammation, irrespective of whether the trigger is immune mediated or of infectious origin (77). PMN-derived mediators, especially reactive oxygen intermediates, have been implicated as the major effector molecules in several animal models (145). Eosinophils can predominate the intraocular infiltrate during parasitic infections of the eye, especially acute endophthalmitis due to toxocariasis (78), and they participate in certain forms of presumed T cell–mediated inflammations of the eye (135). Macrophages are also extremely important effector cells in ocular inflammation. They are often detected during acute ocular infections or immunogenic inflammation, even if other cell types such are neutrophils are more numerous. Macrophage-derived cytokines have been suspected to contribute significantly to the amplification of inflammation (45). Natural killer (NK) cells and other related large, granular lymphocytic cells are also believed to participate in virus infections, but their precise roles have not been well characterized.

Animal Models and Human Disease Relevance

Our understanding of the immunopathogenic mechanisms that operate during the evolution of various ocular diseases in humans has been enhanced significantly by the use of experimental animal model systems. In the following sections, we summarize three experimental animal model systems that have been used to investigate the pathogenesis of ocular diseases in humans that have CNS counterparts: *(1)* autoimmune inflammation of the retina; *(2)* virus-induced retinitis in the immunocompetent host; and *(3)* virus infection of the retina during immunosuppression.

Experimental Autoimmune Uveitis

Uveitis comprises a diverse group of intraocular inflammations that represents a major cause of visual impairment, affecting approximately 10% of visually handicapped persons in the United States. Although the precise etiology of most forms of uveitis is unknown, T cell–mediated autoimmune processes are thought to play a major role in the pathogenesis of certain types of uveitis, especially sympathetic ophthalmia. The best-characterized model for autoimmune ocular inflammation is an animal model for retinal inflammation, experimental autoimmune uveitis (EAU) (68). When compared with human chorioretinitis, however, differences in histopathology, time course, and other features are apparent, raising concerns about the applicability of EAU to human disease. However, until better animal model systems are developed, EAU remains the best model for the study of human intraocular inflammation.

EAU closely resembles a well-characterized T cell–mediated autoimmune disease of the CNS, experimental allergic encephalomyelitis (EAE) (see Chapter 21). EAU is induced by immunization with purified retinal proteins or their peptide fragments which have been emulsified in complete Freund's adjuvant. The most common protein used is retinal soluble protein, or S antigen, a 48,000-kilodalton intracellular protein found in rod outer segments and the pineal gland (17,174). S antigen is probably identical to the membrane-bound photoreceptor, arrestin (143). In addition, a variety of other autoantigens have been purified, including interphotoreceptor retinol binding protein (IRBP) (70), rhodopsin (121), phosducin (57), recoverin (76), and several poorly characterized but highly pathogenic RPE-associated proteins (21,22,109). Synthetic peptides made from these molecules have allowed identification of highly pathogenic epitopes within the whole antigen (1,55,56,63,153,165), some of which are highly uveitogenic, but not necessarily stimulatory to T cells in vitro (110). Of clinical interest is the finding that specific uveitopathogenic regions of S antigen share sequence homology with a variety of peptides derived from various microorganisms (see Molecular Mimicry below).

Models of EAU have been developed in guinea pigs, rats, rabbits, mice, and nonhuman primates, although the uveitogenic responses are varied, suggesting a role for host genetics in disease pathogenesis. Some strains of rats, such as Lewis and PVG, are more susceptible to EAU than other strains (26). In mice, EAU develops following immunization with IRBP (27); surprisingly, S antigen is poorly uveitogenic in this species and fails to induce EAU. While genetic predisposition clearly contributes to the course of EAU, the requirement for genetic predisposition to the disease process remains unknown. Moreover, the observation that PVG rats are highly susceptible to EAU, but not susceptible to EAE (31), suggests that genetic predispositions are not always the same in these diseases, despite their similar immunopathologic features (24).

During early stages of EAU, large numbers of CD4+ T cells infiltrate the retina (29). This is followed by the irreversible destruction of photoreceptor cells and a general loss of retinal architecture, possibly due to DH and/or cytotoxic T-cell activities (125). That CD4+ T cells are the primary mediators of disease was shown initially by adoptive transfer studies in which naive Lewis rats that received antigen-activated CD4+ T cells developed uveitis (28). Uveitis in rats can also be inhibited by anti-Ia or anti-CD4+ antibodies (5,177,146). In contrast, the precise role of CD8+ T cells in the immunopathologic process is not as well defined. Increased numbers of CD8+ T cells appear within the retina at later stages of EAU, an observation suggesting that these cells can down-regulate the disease process (29). However, no change in the course of uveitis is seen in Lewis rats treated with anti-CD8+ antibodies before EAU induction, which suggests that CD8+ T cells are not important in regulating EAU (25). Mast cells, however, may play a role in the pathogenesis of EAU, through direct enhancement of inflammation and/or through facilitation of breakdown of the blood-ocular barrier at the retina (113,116). While both EAU and EAE are clearly mediated by cellular immunity, a role for humoral immunity has also been proposed (42,43).

An evaluation of lymphokines in the pathogenesis of EAU has received considerable attention in recent years (16,30,137). A time-course study (148a) of lymphokine mRNA's expressed during the development and resolution of EAU in mice immunized with IRBP revealed abundant amounts of IL-2 and IFN-γ mRNA in retinas recovered 14 and 21 days after immunization. In contrast, retinas recovered 28 and 35 days after immunization expressed high amounts of mRNA for IL-4 and IL-10. Acute-stage EAU was therefore correlated with the presence of Th1-type lymphokines, whereas resolution of the disease was associated with Th2-type lymphokines. Thus, Th2-type lymphokines might serve as regulatory cells capable of conferring protection from disease, and direct enhancement of the Th2 arm of the immune response might represent a strategy for immunotherapy of ocular autoimmune disease (26a).

Acute Retinal Necrosis

Since the retina represents an extension of the brain, it is not surprising that herpesviruses, long associated with neurological diseases, have been identified as the etiologic agents responsible for a variety of retinal diseases. One such example is HSV-1. While recognized for years as the cause of a potentially life-threatening acute hemorrhagic necrotizing encephalitis in immunocompetent adults (131,178), HSV-1 also has been identified as a possible etiologic agent for a sight-threatening acute hemorrhagic necrotizing retinitis termed *acute retinal necrosis* (ARN) (44,59,115). Clinically, ARN usually occurs in otherwise healthy individuals with the sudden onset of diffuse inflammation, retinal vasculitis, necrotizing retinitis, vitritis, and retinal detachment, all of which often lead to blindness (40,67). Histopathologic features include full-thickness retinal necrosis, arteritis, inflammatory infiltrates consisting of macrophages, lymphocytes, and PMNs, and occasional retinal cells with intranuclear inclusions (40). The disease is unilateral in most cases. Serologic studies have suggested that ARN originates in some patients from recurrent HSV-1 infection, while other cases appear to be due to primary infection (115,117).

The precise pathway whereby HSV-1 invades the retina to produce disease remains unknown. CNS changes may accompany the illness, but surprisingly, in the absence of clinical neurologic disease. CSF recovered from ARN patients may demonstrate a mononuclear pleocytosis and elevated protein levels (115,142,150,159). Antibody to HSV-1 has also been detected in the CSF of some ARN patients (62). Finally, magnetic resonance imaging analysis of the brain of an ARN patient who displayed normal signs upon neurologic examination revealed abnormalities in the regions of the optic tracts and lateral geniculate ganglia (115). Taken together, these findings are consistent with a concomitant subclinical encephalitis during ARN.

Studies utilizing the von Szily animal model for primary HSV-1 retinitis in rabbits (173) and mice (179) indicate that this model shares a number of features with ARN. Among the most intriguing similarities between the animal model and ARN include the development of unilateral retinitis and subclinical encephalitis associated with optic nerve, optic tract, and lateral geniculate ganglia involvement. In the mouse model, inoculation of HSV-1 (KOS strain) into the AC of one eye of a euthymic BALB/c mouse produces a necrotizing retinitis in the uninoculated contralateral eye within 7 to 10 days of infection (179). In sharp contrast, the infected eye appears to be protected from fulminant necrosis, although significant retinal damage does occur as determined by abnormal retinal electrophysiology and other findings (80). Infectious virus can also be recovered from brain tissue in the absence of detectable clinical encephalitis with peak virus titers found on day 5 to 7 postinfection (9). Virus spread from the inoculated eye to the CNS appears to occur via parasympathetic fibers of the oculomotor nerve that supply the iris and ciliary body (9,122,172). Subsequent virus spread within the brain appears to be limited to nuclei of the visual system and the suprachiasmatic area of the hypothalamus, with virus ultimately reaching the contralateral eye from the brain via retrograde axonal transport through the optic nerve (172). Thus, virus spread apparently occurs by neural routes in this animal model rather than by hematogenous ones. One limitation of this animal model of ARN, however, is its apparent virus strain specificity; some HSV-1 strains other than KOS (85,89,92), including a clinical isolate from an ARN patient (51), produce not only bilateral retinitis, but also clinical encephalitis and death following unilateral AC inoculation.

The retinal disease that develops in the contralateral eye of BALB/c mice inoculated intracamerally with HSV-1 (KOS) presents with several unique pathophysiologic features. Retinitis begins with the focal expression of virus genes and virus-induced antigens on infected ganglion cells and/or Müller cells of the retina, followed shortly thereafter by infiltration of PMN and mononuclear leukocytes into the retina. Clinical examination of mouse eyes at this early stage of retinitis resembles findings similar to those associated with human ARN (34). Approximately 3 days after the onset of retinitis, the abrupt appearance of retinal necrosis occurs in association with rapid loss of all retinal architecture. Over time, the inflammation subsides, ultimately leaving a fibroproliferative scar to replace the retinal tissue.

In terms of the pathophysiology of retinal disease in the contralateral eye, the relative contributions of virus replication and host cell infection versus the specific immune response to virus antigens have been extremely difficult to ascertain. This difficulty arises from the inherent complexity of the animal model which involves virus replication at several sites and virus spread over time (days) from the inoculated eye, through the CNS, to the contralateral eye where retinal disease ultimately occurs. Nevertheless, several studies have suggested a role for virus-specific immune responses as mediators of immunopathology during evolution of retinal disease in the contralateral eye (10,11,19,163,187). On the other hand, a role for virus replication in the development of retinal damage has been suggested by studies in athymic nude mice (6). These animals develop bilateral retinal necrosis, although some of the histopathologic features of disease in athymic mice suggest a slower and less explosive course than that observed in euthymic animals. The mechanism(s) whereby retinal necrosis develops remains controversial, although immunopathogenic mechanisms, vascular occlusion, and anatomic factors (schisis) have been implicated (33,47).

In addition to its contribution to retinal injury, the immune system may also regulate the spread of virus from the inoculated eye, into and through the CNS, and into the contralateral eye. Intravenous administration of HSV-1-specific, in vitro-activated, cytotoxic T lymphocytes prior to ocular inoculation apparently limits the spread of virus and protects the animals from contralateral retinitis (12,188). In contrast, a possible protective role for antibody remains unclear. Passive studies using hyperimmune HSV-1 rabbit serum have suggested that neutralizing antibody fails to prevent virus spread and does not influence the development of contralateral retinitis (46); however, protection has been achieved in similar passive transfer studies using a monoclonal antibody to an individual HSV-1-specific glycoprotein (5a).

While immune responses may regulate virus spread in this animal model, immune privilege also appears to facilitate virus spread. Following AC inoculation, BALB/c mice fail to mount a vigorous DH response to HSV-1 due to the development of virus-induced ACAID (161). Consequently, complete and effective maturation of cytotoxic T cells fails to occur within the inoculated eye due to the absence of T-cell help. Without localized HSV-1-specific DH and cytotoxic T-cell responses to contain virus infection within the inoculated eye, virus escapes into the brain, replicates, and eventually invades the contralateral retina. However, a different outcome is observed in mouse strains genetically resistant to HSV-1-induced ACAID, as occurs in HSV-1 (KOS)-infected C57BL/6 mice (103). In these animals, a vigorous DH reaction to HSV-1 is associated with reduced virus spread and the absence of contralateral retinitis. Whether ACAID plays a role in the pathogenesis of ARN in humans remains to be shown.

Cytomegalovirus Retinitis

While CMV has been recognized to infect the brain and spinal cord of persons immunosuppressed by HIV-1 infection and to contribute significantly to neurologic disease during AIDS (31a,47) (see Chapter 22), the virus also produces a sight-threatening retinitis in approximately 40% of the AIDS patient population (87,189a). Indeed, CMV retinitis has become the most common and significant infectious ocular disease associated with HIV-1-induced immunosuppression. It is noteworthy that simultaneous infection of the retina and brain has been documented in some AIDS patients (53,140), although a direct correlation between CMV retinitis and CMV encephalitis remains uncertain (64).

CMV infection of the retina presents clinically as white granular foci of infection usually adjacent to retinal vessels, an observation consistent with hematogenous spread of the virus from extraocular reservoirs of virus infection within the body. The lesions gradually increase in size over weeks to months and may be accompanied by hemorrhage. Histopathologically, CMV produces a full-thickness retinal necrosis associated with abrupt transition zones between areas of necrotic tissue and areas of less-involved retina. A granulomatous choroiditis is often noted subjacent to areas of retinitis. In addition, cytomegalic intranuclear inclusions (cytomegalocytes), which are pathognomonic for CMV infection, are found throughout the infected retinal tissue. A neutrophilic infiltrate is also associated with areas of CMV retinitis during AIDS. Finally, the virus may invade glial cells in the optic nerve.

Unlike HSV-1 (which can induce disease in a variety of animal hosts), human CMV is highly species-specific and fails to replicate in experimental animals and induce typical cytomegalic disease. For this reason, several laboratories have turned to murine CMV (MCMV), a mouse virus related to human CMV in terms of structure, replication scheme, and tropisms (86,124a), to study the virologic and immunologic factors that contribute to the pathogenesis of CMV retinitis in humans. Attempts to induce MCMV retinitis in immunocompetent BALB/c mice by either systemic or intraperitoneal inoculation routes have generally failed to produce characteristic retinal infection (13,14,73,83). While direct intraocular injections into the AC or vitreous cavity of euthymic BALB/c mice succeeded in producing focal retinal necrosis in a small percentage of animals, the characteristic histopathologic features observed during human CMV retinitis were not reproduced (88,144,149). However, ocular infection by subretinal (or supraciliary) injection of MCMV (7) was subsequently found to produce a necrotizing retinitis in both immunocompetent and immunosuppressed BALB/c mice with histopathologic features nearly identical to those observed during AIDS-associated CMV retinitis, i.e., full-thickness retinal necrosis accompanied by virus-induced inclusions and cytomegalocytes in the neurosensory retina and RPE; retinal inflammatory infiltrates consisting predominantly of neutrophils; hemorrhage; and abrupt transition zones between areas of involved and uninvolved retina (138).

Subsequent work with this murine model of CMV retinitis demonstrated that immunosuppression with corticosteroids increases the susceptibility of BALB/c mice to MCMV necrotizing retinitis; typical retinitis developed in animals inoculated by the subretinal route, despite the use of a smaller input dose of virus (8). The efficacy of the subretinal route of inoculation in this animal model is unclear, but it may relate to the role of the RPE as the initial target for MCMV infection during the evolution of disease (7). In addition, studies to explore the protective role of T-cell responses suggest that MCMV retinitis readily develops in animals immunosuppressed by depletion of T cells using cytotoxic antibodies specific for CD4+ or CD8+ subsets (8). Depletion of the CD8+ subset alone, but not of the CD4+ subset alone, was found to be nearly as effective in allowing MCMV retinitis as depletion of both subsets together or nonspecific immunosuppression using steroids. These findings suggest that the CD8+ T cell subset may play an important role in preventing ocular CMV infection in immunosuppressed patients.

Although MCMV retinitis develops in BALB/c mice treated with corticosteroids and/or cytotoxic antibodies to CD4+ and CD8+ T cells, these immunosuppressive protocols do not duplicate the unique complexity of immunosuppression achieved by HIV-1 during the evolution of AIDS. We have therefore attempted to induce MCMV retinitis in mice with murine AIDS (MAIDS), a progressive immunodeficiency syndrome produced by a mixture of murine leukemia viruses (LP-BM5) (128). Many features of MAIDS resemble those observed in individuals infected with HIV-1, including generalized persistent lymphadenopathy, early polyclonal activation of B cells, alterations in cytokine profiles, impairment of T-cell function, increased susceptibility to opportunistic infections, and the development of B-cell lymphomas during late-stage disease (74,82,107,127–129). Results have shown that adult C57BL/6 mice immunosuppressed by murine retrovirus infection exhibit increased susceptibility to MCMV retinitis (49). Moreover, the necrotizing retinitis that develops in MAIDS animals infected with MCMV by subretinal injection has histopathologic features similar to those of AIDS-related CMV retinitis in humans. MAIDS may therefore serve as a useful experimental animal model for investigating several aspects of CMV retinitis in AIDS patients, especially those which relate to pathogenesis of the disease in a setting of retrovirus-induced immunosuppression and immune-based therapeutic strategies (48,50,50a).

Topics of Speculation and Conclusions

Duality of Inflammation: Infection vs. Immunity

Inflammation can be triggered independently by one of at least three initiating mechanisms: infection (i.e., colonization and replication of a microorganism), immune response, and injury. It is noteworthy that inflammation can be triggered by infection even without an immune response. In both the eye and the CNS, the relative contributions to disease of two of these trigger mechanisms, infection and immune response, is often difficult to discern. Differentiation between these two mechanisms is of particular importance in clinical situations, since the rapidity with which devastating tissue destruction takes place often demands rapid institution of effective therapy. For example, both the retina and the brain are susceptible to infection with herpesviruses. Whether treatment should include antiviral therapy to combat virus replication, or immunosuppressive therapy to reduce inflammation, or a combination of both, may be critical to the final clinical outcome. For example, clinical observations (47,141,156) and experimental animal models of disease (2,20,86,91) have implicated a virus-specific T-cell response as a mediator of immunopathology during herpes simplex encephalitis. At the present time, however, the debate over the choice and timing of anti-infection therapy versus immunosuppressive therapy to treat many ocular and CNS infections remains unresolved and controversial.

Immune privilege within the microenvironments of the eye and CNS might also suppress certain aspects of protective immune therapy, allowing the spread of infection and thereby exacerbating the clinical course. This issue is complicated further by microorganisms that are capable of establishing latent or chronic infections. While many viruses are capable of latent infections within the CNS (98), latent virus infection of the retina remains an area of controversy. However, *Toxoplasma* retinitis in the immunocompetent host is thought to originate from reactivation of encysted organisms that remain in a latent form within the retinal tissues following primary infection, possibly for the lifetime of the individual. The factors that allow reactivation of *Toxoplasma* organisms in the ocular compartment of a small percentage of healthy persons are unknown, but they may involve breakdown of immune privilege.

Infection in the Immunosuppressed Host

Impairment of cell-mediated immunity allows for the development of a variety of unique ocular diseases produced by opportunistic microorganisms, many of which also infect the CNS. For example, patients with AIDS often experience CMV retinitis (see above), ocular toxoplasmosis, and herpes zoster ophthalmicus (87). Surprisingly, despite the high incidence of mucocutaneous disease caused by HSV-1 or *Candida albicans* in this patient population, individuals with AIDS seldom suffer from HSV-1 keratitis, HSV-1 retinitis, or *Candida* chorioretinitis. The reason(s) for the seemingly selective nature of the eye to some, but not all, opportunistic microorganisms during AIDS is unknown, but it may be related to issues involving mechanisms of pathogen spread from extraocular sites into the eye. In addition, an understanding of the unique immunologic changes that may occur within the ocular microenvironment during retrovirus-induced immunosuppression, as compared with those induced by immunosuppressive drugs or lymphomas, has received little attention. The murine model for retrovirus-induced immunosuppression described above (i.e., MAIDS) may prove to be useful for such investigations. Finally, the effect of HIV-1 itself on the retina, either through direct infection or through the production of neurotoxic molecules similar to those that have been associated with the development of AIDS dementia complex in the CNS (157), have not yet been fully explored.

Molecular Mimicry

Autoimmunity may play an important role in the pathogenesis of inflammatory ocular diseases. One mechanism whereby autoimmunity to self-antigens in the eye or CNS might be triggered is through molecular mimicry, the immunologic cross-reaction between epitopes of an unrelated foreign antigen and self-epitopes with similar structures (136). Theoretically, these epitopes would be similar enough to stimulate an immune response, but different enough to cause a breakdown of immunologic tolerance. Foreign antigens, such as those present within yeast, viruses, or bacteria, would elicit the formation of antibodies or effector lymphocytes, which in turn would react with similar epitopes of a self-antigen. A dynamic process would then be initiated, causing tissue injury by an autoimmune response that would induce additional lymphocyte responses directed at more self-antigen. Thus, the process would not require either the ongoing replication of a pathogen or the continuous presence of the immunogen (51).

Evidence for molecular mimicry was first demonstrated in the eye experimentally when it was found that the primary amino acid sequence of a variety of foreign antigens (including those of baker's yeast histone, *E. coli,* Group A streptococcus, hepatitis B virus, and certain murine and primate retroviruses) showed sequence homology to a uveitopathogenic site of the ocular autoantigen, S antigen (55,114,152,154,155). Immunization of Lewis rats with crude extracts prepared from these organisms, or synthetic peptides corresponding to the homologous sequences, induced retinal inflammation. In addition, T cells isolated from these rats with foreign substances cross-reacted with autoreactive T cells, thus providing evidence for molecular mimicry between self and non-self proteins (152,154). Molecular mimicry has been implicated in the pathogenesis of EAE, since many viruses such as measles and the coronavirus JHM have been found to induce sensitivity to myelin basic protein (99,176), and homologous sequences have been identified between virus peptides and myelin basic protein (72). Of interest, however, has been the finding that some proteins that share primary amino acid sequence homology with S antigen are not necessarily uveitogenic in animals (55), which suggests that the mechanisms whereby molecular mimicry operates may be more complex than originally thought. At present, there is no definitive clinical evidence to suggest that molecular mimicry contributes to autoimmune diseases of the human eye.

Role of Immune Privilege in Disease Therapeutics

The reason(s) for the existence of immune privilege is controversial. Is it an immunologic side-effect or does it play a vital role in maintenance of tolerance and protection from organ-specific inflammation? Whatever the reason(s), knowledge gleaned from studies of the immunologic mechanisms of immune privilege may provide important information relevant to the development of novel therapeutic strategies. In fact, experiments have already revealed that the induction of ACAID via a single injection of S antigen or IRBP, prior to cutaneous immunization with uveitogenic doses of these autoantigens, successfully suppresses the subsequent expression of autoantigen-specific DH responses, leading to a reduction in the incidence and intensity of EAU (81). Furthermore, if the crucial role of TGF-β on macrophages during ACAID induction (183) is correct, this observation offers a potential mechanism for the generation of macrophages capable of inducing antigen-specific suppressor T cells, but without the necessity of AC inoculation. Thus, in vitro exposure of macrophages plus antigen to TGF-β would be predicted to alter the capacity of macrophages to immunize the host. Confirmation of this prediction has been provided experimentally in mice which develop ACAID-like immunity following intravenous injection with TGF-β-treated macrophages (183). Ultimately, this approach might prove useful clinically for induction of tolerance to transplantation antigens or in the treatment of autoimmune disease.

Studies on immune privilege also suggest another therapeutic concept known as "paracrine immunosuppression." If immunologic tissue microenvironments are indeed subject to regulation, then pharmaceutical agents might be developed that could successfully manipulate the microenvironment, perhaps through the local production of immunosuppressive cytokines by host tissue. With respect to the eye, topical medications could be developed that would target the secretory epithelium to secrete increased levels of TGF-β or neuropeptides. In this way, natural defenses would be activated to suppress inflammation within the ocular compartment and restore a normal immunologic microenvironment.

Final Comments

In this review, we have compared the immunologic microenvironment of the eye with that of the CNS with respect to information derived from in vitro studies, experimental animal models, and clinical observations (Table 18.2). In many ways, studies of the

Table 18-2 Comparison of Immunologic Microenvironment of the Eye and CNS

	Eye	*CNS*
Normal Microenvironment		
Fluid(s)	Aqueous humor; vitreous gel	Cerebrospinal fluid
Lymphatics	No	Yes
Local antigens communicate with lymphoid system	Yes	Yes
Blood-tissue barriers	Yes	Yes
Immune-privileged site	Yes	Yes
Afferent immune deviation	Yes	?
Efferent blockade	Yes	?
Immunosuppressive molecules	Yes	?
Inflammatory Microenvironment		
Local antibody synthesis	Yes	Yes
DH responses	Yes	Yes
Cytotoxic T-cell responses	Yes	Yes
Specific Disease States		
Autoimmune disease		
Experimental	EAU	EAE
Clinical	?	Postinfectious leuko-encephalopathy
HSV-1 infection (immunocompetent host)	ARN	Herpes simplex encephalitis
CMV infection (immunosuppressed host)	CMV retinitis	CMV encephalitis

immunologic microenvironment of the eye have outpaced those of the CNS when exploring such issues as immune privilege and tissue specialization. Conversely, such issues as lymphocyte trafficking, blood-tissue barriers, and cytokine functions have been explored more fully within the CNS. Despite these differences in focus, however, we conclude that the immunologic microenvironment of the eye and that of the CNS are more similar than dissimilar; knowledge derived from studies of one microenvironment can be extrapolated to the other with reasonable confidence. Future investigation of either microenvironment will continue to provide new insights on the pathophysiology of disease that occur in both of these unique immune-privileged sites, leading ultimately to improved diagnostic and therapeutic regimens that may one day impact significantly on sight-threatening and life-threatening diseases of the eye and the brain.

Acknowledgments

This work was supported by NIH grants EY10327 (S.W.C.) and EY10568 (R.D.D.).

References

1. Adamus G, Schmied JL, Hargrave PA, Arendt A, Moticka EJ. Induction of experimental autoimmune uveitis with rhodopsin synthetic peptides in Lewis rats. Curr Eye Res 11:657–667, 1992.
2. Altmann DM, Blyth WA. Protection from herpes simplex virus-induced neuropathology in mice showing delayed hypersensitivity tolerance. J Gen Virol 66:1297–1303, 1985.
3. Aronson SB, McMaster PRB. Passive transfer of experimental allergic uveitis. Arch Ophthalmol 91:60–65, 1971.
4. Aronson SB, Moore TB, O'Day DM. The effect of structural alterations on anterior ocular inflammation. Am J Ophthalmol 70:886–893, 1970.
5. Atalla L, Linker-Israeli M, Steinman L, Rao NA. Inhibition of autoimmune uveitis by anti-CD4 antibody. Invest Ophthalmol Vis Sci 31:1264–1270, 1990.
5a. Atherton SS. Protection from retinal necrosis by passive transfer of monoclonal antibody specific for herpes simplex virus glycoprotein D. Curr Eye Res 11:45–52, 1992.
6. Atherton SS, Altman NH, Streilein JW. Histopathologic study of herpes virus-induced retinitis in athymic BALB/c mice: evidence for an immunopathologic process. Curr Eye Res 8:1179–1192, 1989.
7. Atherton SS, Newell CK, Kanter MY, Cousins SW. Retinitis in euthymic mice following inoculation of murine cytomegalovirus (MCMV) via the supraciliary route. Curr Eye Res 10:667–677, 1991.
8. Atherton SS, Newell CK, Kanter MY, Cousins SW. T cell depletion increases susceptibility to murine cytomegalovirus retinitis. Invest Ophthalmol Vis Sci 33:3353–3360, 1992.
9. Atherton SS, Streilein JW. Two waves of virus following anterior chamber inoculation with HSV-1. Invest Ophthalmol Vis Sci 28:571–579, 1987.
10. Azumi A, Cousins SW, Kanter MY, Atherton SS. Modulation of murine herpes simplex virus type 1 retinitis in the uninoculated eye by CD4+ T lymphocytes. Invest Ophthalmol Vis Sci 35:54–63, 1994.

11. Azumi A, Atherton, SS. Sparing of the ipsilateral retina following anterior chamber inoculation of HSV-1: requirement for either CD4+ or CD8+ T cells. Invest Ophthalmol Vis Sci 35:3251–3259, 1994.

12. Baarsma GS, Luyendijk L, Kijlstra A, de Vries J, Peperkamp E, Mertens DAE, van Meurs JC. Analysis of local antibody production in the vitreous humor of patients with severe uveitis. Am J Ophthalmol 112:147–150, 1991.

13. Bale JF, O'Neil ME, Hogan RN, Kern ER. Experimental murine cytomegalovirus infection of ocular structures. Arch Ophthalmol 102:1214–1219, 1984.

14. Bale JF, O'Neil ME, Lyon B, Perlman S. The pathogenesis of murine cytomegalovirus ocular infection. Anterior chamber inoculation. Invest Ophthalmol Vis Sci 31:1575–1581, 1990.

15. Barker CF, Billingham R. Immunologically privileged sites. Adv Immunol 25:1–54, 1991.

16. Barton K, McLaughlan MT, Calder VL, Lightman S. Interleukin 2, interferon gamma and interleukin 4 production by lymphocytes in the retina in EAU. Invest Ophthalmol Vis Sci (Suppl) 34:1144, 1993.

17. Beneski DA, Donoso LA, Edelberg KE, Magargal LE, Folberg R, Merryman CF. Human retinal S-antigen: isolation, purification, and characterization. Invest Ophthalmol Vis Sci 25:686–690, 1984.

18. Benson JL, Niederkorn JY. In situ suppression of delayed-type hypersensitivity:another mechanism for sustaining the immune privilege of the anterior chamber. Immunology 74:153–159, 1991.

19. Berra A, Rodriguez A, Heiligenhaus A, Pazos B, Rooijen NV, Foster CS. The role of macrophages in the pathogenesis of HSV-1 induced chorioretinitis in BALB/c mice. Invest Ophthalmol Vis Sci 35:2990–2998, 1994.

20. Bishop SA, Hill TJ. Herpes simplex virus infection and damage in the central nervous system: immunomodulation with adjunant, cyclophosphamide, and cyclosporin A. Arch Virol 116:57–62, 1991.

21. Broekhuyse RM, Kuhlmann ED, Winkens HJ. Experimental autoimmune anterior uveitis (EAAU): II. Dose-dependent induction and adoptive transfer using a melanin-bound antigen of the retinal pigment epithelium. Exp Eye Res 55:401–411, 1992.

22. Broekhuyse RM, Kuhlmann ED, Winkens HJ. Experimental autoimmune posterior uveitis accompanied by epitheloid cell accumulations (EAPU). A new type of experimental ocular disease induced by immunization with PEP-65, a pigment epithelial polypeptide preparation. Exp Eye Res 55:819–829, 1992.

23. Brubaker RF. Flow of aqueous humor in humans. Invest Ophthalmol Vis Sci 32:3145–3166, 1991.

24. Calder VL, Lightman SL. Experimental autoimmune uveoretinitis (EAU) versus experimental allergic encephalomyelitis (EAE): A comparison of T cell-mediated mechanisms. Clin Exp Immunol 89:165–169, 1992.

25. Calder VL, Wang Y, Lightman SL. In vitro and in vivo effects of anti-CD8 monoclonal antibody on S-antigen induced uveitis in rats. Invest Ophthalmol Vis Sci (Suppl) 32:612, 1991.

26. Caspi RR. Basic mechanisms in immune-mediated uveitis disease. In: Immunology and Medicine Series, Vol 13, S Lightman, ed. Kluwer Academic Publishers, New York, 1989, pp 61–87.

26a. Caspi RR. Th1 and Th2 lymphocytes in experimental autoimmune uveoretinitis. In: Advances in Ocular Immunology, RB Nussenblatt, SM Whitcup, RR Caspi, I Gery, eds. Elsevier Science B.V., Amsterdam, The Netherlands, 1994, pp 55–58.

27. Caspi RR, Roberge FG, Chan CC, Wigger B, Chader GJ, Rozenszajn LA, Lando Z,

Nussenblatt RB. A new model of autoimmune disease: experimental autoimmune uveoretinitis induced in mice with two different retinal antigens. J Immunol 140:1490–1495, 1988.

28. Caspi RR, Roberge FG, McAllister CG, el-Saied M, Kuwabara T, Gery I, Hanna E, Nussenblatt RB. T cell lines mediating experimental autoimmune uveoretinitis (EAU) in the rat. J Immunol 136:928–933, 1986.

29. Chan CC, Mochizuki M, Nussenblatt RB. T-lymphocyte subsets in experimental auto-immune uveitis. Clin Immunol Immunopathol 35:103–110, 1985.

30. Charteris D, Lightman S. Interferon gamma production in experimental autoimmune uveoretinitis. Invest Ophthalmol Vis Sci (Suppl) 32:790, 1991.

31. Charteris DG, Lightman SL. Interferon-gamma production in vivo in EAU. Immunology 75:463–467, 1992.

31a. Cohen B and Dix RD. Cytomegalovirus and other herpesviruses. In: AIDS and the Nervous System, 2nd ed. J Berger, RM Levy, eds. Lippincott-Raven Press, New York, 1996, in press.

32. Cousins SW. T cell activation within different intraocular compartments during experimental uveitis. Dev Ophthalmol 23:150–155, 1992.

33. Cousins SW, Altman NH, Atherton SS. Schisis contributes to necrosis in experimental HSV-1 retinis. Exp Eye Res 48:745–760, 1987.

34. Cousins SW, Gonzalez A, Atherton SS. Herpes simplex retinitis in the mouse. Clinico-pathologic correlations. Invest Ophthalmol Vis Sci 30:1485–1494, 1989.

35. Cousins SW, McCabe MM, Danielpoor D, Streielin JW. Identification of transforming growth factor-beta as an immunosuppressive factor in aqueous humor. Invest Ophthalmol Vis Sci 32:2201–2211, 1996.

35a. Cousins SW, Rouse BT. Chemical mediators of ocular inflammation. In: Ocular Infection & Immunity, JS Pepose, GN Holland, KR Wilhelmus, eds. Mosby, St. Louis, Missouri, 1995, pp 50–70.

36. Cousins SW, Streilein JW. Immune privilege and its regulation by immunosuppressive growth factors in aqueous humor. In: Ocular Immunology Today, M Usui, S Ohno, K Aoki, eds. Elsevier, Amsterdam, 1990, pp 81–84.

37. Cousins SW, Streilein JW. Transforming growth factor-β and other factors in aqueous humor inhibit the local adoptive transfer of delayed hypersensitivity to the skin. Invest Ophthalmol Vis Sci (Suppl) 34:973, 1993.

38. Cousins SW, Trattler WB, Streilein JW. Immune privilege and suppression of immunogenic inflammation in the anterior chamber. Curr Eye Res 10:287–297, 1991.

39. Crawford JP, Movat HZ, Ranadive N, Hay JB. Pathways to inflammation induced by immune complexes. Federation Proc 41:2583–2587, 1982.

40. Culbertson WW, Blumenkranz MS, Haines H, Gass JDM, Mitchell KB, Norton EWD. The acute retinal necrosis syndrome. Part 2: Histopathology and etiology. Ophthalmology 89:1317–1325, 1982.

41. Davson H. Physiology of the Eye, 5th ed. Peragon Press, New York, 1990.

42. De Kozak Y, Audibert F, Thillaye B, Chedid L, Faure J-P. Effects of mycobacterial hydro-soluble adjuvants on the induction and prevention of experimental uveoretinitis in guinea pigs. Ann Immunol (Paris) 130:29–32, 1979.

43. De Kojak Y, Yuan WS, Bogossian M, Faure J-P. Humoral and cellular immunity to retinal antigens in guinea pigs. Mod Probl Ophthalmol 16:51–58, 1976.

44. De La Paz MA, Young LHY. Acute retinal necrosis syndrome. Semin Ophthalmol 8:61–69, 1993.

45. Dijkstra CD, Dopp EA, Huitinga I, Damoiseaux JGMC. Macrophages in experimental autoimmune diseases in the rat: a review. Curr Eye Res (Suppl) 11:75–79, 1992.

46. Dix RD, Atherton SS, Streilein JW. Effect of passively-administered neutralizing antibody on the development of herpes simplex virus type 1 retinitis. Invest Ophthalmol Vis Sci (Suppl) 27:117, 1986.

47. Dix RD, Baringer JR, Panitch HS, Rosenberg SH, Hagedorn J, Whaley J. Recurrent herpes simplex encephalitis: recovery of virus after Ara-A treatment. Ann Neurol 13:196–199, 1983.

48. Dix RD, Cray C, Cousins SW. Antibody alone does not prevent experimental cytomegalovirus retinitis in mice with retrovirus-induced immunodeficiency (MAIDS). J Gen Virol (in press), 1997.

49. Dix RD, Cray C, Cousins SW. Mice immunosuppressed by murine retrovirus infection (MAIDS) are susceptible to cytomegalovirus retinitis. Curr Eye Res 13:587–595, 1994.

50. Dix RD, Cray C, Cousins SW. Cytomegalovirus retinitis during AIDS: current issues and future directions. Reg Immunol 6:112–118, 1994.

50a. Dix RD, Giedlin M, Cousins SW. Systemic cytokine immunotherapy for experimental cytomegalovirus retinitis in mice with retrovirus-induced immunodeficiency (MAIDS). Invest Ophthalmol Vis Sci (in press), 1997.

51. Dix RD, Hamasaki DI, Hurst L, Culbertson WW, Lewis ML. Bilateral retinal disease following unilateral inoculation of mice with a HSV-1 isolate from a patient with acute retinal necrosis. Invest Ophthalmol Vis Sci (Suppl) 31:314, 1990.

52. Dix RD, Palm SE. Opportunistic infections of the central nervous system during AIDS. Adv Neuroimmunol. 3:81–96, 1993.

53. Dix RD, Resnick L, Culbertson W, Dickinson G, Fisher E, Saenz M. Intraocular HIV-1-specific IgG synthesis in a patient with CMV retinitis. Reg Immunol 2:1–6, 1989.

54. Dorey C, Faure J-P. Isolement et caracterisation d'un antigene retinien de la retine induisant l'uveo-retinite auto-immune experimentale. Ann Immunol (Paris) 128C:229–232, 1977.

55. Donoso LA, Gregerson DS, Fling SP, Merryman CF, Sery TW. The use of synthetic peptides in the study of experimental autoimmune uveitis. Curr Eye Res (Supp) 9:155–161, 1990.

56. Dua HS, Abrams M, Barrett JA, Gregerson DS, Forrester JV, Donoso LA. Epitopes and idiotypes in experimental autoimmune uveitis: a review. Curr Eye Res (Suppl) 11:59–65, 1992.

57. Dua HS, Lee RH, Lolley RN, Barrett JA, Abrams M, Forrester JV, Donoso LA. Induction of experimental autoimmune uveitis by the retinal photoreceptor cell protein, phosducin. Curr Eye Res (Suppl) 11:107–111, 1992.

58. Duke-Elder WS. System of Ophthalmology: Disease of the Uveal Tract, Vol 9. CV Mosby, St. Louis, 1966.

59. Duker JS, Nielsen JC, Eagle RC Jr, Bosley TM, Granadier R, Benson WE. Rapidly progressive acute retinal necrosis secondary to herpes simplex virus, type 1. Ophthalmology 97:1638–1643, 1990.

60. Dussaix E, Cerqueti PM, Pontet F, Block-Michel E. New approaches to the detection of locally produced antiviral antibodies in the aqueous of patients with endogeneous uveitis. Ophthalmologica 194:145–149, 1987.

61. Eichhorn M, Horneber M, Streilein JW, Lutjen-Drecoll E. Anterior chamber-associated immune deviation elicited via primate eyes. Invest Ophthalmol Vis Sci 34:2926–2930, 1993.

62. el Azazi M, Samuelsson A, Linde A, Forsgren M. Intrathecal antibody production against viruses of the herpesvirus family in acute retinal necrosis syndrome. Am J Ophthalmol 112:76–82, 1991.

63. Eto K, Suzuki S, Singh VK, Shinohara T. Immunization with recombinant *Escherichia coli*

expressing retinal S-antigen-induced experimental autoimmune uveitis (EAU) in Lewis rats. Cell Immunol 147:203–214, 1993.

64. Faber DW, Wiley CA, Lynn GB, Gross JG, Freeman WR. Role of HIV and CMV in the pathogenesis of retinitis and retinal vasculopathy in AIDS patients. Invest Ophthalmol Vis Sci 33:2345–2353, 1992.

65. Ferguson TA, Mahendra SL, Hooper P, Kaplan HJ. The wavelength of light governing intraocular immune reactions. Invest Ophthalmol Vis Sci 33:1788–1795, 1990.

66. Fernando AN. Immunological studies with I^{131} labeled antigen in experimental uveitis. Arch Ophthalmol 63:515–539. 1960.

67. Fisher JP, Lewis M, Blumenkranz M, Culbertson WW, Flynn HW Jr, Clarkson JG, Gass JDM, Norton EWD. The acute retinal necrosis syndrome. Part 1: clinical manifestations. Ophthalmology 89:1309–1316, 1982.

68. Forrester JV, Liversidge J, Dua HS, Towler H, McMenamin PG. Comparison of clinical and experimental uveitis. Curr Eye Res (Suppl) 9:75–84, 1990.

69. Fox A. Role of bacterial debris in inflammation of the joint and eye. APMIS 98:957–968, 1990.

70. Fox GM, Kuwabara T, Wiggert B, Redmond TM, Hess HH, Chader GJ, Gery I. Experimental autoimmune uveoretinitis (EAU) induced by retinal interphotoreceptor retinoid-binding protein (IRBP): differences between EAU induced by IRBP and the S-antigen. Clin Immunol Immunopathol 43:456–264, 1987.

71. Friedlander MH. Immunology of the Eye, 2nd ed. Harper & Row, Philadelphia, 1988.

72. Fujinami RS, Oldstone MBA. Amino acid homology between the encephalogenic site of myelin basic protein and virus: mechanism for autoimmunity. Science 230:1043–1045, 1985.

73. Gao E-K, Yu X-H, Lin C-P, Zhang H, Kaplan HJ. Intraocular viral replication after systemic murine cytomegalovirus infection requires immunosuppression. Invest Ophthalmol Vis Sci 36:2322–2326, 1995.

74. Gazzinelli RT, Makino B, Chattopadhyay SK, Snapper CM, Sher A, Hugin AW, Morse HC III. CD4+ subset regulation in viral infection. Activation of Th2 cells during progression of retrovirus-induced immunodeficiency in mice. J Immunol 148:182–188, 1992.

75. Germuth FG, Maumenee AE, Senterfit LB, Pollack AD. Immunohistologic studies on antigen-antibody reactions in the avascular cornea I. Reaction in rabbits sensitized to foreign proteins. J Exp Med 115:919–925, 1962.

75a. Goldman H, Witmer R. Antikurper in Kammerwasser. Ophthamologica 177:323–332, 1954.

76. Gery I, Chanaud NP III, Anglade E. Recoverin is highly uveitogenic in Lewis rats. Invest Ophthalmol Vis Sci 35:3342–3345, 1994.

77. Granstein R, Staszlaski R, Knisely TL, Zeira ERN, Latina M, Albert DM. Aqueous humor contains transforming growth factor-β and a small (<3500 dalton) inhibitor of thymocyte proliferation. J Immunol 144:3021–3026, 1990.

78. Green WR. Uveal tract. In: Ocular Pathology: An Atlas and Textbook, WH Spencer, ed. WB Saunders, Philadelphia, 1986, pp 1792–2013.

79. Greenwood J. The blood-retinal barrier in experimental autoimmune uveoretinitis (EAU): a review. Curr Eye Res (Suppl) 11:25–32, 1992.

80. Hamasaki DI, Dix RD, Atherton SS. Bilateral alterations of the ERG and retinal histology following unilateral HSV-1 inoculation. Invest Ophthalmol Vis Sci 29:1242–1254, 1988.

81. Hara Y, Caspi RR, Wiggert B, Chan CC, Wilbanks GA, Streilein JW. Suppression of experimental autoimmune uveitis in mice by induction of ACAID with interreceptor retinol binding protein. J Immunol 148:1685–1692, 1992.

82. Hartley JW, Fredrickson TN, Yetter RA, Makino M, Morse HC III. Retrovirus-induced murine acquired immunodeficiency syndrome: natural history of infection and differing susceptibility of inbred mouse strains. J Virol 63:1223–1231, 1989.

83. Hayaski K, Kurihara I, Uchida Y. Studies of ocular murine cytomegalovirus infection. Invest Ophthalmol Vis Sci 26:486–493, 1985.

84. Helbig H, Kittredge KL, Coca-Prados M, Davis J, Palestine AG, Nussenblatt RB. Mammalian ciliary-body epithelial cells in culture produce transforming growth factor-β. Graefes Arch Clin Exp Ophthalmol 229:84–91, 1991.

85. Hemady R, Opremcak M, Zaltas M, Berger A, Foster CS. Herpes simplex virus type-1 strain influence on chorioretinal disease patterns following intracameral inoculation in Igh-1 disparate mice. Invest Ophthalmol Vis Sci 30:1750–1757, 1989.

85a. Hendricks RL, Tang Q. Cellular immunity and the eye. In: Ocular Infection & Immunity, JS Pepose, GN Holland, KR Wilhelmus, eds. Mosby, St. Louis, Missouri, 1995, pp 71–95.

86. Ho M. Cytomegalovirus Biology and Infection, 2nd ed. Plenum Press, New York, 1991.

87. Holland GN. Acquired immunodeficiency syndrome and ophthalmology: the first decade. Am J Ophthalmol 114:86–95, 1992.

88. Holland GN, Fang EN, Glasgow BJ, Zaragoza AM, Siegel LM, Graves MC, Saxton EH, Roos RY. Necrotizing retinopathy after intraocular inoculation of murine cytomegalovirus in immunosuppressed adult mice. Invest Ophthalmol Vis Sci 31:2326–2324, 1990.

89. Holland GN, Togni BI, Briones OC, Dawson CR. A microscopic study of herpes simplex virus retinopathy in mice. Invest Ophthalmol Vis Sci 28:1181–1190, 1987.

89a. Holland GN, Tufail A, Jordan MC. Cytomegalovirus diseases: In: Ocular Infection & Immunity, JS Pepose, GN Holland, KR Wilhelmus, eds. Mosby, St. Louis, Missouri, 1995, pp 1088–1129.

90. Hooks JJ, Chan CC, Detrick B. Identification of the lymphokines interferon gamma and interleukin-2 in inflammatory eye disease. Invest Ophthalmol Vis Sci 29:1444–1451, 1988.

91. Hudson SJ, Streilein JW. Functional cytotoxic T cells are associated with focal lesions in the brains of SJL mice with experimental herpes simplex encephalitis. J Immunol 152:5540–5547, 1994.

92. Hurst L, Hamasaki DI, Stewart R, Dix RD. Comparative neuroinvasiveness, neurovirulence, and retinovirulence of two KOS strains of herpes simplex virus type 1. Invest Ophthalmol Vis Sci (Suppl) 32:801, 1991.

93. Igietseme JU, Calzada P, Gonzalez A, Streilein JW, Atherton SS. Protection of mice from herpes simplex virus-induced retinitis by in vitro-activated immune cells. J Virol 63:4808–4813, 1989.

94. James K. Interactions between cytokines and alpha 2-macroglobulin. Immunol Today 11:63–66, 1990.

95. Jampel H, Roche N, Stark WJ, Roberts AB. Transforming growth factor-β in aqueous humor. Curr Eye Res 10:963–970, 1991.

96. Jiang LQ, Streielin JWS. Immune privilege is extended to allogeneic tumor cells in the vitreous cavity. Invest Ophthalmol Vis Sci 32:224–228, 1991.

97. Jiang LQ, Streilein JW. Immunity and immune privilege elicited by autoantigens expressed on syngeneic neonatal neural retina grafts. Curr Eye Res 11:697–709, 1992.

98. Johnson RT. Viral Infections of the Nervous System. Raven Press, New York, 1982.

99. Johnson RT, Griffin DE, Hirsch RL, Wolinsky JS, Roedenbeck S, de Soriano IL, Vaisberg A. Measles encephalomyelitis—clinical and immunologic studies. N Engl J Med 310:137–141, 1984.

100. Kaiser CJ, Ksander BR, Streilein JW. Inhibition of lymphocyte proliferation by aqueous humor. Reg Immunol 2:42–49, 1989.

101. Kaplan HJ, Stevens TR. A reconsideration of immunologic privilege within the anterior chamber of the eye. Transplantation 19:302–309, 1975.

102. Kaplan HJ, Waldrep C, Nicholson JKA. Immunologic analysis of intraocular mononuclear cell infiltrates in uveitis. Arch Ophthalmol 102:572–577, 1984.

103. Kielty D, Cousins SW, Atherton SS. HSV-1 retinitis and delayed hypersensitivity in DBA/2 and C57BL/6 mice. Invest Ophthalmol Vis Sci 28:1994–1999, 1987.

104. Kijlstra A. The value of laboratory testing in uveitis. Eye 4:732–736, 1990.

105. Kijlstra A, Luyendijk L, Baarsma GS, Rothova A, Schweitzer, CMC, Timmerman Z, de Vries J, Breebaar AC. Aqueous humor analysis as a diagnostic tool in toxoplasma uveitis. Int Ophthalmol 13:383–386, 1989.

106. Kijlstra A, van den Horn GJ, Luyendijk L, Baarsma GS, Schweitzer CMC, Zaal MJM, Timmerman Z, Beintema M, Rothova A. Laboratory tests in uveitis: new developments in the analysis of local antibody production. Documenta Ophthalmologica 75:225–231.

107. Klineman DM, Morse HC III. Characteristics of B cell proliferation and activation in murine AIDS. J Immunol 142:1144–1148, 1989.

108. Knisely TL, Anderson TM, Sherwood ME, Flotte TJ, Albert DA, Granstein RD. Morphologic and ultrastructural examination of I-A+ cells in the murine iris. Invest Ophthalmol Vis Sci 32:2432–2440, 1991.

109. Konda BR, Pararajasegaram G, Wu GS, Stanforth D, Rao NA. Role of retinal pigment epithelium in the development of experimental autoimmune uveitis. Invest Ophthalmol Vis Sci 35:40–47, 1994.

110. Kotake S, de Smet MD, Wiggert B, Redmond TM, Chader GJ, Gery I. Analysis of the pivotal residues of the immunodominant and highly uveitogenic determinant of IRBP. J Immunol 146:2995–3001, 1991.

111. Kraus-Mackiw E, Coles RS. Exogenous uveitis: sympathetic uveitis and toxic lens syndrome. In: Uveitis: Pathophysiology and Therapy, 2nd ed, E Kraus-Mackiw, GR O'Connor, eds. Thieme Medical Publishers, New York, 1986, pp 110–154.

112. Ksander BR, Streilein JW. Failure of infiltrating precursor cytotoxic T cells to acquire direct cytotoxic function in immunologically privileged sites. J Immunol 145:2057–2063, 1990.

113. Lee CH, Lang LS, Orr EL. Changes in ocular mast cell numbers and histamine distribution during experimental autoimmune uveitis. Reg Immunol 5:106–113, 1993.

114. Lerner MP, Frick L, Donoso LA, Hargrave PA, Cunningham MW. Uveitogenic proteins share epitopes with group A streptococcal M protein. Invest Ophthalmol Vis Sci (Suppl) 35:1863, 1994.

115. Lewis ML, Culbertson WW, Post JD, Miller D, Kokame GT, Dix RD. Herpes simplex virus type 1. A cause of acute retinal necrosis syndrome. Ophthalmology 96:875–878, 1989.

116. Li Q, Fujino Y, Caspi RR, Najafian F, Nussenblatt RB, Chan CC. Association between mast cells and the development of experimental autoimmune uveitis in different rat strains. Clin Immunol Immunopathol 65:294–299, 1992.

116a. Liesegang TJ. Fuchs uveitis syndrome. In: Ocular Infection & Immunity, JS Pepose, GN Holland, KR Wilhelmus, eds. Mosby, St. Louis, Missouri, 1995, 494–506.

117. Ludwig IH, Zegarra H, Zakov ZN. The acute retinal necrosis syndrome: possible herpes simplex retinitis. Ophthalmology 91:1659–1664, 1984.

118. Luyendijk L, van der Horn GJ, Visser OHE, Suttorp-Schulten MSA, van de Biesen PR, Rothova A, Kijlstra A. Detection of locally produced antibodies to herpes viruses in the

aqueous of patients with acquired immune deficiency syndrome (AIDS) or acute retinal necrosis syndrome (ARN). Curr Eye Res 9 (Suppl):7–11, 1990.

119. Marak GE, Font RL, Alepa FP, Ward PA. Effects of C3 inactivator factor on the development of experimental lens-induced granulomatous endophthalmitis. Ophthalmic Res 9:416–420, 1977.

120. Marak GE, Wacker WB, Rao NA, Jack R, Ward PA. Effects of complement depletion on experimental allergic uveitis. Ophthalmic Res 11:97–107, 1979.

121. Marak GE Jr, Schichi H, Rao NA, Wacker WB. Patterns of experimental allergic uveitis induced by rhodopsin and retinal rod outer segments. Ophthalmic Res 12:165–176, 1980.

122. Margolis TP, LaVail JH, Setzer PY, Dawson CR. Selective spread of herpes simplex virus in the central nervous system after ocular infection. J Virol 63:4756–4761, 1989.

123. McMenamin PG, Holthouse I. Immunohistochemical characterization of dendritic cells and macrophages in the aqueous outflow pathways of the rat eye. Exp Eye Res 55:315–324, 1992.

124. McMenamin PG, Holthouse I, Holt PG. Class II major histocompatibility complex (Ia) antigen bearing dendritic cells within iris and ciliary body of the rat ege. Immunology 77:385–393, 1992.

124a. Mocarski Jr ES. Cytomegalovirus biology and replication. In: The Human Herpesviruses, B Roizman, RJ Whitley, C Lopez, eds. Raven Press, New York, 1993, pp 173–226.

125. Mochizuki M, Kuwabara T, McAllister C, Nussenblatt RB, Gery I. Adoptive transfer of experimental autoimmune uveoretinitis in rats: Immunopathogenic mechanism and histological features. Invest Ophthalmol Vis Sci 26:1–9, 1985.

126. Mondino BJ, Sidaharo Y, Meyer IJ, Sumner HJ. Inflammatory mediators in the vitreous humor of AIDS patients. Invest Ophthalmol Vis Sci 31:798–804, 1990.

127. Morse HC III, Yetter RA, Via CS, Hardy RR, Cerny A, Hayakawa K, Hugin AW, Miller MN, Holmes KL, Shearer GM. Functional and phenotypic alterations in T cell subsets during the course of MAIDS, a murine retrovirus-induced immunodeficiency syndrome. J Immunol 143:844–849, 1989.

128. Mosier DE, Yetter RA, Morse HC III. Retroviral induction of acute lymphoproliferative disease and profound immunosuppression in adult C57BL/6 mice. J Exp Med 161:766–784, 1985.

129. Mosier DE, Yetter RA, Morse HC III. Functional T lymphocytes are required for a murine retrovirus-induced immunodeficiency disease (MAIDS). J Exp Med 165:1737–1742, 1987.

130. Murray PI, Hoekzema R, Van Haren MA, Lyendijk L, Kijlstra A. Aqueous humor analysis of Fuch's heterochromic cyclitis. Curr Eye Res 5:686–693, 1991.

131. Nahmias AJ, Whitley RJ, Visintine AJ, Takei Y, Alford CA Jr. Herpes simplex encephalitis: laboratory evaluations and their diagnostic significance. J Infect Dis 145:829–836, 1982.

132. Niederkorn JY. Immune privilege and immune regulation in the eye. Adv Immunol 48:191–226, 1991.

132a. Niederkorn JY and Ferguson TA. Anterior chamber associated immune deviation (ACAID). In: Ocular Infection & Immunity, JS Pepose, GN Holland, KR Wilhelmus, eds. Mosby, St. Louis, Missouri, 1995, pp 96–103.

133. Niederkorn JY, Streilein JW, Shadduck JA. Deviant immune responses to allogeneic tumors injected intracamerally and subcutaneously in mice. Invest Ophthalmol Vis Sci 20:355–363, 1980.

134. Nussenblatt RB. Experimental autoimmune uveititis: mechanisms of disease and clinical therapeutic indications. Invest Ophthalmol Vis Sci 32:3131–3141, 1993.

135. Nussenblatt RB, Palestine AG. Uveitis: Fundamentals and Clinical Practice. Year Book Medical Publishers, Chicago, 1989.

136. Oldstone MBA. Molecular mimicry and autoimmune disease. Cell 50:819–820, 1987.

137. Pararajasegaram G, Hofman FM, Roa NA. Immunoregulatory molecules present in experimental autoimmune uveitis. Invest Ophthalmol Vis Sci (Suppl) 32:932, 1991.

138. Pepose JS. Cytomegalovirus infections of the retina. In: Retina, Vol 2, SJ Ryan, AP Schachat, RB Murphy, A Patz eds. CV Mosby Press, St. Louis, 1989, pp 589–596.

139. Pepose JS, Flowers B, Stewart JA, Grose C, Levy DS, Culbertson WW, Kreiger AE. Herpesvirus antibody levels in the etiologic diagnosis of the acute retinal necrosis syndrome. Am J Ophthalmol 113:248–256, 1992.

140. Pepose JS, Hilborne LH, Cancilla PA, Foos RY. Concurrent herpes simplex and cytomegalovirus retinitis and encephalitis in the acquired immune deficiency syndrome (AIDS). Ophthalmology 91:1669–1677, 1984.

140a. Pepose JS, Holland GN, Wilhelmus KR. Ocular Infection & Immunity, Mosby, St. Louis, Missouri, 1995.

141. Price C, Chernik NL, Horta-Barbosa L, Posner JB. Herpes simplex encephalitis in an anergic patient. Am J Med 54:222–227, 1973.

142. Price FW, Schlaigel TF. Bilateral acute retinitis. Am J Ophthalmol 89:419–423, 1980.

143. Psfister C, Chabre M, Plouet J, Tuyen VV, De Kozak Y, Faure JP, Kuhn H. Retinal S-antigen identified as the 48K protein regulating light-dependent phosphodiesterase in rod cells. Science 228:891–893, 1985.

144. Rabinovitch T, Oh JO, Minasi P. In vivo reactivation of latent murine cytomegalovirus in the eye by immunosuppressive treatment. Invest Ophthalmol Vis Sci 31:657–663, 1990.

145. Rao NA. Role of oxygen free radicals in retinal damage associated with experimental uveitis. Trans Am Ophthalmol Soc 89:797–850, 1990.

146. Rao NA, Atalla L, Fong SL, Chen F, Linker-Israeli M, Steinman L. Antigen-specific suppressor cells in experimental autoimmune uveitis. Ophthalmic Res 24:92–98, 1992.

147. Raviola G. The structural basis of the blood-ocular barrier. Exp Eye Res 23:27–63, 1977.

148. Resnick L, diMarzo-Veronese F, Schupbach J, Tourtellotte WW, Ho DD, Muller F, Shapshak P, Vogt M, Groopman JE, Markham PD, Gallo RC. Intra-blood-brain-barrier synthesis of HTLV-III-specific IgG in patients with neurologic symptoms associated with AIDS or AIDS-related complex. N Engl J Med 313:1498–1504, 1985.

148a. Rizzo LV, Silver PB, Hakim F, Chan CC, Wiggert B, Caspi RR. Establishment and characterization of an IRBP-specific T cell line that induces EAU in B10.A mice. Invest Ophthalmol Vis Sci (Suppl) 34:1143, 1993.

149. Schwartz JN, Daniels CA, Shivers JC, Klintworth GK. Experimental cytomegalovirus ophthalmitis. Am J Pathol 77:477–492, 1974.

150. Sergott RC, Belmont JB, Savino PJ, Fischer DH, Bosley TM, Schatz NJ. Optic nerve involvement in the acute retinal necrosis syndrome. Arch Ophthalmol 103:1160–1166, 1985.

151. Shinohara T, Singh VK, Tsuda M, Yamaki K, Abe T, Suzuki S. S-antigen: from gene to autoimmune uveitis. Exp Eye Res 50:751–757, 1990.

152. Singh VK, Kalra HK, Yamaki K, Abe T, Donoso LA, Shinohara T. Molecular mimicry between a uveitopathogenic site of S-antigen and viral peptides. Induction of experimental autoimmune uveitis in Lewis rats. J Immunol 144:1282–1287, 1990.

153. Singh VK, Nussenblatt RB, Donoso LA, Yamaki K, Chan CC, Shinohara T. Identification of a uveitopathogenic and lymphocyte proliferation site in bovine S-antigen. Cell Immunol 115:413–419, 1988.

154. Singh VK, Yamaki K, Abe T, Shinohara T. Molecular mimicry between uveitopathogenic

sites of retinal S-antigen and *Escherichia coli* protein: induction of experimental autoimmune uveitis and lymphocyte cross-reaction. Cell Immunol 122:262–273, 1989.

155. Singh VK, Yamaki K, Donoso LA, Shinohara T. Molecular mimicry: yeast histone HS-induced experimental autoimmune uveitis. J Immunol 142:1512–1517, 1989.

156. Sobel RA, Collins AB, Colvin RB, Bhan AK. The in situ cellular response in acute herpes simplex encephalitis. Am J Pathol 125:332–338, 1986.

157. Spencer DC, Price RW. Human immunodeficiency virus and the central nervous system. Annu Rev Microbiol 46:655–693, 1992.

158. Steinman RM. The dendritic cell system and its role in immunogenicity. Annu Rev Immunol 9:271–305, 1991.

159. Sterberg P, Knox DL, Finkelstein D, Green WR, Murphy RP, Patz A. Acute retinal necrosis syndrome. Retina 2:145–152, 1982.

160. Streilein JW. Immune regulation in the eye: a dangerous compromise. FASEB J 1:199–208, 1987.

161. Streilein JW, Atherton S, Vann V. A critical role for ACAID in the distinctive pattern of retinitis that follows anterior chamber inoculation of HSV-1. Curr Eye Res 6:127–131, 1987.

162. Streilein JW, Cousins SW, Bradley D. Effect of intraocular gamma-interferon on the immunoregulatory properties of iris and ciliary body cells. Invest Ophthalmol Vis Sci 33:2304–2315, 1992.

163. Streilein JW, Igietseme JU, Atherton SS. Evidence that precursor cytotoxic T cells mediate acute necrosis in HSV-1-infected retinas. Curr Eye Res 10:81–86, 1991.

164. Streilein JW, Niederkorn JY. Induction of anterior chamber associated immune deviation requires an intact functional spleen. J Exp Med 153:1058–1067, 1981.

165. Sunil S, Eto K, Singh VK, Shinohara T. Oligopeptides of three of five residues derived from uveitopathogenic sites of retinal S-antigen induce experimental autoimmune uveitis (EAU) in Lewis rats. Cell Immunol 148:198–207, 1993.

166. Suttorp-Schulten MSA, Zaal MJW, Luyendijk L, Bos PJM, KIJlstra A, Rothova A. Aqueous chamber tap and serology in acute retinal necrosis. Am J Ophthalmol 108:327–333, 1989.

167. Taylor AW, Streilein JW, Cousins SW. Alpha$_2$-macroglobulin may neutralize ocular immune privilege. FASEB J (Suppl) XX:1042, 1992.

168. Taylor AW, Streilein JW, Cousins SW. Identification of alpha melanocyte stimulating hormone as a possible immunoregulatory factor in aqueous humor. Curr Eye Res 12:1199–1206, 1992.

169. Taylor AW, Streilein JW, Cousins SW. Neuropeptides in aqueous humor may regulate T-lymphocytes within the eye. Invest Ophthalmol Vis Sci (Suppl) 33:1283, 1993.

170. Unger WG, Terenghi G, Ghatei MA, Ennis KW, Butler JM, Zhang SQ, Too HP, Polack JM, Bloom SR. Calcitonin gene-related polypeptide as a mediator of the neurogenic ocular injury response. J Ocul Pharmacol 1:189–199, 1985.

171. van Dooremaal JC. Die Entwickelung der in fremden Grund versetzen lebenden Gewebe. Albrecht von Graefes Arch Ophthalmol 19:359–366, 1873.

172. Vann VR, Atherton SS. Neural spread of herpes simplex virus after anterior chamber inoculation. Invest Ophthalmol Vis Sci 32:2462–2472, 1991.

173. von Szily A. Experimental endogenous transmission of infection from bulbus to bulbus. Klin Monatsbl Augenheilkd 75:593–602, 1924.

174. Wacker WB, Donoso LA, Kalsow CM, Yankeelov JA Jr, Organisciak DT. Experimental allergic uveitis. Isolation, characterization, and localization of a soluble uveitopathogenic antigen from bovine retina. J Immunol 119:1949–1958, 1977.

175. Waldrep JC, Mondino BJ. Humoral immunity and the eye. In: Ocular Infection & Immunity, JS Pepose, GN Holland, KR Wilhelmus, eds. Mosby, St. Louis, Missouri, 1995, pp 33–49.

176. Watanabe R, Wege H, ter Meulen V. Adoptive transfer of EAE-like lesions from rats with coronovirus-induced demyelinating encephalomyelitis. Nature 305:150–153, 1983.

177. Wetzig R, Hooks JJ, Percopo CM, Nussenblatt RB, Chan C-C. Anti-Ia antibody diminishes ocular inflammation in experimental autoimmune uveitis. Curr Eye Res 7:809–818, 1988.

178. Whitley RJ, Soong SL, Linneman C Jr, Liu C, Pazin G, Alford CA. Herpes simplex encephalitis—clinical assessments. JAMA 247:317–320, 1982.

179. Whittum JA, McCulley JP, Niederkorn JY, Streilein JW. Ocular disease induced in mice by anterior chamber inoculation of herpes simplex virus. Invest Ophthalmol Vis Sci 25:1065–1073, 1984.

180. Wilbanks GA, Mammolenti MM, Streilein JW. Studies on the induction of anterior chamber associated immune deviation. II. Eye-derived cells participate in generating blood-borne signals that induce ACAID. J Immunol 146:3018–3024, 1991.

181. Wilbanks GA, Streilein JW. The differing patterns of antigen release and local retention following anterior chamber and intravenous inoculation of soluble antigen: the eye is an antigen depot. Reg Immunol 2:390–389, 1989.

182. Wilbanks GA, Streilein JW. Distinctive humoral responses following anterior chamber and intravenous administration of soluble antigen: evidence for active suppression of IgG2a-secreting B cells. Immunology 71:566–572, 1990.

183. Wilbanks GA, Streilein JW. Fluids from immune privileged sites endow macrophages with the capacity to induce antigen-specific immune deviation via a mechanism involving transforming growth factor-β. Eur J Immunol 22:1031–1036, 1992.

184. Witmer R. Clinical implications of aqueous humor studies in uveitis. Am J Ophthalmol 86:39–43, 1978.

185. Wong VG, Anderson RR, McMaster PRB. Endogenous immune uveitis. Arch Ophthalmol 85:93–102, 1971.

186. Yoshitushi T, Shichi H. Immunosuppressive factors in procine vitreous body. Curr Eye Res 10:1141–1144, 1991.

187. Zaltas MM, Opremcak M, Hemady R, Foster CS. Immunohistopathologic findings in herpes simplex virus chorioretinitis in the von Szily model. Invest Ophthalmol Vis Sci 33:68–77, 1992.

188. Zhao M, Azumi A, Atherton SS. Immune effector cell (IEC)-mediated protection from HSV-1 retinitis occurs in the central nervous system (CNS). Invest Ophthalmol Vis Sci (Suppl) 35:1682, 1994.

189. Zirm M. Proteins in aqueous humor. Adv Ophthalmol 40:100–172, 1980.

V

NEUROIMMUNOLOGY OF DISEASE

19

Autoimmune Demyelinating Diseases of the Central Nervous System

CLAUDE P. GENAIN
STEPHEN L. HAUSER

The demyelinating diseases represent the most important category of noninfectious inflammatory disorders of the CNS. These disorders are characterized by specific pathologic features that include demyelination, relative sparing of axon cylinders, perivenular inflammation and macrophage infiltration. An autoimmune basis for these disorders is suggested by their similarity to experimental allergic encephalomyelitis (EAE) and by supporting clinical immunologic data.

Acute Demyelinating Diseases

Acute disseminated encephalomyelitis (ADEM) may occur without known antecedent or may follow immunization (postvaccinial encephalomyelitis) or infection (postinfectious encephalomyelitis). Pathologically, these disorders are characterized by widespread, scattered small foci of perivenular inflammation and by demyelination (6,38,50). The cellular infiltrate in ADEM is comprised predominantly of mononuclear cells and macrophages. In keeping with the monophasic nature of the disease, all lesions are found to be of the same age in typical cases (36).

Postvaccinal encephalomyelitis may occur after administration of rabies, smallpox, or other vaccines. With rabies immunization, ADEM is most likely to occur from vaccines that are prepared by propagation in brains of adult animals (42) (Semple vaccine). With these vaccines, the risk of ADEM has been estimated at between 1 in 400 and 1 in 5,000. In developed countries, use of newer rabies vaccines prepared from duck embryo or human diploid tissue has dramatically reduced the risk of ADEM, but use of the Semple vaccine continues in some parts of the world. It is an important theoretical point that ADEM can occur with the newer rabies virus vaccines that are not prepared by propagation in myelinated tissue. In addition to rabies vaccines, ADEM may also complicate immunization against smallpox (60), but the disappearance of smallpox has eliminated the need for prophylaxis and thus this complication.

Postinfectious encephalomyelitis may follow any of the common childhood viral exanthems. Natural infection with measles virus is most frequently complicated by ADEM (51) (1 per 500–1,000 cases). In developed countries, the widespread use of measles immunization has dramatically reduced the incidence of ADEM, but in some parts of the world measles infection, and hence this complication, remains common. (Postvaccinial encephalomyelitis may on rare occasions also follow administration of the measles vaccine.) A variety of other viruses, including rubella, varicella, mumps, Epstein-Barr, and influenza, have also been associated with ADEM (6,36,75). Mycoplasma infection represents an important nonviral infectious cause of ADEM (29).

Immunopathogenesis

The mechanism by which such diverse immune stimuli, including vaccination and infection with various DNA and RNA viruses, trigger a similar pattern of tissue injury is unclear. In cases of ADEM that follow rabies immunization, the coadministration of CNS tissue with the viral inoculum almost certainly is responsible for production of an EAE-like disease. Myelin basic protein (MBP) appears to be one target antigen in rabies vaccine ADEM, since autoantibodies can be identified in affected individuals (42). In ADEM associated with measles virus infection, induction of an immune response to a variety of CNS antigens occurs, but only the response to MBP correlates with the development of ADEM (51).

How an immune response against MBP is triggered by measles virus infection is not known, but it might include cross-sensitization due to antigens shared between measles virus and MBP, viral-mediated CNS injury with secondary sensitization to MBP, or nonspecific effects of viral infection on immune regulation. The possibility that molecular mimicry could trigger a cross-reactive response to MBP is suggested by the presence of an amino acid sequence homology between an envelope protein of measles and MBP. Similar stretches of homology exist between other viral proteins and MBP, and also between viruses and proteolipid protein (PLP) (144). Alternatively, an immune response to a neurotropic virus might result in CNS autoimmunity via an anti-idiotypic mechanism. Anti-idiotypic antibodies (or T cells) resembling the "internal image" of the viral receptor that recognizes a CNS cell could result in tissue damage. Experimentally, immunization of rodents with antiserum from measles-infected animals results in encephalomyelitis, suggesting an anti-idiotypic mechanism of disease. Virus-induced autoimmunity might also arise from antigen-nonspecific activation of T cells or macrophages in susceptible individuals, although it is noteworthy that familial aggregation has not been characteristic of ADEM.

Pathologically, the distinguishing characteristic of ADEM is the multiple small foci of perivenous inflammation and demyelination found scattered throughout the cerebral hemispheres, brain stem, and spinal cord (36,38). The inflammatory response is comprised predominantly of lymphocytes and monocytes/macrophages. Large lesions often have irregular edges because they are formed by coalescence of many smaller lesions. This feature helps to distinguish lesions of ADEM from those of chronic multiple sclerosis (MS). In MS, large lesions are thought to be created by concentric outward growth at the leading edge of demyelination, resulting in a smoothly rounded or oval appearance. Another pathologic hallmark of ADEM is that all lesions are of the same age.

Symptoms and Signs

Typically, ADEM is an acute disorder, evolving over the course of hours to several days (6,36,38,51,75). Patients typically complain of fever and headache or neck pain accompanied by evolving visual, motor, or sensory symptoms. In severe cases, lethargy may rapidly evolve to obtundation or coma. Seizures may occur. On examination there are multifocal, long tract signs affecting visual, motor, sensory, cerebellar, or brain stem pathways. This multiplicity of signs is the most characteristic feature of ADEM. Complete transverse myelitis with acute spinal shock (e.g., transient areflexia below the level of the lesion), or bilateral optic neuritis may be present. In general, postinfectious and postvaccinial ADEM are clinically similar, although prominent cerebellar involvement is a distinctive feature of ADEM following natural infection with chicken pox.

Cerebrospinal fluid (CSF) and magnetic resonance imaging (MRI) studies are the most useful paraclinical tests in suspected ADEM (36,55). CSF protein is at normal or mildly elevated levels, but generally by no higher than 150 mg percent. Lymphocytic pleocytosis, up to 200 cells per μl, is found, and early in the course, a mixed CSF infiltrate that includes polymorphonuclear cells may be present. Oligoclonal banding is detected in up to half of the cases of ADEM. In some patients, banding was no longer present at repeat lumbar puncture following recovery from the acute illness. MRI scanning may reveal extensive gadolinium enhancement in the brain and spinal cord (55).

The diagnosis of ADEM may be easy or difficult, depending upon the clinical setting. When onset follows vaccination, or develops during the course of an exanthemous illness, most commonly as the patient is recovering and the skin rash is fading, diagnosis is trivial. More often, there is no recent vaccination, and a history of infection is absent or vague. In such cases, a diagnosis must be inferred from the simultaneous onset of disseminated symptoms and signs referable to the optic nerve, brain, and spinal cord in the presence of inflammatory CSF. Acute viral encephalitis may be considered in some cases. In comatose patients or those with evidence of predominant cerebral involvement, herpes simplex encephalitis is suggested by a clinical prodrome indicating a temporal lobe syndrome, a mixed CSF cell infiltrate containing red blood cells, and MRI findings of destructive lesions surrounding the medial temporal lobes.

The distinction between ADEM, especially mild forms of ADEM, and acute MS may not be possible. In MS, optic neuritis is generally unilateral and transverse myelopathy is incomplete, while in ADEM, optic neuritis may be bilateral and myelitis complete. In MS, CSF protein is normal and the CSF cell count is less than 50 cells/μl. MRI lesions are typically of different ages in MS (i.e., some enhance and others do not), they are asymmetric, and tend to spare the posterior fossa (55).

Treatment of ADEM consists of intravenous methylprednisolone followed by oral prednisone for a total of 4–8 weeks. Prognosis not surprisingly reflects the severity of the acute illness. Measles encephalomyelitis is reported to have an acute mortality of 5–20% and the majority of survivors suffer from permanent neurologic residua. Children with ADEM may recover with little motor disability but have permanent seizure, behavioral, or learning disorders. Survivors from acute ADEM have been followed for decades and found to be free from recurrent disease, indicating that an evolution to chronic demyelinating disease did not occur. On rare occasions, apparent cases of typical ADEM have evolved into a chronic relapsing-remitting disorder simulating MS.

Acute hemorrhagic encephalomyelitis (AHL) of Weston Hurst is a particularly devastating and hyperacute demyelinating disorder. AHL is distinguished pathologically from ADEM by more intense inflammation comprising polymorphonuclear cells and by frank vasculitis resulting in fibrin deposition and multiple small hemorrhages scattered throughout the neuraxis. In some cases, large necrotic white matter lesions may be present at autopsy. The clinical syndrome resembles ADEM but is more acute and severe. Rapid progression to coma and death is common, although cases of complete recovery are also reported. Characteristic CSF changes of AHL consist of marked pleocytosis (up to 3,000 cells/μl), red blood cells, and raised protein content.

It is likely that the underlying etiology of ADEM and AHL are similar. In EAE, demyelinating lesions may resemble either ADEM or AHL, depending upon the genotype of the host, the immunization regimen, and the adjuvant used.

Chronic Demyelinating Diseases: Multiple Sclerosis

In contrast to the self-limited demyelinating diseases AHL and ADEM, MS is characterized by the dissemination of lesions in both time and space. Excluding trauma, MS is the most common cause of acquired neurologic disability arising between early to mid-adulthood. MS affects approximately 350,000 Americans. The etiology of MS is not known, but it is most likely due to an autoimmune response to CNS myelin, triggered by an environmental exposure (presumably a virus) in a genetically susceptible host. The clinical course of MS is variable, ranging from a benign to a rapidly progressive and devastating illness. Proper care of the patient with MS requires an understanding of the natural history, clinical phenotypes, and available therapies to treat symptoms and to modify the long-term course of the disease.

Histopathology

Macroscopic examination of the brain discloses multiple sclerotic areas, termed *plaques,* that are easily distinguished from surrounding white matter tissue (68,70,102). MS plaques vary in size from less than a millimeter to several centimeters. Other characteristics of typical plaques are their sharp edges and location centered around small veins. The temporal sequence of plaque development has been inferred from study of postmortem and biopsy tissue. The acute MS lesion, rarely present at autopsy, consists of perivenular cuffing and tissue infiltration with mononuclear cells, primarily macrophages and T cells (2). B cells and plasma cells are rare, and polymorphonuclear leukocytes are absent from MS lesions. The inflammatory response is associated with demyelination with relative sparing of axis cylinders, and with preservation of,and in some cases, proliferation of oligodendrocytes (104). As lesions progress, large numbers of macrophages and microglial cells scavenge the myelin debris, and proliferation of astrocytes is noted (2,102,103). Oligodendrocytes are scant or absent at this stage. In chronic lesions, complete demyelination and dense gliosis are characteristic; mononuclear cell inflammation may be present (chronic active plaque) or absent (chronic inactive plaque). In some chronic active plaques, the histologic features change from more acute to more chronic as one moves from the edge to the center of the lesion. This finding suggests that they developed by concentric outward growth.

Although classic MS lesions are identified by selective loss of myelin with preservation of the neuropil, in approximately 10% of plaques there is partial or even complete axonal destruction, leading in rare cases to cavitation. Remyelination is lacking in most MS lesions, but may occur. Successive waves of remyelination may produce the characteristic lesion of Balo's concentric sclerosis, an unusual histologic subtype of MS characterized by layers of demyelination and remyelination creating an onion skin pattern.

The correlation between clinical symptoms and plaque location and size is poor in MS (68,70). An extensive plaque burden may be associated with only mild clinical signs, and conversely, some severely disabled patients may have only minor pathologic correlates, a finding also noted when plaque load is estimated in vivo by head MRI (see below). Some of the discrepancy between the pathologic and clinical severity of MS may be explained by differences in the disruption of axonal conduction that results from MS lesions.

Epidemiology

Certain epidemiologic characteristics of MS appear to be present in all populations studied (58,68,70). MS is approximately twice as common in females than in males. Onset is typically during early to middle adulthood. Ten percent of cases begin before age 18. Onset as early as age 2 or as late as the eighth decade of life is reported. Mean age of onset in men is slightly later than in women.

MS is in general a disease of temperate climates. In both the northern and southern hemispheres, the prevalence of MS decreases with decreasing latitude. In the United States and in Europe, similar prevalence rates are present at comparable latitudes. These data support a possible environmental effect on MS, an effect also supported by migration data. Children born to parents who have migrated from a high-risk to a low-risk area for MS appear to have a lower lifetime risk than their parents. Conversely, migration of parents from a low-risk to a high-risk area confers a higher risk for MS in the children (58). Some migration studies, notably those from South Africa and Israel, have suggested that the critical time of the suspected exposure occurred before age 15 years, but these conclusions are based upon small numbers of individuals who have migrated at different ages. The final evidence for an environmental effect on MS is derived from a small number of apparent point epidemics that have been reported. The most convincing evidence of this sort occurred among the native population of the Faroe Islands, located between Iceland and Norway, following the British military occupation during World War II (59).

Genetics

Evidence of a genetic effect on susceptibility to MS is found in different prevalence estimates between ethnic groups that reside in similar environments, from studies of familial aggregation, and from twin studies (84,90).

The highest reported prevalence of MS, estimated at 250 cases per 100,000 population, occurs in the Orkney islands north of the mainland of Scotland (58). MS is also highly prevalent throughout northern Europe, particularly in Ireland and throughout Scandinavia. In the United States, the prevalence is higher among Caucasians than in other racial groups, which is consistent with observations in other parts of the world. MS is extremely uncommon in Japan (2 per 100,000) and among Black Africans. The low risk for these groups has been thought to represent genetic resistance. Japanese-Americans residing in Hawaii are at higher risk for MS than are their ethnic counterparts in Japan, which is consistent with some environmental effect. The prevalence of MS among African-Americans is approximately one-third that for Caucasian Americans.

Familial aggregation results in an increase in the risk for MS among first-, second- and third-degree relatives of patients (110,111). As predicted from a genetic model, the increase in risk decreases successively as the relationship to the affected relative becomes more distant. Analysis of different "multiple affected member" pedigrees raises the possibility of different genetic subtypes; in general, the prevalence among siblings is higher than that among parents or children of MS patients. This raises the possibility of a recessive effect on MS, yet the concordance estimates between non-twin siblings (2–5%) is lower than the 25% predicted by a fully penetrant Mendelian recessive model.

The most compelling data that susceptibility to MS is inherited is derived from twin studies (25,109). The risk of MS to a monozygotic twin of an MS patient is approximately 30%, whereas the risk to a fraternal twin, at 2–9%, is similar to the risk of a non-twin sibling. When monozygotic twin pairs discordant for MS were followed for a 10-year period, MS was found to appear in some of the healthy twins. Furthermore, MRI and spinal fluid examinations of some healthy twins were abnormal, raising the possibility that subclinical MS was present.

Pedigree analysis of multiple affected member families is most consistent with the hypothesis that more than one unlinked gene contributes to susceptibility (9,24,39,43, 90,114,121,133,141). Furthermore, genetic heterogeneity, i.e., independent major genes, may also be present in MS (37). The major histocompatibility complex (MHC) on chromosome 6 has been identified as one genetic determinant for MS (82,128). This complex includes genes encoding the histocompatibility antigens (the histocompatibility leukocyte antigen [HLA] system) and proteins that function in the context of antigen presentation to T cells. Association studies suggest that MS susceptibility is related to certain alleles of the class II (DR, DQ, and DP) region of the MHC (24,43,84, 121). The DR2 (15), DQw1 haplotype is common in Caucasian populations at risk for MS, and some family studies support a genetic effect of the DR2-bearing haplotype on susceptibility. Several studies also implicate DR3-bearing haplotypes as MS-associated. Additional haplotypes appear to be associated with MS in other ethnic populations, but family studies supporting their role have been negative or are lacking. It is of interest that the DR2-bearing MHC haplotypes that are present on MS chromosomes are heterogeneous, suggesting that the genetic effect is due to the class II locus itself and not due to another gene within the MHC in linkage disequilibrium with this region. It should also be emphasized that the MHC confers only a small genetic effect on MS— less than the contribution of this locus to other chronic inflammatory disorders, for example, insulin-dependent diabetes mellitus.

Immunopathogenesis

Most of our knowledge of the putative mechanisms that may cause MS is derived from the study of disease models in laboratory animals. In EAE, CNS inflammation is mediated by CD4+/CD8− T-cells reactive against myelin antigens, and in particular against MBP (97,100,146).

However, the role of MBP-reactive T cells in the pathogenesis of human MS remains uncertain. MBP-reactive T cells exist in the circulation of individuals with MS and healthy controls (48,52,67,146). Initial reports that the frequency of MBP-reactive T cells is increased in the circulation of patients with MS were not confirmed. MBP-reactive T cells appear to carry an increase in the frequency of genetic mutations, which suggests that they have undergone chronic stimulation in vivo (4). These cells also appear to be concentrated in the CSF as compared to their frequency in peripheral blood (92). In most MS patients and controls, a diverse repertoire of circulating T cells is capable of responding to MBP. Clonal diversity has been demonstrated in terms of recognition of different epitopes of MBP, restriction to different class II gene products, and usage of different T-cell receptor (TcR) genes (20,48,52,63,66,74,99,132). In the CSF, some reports suggest that preferential utilization of Vβ5.2 and Vβ6 TcR gene products occurs in MBP-reactive T cells in MS (13,19). Study of TcR RNA from MS brain tissue indicated that DR2+ patients express a hypervariable CDR3 region (comprised of J-D-V sequences) on some Vβ5.2 TcR genes that are similar to those found in encephalitogenic MBP-reactive T cells in the Lewis rat (3,91). These similarities suggested that some brain-infiltrating T cells in MS patients were reactive against an epitope of MBP within the 68–88 amino acid region. These preliminary data await confirmation from studies of larger numbers of MS patients.

By analogy to EAE, it is possible that more than one antigen may trigger disease. In addition to MBP, proteolipid protein (PLP), myelin-oligodendrocyte glycoprotein (MOG), myelin-associated glycoprotein (MAG), glial fibrillary acidic protein (GFAP), the astrocyte S100β, and glycolipids and phospholipids protein can all function as immunogens in various models of EAE (7,49,57,65,79,107,117,125,131,139). In this regard, recent data suggests that specific proliferative T-cell responses to MOG can be detected in MS patients (54,124,143). The T-cell repertoire responsible for EAE may also expand as the disease evolves from an acute into a chronic form. This has been demonstrated by experiments in which EAE induced by a synthetic peptide fragments of either MBP or PLP triggered a T-cell response to other determinants of these proteins (23,62,71,76). Thus, in a chronic disease like MS, it is likely that secondary sensitization to different myelin antigens may occur, and that some of these responses may result in pathologic consequences to the host.

In addition to infiltrating T cells, elevated levels of CNS immunoglobulin (Ig) are characteristic of MS (68,129,130). Some of this antibody can be shown to be oligoclonal, indicating that it is comprised of a small number of different antibody molecules. Oligoclonal Ig is also present in some patients with ADEM and in many chronic inflammatory diseases of the CNS, including infectious diseases. Its presence is thus not specific to MS. It is synthesized by plasma cells that reside locally in the CNS. The specific pattern or fingerprint of oligoclonal Ig is unique to each patient. Numerous attempts to identify a specific antigen against which the majority of oligoclonal Ig is directed have been unsuccessful in MS, in contrast to chronic infections in which some CSF Ig is found to be directed against the specific pathogen.

The mechanism of tissue damage in MS is not known. It has been proposed that cytokine products of activated T cells, macrophages, or astrocytes may contribute to lesion development. For example, the cytokine tumor necrosis factor (TNF)-α has been found in rodents to be selectively toxic to myelin and to oligodendrocytes in vitro (115,120,145). TNF-α is present in brain lesions of MS (44,116), levels of TNF-α in the CSF parallel MS disease activity (10,41,118), and antibodies to or inhibitors of TNF-α block acute EAE (32,78,108). Selective demyelination does not occur in most inflammatory disorders of the CNS, thus it is difficult to explain how a cytokine product of activated Th1 T cells and macrophages could entirely account for the specific immunopathology of MS. A role for antibody-mediated mechanisms of demyelination has been long-postulated (14,16). Recent studies including one in nonhuman primates have provided additional support for this hypothesis, as nondemyelinating forms of EAE can be converted to demyelinating forms by certain antibodies, specially antibodies directed against MOG (31,61). In MS, indirect evidence for antibody participation includes the findings of elevated levels of CSF immunoglobulins, CSF anti-MBP, and anti-MOG antibodies (96,134,143), and detection of the terminal component of complement (C9) in CSF and in MS lesions (21,80,112).

Virology

As noted above, epidemiologic data support the possibility of an environmental exposure in MS (58,68). One hypothesis has suggested that upper socioeconomic groups are at high risk for MS because improved sanitation results in a later exposure to some viruses. Some viruses, poliomyelitis and measles, for example, produce neurologic sequelae more commonly when the initial infection occurs in an older host. Measles virus has long been incriminated, since MS populations consistently have elevated serum titers to the virus, but proof of persistent infection has never been realized. MS has also been reported in individuals with no previous history of exposure to measles. Reports of infection with a human retrovirus related to human T-cell lymphotropic virus (HTLV)-1 have not been confirmed in MS (58); a number of other candidate viruses have been implicated in the pathogenesis of MS (18,50,113), but to date none of these associations has been firmly established (105). Experimental demyelinating disease can result from chronic viral infection of oligodendrocytes (5). Theiler's virus is a murine coronavirus that is similar to measles and to canine distemper virus. Infection with some strains of Theiler's virus results in a chronic CNS disease with multifocal perivascular infiltration and demyelination (64,106,140,144). As is the case for EAE, genetic factors, both MHC-linked and unlinked, influence the susceptibility to CNS disease following infection with Theiler's virus. As an additional possible mechanism for virus-induced disease, environmental exposure to viruses could trigger activation of myelin-reactive T-cells or antibodies by molecular mimicry (8,142,144).

Natural History

It is useful to distinguish between relapsing-remitting and chronic progressive forms of MS (43,68–70,73,127,135,138). *Relapsing-remitting MS* is characterized by discrete attacks of neurologic dysfunction. Relapses typically evolve over several days to weeks and may or may not be followed by recovery. Rarely, an attack may evolve more rapidly over seconds and minutes (94). When recovery occurs, it most often is noted within weeks to months following the acute relapse. The second major form of MS, *chronic progressive MS,* results in gradually progressive worsening without intervening periods of stabilization or remission. Chronic progressive MS most often develops in patients with a prior history of relapsing-remitting MS, and relapses may occur superimposed upon the chronic progressive course. A diagnostic category of primary progressive MS is sometimes applied to cases of chronic progressive MS unaccompanied by relapses at any time.

The clinical course of MS is highly variable, nonetheless, some general prognostic indicators can be defined (69,138). Twenty-five years after the initial symptom, approximately 50% of patients remain ambulatory, and 10% have mild or negligible residua. Favorable prognostic factors include early onset, a relapsing-remitting course, little disability 5 years after onset, and a low relapse frequency (less than one attack per year). Poor prognosis is associated with a late age of onset (40 or older) (45), a chronic progressive course, and a high initial attack frequency. Approximately 50% of patients with relapsing-remitting MS will ultimately develop chronic progressive MS. In chronic progressive MS, disability generally results from progressive paralysis that tends to worsen at a sustained tempo until the patient is paraplegic or bedridden.

Symptoms and Signs

The most common manifestations of MS are sensory symptoms, motor weakness, visual blurring due to optic neuritis, diplopia, ataxia, bladder bowel or sexual dysfunction, and cognitive dysfunction (34,68–70,101). Sensory symptoms usually present as paresthesias—tingling, or pins and needles—and less commonly as hypalgesia or dysesthesias. Some patients may complain of inability to sense bath water temperature with one or both feet. Dysesthesias may include sensations of unpleasant, band-like tightness about the trunk or a limb, shooting pain, or steady, aching pain. Sensory symptoms unaccompanied by detectable abnormalities on neurological examination are common in early MS and should not be dismissed as hysterical in origin. In some patients, the distinction between a central and peripheral origin to acute sensory symptoms may be difficult, and the presence of a spinal cord level symptom is diagnostically helpful in the exclusion of acute neuropathies, for example, acute inflammatory polyneuritis.

The onset of motor symptoms may be insidious or dramatic. Exercise-induced weakness may be noted as clumsiness or stubbing of one great toe. Spasms may occur. Examination may reveal signs of pyramidal tract disease, for example, spasticity, hyperreflexia, extensor plantar responses, absent superficial abdominal reflexes, or a Hoffman sign. Focal areflexia, indicating interruption of the lower reflex arc, may occur from demyelinating lesions of the root entry zone of the spinal cord.

Optic neuritis is a well-recognized symptom of MS. Visual loss may be painless or there may be associated pain from the orbit or supraorbital region. The pain may precede visual loss by 1–2 days, and typically worsens with eye movements. Optic neuritis in MS is typically unilateral but may be bilateral. Examination generally reveals reduced visual acuity, a paracentral scotoma, a Marcus-Gunn pupil (pupillodilation to direct light) detected by a swinging flashlight test, and a swollen disc head. Symptomatic (or asymptomatic) bouts of optic neuritis may be followed by development of optic disc pallor. In patients who present with optic neuritis as the sole manifestation of demyelinating disease, the long-term risk of developing MS is approximately 65%. The risk is higher for patients whose MRI studies suggesting disseminated disease not confined to the optic pathways (81).

Abnormalities of conjugate gaze are common. Diplopia (double vision) in MS is often due to an internuclear ophthalmoplegia (INO) or a sixth-nerve palsy. An INO consists of an impairment of adduction on attempted lateral gaze accompanied by nystagmus in the abducting eye. The preservation of convergence distinguishes the adductor palsy of INO from that of medial rectus palsy. The acute development of a unilateral INO may result from diverse causes, including stroke, but the development of bilateral INO in an awake patient is virtually pathognomonic of MS. More extensive disorders of conjugate gaze may occur in MS, including paralysis of horizontal gaze to one side due to lesions near the abducens nerve nucleus in the lateral pontine tegmentum, and the "1½ syndrome," which is a combination of an INO and lateral gaze palsy.

Cerebellar involvement may result in ataxia of gait and limbs, dysarthria, and tremor. In some patients, severe postural tremor ("rubral tremor") may dominate the clinical picture. When vertigo is the initial manifestation of MS, an incorrect diagnosis of labyrinthitis is often made. The presence of related signs indicative of brain-stem dysfunction, for example, facial numbness or weakness, deafness, diplopia, or vertical nystagmus, indicates a "central" rather than a labyrinthine origin to the vertigo.

A variety of other symptoms may present as the initial manifestation of MS or may develop during the course of the disease. Bladder and bowel dysfunction, resulting in urgency, difficulty in voiding or evacuating, and incontinence, are common. Sexual dysfunction may result in impotence in males, and dyspareunia due to decreased vaginal secretions in women. A variety of facial symptoms may occur, including paralysis simulating idiopathic Bell's palsy, trigeminal neuralgia (lancinating facial pain), or facial myokymia (flickering contractions of the facial muscles). Cognitive dysfunction may result in memory loss or personality change. Patients may appear jocular or indifferent to their condition, and inappropriate emotionality (pseudobulbar palsy) may be noted.

Ancillary symptoms of MS include fatigue, Lhermitte symptom, heat sensitivity, and paroxysmal symptoms. Up to 90% of MS patients experience abnormal or sustained fatigue that is serious enough to interfere with their daily lives. Lhermitte symptom consists of electric shock–like sensations that typically are evoked by neck flexion and radiate down the back or, less commonly, into the arms or legs. Lhermitte symptom, due to disease of the cervical spinal cord, is not specific to MS but also occurs with cervical discs and tumors, among other causes. Heat sensitivity is a core symptom of MS and consists of transient neurologic symptoms that develop following exposure to heat (for example a hot shower) or exercise. Uhthoff's symptom of exercise-induced visual blurring is a manifestation of MS-related heat sensitivity. Finally, paroxysmal symptoms are transient—usually 30 seconds or less—and recurrent stereotyped spells. They may consist of paresthesias, tonic contraction of a limb, opisthotonic spasms, dysarthria and ataxia, or transient focal paralysis. The origin of paroxysmal symptoms is not known, but they are theorized to result from repetitive, seizure-like discharges that arise in demyelinated axons.

Laboratory Diagnosis

Laboratory testing may support a diagnosis of MS and exclude other diseases that mimic the MS phenotype. In most situations, the most useful tests are CSF analysis, magnetic resonance imaging (MRI) studies, and evoked response testing (68,89,98,101,135). CSF abnormalities consist of pleocytosis and an increase in the Ig content. Modest CSF pleocytosis (>5 cells/μl), comprised of mononuclear cells, is present in approximately 25% of patients. Counts above 50 cells/μl are unusual but may occur early in the disease course. Pleocytosis of >75 cells/μl or the presence of polymorphonuclear leukocytes in the CSF makes the diagnosis of MS unlikely. In approximately 80% of MS patients, the CSF content of IgG is increased in the setting of a normal total protein. This results from selective production of IgG in the CNS. Elevated levels of CSF IgG are often expressed as a ratio of CSF IgG:albumin. Two or more bands of oligoclonal IgG (see above) are detected by agarose gel electrophoresis in the CSF of most MS patients, and the presence of oligoclonal bands correlates with raised levels of CSF IgG. Oligoclonal bands may not be present at the time of initial presentation of MS.

MRI scanning detects abnormalities in more than 90% of MS patients, thus MRI has assumed an important role in the evaluation of patients with suspected MS (34,81,85,98,101,127). On inversion-recovery (T1) imaging, the CNS appears normal or may reveal punctate areas of dark signal in white matter regions. The most characteristic MRI changes in MS consist of multiple areas of bright signal on spin-echo (T2) sequences. Abnormal T2 bright regions tend to be multiple, asymmetric, and periventricular in location. Some lesions may appear to extend in a linear fashion outward from the ventricular surface, corresponding to the pattern of perivenous demyelination observed pathologically (Dawson's fingers). T2-bright signal areas may also be detected in the spinal cord by MRI. Administration of the contrast agent gadolinium DTPA is used to detect "active" MS lesions in which the blood-brain barrier is disrupted and extravasation of the injected contrast agent into brain parenchyma occurs (123). Additionally, a number of refinements in MRI techniques designed either to increase lesion contrast or to better understand the pathophysiology of MRI abnormalities (for example distinguish between acute and chronic lesions) are being currently evaluated for the diagnosis and assessment of MS (46). Serial MRI studies in relapsing-remitting MS indicate that new MRI abnormal foci appear far more frequently than predicted on the basis of clinical criteria alone (56,72,81,93). A similar frequency of new abnormal foci occurs in chronic progressive MS, although abnormal foci in these patients tend to be more confluent than in patients with relapsing-remitting disease.

Evoked response testing may detect a slowing or interruption of conduction in visual, auditory, somatosensory, or motor pathways. These techniques employ computer averaging methods to record the electrical responses evoked in the nervous system following repetitive stimulation. One or more evoked responses are abnormal in up to 90% of MS patients (68). Although it is assumed that slowing of responses in MS results from the loss of saltatory conduction secondary to demyelination (135), in fact, slowed evoked responses are noted in many non-MS diseases of the nervous system. It is thus a nonspecific finding. Evoked responses are most useful in the diagnosis of MS when they differ between sides, suggesting an asymmetric disease process, when they document a second abnormality in the setting of a single clinically apparent lesion, or when they indicate an objective finding in a patient with subjective complaints only.

Diagnostic Considerations

A correct diagnosis of MS can be reached easily in some patients, but is exceedingly difficult in others. In young adults with relapsing and remitting symptoms that involve multiple different sites of the nervous system, the diagnosis may be deduced by the sophisticated patient prior to contact with a physician. Diagnosis is more difficult when onset suggests a single localized lesion or when a primary progressive course is present. Particularly problematic are cases of rapid or even explosive onset, which can indicate cerebrovascular disease, progressive brain stem syndromes such as brain stem glioma, cervical myelopathy with coexistent degenerative disc disease, or mild symptoms without objective correlate upon examination.

Because of the diversity of clinical presentations that may be due to MS, the differential diagnosis will vary depending on the specific clinical situation. Some neurologic syndromes are rare in MS and their presence should call the suspected diagnosis into question; these include seizures, an extrapyramidal syndrome resembling Parkinson's disease, chorea, isolated dementia, progressive motor weakness with fasciculations, peripheral neuropathy, or aphasia. Chronic inflammatory disorders that affect the CNS but are not restricted to it may be considered, including systemic lupus erythematosus, Behcet's disease, Sjogren's disease, and sarcoidosis. The distinctive clinical features or laboratory signs of these disorders generally permit their differentiation from MS. Primary CNS lymphoma may produce solitary or multifocal CNS lesions with CSF pleocytosis and may respond transiently to steroid therapy. On occasion, chronic CNS infections, Lyme disease, or meningovascular syphilis may also be considered. A progressive myelopathy may be due to deficiency of vitamin B12, but a coexisting peripheral neuropathy is generally the rule.

Therapy

Therapy for MS can be divided into interventions useful for *(1)* acute relapses of MS; *(2)* prophylaxis for relapses; *(3)* chronic progressive MS; and *(4)* symptomatic treatment.

Acute relapses can be treated with intravenous methylprednisolone (MePDN) or corticotropin (ACTH) (11,22,77,126). Pulse therapy with these agents speeds the tempo of recovery from acute attacks and may modestly improve the degree of recovery occurring over a short follow-up period. Their use is generally reserved for patients with moderate or severe attacks. In a recent trial of MePDN for acute optic neuritis, therapy was associated with a greater reduction in the subsequent development of MS as compared to placebo or oral prednisone therapy (12). This result has raised the possibility that short-term treatment with MePDN may retard the evolution of an initial attack of MS. MRI findings in patients with optic neuritis or other monosymptomatic presentations (e.g., transverse myelitis, brainstem encephalomyelitis) have prognostic implications that are relevant to an evolution to MS over a 2–3-year period. Evidence of disseminated lesions at presentation are associated with a 35–45% evolution to MS, compared with 5–10% in patients with normal or single-lesion MRI scans (12,28,81,98,127). Thus, MePDN might be employed for initial attacks when an MRI scan indicates multifocal disease.

Interferon beta (IFN-β) has recently been found to be effective in the prophylaxis of MS relapses (47). Biweekly subcutaneous injections reduced the relapse rate by one-third and reduced severe relapses by one-half. Treatment was also associated with a marked reduction in the evolution of abnormalities detected by MRI scan, confirming the clinical effect on relapse rate (47,122). IFN-β treatment was also associated with a tendency toward reduced accumulated disability, but this finding did not reach statistical significance. A transient, flu-like syndrome may occur with the initiation of therapy. In some patients, troublesome side effects such as fatigue and depression have occurred (35,86). Based upon these results, IFN-β should be considered for MS patients who ambulate independently and have relapsing-remitting disease with two or more relapses in the preceding 2 years. The mechanism responsible for the effect of IFN-β on MS is unknown. It might work by reducing the expression of MHC molecules on the surface of antigen-presenting cells in the brain or elsewhere, by decreasing the production of inflammatory cytokines (15,87), by other immunosuppressive effects, or by an antiviral effect. MHC expression induced by IFN-γ can be blocked by IFN-β, and it is noteworthy that IFN-γ administration appeared to trigger attacks of MS in an earlier study (95).

Chronic immunosuppression has been advocated as therapy for some MS patients with chronic progressive disease (26,27,40,83,88,136,137). The antimetabolite, azathioprine, given orally is a relatively safe and well-tolerated form of chronic immunosuppression (26,33). Its beneficial effect is modest in controlled trials and must be weighed against potential risks that include hepatitis, susceptibility to infection, and a theoretical cancer risk (27,33). Methotrexate is another antimetabolite that has been used in progressive MS, and additional clinical trials of this drug are in progress. Pulse therapy with the alkylating agent cyclophosphamide is of benefit to young (<40 years) ambulatory patients with rapidly progressive MS (17,40,137). The side effects associated with treatment are considerable and include nausea, hair loss, a risk of hemorrhagic cystitis, and temporary profound immunosuppression. Cyclosporine has also been shown to have a modest effect on the course of chronic progressive MS, but side effects, notably hypertension and reversible renal dysfunction, have limited its widespread use (83). A number of pilot trials are currently investigating efficacy and safety for other immunomodulating drugs, such as cladribine, linomide, or intravenous immunoglobulins (1,53,119), and antigen-specific immunosuppression (88,136).

While beyond the scope of this review, symptomatic therapy is an often neglected but critical component of a comprehensive care plan for patients with MS. Care is maximized in settings that bring together teams of health care professionals experienced with the biology of MS and with the medical and social consequences of the disease. Chronic pain, spasticity, bowel, bladder, and sexual dysfunction, rehabilitation, challenges to job and family, and psychiatric issues are best managed in comprehensive care settings geared to the special problems of the MS population (30,68).

Acknowledgments

C. P. Genain is a Harry Weaver Neuroscience Scholar of the National Multiple Sclerosis Society. We thank Ms. Caroline Figoni for secretarial assistance.

References

1. Achiron A, Barak Y, Goren M, Gabbay U, Miron S, Rotstein Z, Noy S, Sarova-Pinhas I. Intravenous immune globulin in multiple sclerosis: clinical and neuroradiological results and implications for possible mechanisms of action. Clin Exp Immunol 104 (Suppl 1):67–70, 1996.

2. Adams CWM, Poston RN, Buk SJ. Pathology, histochemistry and immunocytochemistry of lesions in acute multiple sclerosis. J Neurol Sci 92:291–306, 1989.

3. Allegretta M, Albertini RJ, Howell MD, Smith LR, Martin R, McFarland HF, Sriram S, Brostoff S, Steinman L. Homologies between T cell receptor junctional sequences unique to multiple sclerosis and T cells mediating experimental allergic encephalomyelitis. J Clin Invest 94:105–109, 1994.

4. Allegretta M, Nicklas JA, Sriram S, Albertini RJ. T cells responsive to myelin basic protein in patients with multiple sclerosis. Science 247:718–21, 1990.

5. Allen I, Brankin B. Pathogenesis of multiple sclerosis—the immune diathesis and the role of viruses. J Neuropathol Exp Neurol 52:95–105, 1993.

6. Alvord EC Jr. Disseminated encephalomyelitis: its variations in form and their relationships to other diseases of the nervous system. In: Handbook of Clinical Neurology, Vol 47(3), Demyelinating Diseases, JC Koetsier, ed. Elsevier, Amsterdam, 1985, pp 467–502.

7. Amor S, Groome N, Linington C, Morris MM, Dornmair K, Gardinier MV, Matthieu JM, Baker D. Identification of epitopes of myelin oligodendrocyte glycoprotein for the induction of experimental allergic encephalomyelitis in SJL and Biozzi AB/H mice. J Immunol 153:4349–4356, 1994.

8. Barnett LA, Fujinami RS. Molecular mimicry: a mechanism for autoimmune injury. Faseb J 6:840–844, 1992.

9. Beall SS, Biddison W, McFarlin DE, McFarland HF, Hood LE. Susceptibility for multiple sclerosis is determined, in part, by inheritance of a 175-kb region of the TcR Vb chain locus and HLA class II genes. J Neuroimmunol 45:53–60, 1993.

10. Beck J, Rondot P, Catinot L, Falcoff E, Kirchner H, Wietzerbin J. Increased production of interferon gamma and tumor necrosis factor precedes clinical manifestations in multiple sclerosis: do cytokines trigger exacerbations? Acta Neurol Scand 78:318–323, 1988.

11. Beck RW, Cleary PA, Anderson MM Jr, Keltner JL, Shults WT, Kaufman DI, Buckley EG, Corbett JJ, Kupersmith MJ, Miller NR, Savino PJ, Guy JR, Trobe JD, McCrery JA, III, Smith CH, Chrouses GA, Thompson HS, Katz BJ, Brodsky MC, Goodwin JA, Atwell CW, and the optic Neuritis Study Group. A randomized, controlled trial of corticosteroids in the treatment of acute optic neuritis. N Engl J Med 326:581–588, 1992.

12. Beck RW, Cleary PA, Trobe JD, Kaufman DI, Kupersmith MJ, Paty DW, Brown CH. The effect of corticosteroids for optic neuritis on the subsequent development of multiple sclerosis. N Engl J Med 329:1764–1769, 1993.

13. Birnbaum G, van Ness B. Quantitation of T-cell receptor V beta chain expression on lymphocytes from blood, brain, and spinal fluid in patients with multiple sclerosis and other neurological diseases. Ann Neurol 32:24–30, 1992.

14. Bornstein MB, Appel SH. Tissue culture studies in demyelination. Ann NY Acad Sci 122:280–286, 1965.

15. Brod SA, Marshall GDJ, Henninger EM, Sriram S, Khan M, Wolinsky JS. Interferon-beta 1b treatment decreases tumor necrosis factor-alpha and increases interleukin-6 production in multiple sclerosis. Neurology 46:1633–1638, 1996.

16. Brosnan CF, Stoner GL, Bloom BR, Wisniewski HM. Studies on demyelination by activated lymphocytes in the rabbit eye. II. Antibody-dependent cell-mediated demyelination. J Immunol 118:2103–2109, 1977.

17. Canadian Cooperative Multiple Sclerosis Study Group. The Canadian cooperative trial of cyclophosphamide and plasma exchange in progressive multiple sclerosis. Lancet 337:441–446, 1991.

18. Challoner PB, Smith KT, Parker JD, MacLeod D, Coulter SN, Rose TM, Schultz ER, Bennett L, Garber RL, Chang M, Schad PA, Stewart PM, Nowinski RC, Brown JP,

Burmer GC. Plaque-associated expression of human herpesvirus 6 in multiple sclerosis. Proc Natl Acad Sci 92:7440–7444, 1995.

19. Chou YK, Buenafe AC, Dedrick R, Morrison WJ, Bourdette DN, Whitham R, Atherton J, Lane J, Spoor E, Hashim GA, Offner H, Vandenbark AA. T cell receptor V beta gene usage in the recognition of myelin basic protein by cerebrospinal fluid- and blood-derived T cells from patients with multiple sclerosis. J Neurosci Res 37:169–181, 1994.

20. Chou YK, Vainiene M, Whitham R, Bourdette D, Chou CH-J, Hashim G, Offner H, Vandenbark AA. Response of human T lymphocyte lines to myelin basic protein: association of dominant epitopes with HLA class II restriction molecules. J Neurosci Res 23:207–216, 1989.

21. Compston DAS, Morgan BP, Campbell AK, Wilkins P, Cole G, Thomas ND, Jasani B. Immunocytochemical localization of the terminal complement complex in multiple sclerosis. Neuropathol Appl Neurobiol 15:307–316, 1989.

22. Cooperative study in the evaluation of therapy in multiple sclerosis: ACTH vs placebo. Final report. Neurology 20:1–59, 1970.

23. Cross AH, Tuohy VK, Raine CS. Development of reactivity to new myelin antigens during chronic relapsing autoimmune demyelination. Cell Immunol 146:261–269, 1993.

24. Ebers GC, Paty DW, Stiller CR, Nelson RF, Seland TP, Carsen B. HLA-typing in multiple sclerosis sibling pairs. Lancet 2:88–90, 1982.

25. Ebers GC, Sadovnick AD. The role of genetic factors in multiple sclerosis susceptibility. J Neuroimmunol 54:1–17, 1994.

26. Ellison GW, Myers LW, Mickey MR, Graves MC, Tourtellotte WW, Nuwer MR. Clinical experience with azathioprine: the pros. Neurology 38 (Suppl):20–23, 1988.

27. Ellison GW, Myers LW, Mickey MR, Graves MC, Tourtellotte WW, Syndulko K, Holevoet-Howson MI, Lerner CD, Frane MV, Pettler-Jennings P. A placebo-controlled, randomized, double-masked, variable dosage, clinical trial of azathioprine with and without methylprednisolone in multiple sclerosis. Neurology 39:1018–1026, 1989.

28. Filippi M, Horsfield MA, Morrissey SP, McManus DG, Rudge P, McDonald WI, Miller DH. Quantitative brain MRI lesion load predicts the course of clinically isolated syndromes suggestive of multiple sclerosis. Neurology 44:635–641, 1994.

29. Fisher RS, Clark AW, Wolinsky JJ, Panhad IM, Moses H, Merdiney MR. Post-infectious leukoencephalitis complicating *Mycoplasma pneumoniae* infection. Arch Neurol 40:109–113, 1983.

30. Fowler CJ, van Kerrebroeck EV, Nordenbo A, Van Poppel H. Treatment of lower urinary tract dysfunction in patients with multiple sclerosis. J Neurol Neurosurg Psychiatry 55:986–989, 1992.

31. Genain CP, Nguyen MH, Letvin NL, Pearl R, Davis RL, Adelman M, Lees MB, Linington C, Hauser SL. Antibody facilitation of multiple sclerosis-like lesions in a non human primate. J Clin Invest 96:2966–2974, 1995.

32. Genain CP, Roberts T, Davis RL, Nguyen MH, Uccelli A, Faulds D, Li Y, Hedgpeth J, Hauser SL. Prevention of autoimmune demyelination by a cAMP-specific phosphodiesterase inhibitor. Proc Natl Acad Sci USA 92:3601–3605, 1995.

33. Goodkin DE, Bailly RC, Teetzen ML, Hertsgaard D, Beatty WW. The efficacy of azathioprine in relapsing-remitting multiple sclerosis. Neurology 41:20–25, 1991.

34. Goodkin DE, Doolittle TH, Hauser SL, Ransohoff RM, Roses AD, Rudick RA. Diagnostic criteria for multiple sclerosis research involving multiply affected families. Arch Neurol 48:805–807, 1991.

35. Goodkin DE, Kanoti GA. Ethical considerations raised by the approval of interferon beta-1b for the treatment of multiple sclerosis. Neurology 44:166–170, 1994.

36. Griffin DE. Monophasic autoimmune inflammatory diseases of the CNS and PNS. In: Immunologic Mechanisms in Neurologic and Psychiatric Disease, BH Waksman, ed. Raven Press, New York, 1990, pp 91–104.

37. Harding AE, Sweeney MG, Miller DH, Mumford CJ, Kellar-Wood H, Menard D, McDonald WI, Compston DAS. Occurrence of a multiple sclerosis-like illness in women who have a Leber's hereditary optic neuropathy mitochondrial DNA mutation. Brain 115:979–989, 1992.

38. Hart MN, Earle KM. Haemorrhagic and perivenous encephalitis: a clinical-pathological review of 38 cases. J Neurol Neurosurg Psychiatry 38:585–591, 1975.

39. Hashimoto LL, Mak TW, Ebers GC. T-cell alpha chain polymorphisms in multiple sclerosis. J Neuroimmunol 40:41–48, 1992.

40. Hauser SL, Dawson DM, Lehrich JR, Beal MF, Kevy SV, Propper RD, Mills JA, Weiner HL. Intensive immunosuppression in progressive multiple sclerosis: a randomized, three-arm study of high-dose intravenous cyclophosphamide, plasma exchange, and ACTH. N Engl J Med 308:173–180, 1983.

41. Hauser SL, Doolittle TH, Lincoln R, Brown RH, Dinarello CA. Cytokine accumulations in CSF of multiple sclerosis patients: frequent detection of interleukin-1 and tumor necrosis factor but not interleukin-6. Neurology 40:1735–1739, 1990.

42. Hemachudha T, Griffin DE, Giffels JJ, Johnson RT, Moser AB, Phanuphak P. Myelin basic protein as an encephalitogen in encephalomyelitis and polyneuritis following rabies vaccination. N Engl J Med 316:369–374, 1987.

43. Hillert J, Gronning M, Nyland H, Link H, Olerup O. An immunogenetic heterogeneity in multiple sclerosis. J Neurol Neurosurg Psychiatry 55:887–890, 1992.

44. Hofman RM, Hinton DR, Johnson K, Merrill JE. Tumor necrosis factor identified in multiple sclerosis brain. J Exp Med 170:607–612, 1989.

45. Hooge JP, Redekop WK. Multiple sclerosis with very late onset. Neurology 42:1907–1910, 1992.

46. Husted C. Contributions of neuroimaging to diagnosis and monitoring of multiple sclerosis. Curr Opin Neurol 7:234–241, 1994.

47. IFNB Multiple Sclerosis Study Group and The University of British Columbia MS/MRI Analysis Group. Interferon beta-1b in the treatment of multiple sclerosis: final outcome of the randomized controlled trial. Neurology 45:1277–1285, 1995.

48. Jingwu ZR, Madaer R, Hashim GA, Chin Y, Van den Berg-Loonen E, Raus JCM. Myelin basic protein-specific T lymphocytes in multiple sclerosis and controls. Precursor frequency, fine specificity and cytotoxicity. Ann Neurol 32:330–338, 1992.

49. Johns TG, Rosbo NKD, Menon KK, Abo S, Gonzales MF, Bernard CCA. Myelin oligodendrocyte glycoprotein induces a demyelinating encephalomyelitis resembling multiple sclerosis. J Immunol 154:5536–5541, 1995.

50. Johnson R. The virology of demyelinating diseases. Ann Neurol 36:S54–S60, 1994.

51. Johnson RT, Griffin DE, Hirsh RL, Wolinsky JS, Roedenbeck S, Lindo de Sorianoi, Vaisberg A. Measles encephalomyelitis—clinical and immunologic studies. N Engl J Med 310:137–41, 1984.

52. Joshi N, Usuku K, Hauser SL. The T-cell response to myelin basic protein in familial multiple sclerosis: diversity of fine specificity, restricting elements, and T-cell receptor usage. Ann Neurol 34:385–393, 1993.

53. Karussis DM, Meiner Z, Lehmann D, Gomori J-M, Schwartz A, Linde A, Abramski O. Treatment of secondary progressive multiple sclerosis with the immunomodulator linomide: a double-blind, placebo-controlled pilot study with monthly magnetic resonance imaging evaluation. Neurology 47:341–346, 1996.

54. Kerlero de Rosbo N, Milo R, Lees MB, Burger D, Bernard CCA, Ben-Nun A. Reactivity to myelin antigens in multiple sclerosis. Peripheral blood lymphocytes respond predominantly to myelin oligodendrocyte glycoprotein. J Clin Invest 92:2602–2608, 1993.

55. Kesselring J, Miller DH, Robb SA, Kendall BE, Moseley IF, Kingsley D, Du Boulaye PG, McDonald WI. Acute disseminated encephalomyelitis. MRI findings and the distinction from multiple sclerosis. Brain 113:291–302, 1990.

56. Khoury SJ, Guttmann CR, Orav EJ, Hohol MJ, Ahn SS, Hsu L, Kikinis R, Mackin GA, Jolesz FA, Weiner HL. Longitudinal MRI in multiple sclerosis: correlation between disability and lesion burden. Neurology 44:2120–2124, 1994.

57. Kojima K, Berger T, Lassmann H, Hinze-Selch D, Zhang Y, Gehrmann J, Reske K, Wekerle H, Linington C. Experimental autoimmune panencephalitis and uveoretinitis transferred to the Lewis rat by T lymphocytes specific for the S100β molecule, a calcium binding protein of astroglia. J Exp Med 180:817–829, 1994.

58. Kurtzke JF. Epidemiologic evidence for multiple sclerosis as an infection. Clin Microbiol Rev 6:382–427, 1993.

59. Kurtzke JF, Hyllested K. Multiple sclerosis in the Faroe Islands. II. Clinical update, transmission, and the nature of MS. Neurology 36:307–328, 1986.

60. Lane JM, Ruben FL, Neff JM, Millar JD. Complications of smallpox vaccination, 1968. National surveillance in the United States. N Engl J Med 281:1201, 1969.

61. Lassmann H, Brunner C, Bradl M, Linington C. Experimental allergic encephalomyelitis: the balance between encephalitogenic T lymphocytes and demyelinating antibodies determines size and structure of demyelinated lesions. Acta Neuropathol (Berl) 75:566–576, 1988.

62. Lehman PV, Forsthuber T, Miller A, Sercarz EE. Spreading of T cell autoimmunity to cryptic determinants of an autoantigen. Nature 358:155–157, 1992.

63. Liblau R, Tournier-Lasserve E, Maciazek J, Dumas G, Siffert OD, Hashim G, Bach MA. T cell response to myelin basic protein epitopes in multiple sclerosis patients and healthy subjects. Eur J Immunol 21:1391–1395, 1991.

64. Lindsley MD, Patick AK, Prayoonwiwat N, Rodriquez M. Coexpression of class I major histocompatibility antigen and viral RNA in central nervous system of mice infected with Theiler's virus: a model for multiple sclerosis. Mayo Clin Proc 67:829–838, 1992.

65. Linington C, Berger T, Perry L, Weerth S, Hinze-Selch D, Zhang Y, Lu HC, Lassmann H, Wekerle H. T cells specific for the myelin oligodendrocyte glycoprotein mediate an unusual autoimmune inflammatory response in the central nervous system. Eur J Immunol 23:1364–1372, 1993.

66. Martin R, Jaraquemada D, Flerlage M, Richert JR, Whitaker J, Long EO, McFarlin DE, McFarland HF. Fine specificity and HLA restriction of myelin basic protein-specific cytotoxic T cell lines from multiple sclerosis patients and healthy individuals. J Immunol 145:540–548, 1990.

67. Martin R, McFarland HF, McFarlin DE. Immunological aspects of demyelinating diseases. Ann Rev Immunol 10:153, 1992.

68. Matthews WB. McAlpine's Multiple Sclerosis. Churchill Livingston, New York, 1991.

69. McAlpine D, Compston N. Some aspects of the natural history of disseminated sclerosis. Q J Med 21:135–167, 1952.

70. McAlpine D, Lumsden DE, Acheson ED. Multiple Sclerosis: A Reappraisal, Churchill Livingston, Edinburgh & London, 1972, Chapt. 3, pp 83–98.

71. McCarron RM, Fallis RJ, McFarlin DE. Alterations in T cell antigen specificity and class II restriction during the course of chronic relapsing experimental allergic encephalomyelitis. J Neuroimmunol 29:73–79, 1990.

72. McFarland HF, Franck JA, Albert PS, Smith ME, Martin R, Harris JO, Patronas N, Maloni H, McFarlin DE. Using gadolinium-enhanced magnetic resonance imaging lesions to monitor disease activity in multiple sclerosis. Ann Neurol 32:758–766, 1992.

73. McLean BN, Zeman AZJ, Barnes D, Thompson EJ. Patterns of blood-brain barrier impairment and clinical features in multiple sclerosis. J Neurol Neurosurg Psychiatry 56:356–360, 1993.

74. Meinl E, Weber F, Drexler K, Morelle C, Ott M, Saruhan-Direskeneli G, Goebels N, Ertl B, Jechart J, Giegerich G, Schönbeck S, Bannworth W, Wekerle H, Hohlfeld R. Myelin basic protein-specific T lymphocyte repertoire in multiple sclerosis. Complexity of the response and dominance of nested epitopes due to recruitment of multiple T cell clones. J Clin Invest 92:2633–2643, 1993.

75. Miller HG, Stanton JB, Gibbons JL. Para-infectious encephalomyelitis and related syndromes: a critical review of the neurological complications of certain specific fevers. Q J Med 25:427–505, 1956.

76. Miller S, McRae B, Vanderlugt C, Nikcevich K, Pope J, Pope L, Karpus W. Evolution of the T-cell repertoire during the course of experimental immune-mediated demyelinating diseases. Immunol Rev 144:225–244, 1995.

77. Milligan NM, Newcombe R, Compston DAS. A double-blind controlled trial of high dose methylprednisolone in patients with multiple sclerosis: I. Clinical effects. J Neurol Neurosurg Psychiatry 50:511–516, 1987.

78. Monastra G, Cross AH, Bruni A, Raine CS. Phosphatidylserine, a putative inhibitor of tumor necrosis factor, prevents autoimmune demyelination. Neurology 43:153–163, 1993.

79. Moore GRW, Traugott U, Farooq M, Norton WT, Raine CS. Experimental autoimmune encephalomyelitis. Augmentation of demyelination by different myelin lipids. Lab Invest 51:416–424, 1984.

80. Morgan BP, Campbell AK, Compston DAS. Terminal component of complement (C9) in cerebrospinal fluid of patients with multiple sclerosis. Lancet II:251–255, 1984.

81. Morrissey SP, Miller DH, Kendall BE, Kingsley DPE, Kelly MA, Francis DA, MacManus DG, McDonald WI. The significance of brain magnetic resonance imaging abnormalities at presentation with clinically isolated syndromes suggestive of multiple sclerosis. Brain 116:135–146, 1993.

82. Multiple Sclerosis Genetics Group. A complete genomic screen for multiple sclerosis. Nature Genetics 13:469–471, 1996.

83. Multiple Sclerosis Study Group. Efficacy and toxicity of cyclosporine in chronic progressive multiple sclerosis: a randomized, double-blinded, placebo-controlled clinical trial. Ann Neurol 27:591–605, 1990.

84. Myrianthopoulos NC. Genetic aspects of multiple sclerosis. In: Handbook of Clinical Neurology, Vol. 47(3), Demyelinating Diseases, JC Koetsier, ed. Elsevier, Amsterdam, 1985, pp 289–317.

85. National Multiple Sclerosis Society Working Group on Neuroimaging for the Medical Advisory Board. Use of magnetic resonance imaging in the diagnosis of multiple sclerosis: policy statement. Neurology 36:1575, 1986.

86. Neilley LK, Goodin DS, Goodkin DE, Hauser SL. Side effect profile of interferon beta-1b in MS: results of an open label trial. Neurology 46:552–554, 1996.

87. Noronha A, Toscas A, Jensen M. Interferon beta decreases T cell activation and interferon gamma production in multiple sclerosis. Journal of Neuroimmunology 46:145–153, 1993.

88. Noseworthy JN. Immunosuppressive therapy in multiple sclerosis: pros and cons. Int MS J 1:79–89, 1994.

89. Offenbacher H, Fazekas F, Schmidt R, Friedl W, Flooch E, Payer F, Lechner H. Assessment of MRI criteria for a diagnosis of MS. Neurology 43:905–909, 1993.

90. Oksenberg JR, Begovich AN, Erlich HA, Steinman L. Genetic factors in multiple sclerosis. JAMA 270:2362–2369, 1993.

91. Oksenberg JB, Panzara M, Begovich AB, Mitchell D, Erlich HA, Murray RS, Shimonkevitz R, Sherritt M, Rothbard J, Bernard CCA, Steinman L. Selection for T-cell receptor Vβ-Dβ-Jβ gene rearrangements with specificity for a myelin basic protein peptide in brain lesions of multiple sclerosis. Nature 362:68–70, 1993.

92. Olsson T, Wang WZ, Hojeberg B, Kostulas V, Jiang Y-P, Andersson G, Ekre HP, Link H. Autoreactive T lymphocytes in multiple sclerosis determined by antigen-induced secretion of interferon. J Clin Invest 86:981–985, 1990.

93. Ormerod IEC, McDonald WI, Du Boulay GH, Kendall BE, Moseley IF, Kriss A, Peringer E, Halliday AM, Kakigi R. Disseminated lesions at presentation in patients with optic neuritis. J Neurol Neurosurg Psychiatry 49:124–127, 1986.

94. Osterman PO, Westerbey CE. Paroxysmal attacks in multiple sclerosis. Brain 98:189–202, 1975.

95. Panitch HS, Bever CT Jr. Clinical trials of interferons in multiple sclerosis. What have we learned? J Neuroimmunol 46:155–164, 1993.

96. Panitch HS, Hooper CJ, Johnson KP. CSF antibody to myelin basic protein. Measurement in patients with multiple sclerosis and subacute sclerosing panencephalitis. Arch Neurol 37:206–209, 1980.

97. Paterson PY. Molecular and cellular determinants of neuroimmunologic inflammatory disease. Fed Proc 41:2569–2576, 1982.

98. Paty DW, Oger JJF, Kastrukoff LF, Hashimoto SA, Hooge JP, Eisen AA, Eisen KA, Purves SJ, Low MD, Brandejs V, Robertson WD, Li DKB. MRI in the diagnosis of MS: a prospective study with comparison of clinical evaluation, evoked potentials, oligoclonal banding, and CT. Neurology 38:180–185, 1988.

99. Pette M, Fujita K, Wilkinson D, Altmann DM, Trowsdale J, Giegerich G, Hinkkanen A, Epplen JT, Kappos L, Wekerle H. Myelin autoreactivity in multiple sclerosis: recognition of myelin basic protein in the context of HLA-DR2 products by T lymphocytes of multiple sclerosis patients and healthy donors. Proc Natl Acad Sci USA 87:7968–7972, 1990.

100. Pettinelli CB, McFarlin DE. Adoptive transfer of experimental allergic encephalomyelitis in SJL/J mice after in vitro activation of lymph node cells by myelin basic protein: requirement for Lyt 1+ 2− T lymphocytes. J Immunol 127:1420–1423, 1981.

101. Poser CM, Paty DW, Scheinberg L, McDonald WI, Davis FA, Ebers GC, Johnson KP, Sibley WA, Silberberg DH, Tourtellote WW. New diagnostic criteria for multiple sclerosis: guidelines for research protocols. Ann Neurol 13:227–31, 1983.

102. Prineas JW. The neuropathology of multiple sclerosis. In: Handbook of Clinical Neurology, Vol 47(3), Demyelinating Diseases, JC Koetsier, ed. Elsevier, Amsterdam, 1985, pp 213–257.

103. Raine CS. Mulitple sclerosis and chronic relapsing EAE. comparative ultrastructural neuropathology. In: Multiple sclerosis. Pathology, Diagnostic and Management, JF Hallpike, GWM Adams, WW Tourtelotte, ed. William and Wilkins Co., Baltimore, 1983, pp 413–460.

104. Raine CS, Scheinberg L, Waltz JM. Multiple sclerosis—oligodendrocyte survival and proliferation in an active established lesion. Lab Invest 45:534–546, 1981.

105. Rice GP. Virus-induced demyelination in man: models for multiple sclerosis. Curr Opin Neurol Neurosurg 5:188–194, 1994.

106. Rodriguez M. Central nervous system demyelination and remyelination in multiple sclerosis and viral models of disease. J Neuroimmunol 40:255–263, 1992.

107. Roth GA, Roytta M, Yu RK, Raine CS, Bornstein MB. Antisera to different glycolipids induce myelin alterations in mouse spinal cord tissue cultures. Brain Res 339:9–18, 1985.

108. Ruddle NH, Bergman CM, McGrath KM, Lingenheld EG, Grunnet ML, Padula SJ, Clark RB. An antibody to lymphotoxin and tumor necrosis factor prevents transfer of experimental allergic encephalomyelitis. J Exp Med 172:1193–1200, 1990.

109. Sadovnick AD, Armstrong H, Rice GP, Bulmer D, Hashimoto L, Paty DW, Hashimoto SA, Warren S, Hader W, Murray TJ, Leland TP, Metz L, Bell R, Duquette P, Gray T, Nelson R, Weinshenker B, Brunet D, Ebers GC. A population-based study of multiple sclerosis in twins: update. Ann Neurol 33:281–285, 1993.

110. Sadovnick AD, Bulman D, Ebers GC. Parent-child concordance in multiple sclerosis. Ann Neurol 29:252–255, 1991.

111. Sadovnick AD, McLeod PMJ. The familial nature of multiple sclerosis: empiric recurrence risks for first, second-, third-degree relatives of patients. Neurology 31:1039–1041, 1981.

112. Sanders ME, Koski CL, Robbins D, Shin ML, Frank MM, Joiner KA. Activated terminal complement in cerebrospinal fluid in Guillain-Barre sydrome and multiple sclerosis. J Immunol 136:4456–4459, 1986.

113. Sanders VJ, Waddell AE, Felisan SL, Li X, Conrad AJ, Tourtellotte WW. Herpes simplex virus in postmortem multiple sclerosis brain tissue. Arch Neurol 53:125–133, 1996.

114. Seboun E, Robinson MA, Doolittle TH, Cirolla TA, Kindt TH, Hauser SL. A susceptibility locus for multiple sclerosis is linked to the T cell receptor β chain complex. Cell 57:1095–1100, 1989.

115. Selmaj KW, Raine CS. Tumor necrosis factor mediates myelin and oligodendrocyte damage in vitro. Ann Neurol 23:339–346, 1988.

116. Selmaj K, Raine CS, Cannella B, Brosnan CF. Identification of lymphotoxin and tumor necrosis factor in multiple sclerosis lesions. J Clin Invest 87:949–954, 1991.

117. Sergott RC, Brown MJ, Lisak RP, Miller SL. Antibody to myelin-associated glycoprotein produces central nervous system demyelination. Neurology 38:422–426, 1988.

118. Sharief MK, Phil M, Hentges R. Association between tumor necrosis factor-α and disease progression in patients with multiple sclerosis. N Engl J Med 325:467–472, 1991.

119. Sipe JC, Romine JS, Koziol JA, McMillan R, Syroff J, Beutler E. Cladribine in treatment of chronic progressive multiple sclerosis. Lancet 344:9–13, 1994.

120. Soliven B, Szuchet S, Nelson D. Tumor necrosis factor inhibits K+ current expression in cultured oligodendrocytes. J Membr Biol 124:127–137, 1991.

121. Stewart GJ, McLeod JG, Basten A, Bashir HV. HLA family studies and multiple sclerosis: a common gene, dominantly expressed. Hum Immunol 3:13–29, 1981.

122. Stone LA, Frank JA, Albert PS, Bash C, Smith ME, Maloni H, McFarland HF. The effect of interferon-beta on blood-brain barrier disruptions demonstrated by contrast-enhanced magnetic resonance imaging in relapsing-remitting multiple sclerosis. Ann Neurol 37:611–619, 1995.

123. Stone LA, Smith ME, Alberts PS, Bash CN, Maloni H, Franck JA, McFarland HF. Blood-brain barrier disruption on contrast-enhanced MRI in patients with mild relapsing-remitting multiple sclerosis: relationship to course, gender and age. Neurology 45:1122–1126, 1995.

124. Sun J, Link H, Olsson T, Xiao BG, Andersson G, Ekre HP, Linington C, Diener P. T and B cell responses to myelin-oligodendrocyte glycoprotein in multiple sclerosis. J Immunol 146:1490–1495, 1991.

125. Tabira T, Kira J-I. Strain and species differences of encephalitogenic determinants of

myelin basic protein and proteolipid apoprotein. In: Myelin: Biology and Chemistry. RE Martenson, ed. CRC Press, Ann Arbor, MI, 1992, pp 783–799.

126. Thompson AJ, Kennard C, Swash M, Summers B, Yuill GM, Shepherd DI, Roche S, Perkin GD, Loizou LA, Ferner R, Hughes RAC, Thompson M, Hand J. Relative efficacy of intravenous methylprednisolone and ACTH in the treatment of acute relapse in MS. Neurology 39:969–971, 1989.

127. Thompson AJ, Kermode AG, Wicks D, MacManus DG, Kendall BE, Kingsley DPE, McDonald WI. Major differences in the dynamics of primary and secondary progressive multiple sclerosis. Ann Neurol 29:53–62, 1991.

128. Tienari PJ, Wikstrom J, Koskimies S, Partanen J, Palo J, Peltonen L. Reappraisal of HLA in multiple sclerosis: close linkage in multiplex families. Eur J Hum Genet 1:257–268, 1993.

129. Tourtelotte WW. Cerebrospinal fluid in multiple sclerosis. In: Handbook of Clinical Neurology, PJ Vinken, GW Bruyn, ed. Amsterdam, North Holland, 1970, pp 324.

130. Tourtelotte WW, Potvin AR, Fleming JO, Murthy KN, Levy J, Syndulco K, Potvin JH. Multiple sclerosis: measurement and validation of central nervous system IgG synthesis rate. Neurology 30:240–244, 1980.

131. Tuohy VK. Peptide determinants of myelin proteolipid protein (PLP) in autoimmune demyelinating disease: a review. Neurochem Res 19:935–944, 1994.

132. Usuku K, Joshi N, Hauser SL. T-cell receptors: germline polymorphism and patterns of usage in demyelinating diseases. Crit Rev Immunol 92:381–393, 1992.

133. Walter MA, Gibson WT, Ebers GC, Cox DW. Susceptibility to multiple sclerosis is associated with the proximal immunoglobulin heavy chain variable region. J Clin Invest 87:1266–1273, 1991.

134. Warren KG, Catz I, Johnson E, Mielke B. Antimyelin basic protein specific forms of multiple sclerosis. Ann Neurol 35:280–289, 1994.

135. Waxsman SG. Clinical course and electrophysiology of multiple sclerosis. In: Advances in Neurology, Vol 47, Functional Recovery in Neurological Disease, SG Waksman, ed. Raven Press, New York, 1988, pp 157–184.

136. Weiner HL, Hohol MJ, Khoury SJ, Dawson DM, Hafler DA. Therapy for multiple sclerosis. Neurol Clin 13:173–196, 1995.

137. Weiner HL, Mackin GA, Orav EJ, Hafler DA, Dawson DM, LaPierre Y, Herndon R, Lehrich JR, Hauser SL, Turel A, Fisher M, Birnbaum G, McArthur J, Butler R, Moore M, Sigsbee B, Safran A, Northeast Cooperative Multiple Sclerosis Treatment Group. Intermittent cyclophosphamide pulse therapy in progressive multiple sclerosis: final report of the Northeast Cooperative Multiple Sclerosis Treatment Group. Neurology 43:910–918, 1993.

138. Weinshenker BG. Natural history of multiple sclerosis. Ann Neurol 36 Suppl:S6–S11, 1994.

139. Wekerle H, Kojima K, Lannes-Vierra J, Lassmann H, Linington C. Animal models. Ann Neurol 36:S47–S53, 1994.

140. Welsh CJ, Tonks P, Borrow P, Nash AA. Theiler's virus: an experimental model of virus-induced demyelination. Autoimmunity 6:105–112, 1990.

141. Wood NW, Sawcer SJ, Kellar-Wood HF, Holmans P, Clayton D, Robertson N, Compston DA. Susceptibility to multiple sclerosis and the immunoglobulin heavy chain variable region. J Neurol 242:677–682, 1995.

142. Wucherpfennig KW, Strominger JL. Molecular mimicry in T cell mediated autoimmunity: viral peptides activate human T cell clones specific for myelin basic protein. Cell 80:695–705, 1995.

143. Xiao BG, Linington C, Link H. Antibodies to myelin-oligodendrocyte glycoprotein in cerebrospinal fluid from patients with multiple sclerosis and controls. J Neuroimmunol 31:91–96, 1991.

144. Yamada M, Zurbriggen A, Fujinami RS. Monoclonal antibody to Theiler's murine encephalomyelitis virus defines a determinant on myelin and oligodendrocytes, and augments demyelination in experimental allergic encephalomyelitis. J Exp Med 171:1893–1907, 1990.

145. Zajicek JP, Wing M, Scolding NJ, Compston DAS. Interactions between oligodendrocytes and microglia. A major role for complement and tumor necrosis factor in oligodendrocyte adherence and killing. Brain 115:1611–1631, 1992.

146. Zamvil SS, Steinman L. The T-lymphocyte in experimental allergic encephalomyelitis. Ann Rev Immunol 8:579–621, 1990.

20

AIDS and the Nervous System

LAWRENCE S. HONIG

In 1981, a new human disease entity, initially characterized by opportunistic infections indicative of acquired immunodeficiency, was described in Los Angeles and New York. The syndrome was named *acquired immune deficiency syndrome* (AIDS). At first, pulmonary and cutaneous manifestations were most evident, particularly *Pneumocystis* pneumonia, mucosal candidiasis, and Kaposi's sarcoma of the skin (60,112). However, it soon became apparent that the nervous system, both central and peripheral, was prominently affected, often early in the course of disease (56a,82,123,132). The underlying systemic defect consisted of a severe decline in the number of T-helper (CD4+) cells, leading to compromised cell-mediated immunity, and a variety of other abnormalities in the immune response. Because of the defect in cell-mediated immunity, opportunistic infections and neoplasms figured prominently in the neurological, as well as systemic, manifestations of AIDS. However, some of the prominent nervous system conditions, such as subcortical dementia and spastic paraparesis, as well as certain neuropathies and myopathies did not appear to be caused by any specific opportunistic pathogens. These conditions were presumably related either to the etiologic agent of AIDS itself, or to the accompanying immune dysregulation. Thus, AIDS has provided impetus for much increased research in the field of neuroimmunology.

The causative agent of AIDS was identified in 1983–1984 as a retrovirus. Various isolates of the virus were called *lymphadenopathy-associated virus* (LAV) (6), *human T-lymphotropic virus III* (HTLV-III) (51), and *AIDS-associated retrovirus* (ARV) (95). The newly identified virus infected CD4+ lymphocytes and macrophages, resulting in the immunodeficiency of AIDS. The virus morphologically was an enveloped C-type particle, and was classified as a member of the *Lentivirinae* retroviral subfamily; by

727

consensus it was named *human immunodeficiency virus* (HIV). The original virus isolated from North America and Europe is presently known as HIV-1, because of the discovery of the related virus, HIV-2 (25). HIV-2 causes acquired immunodeficiency syndrome clinically indistinguishable from that caused by HIV-1, although HIV-2 may be less virulent and have a longer incubation period (109). HIV-2 is very common in parts of Africa but has an extremely low prevalence in North America (109). HIV-1 and 2 are related to other animal lentiviruses, which similarly cause neurological disease in addition to hematological and rheumatological dysfunction in their respective host species (58,66,81). The HIV genome also has structural similarities to the more distantly related retroviruses of the *Oncovirinae* subfamily, including human leukemia/ lymphoma viruses HTLV-I and HTLV-II (50).

The RNA genomes of a number of HIV isolates have been entirely sequenced. As with most retroviruses, there are three major genes that are arranged *gag-pol-env* (50). *Gag* codes for the group-specific proteins (p24, p17, p9, p7) of the ribonucleoprotein viral core. *Env* encodes the viral envelope, or coat, glycoproteins (gp120, gp41). The *pol* gene encodes the polymerase enzyme (p64, p53) that performs reverse transcription of the viral RNA into DNA, as well as the nuclease (p34) that effects integration into the host genome, and the proteinase (p11) involved in processing viral proteins from their precursors. All HIV isolates to date also show at least four other small open reading frames that are sandwiched-in, coding for proteins named *tat, rev, vif,* and *nef* (50). The protein products encoded by these genes have important regulatory properties at transcriptional and translational levels in governing viral expression and function (50).

Infection of cells of the immune system is a major cell tropism of HIV (23), particularly cells with the CD4 surface molecule. CD4+ T lymphocytes experience lytic infection, while human macrophages and their blood-borne precursors, monocytes, show persistent productive viral infection without associated cell death. Viral invasion of the central nervous system (CNS) often occurs very early in the course of disease (33,138). Virus may be cultured from cerebrospinal fluid (CSF), and intrathecal antibody production can be demonstrated. A proportion of patients have clinical symptoms due to this CNS involvement at the time of acute infection (33,36,62,82). Prominent CNS involvement, even in the absence of any secondary disease processes, has given rise to the idea that the HIV retrovirus is also "neurotropic," i.e., it has a special affinity for targeting the nervous system (23,24,145).

The proposition that HIV is neurotropic has led to extensive efforts at identifying virus infection of neuronal or glial cells, in addition to elucidating the wide spectrum of opportunistic infection. Despite some reports discussed below purporting to demonstrate such direct viral infection of neural cells, it is now considered unlikely that such direct viral infection is a significant feature. Thus, search for the neuropathophysiology of "primary" (nonopportunistic) AIDS-associated neurological disease has expanded. There is recognition of likely roles for *(a)* monocytes/macrophages as carriers allowing virus entry into the central nervous system, *(b)* viral proteins and infected macrophage-derived products as neurotoxins, or cytokine- or growth factor–effectors, and *(c)* apparent virus-induced autoimmune phenomena. Not only is understanding of these mechanisms important for developing the necessary therapies to alleviate AIDS-associated neurological disease, but also for furthering understanding of major immune-related neurological diseases such as multiple sclerosis, in which homologous immunological mechanisms may pertain (163).

Basic Scientific Findings

Description of Neurological Disease in AIDS

Secondary Infections of the Nervous System

The profound state of immunodeficiency induced by infection with HIV renders patients susceptible to a wide variety of historically rare or uncommon opportunistic infections or neoplasms. In particular, T-cell dysfunction due to lytic infection, with a decreased number of CD4+ T cells, is a dominant deficit. There is also significant B-cell dysfunction, perhaps due in part to T-cell dysregulation, but also likely due in part to Epstein-Barr virus (EBV) effects on B cells through superinfection with or reactivation of this virus. The appearance of neutropenia in AIDS is most often due to bone-marrow suppression induced by medications (e.g., ganciclovir [GCV], zidovudine [ZDV], or sulfa drugs).

Infection with HIV is ultimately followed by immune dysfunction in nearly all infected individuals. Primary infection may be systemically or neurologically symptomatic or asymptomatic. Subsequently, there is usually a prolonged period of years without systemic symptoms. During this phase, there may be mild nervous system symptoms such as headache. The earliest signs of defective cell-mediated immunity frequently are cutaneous anergy, mucocutaneous candidiasis, and decreases in CD4+ T-cell numbers. Paradoxically, at this stage there is often lymphadenopathy due to lymphoid hyperplasia and commonly, signs of B-cell activation, with polyclonal increases in serum immunoglobulins (IgG, IgM, and later, IgA). This B-cell activation presumably is responsible for clinically evident antibody-mediated phenomena, such as hypersensitivity drug reactions and autoimmune, inflammatory skin, muscle, and peripheral nerve disease. Ultimately, AIDS ensues, with signs of severe immune deficiency, namely the development of opportunistic conditions not commonly afflicting individuals with normal immune function.

The deficit in AIDS is dominantly that of impaired cell-mediated immunity due to CD4+ T-cell depletion. Thus it is not surprising that a variety of parasitic, fungal, mycobacterial, eubacterial, and viral infections occur (8,15,82). Many of these conditions had previously been described only in patients iatrogenically immunosuppressed, for reasons of organ transplantation, oncologic, or rheumatologic disorders. Some of the opportunistic conditions reflect invasion of the immunocompromised host by organisms ubiquitous in the environment but not normally bodily resident (e.g., *Cryp-*

tococcus, Pneumocystis). Others correspond to reactivation of previously resident pathogens. For example, individuals with normal immunity may have occult (asymptomatic) or resolved primary infection by a variety of organisms such as *Toxoplasma gondii, Mycobacterium tuberculosis, Treponema pallidum,* cytomegalovirus (CMV), other Herpesviruses, or JC virus. In these persons, organisms are sequestered or quiescent owing to the normally functioning host immune system, but with deficiencies in the immune response there is recrudescent proliferation of the organisms with ensuing symptomatology.

Parasitic infection of the nervous system with *Toxoplasma gondii* is a common feature of AIDS (15,41,98,99,131). The cumulative prevalence of CNS disease is 10–15%. The general population is often asymptomatically infected with this pathogen; serological prevalences in the USA range from 20 to 70%. (Exposure depends on geographical area, food preparation and hygienic practices, and on contact with cat feces.) Formerly, Toxoplasmosis was most often a problem in oncology and organ transplant patients, as well as during pregnancy, due to the risk of transplacental transmission to the fetus. *Toxoplasma* has a complicated life cycle, but disease is primarily symptomatic in the eyes and brain. Trophozoites reach these areas by hematogenous spread, and in the setting of deficient cell-mediated immunity give rise to inflammatory abscesses. Retinochoroidal disease presents as blurred or decreased vision, and examination commonly shows multiple inflammatory patches, with breakdown of the blood-retina barrier visualizable by angiography. Brain abscesses usually cause symptoms from mass effect, with focal deficits and/or seizures. Lesions are often multiple, with distribution at the gray–white matter junction and in the basal ganglia. Radiographically, there is usually ring contrast-enhancement with significant surrounding edema. Fortunately, treatment by sulfa or other antibiotics is usually successful, although it must be continued for life to prevent recurrent lesions. Other CNS parasitic infections may also occur, depending on the patient's environment, including those due to *Strongyloides, Cysticercosis,* and even *Acanthamoeba,* although these are not proven to be increased in AIDS patients.

Fungal infections are common in AIDS (99). The CNS is most often affected by the common soil fungus *Cryptococcus neoformans,* which causes meningitis in about 5% of AIDS patients in the USA and up to 25% of patients in parts of Africa. Cryptococcal meningitis is an infrequent condition in immunocompetent individuals. It most often presents nonfocally with confusion, depressed mental state, or seizures. Treatment with antifungal medications (e.g. amphotericin, fluconazole) usually suppresses the disease. Meningeal infections with *Histoplasma* and *Coccidioides* also occur in AIDS, mostly in the geographic areas respectively endemic for these fungi. Nervous system involvement by *Candida* or *Aspergillus* species in AIDS is usually seen only in patients who are also neutropenic.

Bacterial infections by atypical bacteria are common in AIDS. *Mycobacterium tuberculosis, Mycobacterium avium intracellulare* (MAI) and other mycobacteria, cause significant disability in AIDS patients. The tuberculosis bacillus is a prominent cause of nervous system pathology in the form of meningitis and tuberculomatous CNS abscesses. CNS involvement by MAI appears to be less common and is less well characterized. Infections with "typical" bacteria were initially not thought to be a prominent feature in AIDS; this was explained in part by antibody- and complement-mediated functions being relatively intact. But, due to a relative paucity of exposure, children with AIDS have fewer existing protective antibodies and thus are very susceptible to recurrent bacterial infections. Also, it is now clear that sepsis, subacute bacterial endocarditis with cerebral embolization and consequent strokes, mycotic aneurysms, and pyogenic abscesses can be features of AIDS in adults, albeit not as commonly as some of the other pathogens discussed here. Common bacterial organisms include *Staphylococcus aureus, Streptococcus pneumonia, Hemophilus influenza, Pseudomonas aeruginosa* and *Salmonella* species. In addition, cat-scratch bacillus (*Rochalimaea*) has also been described in AIDS patients, with demonstration of active organismal involvement in the CNS, and intrathecal antibody production (125).

Viruses cause nervous system symptomatology in the HIV-infected patient. Most prominent of these are members of the Herpesvirus and Papovavirus families. Of the Herpesviruses, CMV is most often responsible for disease. Most people have preexistent infection by this virus, with a seroprevalence in the U.S. population of about 50%. Like other members of the *Herpesviridae* family, it normally is dormant, but in cases of immunosuppression—iatrogenically or due to AIDS—CMV virus proliferates, causing symptomatic involvement of the retina, brain, or spinal roots. Retinopathy presents as painless, gradually progressive, sometimes malignantly accelerating, blindness. Encephalitis causes subacute progressive mental decline. Lumbosacral motor polyradiculopathy causes painless loss of ambulation, sparing the bowel and bladder. Fortunately, medications such as ganciclovir and foscarnet can treat retinopathy or polyradiculopathy with gratifying improvement of visual or ambulatory function. Symptoms of CMV encephalitis are less reversible.

Other Herpesvirus family members include EBV, with which infection is common in AIDS, although it usually only impacts the nervous system indirectly: CNS lymphomas may in part be due to EBV-induced myeloproliferation. Herpes simplex viruses (HSV) I and II, as well as varicella-zoster virus, can cause aseptic meningitis, radiculitis, and necrotizing myelitis in some instances.

Progressive multifocal leukoencephalopathy (PML) is the result of papovaviral infection. This disease consists of devastating destruction of cerebral white matter, sometimes with added involvement of gray matter. Pathology shows typical viral inclusions in oligodendroglia, and in situ hybridization and immunocytochemistry reveal the presence of viral genetic material and protein antigens of the human JC virus (JCV). This virus is a member of the papova virus family which includes close relatives: mouse polyoma, vacuolating monkey DNA tumor, and papilloma viruses. (Papilloma virus infections are also frequent in AIDS, but not in the nervous system.) JCV seropositivity is widespread, as with members of the Herpesvirus family, since the majority of the population is exposed to JCV in childhood. Normally, JCV is dormant, residing in the kidney, bone marrow, and spleen; usually it is only pathogenic in conditions of defective host immunity. Since the virus may proliferate in B lymphocytes, it has been suggested that in the setting of AIDS, altered lymphocyte trafficking into the brain may provide for the multiple foci of productive oligodendroglial infection in PML (77). However, more recent reports identifying JCV in brains of immunocompetent elderly HIV-seronegative individuals (42,118) suggest that the JC genome may already be present in the brain prior to development of PML. JC viral strains found in brains of PML patients show extensive heterogeneity in the noncoding regulatory portion of the genome, in comparison to the relatively dormant virus present in other organs or in non-PML patients which is of an invariant "archetypal" type (4). Thus, perhaps due to viral "adaptation" or uncontrolled proliferation in the immunodeficient host, there is development of viral strains that are more active in producing cytolytic oligodendroglial infection, causing PML (42,118,150).

Secondary Neoplasms in the Nervous System

The CNS malignancy of greatest incidence in AIDS is isolated CNS lymphoma of B cell, non-Hodgkin's type. Much less common is cerebral (particularly meningeal) metastatic involvement from systemic lymphoma which is usually of large-cell immunoblastic, or Burkitt's type, and is likely the product of activation of B-lymphotropic viruses such as EBV. While Kaposi's sarcoma of the skin and gut is a feature of AIDS apparently arising as a consequence of infection with human herpesvirus-8 (HHV-8) (51a), dissemination with involvement of the brain or meninges occurs extremely rarely.

Prior to the onset of AIDS, isolated lymphoma of the CNS was an uncommon condition in normal, immunologically competent individuals, occurring in the elderly and in patients with iatrogenic immunosuppression. But at present, most cases of isolated CNS lymphoma have AIDS as the underlying condition. The disorder presents as a progressive focal or multifocal cerebral deficit. Imaging studies reveal contrast-enhancing mass or masses, reflecting breakdown of the blood-brain barrier, with similar radiographic appearance to the lesions of toxoplasmosis. For this lymphoma, radiotherapy and perhaps chemotherapy may be of some therapeutic value.

"Primary" HIV-associated Neurological Syndromes

Subacute dementia (encephalopathy) afflicts most AIDS patients at some stage of their illness (Table 20-1) (35,123,132,152). It presents as a progressive cognitive decline over months to years that, despite extensive neurological, radiological, and pathological investigations, cannot be attributed to secondary, opportunistic conditions. The encephalopathy goes by several names including *AIDS dementia complex* (123) and HIV-associated dementia (112a). While it may appear in the early years following infection and sometimes precede other AIDS-defining conditions, it most typically

Table 20-1 Frequency of "Primary" HIV-Associated Neurological Disorders at Different Stages of HIV Infection[a]

	Acute HIV Infection	Systemically Asymptomatic	Persistent Lymphadenopathy	Definite AIDS
Acute aseptic meningitis	+ +			
Chronic aseptic meningitis		+ +	+ +	+
Dementia/encephalitis		+	+ +	+ + +
Myelopathy	+	+	+ +	+ + +
Inflammatory neuropathies	+ +	+	+	
Axonal neuropathies		+	+ +	+ + +
Myopathy		+	+ +	+ +

[a]Relative frequency of condition at various stages of disease is indicated by number of plus signs. Inflammatory neuropathy includes acute Guillain-Barré-like illness (AIDP), chronic demyelinating neuropathy (CIDP), and mononeuritis multiplex.

occurs in the larger stages of AIDS. Its hallmarks are that of a "subcortical" dementia. Apathy, decreased drive, personality change, vegetative symptoms, decreased attentiveness, and forgetfulness are common, with relative sparing of orientation, language, and remote memory functions. The precise prevalence of HIV encephalopathy among AIDS patients is controversial, with estimates ranging from 30 to 90% cumulatively, depending in part on the stringency of clinical criteria. Neuroradiological studies frequently show patchy white matter disease. Electrophysiological studies may show nonspecific signs of encephalopathy. Cerebrospinal fluid examination is more likely to show higher concentrations of quinolinic acid, neopterin, or β2-microglobulin. The latter two represent byproducts of activation of the cellular immune response.

Pathologically, gross examination of the brain reveals white matter pallor (Fig. 20-1); this occurs in as many as 90% of AIDS brains at autopsy (35,123). Microscopic examination shows gliosis, demyelination, and infiltration with macrophages and multinucleated giant cells. Neocortical gray matter is also involved. Originally, neuronal dropout was not appreciated, but careful quantitative studies show that there is a significant (20–40%) loss of neurons (44,45,85), as well as loss of dendritic and synaptic complexity (111). The etiology is unknown, although probes for various subtle opportunists such as CMV are usually unrevealing. Molecular techniques show intraparenchymal infection with HIV in microglia, macrophages, and multinucleated giant cells (MGC). Some pathologists now partition the microscopic pathologic findings into two categories: *(a)* multifocal areas with perivascular inflammatory MGC, called *HIV encephalitis,* and *(b)* diffuse areas of noninflammatory white matter gliosis and demyelination, called *HIV leukoencephalopathy* (21). However, these two entities overlap.

Myelopathy refers to disease of the spinal cord. Symptoms and signs referable to the cord, in the absence of diagnosed secondary pathology, occur in about 20% of AIDS patients (3,15,20,21,47,97,100,123,129,32a). Usually the presentation is a subacute or

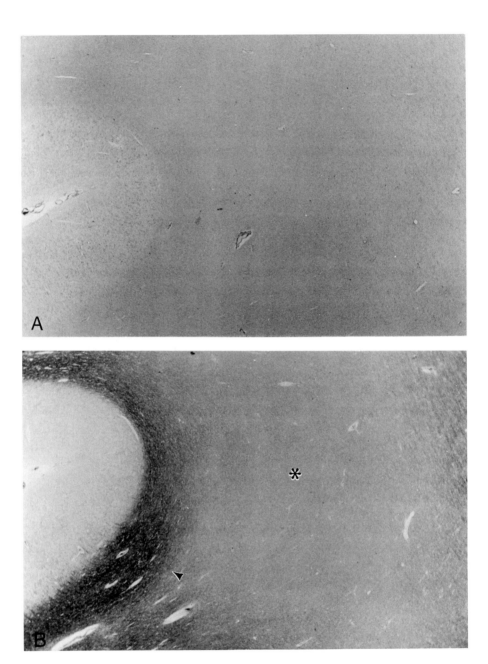

Fig. 20-1. Cerebral pathology of HIV-caused neurological disease. White matter pallor in the brain of an HIV-infected patient may be subtle on standard hematoxylin and eosin-stained section (A). The pallor in this patient with moderate dementia is easily appreciated, however, on the neighboring section (B) which is stained for myelin using Luxol Fast Blue and cresyl violet counterstain; the abnormal, affected area (asterisk) is much lighter than the normal myelin (arrowhead). (From L.S. Honig and D.S. Horoupian, unpublished.)

chronic progressive thoracic myelopathy with spastic weakness of both legs and loss of dorsal column sensory modalities (proprioception and vibration). Bowel and bladder function are less affected. Magnetic resonance imaging discloses no signal changes in the cord, but may show cord atrophy. Pathological examination reveals white matter tract pallor, particularly in the dorsal and lateral funiculi. Microscopic examination reveals a spongy appearance due to vacuolation of variable size and coalescence between lamellae of myelin sheaths; these changes have led to the term *vacuolar myelopathy* (Fig. 20-2). There is preservation of axons, and the myelinated white matter degeneration resembles that seen with vitamin B12 deficiency. While some patients do have mild B12 depletion (87), most do not. Thus, the disorder appears to be associated with HIV, and not a consequence of B12 deficiency. Some reports suggest that the level of HIV expression in macrophages correlates with the extent of the myelopathy (159). Although the prominent vacuolar myelinopathy in the spinal cord is not strictly pathologically homologous to the myelinolysis seen in AIDS subacute leukoencephalitis, the disorders are often correlated and may have common (unknown) pathoetiology. Another type of myelopathy, with degeneration of the gracile tracts without vacuolation, has also been described (136), and may represent tract degeneration due to sensory neuronopathy (loss of dorsal root ganglion neurons).

Neuropathies of various types have been described in the HIV-infected individual (26–29,124,155). These include distal symmetric polyneuropathy (DSPN), acute and chronic inflammatory demyelinating polyneuropathies (AIDP and CIDP), autonomic neuropathy, motor polyradiculopathy, and mononeuritis multiplex. DSPN is in some cases related to nutrition, or to drug toxicity from ddI (dideoxyinosine) or ddC (dideoxycytidine). Likewise, certain neuropathies clearly relate to an opportunistic infection, most notably the lumbosacral motor polyradiculopathy associated with CMV infection. However, a number of neuropathies appear to be intrinsic to HIV infection and unrelated to medication or opportunistic conditions. Sensory-predominant axonal DSPN is common in AIDS, occurring in about a third of individuals, and likely represents a dorsal root ganglionitis. An acute inflammatory demyelinating polyradiculoneuropathy, or Guillain-Barré-like syndrome, most often occurs in the setting of acute HIV infection and serological conversion. This condition, as well as CIDP, appears to be accompanied by a large number of inflammatory endoneurial T cells (27). They may arise as a consequence of the unusual state of immune polyclonal activation, with increased IgG and IgA present, in the initial years following HIV infection.

Myopathy, or muscle disorders, may occur in AIDS patients. Some disorders appear to be of an acquired mitochondrial type, some with nemaline rods, and others are inflammatory polymositis syndromes (14,22,31,38,47,59,86,116,130,154,161). Various etiologies may be responsible including in some cases CMV, in others zidovudine (ZDV, azidothymidine [AZT]) toxicity (130), and less commonly in the United States, coinfection with HTLV-I, which causes a polymyositis-like syndrome. Many cases without ZDV exposure, or CMV or HTLV-I involvement, have been reported (22). Thus, it is likely that an inflammatory muscle condition occasionally arises in AIDS, as

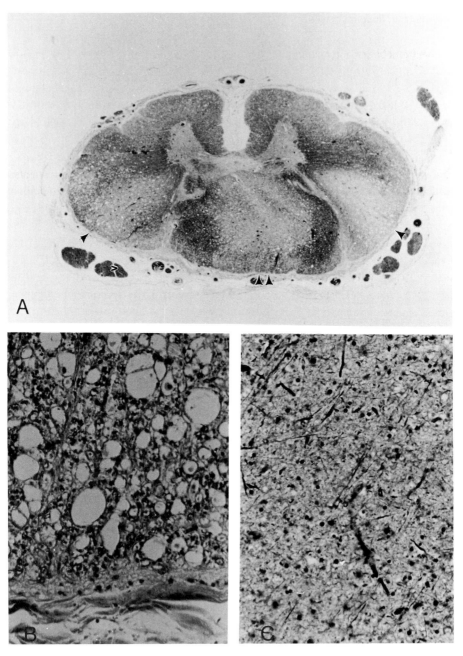

Fig. 20-2. Spinal cord in an AIDS patient with vacuolar myelopathy. A spinal cord section stained for myelin with Luxol Fast Blue and counterstained with cresyl violet shows marked pallor of dorsal (double arrowheads) and lateral (single arrowheads) columns of the cervical cord (A). Higher magnification (B) shows loss of myelin and vacuolar change. However, silver-stained section (C) reveals preservation of axons. (From L.S. Honig and D.S. Horoupian, unpublished.)

do the inflammatory nerve conditions discussed above. Some investigators have reported HIV-virus localization within myofibers, others only within interstitial macrophages (22). The myopathy may be virally provoked by HIV, may be immune-mediated, or possibly is due to elevated cytokine TNF-α, also known as *cachectin.*

Aseptic meningitis is a condition of inflammation of the meningeal coverings of the CNS, without features indicative of the involvement of any apparent organism. Chronic aseptic meningitis without symptoms, or with headaches and malaise, is common throughout the course of HIV infection, occurring in more than one-third of patients. Acute aseptic meningitis, with marked symptoms variably including headache, meningismus, malaise, nausea, vomiting, photophobia, encephalopathy, and ophthalmoplegia, is less common (36,47,98). It occurs in about 1% of HIV-infected individuals and usually reflects primary acute retroviral infection, with concomitant evidence of intrathecal antibody production and systemic seroconversion. The syndrome resembles other aseptic viral meningitides, with a cellular, reactive process in the cerebrospinal fluid. The symptoms are the consequence of inflammation and irritation of meningeal nerves and vasculature.

Mechanisms Underlying Neurological Disease in AIDS

AIDS-associated neurological disease results from a number of secondary conditions as well as from apparent HIV-intrinsic causes. A variety of possible mechanisms may be advanced to explain these latter conditions (Table 20-2). While each of these mechanisms has support from various in vivo and in vitro investigations, multiple mechanisms may actually be operative.

Secondarily Contributing Conditions

Opportunistic infections and neoplasms generally cause focal and pathologically discernible disease as discussed in the previous sections. However, the encephalopathy, myelopathy, and neuropathies of AIDS that do not appear due to opportunistic organisms might nonetheless result from unrecognized infection. A number of researchers have postulated roles for CMV, JC virus, and mycoplasma, as well as more exotic organisms such as *Rochalimaea henselae,* the causative organism of cat-scratch disease. However, pathologically well-studied cases suggest that in most cases subacute encephalitis is not likely due to these known secondary infections (35,123,152).

Malnutrition is another secondary condition that unfortunately occurs frequently among AIDS patients because of decreased appetite from medications, CNS disease, depression, or gastrointestinal disorders. Malabsorption due to gastrointestinal dysfunction from AIDS-related enteric disorders (*Giardia, Cyclospora, Cryptosporidia, Isospora,* visceral Kaposi's sarcoma, etc.) is also common. Resultant malnourishment and vitamin deficiencies can result in nervous system disease. For example, some

Table 20-2 Putative Mechanisms of Neurological Disease in Immunodeficiency

Primary Neuronal or Glial Dysfunction (Related Only to HIV)

Direct viral infection

Effects mediated by infected monocytes/umacrophages:
    Toxic viral products (e.g., gp120, *tat, rev, nef*)
    Toxic macrophage products (e.g., quinolinate, glutamate, other excitotoxins)
    Interference with neurotransmitters (VIP?)
    Interference with growth factors
    Injurious cytokines (e.g., IL-1β, IL-6, TNF-α)
    Blood-brain barrier breakdown

Immune-mediated attack due to
    Nonspecific immune activation
    Superantigen stimulation
    Molecular mimicry
    Innocent bystander
    Blood-brain barrier injury

Secondary Nervous System Dysfunction (Indirectly Related to HIV)

Opportunistic infections

Opportunistic neoplasms

Iatrogenic (drug toxicity)

Nutritional deficiencies

Other coexistent conditions (drug abuse, trauma, etc.)

patients are marginally deficient in vitamin B12, which might possibly play a contributing factor in their neuropathy and myelopathy (87). Other vitamins of putative importance include B1, niacin, and pyridoxine. It has been suggested that due to nutritional disturbances in carrier proteins, coenzymes, and cofactors, some patients may be functionally vitamin-deficient, even with normal-level lab measurements using the usual methods.

Iatrogenic effects in AIDS patients most prominently include drug toxicities reflected as peripheral nervous system disease. Notably, antivirals ddI (2′, 3′-dideoxy-inosine; didanosine), ddC (2′, 3′-dideoxycytidine; zalcitabine) and d4T (2′, 3′-dide-hydro-3′-deoxythymidine; stavudine) cause a distal symmetric polyneuropathy characterized by numbness, tingling, or pain in the feet or hands (145a). Zidovudine (ZDV, AZT) is associated with a mitochondrial myopathy with elevated muscle creatine kinase levels (30a,31), although similar myopathies have also been observed in AIDS patients never treated with ZDV (31).

Coexistent conditions causing neurological disease may also be present in the AIDS patient, although they are not directly related to the HIV virus. Such conditions include traumatic injuries, recreational drug toxicities, such as from alcohol, cocaine, or nitrous oxide, or embolization arising from intravenous drug use–associated endocarditis.

Direct Viral Infection: Cellular Tropisms of HIV

HIV is found in the CNS of infected individuals. Virus has been cultured from the brain and CSF (74,75,96,138), even within the first 2 weeks following HIV infection, and in patients without viremia. HIV has been detected in pathological specimens using southern blot analysis of DNA and by in situ hybridization or PCR for viral specific RNA (1a,145). The exact cellular localization of the virus has been controversial. Originally, several reports suggested localization in astrocytes, oligodendroglia, and neurons (135,146). However, use of double-labeling, with in situ hybridization and immunocytochemical cell markers, mostly has shown that no detectable virus is localized in cells of neuroglial lineage (48,89,123a,153). Thus, a consensus opinion has formed that there is either an extremely low level (43,123a) or no direct infection of neurons with the HIV virus in vivo (21,144a). Astrocytes may be infected in vitro, and HIV has been noted in vivo in pediatric cases (141a,150a); endothelial cells may also be infected (119a). However, the cells that are the primarily HIV infected are microglia, macrophages, their derivatives, the multinucleated giant cells. The developmental origin of microglial cells has been disputed, but it is now accepted that these brain-resident phagocytic cells are, like macrophages, originally bone marrow derived and they migrate into the brain during development (72,126). Unlike CD4+ T cells, which permit productive lytic infection, leading to depletion and resultant cellular immunodeficiency and increased opportunistic infections, the infected monocyte and its derived tissue macrophage are usually nonlytically infected. Fusion of these cells results in syncytial formations termed multinucleated giant cells (MGC).

Despite the lack of evidence for direct neuronal or glial infection with HIV in vivo, the CNS is a preferential (tropic) site for HIV. HIV products or infected macrophage products may be toxic to the nervous system, as discussed below. Thus, the exact mechanisms by which HIV achieves entry into the CNS are important. The *viremic* hypothesis supposes that free, blood-borne virus may penetrate the CNS. Routes of viral invasion might include infection of endothelial cells, which has been reported by some (119a,135,164) but not by others (21,90,153), or passage through the choroid plexus into the CSF. Alternatively, HIV-infected *cells* may infiltrate the CNS, perhaps through altered cell surface or adhesion molecules. For example, HIV-infected T cells show enhanced expression of the adhesion molecule $\alpha5\beta1$-integrin (158). The free passage of infected hematogenous monocytes into the otherwise immunologically privileged CNS may result in a "Trojan horse"-like delivery of virus-infected cells into the brain. Once delivered, virus may spread more diffusely through brain parenchyma into microglial cells for which it may have a special affinity, possibly relating to the CD4 molecule.

Toxic Products of HIV Infection

Since neither primary neuroglial infection nor superimposed secondary opportunistic infection appears to be responsible for the primary retroviral neurological disorders of

AIDS, other HIV-associated mechanisms must be considered. These mechanisms can be grouped functionally by their mediators: excitotoxicity, calcium-influx, reactive oxygen intermediates or peroxides, neurotransmitter modulators or antagonists, growth factor antagonists, injurious cytokines, and cytotoxic cells. Alternatively, putative mechanisms may be characterized by their point of origin: retroviral product, infected macrophage product, glial product stimulated by viral product or infected macrophage, endothelial cell–derived blood-brain barrier breakdown, and "uncontrolled" lymphocyte or macrophage cellular action. Evidence has been discovered in support of a role for a variety of these mechanisms of injury (43,56,56a,83,101,103–105,107,141,148). Elucidation of their relative importance in vivo will be essential for generating rational treatment methods for HIV-related nervous system dysfunction.

HIV retroviral products secreted by HIV-infected macrophages may cause neuroglial dysfunction. Particular attention has been devoted to the envelope glycoprotein gp120, as well as viral products of the *tat, rev* and *nef* genes. The major HIV viral coat protein, gp120, is responsible for the infection of CD4+ cell types through its binding of the CD4 molecule. Injection of gp120 intracerebrally in rats and mice causes abnormalities in behavior and learning (57). A cytocidal effect of gp120 on neurons has been demonstrated in rodent cell cultures, in which addition of picomolar concentrations of viral or recombinant gp120 causes hippocampal or retinal ganglion neuronal death in mixed cultures of neurons, glia, and uninfected monocytoid cells (34,83,103,104,105a,105b). The neurotoxicity may occur via an excitotoxic mechanism that involves direct, or more likely, indirect interaction at the level of the NMDA glutamate receptor (16,34,105,156) and presumably is mediated by calcium influx. One indirect mechanism has been suggested by the observation that the presence of macrophages maybe required for the cell-killing effects of gp120 (104). The role of macrophages might possibly involve proteolytic processing of gp120, or more likely, release of other active factors such as cytokines interleukin-1 (IL-1), tumor necrosis factor-α (TNF-α), kynurenines, other glutamate agonists, or arachidonate (e.g., PAF, LTE4, etc.) metabolites (43,54,167a), although not all investigators have found macrophage-monocyte mediated neurotoxicity (11). For example, gp120 induces IL-1 production when added to human monocytes in vitro (156), or after experimental infusion into rat brain in vivo (147). Astrocytes may also mediate gp120 effects, as gp120 has been shown to cause glutamate efflux from glial cells (7a). In addition to effects on neurons and astrocytes gp120 has been reported to adversely affect oligodendroglia and myelin formation (87a).

Experiments have shown that gp120 toxicity is dependent on, or synergistic with, extracellular glutamate, and that the toxicity can be blocked by specific NMDA antagonists such as dizocilpine (MK801) (16,34,105,156). Activation of the NMDA receptor causes increased intracellular calcium influx and subsequent cell death. Depletion of extracellular calcium or the presence of L-type calcium channel blockers such as nifedipine also prevent gp120 neurotoxicity (34,37,101,102,105). The ultimate mediator of the gp120-induced neurotoxicity may be nitric oxide (NO) and superoxide anions, since inhibitors of nitric oxide synthase as well as depleters of NO or superoxide inhibit cell death (34,105b). Thus, possible effects of gp120 might be that this viral coat protein in the presence of macrophages and extracellular glutamate cause neuronal NMDA receptor activation, with resultant extracellular calcium influx, activation of nitric oxide synthase, NO production, superoxide production, and neuron cell death.

In addition to coat protein, other HIV viral proteins may be toxic to the CNS. The product of the *tat* gene, a transactivating regulator of HIV RNA translation, causes death when injected intracerebrally in mice (61), and it shows neurotoxic effects in vitro (141). Fragments of the product of the *rev* gene, the other positive transactivating element in HIV, also cause lethal neurotoxicity when injected into mice (107). The product of the *nef* gene may also affect neuronal function (107).

Neurotransmitter antagonism is an additional potential mechanism of toxicity for viral products. For example, gp120 antagonizes the activity of the neuromodulatory molecule VIP (vasoactive intestinal peptide) that is important at GABA-ergic synapses (57,127). VIP, or peptide analogs of VIP, have been reported to completely antagonize the cell death–inducing activity of gp120 in culture (16,72a).

Derangements of Immune-related Factors

Macrophage-secreted factors generated by HIV-infected cells or by uninfected cells in response to viral antigens, may be responsible for neuronal dysfunction and death, and oligodendroglial death and demyelination in the white matter. Macrophages are likely components of neural toxicity. Areas of the brain with plentiful macrophages and MGC exhibit gliosis and demyelination (21,111).

Excitotoxins such as kynurenic and quinolinic acids, which are products of tryptophan metabolism, are increased in the CSF of HIV-infected patients (69–71). Higher concentrations have been measured in patients more severely afflicted with HIV-associated cognitive decline (69). Kynureninates are generally increased in a number of inflammatory nervous system diseases and are thought to be the product of increased intracerebral immune stimulation (70,71). Their detrimental action at the NMDA receptor has been hypothesized to be a factor in HIV-associated neuronal loss (69,71).

Cultured HIV-infected macrophages appear to secrete small, heat-stable, protease-resistant molecules that are neuronotoxic in cultured chick ciliary ganglion cells, rat spinal cord cells (56), or human fetal brain aggregates (134). These factors appear to also act through the NMDA receptor, but apparently they are not identical to either glutamate or quinolinate (56). Some investigators have failed to replicate these findings in different systems, either suggesting a corequirement for astrocytes (54), indicating a need for direct monocyte to human neuron cell adhesion (149), or ascribing the toxicity to *Mycoplasma* contamination with associated induction of glial TNF-α production (11).

Cytokines are small secreted molecules that signal cell-to-cell information in the immune system, thus providing control of the immune response. In addition to regulatory roles in the inflammatory response, they may have direct roles in supporting nonimmune cell growth, in neuronal cytotoxicity (53a), and in regulating the proliferation of viral invaders, including the HIV virus. TNF-α, IL-1, and IL-6 are all increased in the sera and CSF of HIV-infected patients (151,162). Brain tissue of AIDS patients shows increases in IL-1, IL-6, transforming growth factor β (TGF-β), TNF-α, and interferon γ (IFN-γ) (151,157). IFN-α, TNF-α, and IL-6 expression are induced in mononuclear cells cocultured with HIV-infected monocytes (53) or human brain cell cultures (167a). TNF-α levels in CSF are particularly increased in AIDS patients with more advanced HIV disease (64). Although there is not a demonstrated correlation between degree of dementia in adults and CSF TNF-α levels (64), children with AIDS have shown an association between elevated serum TNF and the presence of progressive encephalopathy (117).

Human monocytes in vitro challenged with HIV envelope protein gp120 produce increased IL-1, and arachidonate metabolite PGE2 (105b,156). Coculture of HIV-infected macrophages with glial cells results in the secretion of cytokines TNF-β and IL-1β (54). These cytokines also appear to be released via an arachidonate-mediated pathway and are toxic to cultured fetal rat neurons (54). IL-1 can be cytotoxic to certain cells and is a primary mediator of the inflammatory response. TNF-α mediates myelin and oligodendroglial damage in cultured spinal cord tissue (144). It is plausible that it may be a contributing factor to chronic myelopathy and subacute leukoencephalitis in AIDS.

Cytokines or antibodies may possibly function as growth factor antagonists, thus causing dysfunction or death of CNS neurons, particularly if they are already injured. An example of CNS dependence on growth factors includes the cholinergic neurons of the rodent septal nuclei and nucleus basalis, which suffer retrograde degeneration after axotomy unless supplied with exogenous nerve growth factor (NGF) (49). Culture of septal neurons in the presence of anti-NGF causes reduction in the number of cholinesterase-positive cells surviving in vitro (68).

Immune Dysregulation

Abnormal immune function is the hallmark of AIDS. The immune system operates as a network with various soluble cytokines and effector cells having both positive and negative effects. Thus, it has been suggested that despite the overall cellular immune deficiency, particularly in the terminal stages of the disease, aspects of increased immune function such as autoimmune phenomena might occur, and that these might be involved in the apparent primary HIV nervous system disorders.

Neuropathological examinations show that a classical immune response with prominent lymphocytic infiltration is infrequent in the postmortem brains of patients with AIDS, except in cases where there is evidence of concomitant coinfection with other pathogens or viruses. (For example, HTLV-I-related neurological disease includes active signs of perivascular lymphocytic infiltration in the spinal cord and sometimes in nerve and muscle.) The lack of prominent B- or T-cell infiltration in autopsy series does not exclude a direct role for low-level chronic effects from prolonged abnormalities in lymphocyte and monocyte traffic, nor does it exclude a role of lymphocytes in evanescent attacks (prior transient episodic inflammation). This latter scenario is suggested by reports indicating that perivascular mononuclear inflammation may commonly occur in brains of patients who have died (unnaturally) early in the course of AIDS (62). Brains of AIDS patients generally exhibit large numbers of activated macrophages, with elevated levels of expression of class II (HLA-DR) major histocompatibility antigens (1,115). Another observation which suggests that AIDS features not only a decreased immune response is that pharmacological immunosuppressive therapy does not necessarily cause worsening of disease symptoms. Paradoxically, treatments with glucocorticosteroids are usually not accompanied by a decline in neurological function but may even result in improvement, particularly in children (142).

Analysis of CSF, serum, and neuropathological specimens suggests a partial state of immune activation with HIV-infection. Immunoglobulin levels are elevated in peripheral blood and CSF. Oligoclonal banding in the CSF is frequently present, indicating expansion of particular immunoglobulin species. β2-microglobulin (β2M), an 11-kDa peptide chain component of class I histocompatibility molecules, is increased in plasma, which suggests an increased lymphoid cell turnover, and in CSF (13,17,151), where it is likely derived from macrophages, microglia, and possibly astrocytes, possibly owing to up-regulated expression of HLA class I molecules (1,2,151). The concentration of β2M in CSF is correlated with the severity of HIV dementia (17), although it can be high in early stages of HIV infection (13). Neopterin is a marker for activation of cell-mediated immunity. It is generated by IFN-γ-stimulated macrophages during degradation of guanosine triphosphate (GTP). Neopterin is increased in the CSF and serum of patients; the levels correlate with β2-microglobulin (70,128,151). IFN-γ is a marker for the cell-mediated immune response and its level is also increased in AIDS (63,151). The interleukin-2 receptor (IL-2R, CD25) is also up-regulated (63); this receptor probably derives from activated monocytes and possibly from B cells. Other cytokines such as TNF-α, IL-1, and IL-6 are increased in the plasma and CSF of HIV-infected individuals (64,151). TNF-α is produced by macrophages and activated lymphocytes. It may only be a marker of inflammation due to secondary infections, although it can stimulate HIV replication and, as discussed above, may potentially have a direct neurotoxic effect (144) in addition to its recognized role in modulation of the immune response.

Autoimmunity Merchanisms

Several different mechanisms for autoimmune attack in the setting of human HIV infection have been proposed (9,82). These include *(1)* B-cell polyclonal activation with resultant increased levels of antibodies; *(2)* superantigen stimulation of the immune response; *(3)* molecular mimicry of viral products for host proteins; *(4)* innocent bystander attack on self-antigens; and *(5)* blood-brain barrier injury.

Immunoglobulin levels are usually increased in the blood and CSF of HIV-infected individuals (93). However, circulating B lymphocytes are present in normal numbers, and the increased production of IgG and IgM, as well as of IgD and IgA, may be explained by abnormally high percentages of activated B cells. Evidence supporting this observation includes an increased proportion of B cells that produces immunoglobulin spontaneously or with mitogen-induction (93), increased positivity for the transferrin receptor, and a decreased percentage of Leu-8+ cells (110). While as much as 20 to 50% of antibody production may be directed against HIV antigens, there are also broad nonspecific increases in antibody that are reflected as polyclonal and oligoclonal immunoglobulins (138). Some of the latter are directed against common pathogens, and some may be autoantibodies—for example, a prominent Ig band in CSF and serum which was found to be directed against the human insulinoma gene *rig* in an individual coinfected with HIV-1 and HTLV-II (140). HIV-infected patients also demonstrate a number of nonorgan-specific autoantibodies that are conventionally associated with a variety of idiopathic autoimmune disorders, such as systemic lupus erythematosus or Sjogren's syndrome (120). These antibodies include Ig directed against double-stranded DNA, histones, and ribonucleoproteins, and are reportedly present in as many as 44–95% of HIV-infected patients (120). Thus, a general, nonspecific activation of immunoglobulin synthesis may not only contribute to immune deficiency by preventing antigen-induced stimulation of appropriate antibodies to exogenous challenge but may also cause injury, due to increased levels of antibodies against endogenous nervous system antigens. Such antibodies could cause an immune-mediated attack on the nervous system, particularly in the presence of blood-brain barrier dysfunction.

Superantigens have recently been characterized as molecules that cause either profound activation or suppression of large numbers of T lymphocytes with particular T-cell receptor Vα or Vβ sequences (168). While they are selective for groups of T cells (e.g., 5–25% of the cell population), superantigens differ from conventional antigens in that they do not require antigen processing by presenting cells, and restriction by MHC type is absent. Superantigens bind to MHC class II antigens outside of the normal antigen-binding groove, thereby providing a promiscuous interaction with the T-cell receptor of CD4+ or CD8+ T lymphocytes. A variety of bacterial products appear to act as superantigens and provoke inflammatory disease (168). Since an HIV superantigen might explain aspects of the observed immune activation (and also T-cell depletion) in HIV-infected individuals, investigation is proceeding as to whether HIV might indeed encode a superantigen. Additional support for this idea was generated by the discovery that the retrovirus mouse mammary tumor virus (MMTV) encodes a superantigen in the open reading frame of its 3′-long terminal repeat (88,133). Direct evidence for an HIV superantigen is lacking, although there is some indirect supportive data. HIV-infected individuals may exhibit a restricted repertoire of T-cell receptor Vβ sequences, which suggests selective elimination of a defined set of T cells (78). Also, a superantigen effect may cause Vβ12 to be a preferential target for HIV-1 (94). However, other investigators have found results that are inconsistent with superantigen effect and more consistent with stimulation by conventional antigen (perhaps by molecular mimicry), such as an apparent selective expansion of Vβ5.3 expression in AIDS patients (32). They have also found evidence for MHC restriction (108).

Molecular mimicry is a concept in which autoreactive antibodies result from the host response to a foreign (e.g., viral) antigenic epitope that resembles a normal host self-protein (5). Such autoantibodies to alloantigens might be particularly likely to be directed against antigens of the CNS, since these enjoy immunological privilege and are sequestered by the blood-brain barrier. It has been suggested that several regions of the HIV envelope glycoprotein gp160 and its protein derivatives are homologous to portions of the human leukocyte antigen system (HLA), human IgA molecules (12), IL-2 (137), and an astrocyte protein (167). An antibody response against HLA or Ig molecules might cause immune dysregulation, while a response against astrocytes or endothelial cells might contribute towards breakdown of the blood-brain barrier.

Innocent bystander attack refers to a nonspecific immune response towards native privileged CNS structures, triggered by exogenous antigens, such as the HIV virus. In a number of experimental models, immunization or allograft transplant prompts the generation of cytotoxic T cells which are then less discriminate in their attack (76,166). These cytotoxic cells may be neither antigen-appropriate nor MHC-restricted in the inflammatory focus that they create. This model presupposes some breakdown of the blood-brain barrier, and might involve the presence of an opportunist towards which the primary response is directed. Alternatively, the novel accessibility of previously inaccessible CNS antigens may contribute to this type of immune attack.

Blood-brain barrier injury may occur in HIV infection, particularly in children and in adults with opportunistic infections such as tuberculosis (2). It can be demonstrated pathologically (62), by measurement of increased leakage of albumin into the CSF, i.e., an albumin CSF:serum ratio >0.009 (2,18,71,128,139), or by visualization of contrast-enhancement on neuroimaging studies (7). Barrier breakdown may result not only from injury due to opportunistic infections but also from endothelial cell damage due to direct infection with HIV or inflammatory or cytokine responses. Barrier breakdown is significant because it allows increased exposure of previously hidden self-antigens to antigen-presenting cells, and because it allows systemic toxins greater access to the otherwise privileged CNS.

Other Neuroretroviral Diseases in Humans and Animals

There are three subfamilies within the Retrovirus family: *Lentivirinae, Oncovirinae,* and *Spumavirinae* (160). HIV-1 and HIV-2, which are causative agents in AIDS, share with all other known lentiviruses the property of causing immunological and neurological disease (Table 20-3). They do not cause tumors. The oncoviruses cause tumors and include the human leukemia/lymphoma viruses HTLV-I and HTLV-II, which also cause a chronic nervous system disorder. The Spumaviruses have not been definitively associated with any disease states of the nervous or other systems. Spumaviruses cause foamy cytoplasmic degeneration in cultured cells, and transgenic mice expressing Spumavirus genes have been reported to show progressive degenerative disease of the CNS and muscle (14).

Models for AIDS have been sought via a number of routes, including study of human infections by the other, less lethal, retroviruses, HTLV-I and HTLV-II, and through the study of animal models of AIDS, especially retrovirus-infected primates. In chimpanzees, injected HIV-1 causes persistent T-lymphocyte infection but not infection of monocytes or macrophages (40). Since host seroconversion occurs with demonstrable peripheral and intra-blood-brain synthesis of antibody, this may provide a model for vaccination; but it is not a good model for induced neurological disease, since AIDS-like disease is not observed (46,119).

Another alternative is the study of animal lentiviruses in their natural host species in which these viruses indeed cause illness similar to AIDS. However, even the best of these model systems, that of simian immunodeficiency virus (SIV) in macaques, is imperfect. For example, while giant cell encephalitis may be seen in macaques, diffuse white matter pallor or vacuolar myelopathy is not found (91). Finally, HIV may be studied in engineered hybrid animals containing the human immune system. For example the SCID-hu mouse (113) is an experimental rodent that has a severe immunodeficiency that is alleviated by transplantation of a functioning human immune system. While acute infection with HIV can be demonstrated (122), the lack of a human nervous system may prevent these mice from yielding a good model for neurological illness of AIDS.

Table 20-3 Retroviruses Causing Nervous System Disease in Humans and Animals

Human retroviruses	
HTLV-I	Myeloencephalitis, ?neuropathy, ?myopathy
HTLV-II	Possible myelopathy and/or ataxic syndrome
HIV-1, HIV-2	Central and peripheral nervous system disease
Animal retroviruses	
Monkey	Simian immunodeficiency virus (SIV, STLV-III)
Cow	Bovine immunodeficiency virus (BIV)
Cat	Feline immunodeficiency virus (FIV)
Goat	Caprine arthritis-encephalitis virus (CAEV)
Sheep	Visna-Maedi virus (Ovine progressive pneumonia virus, VMV, OPPV)
Horse	Equine infectious anemia virus (EIAV)

Other Human Retroviruses

The lentivirus HIV-2 is rather closely related to HIV-1, although it is also very closely related to the simian immunodeficiency virus. While the neurological features of HIV-2 infection are less well characterized, due to the very small number of cases reported outside of Africa, the clinical syndrome appears to overlap entirely with that of AIDS from HIV-1 infection (25,106,143). The asymptomatic period following viral infection may be of longer duration, and the AIDS syndrome may be somewhat more indolent, but decreased CD4+ T-cell counts with consequent immunodeficiency, and systemic and nervous system opportunistic infections, are characteristic (109). Sub-acute encephalitis has been described with HIV-2 infection, as in AIDS from HIV-1 (19,25,39).

The other known human retroviruses are HTLV-I and HTLV-II. The epidemiology of infection with these viruses is very similar to that of HIV, namely, infection through sexual, maternal, parenteral, or transfusion routes. HTLV-I is the pathoetiologic agent of adult acute T-cell leukemia, and in about 1% of infected individuals causes nervous system disease, namely, a chronic progressive myelopathy. HTLV-II also has been isolated from patients with T-cell leukemia, hairy cell leukemia, although an incontrovertible association of this virus with hematologic disease has not been proven (50). HTLV-II also does not have a proven association with neurological disease. But in patients coinfected with HTLV-II and HIV, a spastic paraparesis like that with HTLV-I may occur (10), and infection with HTLV-II alone has been associated with myelopathy and/or ataxia in a small number of patients (67,73,80,121). Finally, while it now seems unlikely, there has been controversy regarding whether a retrovirus related to HTLV-I or HTLV-II might possibly have a etiologic role in multiple sclerosis.

The chronic progressive myelopathy called *tropical spastic paraparesis (TSP)* in the Caribbean (30), and *HTLV-I-associated myelopathy (HAM)* in Japan (79) eventually develops in about 1% of individuals infected with HTLV-I. This disorder is now known by the World Health Organization (WHO) convention as *TSP/HAM* or *HAM/TSP* (55,79). It occurs more frequently and more severely when infection is acquired by blood transfusion. Hematologic disease, or adult T-cell leukemia, also develops in several percent of patients with HTLV-I infection. Curiously, the hematologic and neurologic presentations are nearly mutually exclusive (30). Typically, TSP/HAM presents as an indolent progressive thoracic myelopathy marked by autonomic dysfunction (bladder, bowel, and erectile dysfunction), spasticity, weakness, and numbness in the legs (30,114). Unlike the degenerative myelopathy associated with HIV, in which there is vacuolar change in the myelinated columns, TSP/HAM cases usually show inflammatory pathology with perivascular lymphocytic collections in the meninges and cord (79). The pathogenetic mechanisms underlying this process are unknown. Proposed mechanisms include molecular mimicry, superantigen, or general immune activation, as discussed above for HIV.

Retroviruses Causing Neurological Disease in Other Species

Animal oncoviruses include avian, murine, feline, bovine, and simian sarcoma or leukemia viruses. The sarcoma viruses of various species can cause brain tumors when injected intracerebrally into experimental animals (81). Murine leukemia virus can cause a polioencephalomyelopathy that is neither spongiform nor exhibits signs of inflammation (52,84,165). A good animal model of TSP/HAM has not yet been discovered.

All animal lentiviruses thus far identified can cause neurological disease in their host species (Table 20-3), as HIV does in humans. The lentivirus family includes agents infecting the goat (caprine arthritis-encephalitis virus [CAEV]), sheep (ovine Visna-Maedi and progressive pneumonia virus [VMV or OPPV]), cow (bovine immunodeficiency virus [BIV]), horse (equine infectious anemia virus [EIAV]), cat (feline immunodeficiency virus [FIV]), and primate (simian immunodeficiency virus [SIV], previously called *STLV-III*) (58,66,84). These genetically related viruses all cause immunodeficiency in their host animal species, with resultant opportunistic infections. They also are associated with encephalopathy and wasting syndromes similar to those caused by HIV in humans. The best-studied is Visna-Maedi, which infects Icelandic sheep and causes a subacute encephalomyelitis characterized clinically by wasting, spasticity, and paralysis (65,84). Neuropathologic examination shows demyelination. Goats infected with CAEV also develop a chronic wasting leukoencephalomyelitis, as well as progressive arthritis and osteoporosis (66). Similarly, cows infected with bovine immunodeficiency virus develop wasting and weakness associated with brain lesions, and EIAV-infected horses develop subacute encephalitis, in addition to bone-marrow suppression (58,66,84). Macaque monkeys experimentally infected with SIV develop a wasting illness with immunodeficiency resembling AIDS and an accompanying subacute encephalopathy (91,92). These animal models require further study and, despite differences from AIDS, hold the potential for greater understanding of pathogenesis and designs for treatment of AIDS-related neurological disease.

Summary

AIDS is characterized by a severe acquired immunodeficiency, owing to infection with the lymphotropic virus, HIV. Neurological disease figures prominently in AIDS. A proportion of the nervous system involvement is due to *secondary* opportunistic infections or neoplasms. However, a set of syndromes cannot be explained by such secondary causative factors. For these syndromes, HIV infection and/or its effects on the immune system appear to have a *primary* etiologic role. HIV-associated dementia, aseptic meningitis, chronic myelopathy, and certain neuropathies and myopathies are in this class. Despite the variety of potential mechanisms discussed in this chapter, the exact means by which such disorders arise is unclear. The importance of increasing our understanding is twofold. Such knowledge is necessary for designing therapeutic strategies to treat HIV-infected individuals. But also these disorders resemble a number of non-HIV related and putatively immune mediated neurological disorders for which we have insufficient understanding. Thus, AIDS-related disease provides a broader outlook on the role of the immune system in causing neuropathology.

References

1. Achim CL, Morey MK, Wiley CA. Expression of major histocompatibility complex and HIV antigens within the brains of AIDS patients. AIDS 5:535–541, 1991.
1a. Achim CL, Wang R, Miners DK, Wiley CA. Brain viral burden in HIV infection. J Neuropathol Exp Neurol 53:284–294, 1994.
2. Alvarez-Cermeno JC, Varela JM, Villar LM, Casado C, Dominguez M, Roy G, Bootello A, Gonzalez-Porque P. Intrathecal synthesis of soluble class I antigens (sHLA) in patients with HIV infection and tuberculous meningitis. J Neurol Sci 100:152–154, 1990.
3. Anders KH, Guerra WF, Tomiyasu U, Verity MA, Vinters HV. The neuropathology of AIDS. UCLA experience and review. Am J Pathol 124:537–558, 1986.
4. Ault GS, Stoner GL. Two major types of JC virus defined in progressive multifocal leukoencephalopathy brain by early and late coding region DNA sequences. J Gen Virol 73:2669–2678, 1992.
5. Barnett LA, Fujinami RS. Molecular mimicry: a mechanism for autoimmune injury. FASEB J 6:840–844, 1992.
6. Barre-Sinoussi F, Chermann JC, Rey F, Nugeyre MT, Chamaret S, Gruest J, Dauguet C, Axler BC, Vezinet BF, Rouzioux C. Isolation of a T-lymphotropic retrovirus from a patient at risk for acquired immune deficiency syndrome (AIDS). Science 220:868–871, 1983.
7. Belman AL, Diamond G, Dickson D, Horoupian D, Llena J, Lantos G, Rubinstein A. Pediatric acquired immunodeficiency syndrome. Neurologic syndromes. Am J Dis Children. 142:29–35, 1988.
7a. Benos DJ, Hahn BH, Bubien JK, Ghosh SK, Mashburn NA, Chaikin MA, Shaw GM, Benveniste EN. Envelope glycoprotein gp120 of human immunodeficiency virus type 1 alters ion transport in astrocytes: implications for AIDS dementia complex. Proc Natl Acad Sci USA 91:494–448, 1994.
8. Berger JR. The neurological complications of HIV infection. Acta Neurol Scand Suppl. 116:40–76, 1988.
9. Berger JR, Levy JA. The human immunodeficiency virus, type 1: the virus and its role in neurologic disease. Semin Neurol. 12:1–9, 1992.
10. Berger JR, Raffanti S, Svenningsson A, McCarthy M, Snodgrass S, Resnick L. The role of HTLV in HIV-1 neurologic disease. Neurology 41:197–202, 1991.
11. Bernton EW, Bryant HU, Decoster MA, Orenstein JM, Ribas JL, Meltzer MS, Gendelman HE. No direct neuronotoxicity by HIV-1 virions or culture fluids from HIV-1-infected T cells or monocytes. AIDS Res Hum Retroviruses 8:495–503, 1992.
12. Bjork RJ. HIV-1: seven facets of functional molecular mimicry. Immunol Lett. 28:91–96; discussion, 97–99, 1991.
13. Bogner JR, Junge-Hulsing B, Kronawitter U, Sadri I, Matuschke A, Goebel FD. Expansion of neopterin and β-microglobulin in cerebrospinal fluid reaches maximum levels early and late in the course of human immunodeficiency virus infection. Clin Invest 70:665–669, 1992.

14. Bothe K, Aguzzi A, Lassmann H, Rethwilm A, Horak I. Progressive encephalopathy and myopathy in transgenic mice expressing human foamy virus genes. Science 253:555–557, 1991.

15. Bredesen DE, Levy RM, Rosenblum ML. The neurology of human immunodeficiency virus infection. Q J Med 68:665–677, 1988.

16. Brenneman DE, Westbrook GL, Fitzgerald SP, Ennist DL, Elkins KL, Ruff MR, Pert CB. Neuronal cell killing by the envelope protein of HIV and its prevention by vasoactive intestinal peptide. Nature 335:639–642, 1988.

17. Brew BJ, Bhalla RB, Fleisher M, Paul M, Khan A, Schwartz MK, Price RW. Cerebrospinal fluid β2 microglobulin in patients infected with human immunodeficiency virus. Neurology 39:830–834, 1989.

18. Brew BJ, Bhalla RB, Paul M, Sidtis JJ, Keilp JJ, Sadler AE, Gallardo H, McArthur JC, Schwartz MK, Price RW. Cerebrospinal fluid β2-microglobulin in patients with AIDS dementia complex: an expanded series including response to zidovudine treatment. AIDS 6:461–465, 1992.

19. Brun-Vezinet F, Rey MA, Katlama C, Girard PM, Roulot D, Yeni P, Lenoble L, Clavel F, Alizon M, Gadelle S. Lymphadenopathy-associated virus type 2 in AIDS and AIDS-related complex. Clinical and virological features in four patients. Lancet 1:128–132, 1987.

20. Budka H. The definition of HIV-specific neuropathology. Acta Pathol Jpn 41:182–91, 1991.

21. Budka H. Neuropathology of human immunodeficiency virus infection. Brain Pathol 1:163–175, 1991.

22. Chad DA, Smith TW, Blumenfeld A, Fairchild PG, DeGirolami U. Human immunodeficiency virus (HIV)-associated myopathy: immunocytochemical identification of an HIV antigen (gp 41) in muscle macrophages. Ann Neurol 28:579–582, 1990.

23. Cheng-Mayer C. Biological and molecular features of HIV-1 related to tissue tropism. AIDS 4(Suppl 1):S49–S56, 1990.

24. Cheng-Mayer C, Levy JA. Human immunodeficiency virus infection of the CNS: characterization of "neurotropic" strains. Curr Top Microbiol Immunol 160:145–156, 1990.

25. Clavel F, Mansinho K, Chamaret S, Guetard D, Favier V, Nina J, Santos FM, Champalimaud JL, Montagnier L. Human immunodeficiency virus type 2 infection associated with AIDS in West Africa. N Engl J Med 316:1180–1185, 1987.

26. Cornblath DR. Treatment of the neuromuscular complications of human immunodeficiency virus infection. Ann Neurol 23:S88–S91, 1988.

27. Cornblath DR, Griffin DE, Welch D, Griffin JW, McArthur JC. Quantitative analysis of endoneurial T-cells in human sural nerve biopsies. J Neuroimmunol 26:113–118, 1990.

28. Cornblath DR, McArthur JC. Predominantly sensory neuropathy in patients with AIDS and AIDS-related complex. Neurology 38:794–796, 1988.

29. Cornblath DR, McArthur JC, Kennedy PG, Witte AS, Griffin JW. Inflammatory demyelinating peripheral neuropathies associated with human T-cell lymphotropic virus type III infection. Ann Neurol 21:32–40, 1987.

30. Cruickshank JK, Rudge P, Dalgleish AG, Newton M, McLean BN, Barnard RO, Kendall BE, Miller DH. Tropical spastic paraparesis and human T cell lymphotropic virus type 1 in the United Kingdom. Brain 112:1057–1090, 1989.

30a. Cupler EJ, Danon MJ, Jay C, Hench K, Ropka M, Dalakas MC. Early features of zidovudine-associated myopathy: histopathological findings and clinical correlations. Acta Neuropathol (Berl) 90:1–6, 1995.

31. Dalakas MC, Pezeshkpour GH. Neuromuscular diseases associated with human immunodeficiency virus infection. Ann Neurol 23:S38–S48, 1988.

32. Dalgleish AG, Wilson S, Gompels M, Ludlam C, Gazzard B, Coates AM, Habeshaw J. T-cell receptor variable gene products and early HIV-1 infection. Lancet 339:824–828, 1992.

32a. Dal Pan GJ, Glass JD, McArthur JC. Clinicopathologic correlations of HIV-1-associated vacuolar myelopathy: an autopsy-based case-control study. Neurology 44:2159–2164, 1994.

33. Davis LE, Hjelle BL, Miller VE, Palmer DL, Llewellyn AL, Merlin TL, Young SA, Mills RG, Wachsman W, Wiley CA. Early viral brain invasion in iatrogenic human immunodeficiency virus infection. Neurology 42:1736–1739, 1992.

34. Dawson VL, Dawson TM, Uhl GR, Snyder SH. Human immunodeficiency virus type 1 coat protein neurotoxicity mediated by nitric oxide in primary cortical cultures. Proc Natl Acad Sci USA 90:3256–3259, 1993.

35. de la Monte SM, Ho DD, Schooley RT, Hirsch MS, Richardson EP. Subacute encephalitis of AIDS and its relation to HIV infection. Neurology 37:562–569, 1987.

36. Denning DW. The neurological features of acute HIV infection. Biomed Pharmacother 42:11–14, 1988.

37. Dreyer EB, Kaiser PK, Offermann JT, Lipton SA. HIV-1 coat protein neurotoxicity prevented by calcium channel antagonists. Science 248:364–367, 1990.

38. Dwyer BA, Mayer RF, Lee SC. Progressive nemaline (rod) myopathy as a presentation of human immunodeficiency virus infection. Arch Neurol 49:440, 1992.

39. Dwyer DE, Matheron S, Bakchine S, Bechet JM, Montagnier L, Vazeux R. Detection of human immunodeficiency virus type 2 in brain tissue. J Infect Dis 166:888–891, 1992.

40. Eibl MM, Kupcu Z, Mannhalter JW, Eder G, Schaff Z. Dual tropism of HIV-1 IIIB for chimpanzee lymphocytes and monocytes. AIDS Res Hum Retroviruses 8:69–75, 1992.

41. Elder GA, Sever JL. Neurologic disorders associated with AIDS retroviral infection. Rev Infect Dis 10:286–302, 1988.

42. Elsner C, Dorries K. Evidence of human polyomavirus BK and JC infection in normal brain tissue. Virology 191:72–80, 1992.

43. Epstein LG, Gendelman HE. Human immunodeficiency virus type 1 infection of the nervous system: pathogenetic mechanisms. Ann Neurol 33:429–436, 1993.

44. Everall I, Gray F, Barnes H, Durigon M, Luthert P, Lantos P. Neuronal loss in symptom-free HIV infection. Lancet 340:1413, 1992.

45. Everall IP, Luthert PJ, Lantos PL. Neuronal loss in the frontal cortex in HIV infection. Lancet 337:1119–1121, 1991.

46. Fultz PN, McClure HM, Swenson RB, Anderson DC. HIV infection of chimpanzees as a model for testing chemotherapeutics. Intervirology 1:51–58, 1989.

47. Gabuzda DH. Neurologic disorders associated with HIV infections. J Am Acad Dermatol 22:1232–1236, 1990.

48. Gabuzda DH, Ho DD, De la Monte SH, Hirsch MS, Sobel RA. Immunohistochemical identification of HTLV-III antigen in brain from patients with the subacute encephalitis of acquired immunodeficiency syndrome. Ann Neurol 20:289–295, 1986.

49. Gage FH, Tuszynski MH, Chen KS, Fagan AM, Higgins GA. Nerve growth factor function in the central nervous system. Curr Top Microbiol Immunol 165:71–93, 1991.

50. Gallo RC. Human retroviruses: a decade of discovery and link with human disease. J Infect Dis 164:235–243, 1991.

51. Gallo RC, Salahuddin SZ, Popovic M, Shearer GM, Kaplan M, Haynes BF, Palker TJ,

Redfield R, Oleske J, Safai B. Frequent detection and isolation of cytopathic retroviruses (HTLV-III) from patients with AIDS and at risk for AIDS. Science 224:500–503, 1984.

51a. Gao S-J, Kingsley L, Hoover DR, Spira TJ, Rinaldo CR, Saah A, Phair J, Detels R, Parry P, Chang Y, Moore PS. Seroconversion to antibodies against Kaposi's sarcoma-associated herpesvirus-related latent nuclear antigens before the development of Kaposi's sarcoma. New Engl J Med 335:223–241, 1996.

52. Gardner MB. Neurotropic retroviruses of wild mice and macaques. Ann Neurol. 23:S201–S206, 1988.

53. Gendelman HE, Baca LM, Kubrak CA, Genis P, Burrous S, Friedman RM, Jacobs D, Meltzer MS. Induction of interferon alpha in peripheral blood mononuclear cells by human immunodeficiency virus (HIV)-infected monocytes: restricted antiviral activity of the HIV-induced interferons. J Immunol 148:422, 1992.

53a. Gendelman HE, Genis P, Jett M, Zhai QH, Nottet HS. An experimental model system for HIV-1-induced brain injury. Adv Neuroimmunol 4:189–193, 1994.

54. Genis P, Jett M, Bernton EW, Boyle T, Gelbard HA, Dzenko K, Keane RW, Resnick L, Mizrachi Y, Volsky DJ, Epstein LG, Gendelman HE. Cytokines and arachidonic metabolites produced during HIV-infected macrophage-astroglial interactions: implications for the neuropathogenesis of HIV disease. J Exp Med 176:1703–1718, 1992.

55. Gessain A, Gout O. Chronic myelopathy associated with human T-lymphotropic virus type I (HTLV-I). Ann Intern Med 117:933–946, 1992.

56. Giulian D, Vaca K, Noonan CA. Secretion of neurotoxins by mononuclear phagocytes infected with HIV-1. Science, 250:1593–1596, 1990.

56a. Glass JD, Johnson RT. Human immunodeficiency virus and the brain. Ann Rev Neurosci 19:1–26, 1996.

57. Glowa JR, Panlilio LV, Brenneman DE, Gozes I, Fridkin M, Hill JM. Learning impairment following intracerebral administration of the HIV envelope protein gp120 or a VIP antagonist. Brain Res 570:49–53, 1992.

58. Gonda MA. Bovine immunodeficiency virus. AIDS 6:759–776, 1992.

59. Gonzales MF, Davis RL. Neuropathology of acquired immunodeficiency syndrome. Neuropathol Appl Neurobiol 14:345–363, 1988.

60. Gottlieb MS, Schroff R, Schranker HE, Weisman JD, Fan PT, Wolf RA, Saxon A. Pneumocystic carinii pneumonia and mucosal candidiasis in previously healthy homosexual men. New Engl J Med 305:1425–1431, 1981.

61. Gourdou I, Mabrouk K, Harkiss G, Marchot P, Watt N, Hery F, Vigne R. Neurotoxicity in mice due to cysteine-rich parts of visna virus and HIV-1 Tat proteins. C R Acad Sci III. 311:149–155, 1990.

62. Gray F, Lescs MC, Keohane C, Paraire F, Marc B, Durigon M, Gherardi R. Early brain changes in HIV infection: neuropathological study of 11 HIV seropositive, non-AIDS cases. J Neuropathol Exp Neurol 51:177–185, 1992.

63. Griffin DE, McArthur JC, Cornblath DR. Neopterin and interferon-gamma in serum and cerebrospinal fluid of patients with HIV-associated neurologic disease. Neurology 41:69–74, 1991.

64. Grimaldi LM, Martino GV, Franciotta DM, Brustia R, Castagna A, Pristera R, Lazzarin A. Elevated alpha-tumor necrosis factor levels in spinal fluid from HIV-1-infected patients with central nervous system involvement. Ann Neurol 29:21–25, 1991.

65. Haase AT. The AIDS lentivirus connection. Microbiol Pathog 1:1–4, 1986.

66. Haase AT. Pathogenesis of lentivirus infections. Nature 322:130–136, 1986.

67. Harrington WJ Jr, Sheremata W, Hjelle B, Dube DK, Bradshaw P, Foung SKH, Snodgrass

S, Toedter G, Cabral L, Poiesz B. Spastic ataxia associated with human T-cell lymphotropic virus type II infection. Ann Neurol 33:411–414, 1993.

68. Hartikka J, Hefti F. Comparison of nerve growth factor's effects on development of septum, striatum, and nucleus basalis cholinergic neurons in vitro. J Neurosci Res 21:352–364, 1988.

69. Heyes MP, Brew BJ, Martin A, Price RW, Salazar AM, Sidtis JJ, Yergey JA, Mouradian MM, Sadler AE, Keilp J. Quinolinic acid in cerebrospinal fluid and serum in HIV-1 infection: relationship to clinical and neurological status. Ann Neurol 29:202–209, 1991.

70. Heyes MP, Brew BJ, Saito K, Quearry BJ, Price RW, Lee K, Bhalla RB, Der M, Markey SP. Inter-relationships between quinolinic acid, neuroactive kynurenines, neopterin and beta 2-microglobulin in cerebrospinal fluid and serum of HIV-1-infected patients. J Neuroimmunol 40:71–80, 1992.

71. Heyes MP, Saito K, Crowley JS, Davis LE, Demitrack MA, Der M, Dilling LA, Elia J, Kruesi MJ, Lackner A, Larsen SA, Lee K, Leonard HL, Markey SP, Martin A, Milstein S, Mouradian MM, Pranzatelli MR, Quearry BJ, Salazar A, Smith M, Strauss SE, Sunderland R, Swedo SW, Tourtellotte WW. Quinolinic acid and kynurenine pathway metabolism in inflammatory and non-inflammatory neurological disease. Neuroreport 3:1249–1273, 1992.

72. Hickey WF, Kimura H. Perivascular microglial cells of the CNS are bone marrow-derived and present antigen in vivo. Science 239:290–292, 1988.

72a. Hill JM, Mervis RF, Avidor R, Moody TW, Brenneman DE. HIV envelope protein-induced neuronal damage and retardation of behavioral development in rat neonates. Brain Res 603:222–233, 1993.

73. Hjelle B, Appenzeller O, Mills R, Alexander S, Torrez MN, Jahnke R, Ross G. Chronic neurodegenerative disease associated with HTLV-II infection. Lancet 339:645–646, 1992.

74. Ho DD, Rota TR, Schooley RT, Kaplan JC, Allan JD, Groopman JE, Resnick L, Felsenstein D, Andrews CA, Hirsch MS. Isolation of HTLV-III from cerebrospinal fluid and neural tissues of patients with neurologic syndromes related to the acquired immunodeficiency syndrome. N Engl J Med 313:1493–1497, 1985.

75. Hollander H, Levy JA. Neurologic abnormalities and recovery of human immunodeficiency virus from cerebrospinal fluid. Ann Intern Med 106:692–695, 1987.

76. Holoshitz J, Naparstek Y, Ben-Nun A, Marquardt P, Cohen IR. T lymphocyte lines induce autoimmune encephalomyelitis, delayed hypersensitivity and bystander encephalitis or arthritis. Eur J Immunol 14:729–734, 1984.

77. Houff SA, Major EO, Katz DA, Kufta CV, Sever JL, Pittaluga S, Roberts JR, Gitt J, Saini N, Lux W. Involvement of JC virus-infected mononuclear cells from the bone marrow and spleen in the pathogenesis of progressive multifocal leukoencephalopathy. N Engl J Med 318:301–315, 1988.

78. Imberti L, Sottini A, Bettinardi A, Puoti M, Primi D. Selective depletion in HIV infection of T cells that bear specific T cell receptor V beta sequences. Science 254:860–862, 1991.

79. Iwasaki Y. Pathology of chronic myelopathy associated with HTLV-I infection (HAM/TSP). J Neurol Sci 96:103–123, 1990.

80. Jacobson S, Lehky TMN, Robinson S, McFarlin D, Dhib-Jalbut S. Isolation of HTLV-II from a patient with chronic, progressive neurological disease clinically indistinguishable from HTLV-I-associated myelopathy/tropical spastic paraparesis. Ann Neurol 33:392–396, 1993.

81. Johnson RT. Retroviruses and nervous system disease. Curr Opin Neurobiol 2:663–670, 1992.

82. Johnson RT, McArthur JC, Narayan O. The neurobiology of human immunodeficiency virus infections. FASEB J 2:2970–2981, 1988.
83. Kaiser PK, Offermann JT, Lipton SA. Neuronal injury due to HIV-1 envelope protein is blocked by anti-gp120 antibodies but not by anti-CD4 antibodies. Neurology 40:1757–1761, 1990.
84. Kennedy PG. Molecular studies of viral pathogenesis in the central nervous system. The Linacre Lecture 1991. J R Coll Physicians Lond 26:204–214, 1992.
85. Ketzler S, Weis S, Haug H, Budka H. Loss of neurons in the frontal cortex in AIDS brains. Acta Neuropathol (Berl) 80:92–94, 1990.
86. Kieburtz K, Schiffer RB. Neurologic manifestations of human immunodeficiency virus infections. Neurol Clin 7:447–468, 1989.
87. Kieburtz KD, Giang DW, Schiffer RB, Vakil N. Abnormal vitamin B12 metabolism in human immunodeficiency virus infection. Association with neurological dysfunction. Arch Neurol 48:312–314, 1991.
87a. Kimura-Kuroda J, Nagashima K, Yasui K. Inhibition of myelin formation by HIV-1 gp120 in rat cerebral cortex culture. Arch Virol 137:81–99, 1994.
88. Knight AM, Harrison GB, Pease RJ, Robinson PJ, Dyson PJ. Biochemical analysis of the mouse mammary tumor virus long terminal repeat product. Evidence for the molecular structure of an endogenous superantigen. Eur J Immunol 22:879–882, 1992.
89. Koenig S, Gendelman HE, Orenstein JM, Dal CM, Pezeshkpour GH, Yungbluth M, Janotta F, Aksamit A, Martin MA, Fauci AS. Detection of AIDS virus in macrophages in brain tissue from AIDS patients with encephalopathy. Science 233:1089–1093, 1986.
90. Kure K, Lyman WD, Weidenheim KM, Dickson DW. Cellular localization of an HIV-1 antigen in subacute AIDS encephalitis using an improved double-labeling immuno-histochemical method. Am J Pathol 136:1085–1092, 1990.
91. Lackner AA, Dandekar S, Gardner MB. Neurobiology of simian and feline immunodeficiency virus infections. Brain Pathol 1:201–212, 1991.
92. Lackner AA, Smith MO, Munn RJ, Martfeld DJ, Gardner MB, Marx PA, Dandekar S. Localization of simian immunodeficiency virus in the central nervous system of rhesus monkeys. Am J Pathol 139:609–621, 1991.
93. Lane HC, Masur H, Edgar LC, Whalen G, Rook AH, Fauci AS. Abnormalities of B-cell activation and immunoregulation in patients with the acquired immunodeficiency syndrome. N Engl J Med 309:453–458, 1983.
94. Laurence J, Hodtsev AS, Posnett DN. Superantigen implicated in dependence of HIV-1 replication in T cells on TCR V beta expression. Nature 358:255–259, 1992.
95. Levy JA, Hoffman AD, Kramer SM, Landis JA, Shimabukuro JM, Oshiro LS. Isolation of lymphocytopathic retroviruses from San Francisco patients with AIDS. Science 225:840–842, 1984.
96. Levy JA, Shimabukuro J, Hollander H, Mills J, Kaminsky L. Isolation of AIDS-associated retroviruses from cerebrospinal fluid and brain of patients with neurological symptoms. Lancet 2:586–588, 1985.
97. Levy RM, Bredesen DE. Central nervous system dysfunction in acquired immunodeficiency syndrome. J Acquir Immune Defic Syndr 1:41–64, 1988.
98. Levy RM, Bredesen DE, Rosenblum ML. Neurological manifestations of the acquired immunodeficiency syndrome (AIDS): experience at UCSF and review of the literature. J Neurosurg 62:475–495, 1985.
99. Levy RM, Bredesen DE, Rosenblum ML. Opportunistic central nervous system pathology in patients with AIDS. Ann Neurol 23:S7–S12, 1988.

100. Levy RM, Bredesen DE, Rosenblum ML. Neurologic complications of HIV infection. Am Fam Physician 41:517–536, 1990.
101. Lipton SA. Calcium channel antagonists and human immunodeficiency virus coat protein-mediated neuronal injury. Ann Neurol 30:110–114, 1991.
102. Lipton SA. Memantine prevents HIV coat protein-induced neuronal injury in vitro. Neurology 42:1403–1905, 1992.
103. Lipton SA. Models of neuronal injury in AIDS: another role for the NMDA receptor? Trends Neurosci 15:75–79, 1992.
104. Lipton SA. Requirement for macrophages in neuronal injury induced by HIV envelope protein gp120. NeuroReport 3:913–915, 1992.
105. Lipton SA, Sucher NJ, Kaiser PK, Dreyer EB. Synergistic effects of HIV coat protein and NMDA receptor-mediated neurotoxicity. Neuron 7:111–118, 1991.
105a. Lipton SA. HIV coat protein gp120 induces soluble neurotoxins in culture medium. Neurosci Res Comm 15:31–37, 1994.
105b. Lipton SA, Yeh M, Dreyer EB. Update on current models of HIV-related neuronal injury: platelet-activating factor, arachidonic acid and nitric oxide. Adv Neuroimmunol 4:181–188, 1994.
106. Livrozet JM, Ninet J, Vighetto A, Touraine JL, Touraine F, Caudie C, Kindbeiter K, Poly H. One case of HIV-2 AIDS with neurological manifestations. J Acquir Immune Defic Syndr 3:927–928, 1990.
107. Mabrouk K, Van RJ, Vives E, Darbon H, Rochat H, Sabatier JM. Lethal neurotoxicity in mice of the basic domains of HIV and SIV Rev proteins. Study of these regions by circular dichroism. FEBS Lett 289:13–17, 1996.
108. Manca F, Newell A, Valle M, Habeshaw J, Dalgleish AG. HIV-induced deletion of antigen-specific T cell function is MHC restricted. Clin Exp Immunol. 87:15–19, 1992.
109. Markovitz DM. Infection with the human immunodeficiency virus type 2. Ann Intern Med 118:211–218, 1993.
110. Martinez-Maza O, Crabb E, Mitsuyasu RT, Fahey JL, Giorgi JV. Infection with the human immunodeficiency virus (HIV) is associated with an in vivo increase in B lymphocyte activation and immaturity. J Immunol 138:3720–3724, 1987.
111. Masliah E, Achim CL, Ge N, DeTeresa R, Terry RD, Wiley CA. Spectrum of human immunodeficiency virus-associated neocortical damage. Ann Neurol 32:321–329, 1992.
112. Masur H, Michelis MA, Greene JB, Onorato I, Stouwe RA, Holzman RS, Wormser G, Brettman L, Lange M, Murray HW. An outbreak of community-acquired Pneumocystis carinii pneumonia: initial manifestation of cellular immune dysfunction. N Engl J Med 305:1431–1438, 1981.
112a. McArthur JC, Hoover DR, Bacellar H, et al. Dementia in AIDS patients: incidence and risk factors. Multicenter AIDS Cohort Study. Neurology 43:2245–2252, 1993.
113. McCune JM, Kaneshima H, Lieberman M, Weissman IL, Namikawa R. The SCID-hu mouse: current status and potential applications. Curr Top Microbiol Immunol 152:183–193, 1989.
114. McFarlin DE, Koprowski H. Neurological disorders associated with HTLV-1. Curr Top Microbiol Immunol 160:100–119, 1990.
115. McGeer PL, Itagaki S, McGeer EG. Expression of the histocompatibility glycoprotein HLA-DR in neurological disease. Acta Neuropathol (Berl) 76:550–557, 1988.
116. Miller RG. Neuropathies and myopathies complicating HIV infection. J Clin Apheresis 6:110–121, 1991.
117. Mintz M, Rapaport R, Oleske JM, Connor EM, Koenigsberger MR, Denny T, Epstein LG. Elevated serum levels of tumor necrosis factor are associated with progressive encepha-

lopathy in children with acquired immunodeficiency syndrome. Am J Dis Child 143:771–774, 1989.

118. Mori M, Aoki N, Shimada H, Tajima M, Kato K. Detection of JC virus in the brains of aged patients without progressive multifocal leukoencephalopathy by the polymerase chain reaction and Southern hybridization analysis. Neurosci Lett 141:151–155, 1992.

119. Morrow WJ, Homsy J, Eichberg JW, Krowka J, Pan LZ, Gaston I, Legg H, Lerche N, Thomas J, Levy JA. Long-term observation of baboons, rhesus monkeys, and chimpanzees inoculated with HIV and given periodic immunosuppressive treatment. Aids Res Hum Retroviruses 5:233–245, 1989.

119a. Moses AV, Nelson JA. HIV infection of human brain capillary endothelial cells—implications for AIDS dementia. Adv Neuroimmunol 4:239–247, 1994.

120. Muller S, Richalet P, Laurent CA, Barakat S, Riviere Y, Porrot F, Chamaret S, Briand JP, Montagnier L, Hovanessian A. Autoantibodies typical of non-organ-specific autoimmune diseases in HIV-seropositive patients. AIDS 6:933–942, 1992.

121. Murphy EL, Engstrom JW, Miller K, Sacher RA, Busch MP, Hollingsworth CG. HTLV-II associated myelopathy in 43-year-old woman. REDS Investigators. Lancet 341:757–758, 1993.

122. Namikawa R, Kaneshima H, Lieberman M, Weissman IL, McCune JM. Infection of the SCID-hu mouse by HIV-1. Science 242:1684–1686, 1988.

123. Navia BA, Cho ES, Petito CK, Price RW. The AIDS dementia complex: II. Neuropathology. Ann Neurol 19:525–535, 1986.

123a. Nuovo GJ, Gallery F, MacConnell P, Braun A. In situ detection of polymerase chain reaction-amplified HIV-1 nucleic acids and tumor necrosis factor-alpha RNA in the central nervous system. Am J Pathol 144:659–666, 1994.

124. Parry GJ. Peripheral neuropathies associated with human immunodeficiency virus infection. Ann Neurol 23:S49–S53, 1988.

125. Patnaik M, Schwartzman WA, Barka NE, Peter JB. Possible role of Rochalimaea henselae in pathogenesis of AIDS encephalopathy. Lancet 340:971, 1992.

126. Perry VH, Gordon S. Macrophages and microglia in the nervous system. Trends Neurosci 11:2273–2277, 1988.

127. Pert CB, Smith CC, Ruff MR, Hill JM. AIDS and its dementia as a neuropeptide disorder: role of VIP receptor blockade by human immunodeficiency virus envelope. Ann Neurol 23:S71–S73, 1988.

128. Peter JB, McKeown KL, Barka NE, Tourtellotte WW, Singer EJ, Syndulko K. Neopterin and beta 2-microglobulin and the assessment of intra-blood-brain-barrier synthesis of HIV-specific and total IgG. J Clin Lab Anal 5:317–320, 1991.

129. Petito CK. Review of central nervous system pathology in human immunodeficiency virus infection. Ann Neurol 23:S54–57, 1988.

130. Pinching AJ, Helbert M, Peddle B, Robinson D, Janes K, Gor D, Jeffries DJ, Stoneham C, Mitchell D, Kocsis AE. Clinical experience with zidovudine for patients with acquired immune deficiency syndrome and acquired immune deficiency syndrome-related complex. J Infect 18(Suppl1):33–40, 1989.

131. Porter SB, Sande MA. Toxoplasmosis of the central nervous system in the acquired immunodeficiency syndrome. N Engl J Med 327:1643–1648, 1992.

131a. Power C, McArthur JC, Johnson RT, Griffin DE, Glass JD, Dewey R, Chesebro B. Distinct HIV-1 env sequences are associated with neurotropism and neurovirulence. Curr Top Microbiol Immunol 202:89–104, 1995.

132. Price RW, Brew B, Sidtis J, Rosenblum M, Scheck AC, Cleary P. The brain in AIDS: central nervous system HIV-1 infection and AIDS dementia complex. Science 239:586–592, 1988.

133. Pullen AM, Choi Y, Kushnir E, Kappler J, Marrack P. The open reading frames in the 3′ long terminal repeats of several mouse mammary tumor virus integrants encode V beta 3-specific superantigens. J Exp Med 175:41–47, 1992.

134. Pulliam L, Herndier BG, Tang NM, McGrath MS. Human immunodeficiency virus-infected macrophages produce soluble factors that cause histological and neurochemical alterations in cultured human brains. J Clin Invest 87:503–512, 1991.

135. Pumarola-Sune T, Navia BA, Cordon-Cardo C, Cho ES, Price RW. HIV antigen in the brains of patients with the AIDS dementia complex. Ann Neurol 21:490–496, 1987.

136. Rance NE, McArthur JC, Cornblath DR, Landstrom DL, Griffin JW, Price DL. Gracile tract degeneration in patients with sensory neuropathy and AIDS. Neurology 38:265–271, 1988.

137. Reiher WE III, Blalock JE, Brunck TK. Sequence homology between acquired immunodeficiency syndrome virus envelope protein and interleukin 2. Proc Natl Acad Sci USA 83:9188–9192, 1986.

138. Resnick L, Berger JR, Shapshak P, Tourtelotte WW. Early penetration of the blood-brain barrier by HIV. Neurology 38:9–14, 1988.

139. Resnick L, diMarzo VF, Schupbach J, Tourtellotte WW, Ho DD, Muller F, Shapshak P, Vogt M, Groopman JE, Markham PD. Intra-blood-brain-barrier synthesis of HTLV-III-specific IgG in patients with neurologic symptoms associated with AIDS or AIDS-related complex. N Engl J Med 313:1498–1504, 1985.

140. Rosenblatt JD, Tomkins P, Rosenthal M, Kacena A, Chan G, Valderama R, Harrington W, Saxton E, Diagne A, Zhao J-Q, Mitsuyasu RT, Weisbart RH. Progressive spastic myelopathy in a patient co-infected with HIV-1 and HTLV-II: autoantibodies to the human homologue of rig in blood and cerebrospinal fluid. AIDS 6:1151–1158, 1992.

141. Sabatier JM, Vives E, Mabrouk K, Benjouad A, Rochat H, Duval A, Hue B, Bahraoui E. Evidence for neurotoxic activity of tat from human immunodeficiency virus type 1. J Virol 65:961–967, 1991.

141a. Saito Y, Sharer LR, Epstein LG, Michaels J, Mintz M, Louder M, Golding K, Cvetkovich TA, Blumberg BM. Overexpression of nef as a marker for restricted HIV-1 infection of astrocytes in postmortem pediatric central nervous tissues. Neurology 44:474–481, 1994.

142. Saulsbury FT, Bringelson KA, Normansell DE. Effects of prednisone on human immunodeficiency virus infection. South Med J 84:431–435, 1991.

143. Schneider J, Luke W, Kirchhoff F, Jung R, Jurkiewicz E, Stahl HC, Nick S, Klemm E, Jentsch KD, Hunsmann G. Isolation and characterization of HIV-2ben obtained from a patient with predominantly neurological defects. AIDS 4:455–457, 1990.

144. Selmaj KW, Raine CS. Tumor necrosis factor mediates myelin and oligodendrocyte damage in vitro. Ann Neurol 23:339–346, 1988.

144a. Sharer LR, Saito Y, Epstein LG, Blumberg BM. Detection of HIV-1 DNA in pediatric AIDS brain tissue by two-step ISPCR. Adv Neuroimmunol 4:283–285, 1994.

145. Shaw GM, Harper ME, Hahn BH, Epstein LG, Gajdusek DC, Price RW, Navia BA, Petito CK, O'Hara CJ, Groopman JE. HTLV-III infection in brains of children and adults with AIDS encephalopathy. Science 227:177–182, 1985.

145a. Simpson DM, Tagliati M. Nucleoside analogue-associated peripheral neuropathy in human immunodeficiency virus infection. J Acquir Immune Defic Syndr Hum Retrovirol 9:153–161, 1995.

146. Stoler MH, Eskin TA, Benn S, Angerer RC, Angerer LM. Human T-cell lymphotropic virus type III infection of the central nervous system. A preliminary in situ analysis. JAMA 256:2360–2364, 1986.

147. Sundar SK, Cierpial MA, Kamaraju LS, Long S, Hsieh S, Lorenz C, Aaron M, Ritchie JC,

Weiss JM. Human immunodeficiency virus glycoprotein (gp120) infused into rat brain induces interleukin 1 to elevate pituitary-adrenal activity and decrease peripheral cellular immune responses. Proc Natl Acad Sci USA 88:11246–11250, 1991.

148. Tardieu M, Hery C, Peudenier S. Neurotoxicity of macrophages infected by HIV1. Cell Biol Toxicol 8:117–121, 1992.

149. Tardieu M, Hery C, Peudenier S, Boespflug O, Montagnier L. Human immunodeficiency virus type 1-infected monocytic cells can destroy human neural cells after cell-to-cell adhesion. Ann Neurol 32:11–17, 1992.

150. Tominaga T, Yogo Y, Kitamura T, Aso Y. Persistence of archetypal JC virus DNA in normal renal tissue derived from tumor-bearing patients. Virology 186:736–741, 1992.

150a. Tornatore C, Chandra R, Berger JR, Major EO. HIV-1 infection of subcortical astrocytes in the pediatric central nervous system. Neurology 44:481–487, 1994.

151. Tyor WR, Glass JD, Griffin JW, Becker PS, McArthur JC, Bezman L, Griffin DE. Cytokine expression in the brain during the acquired immunodeficiency syndrome. Ann Neurol 31:349–360, 1992.

152. Vago L, Trabattoni G, Lechi A, Cristina S, Budka H. Neuropathology of AIDS dementia. A review after 205 post mortem examinations. Acta Neurol (Napoli) 12:32–35, 1990.

153. Vazeux R, Brousse N, Jarry A, Henin D, Marche C, Vedrenne C, Mikol M, Woff M, Michon C, Rozenbaum W, Bureau J-F, Montagnier L, Brahic M. AIDS subacute encephalitis. Identification of HIV-infected cells. AM J Pathol 126:403–410, 1987.

154. Verma RK, Ziegler DK, Kepes JJ. HIV-related neuromuscular syndrome simulating motor neuron disease. Neurology 40:544–546, 1990.

155. Villa A, Foresti V, Confalonieri F. Autonomic nervous system dysfunction associated with HIV infection in intravenous heroin users. AIDS 6:85–89, 1992.

156. Wahl LM, Corcoran ML, Pyle SW, Arthur LO, Harel BA, Farrar WL. Human immunodeficiency virus glycoprotein (gp120) induction of monocyte arachidonic acid metabolites and interleukin 1. Proc Natl Acad Sci USA 86:621–625, 1989.

157. Wahl SM, Allen JB, McCartney FN, Morganti KM, Kossmann T, Ellingsworth L, Mai UE, Mergenhagen SE, Orenstein JM. Macrophage- and astrocyte-derived transforming growth factor beta as a mediator of central nervous system dysfunction in acquired immune deficiency syndrome. J Exp Med 173:981–991, 1991.

158. Weeks BS, Klotman ME, Dhawan S, Kibbey M, Rappaport J, Kleinman HK, Yamada KM, Klotman PE. HIV-1 infection of human T lymphocytes results in enhanced alpha 5 beta 1 integrin expression. J Cell Biol 114:847–853, 1991.

159. Weiser B, Peress N, La ND, Eilbott DJ, Seidman R, Burger H. Human immunodeficiency virus type 1 expression in the central nervous system correlates directly with extent of disease. Proc Natl Acad Sci USA 87:3997–4001, 1990.

160. Weiss RA. Retroviruses and human disease. J Clin Pathol 40:1064–1069, 1987.

161. Wiley CA. Neuromuscular diseases of AIDS. FASEB J 3:2503–2511, 1989.

162. Wiley CA, Achim CL, Schrier RD, Heyes MP, McCutchan JA, Grant I. Relationship of cerebrospinal fluid immune activation associated factors to HIV encephalitis. AIDS 6:1299–1307, 1992.

163. Wiley CA, Johnson RT, Reingold SC. Neurological consequences of immune dysfunction:lessons from HIV infection and multiple sclerosis. J Neuroimmunol 40:115–119, 1992.

164. Wiley CA, Schrier RD, Nelson JA, Lampert PW, Oldstone MB. Cellular localization of human immunodeficiency virus infection within the brains of acquired immune deficiency syndrome patients. Proc Natl Acad Sci USA 83:7089–7093, 1986.

165. Wong PK, Shikova E, Lin YC, Saha K, Szurek PF, Stoica G, Madden R, Brooks BR.

Murine leukemia virus induced central nervous system diseases. Leukemia 6 (Suppl. 3):161S–165S, 1992.

166. Woods G, Kitagami K, Ochi A. Evidence for an involvement of T4+ cytotoxic T cells in tumor immunity. Cell Immunol 118:126–135, 1989.

167. Yamada M, Zurbriggen A, Oldstone MB, Fujinami RS. Common immunologic determinant between human immunodeficiency virus type 1 gp41 and astrocytes. J Virol 65:1370–1376, 1991.

167a. Yeung MC, Pulliam L, Lau AS. The HIV envelope protein gp120 is toxic to human brain-cell cultures through the induction of interleukin-6 and tumor necrosis factor-alpha. AIDS 9:137–143, 1995.

168. Zumla A, Superantigens, T cells, and microbes. Clin Infect Dis 15:313–320, 1992.

21

Tumors of the Central Nervous System

CAROL J. WIKSTRAND
DARELL D. BIGNER

In 1980 we published a review article entitled "Immunobiologic Aspects of the Brain and Human Gliomas" in which we stated that the cumulative toxicity of current modes of therapy and the inability to resect the majority of intracranial tumors completely with surgery had led to the search for "an alternate nontoxic, noninvasive form of therapy . . . to control the last remaining tumor cells" (98). The concluding overview at that time was that the future success of immunotherapeutic approaches would depend on the elucidation of relevant tumor-associated antigenic targets, the development of specific immune effectors (monoclonal antibodies [MAbs], reactive lymphocyte populations), and the development of compartmental versus systemic modes of intervention. Since the appearance of that review, a growing number of investigators have defined targets, effectors, and mechanisms of approach and have, predictably, closed some avenues and opened others. The current overview will not resolve the issue, but an increased understanding of the possibilities and limitations of immunotherapeutic approaches within the intrathecal space has been achieved through directed investigation in recent years.

Historical Perspective: Brain Tumors and the Concept of Immunological Privilege

Classical Investigations of Tumor–Host Interactions and the Central Nervous System (CNS)

The attribution of the CNS as an immunologically privileged site grew out of early observations of intracerebral (IC) growth of tumors that were readily rejected when transplanted subcutaneously (SC) (23,26,53,61,84, reviewed in 98). In a prospective study of CNS tumor induction in rats exposed in utero to ethylnitrosourea, Morantz et al. (59) claimed that the immune privilege of the brain prevented alteration of the incidence of induced tumors through life-long systemic immunosupression by *(1)* thymectomy, *(2)* anti-lymphocyte serum treatment, or by immuno-enhancement *(3)* by administration of *bacille Calmette-Guerin.* These studies suggested that the efferent blockade was due to the lack of direct lymphatic drainage in the CNS, and the afferent block of the immune response resulted from the blood-brain barrier's prevention of the passage of immune cells. These studies were widely quoted in support of the concept of failure of immune surveillance in the CNS. Initial studies that documented glioma patient anergy were taken as further evidence of the absence of a potentially productive immune response to CNS tumors.

Brain tumor patients demonstrate a general depression of cell-mediated immunity as measured by response to common skin test antigens (12,13,45), a general depression in both quantity and function of circulating T cells (13,78,108), and an impairment of serological responses which are moderate but sustained following immunization with tetanus and influenza vaccines (47, review in 98).

Afferent and Efferent Response in the CNS: A Reexamination

Accumulated evidence has shown that the immunological privilege of the normal brain and especially of the injured or neoplastic brain is only partial (78,85,94). Salcman and Broadwell suggest that the localization of radioiodinated serum albumin (RISA) and contrast agents used in computed tomography (CT) and magnetic resonance imaging (MRI) depend on the relative leakiness of brain tumor endothelial cells (79). Electron microscopic anomalies in the vascular endothelium of glioma capillaries as compared to those of normal brain have been described (44,85,94). The abnormalities frequently observed were tight junctions that lacked normal pentalaminar structure and vesicular formations and fenestrations. The existence of leakiness in areas of peritumoral endothelium has also been reported (79). The degree of disruption was higher in areas of tumor infiltration and decreased progressively in brain adjacent to tumor (79). Groothius et al. (25) have developed a method to quantify the rate of transcapillary transport of iodinated compounds in brain tumors using contrast-enhanced CT. Blood-to-tissue transfer constants (K_1) were calculated for tumor and tumor-free brain in 10 patients with primary brain tumors. These studies demonstrated K_1 values ranging from those found in normal brain to 15 times that value in a glioblastoma multiforme. This alteration of transcapillary permeability in brain tumors and the absence of a physical barrier to immunological traffic supports the classical series of experiments by Scheinberg et al. (reviewed in 98). Using the IC transplantable C57BL/6J (mouse) methylcholanthrene-induced ependymoblastoma, these investigators established that IC-inoculated tumor cells could elicit first-set rejection in allogeneic hosts and second-set rejection of SC *or* IC tumor cell implants in syngeneic hosts. They also found that primary SC tumor transplants could confer resistance to subsequent IC or SC challenge. These experiments demonstrated that both efferent and afferent arcs of the immune response were elicited to transplants placed within the CNS. Not only can systemic sensitization by IC antigen occur, but an effective response can also be elicited and can travel to IC sites. These phenomena are not the result of "wounding" the normal brain parenchyma by introduction of inocula, since perivascular accumulations of infiltrating lymphocytes occur in 33–50% of human gliomas (74,92). Initial studies of the inflammatory infiltrate of human CNS tumors implicated host macrophages as the primary effectors (104). More recent studies (reviewed in 80) have identified T cells (predominantly cytotoxic and suppressor cells) as the major tumor-infiltrating lymphocytes (TILs). However, natural killer (NK) cells, macrophages, and B cells are also found, especially at the tumor periphery. Isolation and interleukin-2 (IL-2) expansion of TILs from surgical specimens of gliomas have yielded cytotoxic effector cells consisting of approximately 90% CD3+ T cells, and both CD4+ and CD8+ subpopulations. CD16 positive and/or Leu19 positive NK cells have also been observed in TIL cultures (80). IL-2 expansion of these cells in vitro demonstrated that TILs are not necessarily representative of in vivo effector populations in the vicinity of the tumor, but reflect the lineage of cells of peritumoral accumulation. The number of TILs isolated from gliomas is low as compared to the number found in tumors metastatic to the brain or in non-CNS tumors. Moreover, cells freshly isolated from gliomas are negative for activation antigens. Therefore, it has been postulated that suppression of glioma TILs by glioma cells in situ may be induced by an immunosuppressive factor. Support for this idea was provided by the observations of Wrann et al. (105). An immunosuppressive factor detected in brain tumor cyst fluid and in the supernatant of cultured glioma cell lines has been identified as transforming growth factor-β_2 (TGF-β_2), a 12.5 kilodalton (kDa) peptide capable of inhibiting IL-2-dependent cytotoxic T-cell development (37). It is apparent that the CNS, once considered an immunologically privileged site devoid of efferent and afferent immune pathways, is subject to the same complex interactions of immunoregulatory factors that are active systemically (see Chapters 3,4). Although effector systems in the CNS may vary, and suppressor systems may be intrinsically more active, immune mechanisms are operative in CNS tumors and their functional interactions are significant.

Functional Antigenicity of CNS Tumors

Antigenicity of human brain tumors has been analyzed in sera of brain tumor patients or sera obtained following immunization of rabbits or primates with human glioma cells or tissues (46,86,95,97, reviewed in 98). These studies established the following *(1)* gliomas were capable of inducing a humoral response; *(2)* the majority of induced antibody activity was directed against moieties that are shared by normal mature brain and other tissues of neuroectodermal origin (the "neuroectodermal effect"); *(3)* anti-bodies directed against lymphoid lineage-specific marker antigens were induced; and *(4)* oncofetal or developmental stage-related antigens not expressed by normal adult CNS tissue were expressed by normal gliomas. With the advent of MAb technology, dissection of the antigenic molecules expressed by gliomas became possible. Today, an extensive "marker phenotype" of both normal and neoplastic cells of the CNS is available (52,58,98). Molenaar and Trojanowski provide an excellent and thorough description of the cell-type-specific CNS markers that are elaborated by, and are diagnostic of, tumors of the CNS (58). A current and comprehensive review of human glioma cell antigen expression has recently been compiled (52). Over 100 glioma-associated antigens have been cataloged (52); those that define cell type as either integral membrane proteins, nuclear antigens, or secreted substances have figured prominently in the diagnosis of brain tumors. Only a handful of the immunologically detected molecules in tumor cells have been considered viable candidates as targets of immunotherapeutic intervention. Although many other as yet untested antigens may ultimately prove to be of value, the following discussion will be confined to those antigens and immunoreagents that have been tested in vivo.

Recent Advances and the Current Status of CNS Tumor Immunobiology

The Tumor-associated Target Antigen

Certain criteria must be met for any antigen to be considered a proposed target of immunotherapeutic intervention. The target epitope should *(1)* exhibit sufficient densi-ty or concentration in neoplastic cells vs. surrounding normal cells so that it qualifies functionally as tumor associated; *(2)* be homogeneously expressed throughout the tumor; *(3)* be physically accessible to interaction with the soluble or cell-bound recep-tors specifically reactive with it; and *(4)* have inherent stability to mediate the binding or internalization of the immune effector. The molecules described in Table 21-1 meet these criteria and have served as targets of various immunotherapeutic approaches.

Oncogene-associated products have been proposed as tumor-associated target mole-cules for several types of tumors (7,28). In human tumors, many of the protooncogene-encoded products are directly related to cell proliferation and growth control, thus suggesting an association with either the progression to, or maintenance of, the neo-plastic state. A series of studies by Westermark and co-workers (63,64) have shown that human glioma cells in long-term cultures express both the A and B chains of platelet-derived growth factor (PDGF) and the PDGF receptor (PDGFR)-α and/or PDGFR-β. In situ hybridization of glioma tumor tissue demonstrated expression of PDGFR-β in hyperplastic endothelium (30). Using similar techniques, Maxwell et al. (51) demonstrated PDGFR-α in glioma cells. Through immunohistochemical and in

Table 21-1 Cell Surface/Extracellular Matrix-Associated Molecules of Potential Relevance as Targets of Immunotherapy[a]

Elaborated Molecule	Defining MAb[b]	Antigen Characteristics	Distribution Within CNS[c]	Demonstration of In vivo Utility	Key Reference(s)
Oncogene-associated					
PDGF-R α, β chains	α: PDGFR-7 β: PDGFR-B2	α: 170 kDa β: 180 kDa Transmembrane glycoproteins	α: Normal and neoplastic glia β: Hyperplastic endothelium	Immunohistochemical localization	(63) (29)
EGFR	425	170-kDa transmembrane glycoprotein; extracellular EGF-binding domain	Vascular endothelium, fibroblasts, glioma cells	In vivo patient and xenograft model localization	(5,11,31,102)
EGFRvIII	L8A4	145-kDa deletion variant of EGFR with extracellular EGF-binding domain	Glioma cells	Immunohistochemical localization	(6,32,99)
Developmentally or cell lineage-related					
N-CAM	UJ13A	Multiple isoform (120, 145, 170, 180 kDa) transmembrane glycoprotein	Normal adult and fetal brain, glioma, medulloblastoma cells	In vivo patient localization	(72,73)
L1 (human homologue)	UJ181.4	Multiple isoform (200–230 kDa) transmembrane glycoprotein	Glioma, medulloblastoma, pineoblastoma	In vivo patient localization	(60,71)

Antigen	MAb	Description	Localization	Method	Refs
Ganglioside 3'-isoLM1	SL-50	Terminal epitope available on gangliosides and glycoproteins	Fetal brain, gliomas	Immunohistochemical localization	(62,100)
Ganglioside 3',6'-isoLD1	DMAb-22	Terminal epitope available on gangliosides and glycoproteins	Fetal brain, gliomas	Immunohistochemical localization	(50,101)
ECM-associated					
Tenascin	81C6	Glycoprotein hexamer composed of six identical 340-kDa monomers	Glioma ECM; glomeruloid projections of tumor vasculature	In vivo patient and xenograft model localization	(10,111)
Gp 240	Mel-14	240-kDa Glycoprotein; transmembrane; associated with ECM	Gliomas, melanomas, hyperplastic endothelial cells	In vivo patient and xenograft model localization	(17,17,110)
9.2.27 Antigen	9.2.27	Chondroitin sulfate proteoglycan core protein	Gliomas, melanomas, hyperplastic endothelial cells	Xenograft model localization	(81)

[a]This table is not comprehensive. Target molecules listed are those with some degree of biochemical characterization and demonstration of in vivo relevance as assessed by immunohistochemical localization in human tumor samples or by localization in vivo in either rodent xenograft models or human patients. A more comprehensive list of potential glioma-associated target molecules has been provided (52). Abbreviations: MAb, monoclonal antibody; CNS, central nervous system; PDGFR, platelet-derived growth factor receptor; kDa, kilodaltons; ECM, extracellular matrix; EGFR, epidermal growth factor receptor; N-CAM, neural cell adhesion molecule; 3'-isoLM1, IV^{3}NeuAcLcOse$_4$Cer; 3',6'-isoLD1, IV^{3}NeuAc,III^{6}NeuAcLcOse$_4$Cer.

[b]The antigen-defining MAb pair listed is that for which the most extensive analysis exists. There are, for example, multiple anti-EGFR or anti-N-CAM MAbs available.

[c]Antigen distribution outside the CNS is not described. With the exception of 3'-isoLM1, 3',6'-isoLD1, and Gp 240, systemic sites of antigen have been described. Ganglioside antigens are present on teratomas and Gp 240 on melanoma cells. It is probable that extra-CNS antigen sites exist for these.

situ hybridization analyses of 14 glioma cases Kernohan grades I–IV (29), Hermanson et al. showed expression of PDGFR-α in glioma cells of all the cases and grades of tumors examined (29). Expression of PDGFR-β (very low expression in glioma cells) was frequently observed in the endothelial cells of hyperplastic capillaries and more intensely expressed in the higher-grade tumors. The localization of antibodies to the extracellular portion of the PDGFR in all of these glioma cases (14/14), and the limited expression of these molecules in normal brain parenchyma, suggest that PDGFR-α and -β could serve as targets for immunotherapeutic intervention, either by targeted kill or disruption of autocrine and/or paracrine pathways.

Several groups have documented the amplification and overexpression of the epidermal growth factor receptor (EGFR) gene (*v-erbB* protooncogene) in 30–40% of malignant human gliomas (31,41,102). EGFR is rarely detected in normal brain tissue, and it is not observed in peripheral blood or bone marrow cells (90). MAb 425, directed against "normal" EGFR, has been shown to localize specifically in malignant human glioma xenografts in nude mice (91) and to be therapeutically effective in this system. In addition, MAb 425 was cytotoxic in combination with either murine or human effector cells for cultured human glioma cells (5,76). In malignant gliomas, EGFR gene amplification is often associated with structural gene rearrangement which leads to deletion mutations in segments of the gene corresponding to the extracellular domain of the EGFR protein (32,88,106). The most common inframe deletion mutant is EGFRvIII and is found in approximately 17–20% of all human glioblastomas (32,103). The fusion junction of EGFRvIII mutant protein is an attractive, potentially unique epitope for the generation of MAbs. We have produced and characterized a rabbit polyvalent anti-EGFRvIII antibody that specifically precipitates EGFRvIII and reacts with the mutant receptor, but not the normal receptor, in rodent xenograft and human tissue sections (32); monoclonal antibodies specific to EGFRvIII were recently reported by our group (99).

Developmentally related or cell lineage–related epitopes have great potential for targeting MAbs, provided that the expression of the epitope is sufficiently phase-specific so that targeting of normal tissue in the adult patient does not occur. MAb-epitope pairs that have been used successfully are listed in Table 21-1. Despite the presence of the neural cell adhesion molecule (N-CAM) in normal brain, the MAb UJ13A, which recognizes N-CAM, has been successfully administered intravenously to patients for therapy of gliomas (72,73). The very low background uptake observed in normal brain scintigraphy was attributed to an intact blood-brain barrier in normal brain not adjacent to the tumor. A more epitope-restricted target is the human homologue of the murine L1 cell adhesion molecule (27) that is defined by MAb UJ181.4 (71). Although L1 is an integral membrane glycoprotein expressed on neurons in the murine CNS, it (and presumably the homologue) is primarily expressed during late CNS development when granule neurons migrate in the early postnatal cortex (27). Two recently described ganglioside epitopes, $IV^3NeuAcLcOse_4Cer$ (3′-isoLM1) and $IV^3NeuAc,III^6NeuAcLcOse_4Cer$ (3′,6′-isoLD1) (ganglioside abbreviations according to IUPAC-IUB [34]; Svennerholm [89]) (50,100,101), also diminish during development and show relatively undetectable levels in the human CNS after 2 years of age. The monosialoganglioside 3'isoLM1 is present in 100% of malignant gliomas, as demonstrated by thin-layer chromatography and immunostaining (21). Both 3'-isoLM1 and 3',6'-isoLD1 are present in 50% and 67%, respectively, of a panel of 31 human gliomas as shown by immunohistochemistry with 3'-isoLM1-specific MAb SL-50 and the 3',6'-isoLD1-specific MAb DMAb-22 (100,101).

Epitopes on extracellular matrix molecules are appropriate for localization of radioisotope-tagged MAbs, as long as isotopes with relevant path lengths are selected. Defined molecules of this class that have shown promise in xenograft model studies and/or patient administration protocols include the hexabrachion "glial-mesenchymal extracellular matrix" molecule, tenascin (10); 230–240 kDa glycoprotein (defined by MAb Mel-14) elaborated by gliomas, melanomas, and hyperplastic endothelial cells within gliomas (4,16,17); and the core protein of chondroitin sulfate proteoglycan (defined by MAb 9.2.27) (15,81). Each of these molecules, by virtue of their distribution throughout the tumor matrix, their location in the hyperplastic endothelium in gliomas, and their absence of expression in normal brain parenchyma, have proven to be effective targets in vivo (17,81,111).

Approaches to Active Immunotherapy, Specific and Nonspecific

Historically, approaches to active immunotherapy in human glioma patients have been reviewed (69,98). *Active* immunotherapy is designed to enhance the patient's immune capacity to recognize, react to, and potentially destroy resident tumor cells. In *specific active* immunotherapy, antigenic challenges are administered that are identical or that cross-react with the target tumor to induce a specific immune response. *Nonspecific active* immunotherapy consists of the administration of general stimulants such as adjuvants or lymphokines to elicit a systemic or compartmental immune response. Table 21-2 summarizes studies in this area. It must be stressed that these studies have been hampered by the multiregimen therapies received by most subjects prior to entry into immunotherapeutic protocols. Most patients had had surgery, radiation, and steroid therapy and/or chemotherapy in the interest of best conventional care. Consequently, most patients at the time of immunotherapy were clinically deteriorating, relapsed, or moribund, thus making critical analysis difficult.

Various immunogens, including autologous tumor tissue, cells, and cultured glioma cells selected to be HLA-haplo nonidentical with the immunized patient, have been used with a variety of adjuvants to immunize glioma patients (Table 21-2). No case of active specific immunization has demonstrated a sustained, specific humoral or cellular response to autologous tumor. The possible extended survival of patients in studies by Mahaley et al. (47) and Bullard et al. (14) was attributed to the good health and young age of the responding population relative to the recipient population as a whole.

Table 21-2 Clinical Trials with Active Immunotherapy[a] in Patients with Primary Brain Tumors

Type of Intervention	Immunotherapeutic Regimen	Objective Performance vs. Untreated Controls	Reference(s)
Active specific			
Autologous tumor immunization	Irradiated (15,000 rad) autologous tumor tissue SC	0/62 patients developed DCHR; possible EAE in 1 patient; no extension of survival	(8)
	Viable tumor cells + CFA	25/28 patients developed DCHR; EAE in 1 patient; no extension of survival	(93)
	Tumor cells + BCG; intratumoral PPD	No increase in survival time in 15 patients	(2,68)
Heterologous tumor immunization	Irradiated cultured glioma cells + BCG; levamisole	3/20 developed DCHR to immunogen; 1/20 had significant target humoral cytotoxic antibody; possible extension of survival in immunized patients	(47)
Heterologous tumor immunization	Cultured glioma cells + BCG	2/3 patients developed weak antibody titers to the immunogen	(14)
Active nonspecific			
Systemic immunostimulation	BCG (ID)	17/26 patients with + PPD: 50% survival at 3 year vs. 12% in untreated historical sample	(56)
	IFN-α	7/17 patients had + response by CT; evidence of survival prolongation	(49)
	IFN-β	30% adults, 60% children, with reduction of tumor mass or stable disease	(69,109)
Intrathecal/IC stimulation	rIL-2 (ICAV or ICV), ± α-rIFN (SC)	Short-term (10-week) evaluation for IC toxicity; no tumor progression in 6/9 patients	(55)
	rIL-2 (ICV)[b]	Induction of intrathecal TNF-α, IL-6, IL-1β, and IL-2 receptor over 24-hour period	(24,43)

[a]The reader is referred to each study for details concerning tumor pathology, previous therapy, response rate criteria, and control group identity. All studies share standard treatment control problems; the conclusions reported are those of the authors and primarily subjective (clinical improvement) unless otherwise noted. Abbreviations: BCG, *bacille Calmette Guérin;* CFA, complete Freund's adjuvant; CT, computerized tomography; DCHR, delayed cutaneous hypersensitivity reaction; EAE, experimental allergic encephalomyelitis; ICAV, intracavitary; ICV, intracerebroventricular; ID, intradermal; IFN, interferon; IL, interleukin; IM, intramuscular; IV, intravenous; PPD, purified protein derivative (tuberculin); rIL, recombinant interleukin; SC, subcutaneous.

[b]Short-term (0-24-hour) study of the intrathecal reaction to infusion of rIL-2 only; tumor patients had leptomeningeal carcinomatosis secondary to adenocarcinoma of the lung (2 cases) or melanoma (9 cases).

Systemic immunostimulation studies designed to enhance the immunocompetence of glioma patients have yielded conflicting reports (47,56). Miki et al. (56) reported that patients receiving intradermal inoculation of *bacille Calmette-Guerin* and converting to purified protein derivative (PPD+) enjoyed a higher survival rate at 3 years (50%) as opposed to the 12% of patients who did not convert. Conversely, Mahaley et al. (48) reported that administration of the anti-helminthic adjuvant, levamisole, failed to demonstrate elevation in serum or cell-mediated titers of specific (anti-glioma) or nonspecific (recall antigen) antibodies, nor was survival increased in the levamisole-treated groups.

Immunostimulation using recombinant cytokines such as interferons (IFNs) and ILs has recently been attempted. Several groups (49, 109; reviewed in 69) report that intravenous or intramuscular administration or IFN-α or IFN-β in both adult and pediatric patients results in stabilization or reduction of tumor mass with concomitant prolongation of survival in approximately 30% of adult patients and 40–60% of pediatric patients. However, the heterogeneity of pediatric patients in terms of tumor pathology makes it difficult to analyze the beneficial effects of this treatment. Of great potential would be the intracavitary or intrathecal administration of such agents to potentiate the local immune response. Merchant et al. (55) have completed a short-term (10-week) evaluation of IC toxicity following the IC or intracerebroventricular administration of recombinant IL-2. This treatment protocol was tolerated by patients, and no disease progression was noted in 6/9 patients during the 10-week course of treatment. Grimm et al. (24) and List et al. (43) have recently analyzed the intrathecal cellular and cytokine response to the intraventricular administration of IL-2 over a 24-hour period in patients with leptomeningeal carcinomatosis secondary to adenocarcinoma of the lung or melanoma. Analysis of cerebrospinal fluid samples taken at intervals of 0–24 hours revealed the induction of tumor necrosis factor-α (TNF-α), IL-β, IL-6, IFN-γ, and IL-2 receptor. In addition, a rapid influx, apparently from the peripheral blood of neutrophilic leukocytes, occurred, with the subsequent appearance of lymphocytes. These efforts were transient; the cytokine levels fell to baseline levels within 12–24 hours. Nevertheless, the ability to induce a cytokine cascade and the recruitment of cellular effectors provide a rationale for continued investigation of compartmental administration of such agents in combination with other modes of therapy. In addition, intrathecal administration avoids the side effects produced by systemic IL and IFN administration and results in a rapid cellular response.

Approaches to Passive (Adoptive) Immunolocalization and Therapy

Adoptive therapy involves the administration of antibodies (whole or fragments) or effector cells to recipients in an effort to transfer immunity. As summarized in Table 21-3, both antibody- and cell-mediated approaches have been attempted in the treatment of primary brain tumors and other CNS metastatic tumors (primarily melanoma).

Table 21-3 Clinical Trials with Passive (Adoptive) Immunolocalizations or Immunotherapy[a] in Patients with Primary Brain Tumors

Effector System Administered	Target, If Defined	Treatment Regimen	Objective Performance vs. Untreated Controls	Reference
MAbs				
Systemic administration				
MAb 425	EGFR	3 × 50 mCi/m^2 ^{125}I 425 Days 1, 8, 15 (IV)	Median 18-month survival rate of 45% vs. 10% for untreated controls	(11)
MAb UJ13A	N-CAM	1 × .8–2.5 mCi ^{131}I UJ13A (IV)	Localization only; positive tumor to brain ratios in 6/7 patients of 3–13:1	(73)
MAb 81C6	Tenascin	1 × 1.8–3.5 mCi ^{131}I 81C6 (IV or intracarotid); paired label, nonspecific immunoglobulin	Localization only; positive tumor to brain ratios in 5/8 patients of 2.3–76:1	(111)
MAb Me1-14	gp 240	1 × .2–.3 mCi ^{125}I Me1-14 F(ab')$_2$ fragments (IV or intracarotid)	Localization only; positive tumor to brain ratios in 4/4 patients of 2–18:1 with F(ab')$_2$ fragments	(4)
Intrathecal administration				
MAb UJ181.4	L1 homologue	1 × 24–48 mCi ^{131}I UJ181.4	2/5 patients evaluable; clinical response, no toxicity	(60)
MAb 81C6	Tenascin	1 × 60 mCi ^{131}I 81C6	2/2 patients, progressive disease	(60)
MAb Me1-14	gp 240	1 × 45–55 mCi ^{131}I Me1-14	2/2 patients, clinical response by CSF and CT parameters	(60)

Intratumoral/intracystic administration

MAb BC-2	Tenascin	1 × intratumoral injection (average dose 551 mBq) ^{131}I BC-2	Average 4.9% ID/g; no severe toxicity; 2/10 patients developed HAMA by 90 days; 3/10 partial remission; 3/10 stable disease at 8 months	(75)
MAb ERIC	N-CAM	1 × intracystic injection ^{131}I ERIC (1350–2193 mBq)	Tumor:normal brain ratios of 187–564; no severe toxicity; 5/7 patients with stable disease	(70)
Effector Cells				
LAK	—	15 cycles LAK cells + IL-2 via reservoir	1/9 patients with partial response by CT; cerebral edema and neurological side effects: 9/9	(3)
Autologous LAK		Injection of autologous LAK + rIL-2 in neuropil surrounding tumor excision site	Cerebral edema in 29/29; 4/29, no recurrent tumor after 16 months	(54)
LAK + ASL	—	ICAV LAK + ASL + rIL-2 at surgery; 30 days later, LAK − ASL via reservoir	10/11 patients, no survival prolongation; no adverse side effects	(42)
ASL	—	ICAV ASL + IL-2 at surgery	No toxicity; no significant extension of survival (83 patients)	(33)

[a]The reader is referred to each study for details concerning tumor pathology, previous therapy, response rate criteria, and control group identity. All studies share standard treatment control problems; the conclusions reported are those of the authors and primarily subjective (clinical improvement) unless otherwise noted. For excellent reviews of this area, see Schuster and Bigner (83) and Merchant et al. (54). Abbreviations: ASL, autologous stimulated lymphocytes; CT, computerized tomography; EAE, experimental allergic encephalomyelitis; HAMA, human anti-mouse antibody; ICAV, intracavitary; interleukin; IV, intravenous; LAK, lymphokine-activated killer cells; rIL, recombinant interleukin.

In general, systemic administration of labeled MAbs to brain tumor patients has been disappointing. The percent of injected dose localized per gram of tumor is consistently small (%ID/g = .001–.004%) (109), even when there is a high tumor:normal brain ratio of labeled specific antibody (20,73). Significant survival has been claimed for patients receiving anti-EGFR treatment, but the long-term evaluation of this patient study must be confirmed in a randomized phase II or phase III trial. The use of $F(ab')_2$ fragments has been shown to increase early uptake of MAb as measured by tumor: normal brain ratios, but this treatment does not significantly increase the %ID/g (4,109).

Recent efforts have been focused on increasing specific antibody uptake by the regional delivery of specific MAb through intrathecal, intracavitary, or intratumoral routes. Human anti-mouse antibody elicitation is still an issue in compartmental approaches because the compromised blood-brain barrier within the tumor will allow systemic sensitization. Therefore, current efforts to "humanize" MAbs should have direct application to the therapy of tumors within the CNS, whether they are primary or metastatic. Initial results with intrathecal administration of MAbs tailored to the L1 homologue, tenascin, or gp240 in tumor patients have been promising (60). In studies by Moseley et al. (60), 4/6 patients with primary brain tumors or melanoma metastatic to the brain demonstrated clinical response to MAb treatment as measured by computed tomography and cerebrospinal fluid parameters. Toxic effects of this treatment included reversible transient bone marrow suppression, headaches, and seizures. Preliminary studies (70,75) have been conducted using intratumoral or intracystic cavity injections. Sustained levels of %ID/g of 4.9% have been reported with partial remission and disease stabilization (75). Tumor:normal brain ratios of 187–564:1 have been demonstrated following administration of the antineural cell adhesion molecule MAb ERIC into the cyst cavity of 7 glioma patients (70). In addition, negligible toxicity and disease stabilization in 5/7 patients in this study was reported (70). Continued success using compartmental approaches will depend upon the further refinement of epitope-MAb pairs, in terms of both specificity and distribution throughout the tumor. Since human gliomas show complex antigen heterogeneity, it is possible that the use of mixed or sequential MAb treatments of a tumor-designed combination of epitope-defined MAbs will be the best approach. In addition, selection of the most effective isotope for treatment within a confined space, whether tumor or cyst or intrathecal space, will become crucial. It is controversial as to whether the emission path length (longer-range β-emitters vs. short half-life, short penetration α-emitters) must be considered for optimal tumor penetration and minimal normal brain irradiation (57,87).

Studies employing the administration of effector cells within the intrathecal space arose from observations concerning the cytolytic function of TILs isolated from gliomas (38). Effector cells were reported to be efficacious when passively administered in cases of systemic metastatic disease (77) or in model glioma spheroid systems (35). A comprehensive summary of recent trials with stimulated lymphocytes and rIL-2 in human glioma has been published (54). A consistent clinical observation in in vivo trials with IL-2-activated lymphocytes is cerebral edema, which is often of sufficient magnitude to warrant cessation of therapy (54). Administration of steroids to counteract the edema may depress the anti-tumor activity of IL-2 via suppression of the development or maintenance of lymphokine-activated killer (LAK) cells. Production of transforming growth factor (TGF) by glioma cells has also been shown to suppress the proliferation of IL-2-dependent T cells and the generation of cytotoxic T cells in vitro (19), further adding to the complexity of the induction and maintenance of a stimulated lymphocyte response intrathecally.

Representative clinical trials with passive immunotherapy or immunolocalization are summarized in Table 21-3. Some trials maintain that the treatment regimens are well tolerated (33,42), but the number of objective responses as opposed to historical or untreated controls is small (3,42,54). The current consensus about these treatment approaches is expressed well by Lillehei: "Although adoptive immunotherapy was safe and well tolerated, its therapeutic potential remains in question" (42).

Approaches using targeted LAK cells by bispecific anti-CD3/anti-tumor MAbs are of limited success (67). Extended survival of 8/10 patients receiving targeted LAK cells must be regarded with caution, since this study has been subject to question (65,66).

In summary, adoptive immunotherapy for tumors of, or metastatic to, the CNS has demonstrated successful clinical responses following administration of specific, single epitope-defining MAbs, primarily within the intrathecal or intracystic space. These approaches do not show toxicity when targeted against neural cell adhesion molecules that are expressed by normal glial and neuronal cells. They also provide minimization of adverse systemic effects, as well as the induction of a cytokine cascade and lymphocytic influx following intrathecal administration of cytokines. The problematic areas in the use of both soluble molecules and cellular effectors are the inaccessibility to tumor cells beyond the immediately available superficial tumor in the resection site or superficial intrathecal metastasis, and peritumoral edema in the intrathecal compartment, which has immediate adverse consequences.

Experimental Models for New Approaches to Human Patient Immunotherapy

As summarized in Tables 21-2 and 21-3, the clinical trial results of various immunotherapeutic approaches to treatment of brain tumors suggest the following: *(1)* systemic immunization of patients fails to produce an efficacious cellular or humoral anti-tumor response; *(2)* generalized systemic immunostimulation, while possibly increasing survival time of the most fit patients, has not produced a demonstrable immune response; *(3)* intrathecal administration of various cytokines can be tolerated by recipients and induces a local cytokine response and influx of lymphocytes to the intrathecal space; *(4)* intrathecal, intracystic, or intratumoral administration of MAbs to gliomas is superior to intravenous or intracarotid administration in terms of %ID/g tumor:normal brain ratios, and most probably, human anti-mouse antibody induction (18); and *(5)* current protocols for administration of LAK cells and autologous stimulated lymphocytes are hampered by IL-2-induced cerebral edema and have shown no detectable effect. Improvement in current therapeutic protocols will depend upon the development of new approaches in experimental models, several of which currently show promise.

Animal Models for Malignant Gliomas

Several animal models have been used to study malignant gliomas. The standard SC xenograft model system in athymic mice for the preliminary evaluation of the in vivo behavior of antibody conjugates is well established. Although IC xenografts in athymic mice have been used (9), the IC xenografts in rats have yielded more consistent results (40). Recently, Fuchs et al. (22) established an athymic rat model of human neoplastic meningitis. In this system, a catheter is inserted into the subarachinoid space and extended to the lumbar region which allows infusion of suspension cells for tumor establishment, subsequent administration of various therapeutic cells or solutions, and sampling of cerebrospinal fluid. Our results using the transplantable medulloblastoma cell line D341 Med (Fig. 21-1) show that the rat model mimics leptomeningeal carcinomatosis and displays dissemination of the malignant cells throughout the subarachnoid space. As shown in Fig. 21-2, when medulloblastoma is used in this system, the tumor effectively infiltrates between spinal dorsal nerve roots and dorsal root ganglion cells, but it does not invade the pial surface or parenchyma. This animal model offers numerous applications and allows the investigation of combined protocols against established models in the intrathecal space.

A much-needed model has been developed for the investigation of disseminated tumor cells and their accessibility to antibody or cellular effectors (39). In this system, rat 9L gliosarcoma cells are transfected with the *Escherichia coli lacZ* gene, which encodes β-gal. After injection into the right caudate nucleus of rats, these cells produced a focal tumor with disseminating single cells that are unmistakably identified by histochemical staining with Xgal substrate to stain the β-gal-producing cells. The extent and/or inhibition of dissemination, as well as the trafficking of effector cells following various experimental manipulations, can be readily demonstrated.

Modification of the Target Tumor Cell

Certain tumor epitopes, and the MAbs or effector cells that recognize these epitopes, have been manipulated in therapeutic treatments to reduce gliomas. Efforts have been directed to increase the tumor antigen density and the distribution of target epitope in order to enhance antibody or effector cell targeting (82). Adachi et al. (1) have shown

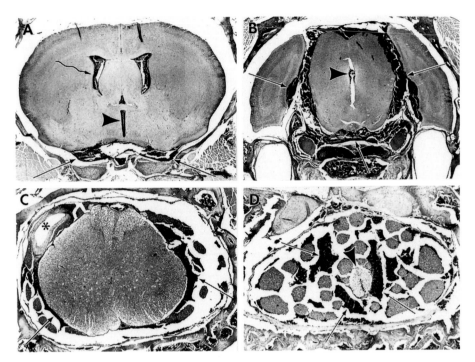

Fig. 21-1. D-341 Med xenograft; whole mount cross sections. A: Cerebrum. Tumor is present in the basilar subarachnoid space (arrows), third ventricle (arrowhead), and lateral ventricles (curved arrow). ×9.5. B: Brain stem. Tumor is in the cerebral acueduct (arrowhead) and in the subarachnoid space encircling the brain stem (arrows). ×8.5. C: Lumbar spinal cord. Tumor is seen in the spinal subarachoid space (arrows). Asterisk shows cateter site. ×32. D: Lumbar cistern. Tumor (arrows) surrounds the nerve roots of the cauda equina and the filum terminale (arrowhead). ×40. (Reprinted by permission of Kluwer Academic Publishers.) Friedman HS, Oakes WJ, Bigner SH, Wikstrand CJ, Bigner DD. Medulloblastoma: tumor biological and clinical perspectives. J. Neuro-oncology 11:1–15, 1991. Kluwer Academic Publishers, The Netherlands.

that recombinant tumor necrosis factor-α (TNF-α) can significantly increase density of EGFR in 3/4 glioma cultured cell lines. Susceptibility to ^{125}I-labeled MAb 425 killing was also increased. Thus, a combination of recombinant TNF-α and MAb 425 conjugate may be an efficacious treatment approach. Wen et al. (96) have shown in the rat 9L model that IFN-γ increased the expression of major histocompatibility complex (MHC) antigens on tumor cells in vitro. However, IFN-γ injected into the tumor increased the number of inflammatory cells within the tumor at the periphery and increased the expression of MHC antigens in endothelial and ependymal cells, but not in the tumor cells. These results suggest that MHC antigen expression inhibition in vivo may be possible, but non-MHC-restricted cell effector mechanisms may be a preferable approach.

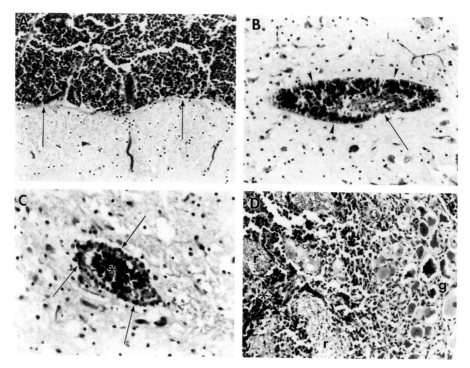

Fig. 21-2. D-341 Med xenograft. A: Tumor present in subarchnoid space (*) does not invade the pial surface (arrows). ×250. B: Tumor within a Virchow-Robin space around a blood vessel (arrow) does not invade the parenchyma (arrowheads). ×325. C: Tumor in the central canal of the cervical spinal cord (*) does not cross the ependymal lining (arrows). ×400. D: Tumor (*) infiltrates between spinal dorsal nerve roots (r) and doral root ganglion cells (g). ×250. (Reprinted by permission of Kluwer Academic Publishers.) Friedman HS, Oakes WJ, Bigner SH, Wikstrand CJ, Bigner DD. Medulloblastoma: tumor biological and clinical perspectives. J. Neuro-oncology 11:1–15, 1991. Kluwer Academic Publishers, The Netherlands.

Improving Localization of Antibodies

Although Riva et al. (75) have shown that compartmental administration of murine MAb BC-2 resulted in weak to moderate human anti-mouse antibody titers in only 2/10 patients 90 days after administration, modification of MAbs by replacement with human nonvariable region frameworks is important to try in order to reduce immunogenicity and generate reagents capable of directing antibody-dependent, cell-mediated cytotoxicity with human effector cells (90). The performance of these altered MAbs is readily measured in the in vitro spheroid glioma model system (36).

Efforts to improve the stability, effectiveness, and dissemination of MAb reagents are currently in progress. Conventionally (iodogen-mediated) radioiodinated MAbs frequently undergo dehalogenation due to the similarity of the MAb protein iodination sites to those of thyroid hormones. Zalutsky et al. (112) have reported decreased dehalogenation, enhanced specific localization, and in vivo stability of the anti-tenascin MAb 81C6 to human glioma xenografts following iodination by ATE (N-succini-midyl-3-(tri-n-butylstannyl)benzoate). Subsequently, Schuster et al. (82) demonstrated improved therapeutic efficacy in the same model with ATE-labeled MAb 81C6.

Immunoglobulin fragments F(ab')$_2$ have been used to increase tumor penetration and clearance of unbound antibody (4,17). Recently, Yokota et al. (107), using quantitative autoradiography, compared the tumor penetration of intact Ig, F(ab')$_2$, Fab', and sFv fragments of a single MAb CC49 which recognizes TAG-72 to target LS-174T human colon carcinoma xenografts in athymic mice. sFv fragments are recombinant proteins (M$_r$, 27,000) composed of a V$_1$ amino acid sequence of a MAb tethered to a V$_H$ sequence by a designed peptide. This study demonstrated that intact IgG was localized predominantly in the area of the blood vessels, while sFv was more evenly distributed throughout the tumor mass. Fab' and F(ab')$_2$ showed intermediate penetration in a size-related manner (107). The reduction in size, coupled with the engineering of desired sequences for labeling or effector function in these studies, can optimize the stability, distribution, and efficacy of these molecules for human therapeutic protocols.

Summary

It is beyond the scope of this chapter to present a comprehensive review of the progress that has been made in glioma immunotherapy since the early 1980s. The representative summaries provided in the tables presented here, however, have identified the exploitable approaches of promise. Intracompartmental administration of effector MAbs and/or cells and immunostimulants is well tolerated, and as early results suggest, it may be capable of extending meaningful survival. Several groups are developing methods to optimize the delivery and stability of the currently identified promising effectors. As additional long-term follow-up data are obtained from ongoing phase I and II trials, the protocols illustrated here that have verifiable long-term benefit will be identified. The evaluation of tumors metastatic to the CNS from systemic primary sites is crucial, since the number of patients presenting with CNS disease secondary to metastasis or acquired immunodeficiency syndrome is constantly increasing as a result of transient success in extra-CNS therapy (43,60). In retrospect, the advances made since the 1980 publication of our review (98) are impressive. With currently known successful approaches and the explosion in molecular engineering, the advances of the coming years will be even more so.

Acknowledgments

Editorial assistance for this chapter was provided by Ann S. Tamariz, E.L.S. This work was supported by NIH grants CA 11898, NS 20023, and CA 56115.

References

1. Adachi K, Belser P, Bender H, Li D, Rodeck U, Benveniste EN, Woo D, Schmiegel WH, Herlyn D. Enhancement of epidermal growth factor receptor expression on glioma cells by recombinant tumor necrosis factor-α. Cancer Immunol Immunother 34:370–376, 1992.

2. Albright L, Seab JA, Ommaya AK. Intracerebral delayed hypersensitivity reactions in glioblastoma multiforme patients. Cancer 39:1331–1336, 1977.

3. Barba D, Saris SC, Holder C, Rosenberg SA, Oldfield EH. Intratumoral LAK cell and interleukin-2 therapy of human gliomas. J Neurosurg 70:175–182, 1989.

4. Behnke J, Mach J-P, Buchegger F, Carrel S, Delaloye B, de Tribolet N. *In vivo* localisation of radiolabelled monoclonal antibody in human gliomas. Br J Neurosurg 2:193–197, 1988.

5. Bender H, Takahashi H, Adachi K, Belser P, Liang S, Prewett M, Schrappe M, Sutter A, Rodeck U, Herlyn D. Immunotherapy of human glioma xenografts with unlabeled, [131]I-, or ^{125}I-labeled monoclonal antibody 425 to epidermal growth factor receptor. Cancer Res 52:121–126, 1992.

6. Bigner SH, Humphrey PA, Wong AJ, Vogelstein B, Mark J, Friedman HS, Bigner DD. Characterization of the epidermal growth factor receptor in human glioma cell lines and xenografts. Cancer Res 50:8017–8022, 1990.

7. Bishop JM. The molecular genetics of cancer. Science 235:305–311, 1987.

8. Bloom HJG. Combined modality therapy for intracranial tumors. Cancer 35:111–120, 1975.

9. Bourdon MA, Coleman RE, Blasberg RG, Groothuis DR, Bigner DD. Monoclonal antibody localization in subcutaneous and intracranial human glioma xenografts: paired-label and imaging analysis. Anticancer Res 4:133–140, 1984.

10. Bourdon MA, Wikstrand CJ, Furthmayr H, Matthews TJ, Bigner DD. Human glioma-mesenchymal extracellular matrix antigen defined by monoclonal antibody. Cancer Res 43:2796–2805, 1983.

11. Brady LW, Markoe AM, Woo DV, Rackover MA, Koprowski H, Steplewski Z, Peyster RG. Iodine-125 labeled anti-epidermal growth factor receptor-425 in the treatment of malignant astrocytomas. J Neurosurg Sci 34:243–249, 1990.

12. Brooks WH, Netsky MG, Normansell DE, Horwitz DA. Depressed cell-mediated immunity in patients with primary intracranial tumors: characterization of a humor immunosuppressive factor. J Exp Med 136:1631–1647, 1972.

13. Brooks WH, Roszman TL, Rogers AS. Impairment of rosette-forming T lymphocytes in patients with primary intracranial tumors. Cancer 37:1869–1873, 1976.

14. Bullard DE, Thomas DGT, Darling JL, Wikstrand CJ, Diengdoh JV, Barnard RO, Bodmer JG, Bigner DD. A preliminary study utilizing viable HLA mismatched cultured glioma cells as adjuvant therapy for patients with malignant gliomas. Br J Cancer 51:283–289, 1985.

15. Bumol TF, Reisfeld RA. Unique glycoprotein-proteoglycan complex defined by monoclonal antibody on human melanoma cells. Proc Natl Acad Sci USA 79:1245–1249, 1982.

16. Carrel S, Acolla RS, Carmagnola AL, Mach J-P. Common human melanoma-associated antigen(s) detected by monoclonal antibodies. Cancer Res 40:2523–2528, 1980.

17. Colapinto EV, Zalutsky MR, Archer GE, Noska MA, Friedman HS, Carrel S, Bigner DD. Radioimmunotherapy of intracerebral human glioma xenografts with ^{131}I-labeled F(ab')$_2$ fragments of monoclonal antibody Mel-14. Cancer Res 50:1822–1827, 1990.

18. Delmonte L. Malignant glioma survival increased by MoAb-guided radioisotope. Oncology Times, May, pp 32–33, 1992.

19. de Tribolet N. Immunology of gliomas. Childs Nerv Syst 5:60–65, 1989.

20. Epenetos AA, Snook D, Durbin H, Johnson PM, Taylor-Papadimitrious J. Limitations of radiolabeled monoclonal antibodies for localization of human neoplasms. Cancer Res 46:3183–3191, 1986.

21. Fredman P, von Holst H, Collins VP, Granholm L, Svennerholm L. Sialyllactotetraosylcera-mide, a ganglioside marker for human malignant gliomas. J Neurochem 50:912–919, 1988.

22. Fuchs HE, Archer GE, Colvin OM, Bigner SH, Schuster JM, Fuller GN, Muhlbaier LH, Schold SC, Friedman HS, Bigner DD. Activity of intrathecal 4-hydroperoxycyclophos-phamide in a nude rat model of human neoplastic meningitis. Cancer Res 50:1954–1959, 1990.

23. Greene HSN. Heterotransplantation of tumors. Ann NY Acad Sci 69:818–829, 1957.

24. Grimm EA, List J, Loudon WG, Bruner JM, Moser RP. Cellular immune response in the human brain: cytokine cascade in the CSF after intraventricular IL-2 injection. J Neuro-oncol 12:252, 1992. [abstr]

25. Groothuis DR, Vriesendorp FJ, Kupfer B, Warnke PC, Lapin GD, Kuruvilla A, Vick NA, Mikhael MA, Patlak CS. Quantitative measurements of capillary transport in human brain tumors by computed tomography. Ann Neurol 30:581–588, 1991.

26. Habel K, Belcher JH. Immunologically privileged sites in studies of polyoma tumor anti-gens. Proc Soc Exp Biol Med 113:148–152, 1963.

27. Harper JR, Prince JT, Healy PA, Stuart JK, Nauman SJ, Stallcup WB. Isolation and sequence of partial cDNA clones of human L1:homology of human and rodent L1 in the cytoplasmic region. J Neurochem 56:797–804, 1991.

28. Hellstrom KE, Hellstrom I. Oncogene-associated tumor antigens as targets for immu-notherapy. FASEB J 3:1715–1722, 1989.

29. Hermanson M, Funa K, Hartman M, Claesson-Welsh L, Heldin CH, Westermark B, Nister M. Platelet-derived growth factor and its receptors in human glioma tissue: expression of messenger RNA and protein suggests the presence of autocrine and paracrine loops. Cancer Res 52:3213–3219, 1992.

30. Hermanson M, Nister M, Betsholtz C, Neldin C, Westermark B, Funa K. Endothelial cell hyperplasia in human glioblastoma: coexpression of mRNA for platelet-derived growth factor (PDGF) B chain and PDGF receptor suggests autocrine growth stimulation. Proc Natl Acad Sci USA 85:7748–7752, 1988.

31. Humphrey PA, Wong AJ, Vogelstein B, Friedman HS, Werner MH, Bigner DD, Bigner SH. Amplification and expression of the epidermal growth factor receptor gene in human glioma xenografts. Cancer Res 48:2231–2238, 1988.

32. Humphrey PA, Wong AJ, Vogelstein B, Zalutsky MR, Fuller GN, Archer GE, Friedman HS, Kwatra MM, Bigner SH, Bigner DD. Anti-synthetic peptide antibody reacting at the fusion junction of deletion-mutant epidermal growth factor receptors in human glioblastoma. Proc Natl Acad Sci USA 87:4207–4211, 1990.

33. Ingram M, Buckwalter JG, Jacques DB, Freshwater DB, Abts RM, Techy GB, Miyagi K, Shelden CH, Rand RW, English LW. Immunotherapy for recurrent malignant glioma: an interim report on survival. Neurolog Res 12:265–273, 1990.

34. IUPAC-IUB Commission on Biochemical Nomenclature (CBN). The nomenclature of lipids. Eur J Biochem 79:11–21, 1977.

35. Iwasaki K, Kikuchi H, Miyatake S-I, Aoki T, Yamasaki T, Oda Y. Infiltrative and cytolytic activities of lymphokine-activated killer cells against a human glioma spheroid model. Cancer Res 50:2429–2436, 1990.

36. Jääskelainen J, Maenpaa A, Patarroyo M, Gahmberg CG, Somersalo K, Tarkkanen J, Kallio M, Timonen T. Migration of recombinant IL-2 activated T and natural killer cells in the intercellular space of human H-2 glioma spheroids *in vitro*. J Immunol 149:260–268, 1992.

37. Kuppner MC, Hamou MF, Bodmer S, Fontana A, De Tribolet N. The glioblastoma-derived T-cell suppressor factor/transforming growth factor-$\beta 2$ inhibits the generation of lymphokine-activated killer (LAK) cells. Int J Cancer 42:562–567, 1988.

38. Kuppner MC, Hamou M-F, de Tribolet N. Activation and adhesion molecule expression on lymphoid infiltrates in human glioblastomas. J Neuroimmunol 29:229–238, 1990.

39. Lampson LA, Wen P, Roman VA, Morris JH, Sarid JA. Disseminating tumor cells and their interactions with leukocytes visualized in the brain. Cancer Res 52:1018–1025, 1992.

40. Lee Y, Bullard DE, Wikstrand CJ, Zalutsky MR, Muhlbaier LH, Bigner DD. Comparison of monoclonal antibody delivery to intracranial glioma xenografts by intravenous and intra-carotid administration. Cancer Res 47:1941–1946, 1987.

41. Libermann TA, Nusbaum HR, Razon N, Kris R, Lax I, Soreq H, Whittle N, Waterfield MD, Ullrich A, Schlessinger J. Amplification, enhanced expression, and possible rearrange-ment of EGF receptor gene in primary brain tumours of glial origin. Nature 313:144–147, 1985.

42. Lillehei KO, Mitchell DH, Johnson SD, McCleary EL, Kruse CA. Long-term follow-up of patients with recurrent malignant gliomas treated with adjuvant adoptive immunotherapy. Neurosurgery 28:16–23, 1991.

43. List J, Moser RP, Steuer M, Loudon WG, Blacklock JB, Grimm EA. Cytokine responses to intraventricular injection of interleukin 2 into patients with leptomeningeal carcino-matosis: rapid induction of tumor necrosis factor-α, interleukin 1-β, interleukin 6, γ-inter-feron, and soluble interleukin-2 receptor (M_r 55,000 protein). Cancer Res 52:1123–1128, 1992.

44. Long DM. Capillary ultrastructure and the blood-brain barrier in human malignant brain tumors. J Neurosurg 32:127–144, 1970.

45. Mahaley MS Jr, Brooks WH, Roszman TL, Bigner DD, Dudka L, Richardson S. Immu-nobiology of primary intracranial tumors: I. Studies of the cellular and humoral general immune competence of brain tumor patients. J Neurosurg 46:467–476, 1977.

46. Mahaley MS Jr, Day ED. Immunological studies of human gliomas. J Neurosurg 23:363–370, 1965.

47. Mahaley MS Jr, Gillespie GY, Gillespie RP, Watkins PJ, Bigner DD, Wikstrand CJ, San-filippo F, McQueen JM. Immunobiology of primary intracranial tumors. Part 8. Serologi-cal responses to active immunization of patients with anaplastic gliomas. J Neurosurg 59:208–216, 1983.

48. Mahaley MS Jr, Steinbok P, Aronin P, Dudka L, Zinn D. Immunobiology of primary intracranial tumors. Part 4. Levamisole as an immune stimulant in patients and in the ASV glioma model. J Neurosurg 54:220–227, 1981.

49. Mahaley MS Jr, Urso MB, Whaley RA, Blue M, Williams TE, Guaspari A, Selker RG. Immunobiology of primary intracranial tumors. Part 10. Therapeutic efficacy of inter-feron in the treatment of recurrent gliomas. J Neurosurg 63:719–725, 1985.

50. Månsson JE, Fredman P, Bigner DD, Molin K, Rosengren B, Friedman HS, Svennerholm L. Characterization of new gangliosides of the lactotetraose series in murine xenografts of a human glioma cell line. FEBS Lett 201:109–113, 1986.

51. Maxwell M, Naber SP, Wolfe HJ, Galanopoulos T, Hedley-Whyte ET, Black PM, An-toniades HN. Co-expression of platelet-derived growth factor (PDGF) and PDGF-

receptor genes by primary human astrocytomas may contribute to their development and maintenance. J Clin. Invest 86:131–140, 1990.

52. McKeever PE, Robertson D, Davenport MD, Shakui P. Patterns of antigenic expression of human glioma cells. Crit Rev Neurobiol 6:119–147, 1991.

53. Medawar PB. Immunity to homologous grafted skin: III. The fate of skin homografts transplanted to the brain, to subcutaneous tissue, and to the anterior chamber of the eye. Br J Exp Pathol 29:58–69, 1948.

54. Merchant RE, Ellison MD, Young HF. Immunotherapy for malignant glioma using human recombinant interleukin-2 and activated autologous lymphocytes. A review of pre-clinical and clinical investigations. J Neurooncol 8:173–188, 1990.

55. Merchant RE, McVicar DW, Merchant LH, Young HF. Treatment of recurrent malignant glioma by repeated intracerebral injections of human recombinant interleukin-2 alone or in combination with systemic interferon-α. Results of a phase I clinical trial. J Neuro-oncol 12:75–83, 1992.

56. Miki Y, Sano K, Takakura K, Mizutani H. Adjuvant immunotherapy with BCG for malignant brain tumors. Neurol Med Chir 16:357–364, 1976.

57. Millar WT, Barrett A. Dosimetric model for antibody targeted radionuclide therapy of tumor cells in cerebrospinal fluid. Cancer Res (Suppl) 50:1043S–1048S, 1990.

58. Molenaar WM, Trojanowski JQ. Biological markers of glial and primitive tumors. In Concepts in Neurosurgery. Vol 4, Neurobiology of Brain Tumors, M Salcman, ed. Williams and Wilkins, Baltimore, 1991, pp 185–210.

59. Morantz RA, Shain W, Cravioto H. Immune surveillance and tumors of the nervous system. J Neurosurg 49:84–92, 1978.

60. Moseley RP, Davies AG, Richardson RB, Zalutsky M, Carrell S, Fabre J, Slack N, Bullimore J, Pizer R, Papanastassiou V, Kemshead JT, Coakham HB, Lashford LS. Intrathecal administration of ^{131}I-radiolabeled monoclonal antibody as a treatment for neoplastic meningitis. Br J Cancer 62:637–642, 1990.

61. Murphy JB, Sturm E. Conditions determining the transplantability of tissues in the brain. J Exp Med 38:183–197, 1923.

62. Nilsson O, Mansson JE, Lindholm L, Holmgren J, Svennerholm L. Sialosyllactotetra-osylceramide, a novel ganglioside antigen detected in human carcinomas by a monoclonal antibody. FEBS Lett 182:398–402, 1985.

63. Nister M, Claesson-Welsh L, Eriksson A, Heldin CH, Westermark B. Differential expression of PDGF receptors in human malignant glioma cell lines. J Biol Chem 266:16755–16763, 1991.

64. Nister M, Libermann TA, Betsholtz C, Pettersson M, Claesson-Welsh L, Heldin C-H, Schlessinger J, Westermark B. Expression of messenger RNAs for platelet-derived growth factor and transforming growth factor-α and their receptors in human malignant glioma cell lines. Cancer Res 48:3910–3918, 1988.

65. Nitta T. Retraction. Int J Cancer 51:163, 1992.

66. Nitta T, Sato K, Okumura K, Steinman L. An analysis of T-cell-receptor variable-region genes in tumor-infiltrating lymphocytes within malignant tumors. Int J Cancer 49:545–550, 1991.

67. Nitta T, Sato K, Yatita H, Okumura K, Ishii S. Preliminary trial of specific targeting therapy against malignant glioma. Lancet (i)335:368–370, 1990.

68. Ommaya A. Immunotherapy of gliomas: a review. Adv Neurol 15:337–359, 1976.

69. Packer RJ, Kramer ED, Ryan JA. Biologic and immune modulating agents in the treatment of childhood brain tumors. Neurol Clin 9:405–422, 1991.

70. Papanastassiou V, Pizer BL, Chandler CL, Zananiri TF, Kemshead JT, Hopkins KI. Phar-

macokinetics and dose estimates following intrathecal administration of ^{131}I-monoclonal antibodies for the treatment of central nervous system malignancies. Int J Radiation Oncology Biol Phys 31:541–552, 1995.

71. Patel K, Kiely F, Phimister E, Melino G, Rathjen F, Kemshead JT. The 200/220 kDa antigen recognized by monoclonal antibody (MAb) UJ127.11 on neural tissues and tumors is the human L1 adhesion molecule. Hybridoma 10:481–491, 1991.

72. Patel K, Rossell RJ, Bourne S, Moore SE, Walsh FS, Kemshead JT. Monoclonal antibody UJ13A recognizes the neural cell adhesion molecule (NCAM). Int J Cancer 44:1062–1068, 1989.

73. Richardson RB, Davies AG, Bourne SP, Staddon GE, Jones DH, Kemshead JT, Coakham HB. Radioimmunolocalization of human brain tumours: biodistribution of radiolabelled monoclonal antibody UJ13A. Eur J Nucl Med 12:313–320, 1986.

74. Ridley A, Cavanagh JB. Lymphocytic infiltration in gliomas: evidence of possible host resistance. Brain 94:117–124, 1971.

75. Riva P, Arista A, Sturiale C, Moscatelli G, Tison V, Mariani M, Seccamani E, Lazzari S, Fagioli L, Ranceschi G, Sarti G, Riva N, Natali PG, Zardi L, Scassellati GA. Treatment of intracranial human glioblastoma by direct intratumoral administration of ^{131}I-labelled anti-tenascin monoclonal antibody BC-2. Int J Cancer 51:7–13, 1992.

76. Rodeck U, Herlyn M, Herlyn D, Molthoff C, Atkinson B, Varello M, Steplewski Z, Koprowski H. Tumor growth modulation by a monoclonal antibody to the epidermal growth factor receptor: immunologically mediated and effector cell-independent effects. Cancer Res 47:3692–3696, 1987.

77. Rosenberg SAL, Lotze MT, Muul LA, Leitman S, Chang AE, Ettinghausen SE, Matory TL, Skibber JM, Shiloni E, Vetto JT, Seipp CA, Shimpson C, Reichert CM. Observations on the systemic administration of autologous lympohkine-activated killer cells and recombinant interleukin-2 to patients with metastatic cancer. N Engl J Med 313:1485–1492, 1985.

78. Roszman TL, Brooks WH. Immunobiology of primary intracranial tumours. III. Demonstration of a qualitative lymphocyte abnormality in patients with primary brain tumours. Clin Exp Immunol 39:395–402, 1980.

79. Salcman M, Broadwell RD. The blood-brain barrier. In: Neurobiology of Brain Tumors. Vol 4, Concepts in Neurosurgery, M Salcman, ed. Williams and Wilkins, Baltimore, 1991, pp 229–249.

80. Sawamura Y, DeTribolet N. Immunotherapy of brain tumors. J Neurosurg Sci 34:265–278, 1990.

81. Schrappe M, Bumol TF, Apelgren LD, Briggs SL, Koppel GA, Markowitz DD, Mueller BM, Reisfeld RA. Long-term growth suppression of human glioma xenografts by chemoimmunoconjugates of 4-desacetylvinblastine-3-carboxyhydrazide and monoclonal antibody 9.2.27. Cancer Res 52:3838–3844, 1992.

82. Schuster JM, Garg PK, Bigner DD, Zalutsky MR. Improved therapeutic efficacy of a monoclonal antibody radioiodinated using N-succinimidyl-3-(tri-n-butylstannyl)benzoate. Cancer Res 51:4164–4169, 1991.

83. Schuster JM, Bigner DD. Immunotherapy and monoclonal antibody therapies. Curr Opin Oncol 4:547–552, 1992.

84. Shirai Y. Transplantations of rat sarcomas in adult heterogenous animals. Jpn Med World 1:14–15, 1921.

85. Shuttleworth EC Jr. Barrier phenomena in brain tumors. Prog Exp Tumor Res 17:279–290, 1972.

86. Siris JH. Concerning the immunological specificity of glioblastoma multiforme. Bull Neurol Inst NY 4:597–601, 1936.

87. Smith DB, Moseley RP, Begent RHJ, Coakham HB, Glaser MG, Dewhurst S, Kelly A, Bagshawe KD. Quantitative distribution of 131-I-labelled monoclonal antibodies administered by intra-ventricular route. Eur J Cancer 26:129–136, 1990.

88. Sugawa W, Ekstrand AJ, James CD, Collins VP. Identical splicing of aberrrant epidermal growth factor receptor transcripts from amplified rearranged genes in human glioblastomas. Proc Natl Acad Sci USA 87:8602–8606, 1990.

89. Svennerholm L. Chromatographic separation of human brain gangliosides. J Neurochem 10:613–623, 1963.

90. Takahashi H, Belser PH, Atkinson BF, Sela B-A, Ross AH, Biegel J, Emanuel B, Sutton L, Koprowski H, Herlyn D. Monoclonal antibody-dependent, cell-mediated cytotoxicity against human malignant gliomas. Neurosurgery 27:97–102, 1990.

91. Takahashi H, Herlyn D, Atkinson B, Powe J, Rodeck U, Alavi A, Bruce DA, Koprowski H. Radioimmunodetection of human glioma xenografts by monoclonal antibody to epidermal growth factor receptor. Cancer Res 47:3847–3850, 1987.

92. Takeuchi J, Barnard RO. Perivascular lymphocytic cuffing in astrocytomas. Acta Neuropathol 35:265–271, 1976.

93. Trouillas P. Immunologie et immunotherapie des tumeurs cerebrales. Etat actuel Rev Neurol 128:23–38, 1973.

94. Vick NA, Bigner DD, Kvedar JP. The fine structure of canine gliomas and intracranial sarcomas induced by the Schmidt-Ruppin strain of the Rous sarcoma virus. J Neuropathol Exp Neurol 30:354–367, 1971.

95. Wahlstrom T, Linder E, Saksela E, Westermark B. Tumor-specific membrane antigens in established cell lines from gliomas. Cancer 34:274–279, 1974.

96. Wen PY, Lampson MA, Lampson LA. Effects of γ-interferon on major histocompatibility complex antigen expression and lymphocytic infiltration in the 9L gliosarcoma brain tumor model: implications for strategies of immunotherapy. J Neuroimmunol 36:57–68, 1992.

97. Wikstrand CJ, Bigner DD. Surface antigens of human glioma cells shared with normal adult and fetal brain. Cancer Res 39:3235–3243, 1979.

98. Wikstrand CJ, Bigner DD. Immunobiologic aspects of the brain and human gliomas. Am J Pathol 98:517–568, 1980.

99. Wikstrand CJ, Hale LP, Batra SK, Hill ML, Humphrey PA, Kurpad SN, McLendon RE, Moscatello D, Pegram CN, Reist CJ. Traweek ST, Wong AJ, Zalutsky MR, Bigner DD. Monoclonal antibodies against EGFRvIII are tumor specific and react with breast and lung carcinomas and malignant gliomas. Cancer Research 55:3140–3148, 1995.

100. Wikstrand CJ, He X, Fuller GN, Bigner SH, Fredman P, Svennerholm L, Bigner DD. Occurrence of lacto series gangliosides 3′-isoLM1 and 3′,6′-isoLD1 in human gliomas *in vitro* and *in vivo*. J Neuropathol Exp Neurol 50:756–769, 1991.

101. Wikstrand CJ, Longee DC, Fuller GN, McLendon RE, Friedman HS, Fredman P, Svennerholm L, Bigner DD. Lactotetraose series ganglioside 3′,6′-iso-LD1 in tumors of central nervous and other systems *in vitro* and *in vivo*. Cancer Research 53:120–126, 1993.

102. Wong AJ, Bigner SH, Bigner DD, Kinzler KW, Hamilton SR, Vogelstein B. Increased expression of the EGF receptor gene in malignant gliomas is invariably associated with gene amplification. Proc Natl Acad Sci USA 84:6899–6903, 1987.

103. Wong A, Bigner S, Bigner D, Vogelstein B. Internal deletions of the EGF receptor gene in primary human gliomas. J Cell Biochem 13B(Suppl):149, 1989 [abstr].

104. Wood GW, Morantz RA. Immunohistologic evaluation of the lymphoreticular infiltrate of human central nervous system tumors. J Natl Cancer Inst 62:485–491, 1979.

105. Wrann M, Bodmer S, de Martin R, Siepl C, Hofer-Warbinek R, Frei K, Hofer E, Fontana A. T cell suppressor factor from human glioblastoma cells is a 12.5 kD protein closely related to transforming growth factor-β. EMBO J 6:1633–1636, 1987.

106. Yamazaki H, Ohba Y, Tamaoki N, Shibuya M. A deletion mutation within the ligand binding domain is responsible for activation of epidermal growth factor receptor gene in human brain tumors. Jpn J Cancer Res 81:773–779, 1990.

107. Yokota T, Milenic DE, Whitlow M, Schlom J. Rapid tumor penetration of a single-chain Fv and comparison with other immunoglobulin forms. Cancer Res 52:3402–3408, 1992.

108. Young HF, Sakalas R, Kaplan AM. Inhibition of cell-mediated immunity in patients with brain tumors. Surg Neurol 5:19–23, 1976.

109. Yung WKA, Castellanos AM, van Tassel P. Intravenous recombinant β-interferon in recurrent malignant gliomas. Neurooncology 5:190, 1987 [abstr].

110. Zalutsky MR, Moseley RP, Benjamin JC, Colapinto EV, Fuller GN, Coakham HP, Bigner DD. Monoclonal antibody and F(ab′)$_2$ fragment delivery to tumor in patients with glioma: comparison of intracarotid and intravenous administration. Cancer Res 50:4105–4110, 1990.

111. Zalutsky MR, Moseley RP, Coakham HB, Coleman RE, Bigner DD. Pharmacokinetics and tumor localization of ^{131}I-labeled anti-tenascin monoclonal antibody 81C6 in patients with gliomas and other intracranial malignancies. Cancer Res 49:2807–2813, 1989.

112. Zalutsky MR, Noska MA, Colapinto EV, Garg PK, Bigner DD. Enhanced tumor localization and *in vivo* stability of a monoclonal antibody radioiodinated using *N*-succinimidyl-3-(tri-*n*-butlystannyl)benzoate. Cancer Res 49:5543–5549, 1989.

22

Immunology of the Peripheral Nervous System

RACHEL GEORGE
JUDITH SPIES
JOHN W. GRIFFIN

Isolated behind its blood-nerve barrier, the peripheral nervous system (PNS) was long considered immunologically privileged, in analogy with the central nervous system (CNS) and the testis. As with these regions, the concept of privilege has undergone radical revision within the past few years, and the differences from other organs now appear more quantitative than qualitative. Circulating lymphocytes can traffic in and out of the peripheral nervous system, and the peripheral nerves contain a collection of immunologically relevant resident cells, including a large population of resident macrophages, numerous mast cells, as well as the endoneurial capillary endothelial cells and their pericytes. When endothelial cells of the peripheral nerve are viewed in cross-section, the peripheral nerve is conveniently divided into the epineurium, perineurium, and endoneurium (Fig. 22-1). The epineurium consists of loose collagenous tissue and fat, and undoubtedly provides shock absorption as well as some tensile strength to the nerves. The larger blood vessels pass through the epineurium. The perineurium consists of several layers of specialized fibroblastic cells, with each layer bounded by a basal lamina, and with tight junctions between adjacent perineurial cells. Interleaved among the perineurial cells are numerous macrophages. The perineurium provides an effective barrier to diffusion of macromolecules from the epineurial space into the endoneurial space. The vascular supply to the endoneurium passes through the perineurium.

The endoneurial space is bounded by the perineurium and contains the nerve fibers and longitudinally oriented collagen, which insures the tensile strength of the individual fascicles. The endothelial cells of the endoneurial vessels form tight junctions with each other, thereby reproducing the blood-tissue barrier system seen in the central nervous system. The resulting blood-nerve barrier, however, is not as tight as the blood-

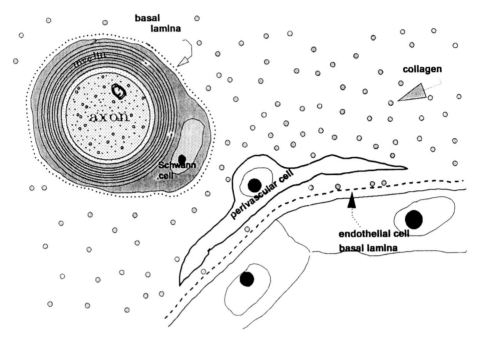

Fig. 22-1. Schematic diagram illustrating the locations of the perivascular macrophages in the PNS. (Reprinted with permission from Griffin et al., J Neuroimmunol 40:153–166, 1992 [39].)

brain barrier. This has been convincingly demonstrated by studies in which high concentrations of circulating horseradish peroxidase can be shown to enter the endoneurial space (6). Similar experiments show no entry past the endothelial tight junctions in the central nervous system (86). The change from blood-nerve to blood-brain barrier occurs within the spinal roots at the CNS–PNS transition zone. Within the surround of endoneurial vessels are the resident macrophages of the peripheral nerve and mast cells. Both lie outside the basal lamina of the endothelium.

Resident Macrophages of the Peripheral Nerve

The number of resident macrophages has only recently been recognised. In the past many of the resident macrophages have undoubtedly been considered endoneurial fibroblasts. The initial recognition of the number of these cells can be traced to a report by Arvidson (6), who demonstrated that if sufficient circulating horseradish peroxidase entered the PNS, it labeled a population of cells within the endoneurial space. This population, constituting 2% to 5% of total cells in the rat sciatic nerve, was correctly interpreted as resident macrophages. One-half to two-thirds of these resident macrophages lie near endoneurial vessels, but outside their basal lamina, and the remainder are distributed throughout the endoneurial space.

The recent availability of macrophage-specific immunoreagents has further delineated this population. Seven to ten percent of the normal endoneurial population is comprised of resident macrophages (39,95). These cells are elongated, longitudinally oriented, and frequently have highly ramified processes (Fig. 22-2). They contain autofluorescent perinuclear granules. A large proportion demonstrates constitutive expression of the major histocompatibility complex (MHC) class II, as well as complement receptor 3 (CR3), and low levels of CD4. They also express the Fc-γ receptor III, a feature they share with the Schwann cells of unmyelinated but not myelinated fibers (127). The available macrophage markers are most extensively developed in the rat (26,95). The resident macrophages are particularly easily demonstrated with the ED2 monoclonal antibody of Dijkstra in the rat (26,39), and they can be seen with F4/80, developed by Austyn and Gordon in the mouse (11). In humans, they are the only MHC class II–positive resident population and are most easily identified with that marker (44).

The bone marrow origin of the resident macrophage population has recently been demonstrated definitively using radiation-induced rat bone marrow chimeras (126). This population is replenished from the circulation in a fashion analogous to that described in the central nervous system (60,76).

The resident macrophages are undoubtedly the primary antigen-presenting cells of the peripheral nervous system. Their extraordinary capacity to sample macromolecules within the endoneurial space was demonstrated by their ability to take up horseradish peroxidase (6). Their location near blood vessels presumably facilitates interaction with trafficking T lymphocytes. Yu and Hickey (136) have demonstrated increased MHC class II expression in isolated nerve segments in cultures and markedly increased expression when the same nerve segments are used for allografts. No similar up-regulation occurs with isografts.

The responses of the resident macrophages to disease within the nerve are not yet fully understood, because in almost all situations circulating macrophages enter the nerve in large numbers and overshadow the resident macrophage population. The resident macrophages have been studied most effectively in short-term organ cultures of peripheral nerve segments from which circulating macrophages are necessarily excluded (25,37). A similar strategy has been used in in vivo cultures in which nerve segments are placed within millipore diffusion chambers and then inserted into the rat peritoneal cavity (13,14,52,107). These preparations demonstrate little or no increase in macrophage numbers, although there is indirect evidence supporting some local proliferation. Goodrum and Novicki (37) have shown that some resident cells become rounded and migrate out of the nerve, suggesting their conversion into motile phagocytic macrophages, but many resident macrophages retain their elongate, ramified morphology.

Mast Cells

There is an extensive mast cell population within the peripheral nervous system, but their normal roles remain largely unexplored. Abrupt, coherent mast cell degranulation

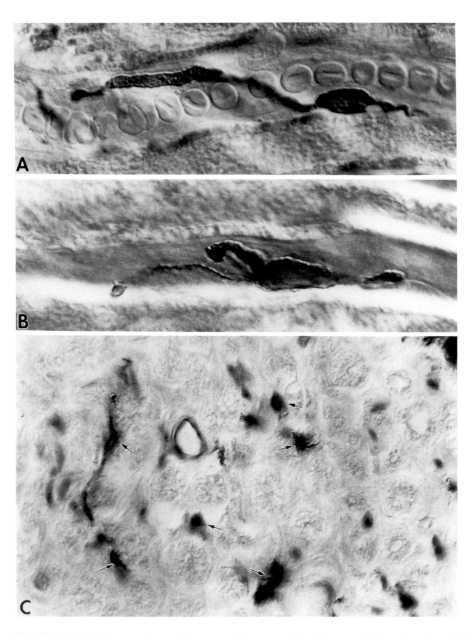

Fig. 22-2. Resident macrophages of the normal human peripheral nerves. A: Teased endoneurial vessel isolated from a normal human sural nerve and immunostained with L243 antibody for MHC class II. Wrapped around the vessel is an elongate resident macrophage. ×1,850. B: A ramified resident macrophage in the endoneurial space. ×2,200. C: Transverse section of a sural nerve from a normal individual who died suddenly. This fresh-frozen cryostat section contains numerous MHC class II–positive resident macrophages (arrows). Most of these profiles represent attenuated, longitudinally oriented processes cut in transverse section. ×11,100. (Reprinted with permission from Griffin JW, George R, Ho T, Macrophage systems in peripheral nerves. A review, Exp Neuropathol Exp Neurol 52:553–560, 1993.)

can produce massive endoneurial edema, apparently associated with breakdown of the blood-nerve barrier. An intriguing aspect of mast cell biology is their apparent contact in the gut with substance P-containing unmyelinated nerve fibers. Bienenstock and colleagues have demonstrated such contacts within the enteric nervous system of the PNS (15,16,115). Their functional significance is not understood.

Immune Responses in Diseases of the Peripheral Nervous System

Wallerian Degeneration

The responses of the immune cells of the PNS have been examined in some detail in Wallerian degeneration, in part because this model is *not* immune mediated. The responses of macrophages and other cells in this system help define the nonspecific behaviors of these cells in disease settings. Wallerian degeneration describes the abrupt breakdown of nerve fibers distal to a site of transection (for reviews see 38,40). In rodents this process is very rapid and the spatiotemporal sequence is well established. In young rats, between 24 and 48 hours after nerve transection, the axon undergoes a characteristic dissolution of the cytoskeleton termed *granular degeneration of the cytoskeleton.* Detailed studies of the spatiotemporal sequence of this change by Lubinska (82,83) have demonstrated that it moves from the site of transection distally along the nerve, with the smallest fibers undergoing axonal breakdown first. An exception to this pattern is seen at the terminals of both motor and sensory fibers; the terminals degenerate earlier than the preterminal axon (91; Hsieh et al., unpublished results). Concomitant with axonal breakdown, there is a characteristic segmentation of the myelin sheaths, culminating in the formation of discrete ovoids—sealed chambers lined by myelin and the surrounding abaxonal Schwann cell. Another very early change within degenerating nerve is breakdown of the blood-nerve barrier, which appears to occur almost synchronously with degeneration of the first affected fibers. The basis for this early change in the endothelial cells is not understood.

By the third day after nerve transection, a large population of circulating macrophages enter the degenerating nerve (39,95). Their numbers dwarf those of resident macrophages and continue to increase for at least 2 weeks. They adhere to degenerating nerve fibers, pass through the basal lamina of the Schwann cell, and enter the fiber, where they participate in phagocytosis and removal of myelin debris (116). In so doing, they generate large amounts of cholesterol esters, and concomitantly produce very large quantities of apolipoprotein E. This arrangement facilitates uptake of cholesterol via the LDL receptor by Schwann cells, as well as endothelial cells, endoneurial fibroblasts, and perineurial cells. The consequence of this process is the removal of most myelin debris within 3 to 4 weeks after nerve transection in laboratory rodents such as the rat.

These infiltrating macrophages play an important role in the production of nerve growth factor (NGF), a factor required for normal maintenance of a population of sensory and autonomic neurons, and normally supplied from the innervated target. Following nerve transection, the Schwann cells of the distal stump (and apparently endoneurial fibroblasts) up-regulate production of NGF. The Schwann cells also produce low-affinity NGF receptor (P75), and the NGF displayed to regenerating axonal sprouts on the surface of denervated Schwann cells provides an attractive pathway for axonal growth. Lindholm and colleagues initially demonstrated the requirement for macrophage-derived interleukin-1 (IL-1) for production of NGF within the transected nerve (59,78,79). Using short-term organ cultures of nerve, they demonstrated that sustained production of NGF only occurred if macrophages were added to the system. This macrophage effect could be replicated by the addition of exogenous IL-1. A similar sequence applies to other neurotrophins, but brain-derived neurotrophic factor (BDNF), at least, represents an exception. (Ciliary neurotrophic factor [CTNF] is normally expressed abundantly within myelin-maintaining Schwann cells, and its levels fall rapidly during Wallerian degeneration.)

Comparison of Wallerian Degeneration in the PNS and the CNS

The differences in the macrophage responses to degeneration in the CNS and PNS are dramatic. It has long been recognized that rounded phagocytic macrophages appear relatively late during degeneration of myelin-bearing CNS tracts. The phenomenon has been studied in an advantageous preparation in which one or more of the lumbar dorsal roots are transected rostral to the dorsal root ganglion, resulting in Wallerian degeneration of the central processes of the primary sensory neurons as they pass through the dorsal root and continue ascending in the dorsal column (33,35,36). Within the dorsal root, the process follows timing similar to that described in peripheral nerves; macrophages enter in abundance within 3 days, and clear myelin debris within 3 weeks (35). Studies of the timing of axonal breakdown have shown that the process is virtually completed within the affected fibers of the dorsal column within 72 hours (in the rat) (36). However, all subsequent aspects of Wallerian degeneration are markedly delayed (35). There is no breakdown of the blood-brain barrier comparable to that seen with the blood-nerve barrier. Circulating macrophages either do not enter or enter in extremely small numbers (35). Those rounded phagocytic macrophages that do participate appear to be derived from conversion of the stellate microglia of the dorsal columns, and this process is relatively slow. For example, only modest numbers of rounded phagocytic macrophages are present at 21 days, and they persist for at least 180 days. The timing is even slower in humans; the macrophages have failed to clear myelin completely from degenerating corticospinal tracts at 2 years following hemispheral cerebrovascular accident (88–90). The basis for this dramatic difference in macrophage entry is not known, but it seems likely that it may reflect differences in expression of endothelial adhesion molecules required for entry of circulating macrophages. In any event, the change occurs precisely at the CNS–PNS transition zone at the level of the dorsal root entry zone.

A recently recognized and intriguing interaction between the peripheral nervous system and cells of the immune system can be found in denervation of the epidermis. Hsieh et al. have recently shown that, in the rat, transection of the sciatic nerve leads to phenotypic changes in the Langerhans cells of the epidermis (67a). The Langerhans cells are bone marrow–derived cells that function as the predominant antigen-presenting cell of the epidermis. The most thoroughly documented phenotypic change is up-regulation of the message as well as gene expression of the neuronal form of ubiquitin carboxy-terminal hydrolase. Present at low levels in normal Langerhans cells, there is a marked up-regulation in denervated rat Langerhans cells. The effect is the consequence of the elimination of the fine epidermal sensory axons (C fibers). A portion of these C fibers approach and appear to contact Langerhans cells (65). These fibers are calcitonin gene-related peptide (CGRP) positive by immunocytochemistry, and Hosoi and co-workers have recently demonstrated that CGRP can alter antigen presentation by Langerhans cells in culture (65). Whether denervation in vivo alters antigen presentation has not been explored.

Experimental Allergic Neuritis

Experimental allergic neuritis (EAN), the most thoroughly studied autoimmune disease of the peripheral nervous system, is a demyelinating disorder that follows sensitization of the animal to whole peripheral nerve myelin or to specific components of peripheral nerve myelin, such as the P_2 protein of myelin or the P_0 glycoprotein (3). In EAN directed against specific myelin proteins, passive transfer using T-cell clones is sufficient to reproduce all features of the disease, providing solid evidence for the long-suspected role of T cells in the pathogenesis of EAN. However, there is increasing interest in the role of antibodies in this disorder, particularly when EAN is generated against whole myelin. Using high-resolution immunocytochemistry of ultra-thin cryosections, Stoll and colleagues demonstrated that one of the earliest changes in whole myelin-induced EAN in the Lewis rat is binding of terminal complement complexes (C5B-9) to the outer surface of the Schwann cell. This change occurs before entry of large numbers of lymphocytes and before any myelin changes are produced. As noted below, very similar findings appear to apply to the acute inflammatory demyelinating form of Guillain-Barré syndrome (GBS) in humans. Similar studies have not yet been done in EAN induced by intrinsic myelin proteins or in T-cell transfer models, but Jung et al. demonstrated that the administration of the soluble complement receptor CR1 ameliorates EAN, consistent with a role of complement (71).

EAN can be induced in a number of animal species by inoculation with peripheral nerve homogenates (130,131), whole peripheral nerve myelin, the myelin proteins P_2 or P_0, or component peptides of these proteins (1,19,20,72,93,111,125). Although EAN is usually considered a monophasic illness, spontaneous exacerbations do occur in several species (17,58,134) and a chronic progressive or relapsing form of the disease which histologically resembles chronic inflammatory demyelinating polyradiculoneuropathy can be induced in some species by repeated inoculation (99,110,129).

The importance of cellular immune mechanisms in the pathogenesis of EAN has long been recognized. Early histopathological studies (75) established that lesions began with a perivascular infiltration of mononuclear cells and the degree of cellular infiltration was subsequently shown to correlate well with the degree of nerve function deficits (119). Moreover, lymph node cells (133) and peripheral blood buffy coat cells (5) from animals with EAN cause demyelination, with preservation of axons, in myelinated peripheral nervous system cultures. However, the most convincing evidence for cell mediated pathogenetic mechanism has come from passive transfer studies. Åstrom and Waksman (10) reported histological lesions corresponding to those seen in very mild, actively induced EAN after intravenous transfer of lymph node cells from rabbits with EAN, and Hughes and colleagues (67b) were subsequently able to passively transfer EAN to naive inbred Lewis rats with lymph node cells from rats immunized with either P_2 or whole myelin.

The central role of T cells in disease pathogenesis was established when Linington et al. (80) were able to transfer disease with a permanent T-cell line (of helper/inducer phenotype) specific for P_2 protein. It has subsequently been shown that T-cell lines specific for P_2 peptides or P_0 and its component neuritogenic peptides are also able to transfer disease (81,96,104). Inactivation and depletion studies have provided further evidence of the significance of T cells. Treatment with monoclonal antibodies reactive to pan T-cell markers prevents the development of EAN after immunization with myelin (64). Similarly, Brosnan et al. (18) have demonstrated that T cell–deficient animals have a reduced susceptibility to EAN and susceptibility can be restored with thoracic duct lymphocytes from normal animals. More specific monoclonal therapy against the CD4+ T-cell subset has also been shown to be effective in disease treatment and prevention (120), as have monoclonal antibodies directed against the α/β T-cell receptor (70) or the IL-2 receptor (53). Helper/inducer T cells recognize antigen in the context of class II MHC antigens, and the presence of CD4+ cells in close proximity to Ia positive macrophages in the endoneurium in EAN (66,97) satisfies the requirements for local T-cell activation. Evidence that this interaction is central to the pathogenesis of EAN is provided by the demonstration that monoclonal antibodies to Ia antigens reduce the severity of EAN in the rat if given before the onset of clinical disease (120). However, the precise mechanism of T-cell action in EAN remains unclear. CD4+ P_2-specific T-cell lines capable of transferring EAN are cytotoxic for cultured Schwann cells (2), but there is little in vivo evidence to support direct T-cell mediated damage to Schwann cells or peripheral nerve myelin. Focal demyelination has been demonstrated after intraneural injection of lymph node cells from animals with EAN (4,63); however, intraneural injection of neuritogenic P_2-specific T-cell lines does not result in electrophysiological or histological evidence of demyelination (114).

The pathogenetic importance of macrophages is also well established. Macrophages are the most prominent cells in the established EAN lesion (57,98), and electron microscopy studies have shown that macrophages strip off myelin lamellae and phagocytose both damaged and apparently intact myelin (12,23,75). Macrophage depletion by intraperitoneal injection of silica dust protects against the development of EAN and slows progression of disease (23,123). Macrophages collected from animals with EAN generate and release increased amounts of arachidonic acid metabolites and toxic oxygen species, and more selective blockade of macrophage function with cyclooxygenase inhibitors (54) and oxygen radical scavengers (55) protects animals from the development of EAN or attenuates the severity of established disease, suggesting that macrophage-derived reactive oxygen intermediates may contribute to myelin damage. Macrophages are also the major source of complement components in inflammatory foci and complement is clearly implicated in EAN pathogenesis. Complement depletion delays development of EAN and reduces the degree of demyelination (30). Stoll and colleagues have demonstrated by immunocytochemistry, transient deposition of terminal complement complex on Schwann cells and myelin sheaths prior to demyelination in EAN, suggesting that complement activation plays a pathogenetic role in the initiation of myelin damage (118).

The presence of activated T cells and macrophages within the inflammatory infiltrates of EAN is associated with the local release of a number of proinflammatory cytokines, including tumour necrosis factor (TNF)-α and interferon-γ (IFN-γ). Both of these cytokines have been demonstrated in acute EAN lesions (108,117), and their pathogenetic significance has been demonstrated by the ability of monoclonal antibody therapy directed against either to reduce the severity of EAN (56,117).

The pathogenetic significance of antibody in EAN has been less clearly established. A role for humoral factors in pathogenesis was suggested by the demonstration that serum from animals with EAN caused demyelination of myelinated peripheral nerve (133,135). Saida et al. (106) subsequently demonstrated demyelination after intraneural injection of rabbit EAN serum into rats and rabbits. Demyelination was complement dependent and was seen only with sera collected after the onset of clinical disease, and the ability of sera to cause in vivo demyelination correlated with in vitro demyelinative capacity. Primary segmental demyelination was associated with macrophages, but no significant lymphocytic infiltrate and myelin vesiculation and splitting occurred before the appearance of macrophages (48,105) as has also been noted in EAN, which suggests that macrophages may be attracted to antibody-sensitized myelin. Serum from rats inoculated with whole nerve or P_2 and rabbit antisera to P_0 have also been shown to cause demyelination when injected intraneurally. Complement-fixing antibodies were described in rabbits by Waksman and Adams (130) after inoculation with sciatic nerve and subsequently, antibodies to peripheral nerve myelin or P_2 have been described in animals immunized P_2 or myelin (21,67b). However, the lack of correlation between antibody titers and clinical course (67b,92,103) combined with the failure of systemic transfer of serum to cause any clinical or histological evidence of EAN (67b,122; K. V.

Toyka, unpublished observations referenced in 124) has resulted in continued uncertainty regarding the role of antibody in pathogenesis. The only evidence of a correlation between circulating anti-myelin antibody levels and the degree of demyelination is found in a study of the peripheral nervous system lesions in EAE in the Lewis rat. Minimal anti-myelin immunoreactivity was found in rats with acute EAE characterized by prominent inflammatory cell infiltrates but little demyelination, whereas animals with chronic EAE with prominent demyelination had high titers of anti-myelin antibodies, suggesting that the anti-myelin antibodies may be causally related to the extent of demyelination (77). More recently it has been demonstrated that systemically administered anti-myelin antibody significantly increases both disease severity and the extent of demyelination in adoptive transfer EAN (47,113) but has no effect on EAN induced by immunization with whole myelin (113), suggesting that humoral mechanisms are already active in the latter model but not in T-cell transfer disease.

Evidence therefore suggests a role for both cell-mediated and humoral factors in EAN. One possible site where these mechanisms may converge is the blood-nerve barrier. Systemic transfer of EAN serum does not cause disease, presumably because of an intact blood-nerve barrier. However, increased blood-nerve barrier permeability is an early feature of EAN (45,100). Activated T cells increase blood-nerve barrier permeability, allowing circulating anti-myelin antibody to enter the endoneurium with consequent focal demyelination at the site where barrier function is deficient (114). This may be one mechanism by which T cells mediate primary demyelination in EAN. A similar effect is also seen with tumour necrosis factor (114), which is of interest, given the demonstrated relationship between TNF levels and blood-brain barrier damage in multiple sclerosis (109).

The Guillain-Barré Syndrome

With the success of the worldwide vaccination program for poliomyelitis, the Guillain-Barré syndrome (GBS) has become the most common cause of acute paralysis on a neuromuscular basis throughout most of the world. It often follows an infection, and several lines of evidence indicate that the disorder is immunologically mediated. GBS can reduce a previously healthy person to severe paralysis requiring respiratory support within a period of a few days.

After steady incremental progress for many decades, studies of the pathogenesis of GBS have produced rapid advances in the past 3 years. The current excitement surrounding this disorder derives from four aspects. First, the immunopathogenesis increasingly appears to be based on shared epitopes between the infectious organism and peripheral nerve, a mechanism often referred to as *molecular mimicry*. Second, it is increasingly clear that there are multiple forms of GBS, and it appears that the target antigen or epitope differs among the different forms. For this reason, throughout the remainder of this discussion GBS should be interpreted as the Guillain-Barré syndromes. Third, there is increasing evidence that glycoconjugates can be important target antigens in the Guillain-Barré syndromes. Finally, in many forms the immune attack appears to be antibody and complement mediated.

Heterogeneity of the Guillain-Barré Syndrome

Normal function of a myelinated peripheral nerve fiber depends on the integrity of both its axon and the myelin sheath. Interruption of conduction can occur as a result of demyelination at a single internode or even paranode. The axon can be lost because of interruption in its continuity somewhere along its course (for example, as a result of mechanical injury), with consequent Wallerian degeneration, or by death of the nerve cell body, with consequent degeneration of the whole neuron. In general, recovery varies with the nature of the injury: because remyelination, a relatively rapid process, is sufficient to restore the security of conduction in demyelination, recovery from this process can be quite rapid. Following Wallerian-like degeneration, recovery depends on regeneration of nerve fibers, a notoriously slow process, and recovery after the death of the whole neuron will not occur unless other neurons are able to take over the function of their missing neighbor.

Classical histologic studies identified demyelination as the characteristic lesion in many autopsied cases of Guillain-Barré syndrome (7). In addition, many cases had extensive lymphocytic infiltration of the affected regions of the peripheral nerves (7), and the clinical diagnosis, Guillain-Barré syndrome, became virtually synonymous with the pathologic diagnosis of acute inflammatory demyelinating polyneuropathy (AIDP) (8,9). A widespread presumption was that Guillain-Barré syndrome represented an immune attack on an antigen of the myelin sheath.

In 1986 Feasby and colleagues (29,31) suggested that in some cases of GBS there was primary axonal degeneration without preceding demyelination, and that the target antigen might lie on the axon. This suggestion was highly controversial. Earlier studies of EAN had shown that the extent of secondary axonal degeneration correlated with the dose of myelin antigen used in immunization and documented that axonal degeneration was a feature of severe inflammatory demyelinating disorders (46). An attractive interpretation of the acute severe cases with extensive evidence of axonal degeneration that were described by Feasby was that they represented very severe cases of typical inflammatory demyelinating neuropathy. However, recent autopsy studies on cases dying between 6 days and 7 months after onset have provided strong pathologic support for a primary attack on the axon with little associated demyelination (28,31,41). The term *acute motor sensory axonal neuropathy* (AMSAN) has recently been suggested for this form of GBS (42).

More recently, a closely related variant, *acute motor axonal neuropathy* (AMAN), has been identified (41–43,87). AMAN is distinguished by normal sensory nerve fibers, as judged clinically, electrodiagnostically, and pathologically. AMAN was first recognized in China, where in some hospitals in northern China it appears in the form of epidemics occurring each summer. This feature has made it possible to study large numbers of cases, and an international collaborative study comprised of investigators from the Second Teaching Hospital of Shijiazhuang, China, the University of Pennsylvania, and the Johns Hopkins University has been underway for the past 5 years (42,85,87). It is now clear that the same pattern of disease has been identified in other parts of Asia (22), North America (69), Europe (132), and Latin America (101) as well.

A final disorder merits inclusion in this discussion, the Fisher syndrome, characterized by acute onset of unsteadiness of gait (ataxia), loss of reflexes (areflexia), and inability to move the eyes, usually associated with nonreactive pupils (internal and external ophthalmoplegia (32). Because the patient's strength was characteristically preserved, these cases did not fit the clinical criteria established by Guillain and Barré, and their relationship to GBS was controversial. However, because of recently recognized similarities in immunopathogenesis, it is appropriate to include the Fisher syndrome within the group of Guillain-Barré syndromes.

Figure 22-3 presents an operational classification of the Guillain-Barré syndromes. This classification is intended to provide a basis for discussion, and undoubtedly, other disorders will require inclusion in the future. In addition, an unanswered question is the extent to which transitional disorders, for example, with both demyelinating and axonal features, may occur in the same patient.

Shared Epitopes with Infectious Agents

The Guillain-Barré syndrome has long been recognized to follow an infectious illness in many patients. Two specific infections identified early were infection with herpes

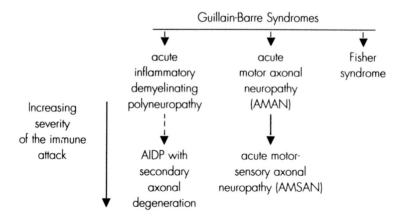

Fig. 22-3. Proposed interrelationships of the forms of GBS. (Reprinted with permission from Griffin et al., Pathology of the motor-sensory axonal Guillain-Barré syndrome, Ann Neurol 39:17–28, 1996 [41].)

virus and with *Mycoplasma pneumoniae,* a bacterial infection of the lung. An important advance was the identification that enteric infection with the gram-negative curved rod, *Campylobacter,* could precede Guillain-Barré. This observation has been replicated in many parts of the world, but the true frequency of post-*Campylobacter* GBS remains uncertain. *Campylobacter* enteritis is usually self-limited, and the organism may be cleared from the gastrointestinal tract by the time the patient develops neurologic sequelae. The serologic tests for *Campylobacter* are difficult both to perform and to interpret, so that the proportion of post-*Campylobacter* remains uncertain, but it appears to range from 15% to 75% in various parts of the world (24,27,61,73,87,94, 112,128,132).

Yuki and co-workers identified cases of post-*Campylobacter* GBS who had immunoreactivity against the sugar epitope *gal(β1-3galNAC),* an epitope present in the ganglioside GM1 (145). This epitope is present in at least some species of *Campylobacter,* including *Campylobacter jejuni,* the most frequently encountered cause of human enteritis (137,140). The *Campylobacter jejuni* strains can be divided into a number of strains on the basis of the carbohydrate antigens in the lipopolysaccharides. Yuki recognized that the lipopolysaccharides of neuritogenic *Campylobacter* strains contained epitopes reactive with anti-GM1 antibodies, and suggested that molecular mimicry might play a role in these acute axonal cases (34,138,141). Supporting evidence for this concept came from the recognition that cases of the distinctive Fisher syndrome had antibodies against the unusual ganglioside GQ1b, and that GQ1b-reactive epitopes were expressed in the lipopolysaccharide of the *Campylobacter* isolated from patients with the Fisher syndrome (139).

These examples provide strong support for the hypothesis that molecular mimicry underlies the immunopathogenesis of postinfectious GBS, and they have directed attention to the neurobiology of specific epitopes in peripheral nerve fibers. In addition, this hypothesis has prompted a search for reactivity against glycoconjugates in other GBS cases. Among the other epitopes toward which antibody has been convincingly demonstrated in GBS are the gangliosides LM1 (68) and GD1a (143), as well as the unusual ganglioside N-acetylamino-GD1a (74a). A recent study has examined 80 GBS sera for reactivity against galactocerebroside (galC) and identified anti-galC antibodies in 4 cases (74b). All 4 followed previous *Mycoplasma pneumoniae* infection (74b), suggesting that a galC-like epitope may be expressed in the organism.

Immunopathogenesis of GBS

AIDP

AIDP was long presumed to be a T cell–mediated disorder. This presumption was based on the lymphocytic inflammation found in many cases (7) and on the analogy to EAN. In AIDP it has recently been possible to reevaluate the pathology of early and unusually well-preserved cases (41–43,84). The number of previous early autopsies appropriate for detailed electron microscopic analysis has been very limited. Three well-preserved cases dying within the first 9 days have been studied in collaboration with the group at Second Teaching Hospital, Shijiazhuang, China (42,84). In a case that died 3 days after onset, the pathologic changes in the spinal roots were very mild, with only occasional fibers undergoing the late stages of demyelination. Staining with markers of complement activation demonstrated complement-activation products on the outermost surface of the Schwann cell. Electron microscopy of these fibers showed that most had early vesicular changes in the myelin sheaths. The vesiculation of myelin tended to begin in the outermost lamellae. The resulting pathologic picture closely resembled the appearance of nerve fibers exposed to anti-galactocerebroside antibody in the presence of complement. They also resembled the effect of lysolecithin on nerve fibers. The lysolecithin effect has been in turn reproduced by application to nerve fibers of the calcium ionofors A23187 and ionomycin. Thus, an attractive reconstruction is that an antibody directed against epitopes on the outermost surface of the Schwann cell (the abaxonal Schwann cell plasmalemma) binds complement, resulting in sublytic complement activation and formation of complement pores. The resulting entry of calcium is sufficient to activate calcium-sensitive enzymes, potentially including phospholipase A2 and proteases capable of degrading myelin proteins.

As the myelin damage proceeds, the Schwann cell perikaryon may amputate the damaged sheath, and itself proliferate, giving rise to daughter Schwann cells. The removal of damaged myelin (as demonstrated in the lysolecithin model) (49–51) is carried out in part by hematogenous macrophages that phagocytose myelin debris. Clearance of myelin from an internode sets the stage for remyelination by multiple daughter Schwann cells.

The nature of the epitope on the abaxonal Schwann cell plasmalemma that may be involved in this form of the AIDP is uncertain, but recent studies of Kusonoki and colleagues suggest the attractive possibility that galactocerebroside can be such an epitope.

Axonal Forms of GBS

The immunopathogenesis of the AMAN cases was evaluated in 7 autopsies. The pattern in the most severe cases consisted of Wallerian-like degeneration of nerve fibers beginning just beyond the ventral root exit zone (42,43,87). As shown in Fig. 22-3, the motor neurons survived but underwent the axon reaction similar to changes seen following mechanical interruption of motor axons. In these cases, the dorsal root fibers remained normal.

Early Changes in Mild Cases

By pathologic criteria, the earliest identifiable changes are in the nodes of Ranvier of motor fibers (43). The nodal gap lengthens at times when the fibers appear otherwise normal. Immunopathologically, this change correlates with the binding of IgG and the activation of complement, as reflected in the presence of the complement activation marker C3d, on those nodes of Ranvier. At early times as well, macrophages are recruited to overlie the node of Ranvier (43), perhaps as a result of the elaboration of C5a and other complement-derived chemoattractants. These macrophages insert processes into the nodal gap, penetrating the overlying basal lamina of the Schwann cell (43). The macrophages then encircle the node and frequently dissect beneath the myelin sheath attachment sites of the paranode to enter the periaxonal space of the internode (Fig. 22-4).

Many fibers express complement activation markers in the periaxonal space—that is, the 11-nm space between the axolemma and the Schwann cell plasmalemma that surrounds the axon (the adaxonal Schwann cell plasmalemma). The periaxonal space is normally extremely regular in its spacing, and it is sealed from both ions and macromolecules of the endoneurial fluid by junctional complexes between the myelin terminal loops and the axolemma. The intrusion of the macrophage probably opens the

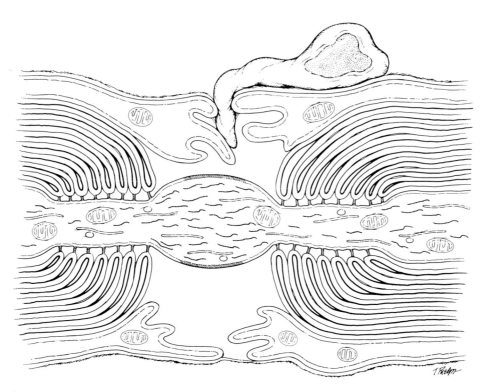

Fig. 22-4. Schematic illustration of the early changes in axonal forms of GBS. Node of Ranvier is lengthened and coated with complement activation products (the terminal complement complex C5b-9 and C3d). Macrophages are recruited specifically to the node and initially extend processes through the overlying Schwann cell basal lamina to contact nodal axolemma.

periaxonal space to endoneurial constituents, allowing antibody and complement to enter the internodal region. Immunocytochemical studies have demonstrated that the epitope to which IgG binds is on the axolemma (as it is in the node of Ranvier). As macrophages also invade the periaxonal space, the axon collapses away from the Schwann cell, resulting in a marked dilatation of the periaxonal space. However, the axon appears to survive for some period of time, even though it is surrounded by macrophages. The end stage of this process is interruption of motor axons with degeneration extending as far up as the ventral root exit zone.

Patients with such extensive Wallerian-like degeneration of ventral root fibers could recover only by regeneration, and very long periods of time would be required. However, many patients with AMAN recover quite rapidly (62a). This suggests that the early stages of antibody binding to nodes may be capable of blocking conduction. Roberts and colleagues have shown that anti-GQ1b antibody-positive sera from patients with GBS are capable of blocking conduction and of eliminating end-plate potentials in mouse phrenic nerve diaphragm preparation without impairing the production of miniature end-plate potentials (102). Takigawa and colleagues (121) have used antibodies made by immunization with GM1 in patch-clamp studies of single nerve fibers. Sera from rabbits immunized with GM1 have altered nodal ion channel function. In the presence of complement, anti-GM1 antibodies suppress the sodium current and cause nonspecific current leakage. The increased sodium conductance results from the channel being held in the open state. In the absence of complement, the anti-GM1 antibodies increase the rate of rise in amplitude of the potassium current, probably by uncovering paranodal potassium channels.

A further stage of change capable of inducing failure of impulse conduction would appear to be opening of the entire periaxonal space, effectively removing the insulating effect of the myelin sheath as just described. Finally, one patient has been studied in whom the motor fiber degeneration appeared largely limited to the distalmost regions of motor fibers, including the motor nerve terminals. Recovery by regeneration over relatively short distances could be accomplished quickly and may be a factor in rapid recovery in AMAN as well. Selective degeneration of distal nerve fiber regions may reflect the lack of a blood-nerve barrier at the motor nerve terminals, and consequent accessibility to circulating antibody (62b).

The Fisher Syndrome

Recent studies have shown that the anti-GQ1b antibodies characteristic of the Fisher syndrome have the ability to alter synaptic release at motor nerve terminals (102). This result at first seems anomalous, because weakness is not a feature of Miller Fisher syndrome. However, this suggests that there is a small amount of epitope present even in motor nerve terminals of somatic musculature, and that the anti-ganglioside antibody has the capacity to block normal quantal release. The motor fibers, which are known to be heavily enriched in GQ1b-reactive epitopes, are the oculomotor fibers—those fibers whose function is affected in the Fisher syndrome. Whether the ataxia is on the basis of sensory abnormalities with loss of proprioception (sensory ataxia) or cerebellar disease (cerebellar ataxia) remains an area of controversy, but anti-GQ1b antibodies are known to stain both sensory neurons in the dorsal root ganglia and a population of cerebellar neurons (139).

In summary, in at least three of the Guillain-Barré syndromes the pathogenesis appears to involve development of antibody to glycoconjugates of the organism that see epitopes on peripheral nerve fibers. The specific fibers affected and the nature of the pathophysiology reflect the epitope attacked. Of special importance is the recognition that the antibodies have the potential to affect physiologic function at times when structural changes are modest.

References

1. Abramsky O, Teitelbaum D, Arnon R. Experiemntal allergic neuritis induced by a basic neuritogenic protein (P_1L) of human peripheral nerve origin. Eur J Immunol 7:213–217, 1977.
2. Argall KG, Armati PJ, Pollard JD, Bonner J. Interactions between CD4+ T cells and rat Schwann cells in vitro. 2. Cytotoxic effects of P2-specific CD4+ T cell lines on Lewis rat Schwann cells. J Neuroimmunol 40:19–30, 1992.
3. Arnason BGW. Idiopathic polyneuritis (Landry-Guillain-Barré-Strohl syndrome) and experimental allergic neuritis: a comparison. Res Publ Assoc Res Nerv Ment Dis 49:156–175, 1971.
4. Arnason BGW, Chelmicka-Szorc E. Passive transfer of experimental allergic neuritis in Lewis rats by direct injection of sensitised lymphocytes into the sciatic nerve. Acta Neuropathol 22:1–6, 1972.
5. Arnason BGW, Winkler GF, Hadler NM. Cell-mediated demyelination of peripheral nerve in tissue culture. Lab Invest 21:1–10, 1969.
6. Arvidson B. Cellular uptake of exogenous horseradish peroxidase in mouse peripheral nerve. Acta Neuropathol 37:35–41, 1977.
7. Asbury AK, Arnason BG, Adams RD. The inflammatory lesion in idiopathic polyneuritis. Medicine 48:173–215, 1969.
8. Asbury AK, Arnason BG, Karp HR, McFarlin DE. Criteria for diagnosis of Guillain-Barré syndrome. Ann Neurol 3:565–566, 1978.
9. Asbury AK, Cornblath DR. Assessment of diagnostic criteria for Guillain-Barré syndrome. Peripheral Neuropathy Association—Program and Abstracts, Oxford, England 1990, p 26 (abstract).
10. Astrom K, Waksman BH. The passive transfer of experimental allergic encephalomyelitis and neuritis with living lymphoid cells. J Pathol Bacteriol 83:89–106, 1962.
11. Austyn JM, Gordon S. F4/80, a monoclonal antibody directed specifically against the mouse macrophage. Eur J Immunol 11:805–815, 1981.
12. Ballin RHM, Thomas PK. Electron microscopic observations on demyelination and remyelination in experimental allergic neuritis. Part 1. Demyelination. J Neurol Sci 8:1–18, 1968.
13. Beuche W, Friede RL. The role of non-resident cells in Wallerian degeneration. J Neurocytol 13:767–796, 1984.

14. Beuche W, Friede RL. Myelin phagocytosis in Wallerian degeneration depends on silica-sensitive, bg/bg-negative and Fc-positive monocytes. Brain Res 378:97–106, 1986.

15. Bienenstock J, Blennerhassett M, Tomioka M, Marshall J, Perdue MH, Stread RH. Evidence of mast cell-nerve interactions. In: Neuroimmune Networks: Physiology and Diseases, EJ Goetzl, NH Spector, eds. Alan R. Liss, New York, 1989, pp 149–154.

16. Bienenstock J, MacQueen G, Sestini P, Marshall JS, Stead RH, Perdue MH. Mast cell/nerve interactions in vitro and in vivo. Am Rev Respir Dis 143:S55–S58, 1991.

17. Brosnan CF, Lyman WD, Neighbour PA. Chronic experimental allergic neuritis in the Lewis rat. J. Neuropathol Exp Neurol 43:302 (abstract) 1984.

18. Brosnan JV, Craggs RI, King RHM, Thomas PK. Reduced susceptibility of T cell-deficient rats to induction of experimental allergic neuritis. J Neuroimmunol 14:267–282, 1987.

19. Brostoff SW, Levitt S, Powers JM. Induction of experimental allergic neuritis with a peptide from myelin P_2 basic protein. Nature 268:752–753, 1977.

20. Carlo DJ, Karkhanis YD, Bailey PJ, Wisniewski HM. Experimental allergic neuritis: evidence for the involvement of the P_0 and P_2 proteins. Brain Res 88:580–584, 1975.

21. Caspary EA, Field EJ. Antibody response to central and peripheral nerve antigens in rat and guinea-pig. J Neurol Neurosurg Psychiatry 28:179–182, 1965.

22. Coe CJ. Guillain-Barré syndrome in Korean children. Yonsei Med J 30:81–87, 1989.

23. Craggs RI, King RHM, Thomas PK. The effect of suppression of macrophage activity on the development of experimental allergic neuritis. Acta Neuropathol 62:316–323, 1984.

24. Crandall JE, Caviness VS Jr. Axon strata of the cerebral wall in embryonic mice. Dev Brain Res 14:185–195, 1984.

25. Crang AJ, Blakemore WF. Observations on Wallerian degeneration in explant cultures of cat sciatic nerve. J Neurocytol 15:471–482, 1986.

26. Dijkstra CD, Dopp EA, Joling P, et al. The heterogeneity of mononuclear phagocytes in lymphoid organs: distinct macrophage subpopulations in the rat recognized by the monoclonal antibodies ED1, ED2, and ED3. Immunology 54:589–599, 1985.

27. Enders U, Karch H, Toyka KV, Michaels M, Zielasek J, Pette M, Heesemann J, Hartung H-P. The spectrum of immune responses to *Campylobacter jejuni* and glycoconjugates in Guillain-Barré syndrome and in other neuroimmunological disorders. Ann Neurol 34:136–144, 1993.

28. Feasby TE, Gilbert JJ, Brown WF, Bolton CF, Hahn AF, Koopman WF, Zochodne DW. An acute axonal form of Guillain-Barré polyneuropathy. Brain 109:1115–1126, 1986.

29. Feasby TE, Gilbert JJ, Brown WF, et al. An acute axonal form of Guillain-Barré polyneuropathy. Brain 109:1115–1126, 1986.

30. Feasby TE, Gilbert JJ, Hahn AF, Neilson M. Complement depletion suppresses Lewis rat experimental allergic neuritis. Brain Res 419:97–103, 1987.

31. Feasby TE, Hahn AF, Brown WF, Bolton CF, Gilbert JJ, Koopman WJ. Severe axonal degeneration in acute Guillain-Barré syndrome: evidence of two different mechanisms? J Neurol Sci 116:185–192, 1993.

32. Fisher M. An unusual variant of acute idiopathic polyneuritis (syndrome of ophthalmoplegia ataxia and areflexia). N Engl J Med 255:57–65, 1956.

33. Franson P, Ronnevi L-O. Myelin breakdown and elimination in the posterior funiculus of the adult cat after dorsal rhizotomy: a light and electron microscopic qualitative and quantitative study. J Comp Neurol 223:138–151, 1984.

34. Fujimoto S, Yuki N, Itoh T, Amako K. Specific serotype of *Campylobacter jejuni* associated with Guillain-Barré syndrome. J Infect Dis 165:183, 1992 [letter].

35. George R, Griffin JW. Delayed macrophage responses and myelin clearance

during Wallerian degeneration in the central nervous system: the dorsal radiculotomy model. Exp Neurol 129:225–236, 1994.

36. George R, Griffin JW. The proximo-distal spread of axonal regeneration in the dorsal columns of the rat. J Neurocytol 23:657–667, 1994.

37. Goodrum JF, Novicki DL. Macrophage-like cells from explant cultures of rat sciatic nerve produce apolipoprotein E. J Neurosci Res 20:457–462, 1988.

38. Griffin JW, George EB, Hsieh S-T, Glass JD. Axonal degeneration and other disorders of the axonal cytoskeleton. In: The Axon, Structure, Function, & Pathophysiology, S Waxman, J Kocsis, P Stys, eds. Oxford University Press, New York, 1995, pp 375–390.

39. Griffin JW, George R, Lobato C, Tyor WR, Li CY, Glass JD. Macrophage responses and myelin clearance during Wallerian degeneration: relevance to immune-mediated demyelination. J Neuroimmunology 40:153–166, 1992.

40. Griffin JW, Hoffman PN. Degeneration and regeneration in the peripheral nervous system. In: Peripheral Neuropathy, 3rd ed, PJ Dyck, PK Thomas, JW Griffin, PA Low, J Poduslo, eds. WB Saunders, Philadelphia, 1992, pp 361–376.

41. Griffin JW, Li CY, Ho TW, Tian M, Gao CY, Xue P, Mishu B, Cornblath DR, Macko C, McKhann GM, Asbury AK. Pathology of the motor-sensory axonal Guillain-Barré syndrome. Ann Neurol 39:17–28, 1996.

42. Griffin JW, Li CY, Ho TW, Xue P, Macko C, Cornblath DR, Gao CY, Yang C, Tian M, Mishu B, McKhann GM, Asbury AK. Guillain-Barré syndrome in northern China: the spectrum of neuropathologic changes in clinically defined cases. Brain 118:577–595, 1995.

43. Griffin JW, Li CY, Macko C, Ho TW, Hsieh S-T, Xue P, Wang FA, Cornblath DR, McKhann GM, Asbury AK. Early nodal changes in the acute motor axonal neuropathy pattern of the Guillain-Barré syndrome. J Neurocytol 25:33–51, 1996.

44. Griffin JW, Wesselingh SL, Griffin DE, Glass JD, McArthur JC. Peripheral nerve disorders in HIV infection: Similarities and contrasts with CNS disorders. In: HIV, AIDS, and the Brain. ARNMD Proceedings, vol 72, RW Price, SW Perry, eds. Raven Press, New York, 1994, pp 159–182.

45. Hahn AF, Feasby TE, Gilbert JJ. Blood-nerve barrier studies in experimental allergic neuritis. Acta Neuropathol 68:101–109, 1985.

46. Hahn AF, Feasby TE, Steele A, Lovgren DS, Berry J. Demyelination and axonal degeneration in Lewis rat experimental allergic neuritis depend on myelin dosage. Lab Invest 59:115–126, 1988.

47. Hahn AF, Feasby TE, Wilkie L, Lovgren D. Antigalactocerebroside antibody increases demyelination in adoptive transfer experimental allergic neuritis. Muscle Nerve 16:1174–1180, 1993.

48. Hahn AF, Gilbert JJ, Feasby TE. Passive transfer of demyelination by experimental allergic neuritis serum. Acta Neuropathol 49:169–176, 1980.

49. Hall SM. Some aspects of remyelination after demyelination produced by the intraneural injection of lysophosphatidyl choline. J Cell Sci 13:461–477, 1973.

50. Hall SM, Gregson NA. The in vivo and ultrastructural effects of the injection of lysophosphatidyl choline into myelinated peripheral nerve fibers of the adult mouse. J Cell Sci 9:769–789, 1971.

51. Hall SM, Gregson NA. The effects of mytomycin C on remyelination in the peripheral nervous system. Nature 252:303–305, 1974.

52. Hann PG, Beuche W, Neumann U, Friede RL. The rate of Wallerian degeneration in the absence of immunoglobulins. A study in chick and mouse peripheral nerve. Brain Res 451:126–132, 1988.

53. Hartung H-P, Schafer B, Diamanstein T, Fierz W, Heininger K, Toyka KV. Suppression of P$_2$-T cell line-mediated experimental autoimmune neuritis by interleukin-2 receptor targeted monoclonal antibody ART 18. Brain Res 489:120–128, 1989.

54. Hartung H-P, Schafer B, Heininger K. Stoll G, Toyka KV. The role of macrophages and eicosanoids in the pathogenesis of experimental allergic neuritis. Serial clinical, electrophysiological, biochemical, and morphological observations. Brain 111:1039–1059, 1988.

55. Hartung H-P, Schafer B, Heininger K, Toyka K. Suppression of experimental autoimmune neuritis by the oxygen radical scavengers superoxide dismutase and catalase. Ann Neurol 23:453–460, 1988.

56. Hartung H-P, Schafer B, van der Meide PH, Fierz W, Heininger K, Toyka KV. The role of interferon-gamma in the pathogenesis of experimental autoimmune disease of the peripheral nervous system. Ann Neurol 27:247–257, 1990.

57. Hartung H-P, Toyka KV. T-cell and macrophage activation in experimental autoimmune neuritis and Guillain-Barré syndrome. Ann Neurol 27 (Suppl):S57–S63, 1990.

58. Harvey GK, Pollard JD, Schindhelm K, Antony J. Chronic experimental allergic neuritis. An electrophysiological and histological study in the rabbit. J Neurol Sci 81:215–225, 1987.

59. Heumann R, Lindholm D, Bandtlow C, Meyer M, Radeke MJ, Misko TP, Shooter E, Thoenen H. Differential regulation of mRNA encoding nerve growth factor and its receptor in rat sciatic nerve during development, degeneration, and regeneration: role of macrophages. Proc Natl Acad Sci USA 84:8735–8739, 1987.

60. Hickey WF, Kimura H. Perivascular microglial cells of the CNS are bone marrow-derived and present antigen in vivo. Science 239:290–292, 1988.

61. Ho TW, Mishu B, Li CY, Gao CY, Cornblath DR, Griffin JW, Asbury AK, Blaser MJ, McKhann GM. Guillain-Barré syndrome in northern China: relationship to *Campylobacter jejuni* infection and anti-glycolipid antibodies. Brain 118:597–605, 1995.

62. Ho TW, Roberts M, Hsieh S-T, Nachamkin I, Willison HJ, Sheikh KA, Kiehlbauch J, Flanigan K, McArthur JC, Cornblath DR, McKhann GM, Newsom-Davis J, Vincent A, Griffin JW. Mechanism of paralysis and recovery in acute motor axonal neuropathy after *Campylobacter* infection. Neurology, in press.

62a. Ho TW, Li CY, Cornblath DR, Gao CY, Asbury AK, Griffin JW, McKhann GM. Patterns of recovery in the Guillain-Barré syndromes. *Neurology* 1996 (In Press).

62b. Ho TW, Hsieh S-T, Nachamkin I, Willison HJ, Sheikh KA, Kiehlbaouch J, Flanigan K, McArthur JC, Cornblath DR, McKhann GM, Griffin JW. Motor nerve terminal degeneration provides a potential mechanism for rapid recovery in acute motor axonal neuropathy after *Campylobacter* infection. *Neurology* (In Press).

63. Hodgkinson SJ, Westland KW, Pollard JD. Transfer of experimental allergic neuritis by intraneural injection of sensitized lymphocytes. J Neurol Sci 123:162–172, 1994.

64. Holmdahl R, Olsson T, Moran T, Klareskog L. In vivo treatment of rats with monoclonal anti-T-cell antibodies. Scand J Immunol 22:157–169, 1985.

65. Hosoi J, Murphy GF, Egan CL, Lerner EA, Grabbe S, Asahina A, Granstein RD. Regulation of Langerhans cell function by nerves containing calcitonin gene-related peptide. Nature 363:159–163, 1993.

66. Hughes RAC, Atkinson PF, Gray IA, Taylor WA. Major histocompatibility antigens and lymphocyte subsets during experimental allergic neuritis in the Lewis rat. J Neurol 234:390–395, 1987.

67a. Hsieh S-T, Choi S, Lin W-M, McArthur JC, Griffin JW. Epidermal denervation and its effects on keratinocytes and Langerhans cells. J Neurocytol 25:513–524, 1996.

67b. Hughes RAC, Kadlubowski M, Gray IA, Leibowitz S. Immune responses in experimental allergic neuritis. J Neurol Neurosurg Psychiatry 44:565–569, 1981.

68. Ilyas AA, Willison HJ, Quarles RH, Jungawala FB, Cornblath DR, Trapp BD, Griffin DE, Griffin JW, McKhann GM. Serum antibodies to gangliosides in Guillain-Barré syndrome. Ann Neurol 23:440–447, 1988.

69. Jackson CE, Barohn RJ, Mendell JR. Acute paralytic syndrome in three American men. Comparison with Chinese cases. Arch Neurol 50:732–735, 1993.

70. Jung S, Kramer S, Schluesener JH, Hunig T, Toyka KV, Hartung H-P. Prevention and therapy of experimental autoimmune neuritis by an antibody against T cell receptors-α/β. J Immunol 148:3768–3775, 1992.

71. Jung S, Toyka KV, Hartung H-P. Soluble complement receptor type 1 inhibits experimental autoimmune neuritis in Lewis rats. Neurosci Lett 200:1–4, 1995.

72. Kadlubowski M, Hughes RAC. Identification of the neuritogen for experimental allergic neuritis. Nature 277:140–141, 1979.

73. Kaldor J, Speed BR. Guillain-Barré syndrome and *Campylobacter jejuni:* a serological study. Br Med J 288:1867–1870, 1984.

74a. Kusunoki S, Chiba A, Kon K, Ando S, Arisawa K, Tate A, Kanazawa I. N-acetylgalactosaminyl GD1a is a target molecule for serum antibody in Guillain-Barré syndrome. Ann Neurol 35:570–576, 1994.

74b. Kusunoki S, Chiba A, Hitoshi S, Takizawa H, Kanazawa I. Anti-Gal-C antibody in autoimmune neuropathies subsequent to *mycoplama* infection. *Muscle Nerve* 18:409–413, 1995.

75. Lampert PW. Mechanism of demyelination in experimental allergic neuritis. Lab Invest 20:127–138, 1969.

76. Lassmann H, Schmied M, Vass K, Hickey WF. Bone marrow derived elements and resident microglia in brain inflammation. Glia 7:19–24, 1993.

77. Lassmann H, Vass K, Brunner C, Wisniewski HM. Peripheral nervous system lesions in experimental allergic encephalomyelitis. Acta Neuropathol 69:193–204, 1986.

78. Lindholm D, Heumann R, Hengerer B, Thoenen H. Interleukin-1 increases stability and transcription of mRNA encoding nerve growth factor in cultured rat fibroblasts. J Biol Chem 263:16348–16351, 1988.

79. Lindholm D, Heumann R, Meyer M, Thoenen H. Interleukin-1 regulates synthesis of nerve growth factor in non-neuronal cells of rat sciatic nerve. Nature 330:658–659, 1987.

80. Linington C, Izumo S, Suzuki M, Uyemura K, Meyermann R, Wekerle H. A permanent rat T cell line that mediates experimental allergic neuritis in the Lewis rat in vivo. J Immunol 133:1946–1950, 1984.

81. Linington C, Lassmann H, Ozawa K, Kosin S, Mongan L. Cell adhesion molecules of the immunoglobulin supergene family as tissue specific autoantigens: induction of experimental allergic neuritis (EAN) by P0 protein-specific T cell lines. Eur J Immunol 22:1813–1817, 1992.

82. Lubinska L. Early course of Wallerian degeneration in myelinated fibers of the rat phrenic nerve. Brain Res 130:47–63, 1977.

83. Lubinska L. Patterns of Wallerian degeneration of myelinated fibres in short and long peripheral stumps and in isolated segments of rat phrenic nerve. Interpretation of the role of axoplasmic flow of the trophic factor. Brain Res 233:227–240, 1982.

84. Hafer-Macko CE, Sheikh KA, Li CY, Ho TW, Cornblath DR, McKhann GM, Asbury AK, Griffin JW. Immune attack on the Schwann cell surface in acute inflammatory demyelinating polyneuropathy. Ann Neurol 39:625–635, 1996.

85. Mato M, Ookawara S, Mato TK, Namiki T. An attempt to differentiate further between

microglia and fluorescent granular perithelial (FGP) cells by the capacity to incorporate exogenous protein. Am J Anat 172:125–140, 1985.

86a. Hafer-Macko C, Hsieh S-T, Li CY, Ho TW, Sheikh K, Cornblath DR, McKhann GM, Asbury AK, Griffin JW. Acute motor axonal neuropathy: an antibody-mediated attack on axolemma. Ann Neurol, in press.

86b. Mato M, Ookawara S, Sugamata M, Aikawa E. Evidences for the possible function of the fluorescent granular perithelial cells in brain as scavengers of high molecular-weight waste products. Experientia 40:399–402, 1984.

87. McKhann GM, Cornblath DR, Griffin JW, Ho TW, Li CY, Jiang Z, Wu HS, Zhaori G, Liu Y, Jou LP, Liu TC, Gao CY, Mao JY, Blaser MJ, Mishu B, Asbury AK. Acute motor axonal neuropathy: a frequent cause of acute flaccid paralysis in China. Ann Neurol 33:333–342, 1993.

88. Miklossy J, Clarke, S, Van der Loos H. The long distance effects of brain lesions: Visualization of axonal pathways and their terminations in the human brain by the Nauta method. J Neuropathol Exp Neurol 50:595–614, 1991.

89. Miklossy J, Van der Loos H. Cholesterol ester crystals in polarized light show pathways in the human brain. Brain Res 426:377–380, 1987.

90. Miklossy J, Van der Loos H. The long-distance effects of brain lesions: visualization of myelinated pathways in the human brain using polarizing and fluorescence microscopy. J Neuropathol Exp Neurol 50:1–15, 1991.

91. Miledi R, Slater CK. On the degeneration of rat neuromuscular junctions after nerve section. J Physiol 207:507–528, 1970.

92. Milek DJ, Cunningham JM, Powers JM, Brostoff SW. Experimental allergic neuritis. Humoral and cellular immune responses to the cyanogen bromide peptides of the P2 protein. J Neuroimmunol 4:105–117, 1983.

93. Milner P, Lovelidge CA, Taylor WA, Hughes RAC. P_0 myelin protein produces experimental allergic neuritis in Lewis rats. J Neurol Sci 79:275–285, 1987.

94. Mishu B, Ilyas AA, Koski CL, Vriesendorp F, Cook SA, Mithen F, Blaser MJ. Serologic evidence of previous *Campylobacter jejuni* infection in patients with the Guillain-Barré syndrome. Ann Intern Med 118:947–953, 1993.

95. Monaco S, Gehrmann J, Raivich G, Kreutzberg GW. MHC-positive, ramified macrophages in the normal and injured rat peripheral nervous system. J Neurocytol 21:623–634, 1992.

96. Olee T, Powell HC, Brostoff SW. New minimum length requirement for a T cell epitope for experimental allergic neuritis. J Neuroimmunol 27:187–190, 1990.

97. Olsson T, Holmdahl R, Klareskog L, Forsum U. Ia-expressing cells and T lymphocytes of different subsets in peripheral nerve tissue during experimental allergic neuritis in Lewis rats. Scand J Immunol 18:339–343, 1983.

98. Ota K, Irie H, Takahashi K. T cell subsets and Ia-positive cells in the sciatic nerve during the course of experimental allergic neuritis. J Neuroimmunol 13:283–292, 1987.

99. Pollard JD, King RHM, Thomas PK. Recurrent experimental allergic neuritis. An electron microscope study. J Neurol 24:365–383, 1975.

100. Powell HC, Braheny SL, Myers RR, Rodriguez M, Lampert PW. Early changes in experimental allergic neuritis. Lab Invest 3:332–338, 1983.

101. Ramos-Alvarez M, Bessudo L, Sabin A. Paralytic syndromes associated with noninflammatory cytoplasmic or nuclear neuronopathy: acute paralytic disease in Mexican children, neuropathologically distinguishable from Landry-Guillain-Barré syndrome. JAMA 207:1481–1492, 1969.

102. Roberts M, Willison H, Vincent A, Newsom-Davis J. Serum factor in Miller-Fisher variant of Guillain-Barre syndrome and neurotransmitter release. Lancet 343:454–455, 1994.

103. Rostami A, Brown MJ, Lisak RP, Sumner AJ, Zweiman B, Pleasure DE. The role of myelin P_2 protein in the production of experimental allergic neuritis. Ann Neurol 16:680–685, 1984.

104. Rostami A, Gregorian SK, Brown MJ, Pleasure DE. Induction of severe experimental autoimmune neuritis with a synthetic peptide corresponding to the 53-78 amino acid sequence of the myelin P_2-protein. J Neuroimmunol 30:145–151, 1990.

105. Saida K, Saida T, Brown MJ, Silberberg DH, Asbury AK. Antiserum-mediated demyelination in vivo. A sequential study using intraneural injection of experimental allergic neuritis serum. Lab Invest 39:449–462, 1978.

106. Saida T, Saida K, Silberberg DH, Brown MJ. Transfer of demyelination by intraneural injection of experimental allergic neuritis serum. Nature 272:639–641, 1978.

107. Scheidt P, Friede RL. Myelin phagocytosis in Wallerian degeneration. Properties of millipore diffusion chambers and immunohistochemical identification of cell populations. Acta Neuropathol 75:77–84, 1987.

108. Schmidt B, Stoll G, van der Meide P, Jung S, Hartung HP. Transient cellular expression of gamma-interferon in myelin-induced and T-cell line-mediated experimental autoimmune neuritis. Brain 115(Part 6):1633–1646, 1992.

109. Sharief MK, Thompson EJ. In vivo relationship of tumor necrosis factor-alpha to blood-brain barrier damage in patients with active multiple sclerosis. J Neuroimmunol 38:27–34, 1992.

110. Sherwin AL. Chronic allergic neuropathy in the rabbit. Arch Neurol 15:289–293, 1966.

111. Shin H, McFarlane EF, Pollard JD, Watson EGS. Induction of experimental allergic neuritis with synthetic peptides from myelin P_2 protein. Neurosci Lett 102:309–312, 1989.

112. Speed B, Kaldor J, Cavanagh P. Guillain-Barré syndrome associated with *Campylobacter jejuni* enteritis. J Infect Dis 8:85–86, 1984.

113. Spies JM, Pollard JD, Bonner JG, Westland KW, McLeod JG. Synergy between antibody and P_2-reactive T cells in experimental allergic neuritis. J Neuroimmunol 57:77–84, 1995.

114. Spies JM, Westland KW, Bonner JG, Pollard JD. Intraneural activated T cells cause focal breakdown of the blood–nerve barrier. Brain 118:857–868, 1995.

115. Stead RH, Dixon MF, Bramwell NH, Riddell RH, Bienenstock J. Mast cells are closely apposed to nerves in the human gastrointestinal mucosa. Gastroenterology 97:575–585, 1989.

116. Stoll G, Griffin JW, Li CY, Trapp BD. Wallerian degeneration in the peripheral nervous system: participation of both Schwann cells and macrophages in myelin degradation. J Neurocytol 18:671–683, 1989.

117. Stoll G, Jung S, Jander S, van der Meide P, Hartung HP. Tumor necrosis factor-alpha in immune-mediated demyelination and Wallerian degeneration of the rat peripheral nervous system. J Neuroimmunol 45:175–182, 1993.

118. Stoll G, Schmidt B, Jander S, Toyka KV, Hartung H-P. Presence of the terminal complement complex (C5b-9) precedes myelin degradation in immune-mediated demyelination of the rat peripheral nervous system. Ann Neurol 30:147–155, 1991.

119. Strigard K, Brismar T, Olsson T, Kristensson K, Klareskog L. T-lymphocyte subsets, functional deficits, and morphology in sciatic nerves during experimental allergic neuritis. Muscle Nerve 10:329–337, 1987.

120. Strigard K, Olsson T, Larsson P, Holmdahl R, Klareskog L. Modulation of experimental allergic neuritis in rats by in vivo treatment with monoclonal anti-T cell antibodies. J Neruol Sci 83:282–291, 1988.

121. Takigawa T, Yasuda H, Kikkawa R. Antibodies agains GM1 ganglioside affect K$^+$ and Na$^+$ currents in isolated rat myelinated nerve fibers. Ann Neurol 37:436–442, 1995.

122. Tandon DS, Griffin JW, Drachman DB, Price DL, Coyle PL. Studies on the humoral mechanisms of inflammatory demyelinating neuropathies. Neurology 30(Abstract):362, 1980.

123. Tansey FA, Brosnan CF. Protection against experimental allergic neuritis with silica quartz dust. J Neuroimmunol 3:169–179, 1982.

124. Toyka KV, Heininger K. Humoral factors in peripheral nerve disease. Muscle Nerve 10:222–232, 1987.

125. Uyemura K, Suzuki M, Kitamura K, Horie K, Matsuyama H, Nozaki S, Muramatsu I. Neuritogenic determinant of bovine P$_2$ protein in peripheral nerve myelin. J Neurochem 39:895–898, 1982.

126. Vass K, Hickey WF, Schmidt RE, Lassmann H. Bone marrow-derived elements in the peripheral nervous system: an immunohistochemical and ultrastructural investigation in chimeric rats. Lab Invest 69:275–282, 1993.

127. Vedeler CA, Nilsen R, Matre R. Localization of Fc-gamma receptors and complement receptors CR1 on human peripheral nerve fibres by immunoelectron microscopy. J Neuroimmunol 23:29–34, 1989.

128. Vriesendorp FJ, Mishu B, Blaser M, Koski CL. Serum antibodies to GM1, peripheral nerve myelin, and *Campylobacter jejuni* in patients with Guillain-Barré syndrome and controls: correlation and prognosis. Ann Neurol 34:130–135, 1993.

129. Waksman BH. Experimental immunological disease of the nervous system. In Mechanisms of Demyelination, AS Rose, CM Pearson, eds. McGraw-Hill, New York, 1963, pp XXX–XXX.

130. Waksman BH, Adams RD. Allergic neuritis: experimental disease in rabbits induced by the injection of peripheral nervous tissue and adjuvants. J Exp Med 102:213–235, 1955.

131. Waksman BH, Adams RD. A comparative study of experimental allergic neuritis in the rabbit, guinea pig, and mouse. J Neuropathol Exp Neurol 15:293–313, 1956.

132. Winer JB, Hughes RAC, Osmond C. A prospective study of acute idiopathic neuropathy. 2. Antecedent events. J Neurol Neurosurg Psychiatry 51:613–618, 1988.

133. Winkler GF. In vitro demyelination of peripheral nerve induced with sensitized cells. Ann NY Acad Sci 122:287–296, 1965.

134. Wisniewski HM, Brostoff SW, Carter H, Eylar EH. Recurrent experimental allergic poly-ganglioradiculoneuritis. Arch Neurol 30:347–358, 1974.

135. Yonezawa T, Ishihara Y, Matsuyama H. Studies on experimental allergic peripheral neuritis. I. Demyelinating patterns studied in vitro. J Neuropathol Exp Neurol 27:453–463, 1968.

136. Yu LT, Rostami A, Silvers WK, Larossa D, Hickey WF. Expression of major histocompatibility complex antigens on inflammatory peripheral nerve lesions. J Neuroimmunol 30:145, 1990.

137. Yuki N, Handa S, Taki T, Kasama T, Takahashi M, Saito K. Cross-reactive antigen between nervous tissue and a bacterium elicits Guillain-Barré syndrome: molecular mimicry between gangliocide GM1 and lipopolysaccharide from Penner's serotype 19 of *Campylobacter jejuni*. Biomed Res 13:451–453, 1992.

138. Yuki N, Sato S, Fujimoto S, Yamada Y, Kinoshita A, Itoh T. Serotype of *Campylobacter jejuni*, HLA, and the Guillain-Barré syndrome. Muscle Nerve 16:968–969, 1992.

139. Yuki N, Sato S, Tsuji S, Ohsawa T, Miyatake T. Frequent presence of anti-GQ1b antibody in Fisher's syndrome. Neurology 43:414–417, 1993.

140. Yuki N, Taki T, Inagaki F, et al. A bacterium lipopolysaccharide that elicits Guillain-Barré syndrome has a GM1 ganglioside-like structure. J Exp Med 178:1771–1775, 1993.

141. Yuki N, Taki T, Takahashi M, et al. Penner's serotype 4 of *Campylobacter jejuni* has a lipopolysaccharide that bears a GM1 ganglioside epitope as well as one that bears a GD1a epitope. Infect Immun 62:2101–2103, 1994.

142. Yuki N, Yoshino H, Sato S, Miyatake T. Acute axonal polyneuropathy associated with anti-GM$_1$ antibodies following *Campylobacter jejuni* enteritis. Neurology 40:1900–1902, 1990.

143. Yuki N, Yoshino H, Sato S, Shinozawa K, Miyatake T. Severe acute axonal form of Guillaine-Barré syndrome associated with IgG anti-GD$_{1a}$ antibodies. Muscle Nerve 15:899–903, 1992.

Index

Acetylcholine receptor
  myasthenia gravis in, 28–30; 339–40;
    Fig. 9-2
AchR. *See* Acetylcholine receptor
ACTH. *See* Adrenocorticotropin
Acute demyelinating disease, 703–06
Acute disseminated encephalomyelitis
  animal models for, 24–25
  definition, 24
Acute hemorrhagic encephalomyelitis, 706
Acute inflammatory demyelinating
    polyneuropathy
  definition, 795
  immunopathogenesis, 797–98
Acute motor axonal neuropathy
  definition and types of, 795–97,
    Fig. 22-3
  treatment of, 800
Acute motor sensory axonal neuropathy
  definition and types of, 795–97,
    Fig. 22-3
Acute retinal necrosis
  definition, 682
  etiology, 682
  pathophysiology, 683
ADC. *See* AIDS Dementia Complex
ADCC. *See* Antibody-dependent
    complement cytotoxicity
Addressins, 204–05
ADE. *See* Acute disseminated
    encephalomyelitis; Antibody-
    dependent enhancement
ADEM. *See* Acute disseminated
    encephalomyelitis
Adhesion molecules. *See also* Selectins
  astrocytes, 378
  changes on endothelial cells, Table 7-1

changes on T cell following activation,
    207–10, Table 7-2
costimulatory functions, 212–13
intracellular adhesion molecules, 83,
    203–05, Table 7-1
lymphocyte function associated antigen,
    203–05, Table 7-1
T cell activation in, 366–67
types of, 203–205, Table 7-1, 7-2
Adoptive therapy
  brain tumor treatment in, 769–73;
    Table 21-3
Adjuvant
  definition, 80
  types of, 80
Adrenocorticotropin
  disease models, 19, 565–67
  effects of cytokines on, 559–61,
    Table 14-3
  effects on immune system, 549–53,
    Table 14-1
  paracrine and autocrine action, 564
  production of, 555–59, 562–64,
    Table 14-4
  receptors on lymphocytes, 553–55,
    Table 14-2
  releasing factor for, 552–53, Table 14-1,
    14-2
AHL. *See* Acute hemorrhagic
    encephalomyelitis
AIDP. *See* Acute inflammatory
    demyelinating polyneuropathy;
    Guillain-Barré syndrome
AIDS
  aseptic menigitis, 737
  CMV retinitis, 684, 687
  drug toxicity, 738

AIDS (*continued*)
immunosuppression, 656
infections associated with, 730–32
myelopathies, 733–35, Fig. 20-2
myopathies, 735
neuropathies, 735
secondary neoplasms, 732, 737
AIDS Dementia Complex
cellular tropism, 739
definition and pathology, 348–49, 729–
32, Table 1-2, Table 20-2
encephalitis in, 733
IL-1 role in, 429
neurological syndromes associated with,
732, Table 20-1
TGF-β role in, 442, 646, 656
TNF-α role in, 429
Alpha-melanocyte-stimulating hormone
aqueous humor in, 113, 117, Table 18-1
α-MSH. *See* Alpha-melanocyte-stimulating
hormone
ALS. *See* Amyotropic lateral sclerosis
Alzheimer's disease
astrocytes in, 184
IL-1 role in, 429
TGF-β role in, 646
AMAN. *See* Acute motor axonal
neuropathy
AMSAN. *See* Acute motor sensory axonal
neuropathy
Amyotropic lateral sclerosis
autoimmunity in; Table 1-1
Anergy, 212
Annexins. *See* Lipocortins
Anterior chamber
cytokines in, 113
definition, 112, 669
immunoglobulins in, 119–21
immunosuppression in, 117, 643
microenvironment, 117, 643
Anterior chamber-associated immune
deviation
definition, 111, 676
efferent limb of neural-ocular system,
117
feature of neural-occular immune system,
121–23
immune deviation in, 116
immunoglobulin production in, 119–21

immunosuppression in, 117–18, 643,
676
Antibody
anti-Hu, 346
anti-MBP, 711
anti-MOG, 711
anti-Yo, 346
classes of, 71–72
humoral response in, 81
monoclonal serotherapy, 72
occular inflammation in, 678–79
oligoclonal, 710
synthesis in brain, 144, 211
Antibody-dependent complement
cytotoxicity, 17
Antibody-dependent enhancement, 591
Antigen
autoantigens, 471–74. *See also*
Autoimmunity
B7.1-7.2, 212
CD antigens, Table 7-1, 7-2
cytotoxic lymphocyte target antigens,
500
encephalitogenic CNS antigens, 461–63
epitope dominance, 463–65
inhibition, 349–50
Lewis^x, Lewis sialo^x, 211
MECA, 204
myelin basic protein as, 461–63
PCD-AA, 346
presentation, concept of, 365–68
recognition of, 70–74
S antigen
superantigen, 470
tumor-associated target antigen, 763–67,
Table 21-1
Antigen presentation. *See also* Antigen
presenting cell
astrocytes by, 377–88, Fig. 10-1,
Table 10-2
cellular interaction in, 78–81, 83–85
CNS in, 211–212
definition and concept of, 72, 499, 365–
68, Table 10-2
microglia by, 384–91, Fig. 10-1,
Table 10-2
nervous system-restricted, 107–09
neurons by, 398–401, Fig. 10-1,
Table 10-2

oligodendrocytes by, 395–98, Fig. 10-1, Table 10-2
perivascular cells by, 368–76, Fig. 10-1, Table 10-2
smooth muscle cells/pericytes by, 368–76, Fig. 10-1, Table 10-2
tissue-restricted, 101
vascular endothelial cells by, 368–76, Fig. 10-1, Table 10-2
Apoptosis, 212, 646–47
Aqueous humor
cytokines in, 113
immunoglobulins in, 119–121
immunosupressive properties, 113–14, 643–44
secreted by, 112, 669
Arginine vasopressin, 552–53
ARN. *See* Acute retinal necrosis
Arrestin. *See* S antigen
ARV. *See* Human immunodeficiency virus
Astrocyte
AIDS in, 740
Alzheimer's disease in, 104
antigen presentation role in, 377–83, Fig. 10-1, Table 10-2
astrogliosis in, 619
colony-stimulating factors, effects on and production by, 443–44, Table 11-6
effects of immune factors on, Table 6-2
experimental allergic encephalomyelitis in, 183
historical aspects, 173
IL-1, effects on, 425; production of, 427
IFN-γ, effects on, 430
MHC expression on, 377–83, Table 10-1
morphology and functions of, 174–76, Fig. 6-1, 6-2
TGF-β, effects on and production by, 440–41, Table 11-5
TNF-α, β, effects on and production by, 433–35, Table 11-3,
prostaglandin production by, 648
reactions to injury, 179
transplantation in, 623
Autoimmunity
AIDS in, 743–45
antigen and peptide inhibition, 349–50
cytokine inhibition, 350–51
CD4+ T cells in, 460–61

EAE role in, 8–19, 460–61
EAN role in, 8–19, 460–61
MOG, 345
multiple sclerosis in, 19–23, Table 1-1
myelin P2, 335
paraneoplastic neurological syndromes in, 345–47
pathogenic T cells in, 468–71
PCD-AA, 346
self vs. nonself, concept of, 76–78
tolerance, 77
AVP. *See* Arginine vasopressin

B-Cell
cellular basis of immune system as, 70–74
cellular interactions of, 81, 83–85
circulation of, 201–05
CNS in, 210–11
memory, 75–76
migration and trafficking of, 82–83, 145, 201–05, 210–11
receptors on, 71–74
BALT. *See* Bronchial-associated lymphoid tissue
BBB. *See* Blood-brain barrier
Bcl-2, 80
BDNF. *See* Brain-derived neurotrohic factor
BIV. *See* Bovine immunodeficiency virus
Blood-brain barrier
breakdown of, 620–21
concept and features of, 140–41, 147, 615
injury in AIDS, 745
regulation of, 147, 163
Blood-nerve barrier, 785
Blood-ocular barrier, 671–74, Fig. 18-2
Bone marrow
innervation of, 238, 285, 250–51, Fig. 8-9, 8-10
Bovine immunodeficiency virus, 748
Brain-derived neurotrophic factor, 790
Bronchial-associated lymphoid tissue, 136

CA. *See* catecholamine
CAEV. *See* caprine arthritis-encephalitis virus

Calcitonin gene-related peptide
  eye in, 675, Table 18-1
  immune response effects on, 280–82
  lymph node in, 247, Fig. 8-24
  peptidergic nerves in, 237
  receptors for on lymphocytes, 261–62
  spleen in, 243, 245, Fig. 8-19, 8-20
  thymus in, 238, Fig. 8-12
Canine distemper virus, 592
Caprine arthritis encephalitis virus, 748
Catecholamine
  effects on immune response, 266–69
CCK. *See* cholecystokinin
CD antigens. *See* Antigen
CDV. *See* canine distemper virus
Cerebrospinal fluid
  AIDS cytokines in, 743
  brain tumors in, 769
  cytokines in, 113–14, 117, 644
  immunosuppressive properties of, 117–
    18, 643–44
  secretion of, 113
Chagas' disease, 34
ChAT. *See* Choline acetyltransferase
Chemokines
  CNS inflammation in, 214
Cholecystokinin
  lymph node in, 247
  spleen in, 243
Choline acetyltransferase
  lymph organs in, 250
Chronic inflammatory demyelinating
    polyradiculoneuropathy
  animal models, 27–28
  definition and description of, 25–27
CIDP. *See* chronic inflammatory
    demyelinating
    polyradiculoneuropathy
Ciliary neurotropic factor, 790
CMV. *See* Cytomegalovirus
Colony-stimulating factor. *See also*
    Cytokine
  actions of, 424, 443
  expression by glia, 443–44, Table 11-6
  viral infections of the CNS in, 585–
    87
Complement
  cerebrospinal fluid in, 135
  decay-accelerating factor binding, 120

Corticotropin-releasing factor
  effects on immune response, 552–53,
    Table 14-1, 14-2
  nerves in, 238
  production of, 556, 563
CRF. *See* Corticotropin-releasing factor
CSF. *See* Cerebrospinal fluid
Cytokines
  biological actions on glial cells, 425–27,
    Table, 11-1, 430–32, Table 11-2,
    433–35, Table 11-3, 438,
    Table 11-4, 440, Table 11-5, 443,
    Table 11-6, 651–52
  CNS viral infections in, 585–87
  definition and functions, 421–25
  expression by glial cells, 427–28, 435–
    36, 438, 440–41, 443
  immune response in, 85–89
  inhibition, 350
  neuroendocrine system effects on, 559–
    61
  neurological disease in, 428–30, 432–33,
    436–38, 439–40, 442–44, 652–53
  proinflammatory, 213–14
  receptors in neuroendocrine system,
    561–62
Cytomegalovirus
  AIDS in, 731, 737
  immune response to, 28, 587–88
  retinitis in, 684–86
Cytotoxic T cells
  cell-cell interactions of, 502, Fig. 13-3
  comparison to NK cells, 509–14
  control in CNS, 522–26
  definition and role in immune system,
    493–94
  graft rejection in, 501, 531–33
  immune network role in, 493–94
  MHC restriction of, 495–97
  migration into the brain, 503, 523
  neural cells against, 518
  specificity and memory of, 495
  target susceptibility, 501
  tumors in CNS against, 528–31
  viral infections in CNS, 526–28,
    Table 13-2

DAF. *See* Decay-accelerating factor
Decay-accelerating factor, 120, 135

Delayed hypersensitivity
  definition, 12
  neurotransmitter effects on, 264
  suppression of, 135, 146, 642–43, 679–80
DH. *See* Delayed hypersensitivity
Dynorphin A
  lymph nodes and nerves in, 247

E-selectin. *See* Selectins
EAE. *See* Experimental allergic
      (autoimmune) encephalomyelitis
EAMG. *See* Experimental autoimmune
      myasthenia gravis
EAN. *See* Experimental allergic
      (autoimmune) neuritis
EAU. *See* Experimental allergic
      (autoimmune) uveitis
EIAV. *See* Equine infectious anemia virus
ELAM-1. *See* Selectins
Endoneurium, 785
Epineurium, 785
Equine infectious anemia virus, 748
Epitope
  autoantigen, 472
  dominance, 464
  encephalitogenic, Table 9-1
  myelin basic protein, 342
  spreading, 464
Experimental allergic (autoimmune)
      encephalomyelitis
  antibody synthesis in, 211
  antigen and peptide inhibition of, 49–50
  astrocytes in, 184, 380
  CD4⁺ T cells in, 460, 471–74, 596
  cell surface antigen changes in, 209–10
  cytokine inhibition, 350–51
  definition and experimental models of,
      8–13, 118
  genetic regulation of, 13–19
  IL-1 role in, 16, 428
  IL-6 role in, 16, 439
  IL-10 role in, 650
  IFN role in, 16, 432–33, 652–53
  immune regulation of, 17–18
  lipocortins in, 649
  myelin proteins in, 791–93
  TcR peptide therapy in, 350
  TGF-β role in, 16, 444, 645–46
  TH1 response, 206–210

TNF-α, β role in, 16, 436–37
vascular endothelial cells in, 370–76
Experimental allergic (autoimmune) neuritis
  CD4⁺ T cells in, 460–61
  defintion and experimental models, 10–
      13, 791–94
  genetic regulation, 13–19
  IFN-γ role in, 793
  macrophages in, 793
  myelin proteins in, 791–93
  myelin P2, 335
  TNF-α role in, 793
Experimental autoimmune myasthenia
      gravis 7, 29–30
Experimental autoimmune uvetis, 347–48,
      680–82
Eye
  anatomy, 670, Fig. 18-1
  anterior chamber, 675
    immune deviation, 116–25, 676–77
  antigen and leukocyte clearance, 674
  blood-ocular barrier, 671–74
  disease and animal models, 680–86
    acute retinal necrosis, 682–84. *See
      also* Acute retinal necrosis
    cytomegalovirus retinitis, 684–86. *See
      also* Cytomegalovirus
    experimental autoimmune uveitis,
      680–82. *See also* Experimental
      autoimmune uveitis
  immunologic microenvironment, 669–77
  immunosuppressive molecules by ocular
      tissues, 117–18, 674, Table 18-1
  inflammation in, 677–78
    antibody and B lymphocytes, 119–21,
      678
    T lymphocytes, and cellular immunity,
      679
  neural-occular immune system. *See also*
      Neural-occular immune system
    features of, 107–16, Table 3-2, 3-3

Fas-FasL pathway, 646–47
Feline immunodeficiency virus, 748
Fisher syndrome, 800–01
FIV. *See* Feline immunodefiency virus

GALT. *See* Gut-associated lymphoid tissue
GBS. *See* Guillain-Barré syndrome

GH. *See* Growth hormone
Glial-stimulating factor, 420
Glioblastomas. *See also* Gliomas
  immunosuppression in, 647–48
Gliomas
  cell surface marker and extracellular
    matrix expression, Table 21-1
  immunosuppression in patients with,
    647–48
  immunotherapy, 767–73
    active, Table 21-2
    animal models, 774
    nonspecific, 767
    passive, 769, Table 21-3
    specific, 767
  target cells, 774–77
Graft
  allograft, 625–27
  host sensitization, 627–28
  sites for transplantation in nervous
    system, 618
  survival and rejection of, 618, 628
  vascularization of, 624–25
  xenografts, 631–633, Table 5-6
Graft-versus-host disease
  immune response in, 370, 629–30,
    Fig. 10-3
  microglia involvement, 384
Growth hormone
  disease models, 567
  effects on immune response, 550–55,
    Table 14-1
  paracrine and autocrine, 564
  production of, 557–59, 562–64,
    Table 14-4
  releasing factor, Table 14-1
GvHD. *See* Graft-versus-host disease
Guillain-Barré syndrome
  axonal forms, 798
  animal models, 27–28, 794–800
  classification, 25–26, Fig. 22-3
  heterogeneity, 795–97
  immunopathogenesis, 797–98
  molecular mimicry, 339, 794, 796–
    97
  myelin P2, 335
Gut-associated lymphoid tissue
  definition of, 236
  innervation of, 236, 249–50, 254

HAM/TSP. *See* Tropical spastic paraparesis
Hapten, 75
Hashimoto's thyroiditis, 4
Herpes simplex virus
  AIDS in, 731
  CNS disease in, 579–81, Table 15-1
  epitope shared with Guillain-Barré
    syndrome, 796
  human herpesvirus 8, 732
  retinitis in, 682–84, 687
  type 1 in ARN, 682
HEV. *See* High endothelial venule
High endothelial venule, 202, 205–06
HIV. *See* Human immunodeficiency virus
HTLV. *See* Human T-cell lymphotrophic
  virus
Human immunodeficiency virus
  Type I
    cellular tropism, 739
    leukoencephalopathy, 733
    neurological disease in, 578, 728–29,
      733, Table 20-3
    toxic products, 739–41
  Type II, 747, Table 20-3
Human JC virus, 731, 737
Human serum albumin
  antibody response in brain to,
    144
  systemic response to, 143
Human T-cell lymphotrophic virus
  Type I, 37–39, 379, 742, 746–47,
    Table 1-2, 20–3
  Type III, 727, 746–47, Table 20-3

ICAM. *See* Adhesion molecules
Immune privilege
  brain, 5–6, 114, 642
  disease therapeutics, 688–89
  eye, 114–116, 642, 674–77
  transplantation experiments, 115, 134,
    613–14
Immune response
  afferent limb of, 116, 135, 141, 143,
    148, Fig. 4-3
    suppression of, 461, 642–43
  AIDS in, 729–32, 741–43
  antigen presentation in, 365–68
  B-T cooperation, 81–82
  brain in, 143, 144–46

calcitonin gene related peptide effects, 280–82
cellular basis of, 70
CTL response. *See* Cytotoxic lymphocyte deviation, 116–119
efferent limb of, 117, 135, 141, 761, Fig. 4-3
epitope dominance in, 463–65
general properties of, 70
immunopathology, 85–89
memory, 74–76, 82
MHC restriction of, 496–97, Figure 13-2
myelin basic protein to, 461–63
neuro-occular immune system in, 121–24
NK response. *See* NK cells
noradrenergic modulation of, 265–72
NPY effects on, 275
opiate peptide effects, 282–85
regional specialization of, 100–01, 106, 136
somatostatin effects, 278–80
substance P effects, 275
specificity of, 70
T cell receptor usage, 465–68
TH1 and TH2 types, 79–80
tolerance, 76–78
  oral, 349
VIP effects, 272–75
Immune system. *See* Immune response
Immunosuppression
  ACAIDS in, 116–18
  afferent limb of immune system of, 642–43
  AIDS in, 656, 729–32
  cytokine involvement, 213–14
  CD4$^+$ self-reactive T cells, 471–74, 657
  efferent limb of immune system of, 643–44
  eye in, 117–18, 674
  measles in, 655
  multiple sclerosis in, 656–57, 717
  oral tolerance, 349
  transplantation, 630–31, 633–34
  tumors of the CNS, 761
Inflammation
  cellular interactions in, 85–89, 201
  chemokines, 214
  cytokines in, 213–14

eye in, 686–87
initiation in CNS, 211–12
substance P effects, 275–78
vascular endothelial cells role in, 370–76
VIP effects, 274
Integrins, 203–05
Interferon alpha/beta
  astrocyte production of, 651
  brain tumors in, 769
  disease role, 652–53
  immunosuppressive properties, 651–52
  viral infections of CNS, 586–87
Interferon gamma. *See also* Cytokines
  biological action on glial cells, 430–32, Table 11-2
  EAE, MS role in, 432–33
  EAN role in, 793
  MHC antigen upregulation by,
  viral infections of CNS, 585–87
Interleukin-1. *See also* Cytokines
  biological action on glial cells, 25–27, Table 11-1; on hypothalamus vs. pituitary, 565
  effects on neuroendocrine system, 559–61, Table 14-3
  expression by glial cells, 427–28
  immune response in, 85–89
  neurological disease in, 428–30, 740
  receptors in neurendocrine system for, 561–62
  viral infections in CNS, 585–87
Interleukin-2
  brain tumors, 769
  effects on neuroendocrine system, 559–61, Table 14-3
  immune response in, 86–89
  viral infections in CNS, 585–87
Interleukin-3
  effects on microglia, Table 11-6
Interleukin-4
  immunosuppressive effects, 650
Interleukin-6
  biological actions on glial cells, 438
  effects on neuroendocrine system, 559–61, Table 14-3
  expression by glial cells, 438, Table 11-4
  involvement in disease, 439–40
  viral infection in CNS, 585–87

Interleukin-10
  immunosuppressive effects, 213, 650
Inteurleukin-12
  immunosuppression in measles, 655–56
Interstitial fluid
  drainage into blood and lymph, 138–40,
      Fig. 4-2
  production and turnover, 136–38,
      Fig. 4-1
  recovery of substances from, Table 4-1
Intracellular adhesion molecules. See
      Adhesion molecules
ISF. See Interstitial fluid

JCV. See Human JC virus
JHM. See J. Howard Muller virus
J. Howard Muller virus, 587, 688
  inhibition of, 588, 590–92, Table 1-2

LAM-1. See Selectins
Lambert-Eaton myasthenia syndrome, 30–32
Langerhan cells, 108
LAT. See Latency-associated transcripts
LAV. See Lymphadenopathy-associated virus
LFA-1. See Adhesion molecules
LCMV. See Lymphocytic choriomeningitis
      virus
LECCAM-1. See Selectins
LEMS. See Lambert-Eaton myasthenia
      syndromes. See also Paraneoplastic
      syndromes
Leprosy, 41, Table 1-2
Leutinizing hormone-releasing hormone,
      558–59, 563–64, Table 14-4
LHRH. See Leutinizing hormone-releasing
      hormone
Lipocortins
  production, 649
  immunosuppressive properties, 649
  multiple sclerosis in, 649
Ly-6 gene product, 654
Lymphatics
  CNS in, 136–40, 615, Fig. 4-1, 4-2,
      Table 4-1
  eye, 104, 111, Fig. 4-2
Lymphocytes
  activation of, 212–13
  antigen presentation, 365–68
  autoimmune effects, 460–61

B-cells. See also B-cells
  B7 protein, 80
  CNS in, 210–11
  occular inflammation in, 678–79
cell surface antigen changes following
      activation, 595–96, Table 7-2
CD4+. See also T-cells
  AIDS in, 729–32
  CMV retinitis in, 685
  definition, 494
  EAE in, 709–11
  EAU in, 681
CD4+/CD8+ in viral infections, 593–95
circulation of, 201–05
diapedesis, 102
encephalitis in, 474–75
homing, 202, 625
inflammation, 85–89
memory, 203
migration of, 82–83
neuro-occular immune system in, 102–
      03, 109, 679
neurotransmitter effects, 264, 475–77
response to antigen, 78
T-cells. See also T-cells
  CNS in, 207–10
  TH1 and TH2, 206, 212–13, 595–96
  tissue tropic, 102–03, 109
  tumor infiltration of, 762
Lymphocytic choriomeningitis virus, 586,
      588, Table 1-2, 15-1
Lymphadenopathy-associated virus, 727.
      See also Human immunodeficiency
      virus
Lyme's disease, 34, Table 1-2
Lymph node
  CNS transplantation in, 615–16
  innervation of, 233, 247–49, 254
  lymphocyte homing to, 204–05
  T-dependent areas

Macrophage
  "activated," 83
  AIDS in, 741
  antigen presentation, Table 10-2
  choroid plexes and leptomeninges, 159,
      162, 384, 394
  distribution, 157
  EAN in, 793

Guillain-Barré syndrome in, 799,
    Fig. 22-4
kinetics, 156–57
MHC antigen expression, Table 10-1
ontogeny, 156
peripheral nerve in, 786–87, Fig. 22-1,
    22-2
perivascular, 159, 384, 391–94
Wallerian degeneration in, 789
MAG. *See* Myelin-associated glycoprotein
MAI. *See* Mycobacterium ovium
    intracellulare
MAIDS. *See* Murine AIDS
MALT. *See* Mucosa-associated lymphoid
    tissues
Mast cells
    IgG E, 85
    peripheral nervous system, 787–89
MBP. *See* Myelin basic protein
MCMV. *See* Murine cytomegalovirus
Measles virus
    cellular response to, 594, 595–97
    immune alterations in, 578, 584–85, 588,
        655, Table 15-1
    immunosuppression, 655
        IL-12 in, 655
    inhibition of, 591, 594
MECA-79 antigen, 204
MEL-14. *See* Selectins
Memory, 74–6, 203
Met-enkephalin, 243, 246
MG. *See* Microglia
MHC molecules
    antigen complex with, 497–99
    antigen presenting cell-T cell interactions
        in, 84–5
    astrocyte expression, 377–83, Table 10-1
        modulation by IFN-γ, 430–32
    cytosolic pathway, 497–99, Fig. 13-2
    endosomal pathway, 497–99, Fig. 13-2
    eye in, 109
    immune response role in, 79, 365–8,
        497–99, Fig. 13-2
    immunosuppression in, 654–55
    macrophages expression in CNS, 391–
        94, Table 10-1
    microglial expression, 385–91,
        Table 10-1
    modulation by IFN-γ, 430–32

Müller cells on, 109
neuron expression, 398–401, Table 10-1
NK response role in, 514–21, Table 13-1
oligodendrocyte expression, 395–98,
    Table 10-1
restriction of, 72–73
smooth muscle pericyte expression, 370–
    76, Table 10-1
transplantation in CNS, 614–15, 621–23,
    629–30, Fig. 16-1
vascular endothelial cell expression,
    370–76, Table 10-1
viral infections in CNS, 587
Microenvironment
brain, 105, 146
comparison of eye and brain, Table 18-2
eye in, 105, 112, 669, 674, 677–78
regulation of, 147, 643–44, 677
Microglia
activation, 164
antigen presentation by, 384–91,
    Table 10-2
colony stimulating factors actions on,
    443–44, Table 11-6
distribution, 157, Fig. 5-1, 5-2
graft-versus-host disease, Fig. 10-3
IFN-γ effects on, 430–432
IL-1 production, 427
IL-3 effects on, Table 11-3
IL-6 effects on, 438, Table 11-4
irradiated bone marrow chimeras, 387–
    91
kinetics, 160
MHC expression, 384–91, Table 10-1
microgliosis, 619
phenotypes, 162, 383
prostaglandin production, 648
response to injury, 165, 167, 384–91,
    Fig. 10-2
TGF-β production and expression, 440–
    441, 644–46, Fig. 11-5
TNF-α actions on, 435, Table 11-3
transplantation in CNS, response to, 623,
    629
MOG. *See* Myelin oligodendrocyte
    glycoprotein
Monoclonal gammopathies, 32–33
Molecular mimicry
AIDS in, 745

Molecular mimicry (*continued*)
    EAE in, 470
    eye in, 687–88
    Guillain-Barré syndrome in, 339,
      794
Mucosa-associated lymphoid tissues
    antibodies in, 106
    features of, 105, 136
    lymphocytes in, 106
Müller cells, 670
Multiple sclerosis
    antibody synthesis, 211
    astrocyte role in, 183
    chronic progressive form, 712
    epidemiology, 201, 708
    genetics, 201, 708–09
    histopathology, 707
    history of, 19–21
    IFN role, 432–33, 652–53
    IL-1 role, 428–29
    IL-6 role, 439
    immunopathogenesis, 21–22, 709–11
    immunosuppression of, 21, 656–57
    laboratory diagnosis, 714–16
    lipcortin role, 649
    MAG in, 336
    MOG in, 345
    myelin basic protein, 19–23
    PLP, 344
    relapsing-remitting form, 712
    symptoms and signs, 14, 712
    TGF-β role, 442, 656
    therapy, 716–17
Murine AIDS, 686–87
Murine cytomegalovirus, 685–86
MV. *See* Measles virus
Myasthenia gravis, 28–30, 340
Mycobacterium
    avium intracellulare, 730–32
    tuberculosis, 730
Myelin P2, 334–36
Myelin-associated glycoprotein, 14, 32,
    336–37, Fig. 9-1
Myelin basic protein
    astrocyte involvement, 380–81
    ADEM in, 704
    anergy of, 471–74
    antibody response in brain, 146, 341,
      Table 9-1

    antigen in systemic immune response,
      143, 341
    CD4$^+$ T cells against, 461–63, 596
    definition and mutants of, 341
    EAN in, 13–19, 701–94
    EAU in, 13–19
    encephalitogenic antigen as, 461–63,
      596
    multiple sclerosis in, 19–23, 709–
      11
    oligodendrocyte involvement, 395
    oral tolerance, 349
    PIE, 24
    T cell receptor gene usage, 465–68
Myelin oligodendrocyte glycoprotein, 14,
    344–45, Fig. 9-1

NA. *See* Noradrenergic
NE. *See* Norepinephrine
Neural-occular immune system
    components of, 107–10, Table 3-2, 3-3
      antigen presenting cells, 107–09, 136
      immunoglobulin production, 119–21
      lymphocytes, tissue-trophic, 102–03,
        109–10
    manifestations, 114–16
    pathology, 119
    rationale for existence, 124–25
    scheme of, 121–24
Neurons
    antigen presenting cells as, 398–
      401, Table 10-2
    cholinergic, 250
    development of, 285–297
    MHC antigen expression, Table 10-1
    neuroendocrine functions on, 7
    noradrenergic, 227–36, Fig. 8-25, 8-30,
      Table 8-1
    peptidergic, 237
Neuropeptide Y
    immune system effects, 275
    lymph nodes in, 247, Fig. 8-23
    lymphocyte receptors for, 259
    peptidergic nerves in, 237
    spleen in, 243, 245, Fig. 8-16
    thymus in, 238, Fig. 8-11
Neurokinin A, B, 238
Neurotensin, 243
NIS. *See* Neural-occular immune system

NK cells. *See also* lymphocytes
   activity in CNS, 518, 534–36; activity in
      immune system, 83, 493–94
   comparison to CTL, 509
   definition, 504–05
   graft rejection in, 508
   heterogeneity of, 504
   recognition, role of MHC, 507, 510–14,
      Table 13-1
   targeted to cells, specificity and memory,
      505–07
Nodes of Ranvier, 798–800, Fig. 22-4
Noradrenergic
   autoimmunity effects on, 297
   development of nerves in lymphoid
      organs, 227–36, 285–91, Table 8-1
   immune system modulation, 265
   neurotransmitter release, 254–56
   receptors on lymphocytes, 256–58
Norepinephrine
   immune system modulation, 265, 267
   nerves in, 244, 246
   release in spleen, 254
NPY. *See* Neuropeptide Y
NT. *See* Neurotensin

Oligodendrocytes
   antigen presentation, 394–98, Table 10-2
   IFN-γ effects on, 430, Table 11-2
   IL-1 production, 427
   MHC expression, 395–98, Table 10-1
   myelin oligodendrocyte glycoprotein,
      344–45
   TNF-α effects on, 433, Table 11-3
Opiate peptides
   immune response effects on, 282–85
   lymphoid organs in, 237
   receptors on lymphocytes, 262–64, 551
   types of, 263
OPPV. *See* Progressive pneumonia virus

PALS. *See* Periarteriolymphatic sheath
Paraneoplastic cerebellar degeneration-
      associated autoantigen, 346
Paraneoplastic neurological syndromes, 30–
      32, 345–47
PCD-AA. *See* Paraneoplastic cerebellar
      degeneration associated autoantigen
Peptide histidine isoleucine, 247

Peptide inhibition, 349–50
Peptidergic
   nerves in lymphoid organs, 237
   receptors on lymphocytes, 258–59
Periarteriolymphatic sheath, 247, Fig. 8-17
Perineurium, 785
Perivascular cells
   antigen presenting capabilities, 371–76,
      Table 10-2
   definition, 391–94
   MHC antigen expression, 392–94, Fig.
      10-4
Peyer's patches, 237
PHI. *See* Peptide histidine isoleucine
PLP. *See* Proteolytic protein
PML. *See* Progressive multifocal
      leukoencephalopathy
PO glycoprotein, 337–39, Fig. 9-1
POEMS. *See* Polyneuropathy,
      organomegaly, hyperpigmentation,
      myeloma and skin change syndrome
Polio virus, 578, 580–81
Polyneuropathy, 336, 338
Polyneuropathy, organomegaly,
      hyperpigmentation, myeloma and
      skin change syndrome, 33
Postinfectious encephalomyelitis, 23–25
Postvaccinal encephalomyelitis, 23–24
Progressive multifocal
      leukoencephalopathy, 731
Progressive pneumonia virus, 748
Progressive rubella panencephalitis, 39–41,
      Table 1-2
PRL. *See* Prolactin
Prolactin
   disease models, 567
   immune system effects, 550–55,
      Table 14-1, 14-2
   production, 555–59, 563–64, Table 14-4
Prostaglandins
   production and immunosuppressive
      properties, 648
Proteolipid protein
   disease in, 342–44, Fig. 9-1, 704, 709–
      11
   encephalitogenic epitopes, Table 9-1
   mutants of, 343–44
P-selectin. *See* Selectins
Psychoneuroimmunology, 6–8

Purkinje cell antigens, 345–47
PVC. *See* Perivascular cell
PVE. *See* Postvaccinal encephalomyelitis

Rabies virus, 585
RANTES, 209
Retinal pigment epithelium, 670
RPE. *See* Retinal pigment epithelium
RV. *See* Rabies virus

SALT. *See* Skin associated lymphoid
     tissues
Schwann cells
     CNTF expression, 790
     NGF expression, 790
     PO glycoprotein production, 337–39
     Wallerian degeneration in, 789–90
Selectins. *See also* Adhesion molecules
     changes following lymphocyte activation,
          207–10
     types of, 203–05, Table 7-1, 7-2
Semliki Forest virus, 590
SFV. *See* Semliki Forest virus
SGLPG. *See* Sulfated glucuronic acid
     lactosaminyl paragloboside
Simian immunodeficiency virus, 207, 578,
     748, Table 1-2
Sindbis virus, 578–89, Table 15-1
SIV. *See* Simian immunodeficiency virus
Skin-associated lymphoid tissues
     definition and features, 107
SLE. *See* Systemic lupus erythematosus
Smooth muscle pericytes
     antigen presentation capacity, 370–76,
          Table 10-2
     antigen recognition in, 368–70, Fig. 10-1
     MHC expression, 370–76, Table 10-1
SM/P. *See* Smooth muscle/pericytes
SOM. *See* Somatostatin
Somatostatin
     immune response effects, 278–80,
          Table 14-1
     peptidergic nerves, 237
     Peyer's patches, 249
     receptors on lymphocytes for, 260–61
S antigen, 347–48
SP. *See* Substance P
Spleen
     aging effects, 292

development of noradrenergic nerves,
     286, Fig. 8-25, 8-26, 8-27
innervation of, 230, 243–47, 253–54,
     Fig. 8-16
Subacute sclerosing panencephalitis, 34,
     39–41, 584–586, Table 1-2
Substance P
     eye in, Table 18-1
     immune system effects, 275–78
     lymph node in, 247
     peptidergic nerves in, 237
     peripheral nerves, 789
     receptors on lymphocytes for, 259
     spleen in, 243, 245, Fig. 8-18, 8-21
     thymus in, 238, Fig. 8-13
Sulfated glucuronic acid lactosaminyl
     paragloboside, 32
Superantigen, 744
Suppressin, 650–51
Sympathectomy, 269–71
Systemic lupus erythematosus, 33–34

T-cell. *See also* Lymphocytes
     activation of, 212
     adhesion molecules, 209
     antigen presentation to, 365–68
     cellular interactions, 83–85, 212–13
          cooperation with B cells, 81
     circulation and migration of, 82–83,
          201–05
     CNS in, 207–10
     immune response in, 70–74
     inflammation in, 85–89
     memory, 75–76
     receptor usage, 70, 72, 465–68
     TCR-CD3 complex, 495
     TH1 and Th2, 79, 206, 212–13, 595–97
     viral infections in, 593–95
Tachykinins, 238
TGF-β. *See* Transforming growth factor-β
TH. *See* Tyrosine hydroxylase
Theiler's murine encephalomyelitis virus,
     578, 582–83, 594, 596, Table 1-2
Thymus
     aging effects, 291
     innervation of, 229, 238–43, 251–53,
          286, Fig. 8-11, 8-12
TIL. *See* Tumor infiltrating lymphocytes.
     See also Lymphocytes

Tissue-restricted microenvironment
cytokines in, 113
definition, 105–06, 112–13
neural-occular immune sytem in, 112–14
TMEV. *See* Theiler's murine
encephalomyelitis virus
Tolerance, 5–6, 77, 349
Tonsils, 237
Transforming growth factor-β. *See also*
Cytokines
biological actions on glial cells, 440
brain tumors in, 762
cerbrospinal fluid in, 114, 147
CNS disease involvement in, 442–43,
645–46
definition, 424
expression by glial cells, 440–41, 644–
46, Table 11-5
immunosuppressive properties, 644–45
interstitial fluid in, 148
multiple sclerosis in, 645, 711
production by ocular tissues and in
aqueous humor, 113, 147, 674,
677–78, Table 18-1
proinflammatory cytokine as, 213–14
viral infections, 585–87
Transplantation
allografting, 625–27
astrogliosis and microgliosis in, 619
blood-brain barrier breakdown in, 620–
21
definition neural, 611
graft sites, Fig. 16-2
graft survival and rejection, 612, 628–29
host sensitization, 627–28
immunosuppression in, 633–34
MHC antigen role in, 614–15, 621–23,
Fig. 16-1
models for, 617–19
tolerance, 5–6
vascularization of grafted tissue, 624–25
xenotransplantation, 631–33
Tropical spastic paraparesis, 37–39, 747
TSH. *See* Thyroid stimulating hormone
TSP. *See* Tropical spastic paraparesis
Tumor necrosis factor. *See also* Cytokines
AIDS in, 437, 740–43
biological action on glial cells, 423,
433–35, Table 11-4

brain tumors, 769
EAE role in, 436, 476
EAN role in, 793
expression by glial cells, 435
inflammation, 213–14
lymphocyte adhesion in, 205
multiple sclerosis in, 436, 711
neuroendocrine system effects, 559–61,
Table 14-3
viral infections of CNS in, 588–87
Tumors. *See also* Gliomas
animal models for study, 774
antigenicity, 762–63
cell surface marker expression, 763–67,
Table 21-1
immunotherapy, 767–73
active, 767, Table 21-2
nonspecific, 767, Table 21-2
passive, 769, Table 21-3
specific, 767
lymphocyte infiltration, 762
target cell, 774–77
TGF-β production, 647–48, 762
Tyrosine hydroxylase, 245

Vascular endothelial cells
adhesion of lymphocytes to, 203–05
antigen presentation by, 370–76,
Table 10-2
antigen recognition, 368–70
MHC expression, 370–71, Table 10-1
transformation to HEV, 205–06
Vasoactive intestinal peptide
aqueous humor in, 113, 117, Table 18-1
gut-associated lymphoid tissue in, 23–26
immune response effects on, 272–75
peptidergic nerves, 237
Peyer's patches, 249
receptors on lymphocytes for, 258
spleen, 244–45, Fig. 8-17
thymus, 238, Fig. 8-14, 8–15
VIP. *See* Vasoactive intestinal peptide
Viruses
acute cytolytic infections, 581–85
cellular interactions in CNS, 578
CNS disease in, Table 15-1
CNS entry, 577–78, Fig. 15-1
humoral response to, 587; enhancement
by, 591–93

Viruses (*continued*)
    inhibition of viral spread, 588–91
    latency associated transcripts, 583
    persistent infections, 581–85
Visna-Maedi virus, 578, 748, Table 1-2
VMV. *See* Progressive pneumonia virus

Wallerian degeneration
    comparison in PNS and CNS, 790–91
    features of, 789–91

Yellow fever virus, 589
YFV. *See* Yellow fever virus